a LANGE medical book

Occupational Medicine

a **LANGE** medical book

Occupational Medicine

Edited by

Joseph LaDou, MD
Clinical Professor of Medicine and Chief
Division of Occupational and Environmental Medicine
Department of Medicine
University of California, San Francisco

APPLETON & LANGE
Norwalk, Connecticut/San Mateo, California

0-8385-7207-3

90 91 92 93 94 / 10 9 8 7 6 5 4 3 2 1

Prentice Hall International (UK) Limited, *London*
Prentice Hall of Australia Pty. Limited, *Sydney*
Prentice Hall Canada, Inc., *Toronto*
Prentice Hall Hispanoamericana, S.A., *Mexico*
Prentice Hall of India Private Limited, *New Delhi*
Prentice Hall of Japan, Inc., *Tokyo*
Simon & Schuster Asia Pte. Ltd., *Singapore*
Editora Prentice Hall do Brasil Ltda., *Rio de Janeiro*
Prentice Hall, *Englewood Cliffs, New Jersey*

ISBN: 0-8385-7207-3
ISSN: 1047-4498

Designer: Steven M. Byrum

PRINTED IN THE UNITED STATES OF AMERICA

Table of Contents

SECTION IV: OCCUPATIONAL EXPOSURES

SECTION V: PROGRAM MANAGEMENT

Preface

Occupational Medicine is a concise, comprehensive resource for health care professionals in all specialties who are called on to diagnose and treat occupational injuries and illnesses. Its broad coverage and emphasis on fundamental concepts also make it an ideal text for students and residents.

COVERAGE AND APPROACH TO THE SUBJECT

The book provides a complete guide to common occupational injuries and illnesses, their diagnosis and treatment, and preventive and remedial measures in the workplace. Our aim is to help physicians understand and deal with the complexities of occupational medicine and at the same time to provide useful clinical information on common illnesses and injuries.

SPECIAL AREAS OF EMPHASIS

- Detailed coverage of diagnosis and treatment of a broad spectrum of occupational injuries and illnesses.
- Basic chapters on toxicology and immunology, providing the foundation necessary for a solid understanding of occupational disease.
- Practical information on toxic properties and clinical manifestations of common industrial materials.
- Accident and illness prevention techniques for the workplace.

SPECIAL SUBJECTS IN SUPPORT

- Although epidemiologic data are not presented, much of the clinical information is drawn from epidemiologic studies, and the reader will learn epidemiologic principles by studying the text. (Prior understanding of these principles is not necessary for an understanding of the information in the various chapters.) A basic introduction to that subject is presented in the Appendix.

- The role of other health and safety professionals and their interaction with physicians is examined; importance of a team effort in developing health and safety programs in the workplace is emphasized.
- Chapters on the legal aspects of occupational medicine and on the relationship of occupational medicine to environmental medicine round out the book's comprehensive approach.

ORGANIZATION AND HIGHLIGHTS OF INDIVIDUAL SECTIONS

Section I (Chapters 1 through 5) discusses the health professional's role on the health and safety team. It provides guidance for identifying workplace and community exposures to toxic materials, putting this information to immediate clinical use, and applying it toward better health and safety practices in the workplace. It also orients physicians to the special nature of disability examinations required for workers' compensation insurance settlements and considers some of the legal issues important to the practice of occupational medicine.

Section II (Chapters 6 through 11) is a concise discussion of common occupational injuries and their treatment and of the physical hazards of heat, cold, and radiation. It also emphasizes the important discipline of ergonomics and discusses how ergonomic principles can be instituted in the workplace in order to prevent further work loss from injury and illness.

Section III (Chapters 12 through 24) is a comprehensive discussion of clinical toxicology arranged by organ system, with special emphasis on the workplace origin of toxic exposures. It provides a thorough review of commonly recognized occupational illnesses and highlights many clinical problems not often thought to be work-related. Chapter 15 on Occupational Infections includes an up-to-date discussion of AIDS and its implications in the workplace.

Section IV (Chapters 25 through 34) presents the most common toxic materials and the diagnostic and treatment recommendations appropriate to them. This section is designed as an immediate reference source and clinical guide for the practicing health care professional. The discussion of pesticides, in particular, emphasizes the environmental as well as occupational exposures that may lead to illness. The chapter on biologic monitoring provides the information necessary for instituting medical surveillance programs and for interpreting data obtained in such programs.

Section V (Chapters 35 through 39) discusses the roles and responsibilities of other health and safety professionals, including the industrial hygienist and the safety professional. The chapter on industrial hygiene includes a discussion of recommended exposure limits for common industrial materials. Chapters on occupational stress and drug and alcohol abuse in the work setting discuss programs for controlling and treating these problems. Chapter 39 introduces environmental medicine and some of the complex societal issues that accompany industrialization and technologic advances throughout the world. Emphasis is placed on recognizing that some common occupational exposures are found also in homes and public locations and require the same high index of suspicion that physicians assume when caring for workers.

The **Appendix** provides concise introductions to biostatistics and epidemiology. These principles are important not only in research but also in clinical practice. Ultimately, all occupational physicians are clinical epidemiologists.

ACKNOWLEDGMENTS

I wish to thank the many *Occupational Medicine* contributors, whose willingness to work together over a protracted developmental process has added so much to the quality of the book.

TO OUR READERS

The guidance of our readers will be essential to our continuing efforts to maintain this book as a major resource for education and reference in this important field of medicine. Suggestions and comments should be addressed to Joseph LaDou, MD, Division of Occupational and Environmental Medicine, UCSF, Box 0924, San Francisco, CA 94143.

San Francisco
March, 1990   —Joseph LaDou

The Authors

Charles E. Becker, MD
Professor of Medicine and Director, Northern California Occupational Health Center, San Francisco General Medical Center, University of California, San Francisco.

Clinical Toxicology, Gases, Substance Abuse & Employee Assistance Programs

Neal L. Benowitz, MD
Professor of Medicine and Chief, Clinical Pharmacology, San Francisco General Medical Center, University of California, San Francisco.

Cardiovascular Toxicology, Smoking & Occupational Health

John M. Bielan, MD, JD
Law Offices, San Francisco, California.

Liability in Occupational Health Practice

Edwin C. Cadman, MD
Professor and Chairman, Department of Internal Medicine, Yale University School of Medicine, New Haven, Connecticut.

Occupational Cancer

William L. Clark, MD
Division of Industrial Accidents, State of California, San Francisco, California.

Disability Evaluation

Richard Cohen, MD, MPH
Associate Clinical Professor, University of California, San Francisco.

Injuries Due to Physical Hazards, Occupational Infections

Lloyd E. Damon, MD
Assistant Professor of Medicine, Cancer Research Institute, University of California, San Francisco.

Occupational Hematology

Susan Desmond, MD
Assistant Professor of Medicine, Cancer Research Institute, University of California, San Francisco.

Occupational Cancer

William J. Estrin, MD
Assistant Professor of Neurology, San Francisco General Medical Center, University of California, San Francisco.

Neurotoxicology

Michael L. Fischman, MD, MPH
Assistant Clinical Professor, University of California, San Francisco.

Occupational Cancer, Building-Associated Illness

Catherine Sonquist Forest, MD, MPH
University of California, San Francisco.

Female Reproductive Toxicology

Douglas P. Fowler, PhD, CIH
Assistant Clinical Professor, University of California, San Francisco.

Industrial Hygiene

Donald F. German, MD
Assistant Clinical Professor, University of California, San Francisco.

Clinical Immunology

Ernest K. Goodner, MD
Clinical Professor and Chief, Department of Ophthalmology, San Francisco General Medical Center, University of California, San Francisco.

Eye Injuries

Robert J. Harrison, MD, MPH
Assistant Clinical Professor and Chief, Occupational and Environmental Medicine Clinic, University of California, San Francisco.

Liver Toxicology, Chemicals, Biologic Monitoring

Franklin T. Hoaglund, MD
Professor of Orthopedic Surgery, University of California, San Francisco.

Musculoskeletal Injuries

William G. Hughson, MD, PhD
Associate Clinical Professor and Chief, Division of Occupational Medicine, University of California, San Diego.

Occupational Lung Diseases

Robert K. Jackler, MD
Assistant Professor of Otolaryngology-Neurotology, University of California, San Francisco.

Occupational Hearing Loss

George A. Kaysen, MD, PhD
Associate Professor and Chief, Renal Division, University of California, Davis.

Renal Toxicology

Joseph LaDou, MD
Clinical Professor and Chief, Division of Occupational and Environmental Medicine, Department of Medicine, University of California, San Francisco.

The Practice of Occupational Medicine, Approach to the Diagnosis of Occupational Illnesses, Environmental Health

Robert C. Larsen, MD
Assistant Clinical Professor of Psychiatry, University of California, San Francisco.

Substance Abuse & Employee Assistance Programs

Gideon Letz, MD, MPH
Associate Clinical Professor, University of California, San Francisco.

Male Reproductive Toxicology

D. Richard Lewis, MD, MPH
Assistant Clinical Professor, University of California, San Francisco.

Metals, Plastics, The Rubber Industry

James R. Nethercott, MD
Professor and Director, Division of Occupational Medicine, School of Hygiene and Public Health, The Johns Hopkins University, Baltimore, Maryland.

Occupational Skin Disorders

Gareth J. Parry, MB, FRACP
Associate Professor of Neurology, Louisiana State University School of Medicine, New Orleans, Louisiana.

Neurotoxicology

Franklyn G. Prieskop, MS, CSP
The Crawford Company, Santa Ana, California.

Occupational Safety

David M. Rempel, MD, MPH
Assistant Clinical Professor, University of California, San Francisco.

Biologic Monitoring

Jon Rosenberg, MD, MPH
Associate Clinical Professor, University of California, San Francisco.

Clinical Toxicology, Solvents, Pesticides, Biologic Monitoring

Linda Rudolph, MD, MPH
Assistant Clinical Professor, University of California, San Francisco.

Female Reproductive Toxicology

Hope S. Rugo, MD
Department of Medicine, University of California, San Francisco.

Occupational Hematology

Susan T. Sacks, PhD
Visiting Lecturer, Epidemiology and International Health, University of California, San Francisco.

Biostatistics & Epidemiology

Marc B. Schenker, MD, MPH
Associate Professor and Chief, Division of Occupational and Environmental Medicine, University of California, Davis.

Biostatistics & Epidemiology

David N. Schindler, MD
Associate Clinical Professor of Otolaryngology, University of California, San Francisco.

Occupational Hearing Loss

James P. Seward, MD, MPP
Assistant Clinical Professor, University of California, San Francisco.

Occupational Stress

Judd Shellito, MD
Associate Professor of Medicine, University of California, San Francisco.

Occupational Lung Diseases

Dean Sheppard, MD
Associate Professor and Director, Lung Biology Center, University of California, San Francisco.

Occupational Lung Diseases

Charles L. Swezey, LLB
California Workers' Compensation Appeals Board, San Francisco, California.

Workers' Compensation Law

David A. Thompson, PhD
Department of Industrial Engineering, Stanford University.

Ergonomics & the Prevention of Occupational Injuries

William Vermere, PhD
Department of Environmental Health and Safety, University of California, San Francisco.

Thomas O. Wildes, MD
Assistant Clinical Professor and Chief, Head and Neck Surgery, San Francisco General Medical Center, University of California, San Francisco.

Facial Injuries

The Practice of Occupational Medicine

Joseph LaDou, MD

The rapid proliferation of new industrial materials, new production methods, and new commercial products in the 20th century—particularly since World War II—has gone forward with too little attention paid to assessment of their effects on the environment and on human health. Only about 10,000 of the estimated 60,000 chemicals used commercially today have been tested for toxicity in animals.

While toxicity testing lags far behind the rate of new developments, the incidence of work- and environment-related illnesses in humans increases. Similarly, the number of trained professionals in occupational safety and health is much lower than what is needed to prevent and treat these illnesses.

The result is that private physicians must assume the burden of diagnosing, treating, and if possible preventing work-related illnesses and injuries. In the USA, there are more than 5 million business establishments with 85 million employees. Nearly 90% of the businesses employ fewer than 100 workers, and it is in these smaller workplaces that many of the more serious occupational safety and health problems exist. The National Institute for Occupational Safety and Health (NIOSH) estimates that only 2% of employees in these businesses have access to industrial hygiene services and workplace monitoring programs, and only rarely is an occupational health nurse available to the small employer.

TRAINING IN OCCUPATIONAL MEDICINE

With additional postgraduate training in occupational medicine, physicians in many specialties could provide the occupational health care required by most employers. NIOSH estimates that industry requires a minimum of 30,000 physicians with short-course training in occupational medicine and 1000 residency-trained occupational health physicians in addition to the estimated 800 practicing physicians currently certified in this specialty. To accomplish the objective of expanding general medical practice to cover the shortage of occupational health professionals, 3 conditions must be met: (1) Primary care physicians must be trained in the disciplines of occupational and environmental medicine; (2) they must be dedicated to learning and practicing new skills in prevention, diagnosis, and treatment of occupational injuries and illnesses; and (3) they must be familiar with the skills provided by other members of the occupational health and safety team and make a commitment to working with those professionals in a team context.

Medical schools generally offer only a few hours of formal instruction in occupational medicine. Only 20 medical schools in the USA offer residency training in occupational medicine, and fewer than that offer postgraduate courses for practicing physicians. This means that most training in occupational and environmental medicine will have to be gained through individual study and practical experience.

Reasons for incorporating occupational health care into the training and practice of general medicine include the following:

(1) Large numbers of people are exposed to toxic materials, and the extent of exposure is important information physicians must have in evaluating their patients' complaints. Millions of workers have exposures sufficient to result in demonstrable health problems. Fortunately, the adverse effects are reversible in a significant number of cases when the toxic material is identified and exposure is held thereafter to an acceptable level.

(2) Early recognition by physicians of unusual patterns of illnesses in their patients can alert the plant authority and local public health officials to the need for further industrial and environmental control measures.

(3) New chemicals introduced into the industrial setting require toxicologic testing as well as the development of a medical literature data base. Physicians can contribute to this data base by reporting their observations in the occupational and environmental health literature. Case reports often prompt industry-wide epidemiologic studies.

(4) A multidisciplinary occupational health and safety team must include physicians with training and experience in recognizing, treating, and preventing occupational illness. When broadly trained and experienced, the physician can serve as the health and safety team leader.

(5) Physicians in general practice will continue to encounter problems in managing patients with work-related health problems. In such cases, the physician must ask questions about all aspects of the patient's life, including the past and present occupational

history. The physician must have the training needed to consult perceptively with specialists in occupational and environmental medicine and with other occupational health professionals, including safety professionals and industrial hygienists.

EVOLUTION OF THE FIELD OF OCCUPATIONAL MEDICINE

Recognition of work-related disease has been slow in evolving. In the early part of this century, efforts to focus attention on occupational health hazards were largely ignored.

> A tunnel was being constructed through a nearby mountain to divert water from 2 rivers to a planned hydroelectric plant farther south. Plans at first called for the tunnel to be 32 ft wide, but when the rock was found to have a high content of quartz, the width was expanded to 46 ft. Dust in the tunnel was so thick that workers often could not see beyond 10 ft, and the silica content of the dust ranged between 90% and 95%. The workers had trouble breathing, and as conditions worsened, they began to drop dead in the tunnel. Within a few months, 50% had died or were suffering from silicosis.

This disaster at Gauley Bridge, West Virginia, in the 1930s—which eventually claimed the lives of 476 men and disabled an additional 1500—focused government and public attention on the neglected problem of occupational disease as a public health concern.

Through much of the 20th century, Dr Alice Hamilton was a pioneer in the field of occupational medicine and environmental toxicology. Her descriptions of lead poisoning in factories, silica exposure in quarries, and mercury poisoning in quicksilver mines—as well as her demands for preventive health care in US industry—served as initial steps toward recognizing occupational diseases and dealing with them.

The pervasiveness of potentially toxic contaminants both in the workplace and in the home and community environment is a source of ongoing concern. Public concern has resulted in the development of a number of governmental activities to protect the health of workers and of the community. Passage of the Occupational Safety and Health Act in 1970 created the Occupational Safety and Health Administration (OSHA) and the National Institute for Occupational Safety and Health (NIOSH). These and other government agencies, including the Environmental Protection Agency (EPA), and private organizations concerned with occupational and environmental health are reviewed in Chapter 2.

PREVENTION OF OCCUPATIONAL & ENVIRONMENTAL ILLNESSES

Preventing work-related and environmental illnesses is made difficult by the following features of life in an industrialized society:

(1) The uninterrupted flow of new and untested chemicals into the workplace and subsequently into the environment.

(2) The paucity of data about the toxicologic and environmental effects of most of these substances, including their interactions, their metabolites, and their cumulative effects.

(3) Diagnostic difficulties related to the sometimes protracted intervals between the exposure and the onset of disease or occurrence of overt symptoms.

(4) The problems of safe disposal of hazardous wastes and the often prohibitive costs of detoxification of the most hazardous materials.

Health Surveillance Techniques

Health surveillance techniques frequently include preplacement and periodic physical examinations of workers. Preventive health examinations—including batteries of screening laboratory tests—are parts of many occupational health and safety programs. In recent years, testing has been expanded to include assessment of genetic predisposition to certain occupational illnesses, eg, G6PD testing of workers exposed to hemolytic agents and testing for serum antitrypsin deficiency in an effort to prevent chronic obstructive pulmonary disease. Debate over the legal and ethical issues inherent in genetic testing is resulting in a slow acceptance of these practices.

Worker Population Surveillance Systems

Studies of illnesses and causes of death of workers in various industries in the USA have often been flawed by failure to sort information by industry or specific occupation or to include information about exposure of workers to toxic substances. Because the death certificates in only about a dozen of the 50 states include information about the deceased worker's occupation and employment history, it is impossible to evaluate occupational mortality patterns at the national level. Work history is not usually part of the hospital record either. This further restricts the efforts of worker health surveillance groups to determine the extent of occupational illnesses and to identify workplace hazards that need to be controlled or eliminated.

Epidemiologic Studies

Epidemiologic methods can be used to (1) identify subgroups of the population at high risk for given diseases and injuries, (2) detect hazardous exposures and their adverse effects, (3) determine the effectiveness of control measures instituted in the workplace, and (4) evaluate the efficiency of screening tests for occupational diseases or substance abuse in the workplace. A brief introduction to basic epidemiologic methods is presented in the Appendix.

OCCUPATIONAL ILLNESSES

Scope of the Problem

Each year in the USA, over 2 million people suffer

permanent or temporary disability from various causes. Although the number of people with disabilities resulting from occupational illness is not known, it has been estimated that there are at least 390,000 new cases of disabling occupational illness and as many as 100,000 deaths from occupational diseases each year. Yet one study suggested that because of the difficulty of diagnosis and the likelihood that occupational illness claims will be disputed by employers, only 3% of workers with occupational illnesses were receiving compensation under the workers' compensation insurance system.

Workers in manufacturing have the highest number of occupational illnesses. Although they constitute only 20% of total employees, they account for 35% of occupational illnesses, with skin rashes and eye disorders representing most cases. The leading cause of occupational illnesses among production workers is exposure to toxic chemicals, such as solvents, acids, and those chemicals found in soaps, petroleum fractions, paints, plastics, and resins. Additional problems occur from exposure to dusts, gases, and metals.

Occupational stress is becoming more widely recognized among workers and, consequently, is beginning to add to the total number of occupational disease cases receiving workers' compensation benefits. Heart disease has become a major source of workers' compensation stress claims in many states, and cerebrovascular accidents and other vascular diseases are common occupational illnesses and suitable claims for compensation in some states. Furthermore, occupational illnesses resulting from repeated exposure to stressors such as noise, heat, repetitive movements, and years of heavy lifting now result in "cumulative injury" claims. Although such cases account for only a small percentage of total claims, their treatment and settlement costs are high.

Major Occupational Illnesses

NIOSH has developed a priority list of the 10 leading work-related illnesses and injuries. Three criteria were used to develop the list: (1) the frequency of occurrence of the illness or injury, (2) its severity in individual cases, and (3) its potential for prevention.

Occupational lung disease is first on the list. NIOSH estimates that 1.2 million workers are exposed to silica dust and that about 60,000 exposed workers will suffer some degree of silicosis. Among some 20 million living men and women exposed to asbestos, between 75,000 and 300,000 are expected to develop exposure-related cancer in the next 50 years. Longitudinal studies of exposed shipyard workers show that 10–18% die of asbestosis. Byssinosis has already disabled an estimated 35,000 current and retired textile workers. About 4000 deaths each year are attributed to legislatively defined "black lung disease." The prevalence of occupational asthma varies from 10% to nearly all of workers in certain high-risk occupations.

NIOSH considers occupational cancer to be the second leading work-related disease, followed by cardiovascular diseases, disorders of reproduction, neurotoxic disorders, noise-induced hearing loss, dermatologic conditions, and psychologic disorders.

Occupational Illnesses Resulting From Exposure to Toxic Materials

A large majority of occupational illnesses are due to exposure to toxic substances. As high-technology industries replace traditional forms of manufacture, the use of new and often toxic materials increases. Microelectronics manufacturers, for example, use hundreds of chemicals developed specifically for their product lines. Industrial hygiene services are in many cases unavailable to workers in these companies, and information on the toxic effects of the materials used is often inadequate or nonexistent.

Although industry spends an estimated 2% of corporate revenues on health and safety programs, very little of this outlay is for toxicologic studies or for worker health problems. As a result, there is little information about the possible toxicity of most of the commonly used industrial chemicals, and the long-term effects of these chemicals on the environment and on community health are generally unknown.

The National Research Council of the National Academy of Sciences concluded from a recent study that toxicologists have fairly complete information on health hazards for only 10% of pesticides and only 18% of drugs in use today. Moreover, at least one-third of pesticides and drugs have never been tested for toxicity. The problem with common commercial chemicals is even more serious, since nearly 80% of them have never been tested, and little is known about many that have been studied.

Occupational health professionals and government officials thus anticipate that there will be more deleterious effects on worker and community health in the future. A further area now being studied by toxicologists is the interaction of toxic materials, in which one substance may potentiate the toxicity of other chemicals or in which new chemicals may be created by interaction with others.

OCCUPATIONAL INJURIES

Every year, American workers suffer an estimated 1 million eye injuries, 400,000 fractures, 21,000 amputations, and more than 2 million lacerations severe enough to require medical treatment. Hospital emergency rooms alone treat at least 3 million occupational injuries each year. Work-related injuries occur at a rate more than twice that of injuries in the home or public places and account for more than 200 million lost workdays annually at a cost in excess of $25 billion.

The most common occupational injuries involve the musculoskeletal system, with over 1 million workers sustaining back injuries each year.

Many studies of injury reporting systems in industry indicate that occupational injuries are grossly underreported. When employers assign injured workers to "light duty," they sometimes feel relieved of the obligation to report the injuries. Similarly, occupational injuries and illnesses are often not reported if no loss of work time occurs. Comparisons of national reporting with that of individual states, such as California, have led some investigators to conclude that occupational illnesses are at least 50% underreported nationally.

There may be as many as 10 million injuries, 30 million separate bouts of illness, between 20,000 and 75,000 deaths, and, cumulatively, 2 million disabled each year in the United States.

Nonetheless, injury rates have been declining as a result of a fundamental change in US industry and employment patterns: The service sector is growing fairly rapidly, while many traditional manufacturing industries are in decline. Because service employment (eg, food and clothing sales, banking, insurance) is generally safer than labor or trade work with heavy equipment and mechanized processes, the injury rate for all industries decreased from 11 injuries per 100 workers in 1973 to 8.7 injuries per 100 workers in 1988. Injury rates may continue to decline because of continuing expansion of the service sector relative to manufacturing.

The major causes of occupational deaths are work-related motor vehicle accidents, falls, trauma, and electric shock. The industries with the highest rates of fatal injury are mining and quarrying, construction, and agriculture.

REFERENCES

Advisory Panel for Preventing Illness and Injury in the Workplace: *Preventing Illness and Injury in the Workplace*. US Congress, Office of Technology Assessment, OTA-F-256, 1985.

American Medical Association: *Occupational Health Service: A Practical Approach*. American Medical Association, 1989.

Association of Schools of Public Health/National Institute for Occupational Safety and Health: *Proposed National Strategies for the Prevention of Leading Work-Related Diseases and Injuries*. Part 1, 1986.

National Institute for Occupational Safety and Health: National Occupational Exposure Survey: Analysis of Management Interview Responses. DHHS (NIOSH) Publication No. 89-103, 1989.

Cullen MR: Occupational medicine: A new focus for general internal medicine. *Arch Intern Med* 1985; **145**:511.

Institute of Medicine, Division of Health Promotion and Disease Prevention: *Role of the Primary Care Physician in Occupational and Environmental Medicine*. National Academy Press, 1988.

National Research Council, National Academy of Sciences: *Toxicology Testing: Strategies to Determine Needs and Priorities*. National Academy Press, 1985.

National Research Council, Panel on Occupational Safety and Health Statistics: *Counting Injuries and Illnesses in the Workplace: Proposals for a Better System*. Pollack ES, Keimig DG (editors). National Academy Press, 1987.

US Department of Labor, Bureau of Labor Statistics: *Occupational Injuries and Illnesses in the United States by Industry*. Bulletin 2308. US Government Printing Office, 1988.

Approach to the Diagnosis of Occupational Illnesses

2

Joseph LaDou, MD

The diagnosis of an occupational illness is often difficult because the history of work exposure is difficult to obtain and interpret. The problem is compounded by the fact that occupational illnesses are generally associated with many years of exposure to a variety of toxic materials rather than to one specific material. Other factors such as heredity, personal life-style, and psychosocial factors may also contribute to the problem of diagnosis.

> A patient has frequent respiratory infections that appear to be caused by long-term exposure to fumes and vapors at work. The problem does not subside during his annual vacations away from the plant. He is also a heavy smoker.

How can the physician determine which contaminant is making the patient ill? When common illnesses are ruled out after thorough assessment, the physician must question whether the patient's problem stems from exposure to toxic materials in the workplace, conditions in the home, or environmental exposure. A useful tool in this regard is the medical history and, more importantly, the occupational and environmental medical history. A visit to the workplace may be in order, as well as a review of the health records maintained by the employer.

THE OCCUPATIONAL MEDICAL HISTORY

The most important diagnostic skill in the practice of occupational medicine is the taking of a comprehensive occupational medical history. The importance of this skill cannot be overemphasized in the training of medical students and in the everyday practice of physicians. As outlined in Table 2–1, the occupational medical history should include a variety of questions not always considered pertinent to general medical histories.

The Occupational and Environmental Health Committee of the American Lung Association has developed a convenient form (Fig 2–1) for obtaining an individual occupational and environmental medical history that can be used both as a data base and for screening purposes. Further history taking and comprehensive evaluation are required for diagnosis. The occupational history can be expanded by also using the follow-up questions listed in Table 2–2.

EMPLOYEE DOCUMENTS

If the physician suspects that the workplace is the source of the health problem, the employer should be asked to produce the patient's records pertaining to sick leave, accidents, and job performance. The person in charge of the company's health and safety program is usually able to accommodate these requests. The physician should also ask to see the workers' compensation insurance underwriter files describing all medical care rendered to the patient for previous occupational illnesses and injuries. Only those with a demonstrated need to know are permitted access to these otherwise confidential health and safety data.

The physician's recommendations after review of the records will be important not only to the worker but also to the employer, since workers' compensation payments are adjusted to reflect the need for further investment in safety and industrial hygiene measures. The physician must indicate on the insurance form whether the illness is related to work. Neglecting to state this opinion early in the course of treatment may cause delays in benefits to the worker and may also create problems with statute of limitations provisions that would later deny payments to the worker.

THE OCCUPATIONAL HAZARD

When a patient's medical history indicates that occupational or environmental factors may be a cause of illness, the physician should identify all potentially toxic materials the worker is exposed to both in the workplace and at home or elsewhere. Technical data pertaining to the chemical properties, uses, and toxicity of many industrial materials are available to treating physicians.

Two excellent books cited below should be in the library of every practicing occupational physician. They are sources of information on potential health hazards of a wide variety of industries and serve as guides to identification or recognition of hazards of hundreds of industrial processes. The industries chosen are major production facilities employing large numbers of workers and representing varying hazard potentials.

Table 2–1. Information to be included in the occupational medical history
(additions to standard medical history questions).[1]

Present illness

Under each individual problem listed in your problem-oriented record, add the following 4 questions:

1. Are the symptoms associated with work? Are these symptoms improved during vacations or weekends?
2. Are other workers similarly affected?
3. Are you currently exposed to any dust, fumes, or chemicals?
4. Was a first report of work injury filed by a physician? (This is an extremely valuable way of identifying the specifics of an occupational injury and also identifying those physicians who evaluated the patient immediately after the suspected injury.)

Work history

1. List in chronologic order all jobs. Describe in detail the work site (a diagram may be helpful). Describe a typical workday and job duties.
2. Was protective equipment issued? Do you have knowledge of safety programs given on the job?
3. Is ventilation in your workplace appropriate?
4. Was a preemployment examination done?
5. Was any specialized periodic testing or medical surveillance done on prior jobs? Is it done on current jobs?
6. Are you aware of industrial hygiene sampling of the workplace?
7. List the total number of days missed on each job. List specific reasons for absence.
8. Has a worker compensation claim ever been filed in your behalf? If so, list the specifics.
9. Have there been special health and safety issues presented by your labor union?
10. In addition to your regular work, have you ever moonlighted? List additional jobs.

Past history

Certain occupational exposure may be subtle and require a specific response:

1. Have you regularly been exposed to loud noises or to excessive vibration or heat?
2. Have you ever been exposed to asbestos?
3. Have you ever been exposed to radioactive chemicals or excessive radiation?
4. Have you been exposed to chemicals?
5. During military service, what were your duties? Did you have any exposure to potentially toxic agents?

Environmental health history

There is increasing recognition of subtle problems in the environment contributing to disease:

1. Are there any new factories located in your neighborhood?
2. Have you been exposed to any hazardous waste sites or toxic spills?
3. List jobs of your spouse or partner.
4. Is there commonly air pollution in your environment?
5. List all hobbies and recreational activities. Specifically, do you work with painting, sculpting, welding, or woodworking? If so, describe the location and ventilation.
6. Describe the insulation and heating in your current and past living areas.
7. What agents are used to clean your home and workplace?
8. Are insecticides used in your home or environment?
9. Do you maintain firearms in your home or workplace?
10. Do you wear seat belts?

Review of systems

It is especially important to recognize high-risk jobs such as fire fighting, mining, and forestry. Special emphasis should be placed on detecting occupational skin and lung diseases, cancer, peripheral neuropathy, and liver disorders. In addition, specific questions should be asked about 2 special areas: working hours and reproductive history.

1. What are your working hours? Has your job schedule required major changes of shift work that have disturbed your sleep? Are you bored on the job?
2. Record the number of miscarriages, children, stillbirths, prior pregnancies, and difficulties in conceiving. Have you noted any change in libido or menses?

[1]Modified and reproduced, with permission, from Becker CE: Key elements of the occupational history for the general physician. *West J Med* 1982;**137:**581.

Burgess WA: *Recognition of Health Hazards in Industry: A Review of Materials and Processes.* Wiley, 1981.

Grayson M (editor): *Kirk-Othner Concise Encyclopedia of Chemical Technology,* 3rd ed. Wiley, 1985.

THE MATERIAL SAFETY DATA SHEET (MSDS)

An important step in obtaining information is often to request an MSDS on each of the suspected materials. The Occupational Safety and Health Administration (OSHA) requires suppliers to include these data sheets with each shipment of industrial materials and requires employers to maintain them and make them available to physicians and workers. An MSDS can be obtained by telephone or by written request to either the employer or the supplier. If the product or process is a trade secret, the physician or worker may be required to sign a confidentiality agreement before receiving sensitive information.

The MSDS primarily assists company personnel in the event of emergencies. Although it seldom provides adequate clinical information for the treating physician, the MSDS often serves as a starting point in the assessment of the worker's possible exposure to toxic substances.

Occupational/Environmental History Form

I. IDENTIFICATION

Name: _____ Soc. Sec. _____

Address: _____ Sex: M F

_____ Birthday: _____

Telephone: home _____ work _____

II. OCCUPATIONAL PROFILE

Fill in the table below listing all jobs at which you have worked, including short-term, seasonal, and part-time employment. Start with your present job and go back to the first. Use additional paper if necessary.

Workplace (Employer's name and address or city)	Dates worked From To	Did you work full time?	Type of Industry (Describe)	Describe your job duties	Known health hazards in workplace (dusts, solvents, etc.)	Protective equipment used?	Were you ever off work for a health problem or injury?

Figure 2–1. Occupational and environmental medical history form. (continued on page 8.) (Modified and reproduced, with permission, from Occupational and Environmental Health Committee of the American Lung Association: Taking the occupational history. *Ann Intern Med* 1983;**99**:641.)

Table 2–2. Additional Questions for the Evaluation of Occupational Associations to the Present Illness[1]

Question	Interpretation
Is your condition better or worse when you are off work for a few days or on vacation?	Identify patterns suggesting either improvement or exacerbation on withdrawal from exposure.
Is your condition better or worse when you return to work after a weekend or vacation?	Identify patterns suggesting return of the condition on reexposure in the workplace.
Does your condition get worse or better after you have been back at work for several days or shifts?	Identify patterns suggesting either tolerance or cumulative effects with multiple exposure.
Describe your workplace. (Please draw a diagram and indicate your work station.)	Evaluate the proximity to exposure, protection available (ventilation or barriers), mobility within the workplace, and location of coworkers who may also be affected.
What ventilation systems are used in your work space? Do they seem to work?	Obtain a general impression of adequacy of ventilation by air movement and odors.
Does the protective equipment you are issued fit properly? Do you receive instructions in its proper use? Do you ever fix or make changes in the equipment to make it more comfortable?	Consider the possibility that protective equipment is not fully effective. In the case of respirators (masks), ask if they are "fit-tested" to comply with Occupational Safety and Health Administration (OSHA) regulations.
Where do you eat, smoke, and take your breaks when you are on the job?	Identify opportunities for food- and cigarette-borne intake, and evaluate the adequacy of rest stations (isolation from heat, noise, fumes).
Where are your (and your spouse's or partner's) work clothes laundered?	Identify possibility of passive exposure at home or of prolonged skin contact.
How often do you wash your hands at work, and how do you wash them?	Identify the potential for contamination of hands or contact with solvents or drying agents.
What is your spouse's or partner's occupation?	Identify the potential for passive exposure (an occupational history for the spouse or partner may be indicated).
Have any of your fellow workers experienced similar conditions?	Identifying others who may have been affected may lead to inquiries that clarify the individual patient's problem. Prevention-oriented interventions or requests for investigation by the state or federal branch of OSHA may be required.
Do you recall a specific incident or accident that occurred on the job? Were others also affected?	Identify unusual or transient conditions that may have resulted in an exposure not reflected in the occupational history, such as leaks, fires, or uncontrolled exothermic chemical reactions.
Are animals (pets, livestock, birds, or pests such as mice) present in the vicinity of the workplace? Has there been a change in their health, appearance or behavior?	Animals (and especially animal wastes) may be a source of infectious or allergic hazards. Animals may also respond to toxic exposures that affect humans.

[1]Modifed and reproduced, with permission, from Occupational and Enviromental Health Committee of the American Lung Association: Taking the occupational history. *Ann Intern Med* 1983;**99**:641.

III. OCCUPATIONAL EXPOSURE INVENTORY

1. Please describe any health problems or injuries you have experienced connected with your present or past jobs:

2. Have any of your co-workers also experienced health problems or injuries connected with the same jobs? ...... No   Yes
   If yes, please describe:

3. Do you or have you ever smoked cigarettes, cigars, or pipes? .... No   Yes
   If so, which and how many per day:

4. Do you smoke while on the job, as a general rule? .... No   Yes

5. Do you have any allergies or allergic conditions? .... No   Yes
   If so, please describe:

6. Have you ever worked with any substance which caused you to break out in a rash? .... No   Yes
   If so, please describe your reaction and name the substance:

7. Have you ever been off work for more than a day because of an illness or injury related to work? .... No   Yes
   If so, please describe:

8. Have you ever worked at a job which caused you trouble breathing, such as cough, shortness of wind, wheezing? No   Yes
   If so, please describe:

9. Have you ever changed jobs or work assignments because of any health problems or injuries? .... No   Yes
   If so, please describe:

10. Do you frequently experience pain or discomfort in your lower back or have you been under a doctor's care for back No   Yes
    problems? ....
    If so, please describe:

11. Have you ever worked at a job or hobby in which you came into direct contact with any of the following substances
    by breathing, touching, or direct exposure? If so, please check the box beside the substance.

☐ Acids	☐ Beryllium	☐ Chromates	☐ Heat (severe)	☐ Nickel	☐ Radiation	☐ Trichloroethylene
☐ Alcohols	☐ Cadmium	☐ Coal dust	☐ Isocyanates	☐ Noise (loud)	☐ Rock dust	☐ Trinitrotoluene
(industrial)	☐ Carbon	☐ Cold (severe)	☐ Ketones	☐ PBBs	☐ Silica powder	☐ Vibration
☐ Alkalis	tetrachloride	☐ Dichlorobenzene	☐ Lead	☐ PCBs	☐ Solvents	☐ Vinyl chloride
☐ Ammonia	☐ Chlorinated	☐ Ethylene dibromide	☐ Manganese	☐ Perchloroethylene	☐ Styrene	☐ Welding fumes
☐ Arsenic	naphathalenes	☐ Ethylene dichloride	☐ Mercury	☐ Pesticides	☐ Talc	☐ X-rays
☐ Asbestos	☐ Chloroform	☐ Fiberglass	☐ Methylene	☐ Phenol	☐ Toluene	
☐ Benzene	☐ Chloroprene	☐ Halothane	chloride	☐ Phosgene	☐ TDI or MDI	

If you have answered "yes" to any of the above, please describe your exposure on a separate sheet of paper.

IV. ENVIRONMENTAL HISTORY

1. Have you ever changed your residence or home because of a health problem? .... No   Yes
   If so, please describe:

2. Do you live next door to or very near an industrial plant? .... No   Yes
   If so, please describe:

3. Do you have a hobby or craft which you do at home? .... No   Yes
   If so, please describe:

4. Does your spouse or any other household member have contact with dusts or chemicals at work or during leisure No   Yes
   activities? ....
   If so, please describe:

5. Do you use pesticides around your home or garden? .... No   Yes
   If so, please describe:

6. Which of the following do you have in your home? (Please check those that apply.)

   ☐ Air conditioner   ☐ Air purifier   ☐ Humidifier   ☐ Gas stove   ☐ Electric stove   ☐ Fireplace   ☐ Central heating

Figure 2–1 (cont'd). Occupational and environmental medical history form. (Modified and reproduced, with permission, from Occupational and Environmental Health Committee of the American Lung Association: Taking the occupational history. *Ann Intern Med* 1983;**99**:641.)

ADDITIONAL SOURCES OF TECHNICAL INFORMATION

Because of the shortcomings of the MSDS, additional information on toxic materials is often needed. Sources include the following:

(1) The employer may have information beyond what is written on the MSDS. As discussed below, it is helpful to establish a line of communication with the person in charge of health and safety at the company.

(2) Poison control centers, county and state health departments, regional offices of the National Institute for Occupational Safety and Health (NIOSH), other

government agencies and local academic institutions with departments of occupational medicine, toxicology, industrial hygiene, or safety engineering may be helpful.

(3) Workers' compensation insurance carriers often employ specialists in safety, industrial hygiene, and occupational medicine and occupational health nursing. They may already be familiar with the workplace where the exposure occurred.

(4) Occupational physicians and industrial hygienists in practice in the area can often assist in evaluating the incident and may have information about other incidents of a similar nature.

(5) Medical libraries in academic centers and local hospitals can provide computer searches regarding toxic materials. The equipment needed to access the National Library of Medicine MEDLARS system is rapidly becoming standard in almost every hospital, medical library, clinic, and doctor's office. All you need is a computer terminal or a personal computer, a modem, a printer, and the appropriate software.

Haynes (1986) has reviewed and compared 17 combinations of software and vendors available to practicing physicians. A simple method of obtaining on-line information services is to subscribe to the American Medical Association AMA/NET. Information is available by calling (800) 426–2873.

The National Library of Medicine will send you an online services application along with a helpful brochure describing *Grateful Med* for people who want easy access to the Library's vast collection of medical and health science information.

DATABASES

The databases described in the following section can be reached through National Library of Medicine, MEDLARS Management Section, 8600 Rockville Pike, Bethesda, MD 20894. (301) 496–1693; (800) 638–8480.

MEDLARS
(MEDical Literature Analysis
and Retrieval System)

MEDLARS is the computerized system of databases based at the National Library of Medicine. The databases may be accessed by more than 20,000 universities, medical schools, hospitals, government agencies, commercial and nonprofit organizations, and private individuals. MEDLARS contains some 11,500,000 references to journal articles and books in the health sciences published after 1965. An individual user may search the store of references to produce a list of them pertinent to a specific question.

A number of online databases are available on the MEDLARS system. Each is described in a section below, beginning with MEDLINE (MEDlars onLINE), the largest and most frequently used, with approximately 700,000 references to biomedical journal articles published in the current and 2 preceding years.

TOXLINE
(TOXicology information onLINE)

TOXLINE and TOXLIT (TOXicology LITerature from special sources) include bibliographic references covering pharmacologic, biochemical, physiologic, environmental, and toxicologic effects of drugs and other chemicals. TOXLINE, TOXLIT, and TOXLIT65 each contain approximately 800,000 citations, almost all with abstracts or indexing terms and CAS Registry Numbers.

CHEMLINE
(CHEMical dictionary onLINE)

An online chemical dictionary with more than 790,000 records. Contains chemical names, synonyms, CAS Registry Numbers, molecular formulas, NLM file locators, and basic ring structure data.

CANCERLIT
(CANCER LITerature)

Sponsored by NIH's National Cancer Institute. Contains more than 580,000 references dealing with various aspects of cancer.

TOXNET
(TOXicology data NETwork)

TOXNET is a computerized system of toxicologically oriented data banks operating under MEDLARS. TOXNET provides information on potentially toxic or otherwise hazardous chemicals. TOXNET contains the following files: HSDB (Hazardous Substances Data Bank), CCRIS (Chemical Carcinogenesis Research Information System), and RTECS (Registry of Toxic Effects of Chemical Substances). Each TOXNET file is described in a section below.

Planning is under way to add additional files to TOXNET in the coming months. These include CDF (Chemical Directory File), the Environmental Protection Agency's IRIS (Integrated Risk Information System), GENE-TOX (Genetic Toxicology), and ATSDR's (Agency for Toxic Substances and Disease Registry) Toxicological Profiles.

For detailed information on TOXNET contact the Specialized Information Services Division, National Library of Medicine, 8600 Rockville Pike, Bethesda, MD 20894. Telephone (301) 496–6531 or (301) 496–1131.

HSDB
(Hazardous Substances
Data Bank)

A scientifically reviewed and edited data bank containing toxicologic information strengthened with additional data related to the environment, emergency situations, and regulatory issues. Contains records for more than 4100 chemical substances.

CCRIS
(Chemical Carcinogenesis
Research Information System)

Sponsored by the National Cancer Institute, CCRIS contains evaluated data and information derived from both short- and long-term bioassays on 1200 chemical substances. Studies relate to carcinogens, mutagens, tumor promoters, cocarcinogens, metabolites and inhibitors of carcinogens, etc.

RTECS
(Registry of Toxic Effects of Chemical Substances)

An online, interactive version of the National Institute of Occupational Safety and Health (NIOSH) publication, *Registry of Toxic Effects of Chemical Substances*. Contains basic acute and chronic toxicity data for more than 92,000 potentially toxic chemicals.

DBIR
(Directory of Biotechnology Information Resources)

DBIR is a multicomponent data bank containing information on a wide range of resources related to biotechnology.

ETIC
(Environmental Teratology Information Center) and
ETICBACK (the back file for ETIC)

These are bibliographic databases covering teratology and developmental toxicology. They are produced by the Environmental Mutagen, Carcinogen, and Teratogen Information Program of the Oak Ridge National Laboratory, Oak Ridge, Tennessee.

ETIC contains citations to articles published since 1989. These records will contain bibliographic citations, abstracts (if available), MeSH (Medical Subject Headings), ETIC keywords, chemical names, and Chemical Abstract Service (CAS) Registry Numbers. ETICBACK contains approximately 46,000 citations to literature published between 1950–1988.

TRI
(Toxic Chemical Release Inventory)

TRI contains information on the annual estimated releases of toxic chemicals to the environment. Based upon data collected by the Environmental Protection Agency (EPA) and mandated by Title III of the SUPERFUND Amendments and Reauthorization Act (SARA) of 1986, the Inventory contains provisions for the reporting, by industry, of data on more than 300 toxic chemicals released into the air, water, and land. Data submitted to EPA include names and addresses of facilities that manufacture, process, or otherwise use these chemicals as well as amounts released to the environment or transferred to waste sites. Title III, also known as the Emergency Planning and Community Right-to-Know Act, calls for the EPA to collect these data nationwide on an annual basis. The law mandates that the data be made publicly available through a computer database. The online TRI file is likely to have a broad-based user audience, including industry, state and local environ-

mental agencies, emergency planning committees, the Federal government, and other regulatory groups. Another important user group is likely to be concerned citizens who, on their own or through public interest groups and public libraries, will use TRI to answer their questions about chemical releases in their communities.

TRI data are arranged in the following broad categories:

Facility identification
Substance identification
Environmental release of chemical
Waste treatment
Off-site waste transfer

The data include the names, addresses, and public contacts of plants manufacturing, processing, or using the reported chemicals; the maximum amount stored on site; the estimated quantity emitted into the air (point and nonpoint emissions), discharged into bodies of water, injected underground, or released to land; methods used in waste treatment and their efficiency; and data on the transfer of chemicals off-site for treatment or disposal, either to publicly owned treatment works or elsewhere.

For further details about the status of the TRI file, contact the TRI Representative, Specialized Information Services, National Library of Medicine, 8600 Rockville Pike, Bethesda, MD 20894. (301) 496–6531.

The American College of Occupational Medicine publishes a *Directory of Occupational Health & Safety Software*. The directory provides descriptions, uses, hardware requirements, training resources, user support, cost, and other computer information for 10 multipurpose, 4 clinic management, 9 health screening and surveillance, 4 disability management, 10 chemical and environmental, 5 decision support-loss control, 6 health promotion-fitness, and 3 miscellaneous software programs. For information, contact Kent W. Peterson, MD, 310 E. Market Street, Charlottesville, VA 22901. (804) 977–3784.

ASSESSMENT OF THE WORKPLACE

The physician should become familiar with the patient's work and the environment in which the work is done. This often necessitates a visit to the workplace. A review of the working conditions requires the cooperation of company managers. Physicians who deal with these problems should learn whom to contact and should have some understanding of their roles in the company's health and safety program.

Working With Safety Professionals

By law, all companies must have a designated safety officer at every office or plant. In small companies, this person may have little or no formal training in safety matters and may have a variety of other responsibilities. In larger companies, the safety professional is more likely to be trained in safety science and to deal solely with health and safety matters. Some companies are large enough to maintain a medical office staffed by one or more physicians and the services of occupational health nurses and other professionals.

The safety professional is the first person the physician should seek out during the visit to the work site. The working relationship between the safety professional and the occupational physician is founded on mutual respect. If the physician shows little respect for the level of professionalism of the health and safety team members, their full cooperation cannot be assured.

The safety professional should be able to provide a description of the company's activities, products, and processes; to give the physician information about past injuries and illnesses in the work force; and to take the physician on a tour of the general work areas and the specific areas where the patient has been working. See Chapter 31 for further information on the role of the safety professional.

Working With Industrial Hygienists

Industrial hygienists are skilled health and safety professionals who are trained to measure and control the levels of exposure of workers to toxic materials, physical hazards, and infectious agents. Only the largest companies with well-developed health and safety programs have an industrial hygienist on the staff. Nonetheless, industrial hygiene data can be made available to smaller companies by consultants or by industrial hygienists from a workers' compensation insurance carrier. If the company employs an industrial hygienist or a consultant, the physician should work with that individual to the maximum extent possible. Industrial hygiene data are invaluable in proving or ruling out many occupational disease possibilities. These data are also important in development of control measures and in the eventual monitoring of the effectiveness of the measures.

Industrial hygiene is discussed further in Chapter 32.

Case Example of the Team Approach to Occupational Safety & Health

A physician observed a number of severe chemical burns in patients who worked for a semiconductor manufacturer in his area. He telephoned the company's safety professional and asked whether a tour of the work area could be arranged. The company was small and did not have an industrial hygienist, but as a result of the rapport developed during the telephone conversation, the safety professional arranged for an industrial hygienist from a larger semiconductor company nearby to join the tour.

When the physician toured the workplace, he was introduced to the occupational health nurse. He learned

that there had been a significant number of burns from hydrofluoric acid, used in an etching process. The nurse explained that the workers were required to immerse racks of silicon wafers into acid tanks and that the resulting burns developed slowly because the acid was diluted with water. Most burns were being seen half a day later by private physicians, who were not always told by the workers that the burns were associated with chemical exposure at work.

The hygienist had previously measured the airborne levels of hydrofluoric acid in the work area, and he gave the physician a copy of these data. Although he had recommended changes in the hoods and vents of the area, he had not found evidence that illness would result from inhalation of vapors at the levels measured. The physician was surprised to learn that the industrial hygienist was familiar with systemic effects of exposure to hydrofluoric acid. The patients seen by the physician showed no evidence of such effects.

The company safety professional gave the physician a copy of the MSDS for hydrofluoric acid and reported that the company had already instituted corrective measures to vent the acid tanks and to provide splash guards over the tanks. Protective clothing and a different type of glove were being distributed to workers.

As a result of his trip to the workplace, the physician learned that he was dealing with an occupational injury and with the possibility of an occupational illness in more severe cases of exposure to hydrofluoric acid. He also learned that the health and safety professionals at the company would begin an education program with the workers and were taking other measures to prevent further injuries.

Most importantly, the physician was included as a member of the health and safety team and was asked to discuss any future cases suspected to be the result of exposure to toxic materials by the company's workers.

ASSESSMENT OF FACTORS OUTSIDE THE WORKPLACE

When a review of the workplace has offered no clues to the source of the patient's health problem, the physician must consider the possibility that the illness is due to exposure to toxic materials or emissions in the home or in various hobby activities. These include disinfectants, cleaning agents, paint removers, wax strippers, solvents, and pesticides; emissions from heating or cooling devices, microwave ovens, and sunlamps; and a wide variety of materials used in painting, ceramics, printmaking, sculpture and casting, welding, stained glass, woodworking, photography, and many forms of commercial art.

The timing of the onset of symptoms is important in determining whether an illness is work-related. Symptoms that occur during the workweek and subside over weekends certainly suggest an occupational cause. Conversely, those that appear only when away from the workplace could well be associated with home exposure or hobby activities.

GOVERNMENT AGENCIES & PRIVATE ORGANIZATIONS CONCERNED WITH OCCUPATIONAL HEALTH

The occupational physician needs to become familiar with government organizations that provide information about occupational health and safety—in particular with OSHA regulations and with technical reports from OSHA and NIOSH dealing with specific questions.

OCCUPATIONAL HEALTH & SAFETY ADMINISTRATION (OSHA)

OSHA—US Department of Labor, Room N3647, 200 Constitution Avenue NW, Washington, DC 20010; (202) 523–8148—is the primary regulatory agency for occupational safety and health. Its standards are law throughout the United States, and its compliance officers can inspect the workplace at any time to determine the status of health and safety and to cite employers for violations of the law. The federal statute governing OSHA makes it possible for states to operate their own compliance plans, and about half of the states have developed such plans. In these states, jurisdiction for all occupational health and safety enforcement is at the state level. After federal OSHA has adopted or changed a regulation, state programs have 6 months to adopt a regulation that is at least as effective as the federal. Most states simply adopt equivalent standards.

In states that do not have approved plans, jurisdiction is at the federal level. Jurisdiction for public employees always rests with the state—even those without state OSHA programs. State OSHA programs can provide safety and health consultants at the worksite. The OSHA Act also requires that each federal agency develop and maintain a safety program consistent with OSHA standards.

OSHA information is generally obtained from the regional offices (see below). OSHA headquarters can assist with some inquiries.

The Department of Labor publishes a document entitled *All About OSHA,* 1985 (Revised), OSHA 2056. The pamphlet is available at any regional OSHA office. The pamphlet explains the provisions of the 1970 Act and the policies of the agency.

The *Federal Register* publishes all federal OSHA standards as well as all amendments, corrections, insertions, or deletions when adopted. The *Federal Register* is available in many public libraries. Annual subscriptions are available from the Superintendent of Documents, US Government Printing Office, Washington, DC 20402. State OSHA standards are available from state governments that have approved programs. (The location of OSHA's regional offices and state offices are provided below.)

The Federal OSHA Subscription Service provides all standards, interpretations, regulations, and procedures in loose-leaf form. The service also is available from the Superintendent of Documents. (Contact the nearest OSHA Office.) Individual volumes of the OSHA Subscription Service are available as follows:

Volume I: General Industry Standards and Interpretations

Volume II: Maritime Standards and Interpretations

Volume III: Construction Standards and Interpretations

Volume IV: Other Regulations and Procedures

Volume V: Field Operations Manual

Volume VI: Industrial Hygiene Field Operations Manual

OSHA Regional Offices

Region I (CT, ME, MA, NH, RI, VT)
133 Portland Street, First Floor
Boston, MA 02114
(617) 565–7164

Region II (NY, NJ, PR)
201 Varick Street, Room 670
New York, NY 10014
(212) 337–2325

Region III (DE, DC, MD, PA, VA, WV)
Gateway Building, Suite 2100
3535 Market Street
Philadelphia, PA 19104
(215) 596–1201

Region IV (AL, FL, GA, KY, MS, NC, SC, TN)
1375 Peachtree Street NE, Suite 587
Atlanta, GA 30367
(404) 347–3573

Region V (IL, IN, MN, MI, OH, WI)
230 South Dearborn Street
32nd Floor, Room 3244
Chicago, IL 60604
(312) 353–2220

Region VI (AR, LA, NM, OK, TX)
524 Griffin Street, Room 602
Dallas, TX 75202
(214) 767–4731

Region VII (IA, KS, MO, NE)
911 Walnut Street, Room 64106
Kansas City, MO 64106
(816) 426–5861

Region VIII (CO, MT, ND, SD, UT, WY)
Federal Building, Room 1576
1961 Stout Street
Denver, CO 80204
(303) 844–3061

Region IX (CA, AZ, NV, HI)
71 Stevenson Street, 4th Floor
San Francisco, CA 94105
(415) 995–5672

Region X (AK, ID, OR, WA)
Federal Office Building, Room 6003,
909 First Street
Seattle, WA 98174
(206) 442–5930

OSHA Training Institute

Office of Training and Education
1555 Times Drive
Des Plaines, IL 60018
(312) 297–4810

Cincinnati Laboratory

USPO Building, Room 108
5th & Walnut Sts
Cincinnati, OH 45202
(513) 684–3721

Salt Lake City Laboratory

OSHA Analytical Laboratory
P.O. Box 15200
Salt Lake City, UT 84115
(801) 524–5287

Health Response Unit

Health Response Unit-OSHA
P.O. Box 15200
1781 South 300 West
Salt Lake City, UT 84115
(801) 524–5896

NATIONAL INSTITUTE FOR OCCUPATIONAL SAFETY & HEALTH (NIOSH)

NIOSH is the federal research agency that conducts studies to develop recommended safety and health standards. It does not have legal authority to adopt or enforce regulations. Rather, OSHA determines which of the standards proposed by NIOSH will be adopted and enforced. Like OSHA, however, NIOSH has the authority to conduct inspections and to question employers and employees and even to include the use of warrants to gain information on workplace conditions and examine workers. NIOSH also provides services to employers and employees, including telephone consultations and on-site evaluations in many areas of the country.

NIOSH Offices

Director's Office
  Center for Disease Control
  1600 Clifton Road NE, Building 1, Room 3007
  Atlanta, GA 30333
  (404) 639–3771
Robert A. Taft Laboratories
  Technical Information Branch
  4676 Columbia Parkway
  Cincinnati, OH 45226
  (513) 533–8328
Division of Standards Development
  and Technology Transfer
  4676 Columbia Parkway
  Cincinnati, OH 45226
  (513) 533–8302
Appalachian Laboratory for Occupational Safety
  and Health

944 Chestnut Ridge Road
Morgantown, WV 26505
Division of Safety Research: (304) 291–4595
Division of Respiratory Disease Studies: (304) 291–4474

Regional Programs Consultants

DHHS Region I
  JFK Federal Building, Room 1401
  Boston, MA 02203
  (617) 565–1446
DHHS Region IV
  101 Marietta Tower, Suite 1110
  Atlanta, GA 30323
  (404) 331–2396
DHHS Region VIII
  1961 Stout St Denver, CO 80294
  (303) 844–6166

NIOSH Information Services

NIOSH produces a considerable literature on occupational health and safety. To select publications, obtain a copy of *NIOSH Publications Catalog,* 7th ed. DHHS (NIOSH) Publication No. 87-115, 1987.

The catalog contains detailed instructions for ordering NIOSH publications. New NIOSH publications are announced regularly. You may subscribe to this service and obtain a copy of the catalog by writing to NIOSH Publications Office, 4676 Columbia Parkway, MS C-13, Cincinnati, OH 45226. (513) 533–8287.

NIOSH is developing a loose-leaf binder filled with textual material from various contributors titled *Evaluation and Control of the Occupational Environment,* intended primarily as reference information for the industrial hygienist and other health and safety professionals. To be included on the mailing list to receive units as printed, contact NIOSH at the above address. If you have questions regarding the additions and removal of units of text, contact NIOSH at (513) 533–8241.

For detailed information on the NIOSH Division of Surveillance, Hazard Evaluation, and Field Studies, contact NIOSH Division of Surveillance, Hazard Evaluation, and Field Studies, 4676 Columbia Parkway, MS R-12, Cincinnati, OH 45226. (513) 841–4428.

NIOSH offers a service providing information helpful in the identification of more than 100,000 chemicals from brand name information. Contact NIOSH Hazard Section, 4676 Columbia Parkway, MS R-19, Cincinnati, OH 45226. (513) 841–4491.

NIOSH offers a toll-free information telephone number, (800) 356–4674, from 8 AM to 4:30 PM (EST) Monday to Friday. The toll-free number is not intended as an emergency response or medical hotline but should make it convenient for the public to request technical information, health hazard evaluation forms, and other information regarding NIOSH activities.

NIOSH Educational Resource Centers provide

training throughout the country. A Schedule of Courses can be obtained from NIOSH Division of Training and Manpower Development, 4676 Columbia Parkway, Cincinnati, OH 45226.

FOOD & DRUG ADMINISTRATION (FDA)

The Food and Drug Administration (FDA) is concerned with the safety and health of workers in those industries producing and distributing foods, drugs, cosmetics, medical devices, animal feed, and biologic and some electronic products. Inquiries can be made to Food and Drug Administration, National Center for Toxicological Research, 5600 Fishers Lane, Rockville, MD 20857. (301) 443–3170.

ENVIRONMENTAL PROTECTION AGENCY (EPA)

The Environmental Protection Agency (EPA) enforces the Toxic Substances Control Act (TSCA); the Federal Insecticide, Fungicide, and Rodenticide Act (FIFRA); and the Noise Control Act (NCA). It is responsible for regulating the quality of air and water and almost all other environmental problems. Through FIFRA, EPA has primary responsibility for regulating the use of pesticides, including the health of agricultural workers, and establishing safe pesticide levels in agricultural products. OSHA has jurisdiction over the manufacturing and formulation of pesticides (see Chapter 29). Through the TSCA, the agency plays a major role in regulating the output of the nation's chemical industry. Thus, it affects the health and safety of workers as well as public health. It also works with other agencies in collecting and disseminating information on hazardous materials. Finally, it has considerable regulatory authority, even to the point of prohibiting the manufacture of materials it considers dangerous to workers or to the public health. Toxicologic reviews are published as health assessment documents and water criteria documents. Inquiries can be made to the Environmental Protection Agency, 401 M Street SW, Washington, DC 20460. (202) 382–2090.

Information on EPA regulatory programs can be obtained from Toxic Substances Control Act Assistance Office (TAO), EPA (TS-799), Washington, DC 20460. TSCA line: (202) 554–1404. RCRA line: (800) 424–9346.

OTHER RELEVANT GOVERNMENT AGENCIES

The Department of Transportation (DOT) enforces the Hazardous Materials Transportation Act (HMTA). DOT also licenses and regulates drivers engaged in interstate commerce. Other agencies with authority in the area of occupational safety and health include the Mine Safety and Health Administration, the Nuclear Regulatory Commission, the Consumer Product Safety Commission, and a variety of state departments of public health as well as other state agencies.

Agencies of interest to those concerned with occupational safety and health are the following:

Agency for Toxic Substances and Disease Registry (ATSDR)
  US Public Health Service
  1600 Clifton Road MS F-38
  Atlanta, GA 30333
  (404) 488–4620
Bureau of Labor Statistics
  Department of Labor/OSHA
  Patrick Henry Building, Room 4014
  601 D Street NW, Washington, DC 20212
  (202) 272–3470
Consumer Product Safety Commission
  5401 West Bard Avenue
  Bethesda, MD 20207
  (301) 492–6800
Department of Transportation
  400 7th Street SW
  Washington, DC 20590
  (202) 366–4000
Department of Energy
  1000 Independence Avenue SW
  Washington, DC 20585
  (202) 586–5000
Mine Safety and Health Administration
  Department of Labor, Room 601
  4015 Wilson Boulevard
  Arlington, VA 22203
  (703) 235–1452
National Cancer Institute
  9000 Rockville Pike
  Bethesda, MD 20892
  (301) 496–5583; (800) 422–6237
National Institute of Environmental Health Sciences
  P.O. Box 12233
  Research Triangle Park, NC 27709
  (919) 541–3212
National Institute of Standards and Technology
  108 North Drive
  Gaithersburg, MD 20899
  (301) 975–2000
Nuclear Regulatory Commission
  Washington, DC 20555
  (301) 492–7000
National Technical Information Services (NTIS)
  (A central source for sale of federal publications.)
  US Department of Commerce
  5285 Port Royal Road
  Springfield, VA 22161
  (703) 487–4600

PRIVATE AGENCIES & ORGANIZATIONS

American College of Occupational Medicine (ACOM)

ACOM is the largest organization of member

occupational physicians. It sponsors an annual meeting in the spring, the American Occupational Health Conference. Numerous committees research topics of interest to members. There are helpful publications available by contacting the American College of Occupational Medicine, 55 West Seegers Road, Arlington Heights, IL 60005. (312) 228–6850. (Membership in the organization provides subscription to the *Journal of Occupational Medicine.*)

American Public Health Association (APHA)

APHA sponsors an Occupational Health and Safety Section that meets annually and receives publications relevant to occupational health. The address is 1015 15th St NW, Washington, DC 20005. (202) 789–5600. (Membership provides subscription to the *American Journal of Public Health.*)

Society for Occupational & Environmental Health (SOEH)

SOEH has a large membership, including occupational physicians and others interested in occupational and environmental health. The organization sponsors an annual conference in the spring. For information on meetings and publications, contact the society at P.O. Box 42360, Washington, DC 20015-0360; (202) 797–8666. (A full subscription to the *Archives of Environmental Health* is included with membership dues. Membership provides reduced-rate subscription to the *American Journal of Industrial Medicine and Annual Reviews of Public Health.*)

International Commission on Occupational Health (ICOH)

ICOH is an international scientific society whose aims are to foster the scientific progress, knowledge and development of occupational health and safety. It sponsors triennial World Congresses on Occupational Health. ICOH issues a quarterly newsletter and offers reduced subscription rates for a variety of international journals. For information on meetings and publications, contact ICOH at 10 Avenue Jules-Crosnier, CH-1206, Geneva, Switzerland.

ICOH publishes the *International Directory of Research Institutions in Occupational Health*, supplement to the *ICOH Quarterly Newsletter* No. 7/4, November 1988. For information contact Professor J. Jeyaratnam, Department of Community, Occupational, and Family Medicine, National University of Singapore, Lower Kent Ridge Road, Singapore 0511.

ICOH publishes the *International Directory of Databases and Data Banks in Occupational Health.* The directory includes 170 databases distributed in 29 countries and 9 international organizations. The majority of the databases are found in Europe and North America. Most use English. For information contact Professor J. Jeyaratnam at the above address.

International Labor Office (ILO)

ILO is a major source of publications in international occupational and environmental health. They are available from the ILO Publications Center, 49 Sheridan Avenue, Albany, NY 12210. (518) 436–9686.

Other National Organizations

The **American Conference of Governmental Industrial Hygienists (ACGIH)** lists various publications in Publications Catalog No. 0489, available from ACGIH at 6500 Glenway Avenue, Bldg D-7, Cincinnati, OH 45211-4438. (513) 661–7881.

The **American Industrial Hygiene Association (AIHA)** provides information and communication services pertaining to industrial hygiene. The address is 475 Wolf Ledges Parkway, Akron, OH 44311. (216) 762–7294.

The **American Society of Safety Engineers** is the major association of safety professionals in the USA. It publishes a monthly magazine, *Professional Safety*, and sponsors many meetings and training sessions. The address is 1800 E. Oakton Street, Des Plaines, IL 60018–2187. (312) 692–4121.

The **National Safety Council** also publishes numerous books and pamphlets and sponsors training programs and an annual conference. The address is 444 North Michigan Avenue, Chicago, IL 60611. (312) 527–4800.

The **Chemical Manufacturer's Association** provides information on most widely used chemicals. The address is 2501 M Street NW, Washington, DC 20037. (202) 887–1100. The **Chemical Research Center Hotline** for toxic information and treatment recommendations is (800) 262–8200. The **Chemical Transportation Emergency Center (CHEM-TREC)**, (800) 424–9300, provides information for emergencies involving hazardous materials.

The **National Council for Radiation Protection and Measurements (NCRP)**, provides information on the common sources of radiation exposure. The address is 7910 Woodmont Avenue, Suite 800, Bethesda, MD 20814. (301) 657–2652.

The **National Pesticide Telecommunications Network (NPTN)** provides pesticide product information, information on recognition and management of pesticide poisonings, safety information, health and environmental effects, and cleanup and disposal procedures. The network is located at Texas Tech University Health Sciences Center, School of Medicine, Department of Preventive Medicine and Community Medicine, Lubbock, TX 79430. (806) 743–3091; (800) 585–7378.

SOURCES OF INFORMATION ON OCCUPATIONAL HEALTH

A complete list of information sources is available in *Fundamentals of Industrial Hygiene*, 3rd ed. Appendix A: Sources of Help. National Safety Council, 1989.

Recommended reading is included with each chapter of this book. A recommended library of textbooks and reference materials for physicians practicing in the field of occupational medicine is as follows:

Books

Adams RM: *Occupational Skin Disease*, 2nd ed. Saunders, 1989.

Burgess WA: *Recognition of Health Hazards in Industry: A Review of Materials and Processes*. Wiley, 1981.

Clayton GD, Clayton FE (editors): *Patty's Industrial Hygiene and Toxicology*, 3rd ed. 3 vols. Wiley, 1978–1985.

Ellenhorn MJ, Barceloux DG: *Medical Toxicology: Diagnosis and Treatment of Human Poisoning*. Elsevier, 1987.

Finkel AJ: *Hamilton & Hardy's Industrial Toxicology*, 4th ed. PSG, 1983.

Grayson M (editor): *Kirk-Othmer Concise Encyclopedia of Chemical Technology*, 3rd ed. Wiley, 1985.

Haddad LM, Winchester J: *Clinical Management of Poisoning and Drug Overdose*, 2nd ed. Saunders, 1990.

Klaassen CD, Amdur MO, Doull J (editors): *Casarett and Doull's Toxicology: The Basic Science of Poisons*, 3rd ed. Macmillan, 1986.

Maibach HI, Gellin GA: *Occupational and Industrial Dermatology*. Year Book, 1987.

Morgan WK, Seaton A: *Occupational Lung Disease*, 2nd ed. Saunders, 1984.

NIOSH Registry of Toxic Effects of Chemical Substances 1985–86. DHHS (NIOSH) Pub. No. 87–114. Government Printing Office, 1987. Available from Superintendent of Documents, USGPO, Washington, DC 20402 S/N 17-32-00431-5.

Parkes RW: *Occupational Lung Disorders*, 2nd ed. Butterworths, 1982.

Proctor NH, Hughes JP, Fischman ML: *Chemical Hazards in the Workplace*, 2nd ed. Lippincott, 1988.

Raffle PA et al: *Hunter's Diseases of Occupations*, 7th ed. Little, Brown, 1988.

Rom WN: *Environmental and Occupational Medicine*. Little, Brown, 1982.

Sax NI, Lewis RJ: *Rapid Guide to Hazardous Chemicals in the Workplace*. Van Nostrand Reinhold, 1986.

Slote L, Dalton WF (editors): *Handbook of Occupational Safety and Health*. Wiley, 1987.

Threshold Limit Values for Chemical Substances and Physical Agents in the Work Environment. ACGIH, 1989–1990.

Zenz C (editor): *Occupational Medicine: Principles and Practical Applications*, 2nd ed. Year Book, 1988.

Journals

American Industrial Hygiene Association Journal. American Industrial Hygiene Association, 475 Wolf Ledges Parkway, Akron, OH 44311. Monthly.

American Journal of Epidemiology. Society for Epidemiologic Research, 624 N. Broadway, Room 225, Baltimore, MD 21205. Monthly.

American Journal of Industrial Medicine. Alan R. Liss, 41 E. 11th Street, New York, NY 10003. Monthly.

American Journal of Public Health. Journal of the American Public Health Association, 1015 Fifteenth Street, NW, Washington, DC 20005. Monthly.

Archives of Environmental Health. Society for Occupational and Environmental Health. Heldref Publications, 4000 Albemarle Street, NW, Washington, DC 20016. Bimonthly.

British Journal of Industrial Medicine. British Medical Association, Tavistock Square, London WC1 H9JR, England. Quarterly.

Journal of Occupational Health and Safety. CCH International, Talavera and Khartoum Roads, North Ryde, NSW 2113, Australia. Monthly.

Journal of Occupational Medicine. American College of Occupational Medicine, 428 East Preston Street, Baltimore, MD 21202. Monthly.

Journal of the Society of Occupational Medicine. John Wright & Sons Ltd., 823–825 Bath Road, Bristol, BS4 5NU, England. Quarterly.

Occupational and Environmental Medicine Report. OEM Health Information Inc., Oyster Shell House, 12 Marshall Street, Boston, MA 02108. Monthly.

Occupational Medicine: State of the Art Reviews, Hanley & Belfus, Inc., 210 S. 13th Street, Philadelphia, PA 19107. Quarterly.

Scandinavian Journal of Work, Environment & Health. Topeliuksenkatu 41aA, SF-00250 Helsinki, Finland. Monthly.

REFERENCES

Becker CE: Key elements of the occupational history for the general physician. *West J Med* 1982;**137**:581.

Goldman RH, Peters JM: The occupational and environmental health history. *JAMA* 1981;**246**:2831.

Himmelstein JS, Frumkin H: The right to know about toxic exposures: Implications for physicians. *N Engl J Med* 1985;**312**:687.

Levy BS, Wegman DH: The occupational history in medical practice: What questions to ask and when to ask them. *Postgrad Med* (June) 1986;**79**:301.

Occupational and Environmental Health Committee of the American Lung Association: Taking the occupational history. *Ann Intern Med* 1983;**99**:641.

Medical Informatics

Bresnitz EA, Rest KM, Miller N: Clinical industrial toxicology: An approach to information retrieval. *Ann Intern Med* 1985;**103**:967.

DeTore AW: Medical informatics: An introduction to computer technology in medicine. *Am J Med* 1988;**85**:399.

Haynes RB et al: How to keep up with the medical literature. 5. Access by personal computer to the medical literature. *Ann Intern Med* 1986;**105**:810.

Workers' Compensation Law

3

Charles L. Swezey, LLB

Although the primary function of a physician in occupational medicine is treatment and cure, he also plays an important role in beginning and maintaining the flow of benefits to the worker. This function requires at least basic familiarity with the workers' compensation system. The physician must be able to recognize a compensable disability and be aware of what is required of him by the law.

In the USA, there are several federal systems and as many different workers' compensation systems as there are states, but all have certain basic features in common. The principles that have received legislative expression in all systems are as follows: (1) limited liability without fault; (2) compulsory insurance; (3) automatic benefits; (4) medical care; (5) income protection, including death benefits; and (6) expeditious resolution of disputes. Each system is designed to ensure the injured worker prompt but limited benefits and to assign to the employer sure and predictable liability.

Definitions

The words "accident," "injury," "disability," and "disease" as used in workers' compensation practice do not have scientifically precise definitions. In general, however, "injury" is the cause and "disability" the result of work-related damage to workers' bodies.

An injury that activates or aggravates ("precipitates," "lights up," "accelerates," etc) a preexisting condition may be compensable if it arises out of and in the course of the employment.

A "recurrence" is disability manifested later that comes about as a natural result of an earlier injury and not due to any later injury. If the original injury was compensable, the recurrence is compensable.

"Medical treatment" broadly denotes the services of physicians, surgeons, and nurses and the costs of diagnostic procedures, hospitalization and medicines, and supplies and appliances (eg, crutches, artificial limbs). An injured worker may also be entitled to expenses of transportation, lodging, meals, and other costs incidental to diagnosis and treatment. In most states, treatment may be provided not only by medical doctors and dentists but also by optometrists, podiatrists, osteopaths, psychologists, physical therapists, and chiropractors as long as treatment is within the scope of their licensure. It may be a condition of compensation that treatment be supervised by a medical doctor.

Curing or relieving the effects of an injury may require such rehabilitative treatment as physical therapy and training in the use of injured limbs or prostheses. And in appropriate circumstances, home alterations, specially equipped automobiles, swimming pools, and the costs of relocation in areas with more salubrious climates have been awarded as part of medical care.

LIABILITY WITHOUT FAULT

A covered worker injured under statutorily defined conditions is automatically entitled to compensation and treatment. The question of who is "to blame" for the injury is not a relevant concern. For example, if a regularly employed painter falls from a ladder and breaks his arm, the employer has an immediate duty to provide medical treatment and to compensate the worker for lost wages without regard to why the worker fell.

The idea of liability without fault is often difficult for persons familiar with the negligence (tort) system of damages to understand. As a matter of social policy, nearly all Western governments require that occupationally injured workers be appropriately compensated and cared for without regard to who was at fault. Like depreciation and amortization of equipment, premiums paid to insurers who provide coverage for injured workers—and the costs of self-insurance—are regarded as business costs ultimately borne by the consumer.

Before adoption of the workers' compensation laws, seriously injured workers often became public charges or wards of charitable organizations. Lawsuits against the employer were seldom successful, and hard-won recoveries were often received too late and after deductions for lawyer's fees and litigation expenses. The employer against whom negligence could be proved, moreover, was in many cases subject to extravagant or even ruinous jury verdicts.

Against this background, workers' compensation laws can be thought of as a reasonable compromise between workers and employers. The employers, in exchange for limited and predictable liability, now pay claims they were not formerly required to pay; and the workers, in exchange for lesser amounts paid promptly and automatically, give up the possibility of winning large jury verdicts.

The reduced cost of insurance for employers who

report fewer injuries provides an incentive for employers to maintain safe working environments.

Although workers' compensation systems uniformly provide for liability without fault, not every disability suffered by a worker is compensable. The worker must be an employee of a covered employer, and the cause of the disability must meet certain conditions. Not every case is as clear as that of the painter who fell from the ladder.

Covered Employers & Workers

In some states, certain employers (eg, farmers, small businesses, charities, and public agencies) are not required to provide workers' compensation coverage. Other state laws exclude various classes of workers (eg, household servants, casual employees, gardeners). The trend of recent legislation, however, has been to eliminate exemptions from coverage.

Employers and independent contractors are not ordinarily entitled to compensation. Whether a given worker is an employee or an independent contractor is frequently disputed. A person performing services for another is probably an employee if the one for whom the services are being provided has the right to control the manner in which the work is being done and the worker does not appear to be engaged in a separate business.

Compensable Claims

A. Injury: Not every injury is compensable. As stated in California Civil Code Section 3600, the injury must "arise out of and in the course of the employment." Almost all states use similar language, and some states add the requirement that it be a personal injury that occurs "by accident." Accidental in its broadest sense means unusual or unexpected, but the concept may include an element of "suddenness" in either the cause or the result.

The words "arising out of the employment" connote a causal relationship between the employment and the disability. "In the course of employment" refers to the time and space limitations of the employment. For example, if a worker has a heart attack while at work, it occurs in the course of the employment but does not arise out of employment unless the work in some way caused the attack.

If a worker sustains an injury while performing an assigned task on the employer's premises during working hours, the injury clearly arises out of and in the course of the employment. The employer's premises, for the purpose of workers' compensation coverage, may extend beyond the company premises. Under some circumstances, injuries sustained while going to or from work or while subject to special risks created by the employment may be compensable. An example would be an automobile accident occurring when a worker is making a left turn across traffic into the employer's parking lot.

If the injury occurs away from the premises or while the worker is doing something not contemplated by the employer, its compensability will depend upon judicial decisions in the jurisdiction. Injuries away from the premises are generally compensable if the employment caused the worker to be where the injury occurred but not if the worker was engaged in purely personal pursuits.

Some injuries may be exempted from coverage even though incurred in the course of the employment. Intentionally self-inflicted injuries, suicides, and injuries caused by willful intoxication are examples.

B. Disease: In addition to traumatic episodes, occupational injuries may consist of diseases, emotional disorders, or a series of minor insults (perhaps unnoticed) cumulative in effect. Diseases related to employment may be categorized as follows: (1) occupational diseases, (2) other diseases arising out of the employment, (3) diseases resulting from traumatic injury, and (4) existing diseases aggravated by traumatic injury or other work-related factors. Diseases may also cause traumatic injury, as when an epileptic chemical worker has a seizure while holding a flask of caustic liquid.

The term "occupational disease" is usually defined as one arising out of exposure to some condition peculiar to a given occupation. In some states, only specified diseases are compensable; in others, the definition is broad enough to include any disease arising out of and in the course of the employment.

"Other diseases arising out of the employment" are those resulting from some risk the worker must bear that is greater than the risk of the general public. Examples are cases in which the work exposes the worker to an epidemic or endemic disease or such commonplace things as impure drinking water, tinea, or poison oak.

A disease that under normal conditions is likely to progress to disability is not compensable merely because it reaches the point of disability while the affected worker is at work. If, however, an employment condition or injury aggravates or activates an underlying disease process, the resultant disability will ordinarily be compensable. In some jurisdictions, the employment condition must be unusual.

C. Cumulative Trauma: Similar to occupational diseases are injuries caused by repetitive minor trauma. Breakdown of an intervertebral disk from repetitive heavy lifting and jarring and bending of the spine is typical of this type of injury.

Role of the Physician

Physicians are not expected to be experts on all the nuances of workers' compensation law. If it appears to the physician that a worker's employment may have contributed in more than an inconsequential way to the condition being treated, the matter should be handled as an occupational injury or disease. The final determination of compensability will be made by the claims adjustors, lawyers, administrative tribunal, or court.

The determination of whether an injury is compensable, however, is frequently dependent upon the facts surrounding its occurrence. In making this determination, finders of fact often rely on the history of injury recorded by the treating physician. The importance of a complete and accurate history cannot, therefore, be overstressed.

COMPULSORY INSURANCE

All workers' compensation laws either directly or indirectly compel every covered employer to make certain that compensation will be paid to workers entitled to receive it regardless of the employer's solvency. This may be done through insurance with a government fund, insurance with a private carrier, or self-insurance. Penalties for failure to secure payment of compensation in some states are as severe as imprisonment or closing of the business.

State Funds

In some states, insurance may be obtained only from a state compensation fund. Other states have funds that operate in competition with and in the same manner as private insurance companies.

The Insurance Contract

Whether the insurance policy is issued by a state fund or by a private insurance carrier, the insurer has an independent liability to the workers employed by the insured. If the policy is in effect on the date of injury, the insurer must provide all benefits regardless of any defenses it may have against the employer on the insurance contract. Insolvency or demise of the employer has no effect on the liability of the carrier.

Self-Insurance

A large employer may be self-insured. Self-insured employers assume the responsibility for adjusting claims and paying benefits. They may contract with adjusting agencies to provide safety and claims adjusting services. They may also reinsure a portion of the risk to prevent excessive losses.

Permission to self-insure must be obtained from a designated state agency, which requires the employer to demonstrate financial ability to pay all reasonably anticipated claims. A bond or other security to guarantee this ability may also be required.

Role of the Physician

When an occupational injury is reported to an employer or insurance company, some individual or department is assigned the task of adjusting the claim. The adjustor will be in communication with the physician about the worker's claim and is responsible for paying compensation and medical bills and for obtaining from the physician periodic status reports as treatment progresses.

AUTOMATIC BENEFITS

A fundamental objective of workers' compensation laws is to provide the injured worker with medical treatment and money to live on without delay. In the great majority of cases, the employer or insurance carrier begins providing benefits as soon as notice of the injury is received. If the employer is aware of the injury, the worker is ordinarily not required to do anything to start the flow of benefits.

In many states, there are penalties for unreasonable delay in payment of benefits. In a few states, the employer is not required to pay benefits until the employer and the injured worker reach agreement regarding the benefits to be paid.

Reporting Requirements

A. Reporting by the Worker: In order to enable the employer to arrange for prompt medical treatment and to determine the extent of liability, most states require an injured worker to notify the employer about the injury within a specified period—commonly 30 days. If the employer has knowledge of the injury from any source (eg, from a physician or fellow worker), formal notice by the injured worker is usually not a prerequisite to receipt of benefits.

B. Reporting by the Employer: The employer is required to report an occupational injury or death to a state agency within a prescribed period ranging from immediately to 30 days. It may not, however, be necessary to report injuries that do not cause any lost time from work.

C. Reporting by the Physician: Most workers' compensation laws require the treating physician to file a doctor's first report of work injury with the employer (or the employer's insurance company) and with the workers' compensation agency of the state. Independently of any legal compulsion, a physician treating an injured worker should report the injury promptly because the doctor's first report of work injury is often the employer's first knowledge of the injury. No benefits can be provided until the employer or insurance carrier learns of the injury.

Reports from the physician are essential for the initiation of workers' compensation benefits. Continuation of benefits is dependent upon periodic reports from the physician because it is primarily from information contained in these reports that claims adjustors determine the injured worker's right to compensation and the amount and duration of payments (see Chapter 4). Reporting guidelines and requirements are frequently made available to physicians by state agencies or insurance organizations. Physicians who expect to treat occupational injuries should keep on hand a supply of the forms required by these agencies and organizations, and clerical personnel should be familiar with the reporting requirements and where the reports must be sent. (For addresses of workers' compensation agencies, see Table 3–1.)

Table 3–1. Workers' compensation administrators' directory, 1988.

Alabama
Workmen's Compensation Division, Department of Industrial Relations, Industrial Relations Building, Montgomery, AL 36130. (205) 261–2868

Alaska
Workers' Compensation Division, Department of Labor, P.O. Box 1149, Juneau, AK 99802. (907) 465–2790

Arizona
Industrial Commission, 800 West Washington, P.O. Box 19070, Phoenix, AZ 85005–9070. (602) 255–4661

Arkansas
Workers' Compensation Commission, Justice Building, State Capitol Grounds, Little Rock, AR 72201. (501) 682–3930

California
Division of Industrial Accidents, P.O. Box 603, Room 103, San Francisco, CA 94101. (415) 557–3542

Colorado
Workers' Compensation Section, Division of Labor, 1313 Sherman Street, Room 314, Denver, CO 80203. (303) 866–2861

Connecticut
Workers' Compensation Commission, 1890 Dixwell Avenue, Hamden, CT 06514. (203) 789–7783

Delaware
Industrial Accident Board, State Office Building, 6th Floor, 820 North French Street, Wilmington, DE 19801. (302) 571–2885

District of Columbia
Department of Employment Services, Office of Workers' Compensation, P.O. Box 56098, Washington, DC 20011. (202) 576–6265

Florida
Division of Workers' Compensation, Department of Labor and Employment Security, 1321 Executive Center Drive-East, Tallahassee, FL 32399-0680. (904) 488–2548

Georgia
Board of Workers' Compensation, South Tower, Suite 1000, One CNN Center, Atlanta, GA 30303-2705. (404) 656–3875

Guam
Workers' Compensation Commission, Department of Labor, Government of Guam, P.O. Box 9970, Tamuning, GU 96911.

Hawaii
Disability Compensation Division, Department of Labor and Industrial Relations, 830 Punchbowl Street, Room 209, Honolulu, HI 96813. (808) 548–4131

Idaho
Industrial Commission, 317 Main Street, Boise, ID 83720. (208) 334–6000

Illinois
Industrial Commission, 100 West Randolph Street, Suite 8-200, Chicago, IL 60601. (312) 917–6555

Indiana
Workers' Compensation Board, 601 State Office Building, 100 North Senate Avenue, Indianapolis, IN 46204. (317) 232–3808

Iowa
Division of Industrial Services, Department of Employment Services, 1000 E. Grand Avenue, Des Moines, IA 50319. (515) 281–5934

Kansas
Division of Workers' Compensation, Department of Human Resources, Landon State Office Building, 900 SW Jackson, Room 651-S, Topeka, KS 66612-1276. (913) 296–3441

Kentucky
Department of Workers' Compensation, Perimeter Park Width, 1270 Louisville, Building C, Frankfort, KY 40601. (502) 564–5550

Louisiana
Department of Labor, Office of Workers' Compensation Administration, P.O. Box 94040, Baton Rouge, LA 70804-9040. (504) 342–7555

Maine
Workers' Compensation Commission, State Office Building, State House Station 27, Augusta, ME 04333. (207) 289–3751

Maryland
Workers' Compensation Commission, 6 North Liberty, Baltimore, MD 21201. (301) 333–4700

Massachusetts
Department of Industrial Accidents, 60 Washington Street, 7th floor, Boston, MA 02111. (617) 727–4300

Michigan
Bureau of Workers' Disability Compensation, Department of Labor, P.O. Box 30016, 309 North Washington Square, Lansing, MI 48909. (517) 373–3480

Minnesota
Workers' Compensation Division, Department of Labor and Industry, 443 Lafayette Road, St. Paul, MN 55101. (612) 296–6107

Mississippi
Workers' Compensation Commission, 1428 Lakeland Drive, P.O. Box 5300, Jackson, MS 39296-5300. (601) 987–4200

Missouri
Division of Workers' Compensation, Department of Labor and Industrial Relations, P.O. Box 58, Jefferson City, MO 65102. (314) 751–4231

Montana
Division of Workers' Compensation, 5 South Last Chance Gulch, Helena, MT 59601. (406) 444–6518

Nebraska
Workers' Compensation Court, State House, 12th Floor, Lincoln, NE 68509. (402) 471–2568

Nevada
State Industrial Insurance System, 515 East Musser Street, Carson City, NV 89714. (702) 885–5284

New Hampshire
Department of Labor, 19 Pillsbury Street, Concord, NH 03301. (603) 271–3171

New Jersey
Division of Workers' Compensation, Department of Labor, Call Number 381, Trenton, NJ 08625. (609) 292–2414

New Mexico
Workers' Compensation Division, Department of Labor, 700 4th Street, SW, P.O. Box 27198, Albuquerque, NM 87102. (505) 841–8787

New York
Workers' Compensation Board, 180 Livingston Street, Brooklyn, NY 11248. (718) 802–6600

North Carolina
Industrial Commission, Dobbs Building, 430 North Salisbury Street, Raleigh, NC 27611. (919) 733–4820

North Dakota
Workers' Compensation Bureau, Russell Building, Highway 83 North, 4007 North State Street, Bismarck, ND 58501. (701) 224–2700

Ohio
Bureau of Workers' Compensation, 246 North High Street, Columbus, OH 43266-0581. (614) 466–2950

Oklahoma
Oklahoma Workers' Compensation Court, 1915 North Stiles, Oklahoma City, OK 73105. (405) 557–7600

Oregon
Department of Insurance & Finance, Labor and Industries Building, Salem, OR 97310. (503) 378–4100

Pennsylvania
Bureau of Workers' Compensation, Department of Labor and Industry, 3607 Derry Street, Harrisburg, PA 17111. (717) 783–5421

Table 3–1 Workers' compensation administrators' directory, 1988. **(cont'd).**

Puerto Rico
Industrial Commissioner's Office, G.P.O. Box 4466, San Juan, PR 00936. (809) 783–2028

Rhode Island
Department of Workers' Compensation, 610 Manton Avenue, P.O. Box 3500, Providence, RI 02909. (401) 272–0700

South Carolina
Workers' Compensation Commission, 1612 Marion Street, P.O. Box 1715, Columbia, SC 29202. (803) 737–5700

South Dakota
Division of Labor and Management, Department of Labor, Kneip Building, Third Floor, 700 Governors Drive, Pierre, SD 57501–2277. (605) 773–3681

Tennessee
Workers' Compensation Division, Department of Labor, 501 Union Building, Second Floor, Nashville, TN 37219. (615) 741–2395

Texas
Industrial Accident Board, 200 East Riverside Drive, First Floor, Austin, TX 78704. (512) 448–7900

Utah
Industrial Commission, 160 East 300 South, Salt Lake City, UT 84111. (801) 530–6800

Vermont
Department of Labor and Industry, 120 State Street, Montpelier, VT 05602. (802) 828–2286

Virgin Islands
Department of Labor, 22 Hospital Street, Christiansted, St. Croix, VI 00801. (809) 773–6200

Virginia
Industrial Commission, 1000 DMV Building, P.O. Box 1794, Richmond, VA 23214. (804) 257–8600

Washington
Department of Labor and Industries, General Administration Building, HC 101, Olympia, WA 98504. (206) 753–6307

West Virginia
Workers' Compensation Commissioner's Office, P.O. Box 3151, Charleston, WV 25332. (304) 348–2580

Wisconsin
Workers' Compensation Division, Department of Industry, Labor, and Human Relations, P.O. Box 7901, Room 161, 201 East Washington Avenue, Madison, WI 53707. (608) 266–1340

Wyoming
Workers' Compensation Division, State Treasurer's Office, 122 West 25th Street, 2nd Floor, East Wing, Herschler Building, Cheyenne, WY 82002. (307) 777–7441

•

United States
Department of Labor, Employment Standards Administration, Washington, DC 20210. (202) 523–6191
Office of Workers' Compensation Programs. (202) 523–7511

Division of Coal Mine Workers' Compensation. (202) 523–6692
Division of Federal Employees' Compensation. (202) 523–7552
Division of Longshore and Harbor Workers' Compensation. (202) 523–8572
Office of State Liaison and Legislative Analysis. (202) 523–9575
Division of State Workers' Compensation Programs. (202) 523–9575
Benefits Review Board, 1111 20th Street, NW, Suite 757, Vanguard Building, Washington, DC 20036. (202) 653–5060

Alberta
Workers' Compensation Board, P.O. Box 2415, 9912 107th Street, Edmonton, AB T5J 2S5. (403) 427–1100

British Columbia
Workers' Compensation Board, 6951 Westminster Highway, Richmond, BC V7C 1C6. (604) 273–2266

Manitoba
Workers' Compensation Board, 333 Maryland Street, Winnipeg, MB R3G 1M2. (204) 786–5471

New Brunswick
Workers' Compensation Board, P.O. Box 160, Saint John, NB E2L 3X9. (506) 632–2200

Newfoundland
Workers' Compensation Commission, P.O. Box 9000, Station B, St. John's NF A1A 3B8. (709) 778–1000

Northwest Territories
Workers' Compensation Board, P.O. Box 8888, Yellowknife, NT X1A 2R3. (403) 873–7745

Nova Scotia
Workers' Compensation Board, 5668 South Street, P.O. Box 1150, Halifax, NS B3J 2Y2. (902) 424–8440

Ontario
Workers' Compensation Board, 2 Bloor Street East, Toronto, ON M4W 3C3. (416) 927–5144

Prince Edward Island
Workers' Compensation Board, 60 Belvedere Avenue, P.O. Box 757, Charlottetown, PE C1A 7L7. (902) 566–4420

Quebec
Commission de la Sante et de la Securite du Travail, 524 Bourdages Street, Quebec, PQ G1K 7E2. (418) 643–5850

Saskatchewan
Workers' Compensation Board, 1840 Lorne Street, Regina, SK S4P 2L8. (306) 787–4370

Yukon Territory
Workers' Compensation Board, 4114 4th Avenue, Suite 300, Whitehorse, YT Y1A 4N7. (403) 667–5645

Canada
Labour Canada, Occupational Safety and Health Branch, Injury Compensation Division, Ottawa, ON K1A 0J2. (613) 997–2281
Merchant Seamen Compensation Board, Labour Canada, Ottawa, ON K1A 0J2

MEDICAL CARE

The first—often the only—benefit an occupationally injured worker receives is medical care, as defined at the beginning of this chapter. There are no effective time or total cost limitations on this benefit. Although there are minor variations in statutory language, the employer must provide or pay for all medical care reasonably required to cure or relieve the effects of an occupational injury or disease.

Control of Treatment

Historically, almost all workers' compensation laws allowed the employer to control medical treatment as long as adequate treatment was provided. The theory to justify this practice was that because the fastest possible recovery and return to work were in the employer's interest, the employer would arrange for the best possible care. In recognition of the many advantages of a mutually established doctor-patient relationship, however, over half of the states now allow the injured worker to make the choice of physician. In a few states, the selection must be from a list prepared by the state workers' compensation agency or maintained by the employer. In other states, the employer controls the treatment choice of physician initially, but the worker has free choice after a specified period (eg, 30 days). In about a dozen states, the employer retains the traditional full control.

Self-Procured Treatment

Regardless of who has the right to select the physician, it is the employer's responsibility to make certain that an injured worker receives prompt and adequate care. If the employer fails to do so, the worker may obtain treatment at the employer's expense. The employer must have notice of the worker's need for treatment before this duty arises except in cases of emergency or when it is not yet known that the condition being treated arose out of the employment.

Change of Physician

Depending on who selected the treating physician, the other party may be entitled to demand a change to a different physician. The means by which a change is effected varies in different states. In some jurisdictions, an injured worker has an automatic right to select a physician other than members of a panel nominated by the employer. In others, a change may be ordered by the workers' compensation agency. Although it is not unusual for an injured worker to be allowed at least one change of physician for any reason, an employer may be required to show good cause for taking a patient from a physician selected by a worker. Examples of good cause are inappropriate treatment and failure to provide timely and adequate reports regarding the worker's treatment and condition.

Responsibilities of the Worker

An injured worker is usually required to cooperate with the treating physician and to submit to whatever treatment appears reasonably necessary. Unreasonable refusal to accept surgery or other treatment that is comparatively safe and likely to be successful relieves the employer of liability for any disability resulting from the refusal.

Fee Schedules

In some states, the workers' compensation agency issues a schedule setting forth amounts the physician may charge. When a physician undertakes to treat an injured worker, the fee schedule is binding, and the worker may not be charged for the difference between the physician's usual charge and the amount the employer pays under the fee schedule. Studies have failed to establish that fee schedules divert competent physicians from practice in this field.

Role of the Physician

In states where the worker has free choice of physician, the physician will ordinarily direct treatment just as in treating other patients. Where the employer controls the treatment, the physician usually—if time permits—seeks authorization from the employer or the employer's insurance company by contacting the claims examiner before arranging consultations or undertaking major surgery or other costly treatment. In any case, the physician must keep the claims adjustor advised of the patient's progress by periodic reports. Changes in the patient's condition, ability to return to work, hospitalization, and similar matters should be promptly reported.

In treating an occupationally injured worker, the physician must bear in mind that the worker is subjected to numerous types of stress. The stress may be internal, such as anxiety about health, job, and family; or it may be external, such as stress arising from the conflicting purposes and advice of lawyers, supervisors, claims adjusters, friends, union representatives, and family members. If stress is not dealt with, it can result in some degree of psychologic reaction and, in some cases, chronic incapacity to work. Whether the effect of stress is minimal or profound will depend in large measure on how the worker's treatment is handled and how the claim is adjusted.

INCOME PROTECTION

In addition to medical treatment, workers' compensation systems provide some protection against loss of income. Temporary disability indemnity partially replaces wages lost during the healing period. If it appears that the worker will be unable to return to the same occupation, vocational rehabilitation services may be provided. If maximum recovery is incomplete, permanent disability indemnity is paid.

If the injury is fatal, the dependents of the injured worker are compensated for their loss of support by death benefits.

Compensation Rate

The amount of disability indemnity an injured worker receives is based on average weekly earnings. Ascertaining average weekly earnings is not difficult in the case of a full-time permanent worker who is paid a fixed wage in money. Compensation in most states is two-thirds of actual weekly pay at the time of injury up to a maximum limitation.

Income from intermittent employment, piecework, and commissions varies from week to week. Tips or emoluments other than cash may also be part of the worker's pay. In these situations and others in which the compensation rate cannot be fairly based on what the worker earned the week the injury occurred, it is necessary to ascertain the worker's average weekly earning capacity.

Although compensation laws and their interpretations vary, a typical statutory provision for determining average weekly earnings will provide the following: (1) If the worker is steadily employed at a fixed wage, his or her average earnings are the actual weekly earnings on the date of injury. (2) If the worker's earnings are irregular, the average weekly earnings will be computed by averaging the earnings over some convenient period (eg, the preceding year). (3) If earnings are irregular and the worker was not in the labor market during the preceding year, average weekly earnings may be determined by comparison with other similarly situated workers. (4) If none of the foregoing methods can be reasonably or fairly employed, average weekly earnings will be the worker's average weekly earning capacity.

Average earning capacity is not determined simply by averaging past earnings. Consideration is given to all relevant facts, including willingness and ability to work, skill and training, the condition of the labor market, and the employment opportunities for similar workers. In the case of students, apprentices, teenagers, and others who actually anticipate an increase in wages, probable future earnings are sometimes considered.

Average earnings include tips and bonuses; board, lodging, and similar benefits provided by the employer; overtime and vacation pay; and wages from other employers when the worker has more than one job. To be earnings, however, payments from the employer must be in exchange for services. Gifts, reimbursements for expenses, and investment income are examples of payments that are not earnings.

Within maximum and minimum limitations, the weekly compensation rate in most states is two-thirds of the average weekly earnings. However, there is a trend toward using 80% of "spendable" earnings (ie, after-tax income). Maximum and minimum rates depend upon the type of indemnity (temporary, permanent total, or permanent partial) and the jurisdiction. The maximum weekly compensation rate for temporary disability indemnity in 1988 varied from under $140 in Mississippi to over $1000 in Alaska, and the median was approximately $345 (Table 3–2). In an increasing number of states, the maximum weekly benefit is pegged at twice the amount obtained by averaging the weekly wages of all workers in the state during the last year for which statistics are available.

Table 3–2. Maximum weekly compensation rates for temporary disability indemnity in the USA (January 1, 1988).[1]

Maximum Weekly Rate		State
Highest	$1094.00	Alaska
High median	357.00	Colorado
Low median	331.00	Alabama
Lowest	140.00	Mississippi

[1]Modified and reproduced, with permission, from *Analysis of Workers' Compensation Laws.* US Chamber of Commerce, 1988.

Temporary Disability Indemnity

Temporary disability indemnity is paid to injured workers during the "healing period" if they are unable to work. The healing period lasts as long as treatment can reasonably be expected to eliminate or materially reduce the disability.

If temporary disability lasts only a few days or weeks, compensation may not be paid for the first few days of disability. The interval between the injury and the first payment of compensation is called the waiting period. The commonest waiting period is now 3 days, though it is still as long as a week in several states. The purpose of the waiting period is to eliminate the excessive administrative expense of paying a multitude of small claims. If the disability lasts longer than a certain number of days (4–42 days, depending upon the state), compensation for the waiting period is paid retroactively. In some states, there is no waiting period if the injured worker is hospitalized.

Temporary disability continues until the worker is able to return to work or until a decision is reached that further treatment will probably not change the disability status. In some states, however, there is a limit on the number of weeks for which temporary disability indemnity is payable. Where these time limits exist, they vary from 208 to 600 weeks.

It often happens that an injured worker is able to perform some type of work (eg, light work) but cannot return to "regular" work. Under these circumstances, the worker is said to be temporarily partially disabled. Temporary disability indemnity for a partially disabled worker is based on the wage loss caused by the injury. If the worker is actually working, the payment will be a percentage of the difference between what the worker earns each week and the worker's statutory average weekly earnings if the latter is greater. Thus, a partially disabled worker does not lose income by returning to work. If the worker does not return to work, the wage loss must be estimated and will be considered to be total if there is no real market for the type of work he or she can do.

Regardless of whether an injured worker returns to work, temporary disability indemnity terminates when the healing period is over. The disability is considered permanent when maximum improvement has been achieved and the disabling condition has been stationary for a reasonable period of time. Disability is permanent and stationary when it is expected to remain substantially the same for the rest of the worker's life—ie, when no major improvement or worsening is expected.

Vocational Rehabilitation

Whenever it appears unlikely that an injured worker will be able to return to his or her usual occupation, vocational rehabilitation should be considered, because continued employment is usually more valuable both to society and to the worker than the permanent disability income the worker can expect to receive even for total disability. Vocational rehabilitation should be started as soon as the worker is physically able to participate in a suitable program. The earlier such a program is started, the more likely it is to be successful.

Some form of vocational rehabilitation is available in every state. In an increasing number of states, the employer is required to pay for vocational rehabilitation if an injured worker is unable to return to his or her usual occupation and can reasonably be expected to be returned to suitable employment by vocational rehabilitation services. In other states, vocational rehabilitation is provided by special funds supported by premium taxes, appropriations, or transfers from other compensation funds. A few states leave vocational rehabilitation to state departments of rehabilitation or education.

Rehabilitation has been defined as a coordinated medical and vocational effort to restore a permanently disabled worker to a reasonable level of economic self-sufficiency. Ideally, the physician in charge of the rehabilitation program determines as early as possible whether the worker is likely to be precluded from returning to the same occupation and reports this fact to the claims adjustor. The physician's report includes a detailed description of the worker's physical and mental limitations and recommendations about the type of work the worker can perform. The claims adjustor then makes whatever arrangements for vocational rehabilitation the law requires. Some insurance companies and larger self-insured employers provide rehabilitation services beyond what the law requires.

Vocational rehabilitation is not limited to formal retraining. In fact, at least one study has shown that formal schooling, even when combined with on-the-job training, is not only the most expensive but also the least productive form of rehabilitation. Modified or alternative employment with the same employer is the most efficient method of returning a disabled worker to suitable gainful employment. If this is impractical, counseling and job placement assistance will often enable a worker to utilize past training and existing skills in another segment of the labor market. If the worker has a marketable skill or product, self-employment may be considered. Having had extensive contact with the injured worker after the injury, the physician is in an excellent position to recommend the type of rehabilitation that is most likely to be successful.

Rehabilitation services are usually coordinated by a counselor, who may be an employee of the employer, the insurance company, the government, or an independent rehabilitation organization. A rehabilitation program is more likely to be successful if the counselor consults and works with the physician and the physician encourages the worker's participation in the program. Vocational rehabilitation services include evaluation, counseling, retraining, and placement assistance. The physician's advice is essential

to proper evaluation, and encouragement is valuable in the other phases.

Permanent Total or Permanent Partial Disability Indemnity

If maximum improvement has been achieved and the worker still has a permanent disability or impairment that affects ability to compete in the labor market, he or she is entitled to be compensated for this disability. If the disability is total, permanent disability indemnity is paid for the remainder of the worker's life at the weekly rate for temporary disability indemnity in the great majority of states. A worker is totally disabled who cannot engage in any substantial gainful employment for a sustained period. Certain disabilities, such as blindness, loss of both arms, or incurable insanity, are defined as total by some statutes.

Some statutes define total disability as totally incapacitating the worker from working in any occupation. Ability to work part-time on occasion or to work in a sheltered workshop, however, is not inconsistent with total disability status. A worker is totally disabled if working ability is essentially unmarketable.

When a permanently disabled worker's ability to compete in the labor market is not totally destroyed, disability is said to be permanent partial. Amounts of compensation for permanent partial disability vary widely among states, as shown in Table 3–3. All states attempt, in a limited way, to compensate the worker for one or more of the following: (1) impairment of bodily functions, (2) loss of earning capacity, and (3) loss of future wages. Although the terms ''impairment'' and ''disability'' are often used interchangeably, an impairment such as a minor amputation or loss of motion may not affect a worker's ability to compete in the labor market. Conversely, a worker with no loss of limb or motion may be seriously disabled because of pain or debilitation.

A common method of compensating permanent partial disability is based on a statutory schedule listing bodily impairments (eg, loss of a limb or loss of vision). The number of weeks during which permanent disability indemnity will be paid is assigned to each impairment. If a disability is not listed in the schedule, the number of weeks for which

Table 3–3. Maximum award of permanent disability indemnity for loss of an arm at the shoulder in the USA (January 1, 1989).[1]

Total Award		State
Highest	$163,590.00	Pennsylvania
High median	55,230.00	Kansas
Low median	53,400.00	Louisiana
Lowest	19,101.00	Massachusetts

[1]Modified and reproduced, with permission from *Analysis of Workers Compensation Laws.* US Chamber of Commerce, 1989.

permanent partial disability indemnity will be paid is determined by analogy to the schedule or on the basis of estimated loss of earning capacity. In some states, a percentage of partial disability is calculated using the percentages of disability of the whole man or woman in the American Medical Association's Guides to Evaluation of Permanent Impairment. A given number of weeks of compensation is paid for each percent of disability.

In varying degrees, some jurisdictions attempt to compensate for actual wage loss. After the healing period is over, the worker is paid a fraction of the difference between the average earnings before the injury and the average amount the worker is able to earn with the disability during the same period; this amount is subject to a statutory maximum. If the worker cannot find work within his or her capabilities, the wage loss is based on the nature of the disability and on an estimate of the extent to which earning capacity has been reduced.

In California, a complex schedule has been administratively adopted to determine the percentage of permanent partial disability. The number of weeks of compensation to be paid for each percentage point of disability is determined by statute and varies from 3 to 8 weeks depending upon the seriousness of the disability. If disability is greater than 70%, a reduced amount is paid weekly for the rest of the worker's life after the number of weeks of regular permanent disability indemnity is paid.

Regardless of how a worker is to be compensated for permanent partial disability, the starting point is a description of the disability. To a large extent, the description of the disability is obtained from reports of treating and examining physicians.

State Funds for a Second Injury

Nearly every state has a fund that provides compensation for serious cases in which the disability resulting from an injury combines with a preexisting disability to cause a disability substantially greater than either disability alone. For example, loss of vision in one eye rates 25% under the California schedule and is considered a 24% impairment under the American Medical Association's guidelines. If, however, the injured worker is already blind in one eye, the loss of sight in the other eye will leave him or her totally blind and totally disabled under the California schedule.

In some states, the employer is liable only for the disability caused by the injury without regard to any preexisting disability. In order to obviate the injustice to the injured worker, the second-injury fund will, in serious cases, pay the difference between the compensation for the occupational disability and the compensation for the combined disability.

In many states, the employer is required to pay for the entire disability but is reimbursed from the second-injury fund for the compensation in excess of what the law requires for the occupational disability.

The employer may, however, be required to establish that it had knowledge of the prior disability before the injury in order to recover from the fund. In some states, benefits are payable from the fund for total disability only.

Death Benefits

A death benefit is payable to the injured worker's dependents when an occupational injury results in death. The dependents to whom the death benefit is payable are not necessarily the worker's legal heirs but are persons, usually close relatives, listed in the statute. Spouses and minor children are often conclusively presumed to be dependent. Other persons must establish that they were in fact dependent on the deceased worker for support. If a person is included in the statutory enumeration and depended upon the deceased worker for maintenance of his or her accustomed standard of living, he or she probably qualifies as a dependent.

In the great majority of states, the death benefit is paid at a weekly rate comparable to the rate at which the state pays temporary disability indemnity. Payments continue until the surviving spouse remarries and minor children reach the statutory age of majority. Some states provide for a lump sum payment to the spouse on remarriage and for continuing payments beyond the age of 18 years for children who are disabled or still in school.

In other states, the weekly payments are made for a fixed number of weeks (commonly 500) or until a fixed amount has been paid (eg, $95,000 for a total of 2 dependents in California in 1989).

There is also a burial allowance. The person who incurred the burial expense is entitled to reimbursement for the amount actually incurred but not exceeding the statutory maximum amount, which may be as little as $400 or as much as $5000, depending on the state. The burial allowance is usually payable regardless of whether there are dependents. If there are no dependents, many states require that the death benefit be paid to the second-injury fund or a rehabilitation fund.

Role of the Physician

The primary role of the physician with regard to income protection is to restore the worker's earning capacity as quickly and as fully as medically possible. Equally important, however, is the physician's role in initiating and continuing the flow of wage replacement benefits to the injured worker. Unless the claims adjustor knows that the worker is unable to work and has detailed information about the nature and extent of disability, it is unlikely that disability indemnity will be provided on a timely basis.

In addition to keeping the employer or insurance carrier fully advised of the status of the worker's disability, the physician can provide encouragement and emotional support. Recovery is enhanced when the worker's anxiety about the future is allayed. This is particularly true if the worker is unlikely to be able to return to his or her usual occupation.

As soon as it appears that an injured worker is likely to have a permanent disability that will prevent a return to the same job, the physician should advise the claims adjustor of the need for vocational rehabilitation and encourage the injured worker to participate in a plan. Follow-up and cooperation with the rehabilitation counselor are necessary to ensure that a suitable plan for vocational rehabilitation is developed.

The physician's role with regard to permanent disability indemnity is to provide a detailed description of the disability (see Chapter 4).

EXPEDITIOUS RESOLUTION OF DISPUTES

Nature of Disputes

Although workers' compensation laws are designed to be largely self-executing (ie, benefits are provided automatically on notice of the injury and the need for treatment), disputes inevitably arise. At the outset, the employer may deny that the injury even occurred. In occupational disease and cumulative injury cases, the employer frequently contends that the exposure at the work site was not harmful. Cases of mental or cardiac stress are almost always contested.

Even if the injury is admitted, as in the case of a painter falling from a ladder in full view of witnesses, questions may arise about insurance coverage or the proper compensation rate. If the worker has already sought medical treatment, the employer may protest that there was not a reasonable opportunity to provide treatment or that the treatment was not reasonably required to cure or give relief from the effects of the injury. In death cases, the fact or extent of dependency is frequently an issue.

The commonest source of dispute is the nature and extent of the disability resulting from the injury. Not infrequently, an injured worker will claim to be still unable to work when the treating physician releases the worker for return to work. Similarly, an injured worker may assert that permanent disability is greater than the employer estimates from the reports of the treating physician.

Machinery for Resolving Disputes

Most of the disputes that arise in the adjustment of a workers' compensation case require prompt and expeditious decision if the purposes of the law are to be effectuated. Difficult cases may require additional decisions from time to time as treatment progresses or conditions change. The civil courts are not equipped to provide this kind of service, and all but a very few states, therefore, have an administrative tribunal that specializes in deciding workers' compensation cases.

The commonest type of tribunal is a board or commission of 3–15 members. It may be called an industrial commission, an industrial accident board, a workers' compensation commission, a workers' compensation appeals board, or by some other similar title. In the less populous states, the commission or one of its members will hear the case initially. In the larger states, hearing officers (sometimes called administrative law judges, referees, workers' compensation judges, deputy commissioners, or trial examiners) are employed to conduct the initial hearing and to make the decision. The tribunals are designed to provide prompt and reasonable awards and to ensure that the proceedings are as inexpensive, uncomplicated, and informal as possible without infringing on the rights of the litigants to due process of law.

Exclusive Remedy

In states with administrative tribunals, the jurisdiction of the tribunal is exclusive: An injured worker cannot sue the employer in civil court if the injury is compensable under the workers' compensation law and the employer has secured the payment of compensation. This does not mean, however, that the worker is wholly precluded from bringing a civil action.

If the negligence or other fault of someone other than the employer or a fellow worker causes the injury, the worker may bring a civil action against that person. The recovery may, however, be reduced by the amount of the compensation received from the employer. The employer or the employer's insurance carrier may also recover from the negligent third person the cost of the benefits provided to the worker.

Under unusual circumstances, it may be possible for a worker to sue the employer in civil court. The commonest example of this is when the employer is uninsured. Civil suits are sometimes permitted when the employer intentionally inflicted the injury or when the injury is caused or the disability is increased by the employer while acting in some other capacity. An example of the latter is the case of a chiropractor who was guilty of malpractice while treating one of his own injured workers. When a worker recovers costs from the employer in such a suit, the employer is usually entitled to credit for all past expenditures and payments under the compensation system.

Procedures for Resolving Disputes

Initiating proceedings before a workers' compensation tribunal is a simple matter. Anyone who questions a determination made by the person responsible for paying benefits may file a claim or an application for a hearing with the tribunal. The claim form is usually short and nontechnical. No special skill is required to fill it out, and it will be considered adequate to initiate proceedings before the tribunal if the information provided is sufficient to inform the adverse parties that a claim is being made.

If the claim or any response to it raises factual or legal issues, a hearing is scheduled as soon as—and in a location as convenient as—administrative considerations permit. Some acts provide for a hearing within 10–30 days, but that goal is frequently unattainable.

The hearings are informal, but evidence is received in an orderly manner, and each party is given an opportunity to present any relevant evidence it may have. Medical evidence is usually received in the form of written reports rather than oral testimony. Although the hearing in some states may resemble a nonjury civil court trial, most states do not adhere strictly to common law and statutory rules of procedure and evidence. The hearing officer may make inquiry in the manner best calculated to ascertain the substantial rights of the parties without necessarily applying technical rules of evidence.

The parties ordinarily agree to everything that is not seriously disputed, and evidence is produced only on those matters actually at issue. When all of the evidence the parties have to offer is in the record, the parties submit the case for decision by the hearing officer. A decision is ordinarily sent by mail in the weeks that follow. Some statutes specify the time (eg, 30 days) in which a decision must be made.

Appeal of the Case

A party who is dissatisfied with the decision of a hearing officer can usually seek review of that decision by the entire board or commission. If the board is large, a panel of 3 of its members may be authorized to act on behalf of the entire board.

In the USA at least, review of the decision of the board or commission may take place in the civil courts. In most states, however, the findings of the administrative tribunal on factual issues are final, and the appellate courts may reverse a decision only when it constitutes an error of law. It is an error of law, however, for an administrative body to base a finding of fact on evidence that is not "substantial."

Reopening of the Case

An important feature of workers' compensation systems is the power of the adjudicatory body to alter its awards if conditions change or if other good cause exists. Thus, if a worker receives an award of permanent disability and the disability later becomes substantially worse, the worker may be able to reopen the case and obtain an increased award. Such changes in condition are sometimes referred to as "new and further disability." It may also be possible to reopen a claim if later-discovered facts (eg, findings at surgery) establish that the original decision was unjust.

A claim may not ordinarily be reopened, however, merely because the adjudicatory agency changes its mind. Its power to amend the awards is subject to limitations imposed by statute. Unless the party seeking modification of an award brings itself within the provisions of the statute, a final decision of a workers' compensation tribunal is just as binding as a decision in any judicial proceeding.

Time Limitations

Nearly all statutes provide limitations on the time during which proceedings for the collection of compensation may be started. These time limits are called statutes of limitations. A common provision is that proceedings must be commenced within 1 year from the date of injury or 1 year from the date benefits were last provided, whichever is later. Claims filed after 1 year will ordinarily be dismissed. Similarly, most states have limits on the time in which an award of benefits may be reopened (eg, 5 years from the date of injury).

Because of these time limits, injured workers must act promptly when they are denied benefits to which they believe they are entitled and there is no likelihood of an immediate informal resolution of the dispute. It is to everyone's advantage, moreover, to resolve disputes while witnesses are still available and memories are fresh.

Time limitations vary from state to state and can sometimes be waived. Although the law does not favor stale claims, it does favor determination of issues on their merits rather than on technicalities. An injured worker who has inadvertently failed to file a timely claim should, therefore, seek legal advice.

Role of the Physician

Unless there is some question about the reasonableness of charges or the necessity for the treatment provided, the treating physician's only role in the litigation phase of a workers' compensation case is likely to be as a witness. The possibility of being subpoenaed will be reduced if the physician's reports and records are clear and complete. Interference with the physician's practice is minimized when testimony is taken by deposition in the medical office, but in that case the hearing officer is deprived of the opportunity of evaluating the physician's demeanor and asking clarifying questions.

Physicians specializing in forensics frequently make special examinations and prepare reports specifically directed to the matters in dispute. They are sometimes retained to assist one party or the other in preparing for trial. The parties may also agree to abide by the opinion of a forensic examiner whom they mutually select.

Even if the physician is not called upon to take part in the litigation process, he or she should be sensitive to its effect on the patient's progress. A person's first experience with lawyers and courts is bound to cause anxiety. There may be a conscious or unconscious tendency to exaggerate symptoms. A treating physician who has established a good doctor-patient relationship can be helpful in reducing the anxiety and persuading the worker that maximum recovery is to the worker's long-term advantage.

REFERENCES

Analysis of Worker's Compensation Laws: US Chamber of Commerce, 1987.

LaDou J: Cumulative injury in workers' compensation. *Occup Med: State Art Rev* 1988;**3**:611.

LaDou J: *Occupational Health Law: A Guide for Industry.* Marcel Dekker, 1981.

Larson A: *The Law of Workmen's Compensation.* Bender, 1985. [Supplemented annually.]

London BL et al: Workers' compensation and psychiatric disability. *Occup Med: State Art Rev* 1988;**3**:595.

Medical Treatment and Workers' Compensation: A Physician's Guide. California Workers' Compensation Institute, 1983.

State Workers' Compensation Laws. US Department of Labor, 1985.

Swezey CL: *California Workers' Compensation Practice,* 3rd ed. Univ of California Press, 1985. [Supplemented annually.]

Swezey CL: Repetitive trauma as industrial injury in California. *Hastings Law J* 1970;**21**:631.

Disability Evaluation

4

William L. Clark, MD

A physician may be asked to assess ability to work for a variety of reasons, including eligibility for employment, Social Security disability benefits, disability insurance benefits, unemployment insurance benefits, vocational or other forms of rehabilitation, and retirement. This chapter is primarily concerned with evaluation that helps to determine the worker's right to the following benefits, which are outlined in Chapter 3: partial wage replacement for temporary or permanent disability, vocational rehabilitation, or death benefits to which certain designated surviving dependents have a right. The suggestions made here, however, are generally applicable to all types of disability evaluation.

PRELIMINARY CONSIDERATIONS

The line between impairment and disability is not always understood. Impairment is measured by anatomic or physiologic loss, which may produce disability, defined as the inability to pursue the activities of everyday living or the activities of work. Whether a worker is considered "legally disabled" is determined by workers' compensation judges, commissioners, or hearing officers; but unless proper evidence is supplied by physicians, those decisions will not be medically sound.

In stating a medical opinion for legal purposes, the physician need not feel the same degree of certainty as when arriving at an opinion for the diagnosis and treatment of a patient. In diagnosis prior to surgery, 90% or better accuracy is desirable. For legal purposes, a preponderance of the evidence (ie, more than 50% certainty) is all that is required. Use of the terms "50.1%," "more likely than not," and "probably" will establish a legally sufficient basis for a "medically probable" opinion. Use of qualifying terms such as "possibly," "maybe," "could be," or any other words suggesting speculation or guesswork will not raise the physician's opinion to a legally acceptable level.

STANDARDS FOR DISABILITY EVALUATION

Standards for disability evaluation vary. Some states of the USA use the American Medical Association's *Guides to Evaluation of Permanent Impair-* *ment,* and others have their own evaluation schedules. The Veterans Administration and the Social Security Administration also have their own schedules. Physicians who perform disability evaluations should make sure they know which schedule is applicable in each case.

Many states have disability rating schedules that list the percentage of disability and arbitrarily fix the award for a given impairment or loss of function. Comparison of various schedules shows such disparity that the validity of any schedule may be questioned. In addition, no schedule includes all of the possible impairments that might result in limitation of activities. The result is that many physicians feel uncomfortable with the concept of disability rating.

ROLE OF THE PHYSICIAN

Employers, insurance companies, lawyers, and government agencies frequently ask physicians questions that are difficult to answer from a strictly medical and scientific viewpoint. A common example is the request for an assessment of percentage of disability. Percentage of disability may reflect one or more of several types of loss, such as decreased ability to perform a specific job, decreased ability to compete for employment, and work-incurred impairment even though this may not produce disability. A physician who has experience in disability evaluation, is trained in ergonomics, has access to sophisticated strength- and movement-measuring devices, and has done a thorough analysis of the worker's job may be able to determine the worker's ability to perform in that specific job. It is questionable whether the training of most physicians equips them to state what competitive handicap in the open labor market is represented by a given impairment. Physicians performing disability evaluations should therefore avoid using percentages to describe the extent of disability unless they are required by law to do so. At the conclusion of the evaluation, it is preferable to characterize the factors producing disability as follows:

(1) Describe anatomic and physiologic deficiencies, ie, objective *signs* of disability.

(2) Describe the subjective *symptoms* that limit function. *Guides to Evaluation* and some state schedules require that specifically defined terms be used in this description (eg, "slight," "moderate," or

"severe"), and the physician should make sure the words are used in accordance with their assigned definitions. Note that the physician—not the patient—decides which word will be used to describe the symptoms in this portion of the report.

(3) Describe work limitations that should be observed in order to prevent future injury. Be specific in these recommendations. For example, instead of "no heavy lifting," specify "no lifting over 50 pounds at any time, and no repetitive lifting of more than 25 pounds."

ROLE OF THE SYSTEM ADMINISTRATORS

After the above information is provided, a layman trained as a disability rating specialist should be able to determine disability percentages according to the law of the jurisdiction. Sometimes, however, the law requires that a physician must decide the percentage figures, and in such circumstances the physician or other examiner must comply.

Unless the physician happens to be an expert on vocational rehabilitation, his or her comments on this subject should be limited to identifying possible need for rehabilitation services for the worker, and it should be left to vocational rehabilitation specialists to determine whether the worker will benefit from such services. If the physician's conclusions about the extent of disability have been stated clearly, experts on the physical requirements of various occupations will be able to make decisions regarding rehabilitation.

MEDICAL & LEGAL QUESTIONS

Whether a given disability is work-related is partly a medical and partly a legal determination, and physicians should not assume that they can make the determination themselves. As explained in Chapter 3, the disability must "arise out of employment" and "in the course of employment" to be considered a work-related disability. The physician is the expert on the first part of the definition, which relates to medical causation. The second part often involves legal questions that need not concern the physician. Nevertheless, the medical and occupational histories may have a profound effect on the system administrator's judgment about whether the injury occurred in the course of employment.

Apportionment
The person being examined may have disability other than that resulting from the work injury. There may be disability resulting from congenital defects, from previous work or nonwork injuries, from aging, or from the natural progression of preexisting non-disabling conditions. When physicians attempt to apportion responsibility for disability between

employers or between work-related and non-work-related causes—either on their own initiative or because they have been asked to do so—there is a relatively simple way to do it that avoids legal complications.

What the physician should do is write 2 paragraphs. The first should describe the existing disability factors (objective and subjective) and work restrictions. The second paragraph should describe the disability factors and work restrictions that would exist in the absence of the occupational injury. The hearing officer can decide the extent of the disability represented by each of the 2 paragraphs and, by subtraction, can decide the disability the employer is responsible for.

Difference BetweenTreatment Examinations & Disability Evaluations
The physician's role in performing a medical examination for the purpose of treating a patient and forwarding progress reports to an insurance company differs in important ways from the examination undertaken to determine whether an injury is work-related, whether there will be permanent disability, whether vocational rehabilitation is appropriate, etc. Many feel it is not a good practice for physicians to perform disability evaluations on patients they are treating, because (1) the physician cannot be objective; (2) things the physician must say in the report may put at risk the doctor-patient relationship; and (3) performing a disability evaluation puts the physician in the position of having 2 legal relationships, one the doctor-patient relationship with the person being treated and another with the entity to which the physician is reporting; and in some ways the legal requirements of the 2 relationships may be in conflict and create problems for the physician.

Informed Consent
The physician must obtain the worker's informed consent to perform any ancillary procedures, tests, x-rays, etc, and the worker has the right to refuse anything. If the worker refuses procedures or tests the physician thinks are needed, the physician should complete the examination as well as possible, noting why the procedure or test was not done and what the possible significance of it would have been if it had been done and the results had been positive.

Release of Records
Confidentiality of records and disclosure of information are legal areas in which there is considerable uncertainty and in which the law varies from place to place. Before releasing any medical records or medical information to anyone, including the worker, physicians should make certain they are fully acquainted with applicable law (see also Chapter 5).

Records should not be released merely on the basis of a letter or request from an employer's representative or a lawyer. If a subpoena for medical records is received, all records must be released whether or not they seem to be relevant to the case. Before responding to a subpoena from someone other than the worker's lawyer and sending the records, the physician should get in touch with the injured worker or, preferably, the worker's lawyer to indicate that a subpoena was received.

Many physicians are uneasy about sending records, because records in a litigated case are open to public inspection, and there may be things in the records that could be harmful for the worker to read or which should not be read by other people. In such a case, it is always possible to seal part of the records in a separate envelope and attach a letter explaining why this information should be kept separate from other records. A workers' compensation judge or commissioner will evaluate the request and, if appropriate, will make sure the sealed part of the records is not available to the public.

Some records are protected even further. Records of medical care related to certain government-financed programs for mental health and developmental disabilities, communicable diseases, or substance abuse may be released only with the permission of the agency involved. If the physician has such records and receives an order to produce them, a medical society lawyer should be consulted for advice before the records are released.

THE PROCESS OF EVALUATION

Preparation

Before an examination to evaluate disability is undertaken, the physician must understand exactly what the requesting party wants to know. If the form or letter requesting the examination is unclear, clarification should be requested before the examination. Copies of all relevant medical records, reports, and test results should also be requested.

History & Review of the Records

The most important and most often neglected part of the medicolegal report is the history. More reports are disregarded as evidence because of an inadequate history than for any other reason. The history of injury should be taken by the physician and not by an office assistant. It is useful to quote the complaints of the patient verbatim.

The history of the injury or exposure to toxic materials at work should be detailed, and there should be a complete and careful description of the activities of the job. For vocational rehabilitation, it may be useful to request a job analysis performed by a specialist (eg, a human factors engineer, work physiologist, or ergonomist) who is trained to analyze all of the job activities and conditions in specific terms. The history should also include information about all previous employment and all nonwork activities, with particular attention to factors that might have some relation to the present complaints. See Chapter 2 for further information about history taking.

Available medical records should be reviewed carefully. In writing a report, list the records reviewed, but do not summarize or quote from them unless the information is relevant.

Physical Examination

Every physical examination should be a complete one. Physical findings should be quantified, if possible, rather than estimated. For motion testing, for example, use a goniometer and mechanical strength-measuring devices, and measure active motion only. The methods of Macrae (1969) and Moll (1971) can be used for measurement of flexion and extension in the back. The method of Mayer (1984, 1985) is more refined and requires the use of an inclinometer but gives even more information.

Part of every physician's evaluation of the patient is an attempt to validate symptoms. Waddell (1980), Dzioba (1984), and Capra (1985) offer practical suggestions for doing so without the use of psychologic testing.

Ancillary Tests

Laboratory tests and x-rays or other imaging techniques that will help the physician establish the extent of disability should be performed; however, unnecessary testing (particularly the repetition of potentially harmful x-rays) should be avoided.

When there is a graphic representation of test results (as with electrocardiograms, pulmonary function tests, and electroencephalograms), the tracings should be attached to the report for the benefit of physicians who may be reading it and who may want to make their own interpretations.

Written Report

In a workers' compensation case, the patient will probably see reports written by the physician. This should not prevent the physician from writing honest, complete reports but should remind him or her not to make statements that might be misunderstood.

The complete history and physical examination should be reported in appropriate detail. Statements such as ''system review essentially negative'' and ''head and EENT normal'' do not really tell what questions were asked or how carefully the parts were examined, and these considerations are important in a legal document.

Reasons should be given for the diagnosis and for opinions on whether there is disability, what the medical cause of the disability is, whether some of the disability would now be present in the absence of the injury, whether medical treatment is needed now or will be needed in the future, and whether the condition is at this time for practical purposes ''permanent and stationary.'' (See Chapter 3 for a discussion of the importance of these factors and their definitions.) Other physicians reading the report will have noted the items in the history, examination, and laboratory tests that supported the reporting physician's conclusions. However, for nonmedical readers, the reporting physician should briefly summarize the evidence that led to the conclusions.

Since the report will be read primarily by nonmedical personnel, the physician writing it should use clear language and avoid professional jargon. Be sure to explain technical terms, describe specific tests (eg, Romberg's test), and explain the significance of a positive or negative result.

Avoid the appearance of bias, and do not criticize other physicians—though honest disagreement with their opinions is acceptable.

Do not include differential diagnoses in the report. Nonmedical readers are in no position to decide which diagnosis is the correct one, and they expect the reporting physician to give the probable diagnosis. The other possible diagnoses are immaterial. Do not equivocate; state the conclusions quite clearly and in terms of "probable" rather than "possible."

If in your opinion the patient is not telling the truth about something, you should so state, explaining the basis for your opinion.

Make sure that the report is internally consistent, ie, that statements in one part do not contradict those in another part. There are 2 useful techniques for catching this and other kinds of errors. First, read the report carefully 2 or 3 days after it was written. Second, ask a trained person in the office (eg, a secretary) to read the report. If the report has been written properly—so that an administrative law judge, for example, can understand it—the office secretary can certainly understand it also and will be able to identify unclear or contradictory language that should be dealt with.

Be sure to note who contributed to the history taking and physical examination and to preparation of the report. In most cases, the physician should have done it all personally. If someone else assisted (eg, a nurse measured the blood pressure, height, and weight), be sure to indicate this.

A note should be made of the total time spent with the patient. It is common for patients to report that the physician "spent only a few minutes" with them and "never even examined" them (particularly if they are unhappy with the physician's conclusions).

The final report and its conclusions should do the following: (1) answer all questions raised by the requesting party or agency; (2) provide a thorough evaluation and description of the disability; (3) establish the medical cause of the disability; (4) indicate whether the disability is permanent or temporary (see Chapter 3 for details and definitions); (5) indicate whether further treatment is required; and (6) offer logical and adequate reasons for each opinion and conclusion.

REFERENCES

Capra P: Adding psychological scales to your back pain assessment. *Musculoskeletal Med* 1985;**2**:41.

Diorio PB, Fallon LF: Workers' compensation, impairment and disability. *Occup Med: State Art Rev* 1989;**4**:145.

Dzioba RB: A prospective investigation into the orthopedic and psychologic predictors of outcome of first lumbar surgery following industrial injury. *Spine* 1984;**9**:614.

Fox RM: *The Medicolegal Report.* Little, Brown, 1969.

Lasky H: *How to Handle Psychiatric Claims Under the California Workers' Compensation System.* Lex-Com, 1983.

Macrae IF: Measurement of back movement. *Ann Rheum Dis* 1969;**28**:584.

Mayer TG: Use of noninvasive techniques for quantification of spinal range-of-motion in normal subjects and chronic low-back dysfunction patients. *Spine* 1984;**9**:588.

Mayer TG: Using physical measurements to assess low back pain. *Musculoskeletal Med* 1985;**2**:44.

Moll JM: Normal range of spinal mobility. *Ann Rheum Dis* 1971;**30**:381.

Occupational and Environmental Health Committee of the American Lung Association: Taking the occupational history. *Ann Intern Med* 1983;**99**:641.

Prior JA et al: *Physical Diagnosis: The History and Examination of the Patient.* Mosby, 1981.

Waddell G: Nonorganic physical signs in low-back pain. *Spine* 1980;**5**:117.

Liability in Occupational Health Practice

5

John M. Bielan, MD, JD

THE PHYSICIAN IN PRIVATE PRACTICE

The Physician-Patient Relationship

Traditionally, the physician and the patient enter into a contract whereby the physician agrees to provide professional services, using the knowledge and skill of a reasonably prudent practitioner of similar training in the community, and the patient agrees to pay the physician's professional fees. In legal terminology, the physician promises to provide services in conformity with the standard of ordinary care in the community. The *Book of Approved Jury Instructions (BAJI)*, 7th ed, 1986, section 6.00, used in California courts, defines the physician's "duty of care" as follows:

> In performing professional services for a patient, a physician or surgeon has the duty to have that degree of learning and skill ordinarily possessed by reputable physicians and surgeons, practicing in the same or a similar locality and under similar circumstances.
>
> The further duty of the physician is to use the care and skill ordinarily exercised in like cases by reputable members of the profession practicing in the same or a similar locality under similar circumstances, and to use reasonable diligence and his or her best judgment in the exercise of skill and the application of learning, in an effort to accomplish the purpose for which the physician is employed.
>
> A failure to fulfill any such duty is negligence.

The patient in turn places himself or herself "in the physician's hands," relying upon the physician's knowledge, judgment, and skill, and pays the physician for services, either directly or, more often, indirectly, through a third party (eg, an insurance carrier).

Professional Negligence (Malpractice)

Like any negligence action, a malpractice complaint of physician negligence must plead and prove 4 elements: (1) a duty on the part of the physician; (2) a breach of that duty; (3) proximate cause, ie, that the breach is responsible for harm resulting to the patient; and (4) damages (harm) to the party to whom the duty is owed. Professional negligence, or malpractice, occurs when the physician fails in the duty of care to the patient and the patient is harmed as a result.

The purpose of a malpractice lawsuit is not to "do justice" or to "right a wrong" but to compensate the plaintiff for injuries suffered and to "make the patient whole." Inadequate as it may be, the law makes provision only for monetary compensation.

The Physician's Legal Defenses

The physician defending an action grounded in negligence has several common law defenses available: (1) That no actual physician-patient relationship existed. (2) That the physician met the standard of care and there was therefore no breach of duty. (3) That the plaintiff's injuries are not causally related to the alleged negligence. (4) That the injuries are trivial. (5) That the plaintiff contributed to the injury (eg, by refusing treatment, failing to follow the physician's instructions, or failing or refusing to take prescribed medications), in which case the patient's own negligence would diminish the physician's negligence.

Most states follow a scheme of proportionate fault, or comparative negligence, whereby fault is allocated between physician and patient. In some states, if the patient is more than 50% at fault, the suit is completely nullified. Other states (eg, California) follow a more generous rule whereby the patient may recover for the percentage of the injury caused by the physician's negligence even if the patient's own negligence is responsible for almost the entire injury.

THE PHYSICIAN IN THE WORKPLACE

With the advent of physicians in the workplace, the above analysis of physician liability is markedly altered.

Physician-Employee Relationship

In the occupational setting, the physician does not enter into a direct contract with the patient (worker). The physician contracts with the employer to provide care for the worker, and the worker is the third-party beneficiary of that contract.

The nature of the physician-employer relationship is paramount in determining the physician's own liability for alleged negligence. The essential question is whether the physician is an employee or an independent contractor. If the physician is clearly an employee, negligence toward a fellow employee is encompassed by workers' compensation. If the physician is an independent contractor, the common law negligence principles outlined above apply, and the physician can be sued directly by a worker who alleges physician negligence.

In many cases, however, the "fellow employee" concept indeed does not immunize the physician against actions for negligence, and the courts have not been eager to incorporate medical malpractice into the traditional areas encompassed by the workers' compensation scheme. Only if the physician is *clearly and unequivocally* a fellow employee are the courts likely to apply the exclusive remedy provision of the workers' compensation system.

Workers' Compensation & Liability of the Physician

Prior to the advent of workers' compensation, the worker was forced to sue the employer for negligence in the workplace. However, the common law defenses of assumption of the risk and contributory negligence raised by employers frequently prevented the worker from receiving any compensation for the injury. To prevent this inequity and to save industry from being awash in litigation, workers' compensation was adopted in the USA.

As a legal doctrine, workers' compensation holds employers strictly liable for injuries sustained by their workers in the course and scope of employment. As discussed in Chapter 3, fault or negligence need not be proved and need not even exist. Workers are guaranteed compensation for their job-related injuries.

Employers also benefit from workers' compensation. They are saved the costs of litigation, and the compensation actually paid to their injured workers is less than would probably be awarded in civil law suits. Furthermore, the financial burden upon the employer for workers' compensation insurance is "diluted" by being passed on to the consuming public.

The workers' compensation system is the exclusive remedy available to injured workers (see Chapter 3), and they cannot ordinarily sue their employers for injuries sustained on the job.

If the occupational physician is clearly an employee, his or her professional negligence is employee negligence, and workers' compensation is the exclusive remedy of the employee injured as a consequence of that negligence. However, this is true only if the employee-physician is working within the course and scope of his or her employment. If the physician assumes responsibilities in relation to the patient that are outside the physician's employment

parameters, the physician can then be held personally liable for negligent harm that may follow.

Employee Versus Independent Contractor

The courts have evolved 2 tests to resolve the question of whether an occupational physician is an employee or an independent contractor.

The **control test** asks how much independent decision making and control of actions is exercised by the health professional. For example, the physician who is conducting a routine predetermined physical examination or providing care as predetermined and formulated in conjunction with management is deemed to be acting under the control of the employer and is therefore an employee. The physician who is making independent judgments as any physician in private practice does and who is not following preapproved functions or procedures is deemed an independent contractor.

The **indicia test** is simply another way of approaching this question of independent judgment and control. The court seeks indicia (indications) that the health professional is treated as and functions as an employee and so is under company control. Indicia of employee status are present if health professionals are required to keep regular working hours, are receiving the same benefits received by other employees, are required to report regularly to superiors, and must request and obtain authorization before acting outside existing protocols.

Insurance

The nature of medical practice is such that health professionals must and do exercise some independent professional judgment. Therefore, it is unwise for any physician providing occupational health services to rely solely upon the workers' compensation policy of the company to protect against personal liability for professional negligence. Every occupational physician should be personally insured against professional negligence claims, over and above the employer's own workers' compensation coverage.

Employee Health Records

Employee health information obtained through the efforts of the occupational health professional at the request of the company is the property of the company. However, the occupational physician has certain responsibilities in regard to confidentiality and the obligation to inform workers of the results of their medical examinations.

A. Informing the Worker:

1. Ethical obligations–The American College of Occupational Medicine's Code of Ethical Conduct of Physicians Providing Occupational Medical Services (1976) states that occupational physicians should "communicate understandably to those they serve any significant observations about their health, recommending further study, counsel or treatment when indicated."

2. Legal obligations—Courts in the large industrial states of California, Michigan, New York, and Ohio have recognized that the consensual relationship between company physician and worker comes into being for the benefit of the actual or prospective employer. Thus, the courts have uniformly imposed a lower standard of care on the occupational physician than that owed by a physician to a private patient. These states have held that the occupational physician does not have a legal duty to workers to inform them of medical findings. Rather, it is the employer who bears the obligation to inform the workers.

A federal court has held also that an examinee reasonably assumes he or she will be informed of abnormal findings, and this imposes a duty upon the examining physician to so inform the examinee.

3. Recommendations—The legally safest course for the health professional would appear to be to inform the worker of abnormal examination findings. The employer also has an independent duty to so inform, but that duty would be met when the company's occupational health professional has informed the worker. This position is consistent with the ethical recommendations of the American College of Occupational Medicine.

B. Confidentiality of Records: Employee medical information is not to be disclosed to third parties without consent, actual or implied, of the worker. Releasing information from a patient's medical records without the patient's permission or legal justification can result in revocation of a physician's license in about half the states.

1. Ethical obligations—The ethical code of the American College of Occupational Medicine (1976) prescribes that the occupational physician "treat as confidential whatever is learned about individuals served, releasing information only when required by law or by over-riding public health considerations, or to other physicians at the request of the individual according to traditional medical ethical practice; and should recognize that employers are entitled to counsel about the medical fitness of individuals in relation to work, but are not entitled to diagnoses or details of a specific nature." The ethical code of the American Association of Occupational Health Nurses (1977) requires that the nurse "safeguard the employee's right to privacy by protecting information of a confidential nature; releasing information only as required by law or upon written consent of the employee."

2. Employer's right to know—The employer provides employee medical examinations for the employer's own purposes, ie, to gauge and to maintain the "workability" of the employees. Therefore, information divulged to the employer should be limited to workplace-related health. The employees, by acquiescing to examination by company health professionals and by availing themselves of these health services, agree by implied consent to such disclosure. Implied consent to disclose medical information is unrelated to the physician's contractual status. Limitations on disclosure of a professional confidence

apply equally to all physicians as a legal requirement of practice (often statutory).

a. Information about the prospective employee—The health professional should, of course, thoroughly examine and evaluate the job applicant. However, the employer should be informed only of examination results that would either make the applicant unable to perform the job or place him or her at serious risk of harm in the job.

b. Information about the current employee—The employer has a right to know if a current worker is injured or disabled, if the disability is work-related, what the estimated length of disability is, and whether the worker's activities should be temporarily restricted upon his or her return.

C. Employee Access to Medical Records: As discussed above, employee medical records are the property of the employer, but employer access to employee medical records in many states is controlled and restricted by statute (eg, see California Civil Code, sections 56.10 and 56.11). As with employer access to medical records, in many states the employee's own access to health records is provided for by statute (eg, see California Health and Safety Code, sections 25250–25258).

1. Regulations of the Occupational Safety and Health Administration (OSHA)—The OSHA regulation of 1980 requires employers dealing with toxic materials to make their records available to employees within 15 days after an employee's request to examine them. Documents to be made accessible include not only the employee's medical records but also environmental data about the workplace. An employee may even have access to the toxic exposure record of a fellow employee if such information is relevant to his or her own likelihood of toxic exposure.

2. Defamation and the right to privacy—The employer who permits false or confidential employee information to be disseminated in the company can be liable to the employee for defamation or invasion of the employee's right to privacy. The health professional should be advised that if confidential information is "leaked" from the company medical department, both the company and the responsible health professional may be held liable for defamation or invasion of privacy.

THE OCCUPATIONAL HEALTH NURSE

Nurses practicing in occupational settings are usually company employees. However, they commonly have more autonomy than hospital-based nurses and frequently act in the absence of a physician.

The above discussions of the legal obligations and liabilities of occupational physicians apply also to occupational health nurses because the nurses' activities may approach the independent practice of medicine. To ensure that occupational health nurses are not operating outside the scope of licensed nursing practice or outside the umbrella of workers' compensation, the following guidelines should be followed:

(1) The course and scope of the occupational health nurse's professional duties and activities should be defined by protocols outlining standardized nursing procedures. Each protocol should be in writing and should be jointly approved, dated, and signed both by a physician and by a company executive.

(2) Each function or duty of the occupational health nurse should be defined in a protocol. The specific procedure and the circumstances under which the procedure may be performed should be clearly described.

(3) Protocols for occupational health nurses should not include functions that are restricted by law to other health care professionals, such as prescribing or dispensing drugs or performing surgical procedures.

(4) Any special training or experience required of the occupational health nurse in order to perform a particular function or procedure should be stipulated.

(5) Procedures that require direct physician supervision should be identified.

(6) A list should be maintained of all persons authorized to perform the specified functions and procedures.

(7) Protocols should be reviewed on a scheduled periodic basis.

REFERENCES

American Academy of Industrial Hygiene: Code of Ethics for the Professional Practice of Industrial Hygiene, adopted 1979.

American Association of Occupational Health Nurses: Code of Ethics, adopted 1977.

American College of Occupational Medicine: Code of Ethical Conduct of Physicians Providing Occupational Medical Services, adopted 1976.

American Society of Safety Engineers: Code of Ethics for the Safety Profession, adopted 1974.

Harney DM: *Medical Malpractice.* Allen Smith, 1973.

Keeton WP et al (editors): *Prosser and Keeton on Torts,* 5th ed. West Publishing Co, 1984.

King JH: *The Law of Medical Malpractice.* West Publishing, 1977.

LaDou J (editor): *Occupational Health Law: A Guide for Industry.* Marcel Dekker, 1981.

Occupational Safety and Health Administration: Access to employee exposure and medical records, final rule. Federal Register, May 23, 1980 (45 FR 35212).

Strasser AL: Medical relationships with unions and management. In: American Medical Association Congress on Occupational Health: Occupational Safety & Health Symposia, 1976. NIOSH Publication No. 77-179. US Department of Health, Education, and Welfare, 1977.

LEGAL CASES

Ahnert v Wildman, 376 NE 2d 1182 (1978). (The relation between physician and patient is based on contract. The company's "examining physician" does not enter into a contract with the employee. The rights and liabilities of the parties are governed by the law of contract.)

Garcia v Iserson, 309 NE 2d 420 (1974). (Employee received injection in a negligent manner from a physician employed by the company, causing injuries. Worker's compensation was the exclusive remedy, since the physician was a fellow employee— citing New York statute.)

Golini v Nachtigall, 343 NE 2d 762 (1975). (Executive treated and negligently injured by a company physician had no direct action against the physician—citing authority of Iserson supra.)

Hoesl v United States, 451 F Supp 1170 (1978). (Suit for defamation against navy psychiatrist barred by Federal Tort Claims Act. Recovery possible under California law, but not in this case since the physician's communication about employee to employer was privileged and properly made.)

Kofron v Amoco Chemicals Corporation, 441 A 2d 226 (1982). (Asbestos case. Claims for gross negligence against employer dismissed. Workers' compensation was the only remedy.)

Lotspeich v Chance Vought Aircraft, 369 SW 2d 705 (1963). (No cause of action for failure to diagnose tuberculosis on preemployment physical. Neither the physician nor the employer had a duty to diagnose the disease—thus no actionable negligence.)

Mrachek v Sunshine Biscuit, Inc, 123 NE 2d 801 (1954). (Negligent venipuncture of applicant for employment. The physician was an employee, not an independent contractor, and the employer was therefore liable under the doctrine of respondeat superior.)

New York Central R R Co v Wiler, 177 NE 205 (1937). (Rough examination caused hernia. However, submission by the employee to physical examination by a railroad physician did not create a physician-patient relationship—thus no action for negligence.)

Proctor v Ford Motor Co, 302 NE 2d 580 (1973). (Negligent diagnosis and treatment. Fellow employees' immunity statute immunizes physician from personal tort liability "on the condition that such injury . . . is found to be compensable under . . . [the Workers' Compensation Act].")

Rogers v Hovarth, 237 NW 2d 595 (1976). (Suit for malpractice, fraud, and libel. Company physician called plaintiff a "malingerer." Complaints for malpractice and fraud dismissed because no doctor-patient relationship existed.)

Ross v Schubert, 388 NE 2d 623 (1979). (Indiana case contrary to Iserson supra. In enacting the fellow employee immunity provisions of the Workers' Compensation Act, it was not the intent of the legislature to interfere with the traditional doctor-patient relationship. The employer does not control the physician employee in the sense of telling him how to diagnose or treat.)

Tumbarella v Kroger Company, 271 NW 2d 284 (1978). (Employer published defamatory letter regarding theft by cashier. Suit was for false imprisonment, slander, and libel. Complaint states a cause of action for negligent dissemination of unproved allegations and should not have been dismissed. This case warns against careless disclosure of possibly defamatory facts about employees.)

Union Carbide & Carbon Corporation v Stapleton, 237 F 2d 229 (1956). (Employer who had employee examined was negligent for failing to inform him of dangerous condition—tuberculosis.)

Wilcox v Salt Lake City Corporation, 484 P 2d 1200 (1971). (Physician's duty was to the city, and he therefore had governmental immunity from liability for failure to diagnose tuberculosis.)

6

Ergonomics & the Prevention of Occupational Injuries

David A. Thompson, PhD

Ergonomics—also called human factors engineering—is the study of the behavior and activities of people working with mechanical and electronic machines and tools. The function of specialists in ergonomics is to design or improve the workplace, equipment, and procedures of workers to ensure the safe, healthy, and efficient achievement of personal and organizational goals.

Approach to Job Design

Ergonomists, occupational physicians, and other health and safety professionals frequently work together to improve the design of jobs and work stations that appear unsafe or have caused injury. The principles of job design and redesign discussed in this chapter are relevant to both the office and the factory floor, and examples are drawn from both areas. Specific physical conditions and injuries that may result from poor job design are listed, along with suggestions for redesign to alleviate the problems.

Approach to Prevention of Occupational Injuries

Health professionals should seek frequent opportunities to tour work areas and evaluate job procedures, equipment, and working conditions. The concepts and suggestions presented in this and related chapters should be kept in mind during these tours, and problem areas and activities should be noted for later study and possible job redesign. Such tours should be made at least quarterly, with emphasis on work areas where injuries are most often reported.

In addition to redesigning unsafe and unhealthy jobs, consideration might be given to restructuring a job at a new skill level or new mechanization level. This may involve employing the techniques of job simplification (reduction of physical complexity of the job) and job enlargement (broader use of skills or greater variety of tasks), and the aid of an ergonomist or an industrial engineer will often be necessary. These professionals are concerned with employee health and safety as well as productivity, since the two are closely interrelated.

The health professional should also establish a committee within the organization to plan health and safety reviews and follow-up activities and to act as a resource for management. Ergonomists, industrial engineers, safety engineers, human resources personnel, and risk management personnel should all be encouraged to participate in these activities.

Cost-Effectiveness of Preventive Activities

The amount of money budgeted for health needs is becoming large in most organizations, and the health and safety committee can offer advice on the effective use of these funds. Health professionals within the organization might also plan special programs (eg, supervisory training in ergonomics) to dramatically reduce costs related to injuries and workers' compensation insurance premiums. Ergonomic studies have shown that it is not cost-effective to supply employees with low-cost tools and equipment or to place them in work spaces that are poorly designed or overcrowded or in any way cause physical or mental stress.

PHYSICAL STRESS DUE TO POOR WORKPLACE OR EQUIPMENT DESIGN

Use of Anthropometric Data

One of the primary reasons for physical stress on the job is the mismatch in size between the worker and the workplace, equipment, or machinery. This mismatch may result in having to work bent over, having to work with one or both arms and shoulders held high for long periods, having to hold a power tool at some distance for long periods, or having to sit on a stool or bench that is too low or too high.

Figs 6–1 and 6–2 show the body dimensions of adult men and women in the USA. Workplaces and machines are typically designed so that larger workers (up to the 95th percentile) and smaller workers (down to the 5th percentile) can function appropriately. That is, an ideal work space not only accommodates the larger workers' body size, height of viewing, location of hands and feet, etc, but it also keeps control levers within comfortable reach and activation of the smaller workers and accommodates their height of viewing.

Improvement of Work & Workplace Design

A. Elimination of "Waist Motion": The most important physical design rule for a sedentary job is

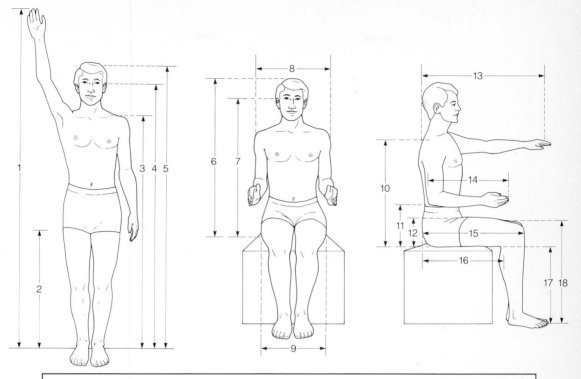

Male Body Dimensions (cm)

Dimension Number	Dimension Name	5th Percentile	50th Percentile	95th Percentile	Standard Deviation
1	Vertical reach	195.6	209.6	223.5	8.46
2	Crotch height	75.4	83.1	90.7	4.67
3	Shoulder height	133.6	143.6	154.1	6.22
4	Eye height	152.4	163.3	175.0	15.29
5	Stature	163.8	174.4	185.6	6.61
6	Height, sitting	84.5	90.8	96.7	3.66
7	Eye height, sitting	72.8	78.8	84.6	3.57
8	Shoulder breadth	41.5	45.2	49.8	2.54
9	Hip breadth, sitting	30.7	33.9	38.4	2.38
10	Shoulder height, sitting	57.1	62.4	67.6	3.18
11	Elbow height, sitting	18.8	23.7	28.0	2.78
12	Thigh clearance	13.0	14.9	17.5	1.36
13	Thumb tip reach	74.9	82.4	90.9	4.85
14	Elbow-fingertip length	44.3	47.9	51.9	2.31
15	Buttock-knee length	54.9	59.4	64.3	2.85
16	Buttock-popliteal length	45.8	49.8	54.0	2.50
17	Popliteal height	40.6	44.5	48.8	2.50
18	Knee height, sitting	49.7	54.0	58.7	2.73

Figure 6–1. Body dimensions for men. Corresponding weights are as follows: 5th percentile, 57.4 kg (126.3 N); 50th percentile, 71 kg (156.2 N); and 95th percentile, 91.6 kg (201.5 N). Appropriate weights must be added for clothing and shoes. (Source of data: *Anthropometry of US Military Personnel.* DOD Handbook–743, 3 October 1980.)

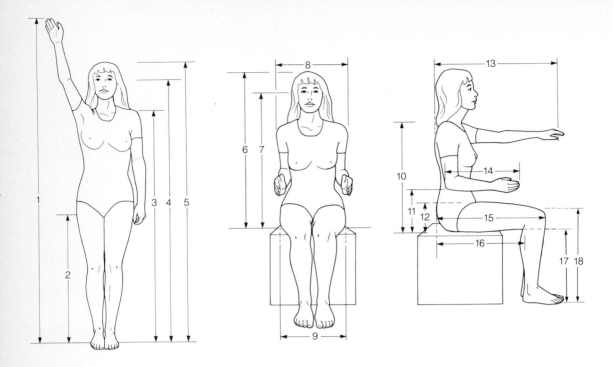

Female Body Dimensions (cm)

Dimension Number	Dimension Name	5th Percentile	50th Percentile	95th Percentile	Standard Deviation
1	Vertical reach	185.2	199.1	213.4	8.64
2	Crotch height	68.1	74.4	81.3	4.06
3	Shoulder height	123.9	133.3	143.7	6.00
4	Eye height	142.2	149.9	158.8	6.35
5	Stature	152.6	162.8	174.1	6.52
6	Height, sitting	79.0	85.2	90.8	3.59
7	Eye height, sitting	67.7	73.8	79.1	3.46
8	Shoulder breadth	38.4	42.0	45.7	2.24
9	Hip breadth, sitting	33.0	38.2	43.9	3.27
10	Shoulder height, sitting	53.7	57.9	62.5	2.66
11	Elbow height, sitting	16.1	20.8	25.0	2.74
12	Thigh clearance	13.2	15.4	17.5	1.31
13	Thumb tip reach	67.7	74.2	80.5	3.88
14	Elbow-fingertip length	40.0	43.4	47.5	2.28
15	Buttock-knee length	53.1	57.7	63.2	3.06
16	Buttock-popliteal length	43.5	47.5	52.6	2.76
17	Popliteal height	38.0	41.6	45.7	2.35
18	Knee height, sitting	46.9	50.9	55.5	2.60

Figure 6–2. Body dimensions for women. Corresponding weights are as follows: 5th percentile, 46.6 kg (102.5 N); 50th percentile, 59.6 kg (131.1 N); and 95th percentile, 74.5 kg (163.9 N). Appropriate weights must be added for clothing and shoes. (Source of data: *Anthropometry of US Military Personnel.* DOD Handbook–743, 3 October 1980.)

that the operator be able to reach all parts and supplies, keyboards, tools, controls, etc, without leaning, bending, or twisting at the waist. Reaching should be restricted to movements of the forearm if possible. Fig 6–3 illustrates the forearm-only (preferable) and full-arm (satisfactory) reach limits for men and women in the USA. Task designs that require movements outside the full-arm reach limits are generally unsatisfactory. These reach limits, called reach envelopes, are based on the dimensions outlined in Figs 6–1 and 6–2 and thus must be modified for special applications or different populations.

The reach envelope rules are particularly important if forces or weights are involved, though repetitive movement of the upper body not against resistance may also become fatiguing and injurious to the lower back. Employees at risk include assembly line work-

ers who must reach to a high shelf or reach behind them to retrieve parts and bus drivers who must lean forward across a steering wheel and then pull it laterally in the direction they wish to turn.

Although some movements of the waist and shoulders may be unavoidable even in well-designed jobs, the design rule still applies: the less required bending and twisting of the waist and torso, the better the job design.

Example: Women of average dimensions (50th percentile) can reach horizontally only about 74 cm (29 in), and short women (5th percentile) can reach horizontally only about 69 cm (27 in), as measured from the back of the chair when they are seated in an upright position. If a shelf of supplies or a panel of controls is 91 cm (36 in) in front of them (also measured from the back of the chair), they will have difficulty obtaining the supplies or manipulating the controls even with bending and twist-

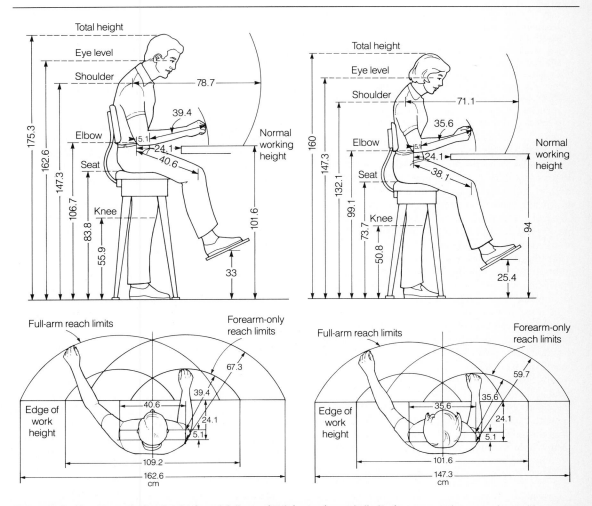

Figure 6–3. Forearm-only (preferable) and full-arm (satisfactory) reach limits for men and women in working areas shown in the horizontal and vertical planes. All dimensions are in centimeters. (Adapted from Farley, 1955. Modified and reproduced, with permission, from Das B, Grady RM: Industrial workplace layout and engineering anthropometry. In: *Ergonomics of Workstation Design.* Kvalseth TO [editor]. Butterworths, 1983.)

ing at the waist. If these activities are frequent, a potential health and safety problem exists resulting from the repetitive strain on back muscles weakened by fatigue. Productivity will also be affected. The work area should be redesigned to reduce the required reaching distances to within comfortable ranges.

B. Avoidance of Static Positions:

1. Static holding positions–An assembly line task might involve holding an object rigidly in one hand and working on it with the other, or a maintenance job might involve holding a hand tool or power tool tightly in one hand for extended periods. In either case, muscle tension reduces vascular flow to the muscles and thus hastens the onset of local fatigue caused by the buildup of lactic acid. Release of tension may be accomplished by using a holding clamp or bench vise or, in the case of hand or power tools, by alternating hands or using self-locking tools. When some holding is still necessary, redesigning the tools or tool handles to achieve maximum comfort is helpful.

> *Example:* In a quality control task, each part being checked was picked up and supported by the worker's left hand and forearm while testing clamps were attached and adjustments made. The job was redesigned so that each part was placed on a waist-high rolling rack that was pulled along by the worker, who then made attachments and adjustments with both hands. Muscle cramping in the left wrist, forearm, and hand was eliminated, and the pace of work increased.

2. Static body positions–Workers who operate typewriters, word processors, adding machines, laboratory equipment, telephone control panels, etc, tend to hold their bodies in a fixed position for protracted periods in order to maintain a consistent physical relationship with the equipment. For example, typists must maintain a fixed spatial relationship between their shoulders and the keyboard in order to strike the proper key each time without looking. In addition to maintaining a fixed shoulder position, they often maintain a rigid neck position required by looking for long periods at the copyholder.

In jobs of this sort, measures must be taken to prevent chronic pain and cumulative trauma disorders resulting from poor circulation and muscle fatigue in the shoulders, neck, and upper back. Workers should be encouraged to exercise, particularly the muscle groups that remain most static, eg, by an occasional bend at the waist. It may be preferable for workers to leave their chairs periodically to collect the next batch of work rather than have it delivered. In-chair exercises designed to move and stretch important muscle groups help maintain muscle tone and alertness.

> *Example:* Keyboard operators in a large office selected a set of simple physical movements—mostly joint manipulation and stretching—that would exercise the muscles held most rigid during keying. Operators were given written descriptions and sketches of the exercises and were instructed in their use. Two short, paid time periods were set aside daily for doing the exercises.

Operators were encouraged to take their regular rest breaks also and to break for a few quick stretching exercises whenever a shoulder, wrist, or other part of the body started to bother them.

Improvement of Equipment Design

Machine operation is most productive and least stressful when the machine does the work and the operator does the thinking.

A. Proper Design of Controls: Controls (eg, levers, switches, joysticks, and pedals) enable the operator to give a machine "orders" or feed it information. They also provide feedback to the operator. Primary controls—those of greatest importance or used most often—should be located within the forearm-only (preferable) reach limits, and other controls should be located within the full-arm (satisfactory) reach limits of the workstation, as shown in Fig 6–3.

B. Proper Design of Displays: Primary displays should be located in front of the operator and slightly (not more than 30 degrees) below eye level. This allows the operator to monitor the displays from a position most comfortable for the head, ie, with the head balanced on top of the spine. Positioning the display higher or lower tends to cause tension of the muscles of the back of the neck, which exacerbates tension in the back muscles. Locating the display to one side or the other of the operator causes stress on the rotation muscles of the neck.

C. Appropriate Control-Display Relationships: The design rules for controls and displays generally allow them to be placed in the most convenient position for the operator, but they also must be integrated with each other on a logical basis.

> *Example:* If a steam turbine is to be monitored and operated, the displays will be in front of and below the eye level of the operator, and the turbine controls generally will be in front of and near the operator's hands. However, the control for rotational speed should be adjacent to and linked logically with its speed indicator display (eg, the control and display should both be contained in a box on the panel or linked by means of a color-coded line). Movement of the speed control upward or to the right should move the speed indicator display also upward or to the right. This will increase the stimulus-response compatibility of the 2 devices and improve the control capability of the operator.

Logical linkages of this sort suggest simple responses to the information displayed to the operator, and more sophisticated logical linkages can indicate more complex responses. In this manner, the control-display relationships can reduce the information-processing load on the operator and thus reduce stress and the rate of errors.

VISUAL PROBLEMS DUE TO POOR ILLUMINATION OR TO GLARE

One or more of the following symptoms and signs may accompany a general feeling of tiredness of the eyes: oculomotor changes (esophoria, exophoria), ocular pain, itching, tearing, reduced ability of the eyes to accommodate and converge properly, headache, and complementary color reversals. "Visual fatigue" often results from visual stress due to rapid accommodation, extended viewing at short focal lengths, poor contrast between target and background, direct or reflected glare, or wrongly fitted corrective lenses. It is commonly associated with extended use of video display terminals (see below) whose screens have reduced contrast and occasionally flicker because of the type of phosphor used in them. Poor working postures and extended static positions of the head and shoulders during working hours may exacerbate visual problems.

Ocular symptoms from overwork do not cause permanent eye damage. However, to provide relief in visually demanding jobs, the workstation must be adequately illuminated and the amount of glare reduced.

Adequate Illumination of the Workstation

The amount of light required to perform a specific task without feeling visual fatigue is a function of the visual difficulty of the task at the desired work speed and quality and the visual acuity of the worker. Degree of visual difficulty is typically determined by (1) the contrast between the target and its background and (2) the spatial resolution or size of the target. Visual acuity, even with corrected vision, varies with age. The recommended ranges of illumination for various types of tasks are shown in Table 6-1.

Reduction of Workstation Glare

Glare may emanate directly from a bright source or may be reflected off the shiny surfaces of machines, work tables, windows, displays, tools, etc. It can be reduced or eliminated by moving the source of the light, changing the orientation of the worker in relation to the shiny surfaces, or covering these surfaces with dull or nonreflective coatings.

Example: In a garment plant, sewing machine operators complained of headaches and tired and itching eyes after lamps were installed on the other side of their machines. The purpose of the lamps was to improve visibility, but they had the opposite effect because their light reflected off the polished wood and metal sewing tables and the sewn material. Moving the lamps eliminated the glare and relieved the visual symptoms and headaches.

Table 6-1. Recommended ranges of illumination for various types of tasks.[1]

Type of Activity or Area	Range of Illumination[2]	
	Lux	Footcandles
Public areas with dark surroundings	20–50	2–5
Simple orientation for short temporary visits	>50–100	>5–9
Working spaces where visual tasks are only occasionally performed	>100–200	>9–19
Performance of visual tasks of high contrast or large size: reading printed material, typed originals, handwriting in ink, good xerography; rough bench and machine work; ordinary inspection; rough assembly	>200–500	>19–46
Performance of visual tasks of medium contrast or small size: reading pencil handwriting, poorly printed or reproduced material; medium bench and machine work; difficult inspection; medium assembly	>500–1000	>46–93
Performance of visual tasks of low contrast or very small size: reading handwriting in hard pencil on poor-quality paper, very poorly reproduced material; very difficult inspection	>1000–2000	>93–186
Performance of visual tasks of low contrast and very small size over a prolonged period: fine assembly, highly difficult inspection, fine bench and machine work	>2000–5000	>186–464
Performance of very prolonged and exacting visual tasks: the most difficult inspection, extra fine bench and machine work, extra fine assembly	>5000–10,000	>464–929
Performance of very special visual tasks of extremely low contrast and small size: some surgical procedures	>10,000–20,000	>929–1858

[1]Adapted from Flynn, 1979. Reproduced, with permission, from Eastman Kodak Company: *Ergonomic Design for People at Work.* Vol 1. Lifetime Learning Publications, 1983.

[2]The choice of a value within a range depends on task variables, the reflectance of the environment, and the individual's visual capabilities.

FATIGUE, PAIN, & CIRCULATION PROBLEMS DUE TO IMPROPER SEATING

Common complaints that stem from improper seating include poor circulation in the lower legs or thighs and pain in the gluteal muscles, lower back, or upper back (Table 6–2).

The primary purpose of a chair is to support the weight of the body comfortably with minimal restriction of circulation. Shifting about, leaning to one side, etc, are natural ways to maintain circulation in the buttocks and thighs, and chair design needs to accommodate these postural variations.

Proper Design of Chairs

Chair design affects blood circulation in the legs. If the seat pan is too long (>41 cm [16 in]), it cuts off circulation at the popliteus muscle, particularly in

Table 6–2. Common complaints that stem from improper seating.

Complaint	Possible Causes
Pain in the gluteal muscles	1. Extended sitting without break, especially constrained sitting. 2. Chair padding too hard, especially under ischial tuberosities and trochanters. 3. Seat not contoured (flat). 4. Chair design restricting movement and periodic adjustment of position.
Pain in the lower back	1. Inadequate lumbar support. 2. Improper adjustment of chair for lumbar support. 3. Excessive turning and twisting of worker while seated (poor location of chair in work space or poor location of some job items off to the sides of normal sitting area). 4. Lifting while seated.
Pain in the upper back	1. Chair too low for work area. 2. Frequent reaching from chair location, particularly at or above the shoulder. 3. Sitting in a static, rigid position for extended periods of time. 4. Armrests too high. 5. Chair back too small, poorly contoured, or improperly adjusted.
Poor circulation in the lower legs	1. Anterior edge of seat pan cutting off circulation because edge too sharp (not curved or "waterfall" design), seat adjusted too high, or lack of footrest to prevent short legs from dangling. 2. High-heeled shoes causing hyperextension of feet. 3. Inadequate foot and leg room causing excessive flexion at knees.
Poor circulation in the thighs	1. Anterior edge of seat pan cutting off circulation (see above). 2. Seat padding too soft. 3. Excessive seat pan contouring in frontal plane (rolls thighs inward).

short women. It is helpful if the edge of the seat under the knees is smoothly curved in a "waterfall" design so there will be no pressure points. The seat should be soft enough to be comfortable but not so soft that changing posture or standing up is difficult. The seat pan should be relatively flat rather than concave so the thighs of heavier people do not roll inward. Some recent chair designs improve comfort by providing additional support under the area of the ischial tuberosities.

Seat design must also provide sufficient lumbar support to maintain a comfortable degree of lordosis of the spine and assist in supporting the weight of the back. A chair should be easily adjustable from a sitting position to conform to the full range of back curvatures, popliteal heights, and buttock sizes. Without such support, general fatigue is much more likely, muscular stress in the upper back tends to occur, and lower back pain may result.

Chairs designed to be safe have 5 legs to reduce the likelihood of tipping over if the occupant leans backward. For comfort, the texture of material on the back and seat should be rough or nubby to allow some air circulation between the material and the body. If the chair has arms, they should be short enough so as not to strike the work table or bench during normal chair movements.

If it is necessary to adjust the chair to such a sitting height that short people's feet do not touch the ground, a sturdy footrest must be provided to prevent the legs from dangling, which puts pressure on the popliteus and restricts circulation to the lower legs.

Types of Chairs

A. Traditional Chairs and Stools: People generally prefer to sit for extended periods in low chairs (seat height of 38–46 cm [15–18 in]), while occasional sitting for a mobile worker is best done on a high stool (seat height of 74–81 cm [29–32 in]) with footrests. For people who move about frequently, it saves a lot of effort to perch on a stool whose height is about the length of the legs, so that the torso, arms, and head are not repeatedly raised and lowered whenever they sit and stand. The advantages of this type of sit-stand stool are reduced fatigue and reduced compression on the spine. Sometimes even stationary workers prefer to alternate between standing and sitting on a high stool, since standing improves leg circulation and may improve spinal lordosis, whereas sitting rests the legs temporarily.

B. Kneeling Chairs: There are several new types of chairs that have forward-sloping seats with a knee rest but no back support. Although some people like these kneeling chairs, many complain of 3 distinct disadvantages: (1) Weight on the knees causes pressure that cuts off circulation to the lower legs and makes getting up and walking difficult. (2) The toes are either flexed or hyperextended—uncomfortable positions to maintain for long periods. (3) It is not possible for users to change sitting positions from time to time as they do in traditional chairs.

C. Chairs With Forward-Sloping Seats: The new chairs that have forward-sloping seats and backrests but do not use knee rests to support the legs hold promise for various classes of jobs and preferences of users. Forward-sloping seats are especially advantageous for users who must be extremely close to or hovering over their work, as is the case with some repairmen, air traffic controllers, dentists, surgeons, etc. In addition to having adjustable heights and back positions, these chairs should have an easily adjustable degree of slope and should provide for additional support to prevent slipping out of the chair (seat pan contouring, "saddle" or "tractor seat" shaping, etc).

Proper Selection of Chairs

There are many well-designed types and models of chairs. The employer should obtain samples of 2 or 3 appropriate chairs (with or without arms, etc) that meet the requirements of the workers and ask the workers to try them out for at least a week. A briefer period for chair testing is usually not sufficient, since initial impressions often differ from long-term impressions. The opinion of the workers should be considered when a supply of new chairs is ordered. If opinions are divided, it is best to order some of each type of chair.

PHYSICAL STRESS & VISUAL PROBLEMS ASSOCIATED WITH VIDEO DISPLAY TERMINAL (VDT) USE

VDT operators often complain of muscle stress in the neck, upper back, shoulders, or wrists, and they frequently experience visual problems from long-term viewing of the VDT screen.

Proper Workstation Layout

The VDT will usually be placed directly in front of the operator, with the display screen below eye level and the keyboard below it and within easy reach. This works well for data acquisition, editing, and programming tasks in which the VDT is the primary source of information.

For word processing and data entry, in which the VDT may not be the primary source of information, the workplace layout will vary. Operators of word processors may require primary visual access to the copy, and data entry clerks may look almost exclusively at the original data records (invoices, checks, etc) they are recording. In this situation, it is the copy stand or the pile of data records that should be in front of the operator, and the VDT should then be positioned to one side or the other. Continual looking to one side to view copy may result in muscle stress and pain in the neck and upper back.

For word processors, the copy stand should be directly adjacent to the VDT, at about the same height (up to 30 degrees below horizontal) and at the same

viewing distance. This will reduce head rotation (side to side and up and down) and eliminate the need for accommodation.

For data entry clerks, manual handling is often required to turn pages, lay aside checks or invoices, etc. In this case, it is necessary to compromise between optimal handling location and optimal viewing area.

> *Example:* In a data processing office, checks were turned over one by one with the left hand while their amounts were entered on a computer keyboard with the right hand. The pile of checks was placed in front of the operator and near the screen. However, in order to turn the checks, the operators had to reach over the keyboard and suspend their arms in space, which caused shoulder pain. Moving the checks closer to the operator would have meant more twisting to the left. Instead, padded armrests were provided to support the left forearm and take the load off the shoulder.

Improvement of Keyboard Design

Most VDTs now have detachable keyboards, which allow more freedom in workplace arrangement, but most have linear keyboard layouts (keys in straight rows) that can eventually cause ulnar deviation of the wrist, which can contribute to the development of tendinitis or carpal tunnel syndrome in long-term keyboard users. Modeled after the typewriter, these keyboards utilize the Scholes (QWERTY) layout. A recent proposal to prevent wrist deviation and such problems as carpal tunnel syndrome and tendinitis is to arrange the keyboard in a V shape so that the keys operated by each hand are in rows perpendicular to the long axis of each forearm.

To prevent radial deviation of the right wrist, for clerks who work mostly with numbers, the keyboard should include a 10-key numeric keypad arranged in adding-machine format on the right side of the alphabetic keys. The keypad may be part of the primary keyboard or may be on a separate keyboard off to the right but directly in front of the right shoulder. The keypad on the right saves the clerk from having to reach up and down a single row of numbers on the top row of a standard keyboard.

If frequent telephone calls must be placed while using the keyboard, a 10-key telephone keypad should also be included. However, since the adding-machine layout differs from the telephone layout, the keypad chosen will probably depend on the relative frequency of data entry and telephone calls, operator preference, and other factors.

Improvement of Display Screen Illumination

VDTs provide their own illumination from the intensity of the cathode ray impinging on the phosphor used in the display screen. Because of technical limitations of this illumination, the brightness of the screen is often lower than that of a printed page, and the contrast may be much lower (about 3:1 for the screen compared to 10:1 for the printed page). In addition, the screen's characters consist of a matrix of tiny dots rather than continuous lines, and thus the characters may appear fuzzy to some VDT operators. Since the screen refreshes itself 60 times every second, operators with sensitive vision may detect some flicker, especially with their peripheral vision, when looking away or looking back at the screen.

The McCullough effect, which causes white horizontal lines to appear reddish after continued exposure to a green screen, may be a persistent problem for some VDT operators, who report seeing reddish lines for as long as a week after exposure. (Some have described traffic signal color confusion when driving home from work and other color-related problems throughout the evening.) Although these problems are rare, they can be reduced by putting a cardboard border of a complementary color around the screen (eg, a red border around a green screen).

Light from sources as bright as or brighter than the screen can cause glare. Not only is this irritating to the eyes, but it also represents "visual noise" that interferes with perception of the information on the screen. The operator must either try to "read through" this glare by focusing behind it or try to ignore it.

There are several ways to reduce the glare:

(1) Reduce the general illumination in the room to about 500 lux. This can be achieved by reducing the amount of overhead lighting (eg, removing every other bulb or fluorescent tube); by installing parabolic louvers over the fluorescent lights to direct the illumination straight downward; or by controlling window illumination with shades, louvered blinds, or tinted window film.

(2) Provide more illumination where needed with desk lamps ("task lighting").

(3) Use glare-reducing filters on VDT screens. These filters are available in several designs, although the principal 2 are coated filters (eg, Polaroid filters) and fine black nylon mesh filters. Polaroid filters trap light reflections internally but should have etched surfaces to prevent their own reflections. Both types of filters also improve visibility by increasing character contrast on the screen. Personal preference seems divided, and both types should be made available to VDT operators.

Another source of visual irritation is bright lights or unshaded windows. Looking up from the screen then causes pupillary constriction, and looking back at the screen requires another adjustment to the lower light level. In addition to taking measures to reduce glare, employers should encourage VDT operators to look up from the screen from time to time to allow the ciliary muscles to relax and thus prevent visual fatigue and pain.

Exercises to Relieve Musculoskeletal Stress

Exercises designed specifically to relieve physical stress and strain and to be conducted at the worksta-

tion have been helpful in preventing injuries due to the cumulative effects of repetitive motion and have hastened healing in injured workers recently returned to their jobs. Specific exercises chosen for a given work area should be based on the particular motions and stresses involved. General guidelines, based on a report by Sauter (1988), include the following:

(1) Exercises should be designed to relieve stress associated with awkward postures, highly repetitive tasks, and sedentary work or static effort.

(2) Exercises should target musculoskeletal stress in the upper and lower extremities, the shoulder girdle, the neck, and the lumbar and thoracic regions of the back.

(3) Exercises should be designed to be performed at the workstation. They should not be so conspicuous that they call attention to the worker or cause embarrassment, nor should they significantly disrupt task performance.

(4) Exercises should be performed during the times the musculoskeletal stress builds up, so that stress relief is timely and continuing. It is better to have many short exercise breaks than to have a few longer breaks; a scattering of micropauses as short as 90–120 seconds is considered healthy. If exercises are performed only at the beginning of the day or at lunchtime, there can be considerable stress buildup before relief.

(5) Exercises should not present any obvious biomechanical or safety hazards. In the absence of musculoskeletal disease, there should be no contraindications.

The assistance of an exercise physiologist is often helpful in prescribing exercises for a particular application. Lee et al (1987) provide a critical review of 9 different exercise routines (see References, below).

CUMULATIVE TRAUMA DISORDERS ASSOCIATED WITH HAND TOOL USE

Table 6–3 provides a list of work-related cumulative trauma disorders of the hand and arm. Most of these disorders are associated with the use of hand tools, and their diagnosis and treatment are discussed in Chapter 7.

Avoidance of Factors Causing Physical Stress

Tool design should be determined by the anatomy of the hand as well as by the task to be accomplished. The following can cause cumulative trauma disorders and should be avoided.

A. Ulnar Deviation: The wrist can be quite strong when held rigid and straight. It loses strength when it is flexed or extended, and damage to the nerves or tendon sheaths may result in carpal tunnel syndrome or tenosynovitis. Consequently, ulnar deviation should be avoided in both tool design and task design.

Table 6–3. Work-related cumulative trauma disorders of the hand and arm.

Disorder	Examples of Workers at Risk	Factor Responsible for Disorder
Carpal tunnel syndrome	New employee, trainee for new task.	Unaccustomed repetitive work with the hands.
Epicondylitis	Carpenter, blacksmith, plasterer, carpet layer.	Radial deviation with inward wrist rotation.
Ganglionic cysts	New employee, trainee for new task.	Unaccustomed use of tendon or joint.
	Brusher, scrubber.	Repeated manipulations with extended wrist.
	Carpenter, meat packer.	Repeated twisting of wrist.
Neuritis in the fingers	Paint scraper, wire clipper, screw tightener.	Contact with hand tools over a nerve in the palm or sides of the fingers.
Tenosynovitis of the finger extensor tendons	Typist, electronic equipment assembler.	Ulnar deviation with outward rotation.
Tenosynovitis of the finger flexor tendons	Painter, paint scraper, cleaner.	Exertions with a flexed wrist.
Tenosynovitis and peritendinitis crepitans of the radial styloid housing the abductor pollicis longus and extensor pollicis brevis	New employee, trainee for new task.	Unaccustomed repetitive work with the hands.
	Data processor, polisher, packager.	Work that involves more than 2000 manipulations per hour.
	Carpenter, metal worker.	Direct local blunt trauma.
	Packager, small parts assembler.	Simple, repetitive movement that is forceful and fast.
	Package wrapper, meat cutter.	Repeated radial or ulnar deviation, particularly with forceful exertions of the thumb.

B. Ulnar Deviation and Supination: Repetitive motions involving ulnar flexion-extension and supination in a task (eg, turning a rotary control to the right and downward, or tightening a bolt or screw) can cause impact shocks and increase the likelihood of tenosynovitis.

C. Palmar Flexion: Although grip strength is generally reduced for any flexion or deviation of the wrist, this is particularly true for palmar flexion. In addition to impeding the intended job performance or its speed, the reduced grip strength may also increase the likelihood that the user will lose control of the tool and drop it. This can result in injury or product damage and will certainly result in increased fatigue.

D. Ulnar Deviation and Palmar Flexion: When ulnar deviation is combined with palmar flexion in a task (eg, wringing clothes, tightening screws, operating "motorcycle-like" controls, looping wire with pliers), the tendons tend to bend and bunch up in the wrist's carpal tunnel. If this occurs frequently, tenosynovitis may develop.

E. Dorsiflexion: Dorsiflexion that is repeated over extended periods can cause tenosynovitis in the back of the hand. Typical activities involving dorsiflexion are polishing with a hand brush and scrubbing with rags or towels. If the brush handle is changed to permit polishing with a straight wrist (ie, the handle grip is at an angle appropriate to the work being done) and if a comparable rag or cloth pad holder is used, tenosynovitis can be prevented.

F. Dorsiflexion and Pronation: While any extended bending of the wrist during tool manipulation may lead to tenosynovitis, tendinitis, or carpal tunnel syndrome, use of the 2 wrist positions of dorsiflexion and pronation together places the worker at increased risk and thus should be avoided whenever possible. During rapid and repetitive motions, there is added pressure between the head of the radius and the capitulum of the humerus in the elbow, and the pressure in this joint can cause friction and heat. Any forces of lifting, pushing, or pulling exacerbate the condition.

G. Arm Flexion and Inward Rotation of the Hand: Arm flexion that occurs in lifting a heavy weight or pulling against resistance will pull the head of the radius tightly into the capitulum of the humerus. When arm flexion is combined with inward rotation of the hand, additional pressure and twisting forces are applied to the head of the radius because of the biceps's secondary function as an outward rotator of the hand. For this reason, inward hand rotation while lifting or pulling is to be avoided.

H. Radial Deviation, Pronation, and Dorsiflexion: Although radial deviation occurs less frequently than ulnar deviation, it may also cause bunching and compression of the tendons and nerves in the wrist. When combined with pronation and dorsiflexion, radial deviation increases the pressure on the head of the radius in the same manner as discussed for arm flexion (see above). Because the general result of extensive radial deviation is epicondylitis, it should be avoided in tool and task design.

I. Use of the Hand as a Tool: The palm of the hand should never be used as a hammer. Even frequent light tapping with the heel of the hand can cause injury to the nerves, arteries, and tendons of the hand and wrist. In addition, the shock waves may travel up the arm to the elbow and shoulder, causing additional physical problems. In assembly work, for example, the palm of the hand has been used for hitting electrical parts to tighten them after inserting and for hitting cabinet doors to align them after assembly. A mallet should be used instead.

J. Repetitive Finger Action: Excessive use of the index finger for operating triggers on hand tools causes local fatigue and may result in a condition called ''trigger finger.'' This condition occurs most frequently if the tool handle is so large that the distal phalanx of the finger has to be flexed while the middle phalanx must be kept straight, but it may also occur with smaller handles.

K. Repetitive Vibration of the Hand and Arm: Vibration of the hand and arm for extended periods, as occurs in the operation of hand power tools such as hand saws, riveting hammers, sanders, pneumatic drills, and grinders, may be a continuing source of pain and physical trauma. While not all workers exposed to vibratory hand tools experience trauma, some develop vibration-induced whitefinger disease. In this disease, constriction of the blood vessels leads to a reduction in blood flow to the fingers and hand and causes them to blanch, tingle, and feel numb. Such vascular attacks seem to be exacerbated by cold working conditions. Workers afflicted with whitefinger disease have reduced blood flow to the skin and reduced skin temperature even when no longer working with vibratory tools, and they may also have a decrease in touch sensitivity, fine finger dexterity, and grip strength. Although the disease usually is not debilitating, advanced cases have led to gangrene of the fingertips. Diagnosis, prevention, and treatment of vibration-induced whitefinger disease are discussed in Chapter 11.

Other conditions linked to the use of vibratory hand tools include neuritis and decalcification and cysts of the radial and ulnar bones.

Proper Design of Tool Handles

To avoid tissue compression stress in the hands, tool handles should be designed so that the force-bearing area is as large as practicable and there are no sharp corners or edges. This means that handles should be either round or oval. A compressible gripping surface is best, but handles should at least have a high coefficient of friction in order to reduce hand-gripping forces needed for tool control. Pinch points should be eliminated or guarded.

Rigid, form-fitting handles with grooves for each finger usually do not improve the grip function unless they are sized to the individual's hand. Form-fitting handles, which presumably are designed for the hand of a worker in the 50th percentile, will spread the fingers of a small (5th percentile) hand too far apart for efficient gripping and will cause uncomfortable ridges under the fingers of a large (95th percentile) hand. If finger grooves are on both handles of a tool held in one hand (eg, grass trimmers), the handle that fits into the palm of the hand causes added discomfort because of the ridges between the grooves.

The use of some tools, such as chisels and paint scrapers, involves application of a lot of force. When the force is transmitted through the pressure-sensitive areas overlying critical blood vessels or nerves in the hand, pain and chronic injury may result. Particularly to be avoided are the radial and ulnar arteries, such as the ulnar artery in the palm of the hand. The obstruction of blood flow leads to numbness and tingling of the hands, and thrombosis of the ulnar artery has also been reported. To prevent these problems, the handle design should be modified to transmit the force through the tough tissues between the thumb and index finger, thereby preventing damage to the more sensitive palm.

Many power tools (eg, drills, sanders, and chain saws) are operated and controlled with 2 hands, and there is generally a primary handle with a trigger to provide for gripping by the dominant hand. If there is a secondary, stabilizing handle, it should be adjustable to either side of the tool to permit use by either left-handed or right-handed people. It will also have the added advantage of permitting the user to change the trigger hand from time to time to reduce fatigue.

BIOMECHANICS OF LIFTING, PUSHING, & PULLING

Although a detailed biomechanical analysis of lifting, pushing, and pulling is beyond the scope of this chapter, some principles of these movements are included here to illustrate basic muscular activity of the body and suggest ways to prevent injuries.

Principles of Lifting

Fig 6–4 illustrates the forces on the base of the spine (L5/S1 forces) that result from 2 different methods of lifting a load weighing 130 N. When the lifting is done with the legs relatively straight (lifting in a stooped position), there is an L5/S1 shear force of 500 N and a spinal compression force of 1800 N. When the lifting is done with the knees bent (lifting in a squatting position, or ''lifting with the legs''), the L5/S1 shear force is only 340 N, but the spinal compression force is 2700 N. (This assumes that the load is too bulky to fit between the knees, as is often the case in practice.) A general safety rule is to ''lift with the legs'' and keep the load as close to the body as feasible in order to reduce the lateral distance between the load and the base of the spine (H in Fig 6–4). However, in the case illustrated, this would not make the job safer or easier. In fact, there is as yet no

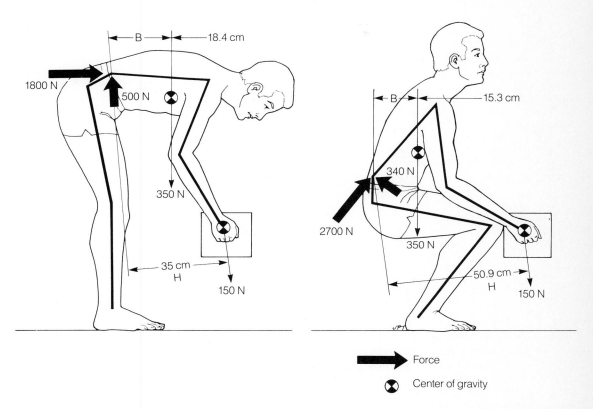

130 N Dead load   0.07$_g$ Horizontal acceleration

3.3° Acceration vector angle

1.15$_g$ Vertical acceleration   150 N Live load

Force

Center of gravity

Figure 6–4. Forces on the base of the spine (L5/S1 forces) that result from 2 different methods of lifting a load weighing 150 N. When the lifting is done with the legs relatively straight, there is an L5/S1 shear force of 500 N and a spinal compression force of 1800 N. When the lifting is done with the knees bent, the L5/S1 shear force is only 340 N, but the spinal compression force is 2700 N. B = horizontal distance from the L5/S1 joint to the body's center of gravity. H = horizontal distance from the L5/S1 joint to the load's center of gravity. (Adapted from Park and Chaffin, 1974. Modified and reproduced, with permission, from Chaffin DB, Andersson GB: *Occupational Biomechanics.* Wiley, 1984.)

clear biomechanical rationale for recommending either lifting posture as being safer.

In general, to prevent lifting injuries, materials handlers should do the following: (1) Have their personal strength limits tested (see below), and make sure the load to be lifted is below 50% of their limit. (2) Avoid lifting loads that exceed the general strength limits calculated for various types of lifting (see below). (3) Minimize twisting with a load, and, when it is necessary to twist, rotate the pelvis. (4) Keep the load close to the body when lifting it. (5) Exercise caution when working in slippery or cluttered areas. (6) Follow the suggestions for safe lifting shown in Fig 6–5.

Principles of Pushing & Pulling

The forces involved in pushing and pulling loads are illustrated in Fig 6–6. As is shown, pulling a load causes more strain on the lower back than pushing a load. Pulling a force of 350 N (the weight of the cart times its coefficient of rolling friction) at a height of 66 cm (26.4 in) above the floor causes a compression force on the lower spine of about 8000 N, which is substantially above the highest value (6400 N) that most workers can tolerate without injury.

The following are general guidelines to prevent injuries when pushing or pulling heavy loads: (1) Make certain that the area ahead of the load is level and clear of obstacles. If it is not level, some system

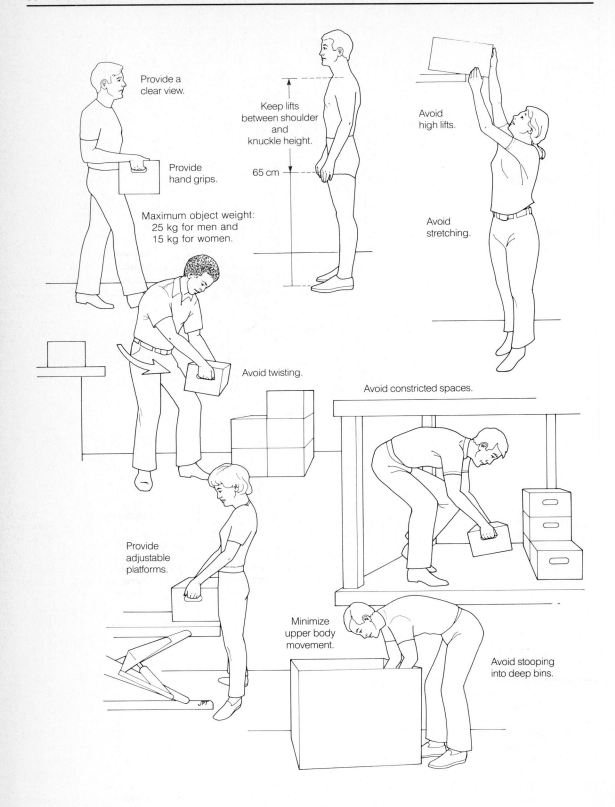

Figure 6–5. Suggestions for safe lifting. (Modified and reproduced, with permission, from Webb RD: *Industrial Ergonomics.* Industrial Accident Prevention Association, 1982.)

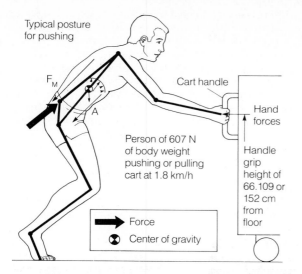

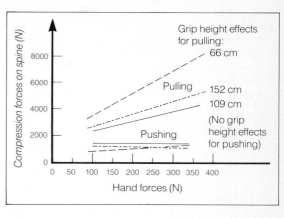

Figure 6–6. Forces involved in pushing and pulling loads. Pulling a force of 350 N (the weight of the cart times its coefficient of rolling friction) at a height of 66 cm above the floor causes a compression force on the lower spine of about 8000 N, which is substantially above the highest value (6400 N) that most workers can tolerate without injury. (Adapted from Lee, 1982. Modified and reproduced, with permission, from Chaffin DB, Andersson GB: *Occupational Biomechanics.* Wiley, 1984.)

of braking should be available. (2) Push the load, rather than pull it. This will reduce spinal stress, and in most cases will improve the visibility ahead. (3) Wear shoes that provide good foot traction. The coefficient of friction between the floor and the sole of the shoes should be at least 0.8 wherever heavy loads are moved. (4) When starting to push a load, brace one foot and use the back, rather than the hands and arms, to apply force. If the load does not start to move when a reasonable amount of force is applied, get help from a coworker or use a powered vehicle. (5) Pushing or pulling is easier when the handles of the loaded cart are at about hip height (91–114 cm, or about 36–47 in, for men) than when they are at shoulder height or above. Handles lower than the hips are awkward and unsafe to use.

EVALUATION OF STRENGTH & WORK CAPACITY

Estimating General Strength Limits

A. Action Limit: The following formula may be used to establish general lifting limits for a group of materials handlers. Most workers (99% of men and 75% of women) should be able to lift loads calculated as follows:

$$AL = 392 \left(\frac{15}{H}\right) [1 - (0.004 |V - 75|)] \left(0.7 + \frac{7.5}{D}\right) \left(1 - \frac{F}{F_{max}}\right)$$

where AL =   action limit, defined as the maximum weight-lifting value (expressed in newtons [N]) above

which management action must be taken to reduce lifting parameters or simplify the job.

H =   horizontal lever arm of the load (horizontal distance [cm] from the load center of mass at the origin of the vertical lift to the midpoint of the ankles); between 15 and 80 cm.

V =   height of the load at the beginning of the lift (vertical distance [cm] from the floor to the load center of mass); between 0 and 175 cm. $|V - 75|$ represents the absolute value of $V - 75$.

D =   vertical travel distance of the load; between 25 cm and 200 − V cm.

F =   average frequency of lifting (lifts ÷ min); between 0.2 and F_{max}.

F_{max} =   maximum frequency of lifts ÷ min, defined by the length of the work period and the body position when lifting. For a 1-hour work period, the F_{max} is 18 when standing and 15 when stooped. For an 8-hour work period, the F_{max} is 15 when standing and 12 when stooped.

The above equation assumes smooth, 2-handed lifting in the sagittal plane of objects that have a moderate width and can be held with relative ease (eg, objects that are not sharp, hot, or slippery). Moreover, it assumes that there are no physical barriers to a direct origin-to-destination lift, that the floor is uncluttered and not slippery, and that there are favorable temperature conditions in the work area. Any departure from these assumptions will lessen the effective lifting ability below the action limit by some appropriate amount.

An ergonomic lifting calculator in the form of a cardboard slide rule is available from the National Safety Council and allows for rapid computation of these lifting limits.

The action limit is intended to protect most workers from injuries, including physical strain and overexertion. Calculation of the action limit is based on limiting the L5/S1 disk compression forces to 3400 N, which biomechanical studies indicate can be tolerated by most people. The action limit also assumes that the average metabolic energy requirement would be no more than 3.5 kcal/min, which most workers can sustain for reasonable periods of time.

B. Maximum Permissible Limit: The National Institute for Occupational Safety and Health (NIOSH) defines a maximum permissible limit which is equal to 3 times the action limit and above which

lifting is not considered safe. Between the action limit and the maximum permissible limit, administrative controls are required and must be enforced. These controls involve higher standards for worker selection and job placement and improved worker training.

When materials handlers work at the maximum permissible limit, they experience L5/S1 disk compression forces of about 6400 N, which is the highest value that most workers can tolerate without injury. They are also exerting energy on the job of at least 5 kcal/min, which is more than most workers can tolerate for very long. In general, only about 25% of men and less than 1% of women can work at or above the maximum permissible limit. Lifting tasks above this limit are clearly unacceptable for most workers, and the tasks should be redesigned. The relationship between the action limit and the maximum permissible limit is shown in Fig 6–7.

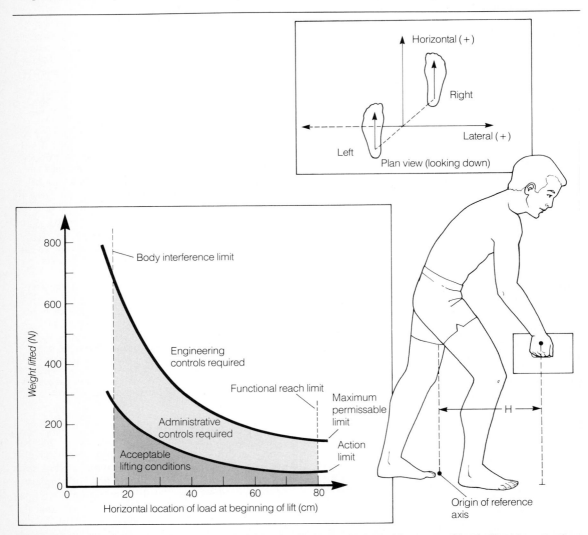

Figure 6–7. Action limit and maximum permissible limit for different horizontal locations of loads lifted from the floor (V = 15 cm) to knuckle height (D = 60 cm) on an infrequent basis (F 0.2). H = horizontal distance from the L5/S1 joint to the center of gravity of the load. (Modified and reproduced, with permission, from Chaffin DB, Andersson GB: *Occupational Biomechanics.* Wiley, 1984.)

Measuring Personal Strength Limits

The most relevant lifting limits for a specific worker are those established directly from that worker's strength and endurance. The worker who lifts correctly within the limits thus established by his or her own ability and within a safe environment (no slippery floors, no unguarded moving machinery, etc) should be relatively safe from injury.

A. Techniques of Measuring Strength: Of the several strength-measuring approaches that are available, the one most often used is the test of static strength of localized muscles (as in lifting with the elbow-shoulder system). At the other extreme, dynamic whole-body strength (as in pushing a cart or lifting to a high shelf) is generally considered more realistic and predictive of lifting ability, but it is harder to determine and standardize.

1. Static strength–Static strength of specific muscle groups is usually tested in 3 standard body positions: with the legs in a partial squat position, with the torso stooped over, and with the arms flexed. The mean static strengths demonstrated by male and female workers when lifting, pushing, and pulling in these 3 positions and in additional positions are shown in Table 6–4.

2. Dynamic strength–The most thoroughly investigated technique of measuring voluntary, dynamic whole-body strength is the psychophysical strength method. Work capacity norms from experienced materials handlers are elicited using an established protocol and then tested for realism over a given period of work. The result is a load limit that a representative population of materials handlers is willing to lift at a specific frequency (eg, once a minute) from one particular height (eg, the floor) to another height (eg, the shoulder). Representative

limits for loads that male and female workers are willing to lift repeatedly are shown in Table 6–5.

B. Interpretation of Strength Measurements: The static strength of a particular muscle group (eg, elbow-shoulder system) is about 50% greater than the comparable dynamic strength (eg, knuckle-shoulder lift) and may even be double the comparable dynamic strength. The reason for this is that dynamic strength involves musculature over a range of joint efficiencies, and the dynamic lifting involves overcoming the load's inertia in its upward acceleration as well as lifting the weight. For this reason, "strength" as measured by the standardized static strength tests cannot be used directly to predict the weight of loads that may be safely lifted by the person being tested. Comparison of standard measures of static strengths with loads actually handled has shown that whenever the actual load is much more than 50% of the relevant static strength measure, the likelihood of injury increases dramatically. Consequently, if standardized static strength testing is incorporated in a job screening program, the results must be discounted to approximately 50% of their measured values when used to estimate safe load-handling capabilities by the tested muscle groups. Whenever possible, the static strength tests should be used in conjunction with dynamic strength tests.

C. Validity of Strength Tests: For jobs requiring strength for materials handling or other tasks, preemployment screening tests may be established to determine which applicants are likely to possess sufficient physical size, strength, and work capacity to perform the necessary tasks without injury to themselves or others. However, any such screening tests must evaluate size, strength, and work capacity traits relevant to the tasks actually to be performed by the applicants. Otherwise, the test may be discriminatory

Table 6–4. Static strengths demonstrated by workers when lifting, pushing, and pulling with both hands on a handle placed at different locations relative to the midpoint between the ankles on the floor.[1]

Test Description	Handle Location[2] (cm)		Mean Strength (N)	
	Vertical	Horizontal	Men	Women
Lift—legs in partial squat	38	0	903	427
Lift—torso stooped over	38	38	480	271
Lift—arms flexed	114	38	383	214
Lift—shoulder high and arms out	152	51	227	129
Lift—should high and arms flexed	152	38	529	240
Lift—shoulder high and arms close	152	25	538	285
Lift—floor level, close (squat)	15	25	890	547
Lift—floor level, out (stoop)	15	38	320	200
Push down—waist level	118	38	432	325
Pull down—above shoulders	178	33	605	449
Pull in—shoulder level, arms out	157	33	311	244
Pull in—shoulder level, arms in	140	0	253	209
Push out—waist level, stand erect	101	35	311	226
Push out—chest level, stand erect	124	25	303	214
Push out—shoulder level, lean forward	140	64	418	276

[1]Modified and reproduced, with permission, from Chaffin DB, Andersson GB: *Occupational Biomechanics.* Wiley, 1984.

[2]Handle locations are measured in midsagittal plane, vertical from the floor and horizontal from the midpoint between the ankles.

Table 6–5. Psychophysical limits for load lifting.[1]

Height of Lift (cm)	Sagittal Plane Box Dimensions (cm)	Mean Lifting Limits[2] (N)	
		Men	Women
Floor to knuckle height when erect	30.5	296	194
	45.7	261	171
	61.0	236	152
Knuckle to shoulder height when erect	30.5	263	141
	45.7	233	129
	61.0	205	127
Shoulder to reach height when erect	30.5	221	120
	45.7	204	110
	61.0	195	112

[1]Reproduced, with permission, from Ayoub MM et al: Development of strength and capacity norms for manual materials handling. *Hum Factors* 1980;**22:**271.
[2]The values represent acceptable lifting limits (N) based on lifting frequency of once per minute sustained for 8 hours.

against women or other physically small applicants. Validation studies may be conducted to establish job relevance for tests or other hiring criteria.

Estimating Work Capacity

For workers who must expend high levels of energy (eg, materials handlers, sanitation crews, and furnace tenders), maximum work capacity is usually defined in terms of their aerobic capacity. Maximum aerobic capacity, or maximum aerobic power, can be determined by measuring heart rate or oxygen uptake. Table 6–6 lists the maximum heart rate and oxygen uptake for men and women in average physical condition.

If there is ever a question about whether an observed employee is exceeding his or her maximum work capacity on a given job, attention should also be paid to simplifying the task, improving the work environment, or both.

THE ROLE OF ENVIRONMENTAL FACTORS IN OCCUPATIONAL INJURIES

The environment affects worker performance, health, and safety in a variety of ways. This discussion will focus primarily on physical aspects of the environment, although the social characteristics of

the workplace (eg, isolation versus overcrowding, being undervalued versus being appreciated, organizational flexibility versus rigidity) often play a significant role in stress-related injuries. For additional information on injuries due to noise, temperature, and vibration, see Chapters 10 and 11.

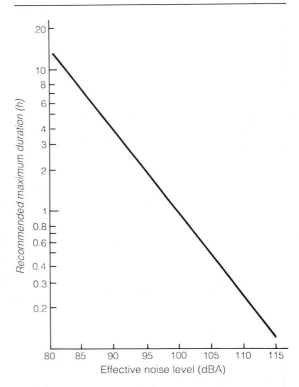

Figure 6–8. Recommended maximum duration of human exposure to various noise levels. Workers should not be exposed to sounds above 115 dBA. (Adapted from the American Conference of Governmental Industrial Hygienists, 1982; National Institute for Occupational Safety and Health, 1972. Reproduced, with permission, from Eastman Kodak Company: *Ergonomic Design for People at Work.* Vol 1. Lifetime Learning Publications, 1983.)

Table 6–6. Maximum heart rate and oxygen uptake for men and women in average physical condition.

Age (yr)	Heart Rate (beats/min)		Oxygen Uptake (mL/kg/min)	
	Men	Women	Men	Women
20–29	190	190	34–42	31–37
30–39	182	182	31–33	25–33
40–49	179	179	27–35	24—30
50–59	171	171	25–33	21–27
60–69	164	164	23–30	18–23

Physical Hazards

Hazards come in many forms, including unguarded moving machinery or equipment, missing or poorly designed railings to protect workers from dangerous areas, and slippery or obstructed floors. The safety and health standards prepared by the Occupational Safety and Health Administration (OSHA) outline the requirements for hazard elimination, as do most company safety regulations. Rigid and consistent enforcement of these safety standards is essential.

Noise

Workers frequently complain that there is too much noise and that this distracts them from their jobs. Loudness is directly related to the mechanical pressure transmitted to the eardrum, although the sound frequency and other characteristics of sound determine the degrading effect it has on performance. At a given intensity, lower frequencies are more likely to produce hearing impairments while high frequencies are more apt to interfere with concentration and

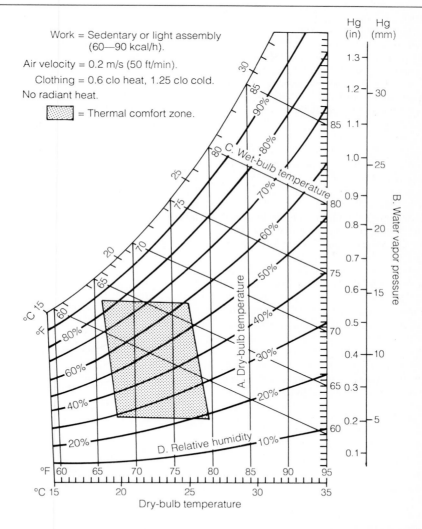

Figure 6–9. Thermal comfort zone. The dry-bulb temperature and humidity combinations that are comfortable for most people doing sedentary or light work are shown as the shaded area on the psychometric chart. The dry-bulb temperature range is 19–26 °C (66–79 °F), and the relative humidity range (shown as parallel curves) is 20–85%, with 35-65% being the most common values in the comfort zone. On this chart, ambient dry-bulb temperature (A) is plotted on the horizontal axis and indicated as parallel vertical lines; water vapor pressure (B) is on the vertical axis. Wet-bulb temperatures (C) are shown as parallel lines with a negative slope; they intersect the dry-bulb temperature lines and relative humidity curves (D) on the chart. In the definition of the thermal comfort zone, assumptions were made about the work load, air velocity, radiant heat, and clothing insulation levels. These assumptions are given in the top left corner of the chart. (Adapted from Rodgers, 1975; based on information from the American Society of Heating, Refrigerating, and Air-Conditioning Engineers [ASHRAE], 1972, 1974; Fanger, 1970. Reproduced, with permission, from Eastman Kodak Company: *Ergonomic Design for People at Work.* Vol 1. Lifetime Learning Publications, 1983.)

thought processes. The less predictable and controllable the sound, the more annoying it is.

In quiet areas, some sound (eg, soft music) may be preferable as a means of masking nearby conversations that might otherwise be distracting. "White noise" (sound spread uniformly over the full hearing spectrum) is sometimes used successfully in lieu of music but is occasionally found to be objectionable.

Sound levels above 50 dB may become increasingly intrusive, objectionable, and fatiguing, depending on their frequency and predictability. Sound levels that exceed 85 dBA (as recorded on a sound level meter's A-weighted scale of frequency bands) and continue for as long as 8 hours may cause hearing loss. If noise levels routinely exceed 85 dBA, it is necessary to control the sound source or provide other means of hearing protection. Fig 6–8 shows the recommended maximum duration of human exposure to various noise levels. Workers should not be exposed to sounds above 115 dBA. Table 6–7 lists examples of the sound levels satisfying various communications needs.

Lighting

See Visual Problems Due to Poor Illumination or to Glare (above) and Table 6–1.

Temperature & Humidity

An elevated ambient temperature or humidity level increases the cardiovascular load of a materials handler, and a low temperature can substantially reduce finger flexibility and accuracy. The thermal comfort zone is characterized by the ideal temperature and humidity conditions for work. An example of this zone for sedentary work, including light assembly work in factories, is given in Fig 6–9. The comfort zone is affected by a number of factors in addition to temperature and humidity. Among these are air velocity (producing a windchill effect), work load, radiant heat sources, and amount and type of clothing. In general, the body's core temperature should not vary by more than 1°C in either direction, and the above factors should be adjusted to accommodate this range.

Vibration

With the increasing interaction between workers and mechanical tools, vibration at critical frequencies and accelerations has become an important source of injury, producing chest and abdominal pain, loss of equilibrium, nausea, Raynaud's phenomenon, muscle contractions, shortness of breath, and carpal tunnel syndrome. In addition, truck drivers and heavy equipment operators have a high incidence of lumbar spinal disorders, hemorrhoids, hernias, and digestive and urinary tract problems, which may be due to a combination of vibration, extended sitting, and truck loading and unloading.

The types of vibration that are of most concern to occupational health and safety analysts are those associated with operation of vehicles (eg, buses, forklifts, and heavy construction equipment) and with operation of machinery (eg, large punch presses, conveyors, and furnaces). The effect of vibration depends on its frequency, acceleration, duration, and direction (vertical or lateral).

Fig 6–10 illustrates the maximum acceptable whole-body vertical vibration exposure times to various frequencies and accelerations, as established by the International Organization for Standardization (IOS). The lower intensities (measured by surface-mounted accelerometers) can be tolerated for longer periods without pain or injury than the high intensities can, and low-intensity vibrations of less than 1 Hz may in fact have a soothing effect.

Whole-body vertical vibration is a continuing problem for vehicle operators. The critical range of the torso's natural resonant frequency is 3–5 Hz, but discomfort can occur in the range of 2–11 Hz. Well-designed seats for bus and truck drivers will diminish the vibration in this critical frequency range by as much as 70%, but many older seats tend to have an amplification effect of as much as 20%. Moreover, the lateral acceleration intensity may be twice the vertical intensity in some buses or trucks. Visual performance is generally impaired in the range of 10–25 Hz. Truck and bus seats usually do not transmit vertical vibrations in this frequency range, but other equipment (eg, overhead cranes, lumber mill saws, and conveying machinery) may do so.

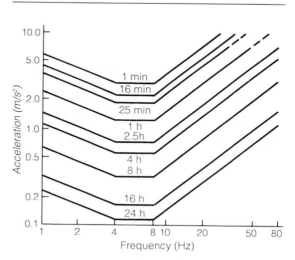

Figure 6–10. Maximum acceptable whole-body vertical vibration exposure times to various frequencies and accelerations. The shorter the vibration exposure, the higher the acceleration levels that can be tolerated. The least acceptable range of frequencies at all accelerations and durations of exposure is from 4 to 8 Hz. (Adapted from the International Organization for Standardization, 1974; Sandover, 1979. Reproduced, with permission, from Eastman Kodak Company: *Ergonomic Design for People at Work.* Vol 1. Lifetime Learning Publications, 1983.)

Table 6–7. Preferred noise criterion (PNC) curves and sound pressure levels recommended for several categories of activity[1]

	PNC Curve[2]	Approximate Sound Pressure Level (dBA)[3]
Listening to faint musical sounds or using distant microphone pickup	10–20	21–30
Excellent listening conditions	≤ 20	≤ 30
Close microphone pickup only	≤ 25	≤ 34
Good listening conditions	≤ 35	≤ 42
Sleeping, resting, relaxing	25–40	34–47
Conversing or listening to radio or TV	30–40	38–47
Moderately good listening conditions	35–45	42–52
Fair listening conditions	40–50	47–56
Moderately fair listening conditions	45–55	52–61
Just acceptable speech and telephone communication	50–60	56–66
Speech not required but no risk of hearing damage	60–75	66–80

[1]Adapted from Beranck, Blazier, and Figwer, 1971. Modified and reproduced, with permission, from Eastman Kodak Company: *Ergonomic Design for People at Work*, vol 1. Lifetime Learning Publications, 1983.
[2]PNC curves are used in many installations for establishing noise spectra.
[3]Voice sound frequencies are used to determine the approximate sound pressure levels. These levels are to be used only for estimates, since the overall sound pressure level does not give an indication of the spectrum.

REFERENCES

Alexander DC, Pulat BM: *Industrial Ergonomics: A Practitioner's Guide*. Industrial Engineering and Management Press, 1985.

Astrand P, Rodahl K: *Textbook of Work Physiology*, 2nd ed. McGraw-Hill, 1977.

Chaffin DB, Andersson GB: *Occupational Biomechanics*. Wiley, 1984.

Eastman Kodak Company: *Ergonomic Design for People at Work*. Vol 1, Lifetime Learning Publications, 1983; Vol 2, Van Nostrand Reinhold, 1986.

Grandjean E (editor): *Ergonomics and Health in Modern Offices*. Taylor & Francis, 1984.

Handbook of Fundamentals. American Society of Heating, Refrigerating, and Air-Conditioning Engineers (ASHRAE), 1989.

Lee KS et al: *Evaluation of Identified Exercises and Development of Exercises for VDT Operators*. Contract No. 87–12182. National Institute for Occupational Safety and Health, 1987.

National Institute for Occupational Safety and Health: *Preemployment Strength Testing*. US Department of Health, Education, and Welfare, 1977.

National Institute for Occupational Safety and Health: *A Work Practices Guide for Manual Lifting*. Technical Report No. 81–122. US Department of Health and Human Services, 1981.

Salvendy G (editor): *Handbook of Human Factors*. Wiley, 1987.

Sauter SL, Gottlieb MS, Knutson SJ: *Improving VDT Work: Causes and Control of Health Concerns in VDT Use*. Univ of Wisconsin Press, 1984.

Sauter SL: *Stress Control Measures in Computer-Mediated Work*. Unpublished research protocol for the National Institute for Occupational Safety and Health, 1988.

Thermal Environmental Conditions for Human Occupancy. ASHRAE Standard 55–74 (ANSI B193.1–76). American Society of Heating, Refrigerating, and Air-Conditioning Engineers (ASHRAE), 1974.

Tichauer ER: *The Biomechanical Basis of Ergonomics: Anatomy Applied to the Design of Work Situations*. Wiley, 1978.

Woodson WE: *Human Factors Design Handbook*. McGraw-Hill, 1981.

Franklin T. Hoaglund, MD

Definitions of Common Orthopedic Conditions

Most occupational injuries are orthopedic in nature. Musculoskeletal injuries, though of common occurrence in the work setting, generally lack precise definitions. For that reason, the following definitions are suggested to the reader before the common musculoskeletal injuries are discussed in detail.

A. Strain: A strained muscle, ligament, or tendon insertion is one that has been pushed or pulled to its extreme by forcing the joint beyond its normal range of motion. It commonly results from lifting a heavy weight or bearing an external force—usually traction force. By definition, the symptoms of strain should resolve within a few days to a week.

B. Sprain: A sprain is an injury in which a ligament has been stretched so far that a few fibers within the substance of the ligament or its attachment may be torn. A complete tear of the ligament is sometimes called a third-degree sprain.

C. Tendinitis: Tendinitis is inflammation of a tendon. It may be the result of a primary inflammatory lesions, such as rheumatoid arthritis, or it may be secondary to a mechanical injury.

D. Tenosynovitis: Tenosynovitis is inflammation of a tendon sheath.

E. Bursitis: Inflammation of a bursa is known as bursitis. A common site is the subacromial bursa (the bursa between the rotator cuff and the coracoacromial ligament).

F. Myositis: Myositis is inflammation of muscle. The inflammation may be primary, as in polymyositis, or secondary to mechanical injury, as when a muscle has been overstretched.

G. Arthritis: Arthritis is a condition in which a joint is inflamed or abnormal. Examples include posttraumatic arthritis, osteoarthritis, and rheumatoid arthritis.

INJURIES OF THE NECK & SHOULDER

1. CERVICAL DEGENERATIVE DISK DISEASE

Cervical degenerative disk disease is common in both men and women after age 40. Symptoms may be first noted after a whiplash injury or after an incident in which the neck has been put in an extreme position or held flexed or extended for long periods. Most patients with complaints of neck pain have underlying degenerative disk disease.

The cause is unknown. The most common site of degenerative change is at C5–6, the point of greatest flexion. Neck motion is restricted by progressive changes in the disk and facet joints and by the presence of osteophytes. In patients over 40, pain usually occurs long after radiographic changes are evident. Soft disk protrusion can account for true radiculopathy, with resulting pain in the arms. Long-standing and more severe changes can eventually produce encroachment on the spinal canal and cervical myelopathy.

Clinical Findings

A. Symptoms and Signs: A common symptom is posterior neck pain or high interscapular pain after prolonged sitting with the head fixed in one position. Symptoms may be severe at night during recumbency. There is often little in the way of physical findings. Upper extremity reflexes, circulation, and sensation are usually normal. Patients demonstrate some restriction of motion and pain with the head in extreme extension, in full flexion, in chin rotation, or in lateral flexion. Local tenderness in the posterior cervical spine is not usually present with disk irritation of a nerve root. Upper extremity symptoms and reflex changes are infrequent but may be present.

B. Imaging: A lateral x-ray view of the cervical spine will reveal narrowing of the disk space and anterior production of osteophytes. The most frequently affected levels are C5 and C6, but any level may be affected. Patients in their 30s occasionally have symptoms before radiographic signs are present; this is especially true for patients who have sustained rear-end auto collisions.

Differential Diagnosis

In patients with pain limited to the interscapular area, the possibility of dorsal spine disease, tumor, or infection should be considered. Bone tenderness over the dorsal spine processes should alert the examiner to the need for a dorsal spine x-ray. Tumors or infection of the cervical spine can produce symptoms but are much less common. Pancoast's tumor or brachial neuritis may produce upper extremity radiculopathy.

Treatment

Patients should be instructed to avoid prolonged sitting with the neck in a fixed position, extreme positions of the head or neck, and activities that bring on symptoms, such as driving, which sometimes requires sudden and extreme head movement. They should be taught to perform gentle range-of-motion exercises while at work, and, as symptoms abate, to do resistance exercises.

A soft cervical collar provides rest for neck muscles by supporting the head, especially late in the day, and will also limit extremes of motion.

In more severe cases, cervical traction in slight flexion is helpful. A nonsteroidal anti-inflammatory drug in conjunction with heat and massage is generally useful. Occasionally, the patient needs acetaminophen with 30 mg of codeine at bedtime. Sleeping in an easy chair, sitting up or with the torso at a 45-degree angle, minimizes discomfort associated with turning over from the recumbent position. Pain usually subsides with time and proper rest.

Cervical spine fusions for cervical degenerative disk disease have unpredictable results. When patients have upper extremity radiculopathy and do not respond to conservative treatment, disk excision and anterior interbody fusion are helpful.

2. PAINFUL SHOULDER ASSOCIATED WITH ROTATOR CUFF DISEASE

Painful shoulder associated with rotator cuff disease is common in both sexes after age 40. The onset of symptoms often coincides with the start of new, repetitive-motion work activities involving the shoulders.

In the normal shoulder, the coracoacromial ligament crosses the supraspinatus and infraspinatus tendon portions of the rotator cuff. In some individuals, contact pressure from this ligament produces an ischemic lesion of the cuff and can produce tendinitis with intervening bursitis in the subacromial bursa. In more chronic situations, there is degenerative rupture of the tendon. If acute mechanical trauma occurs in a preexisting degenerative area, frank disruption of the cuff may result. Impingement of the inflamed area occurs in the middle range of abduction during normal shoulder elevation, but the impinged area is out of the way during full elevation.

Clinical Findings

A. Symptoms and Signs: The onset of anterior shoulder pain may be gradual or acute. In some cases, pain is limited to the lateral arm about the deltoid insertion on the humerus (referred pain). All levels of pain occur, including severe pain at rest due to a tense subacromial bursa. Night pain is a frequent complaint. Tenderness over the greater tuberosity is usually present.

Patients begin to experience anterior shoulder pain when the arm is abducted at 30–40 degrees of elevation. As shoulder elevation beyond 120 degrees is reached, the pain may resolve. Active internal and external rotation is usually associated with discomfort. With significant disruption of the rotator cuff, a patient may have no active elevation past mid range because of lost cuff function.

B. Imaging: Plain film x-rays of the shoulder in internal and external rotation may show some sclerotic change at the site of the greater tuberosity. With disruption of the cuff, the humeral head is elevated in relation to the glenoid cavity.

Disruption of the cuff will be clearly demonstrated by arthrography. The dye injected into the joint easily escapes into the subacromial space and is seen lateral to the greater tuberosity, indicating cuff disruption or tear.

Differential Diagnosis

Acute shoulder sepsis may mimic acute bursitis because of the comparable severity of pain. Sepsis is usually associated with systemic signs, such as an elevated sedimentation rate and white blood cell count. Bursitis may be difficult to distinguish from acute monarticular arthritis and should be diagnosed on the basis of the patient's history and possible other joint involvement. Plain x-rays should rule out preexisting tuberculosis and bone tumors.

Treatment

When patients are comfortable at rest, immobilization of the shoulder by sling and swath and use of analgesics or nonsteroidal anti-inflammatory drugs may be sufficient to relieve pain. Aspiration is indicated in patients not relieved by immobilization.

For patients with acute bursitis, dramatic relief of symptoms may occur with aspiration, lavage, and injection of lidocaine and cortisone. Cortisone is injected with aseptic technique approximately 2.5 cm lateral to the midpoint of the tip of the acromion. A 25-gauge needle is inserted through the deltoid into the subacromial bursa. Injection under pressure should be avoided because it may indicate direct penetration of cortisone into the substance of the rotator cuff. Patients not responding to the first injection of cortisone should receive another injection 2–3 weeks later.

All patients should be taught pendulum exercises, in which the individual flexes at the waist, relaxes all shoulder girdle musculature, and dangles the involved arm in a pendulumlike fashion.

In the few patients who do not respond to conservative treatment or who have frank cuff rupture, surgical treatment may be necessary following double-contrast arthrography to confirm the diagnosis and rule out other disorders. The goal of surgery is to relieve coracoacromial and acromial undersurface pressure (impingement) on the cuff or to repair a torn cuff.

3. FROZEN SHOULDER SYNDROME

In patients with frozen shoulder syndrome, there is marked restriction of glenohumeral joint motion, presumably in response to diffuse inflammation that can be associated with a cuff lesion or local tendinitis. These patients are usually comfortable at rest, and symptoms are produced only when they attempt to move the glenohumeral joint beyond that allowed by the inflammation and adhesions.

Treatment for frozen shoulder syndrome is immobilization to accomplish complete pain relief, followed by range-of-motion exercises that will allow shoulder motion to recover gradually over the next 6–18 months. Occasionally, intra-articular cortisone may be necessary for initial pain relief.

4. ACROMIOCLAVICULAR JOINT SEPARATION

Acromioclavicular joint injuries may result from falls or from direct trauma to the arm or shoulder. They are common in contact sports such as ice hockey and football.

Stability across the acromioclavicular joint is provided primarily by the conoid and trapezoid ligaments. These ligaments, which are connected to the undersurface of the clavicle, suspend the scapula in the upright position by their attachment at the base of the coracoid process. The less robust acromioclavicular ligaments and the attachments of the deltoid musculature between the clavicle and the arm provide additional stability. In minor injuries, the ligaments of the acromioclavicular joint are stretched, and with increased force the coracoacromial ligaments are injured as well. In severe injuries, the deltoid can be partially avulsed from its origin at the clavicle or acromion.

Clinical Findings

Symptoms and signs include pain and tenderness over the acromioclavicular joint and deformity of the joint.

X-rays of the injured shoulder will rule out fracture of the clavicle or proximal humerus. Displacement of the acromioclavicular joint can be demonstrated on an anteroposterior view of the joint and shoulder taken with the patient holding a weight or with traction applied to the humerus.

Treatment

Treatment for most injuries consists of relieving symptoms by using a sling to immobilize the shoulder and support the weight of the arm. Patients may resume activity as comfort returns.

If there is severe disruption of the acromioclavicular joint with detachment of the deltoid, surgery may be indicated. One repair option is the Weaver-Dunn procedure, in which the coracoacromial ligament is detached from the acromion and inserted into the distal end of the clavicle, which has been shortened by 1–2 cm. There is no urgency in deciding whether to operate if the Weaver-Dunn procedure is the surgical option, since this particular repair need not be done immediately. In general, the conservative and surgical approaches to treatment yield equivalent results, at least for the less severe disruptions.

INJURIES OF THE ELBOW, WRIST, & HAND

1. LATERAL HUMERAL EPICONDYLITIS (Tendinitis of Common Extensor Origin, or Tennis Elbow)

Lateral humeral epicondylitis received the designation "tennis elbow" because it was a common complaint among tennis players. The lesion can occur with any type of repetitive wrist dorsiflexion activity, as may be suffered by any worker whose work calls for repeated forceful wrist extension. The pathologic process is thought to represent collagen necrosis at the attachment of the common extensor tendon to the lateral humeral epicondyle or at the origin of the extensor carpi radialis brevis tendon.

Clinical Findings

Patients may have ill-defined elbow symptoms or pain radiating into the dorsal aspect of the forearm. Symptoms may occur at night and at rest, but they usually are related to activity, especially grasping or wrist dorsiflexion. There is local tenderness over the lateral humeral epicondyle or distal to it in the common extensor origin.

On clinical examination, symptoms can be reproduced by asking the patient to dorsiflex the wrist against resistance (as in grasping the back of a chair and lifting) or to apply resistance against wrist dorsiflexion. X-ray findings are normal.

Differential Diagnosis

The symptoms of radial head osteoarthritis, which is rare, can resemble those of tennis elbow. Plain films will usually distinguish the 2 disorders.

A fractured radial head or neck caused by falling on an outstretched hand may cause similar symptoms. The history of the injury and plain film anteroposterior and lateral x-ray views will establish the diagnosis of fracture.

Prevention

General strengthening of elbow and forearm musculature and proper instruction in the use of hand tools may prevent lateral humeral epicondylitis in workers at risk (see Chapter 6).

Treatment

A. General Measures: The lesion usually heals if the harmful activity is eliminated. Patients should be instructed to avoid dorsiflexion activities and carrying heavy objects with the elbow extended (some women carry their purses in that manner). Nonsteroidal anti-inflammatory drugs are helpful, especially for patients with night pain.

B. Specific Measures: A 40-mg injection of triamcinolone acetonide or hydrocortisone into the most tender area of the epicondyle or common extensor origin is usually effective in relieving symptoms. Occasionally, a second injection is necessary. Complications of this treatment include fat necrosis and local skin atrophy. Loss of pigmentation (usually temporary) in darker-skinned patients may result from the injection.

Rarely is release of the common extensor origin or extensor carpi radialis brevis necessary. As patients recover from an acute episode, forearm muscle strengthening is helpful. A Velcro sleeve around the proximal forearm to minimize contraction of the extensor tendon of the extensor muscle mass, as used by some tennis players, also appears to be beneficial.

2. OLECRANON BURSITIS

Olecranon bursitis is irritation and swelling in preexisting (normally occurring) bursa over the olecranon prominence. It is much more common in men, and trauma is usually a factor. Occasionally, the cause of the swelling is a low-grade infection, which must be considered prior to treatment. Swelling that develops over the olecranon process after surgery may be gouty in origin.

Patients usually present with a history of gradual swelling and pain, though these symptoms may be acute after a direct blow to the olecranon process. Signs of increased warmth suggest a septic process. Sepsis can be present when symptoms are quite mild. Localized fluctuant swelling will be present with or without sepsis.

The use of a protective pad to avoid reinjury is sufficient treatment in most cases, and simple immobilization is adequate in mild cases. Aspiration and culture are indicated when sepsis is suspected. Aspiration is best performed by introducing the needle at least 2.5 cm away from the bursa and then tunneling beneath the skin before actual penetration. This technique may prevent secondary infection of a sterile bursa, which is a risk when direct penetration through overlying skin is used.

3. DE QUERVAIN'S TENOSYNOVITIS (First Dorsal Wrist Extensor Compartment Tenosynovitis)

De Quervain's tenosynovitis involves the first dorsal compartment of the wrist. Onset is usually associated with overuse of the thumb, as in repetitive grasping. Rarely, an aberrant or extra tendon may be present in the sheath, which normally contains the abductor pollicis longus and the extensor pollicis brevis. The tenosynovial lining will show low-grade inflammation.

Clinical Findings

Patients in new job activities or those who engage in repetitive grasping complain of pain in an ill-defined area along the radial side of the thumb, occasionally extending as far as the distal interphalangeal joint. Local swelling is usually present over the lateral aspect of the distal radius and may be present in the absence of pain. When the patient grasps the fully flexed thumb into the palm and then deviates the hand ulnad at the wrist, exquisite pain develops and reproduces the patient's complaint (a positive Finkelstein test). Crepitus is frequently present over the involved tendon sheath. There are no specific laboratory or x-ray findings.

Differential Diagnosis

Old nonunion of the navicular bone occasionally produces similar symptoms. Pain associated with osteoarthritis of the first carpometacarpal joint, which occurs in about 15% of white women over the age of 55 years, may mimic De Quervain's tenosynovitis, which occurs in younger patients. Plain film anteroposterior x-rays of the wrist will rule out carpometacarpal osteoarthritis (see below) and nonunion of the navicular bone.

Treatment

Most patients learn to limit their grasping activities, and the symptoms then resolve.

The standard treatment is 1 mL of lidocaine delivered locally with a 25-gauge needle to the common first dorsal extensor sheath; this is followed by 20 mg of triamcinolone acetonide. Injection should not be performed with excessive pressure, since this may damage either of the tendons. With the needle in the proper position, no resistance to injection is encountered. Immobilization of the thumb in a splint is helpful, as are nonsteroidal anti-inflammatory drugs.

In the rare patient who does not respond to local injection, surgical decompression of the common extensor sheath by incision may be necessary. This procedure may inadvertently injure the sensory branch of the radial nerve, even when it is performed with the aid of magnification. Pain associated with a sensory branch radial nerve neuroma is at least as bad as and usually worse than the original tenosynovitis. Symptoms in the majority of patients with tenosynovitis resolve after one cortisone injection.

4. CARPAL TUNNEL SYNDROME

Carpal tunnel syndrome is a traumatic or pressure neuropathy of the median nerve as it passes through the carpal tunnel volar to the 9 flexor tendons. The canal boundaries are the rigid transverse carpal ligament on the volar side and the carpal bones on the dorsal side.

Carpal tunnel syndrome affects patients of any age or either sex. Symptoms may appear after an injury, such as a direct blow to the dorsiflexed wrist or an injury associated with Colles' fracture. Rheumatoid arthritis, which causes inflammation in the sheath surrounding the flexor tendons, is one example of a space-occupying lesion that produces the encroachment. Rare hypothyroid patients with myxomatous tissue in this area are at risk for bilateral symptoms. While the cause of the syndrome is unknown in most cases, repetitive wrist and finger movements involved in work and hobby activities have been implicated.

Clinical Findings

In the absence of injury, patients can gradually and spontaneously develop paresthesias in the median nerve distribution (the distribution in the volar surface of the thumb and the index and long fingers). With progression of the syndrome, patients may be awakened at night with pain or paresthesia. Characteristically, they tend to stand up and massage the area or shake the wrist and fingers. Untreated carpal tunnel syndrome with progressively worsening symptoms may result in permanent damage to the median nerve with consequent persistent skin sensory deficit and thenar motor weakness.

When patients are seen early, there is no evidence of thenar atrophy, and sensation remains intact. If a blood pressure cuff on the arm is inflated midway between arterial and venous pressure, venous engorgement occurs and elicits the symptoms. Patients who hold their wrists maximally flexed will also develop symptoms (Phalen's sign). The diagnosis is confirmed by nerve conduction studies performed in an electrodiagnosis laboratory.

Differential Diagnosis

Pain in the median nerve distribution with compression of the carpal tunnel should be distinguished from full median nerve compression. Occasionally, C6 radiculopathy from cervical disk disease may resemble this condition, but a properly performed neurologic examination should distinguish the two.

Treatment

Use of anti-inflammatory drugs and wrist splints may minimize local inflammation. Injections of cortisone into the carpal tunnel (with care to avoid injection into the median nerve) are also occasionally helpful. Patients who fail to respond to the preceding measures may require surgical carpal tunnel release, which is a well-documented and standardized procedure.

5. OSTEOARTHRITIS OF THE FIRST CARPOMETACARPAL JOINT

Osteoarthritis of the first carpometacarpal joint occurs in about 15% of women over the age of 55

years. The cause is unknown. Although the condition is frequently asymptomatic, some patients are aware of pain at the base of the thumb when grasping, as when unscrewing large glass jars, and there may be a clinical deformity of "squaring" of the base of the thumb at the carpometacarpal joint. Plain film x-rays will demonstrate the osteoarthritic changes in the joint.

The differential diagnosis includes De Quervain's tenosynovitis (see above), in which tenderness and swelling are more proximal, and old nonunions or fractures of the navicular bone. These conditions occur in younger patients and can be ruled out by plain films.

Wearing an orthosis to immobilize the thumb can minimize symptoms. Anti-inflammatory drugs are helpful for patients who experience pain at night. For those who do not respond to conservative treatment, a surgical procedure such as fusion of the first carpometacarpal joint or arthroplasty must be considered.

INJURIES OF THE SPINE

1. LOW BACK PAIN DUE TO DISK DISEASE OR INJURY (Spinal Degenerative Disk Disease)

Injuries to the lower lumbar intervertebral disks, preexisting degenerative disk disease, or both are responsible for most low back problems, occupational or otherwise. In the United States, a specific identifiable injury is associated with the onset of symptoms in only 15% of workers. Symptoms may begin at any age, with a peak incidence in the third or fourth decade. Over half of the population under the age of 65 have had experience with backache, with half of those having lost time from work. By 60 years of age, two-thirds of all adults have some radiographic evidence of degenerative disk disease.

Disks become increasingly less resilient with age, and degeneration may cause the posterior annulus to bulge into the spinal canal. The nucleus pulposus within the annulus may also protrude or herniate through a weakened portion of the annulus or be frankly sequestered in the spinal canal. Pressure of a disk or disk fragment on a nerve root may produce pain or sensorimotor weakness in the distribution of the nerve root. The cause of pain in the absence of direct nerve root pressure is not well understood; it may be due to inflammation in response to injury to the degenerated disk. There are free nerve endings in the posterior third of the annulus.

Clinical Findings

A. Symptoms and Signs: The onset of symptoms may be gradual or sudden. Patients sometimes wake with back pain after a day of strenuous activity, or symptoms may be directly related to a specific fall or lifting incident. Pain is usually but not always associated with motion and may be located in the lower lumbar region, the lumbosacral angle midline, the sacroiliac joint region, or the medial buttock. With associated radiculopathy, patients may experience leg pain independently of back pain. Pain from an S1 radiculopathy may be felt in the posterior calf and lateral border of the foot. L4 radiculopathy produces pain below the knee or in the medial part of the leg, and L5 radiculopathy produces pain in the lateral calf and dorsum of the foot or in the great toe.

Restriction of back motion, common to all patients, is demonstrated on forward bending. Sciatic scoliosis, which is a list to the opposite side of a disk protrusion, may occur. Patients with severe disk problems avoid sitting and prefer standing or recumbency because intradisk pressure is lower in the latter 2 positions.

With a disk that produces radiculopathy, straight leg raising carried out passively by the examiner with the patient recumbent will cause back or leg pain, and the patient will guard against further elevation of the leg; this is considered a positive test. The degree of positivity is the angle of the elevated leg from the table, eg, 45 degrees. S1 radiculopathy causes decreased or absent ankle jerk or decreased sensation along either the lateral border of the foot or the lateral 3 toes. L4 radiculopathy, which is less common, causes decreased or absent knee jerk or decreased sensation in the medial surface of the leg or pretibial region. L5 radiculopathy produces weakness of dorsiflexion of the great toe or hypoesthesia on the dorsum of the foot or great toe.

B. Imaging: Plain film lateral and anteroposterior x-ray views of the entire lumbar spine are obtained with the patient standing. In addition, spot anteroposterior and lateral views of the 2 lowest disks are obtained with the patient recumbent and are used to rule out infection, tuberculosis, tumor, or fracture. CT scan, MRI, or myelography may be performed to define the level of the lesion prior to surgery.

Differential Diagnosis

Almost any pathologic process involving the spine, meninges, abdomen, pelvis, or retroperitoneal area can cause low back pain. Physical examination should include evaluation for costovertebral angle tenderness, urinalysis to rule out renal disorders, abdominal examination for aneurysm, and evaluation of peripheral pulses to determine if there are vascular causes of back pain. If pyogenic infection of the disk space is suspected, gallium and technetium bone scans and an erythrocyte sedimentation rate are helpful in making this diagnosis; plain film x-rays usually show no pathologic changes during the first 2 weeks of back pain due to pyogenic sepsis. In tuberculosis of the spine, which has an insidious onset, plain films will show disk space collapse and endplate loss at the initial examination.

Ankylosing spondylitis (see below), which is more common in males, may start in the latter part of the

second decade. Chest expansion measured at the nipple line will be less than 5 cm. Plain x-rays will show sacroiliitis or early ''squaring'' of the lumbar vertebral bodies.

Deposits of tumor or multiple myeloma in the pedicles of vertebral bodies usually present with an early compression fracture. Technetium bone scans will reveal the former, and immunoelectrophoresis can be used to diagnose the latter.

A large or massive disk protrusion may produce cauda equina syndrome. Symptoms include urinary retention, sphincter paralysis, and perineal numbness. Patients with suspected cauda equina syndrome should be hospitalized and studied by myelography.

Prevention

Proper instruction about prevention of symptoms of degenerative disk disease should be mandatory for all new employees, regardless of their activity level. Education about body mechanics, lifting, bending, the hazards of prolonged sitting, and the deleterious effects of lack of exercise should be emphasized (see Chapter 6). Industrial workers with any degree of low back pain should be given an opportunity for early medical evaluation to minimize progressive changes. Job activity should be designed to minimize prolonged sitting or standing and to avoid sitting while leaning forward and rotating. Employee selection using strength performance criteria may be useful (see Chapter 6). There is no evidence that preemployment x-rays are helpful to either the employer or the employee in identifying individuals who may be at risk for developing low back injuries. However, appropriate evaluation and counseling of individuals with previous back injury or surgery are valuable.

Treatment

A. Conservative Measures: Symptoms in 80–90% of patients with acute low back pain or radiculopathy secondary to disk disease will resolve with conservative measures—temporary bed rest, time, and avoidance of reinjury. Patients with severe pain should be instructed to remain in bed in the semi-Fowler position for 1 week, to eat while lying on one side, to use a bedpan or urinal for urination, to get up only for bowel movements, and, if necessary, to take acetaminophen with 30 mg of codeine or 5 mg of diazepam twice a day. Patients who improve in 1 week can be allowed up half the time for a second week but should avoid sitting. For any patient with significant initial radiculopathy, return to full-time work before 3–6 weeks should be avoided; for those who perform heavy labor, this proscription may be as long as 3–4 months.

Patients whose occupations involve light labor or who are self-employed and can adjust their work schedules may be allowed to work part-time and then be encouraged to be recumbent during leisure time. Initial use of a lumbosacral corset is especially helpful for those whose occupations call for prolonged sitting or driving. As symptoms resolve, corset use is gradually tapered, and patients are taught abdominal strengthening exercises as well as straight leg raising and stretching.

Manipulation, ultrasound, acupuncture, acupressure, heat, and massage provide no long-term benefits. The best results are obtained when mechanical and gravitational stresses are relieved long enough to allow healing and exercise is then gradually resumed. At the appropriate point, a swimming program in which the individual uses either the backstroke or the sidestroke (not the crawl, because it causes extension) is encouraged.

B. Surgical Measures: Patients who fail to respond to conservative treatment (as evidenced by persistent pain and persistently positive results in the straight leg raising test or by sciatic scoliosis with evidence of disk protrusion) are candidates for surgery. Surgery may consist of percutaneous nucleotomy, laminotomy, or diskectomy to relieve nerve root pressure. In rare cases, spinal fusion is added to the procedure.

2. SPINAL STENOSIS

Spinal stenosis may be the result of congenitally short pedicles but is more frequently due to progressive degenerative disk disease in the lumbar spine. It may be the most common cause of leg pain in the elderly.

Disk degeneration at multiple levels with secondary hypertrophy of the ligamenta flava and facet joints causes encroachment on the thecal sac and nerve root impingement. Although involvement at more than one level is evident radiographically, patients usually present with single-root involvement. Standing and walking with the lumbar spine in extension further decrease the already compromised space in the spinal canal. With the spine flexed, as it is when seated, there is more space for the neural contents and relief of symptoms.

Clinical Findings

A. Symptoms and Signs: Neurogenic claudication may be accompanied by an ill-defined pain in the lower extremity or by pain that is distributed along a specific nerve root and felt while walking. Patients may experience difficulty in standing, as when shopping or waiting in line. The symptoms are typically relieved with sitting, recumbency, or even standing with one hip and knee flexed and one foot raised on a stair or footstool.

There may be unilateral reflex changes affecting the involved root, such as decreased ankle jerk (S1), decreased knee jerk (L3 or L4), or decreased power in the great toe extensor (L5). In some cases, there are symmetric signs with generalized areflexia. Patients should be asked to walk to reproduce symptoms and then be reexamined for reflex changes (the Gill walk test). They may not have limitation of spine motion and usually have negative results in the straight leg raising test.

B. Imaging: Plain film x-rays may show scoliosis or degenerative disk changes with associated osteophytic hypertrophy of the facet joints at one or more levels. In younger patients with congenital spinal stenosis, shortening of the pedicles may be seen on lateral x-ray views of the spine; however, this shortening may best be seen on CT scans.

CT scan or MRI of the spine will show encroachment on the theca or nerve roots caused by a combination of disk degeneration, osteophytic overgrowth of the facet joints, and ligamentous hypertrophy at one or more levels. Myelography will show stenosis at one or more levels or even spinal block.

Differential Diagnosis

Patients with degenerative disease of the spine may also have degenerative arthritis of the hips or knees. The source of groin pain upon hip motion is more likely to be the hip joint rather than lower lumbar spinal stenosis. Knee pain associated with degenerative arthritis is more localized. Vascular claudication can mimic neurogenic claudication but is associated with altered pulses and will require assessment by Doppler ultrasound and treatment by vascular surgery. Tumors or infections of the spine may produce leg pain from radiculopathy.

Patients who have bladder or bowel dysfunction and are suspected of having cauda equina syndrome will require immediate investigation. If the diagnosis is confirmed, surgical decompression must be started.

Treatment

Epidural corticosteroids or braces that keep the spine in flexion during walking or standing may be tried. The results vary among patients. Those who do not respond to these measures require surgical decompression. Laminotomy, laminectomy, foraminotomy, or facetectomy may be necessary at one or more levels. Preoperative spinal instability with spondylolisthesis or postdecompression instability must be assessed. If instability is significant, single- or multiple-level spinal fusion should be carried out by the lateral transverse process fusion technique. In rare instances, marked postdecompression or postoperative instability may require internal fixation.

3. COCCYGODYNIA

The coccyx consists of 3 small segments of bone with articulations between them. The segments are connected to the sacrum by the sacrococcygeal joint. A direct fall onto the coccyx or a direct blow to the area can injure any of the articulations and cause coccygodynia. Pain at the lower tip of the spine may persist if the joint is aggravated by sitting. Symptoms can be reproduced by manual palpation of or direct pressure over the coccyx. Plain films will rule out fracture.

Patients should be instructed to sit with a small

pillow under the mid thighs so that the buttocks are raised from the chair. Anti-inflammatory drugs are helpful in relieving pain at night. A few patients require local anesthesia delivered into the articulation, followed by local injection of cortisone.

4. SPONDYLOLYSIS & SPONDYLOLISTHESIS

Spondylolysis, a defect in the pars interarticularis, may develop during childhood when the cartilage there fails to ossify. The defect tends to be familial, but some cases are associated with trauma (as when a football lineman performs a blocking maneuver and puts the spine into forceful extension). This may allow spondylolisthesis, or forward displacement of one vertebra on the next. Spondylolisthesis may also result from degenerative disk disease or facet arthritis. Displacement of L5 on S1 is the most common level seen in isthmic spondylolisthesis; displacement of L4 on L5 is most common in degenerative spondylolisthesis. Individuals with backache have no greater incidence of isthmic spondylolysis and spondylolisthesis than do individuals without backache. The presence of the lesion may not necessarily be the cause of the patient's back pain.

Clinical Findings

A. Symptoms and Signs: Spondylolysis and spondylolisthesis may cause symptoms similar to those of degenerative disk disease. Patients with spondylolisthesis occasionally have bilateral posterior thigh pain and may experience radiculopathy caused by irritation of the nerve root as it passes the fibrocartilaginous buildup at the pars interarticularis (most commonly, the fifth root in L5–S1 spondylolisthesis).

Patients may have tight hamstring muscles in both legs, as demonstrated on straight leg raising. Local point tenderness over the spinous process of the involved vertebrae may produce exquisite tenderness or even radiation of pain in the distribution of the fifth nerve root (doorbell sign).

B. Imaging: An angled anteroposterior x-ray (upshot view) of the 2 lowest vertebrae should demonstrate the defect in the pars interarticularis. Oblique views can also demonstrate the pars defect, but they expose the patient to a large amount of radiation. Spondylolisthesis is obvious on lateral view x-rays.

CT scans will show the pars defect (double facet sign) in spondylolysis and the elongated spinal canal in spondylolisthesis.

Treatment

Patients with spondylolysis or spondylolisthesis should be treated with conservative measures similar to those recommended for patients with disk disease (see above). For those who do not respond to conservative treatment, surgery is indicated. This may consist of the Gill procedure (removal of the spinous process and lamina of each involved vertebra), decompression of the root, transverse process fusion of one or perhaps 2 levels, or a combination of these procedures.

5. ANKYLOSING SPONDYLITIS

Ankylosing spondylitis affects about 1% of the white population and may be more prevalent in other groups such as the southern Chinese. It is much more prevalent among males than females. About 90% of affected patients have a genetic predisposition to the disease, as evidenced by the presence of HLA-B27, and symptoms develop in one out of 7 white patients who test positive for HLA-B27.

Clinical Findings

A. Symptoms and Signs: Patients experience spontaneous and gradual onset of low back pain with associated restriction of spine motion. Symptoms frequently begin during the second decade and, apparently, are more frequently missed during this period. Occasionally, patients will develop a markedly stiffened spine and not remember experiencing any pain. Rarely, the disease presents like sciatica, with back and leg pain.

Restricted back motion can usually be demonstrated on forward flexion, but muscle spasm from disk disease may also do this and is more common. Even in the early stages of disease, maximal chest expansion measured at the nipple line will be less than 5 cm. Stiffening of the spine becomes more obvious as the disease progresses, and normal dorsal kyphosis increases with flattening of the lumbar region and reduction of the normal lumbar lordosis. There may be involvement of the glenohumeral joints or hip joints, and, rarely, a patient will have more peripheral involvement.

B. Imaging: On plain film x-rays of the back, the sacroiliac joints show erosions, sclerosis, and, in more advanced cases, frank bony fusion. Lateral views of the lumbar spine in the early stages show "squaring" of the vertebrae (in which the normal slight anterior concavity has been filled with new bone as a result of inflammation beneath the anterior longitudinal ligament). In later stages, the classic bony bridging, or "bamboo spine," is evident.

Differential Diagnosis

A patient with a stiff, ankylosed spine who complains of pain after a fall should be considered to have a fracture until it is proved otherwise. The fracture could increase the patient's spinal deformity, usually in flexion. Common fracture locations are the dorsolumbar junction and the cervicothoracic junction. It is necessary to obtain bone scans or repeat x-rays or to take special views and immobilize the patient to protect against flexion deformity. Immobilization may involve use of a halo jacket device at the cervicothoracic junction or a brace at the dorsolumbar junction.

Treatment

Treatment is aimed at relieving pain and preventing deformity. Patients should be given anti-inflammatory medication (eg, aspirin, naproxen, piroxicam) and instructed to sleep in an appropriate position without pillows and seek evaluation if they experience pain after an injury. This pain may indicate stress fracture or traumatic fracture, either of which requires protection against flexion deformity.

INJURIES OF THE HIP

1. TROCHANTERIC BURSITIS

Trochanteric bursitis is an uncommon disorder which may be due to local contusion that causes bleeding into the trochanteric bursa. More commonly, however, the onset of symptoms is spontaneous. Symptoms consist of local tenderness and persistent pain with activity.

Trochanteric bursitis is often confused with hip arthritis because of referred joint pain from the latter. The diagnosis can be confirmed by administering an anesthetic into the trochanteric bursa.

Local cortisone injection is usually successful in resolving the symptoms.

2. AVASCULAR NECROSIS OF THE FEMORAL HEAD

Classic avascular necrosis was described in caisson workers subjected to severe atmospheric pressure changes. However, standards for the rate of barometric pressure change (from data on navy divers) have been effective in eliminating pressure change as a cause. Today, avascular necrosis occurs in several groups: in patients with subcapital fractures that interrupt the blood supply; in a small number of patients taking high doses of cortisone (eg, in 15% of those who undergo renal transplantation with concurrent cortisone therapy) and, less frequently, in patients taking low doses of cortisone; in patients with asthma; in patients with lupus erythematosus; and in drug abusers. It also occurs idiopathically. An association with high alcohol consumption has been suggested but seems unlikely.

One theory of pathogenesis is that some abnormality related to the metabolism of cortisone exists in affected individuals. Because only a small number of patients taking cortisone develop the condition, additional idiosyncratic factors are thought to be involved. Changes in marrow pressure of the proximal femur have been documented in early avascular necrosis. As revascularization of the ischemic bone occurs, weakening of subchondral bone produces a fracture and accounts for the mechanical symptoms.

Clinical Findings

A. Symptoms and Signs: The onset of pain associated with activity is usually insidious. Occasionally, a specific event (eg, putting the lower extremity in an extreme position) will precipitate pain. Infrequently, pain occurs at night. Patients limp with an antalgic gait on the affected side, and hip motion may be slightly restricted compared with a lesser involved or uninvolved opposite side. Symptoms can be elicited by movements at the extremes of hip motion—especially rotation.

Some patients with avascular necrosis have involvement of the opposite hip, the knees, or the shoulders. Involvement of both knees and shoulders may occur in the absence of hip disease.

B. Imaging: An anteroposterior x-ray of the pelvis in the early stages of avascular necrosis will show mottling changes in the femoral head. Findings on plain film x-rays are rarely normal. With progression of the disease, there is flattening of the femoral head. This flattening is due to settling of a quadrant of the head—because of the fracture—between the vascular and avascular bone. The cartilage, which receives its nutrients via the surface from the synovial fluid, remains normal until late and secondary osteoarthritic changes occur.

MRI may show abnormalities before they are evident on CT scans but after they are evident on technetium bone scans.

Differential Diagnosis

Symptoms of avascular necrosis may be confused with those of early degenerative arthritis of the hip. The 2 disorders can be distinguished with plain films.

Treatment

Partial relief of symptoms may result from use of measures such as body weight reduction, walking with a cane in the hand on the unaffected side, or walking with crutches.

Attempts to decompress the proximal femur by early drilling and bone grafting of the femoral head and neck, which revascularizes the head and enables it to support the necrotic and compressed area, have been tried and found ineffective.

Surgical treatment is indicated in symptomatic patients in whom the weight-bearing dome of the femoral head has collapsed. At the time of surgery, it is difficult to be certain of the damage to the acetabular cartilage, which, if present, would necessitate total hip replacement. Bipolar hemiarthroplasty, cemented or uncemented, can also be used.

The complications of hip replacement and hemiarthroplasty include loosening, which is the most frequent adverse consequence, and infection on rare occasions. Loose prostheses can be revised. An infected arthroplasty requires debridement of the prosthesis, appropriate antibiotics, and, depending on whether or not the infection has been eradicated, reinsertion of a prosthesis.

3. OSTEOARTHRITIS OF THE HIP

The cause of primary osteoarthritis of the hip is unknown. Secondary osteoarthritis results from mechanical stress related to deficient acetabular coverage, as in congenital hip disease, the femoral head deformity in Legg-Perthes disease, or slipping capital femoral epiphyses. The disease is unrelated to occupation, but it may be first noticed in the workplace. There is no evidence that repeated subliminal trauma to or overuse of the hip is a causative factor.

Osteoarthritis of the hip occurs in 3–8% of whites, in whom most cases are primary. It is rare among southern Chinese and blacks. Osteoarthritis secondary to congenital hip disease is quite common among native Japanese and is more likely to be symptomatic in the fourth, fifth, and sixth decades.

The earliest pathologic changes occur in the articular cartilage, with fibrillation, fissuring, and surface cartilage loss. This is followed by the body's attempt at repair through proliferation and replication of existing chondrocytes. Low-grade inflammatory changes occur in the synovium secondarily and in response to the cartilage surface degeneration. As the disease progresses, osteophytic projections occur at the margins of the articular cartilage and the periosteum, and there is cartilage loss down to eburnated subchondral bone. This results in an incongruous relationship between the femoral head and acetabulum. Synovial and capsular thickening, occurring along with the incongruous bony relationship, contributes to restricted joint motion.

Clinical Findings

A. Symptoms and Signs: Patients gradually become aware of pain with activity. The pain may be felt in the groin, proximal thigh, trochanteric region, or lateral buttock. Rarely, patients complain of pain only in the distal thigh or knee. Early in the course of the disease, patients may not be aware of a subtle hip limp (antalgic gait, or abductor lurch over the affected side). As the disease progresses, they may be awakened at night with hip pain, which is usually what causes them to seek medical evaluation.

Restricted hip motion is seen on clinical examination. The earliest loss is internal rotation, followed by loss of abduction and flexion. With long-standing symptoms, patients may have obvious thigh atrophy.

B. Imaging: Plain film x-rays demonstrate the characteristic changes of osteoarthritis, (ie, joint space narrowing, subchondral sclerosis, and marginal osteophytes).

Treatment

In the early stages of the disease, an anti-inflammatory drug such as naproxen (375 mg twice daily) or ibuprofen (800 mg 3 times daily) may provide symptomatic relief. Using a cane in the hand on the unaffected side or protecting the hip by using 2 crutches is beneficial. Patients who experience unrelieved pain at night or increasing symptoms will require total hip replacement.

INJURIES OF THE KNEE, ANKLE, & FOOT

1. KNEE LIGAMENT INJURIES

Knee ligament injuries can result from indirect force such as a fall or misstep or from a direct blow. They are seen most commonly in young athletes who engage in contact sports, but they also occur in the workplace. The injuries range from simple strain to frank disruption in which the ligament is torn in its substance or avulsed from its bony attachment.

First-degree injury is a tear involving a few fibers of the ligament. The knee is tender on palpation but shows no instability and demonstrates no excessive motion when force is applied. **Second-degree injury,** which is a partial tear of the ligament, also causes no instability. **Third-degree injury** is a complete tear or disruption of the ligament and does result in joint instability. The different ligaments of the knee can be injured individually or in combination.

Diagnosis

Accurate diagnosis of knee ligament injuries requires considerable experience and depends on a careful history, a detailed physical examination of the joint, and special imaging techniques. Severe pain may interfere with proper examination, in which case the procedure must either be performed with the patient under anesthesia or be postponed for a few days.

The most common knee ligament injuries are to the medial collateral and anterior cruciate ligaments or some combination of the two. Lateral collateral ligament and posterior cruciate ligament injuries are less common. Plain film x-rays are obtained and are usually negative for bone injury. MRI can specify the nature and location of ligament disruption as well as provide evidence of injury to the meniscus, articular cartilage, and bone.

In addition to the usual evaluation of knee motion, which will detect the presence of ecchymosis and local swelling, the various ligaments in the knee are tested by stressing the joint in different directions. Such stress can manifest instability and indicate which ligaments are involved. Valgus and varus stresses test the medial and lateral collateral ligaments, respectively. Anterior cruciate stability is tested by the anterior drawer, Lachman, and pivot-shift tests. The posterior drawer test is specific for the posterior cruciate ligament. Stress tests that can demonstrate opening of the joint may also be necessary. The reader is referred to *Campbell's Operative Orthopedics* (1987) for the technique of test administration and the interpretation of test results.

Common Types of Knee Injury

A. Injuries of the Medial Collateral Ligament:
The most frequent mechanism of injury is indirect force that applies valgus stress to the knee. On examination, there may be evidence of local hemorrhage or effusion into the joint. Tenderness can usually be demonstrated at the site of ligamentous injury, at the site of attachment of the ligament in the region of the medial epicondyle, or along the ligament one handbreadth below the joint line at its distal attachment on the tibia. The degree of instability can be determined by applying valgus stress to the joint in full extension and at 20 degrees of flexion. Any instability detected by opening of the medial joint space is indicative of medial collateral ligament injury. Instability noted in full extension indicates medial collateral ligament injury plus additional injury involving the anterior cruciate ligament, the posterior capsule, or both.

B. Injuries of the Anterior Cruciate Ligament:
An injury that is limited to the anterior cruciate ligament can result either from anterior force on a knee that is in extension or from forcing the joint into hyperextension. If the force is great enough, injury to both the anterior and the posterior cruciate ligaments may occur. Anterior cruciate ligament injuries commonly accompany medial collateral ligament injuries in the presence of abduction, flexion, and internal rotation forces on the femur. The medial meniscus may be injured along with the medial collateral and anterior cruciate ligaments. An isolated anterior cruciate ligament injury may appear to have effusion only. However, careful testing performed with the knee held in 20 degrees of flexion may demonstrate forward displacement of the tibia on the femur (Lachman's test).

Treatment

First- and second-degree injuries can be treated symptomatically with crutches and a knee immobilizer. Third-degree injuries of the medial collateral ligament have been effectively treated with cast immobilization or cast bracing and are rarely treated by open surgical repair. The decision to undertake surgery for a complete tear or avulsion of the anterior cruciate ligament depends on the degree of joint instability, the patient's age and athletic habits, and the presence of other ligamentous injuries.

2. PREPATELLAR & INFRAPATELLAR BURSITIS

Local trauma, such as that resulting from a direct blow or from kneeling repeatedly (eg, scrubbing floors), can produce prepatellar bursitis, characterized by pain, tenderness, and irritation of or bleeding into the pancake-shaped bursa overlying the patella. In no form of prepatellar bursitis is there evidence of knee joint effusion indicating intra-articular involvement.

Priests, carpenters who lay flooring, and other workers who kneel over the region of the tibial tubercle may experience similar trauma resulting in infrapatellar bursitis. Superficial infrapatellar bursitis causes diffuse swelling over the tibial tubercle and lower portion of the patellar ligament. Deep infrapatellar bursitis is dumbbell-shaped because the patellar ligament compresses its center.

The treatment of prepatellar or infrapatellar bursitis is usually symptomatic. Knee flexion and kneeling are avoided, and the knee may be splinted in extension when symptoms are severe. Occasionally, prepatellar bursitis may be septic and require diagnostic aspiration, antibiotic treatment, and surgical drainage.

3. CHONDROMALACIA PATELLAE

Chondromalacia patellae is characterized by fibrillation or roughening of the undersurface of the patellar articular cartilage, usually on the medial facet. It occurs much more frequently in growing females than in growing males, but it may also occur during the young adult years. The articular cartilage changes are generally nonprogressive.

Symptoms of anterior knee pain may begin with a direct blow to the patella. They tend to be intermittent and are not usually associated with knee joint effusion. The pain occurs with activity, is usually more severe when descending than when ascending stairs, and is relieved by rest. It can be reproduced during clinical examination by depressing the patella at the patellofemoral groove against active quadriceps contraction. Other causes of knee disorders need to be ruled out by physical examination of the knee and plain film x-rays.

For treatment of most cases of chondromalacia, patients should be instructed to do active isometric quadriceps exercises with the knee in extension and to protect the knee by avoiding kneeling, squatting, and activities that cause discomfort. Symptoms are generally self-limited, lasting for just a few weeks. However, if the patella is frankly subluxing and causing articular damage at the patellofemoral joint, patellar realignment surgery may be necessary.

4. TEARS & INTERNAL DERANGEMENTS OF THE MENISCUS

Traumatic injury to the meniscus may occur at any age, though it occurs most commonly in young male athletes. Some meniscal injuries result from an apparent minor twisting of the lower extremity or even from sudden twisting of the knee while squatting. Injuries are much more common in the medial than in the lateral, more mobile meniscus and can range in severity from those which cause little damage and manifest relatively minor pain to those that displace the large bucket handle of the meniscus and cause frank catching and locking of the joint. The meniscus becomes stiffer with age, and symptoms may result from degenerative tears that occur in the fourth or fifth decade.

About 20% of patients with excised menisci develop radiographic changes of joint space narrowing, and some progress to degenerative arthritis in the vacant compartment. The postmortem studies of Noble (1977) demonstrated that torn menisci left in place are unrelated to degenerative arthritis of the knee joint—and, conversely, that degenerative arthritis of the knee joint can occur in the absence of meniscal injury. Therefore, there is no late risk of osteoarthritis from leaving a torn but asymptomatic meniscus in place.

Clinical Findings

Symptoms and signs of a torn meniscus include pain at the extremes of motion and local tenderness at the joint line over the involved meniscus. McMurray's sign (rotation of the tibia on the femur when moving the knee from flexion to extension) is rarely positive. Diagnosis can be confirmed by MRI and, more definitively, by arthroscopic examination.

Treatment

Patients who continue to manifest symptoms after a prolonged period of rest require surgery. The current trend is to repair the torn meniscus when the tear is located peripherally, where there is vascularity and healing is possible; this can be accomplished through arthroscopy and open repair, followed by immobilization with a cast or brace. Arthroscopic debridement is performed for marginal lesions.

Because long-term osteoarthritis has been associated with total meniscal excision, this procedure should be avoided.

5. ANKLE SPRAINS (Sprains of the Lateral Collateral Ligament Complex)

The lateral collateral ligament complex of the ankle consists of 7 ligaments that attach the fibula to the tibia, talus, and calcaneus. An inversion injury with or without the foot in plantar flexion may strain or sprain the anterior talofibular ligament, which is the ligament most commonly injured. When this happens, tenderness will be present, as will local swelling at either the anterior lateral neck of the talus or the tip of the fibula. A stronger external force may disrupt the posterior talofibular ligament, the calcaneofibular ligament, or the tibiofibular ligaments that account for the ligamentous stability of the ankle mortise.

Clinical Findings

Depending on the seriousness of the injury, pain can range in severity from minimal upon weight bearing to that which is severe enough to make walking impossible. Local swelling and tenderness will be present at the site of ligament damage. Fibular fractures or tibiofibular ligament disruptions can be ruled out with plain film x-rays. The only way to determine the precise degree of ligament disruption is by direct surgical exploration, but this is not indicated. Stress films of the ankle to determine the degree of tilt of the talus can be obtained but are not usually indicated.

Treatment

Treatment of ankle sprains usually consists of relieving the symptoms by supporting the ankle with an elastic bandage or adhesive strapping. In more severe cases, the patient is immobilized for 4–6 weeks in a short leg walking cast. Surgery does not achieve results superior to those attained by conservative treatment.

Ligamentous injury causing disruption of the ankle mortise usually requires surgical treatment.

In rare cases, a patient will have a persistent instability that is impossible to predict at the initial evaluation. When this instability occurs, secondary end-to-end repair of the ankle ligaments may be necessary, or else a secondary ligament reconstruction is required (Chrisman-Snook reconstruction).

6. AVULSION FRACTURES OF THE FIFTH METATARSAL

Avulsion fractures of the tip of the fifth metatarsal are produced by inversion injuries to the foot and the ankle, usually when the ankle is flexed. They occur commonly in athletes and dancers but may also occur in anyone who, for example, steps into a hole or trips.

In contrast with ankle sprain, avulsion fracture does not cause tenderness about the fibular malleolus. Instead, it causes local tenderness and swelling over the base of the fifth metatarsal. Location of the fracture site can be confirmed by x-ray.

Treatment consists of relieving symptoms. Wearing a stiff-soled shoe is sufficient for patients whose symptoms are minimal. More severe injuries and symptoms may call for immobilization in a short leg walking cast for 4–6 weeks. Nonunion of this fracture is rare, though a true Jones fracture—a transverse fracture across the full base of the metatarsal—can result in delayed union and even nonunion.

7. PLANTAR FASCIITIS (Medial Calcaneal Tubercle Bursitis)

Pain affecting the plantar aspect of the medial heel may develop spontaneously or may occur after direct trauma to the area or after impact on the heel. Patients are comfortable at rest, but pain returns with weight bearing and is especially severe when the patient gets out of bed in the morning.

Clinical examination reveals exquisite local tenderness over the medial calcaneal tubercle, which is the site of plantar fascial attachment. Lateral x-rays usually show a spur that projects from the calcaneus and has been present for many years. This suggests that the more recent local symptoms are due to bursitis in the area or to traction on the plantar fascia.

Wearing heel cushions can minimize impact on the heel and relieve symptoms. Use of a soft heel cup is helpful, as is the use of a shoe insert, which maintains the heel in a slightly varus angle and reduces traction on the plantar fascia.

8. MORTON'S NEUROMA

Morton's neuroma is usually found on the common plantar digital nerve branches to the third and fourth toes. It occurs more frequently in women. Pain is produced by direct pressure on the neuroma, which is located between the third and fourth metatarsal heads, and is aggravated by dorsiflexing the toe, as during the push-off phase of gait or when wearing high-heeled shoes. Patients frequently describe the pain as radiating into the toes.

On clinical examination, a small "click" can usually be felt as pressure is applied to the third and fourth metatarsal heads while the the patient dorsiflexes the toes. The click may temporarily disappear after the initial manipulation. Diagnosis can sometimes be confirmed by local nerve block.

Treatment with metatarsal bars or low-heeled, well-fitting shoes is rarely rewarding but should be tried. Surgical excision of the neuroma is frequently necessary.

REFERENCES

Injuries of the Neck & Shoulder

Post M: The Shoulder: *Surgical and Nonsurgical Management.* Lea & Febiger, 1978.

Sherk HH, Watters WC, Zeiger L: Evaluation and treatment of neck pain. *Orthop Clin North Am* 1982;**13**:439.

Weaver JK, Dunn HK: Treatment of acromioclavicular injuries, especially complete acromioclavicular separation. *J Bone Joint Surg [Am]* 1972;**54**:1187.

Injuries of the Elbow, Wrist, & Hand

Birkbeck MQ, Beer TC: Occupation in relation to the carpal tunnel syndrome. *Rheumatol Rehabil* 1975;**14:** 218.

Cannon LJ, Bernacki EJ, Walter SD: Personal and occupational factors associated with carpal tunnel syndrome. *J Occup Med* 1981;**23**:225.

Green DP (editor): Operative Hand Surgery. Churchill Livingstone, 1982.

Kashiwagi D: The tennis elbow: Statistical and EMG studies. In: *Elbow Joint.* Kashiwagi D (editor). Elsevier/North-Holland, 1985.

Moskowitz RW et al (editors): *Osteoarthritis: Diagnosis and Management.* Saunders, 1984.

Wood MR: Hydrocortisone injections for carpal tunnel syndrome. *Hand* 1980;**12**:62.

Injuries of the Spine

Calin A, Fries JF: Striking prevalence of ankylosing spondylitis in "healthy" w27 positive males and females. *N Engl J Med* 1975;**293**:835.

Chaffin DB, Herrin GD, Keyserling WM: Preemployment strength testing: An updated position. *J Occup Med* 1978;**20**:403.

Genant HK (editor): *Spine Update 1984.* Radiology Research and Education Foundation, 1983.

Gibson ES, Martin RH, Terry CW: Incidence of low back pain and pre-placement x-ray screening. *J Occup Med* 1980;**22**:515.

Harber P, SooHoo K: Static ergonomic strength testing in evaluating occupational back pain. *J Occup Med* 1984;**26**:877.

Macnab I: The classic: Disc degeneration and low back pain. *Clin Orthop* 1986;**208**:3.

Maurice-Williams RS: *Spinal Degenerative Disease.* John Wright & Sons, 1981.

Nachemson AL: Advances in low-back pain. *Clin Orthop* 1985;**200**:266.

Pytel JL, Kamon E: Dynamic strength test as a predictor for maximal and acceptable lifting. *Ergonomics* 1981;**24**:663.

Rowe ML: Low back pain in industry: A position paper. *J Occup Med* 1969;**11**:161.

Simmons EH: Kyphotic deformity of the spine in ankylosing spondylitis. *Clin Orthop* 1977;**128**:65.

Snook SH, Campanelli RA, Hart JW: A study of three preventive approaches to low back injury. *J Occup Med* 1978;**20**:478.

Undeutsch K et al: Back complaints and findings in transport workers performing physically heavy work. *Scand J Work Environ Health* 1982;**8(Suppl 1)**:92.

Yu TS et al: Low-back pain in industry: An old problem revisited. *J Occup Med 1984;***26**:517.

Injuries of the Hip

Amstutz HC, Kim WC: Osteoarthritis of the hip. In: *Osteoarthritis: Diagnosis and Management.* Moskowitz RW et al (editors). Saunders, 1984.

Cruess RL: Osteonecrosis of bone: Current concepts as to etiology and pathogenesis. *Clin Orthop* 1986; **208**:30.

Jaffe HL: *Metabolic, Degenerative, and Inflammatory Diseases of Bones and Joints.* Lea & Febiger, 1972.

Injuries of the Knee, Ankle, & Foot

Campbell JW, Inman VT: Treatment of plantar fasciitis and calcaneal spurs with the UC-BL shoe insert. *Clin Orthop* 1974;**103**:57.

Chrisman OD, Snook GA: Reconstruction of lateral ligament tears of the ankle: An experimental study and clinical evaluation of seven patients treated by a new modification of the Elmslie procedure. *J Bone Joint Surg [Am]* 1969;**51**:904.

Crenshaw AH (editor): *Campbell's Operative Orthopedics,* 7th ed. Mosby, 1987.

Mann RA: Interdigital neuroma. In: *Surgery of the Musculoskeletal System.* 4 vols. Evarts CM (editor). Churchill Livingstone, 1983.

Noble J: Lesions of the menisci: Autopsy incidence in adults less than fifty-five years old. *J Bone Joint Surg [Am]* 1977;**59:**480.

Noble J, Hamblen DL: The pathology of the degenerate meniscus lesion. *J Bone Joint Surg [Br]* 1975;**57:**180.

Pickett JC, Radin EL: *Chondromalacia of the Patella.* Williams & Wilkins, 1983.

Quayle JB, Robinson MP: An operation for chronic prepatellar bursitis. *J Bone Joint Surg [Am] 1973;* **55:**287.

Rockwood CA, Green DP: *Adult Fractures.* Vols 1 and 2 of: *Fractures,* 2nd ed. Lippincott, 1984.

Scott GA, Jolly BL, Henning CE: Combined posterior incision and arthroscopic intra-articular repair of the meniscus: An examination of factors affecting healing. *J Bone Joint Surg [Am]* 1986;**68:**847.

8

Facial Injuries

Thomas O. Wildes, MD

Injuries of the face occur with alarming frequency in the workplace. The severity of a facial injury is usually directly correlated with the type, direction, and energy of the injuring force. Superficial abrasions or lacerations are commonly associated with low-energy forces and are usually preventable by use of appropriate protective devices. More severe injuries are commonly associated with equipment failure or improper use of high-speed or pressurized machinery. For example, the disruption of an air compressor or high-speed saw can result in dispersion of heavy particles at high energy, and the improper use of a sandblaster can result in penetration of the skin and eyes by small particles. Chain saws and other cutting tools can cause deep lacerations if protective gear is not used or if improper technique is employed.

Not only do these occupational injuries of the face have the potential for severe deformity and disability, but major facial scars have long-lasting psychologic effects on the workers.

This chapter focuses on management of soft tissue injuries and fractures of the face. For prevention of occupational injuries, see Chapter 6.

COMPREHENSIVE EARLY MANAGEMENT OF TRAUMATIC INJURIES

Steps for the management of traumatic injuries are as follows:

(1) Stabilize the airway: The airway may be obstructed by blood, debris, loose dentures, teeth, or foreign bodies. An attempt should be made to remove these obstructions by suction or by direct instrumentation. The airway may be stabilized by positional changes if the patient is mobile (but bear in mind possible cervical spine injuries, as discussed below). In the event positional changes are not adequate, a forward thrust of the tongue, either by direct traction on the tongue or by forward traction of the symphysis or angles of the mandible, may be adequate to open the airway. If the airway cannot be satisfactorily maintained, intubation or tracheostomy may be required.

(2) Control massive hemorrhage: Massive hemorrhage is ordinarily best controlled by the application of packing or pressure. Careful clamping of bleeding vessels should be undertaken only if packing or pressure does not suffice.

(3) Rule out fracture of the cervical spine: Prior to manipulation of the head and neck, reasonable certainty of stability of the cervical spine should be ensured. The head should be stabilized with sandbags or kept in a neutral position until a cervical fracture is ruled out.

(4) Rule out or treat any major neurologic, thoracoabdominal, and orthopedic injuries after performing the above emergency procedures: The patient's overall condition must not be jeopardized by undue attention focused on maxillofacial injuries.

MANAGEMENT OF SOFT TISSUE INJURIES

Soft tissue may be damaged by blunt trauma or penetrating injury. The degree of damage is usually related to the amount of energy applied to the soft tissue and varies with the injuring instrument (an explosive, a sandblaster, etc). High-velocity, penetrating instruments frequently cause more massive soft tissue injury than is immediately apparent.

Diagnosis

A. Facial Nerve Injury: The patient may complain of difficulty in moving parts of the face. All important facial motions must be evaluated. Ask the patient to wrinkle the forehead, close the eyes tightly, smile, and purse the lips. Failure to perform any of these movements in an otherwise cooperative patient suggests transection of the nerve. The nerve should be examined throughout its entire course to determine the site of injury. A central or temporal bone injury is evaluated by CT scan. Peripheral injury in association with a laceration requires direct exploration and repair of the nerve at the site of injury.

B. Medial Canthus Injury: A laceration that involves the medial canthal area may involve the lacrimal drainage system. Integrity of the ducts must be assured by direct cannulation. Lacerations of the drainage system must be repaired and stented.

C. Parotid Duct Injury: By massaging the parotid gland, saliva can be obtained through the caruncle located opposite the second maxillary molar. Blood in the saliva flowing through this caruncle is a sign of injury to the parotid duct.

D. Eye Injury: See Chapter 9.

E. Ear Injury: See Chapter 10.

Treatment

A. Care of Lacerations: The major goal of treatment of lacerations is to convert a contaminated wound into one that is as clean as a surgical incision. Sterile technique should be used.

1. Emergency measures–As outlined above (see Comprehensive Early Management of Traumatic Injuries), hemorrhage should be arrested by pressure or by careful clamping of vessels if pressure is not adequate.

2. Anesthesia–Sensory and motor function of the nerves of the face and neck must be assessed prior to induction of local or general anesthesia. An anesthetic should be administered before the wound is cleaned. Local anesthesia is best achieved by infiltration of a solution such as 1% lidocaine with 1:100,000 epinephrine. Regional anesthesia (field blocks of specific nerves) can also be used for facial wound repairs.

3. Wound cleaning and repair–After larger foreign bodies are mechanically removed from the wound, it is irrigated with copious amounts of normal saline solution to remove occult debris and bacteria. This can be done by using a blunt needle on a large syringe (eg, a 19-gauge blunt needle on a 60-mL syringe) to forcefully irrigate the depths of the wound.

Because the blood supply to the face is excellent, only obviously necrotic tissue should be removed. The wound is sharply debrided so that macerated edges are excised, and this usually requires excision of some skin. Even a millimeter of debridement provides more viable uninjured tissue for closure. Debridement makes undermining of wound edges a prerequisite so that tissue can be advanced to achieve closure. The edges are undermined in a plane between the dermis and subcutaneous tissue to a distance of 1–2 cm horizontally from the wound edge. No attempt should be made to straighten lacerations unless the laceration can be made to lie completely within or parallel to resting skin tension lines (ie, lines that appear as the lines of aging and are ordinarily directed in a perpendicular direction to the pull of facial muscles). A jagged laceration is eventually less apparent than one that is straight but crosses resting skin tension lines. Prior to wound closure, hemostasis must be meticulous.

4. Wound closure–Subcutaneous tissues are closed with absorbable suture of a suitable size (eg, 3-0 or 4-0 chromic). The skin is closed next with a subcuticular stitch. The needle enters the dermis and exits between the epidermis and dermis on one side, and then it enters between the epidermis and dermis on the opposite side and exits the dermis on that side. The knot is then tied. This technique results in the knot being placed below the surface and therefore not protruding between the skin edges. The wound should already be precisely approximated following suture of the subcuticular layer. The cuticular layer is then sutured with 6-0 monofilament nylon to achieve final closure. There should be no tension on the wound edges, and the cuticular stitch should not be used to close defects of more than 1 mm of skin. Larger defects require placement of more subcuticular sutures to remove all tension from the edges of the skin.

5. Wound dressings and follow-up care–The wound is dressed with an antibiotic ointment, and a tetanus toxoid booster should be given if appropriate. Thereafter, the wound is cleaned 3 times daily with a saline solution or hydrogen peroxide. Antibiotic ointment or petrolatum is applied to help loosen eschars and facilitate epithelialization.

After the cuticular sutures have been in place for about 3–5 days, they are removed. Wound edges are treated with a substance that promotes adhesion (eg, tincture of benzoin), and adhesive strips (eg, Steri-Strips) are applied in a crisscross fashion to the wound edges. These strips should be replaced every 3 days for about 10 days, after which time tissue strength begins to develop as a result of maturation of collagen.

6. Delayed treatment–The delayed treatment of facial lacerations is similar. If infection occurs, sutures are removed, the wound is opened, and wet-to-dry dressings are applied. When the wound has been cleansed of all purulent material and healthy granulation tissue is present, the above steps are used to reclose the wound.

B. Care of Abrasions: Abrasive injuries cause partial-thickness to full-thickness loss of the epidermis. A full-thickness loss of skin results in an anesthetic area similar to that of a third-degree burn.

1. Anesthesia–Anesthesia of a large abraded area can be achieved by local infiltration of an anesthetic solution such as lidocaine with epinephrine, by topical application of an anesthetic gel such as 4% lidocaine jelly, or by field block of specific nerves.

2. Wound cleaning and repair–The wound is cleaned by irrigation. Scrubbing with a soft scrub brush may be required to remove small embedded particles, but scrubbing should be undertaken carefully to avoid causing further injury. Small areas of avulsion (< 3 cm in diameter) can usually be treated by advancement of adjacent tissue or rotation or advancement of local flaps. Larger areas of avulsion require skin grafting.

3. Wound dressings and follow-up care–Partial-thickness abrasions are covered with antibiotic ointment and cleaned 2–3 times daily. For wounds covered with a semiocclusive dressing, the dressing is changed as recommended by the manufacturer of the dressing. No treatment is needed for pigmentary changes that occasionally occur after injury, since the pigment usually reverts to normal within 6–12 months.

C. Care of Skin Penetrated by Foreign Bodies: Foreign bodies that have penetrated the skin (eg, asphalt from a road burn or sand particles from a sandblast injury) must be removed or they will result in a permanent tattoo.

1. Wound cleaning and repair–Sparsely placed

foreign bodies can usually be removed mechanically with a fine forceps. Magnification provided by a loupe or microscope is frequently necessary to achieve adequate removal. Diffusely placed foreign bodies (eg, sand particles) may require removal by dermabrasion, which should be continued only to the depth necessary to remove the particles without causing a full-thickness injury. It is sometimes preferable to perform dermabrasion in a symmetric fashion so that the resulting pattern will be less noticeable.

2. Wound dressings and follow-up care—Care of these injuries following their repair is the same as care of partial-thickness abrasions (see above).

D. Care of Scarred Facial Tissue: Scarring that results from facial injuries may require secondary revision. It is usually best to delay reconstructive measures (eg, Z-plasty, running W-plasty, and geometric broken-line closures) until the scar revision stage of treatment. Scar revisions can be done if necessary after the signs of acute inflammation have resolved (ie, edema and erythema), usually 6–12 months after injury.

MANAGEMENT OF FACIAL FRACTURES

Most facial fractures can be diagnosed on the basis of physical symptoms and signs alone. A hematoma points to a specific site of injury. Facial deformities secondary to depression of facial bone structures are a sign of fracture, and impairment of sensory and motor functions of adjacent nerve structures may also signify a fracture.

General examination should include the following: assessment of facial symmetry and extraocular motility; palpation of the orbital rims, frontozygomatic areas, zygomatic arches, and mandible; determination of the stability and configuration of the nasal dorsum; and evaluation of the 3 major cutaneous branches of the trigeminal nerve, particularly the infraorbital branch.

1. NASAL FRACTURES

The nose is the most commonly fractured structure in the facial skeleton.

Clinical Findings

Epistaxis may be present following injury. The nasal dorsum is obviously deviated to one side or collapsed, and crepitation may be noted. Inspection of the nasal vault shows an impaired airway on one side of the nasal septum, and there may be a septal hematoma. A convexity on one side of the septum should be opposed by a corresponding concavity on the other side. Symmetric convexities that are bluish in color and slightly soft suggest septal hematoma.

Lateral soft tissue x-rays will usually confirm the diagnosis of nasal fracture.

Treatment & Prognosis

Septal hematomas require immediate treatment to prevent infection and secondary necrosis of the septal cartilage, which can result in a saddlenose deformity. Treatment consists of draining the hematoma and using nasal packing to reapproximate the septal mucosa to the septal cartilage. Phenoxymethyl penicillin is usually prescribed as prophylaxis.

Nondisplaced nasal fractures do not require treatment, but a small splint may be helpful for comfort.

Displaced nasal fractures are treated by closed reduction. Some surgeons prefer to wait until swelling has subsided, since they feel that more precise realignment of the nasal dorsum can be achieved at that time. However, performing closed reduction as soon as possible rehabilitates the patient more rapidly and is likely to produce better results, since healing in the displaced position has not begun.

Dislocation of the nasal septum may not be correctable by closed reduction. Immediate or delayed septoplasty may be required to reestablish an adequate nasal airway.

A 7- to 10-day period of disability is expected after reduction of a nasal fracture. A nasal splint is worn for approximately 7 days. Pressure or further injury to the nose must be avoided for at least 3 months following a nasal fracture.

2. MANDIBULAR FRACTURES

Mandibular fractures usually occur from direct trauma to the jaw. The most common site of fracture is the region of the condylar process (Fig 8–1).

Clinical Findings

Malocclusion is the cardinal sign of a mandibular fracture, and multiple fractures are frequently seen. Displacement of fracture fragments results from the pull of the muscles of mastication.

In addition to malocclusion, symptoms and signs may include pain, step-off deformity or instability of the dental arch, hypoesthesia of the mental nerve, foul-smelling breath, trismus or deviation of the jaw on opening, hematoma, and laceration of the oral mucosa. Particular attention should be paid to the patient's dentition. Fractured, chipped, or loosened teeth should be noted. Any avulsed teeth should be located, since they might have been aspirated. Chest x-ray should be done if the teeth cannot be found immediately.

The following facial x-rays should be obtained to confirm the diagnosis of mandibular fracture: right and left oblique views, posteroanterior views of the mandibular symphysis and rami, and modified Towne views in a plane that is parallel to the skull and demonstrates both condyles.

Treatment & Prognosis

If bilateral fractures of the mandibular body cause posterior displacement of the mandible and occlusion

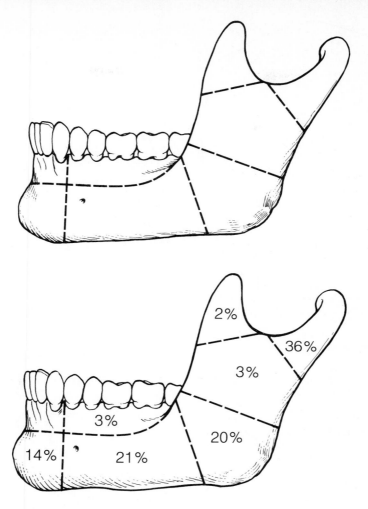

Figure 8–1. Regions of the mandible, showing fracture sites by frequency of involvement. (Redrawn and reproduced, with permission, from Dingman RD, Natvig P: *Surgery of Facial Fractures.* Saunders, 1964.)

of the airway, anterior traction of the angles of the mandible or the tongue may be required to restore an adequate airway. Blood may obstruct the airway and should be removed by suction.

Definitive treatment of mandibular fractures usually consists of intermaxillary fixation for 3–6 weeks, but alternative techniques that utilize compression plating may eliminate the need for fixation in some cases. Open reduction is sometimes required when the muscles of mastication cause diastasis at the fracture site or when a combination of the pull of masticatory muscles and intermaxillary traction causes displacement of the fracture.

Chipped teeth require temporary coverage of pulp and dentin at the time of fracture therapy. Definitive repair of damaged teeth can be done later. Avulsed teeth should be replanted within the first 2 hours of avulsion. They can be stabilized to adjacent teeth during the period of intermaxillary fixation to allow them to heal.

The prognosis for return to function of the mandible following proper treatment is excellent. Subcondylar fractures that remain displaced may cause temporomandibular joint pain on chewing and ultimately result in abnormal mobility of the joint. The period of disability after mandibular fractures is usually 3–6 weeks. If intermaxillary fixation is used, it is maintained for 6 weeks. Return to active heavy labor may not be for 6–8 weeks. If rigid internal fixation techniques are used, return to active heavy labor can be earlier (eg, 4–6 weeks). Return to work times requires individualization based upon the type of injury, the type of repair, the job description, and associated injuries.

3. MAXILLARY (LE FORT) FRACTURES

Maxillary fractures are classified as Le Fort I, II, and III fractures (Fig 8–2). A Le Fort I fracture is a

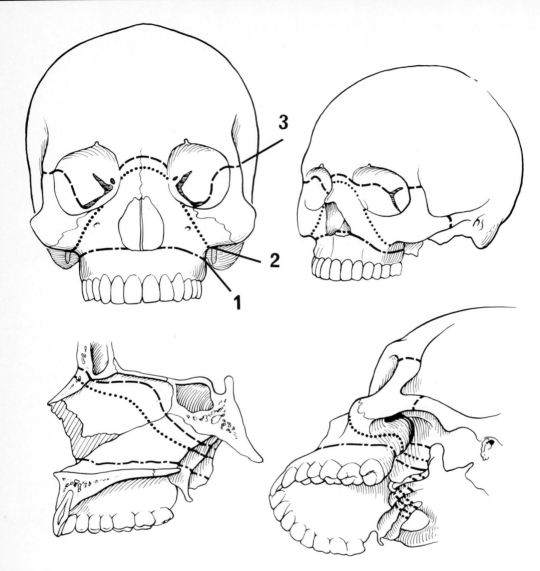

Figure 8–2. Fractures of the maxilla. The numbers 1, 2, and 3 indicate Le Fort I, II, and III fractures, respectively. (Redrawn and reproduced, with permission, from Dingman RD, Natvig P: *Surgery of Facial Fractures.* Saunders, 1964.)

horizontal fracture of the palate and does not involve the orbits. A Le Fort II fracture traverses the infraorbital rim, the orbital floor, the medial wall of the orbit, and the perpendicular plate of the ethmoid bone. A Le Fort III fracture has the characteristics of a Le Fort II fracture with the addition of a zygomatic fracture and is known as craniofacial disjunction.

Clinical Findings

In patients with maxillary fractures, the mid face is displaced posteriorly and inferiorly. This results in malocclusion with the molar teeth meeting prematurely but the incisor teeth meeting with an open bite (apertognathia). The entire mid face appears to be flattened, and there may be epistaxis along with facial

pain. The level of mobility in the mid face depends on the type of fracture. To test for mobility, the forehead is stabilized by the palm of one hand, and the opposite thumb and forefinger are used to grasp the incisor teeth or palate. An attempt is then made to move the palate. In Le Fort I fractures, only the palate is mobile. In Le Fort II and III fractures, findings may include mobility of the nasal dorsum, hypoesthesia of the infraorbital nerve, an associated nasal fracture, and cerebrospinal fluid rhinorrhea resulting from associated fracture of the cribriform plate.

Standard Waters and Caldwell x-ray views of the face should be obtained. Demonstration of fractures through the walls of the maxillary sinuses and orbital rims usually allows for accurate diagnosis. CT scans are usually done to define the exact nature of the injury and to accurately assess the injury of the orbital floor.

Treatment & Prognosis

Adequate cleansing of the upper airways to allow respiration is important. Stabilization of the airway by nasal intubation should be avoided, since intubation may cause further damage to the skull base if it has been fractured. In cases involving a significant nasal fracture, tracheostomy may be required to provide a secure airway. Uncontrolled bleeding is best treated by packing. If packing does not control bleeding, an emergency reduction of the fractures usually does.

Definitive treatment consists of mobilizing the fractured segments and placing them in their anatomic positions. Normal occlusion is obtained by intermaxillary fixation. Fractures at the orbital rim and frontozygomatic areas are treated by direct interosseous wiring. To preclude lengthening of the mid face, the mid face is suspended from the lowest stable portion of the face, which is usually the frontozygomatic suture area. Maxillary fractures complicated by an associated mandibular fracture may require maxillofacial traction with an external headframe appliance. Techniques of rigid internal fixation can be used to obviate the need for intermaxillary fixation and to provide more secure fixation.

Intermaxillary fixation and suspension wires—if used—remain in place for 4–6 weeks. A tracheostomy may be maintained during this entire time if significant obstruction of the nasal airways is caused by packing. A further period of rehabilitation of 1–2 months following maxillofacial injuries is usually necessary. Associated injuries commonly require more prolonged rehabilitation.

4. ZYGOMATIC FRACTURES

The malar eminences provide projection of the cheeks. In a fracture of the zygoma (Fig 8–3), the entire bone is dislocated posteriorly, inferiorly, and medially. The prominence of the zygoma is thus lost, and this will result in an unsightly deformity if allowed to heal without reduction.

Clinical Findings

Symptoms and signs include pain over the malar area; hypoesthesia of the infraorbital nerve; step-off deformity of the infraorbital rim; lateral subconjunctival hemorrhage; downward slant of the palpebral fissure, which is due to inferior displacement of the attachment of the lateral tendon of the canthus; limited extraocular motility; hematoma or crepitation in the gingivobuccal sulcus; and flattening of the malar eminence. Occasionally, fracture of the orbital

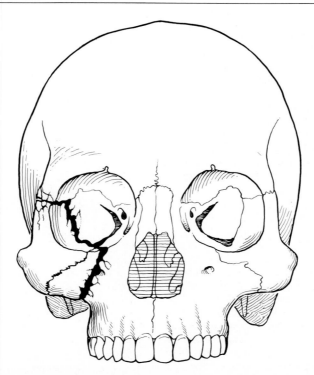

Figure 8–3. Zygomatic compound fracture. (Redrawn and reproduced, with permission, from Dingman RD, Natvig P: *Surgery of Facial Fractures.* Saunders, 1964.)

floor causes entrapment of the inferior rectus muscle, and this results in diplopia on upward gaze. Muscle contusion or neuropraxia of the third cranial nerve can also result in diplopia. In some cases, the eye is displaced backward or recessed in the orbit (enophthalmos) as a result of a relative increase in the volume of the orbit. The zygomatic arch may be displaced medially and impinge on the coronoid process, which can result in trismus or inadequate closure of the jaw.

Standard Caldwell, Waters, submentovertex, and lateral x-ray views should be obtained. A Waters view will usually show infraorbital rim fractures and frontozygomatic suture separations, and it may also show fractures of the lateral maxillary sinus walls. An underpenetrated submentovertex ("bucket-handle") view will demonstrate a fracture of the zygomatic arch. A CT scan of the mid face should be obtained. Direct coronal scans or coronal reconstructions are obtained to assess the integrity of the orbital floor. The integrity of the orbital floor cannot be adequately assessed on the basis of routine x-rays.

Treatment & Prognosis

Emergency treatment of zygomatic fractures is usually not required. Although zygomatic fractures that are minimally displaced require no treatment, those that are more severely displaced should be treated by open reduction. Incisions are usually made at the infraorbital rim and frontozygomatic area. The zygoma is placed in its normal position, and interosseous wires are used to maintain reduction. Instability may require a Caldwell-Luc operation with packing of the maxillary sinus to maintain the normal position of the zygoma.

The orbital floor must also be carefully evaluated, and significant fractures should be treated by bone or cartilage grafting to prevent subsequent enophthalmos or globe ptosis.

The prognosis for return to full function after a zygoma fracture is excellent. Swelling has usually resolved by 2 weeks after the injury. Light work can be resumed at that time. Heavy labor is best delayed until 4 weeks after repair. The malar area should be protected from possible recurrent injury for 3 months after repair.

5. ORBITAL FLOOR ("BLOWOUT") FRACTURES

Clinical Findings

In orbital floor fractures, entrapment of the inferior rectus muscle causes diplopia and fixation of the globe when the patient attempts to look upward. If there is significant displacement of the orbital floor into the maxillary sinus (Fig 8–4), enophthalmos may result. The Waters x-ray usually demonstrates an orbital floor fracture. Disruption of the orbital floor can be seen. The orbital rim remains intact. A teardrop deformity may appear beneath the orbital floor resulting from herniation of the orbital contents

into the maxillary sinus below or hematoma formation in the mucosa of the sinus roof. A CT scan is necessary to determine the exact extent of injury.

Treatment & Prognosis

Surgical reconstruction of the orbital floor is required for entrapment of extraocular muscles or enophthalmos or globe ptosis due to the size of the orbital floor defect. In questionable cases, repair is delayed 10–14 days in order to obtain a more accurate assessment of the degree of deformity or impairment of function.

Measures to explore and treat blowout fractures consist of elevating the orbital floor and inserting an autogenous graft or packing the antrum in an effort to reposition the floor.

If intermaxillary fixation is required, a liquid diet must be followed for about 6 weeks. It is difficult to perform significant physical labor during this time period owing to the inability to open and close the jaws. It is also difficult to sustain an adequate caloric intake, and weight loss is common. If rigid internal fixation techniques are used, an earlier return to work can be anticipated and a normal diet can usually be resumed by the third week. Periods of disability must again be individualized.

6. NASOETHMOIDAL COMPLEX FRACTURES

Clinical Findings

The entire nasal complex can be displaced poste-

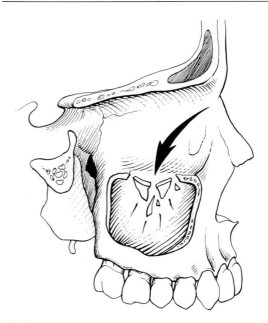

Figure 8–4. Depressed fracture of the orbital floor with displacement into the maxillary sinus. (Redrawn and reproduced, with permission, from Dingman RD, Natvig P: *Surgery of Facial Fractures.* Saunders, 1964.)

riorly, causing collapse of the nasal bones into the ethmoidal sinuses. There may be an associated fracture of the cribriform plate.

Common symptoms and signs of nasoethmoidal complex fractures include facial pain, anosmia, watery rhinorrhea, flattening of the nasal dorsum, widening of the medial canthal area, and downward, lateral, and anterior displacement of the canthus. A torn cribriform plate can cause cerebrospinal fluid rhinorrhea. Disruption of the medial canthal area, with failure of apposition of the inferior lacrimal caruncle to the glove, may result in epiphora (the uncontrolled flow of tears).

A CT scan of the nasal area is the most definitive diagnostic imaging procedure. Waters and Caldwell x-ray views of the area will demonstrate associated fractures.

Treatment & Prognosis

Emergency reduction of nasoethmoidal complex fractures is only necessary in the event of uncontrolled bleeding or persistent cerebrospinal fluid rhinorrhea. Otherwise, treatment may be delayed until 7–10 days after injury; this will allow adequate resolution of edema so that the medial canthal area can be restored to its normal position. Direct wiring of the nasal and lacrimal bones is necessary. Nasal packing may also be required to maintain the normal position of the nasal bones.

The prognosis for return to normal function after nasoethmoidal fractures is excellent. A significant number of patients have persistent slight widening of the intercanthal distance which, however, is not usually functionally significant. The period of disability is usually 6–8 weeks and is often not as long as the disability from associated injuries.

7. FRONTAL SINUS FRACTURES

Clinical Findings

A contusion or laceration over the glabella may be the sign of an underlying fracture of the frontal sinus. Other symptoms and signs include pain, cerebrospinal fluid rhinorrhea or bloody rhinorrhea, and flattening of the glabella.

Caldwell x-ray views usually reveal fractures of the frontal sinus, but CT scans are essential for the diagnosis of fractures of the posterior sinus wall.

Treatment & Prognosis

Emergency therapy is not ordinarily required. In some cases, open reduction may be needed to restore fractured segments to their normal positions. If the fracture is severe, the entire sinus may be removed and the frontonasal ducts plugged.

The period of recuperation after treatment of frontal sinus fractures is usually 4–6 weeks. The period of disability is again usually more related to associated injuries than the facial injury.

Long-term follow-up studies indicate that a mucocele can form many years following injury and may present as a brain abscess or as a mass with erosion of the frontal bones. Secondary treatment of these complications is usually accomplished by obliteration of the frontal sinuses with fat.

REFERENCES

Cook TA: *Basic Soft Tissue Surgery.* Academy of Facial Plastic and Reconstructive Surgery, 1982.

Dingman RO, Natvig P: *Surgery of Facial Fractures.* Saunders, 1964.

Kassell EE: Traumatic injuries of the paranasal sinuses. In: Valvassori GE, Mafee MF (editors): Diagnostic imaging in otolaryngology. *Otolaryngol Clin North Am* 1988; **21:**455.

Kellman RM (editor): Facial plating. *Otolaryngol Clin North Am* 1987;**21:**425.

Maniglia AJ (editor): Trauma to the head and neck. *Otolaryngol Clin North Am* 1983;**16:**471. [Entire issue.]

Mathog RH: *Maxillofacial Trauma.* Williams & Wilkins, 1983.

Prendergast ML, Wildes TO: Evaluation of the orbital floor in zygoma fractures. *Arch Otolaryngol Head Neck Surg* 1988;**114:**446.

Wildes TO: Maxillofacial trauma and surgical repair. (Part 1.) *Hosp Phys* (April) 1988;**24:**18.

Wildes TO: Maxillofacial trauma and surgical repair. (Part 2.) *Hosp Phys* (May) 1988;**24:**27.

9

Eye Injuries

Ernest K. Goodner, MD

The personal tragedy and economic loss associated with impaired vision or even blindness due to occupational eye injuries can be prevented by identifying workers at risk and instituting appropriate safety programs. Proper maintenance of tools and equipment by the employer and effective use of protective devices such as safety glasses or face shields by the employee will reduce the number of injuries such as ocular contusions, trauma due to penetrating and nonpenetrating foreign bodies, conjunctival and corneal abrasions, lid lacerations, and optic nerve damage.

Recognition of the toxic effects of chemical agents and protection from those that may be splashed into the eyes are vital for prevention of visual damage. The ready availability of facilities for cleansing and irrigation of the face and eyes in the workplace is of the utmost importance, since initial steps for treatment of chemical burns—especially those due to strong alkalis and acids—must be carried out immediately by the employee, fellow workers, or anyone else near at hand. There is no time to wait for specialized medical care, so employee education programs for emergency care of chemical burns are essential.

The risks of ocular damage for x-ray technicians, glassblowers, welders, and other workers exposed to ionizing, infrared, and ultraviolet radiation have long been known, but damage due to exposure to excessive amounts of visible light has only recently been recognized. Wearing protective lenses that filter the most offending wavelengths of visible light may become commonplace in the future.

Anatomy & Physiology
(Fig 9–1)

A brief review of ocular anatomy and function will be helpful in understanding the mechanisms of several kinds of eye injuries and how they affect the visual system.

The orbit, eyelid, and conjunctiva are protective mechanisms for the eye. The **orbit** and its bony rim offer excellent mechanical protection from injuries with the exception of those coming from the direct anterior or temporal directions. The **eyelid** and **conjunctiva** are essential for normal maintenance of the smooth, moist, clear anterior surface of the **cornea,** which in turn is essential for clear vision. The normal blinking mechanism depends on the third cranial nerve to open the lids and the seventh to close them.

Moistening of the conjunctiva by lacrimal fluid depends in part on activation of the reflex arc between the sensory fifth innervation of the anterior eye and the parasympathetic secretomotor fibers that accompany the seventh cranial nerve along the petrous temporal bone into the middle fossa and thence to the orbit. Moistening of the **corneal epithelium** is aided by mucus from the goblet cells of the conjunctiva, particularly those on the tarsus of the upper lid. Reflex tear production by the **lacrimal gland** helps dilute and wash away irritating substances that find their way into the conjunctival sac. The rich blood supply of the conjunctiva and lid also helps in resisting and limiting infections of the anterior eye.

Internal structures of the eye can be conveniently divided into anterior and posterior segments. The **anterior segment** includes the cornea, anterior chamber, iris, lens, and ciliary body. These structures comprise the essential optical elements of the eye. The regular pattern of the collagen fibers and posterior endothelial layer of the **cornea** maintain its optical clarity. Since the cornea and **lens** are avascular, they require a specialized source of nutrition, which is provided by aqueous humor. The **ciliary body** produces aqueous humor at a nearly constant rate, bathing the lens and posterior surface of the cornea and then draining near the base of the cornea through the structures associated with Schlemm's canal. A normal rate of production and drainage of aqueous humor maintains the intraocular pressure between 10 and 21 mm Hg. Injuries causing elevation of the pressure can lead to significant loss of vision. The **iris** and its **pupil** adjust the amount of light entering the eye, thereby allowing for accommodation (adjustment of focusing for seeing at different distances).

The **posterior segment** of the eye is the light-sensing portion of the visual system and contains the **retina** and its supporting vascular layer, the **choroid.** The retina has over 1 million nerve fibers that arise from the ganglion cells and collect in the optic disk to form the **optic nerve,** which transmits visual information to the posterior visual system. These nerve fibers are second-order neurons similar to the myelinated sensory tracts of the spinal cord and are not capable of healing with restoration of visual function following injuries such as penetrating wounds of the orbit or posterior orbit fractures involving the optic canal. Depending on the nature of the injury, the fibers may disappear completely (as in the case of

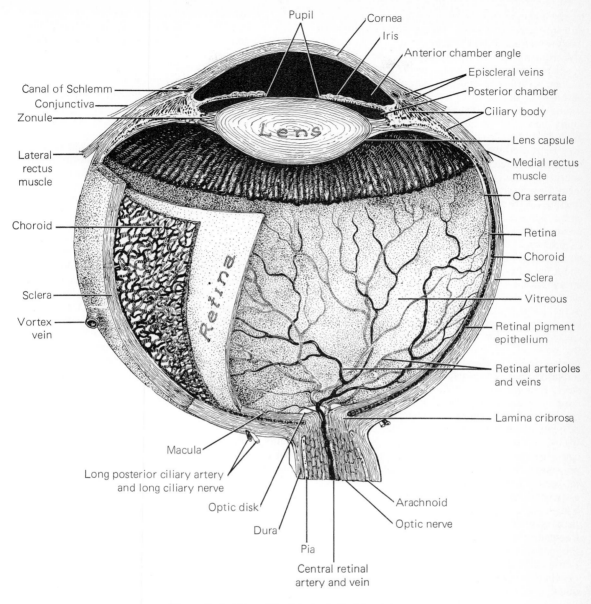

Figure 9–1. View of the inferior half of the right eye.

glaucomatous atrophy of the optic disk) or be replaced with scar tissue (as occurs following acute inflammation such as optic neuritis). The optic chiasm, optic tracts, and visual radiations to the cortex usually are not involved directly in eye injuries except those involving the bones of the head and the intracranial structures.

Visual acuity depends on the optical clarity of the cornea, lens, and vitreous and proper functioning of the **fovea,** which is the avascular center of the retinal **macula** and is composed entirely of specialized cones that are color-sensitive and capable of resolving the finest images. If this small area (< 0.5 mm in diameter) is damaged, no adjacent portion of the retina is capable of assuming the fine function that provides maximum visual acuity.

Eye injuries causing retinal detachment or vitreous hemorrhage can lead to loss of peripheral vision, and injuries of the extraocular muscles or their nerves can produce diplopia (''double vision'').

History & Eye Examination

Caution: For chemical burns (see page 84), emergency treatment should be started immediately, and the history and examination of the patient can proceed in due course. In cases of suspected ruptured or lacerated globe (see below), care must be taken to prevent further damage to the eye during transport to the hospital and initial evaluation.

A. History: As outlined in Table 2–1 and discussed in Chapter 2, the occupational medical history should include a variety of questions not always considered pertinent to general histories. In addition, the worker should be asked about vision before and after the injury and whether any visual loss was sudden or gradual. Sudden loss of vision without obvious injury may be caused by central retinal artery occlusion or ischemic damage to the optic nerve due to giant cell arteritis. These problems require emergency treatment. Progressive loss of vision following facial bone fractures or head injuries is sometimes due to optic nerve damage, which may respond to surgery if recognized in time.

In cases of mechanical injury, the worker should be asked about previous tetanus inoculations and about the nature of the forces involved. Was the eye struck with a small, rapidly moving object that may have penetrated the globe, as sometimes occurs when a steel hammer strikes a steel tool? Or was the eye hit by a large, slowly moving object that may have caused a contusion injury or rupture of the globe? If the presence of a foreign body is suspected, the worker should be asked about the type of material that might be involved (a magnetic metal such as iron or steel, a nonmagnetic metal such as aluminum or copper, or an organic material such as wood), since this information is helpful for determining the method of treatment and for prognosis. Soluble metallic salts from iron- or copper-containing foreign bodies can cause irreversible toxic damage to the retina, best prevented by their prompt removal. Less soluble materials such as aluminum, plastic, or glass are associated with a better prognosis. Organic foreign bodies such as pieces of wood or splinters of plant material may introduce an intraocular infection that is frequently difficult to treat and has a very poor prognosis.

If a chemical burn is present or suspected, the type of chemical (alkali or acid) will influence how quickly and deeply it penetrates the eye. If eye injuries are thought to be due to long-term exposure to chemicals, the various substances to which the worker is exposed should be identified and a material safety data sheet (MSDS) obtained for each, as described in Chapter 2. The worker should also be asked about exposure to aerosols, surfactants, detergents, dust, and smoke, which can damage the corneal epithelium.

B. Examination: Even if an injury is thought to have affected only one eye, both eyes should be carefully examined. If swelling prevents easy opening of the eyes for inspection, a sterile topical anesthetic can be instilled through nearly closed eyelids by applying the drops along the lid fissure. After a few minutes, smooth sterile retractors may be carefully used to lift the lids for eye examination.

1. External eye examination–

a. Eyelids–Note symmetry of the lids of both eyes. Look for lacerations that cross the lid margins and for perforating wounds through the skin of the lid above or below the lid margin. Except in the case of a suspected ruptured or lacerated globe, the lid can be everted to search for foreign bodies on the upper tarsus. To evert the lid, the patient is asked to look down while the physician pulls gently on the lashes and applies mild pressure on the upper surface of the lid.

b. Orbits–Palpate the orbital rims, and note discontinuities and crepitus due to subcutaneous air from fractures of the paranasal sinuses. In orbital fractures, injury to the inferior or superior orbital nerves as they pass through the floor or roof of the orbit can cause decreased sensibility of the lids and face.

c. Conjunctiva–To examine the conjunctiva, evert the lids by applying gentle pressure over the superior orbital rim of the upper lid or over the malar eminence of the lower lid, thereby avoiding direct pressure on the globe. Look for foreign bodies, hemorrhage, laceration, and inflammation.

d. Corneas–With a bright light, look at the light reflection on the normally smooth corneal surface. Irregularities indicate disruptions of the corneal epithelium. Because the cornea is normally clear and lustrous, the surface texture of the iris is easily and clearly seen. A corneal wound with incarceration of the iris may also be indicated by asymmetry of the pupil. A fluorescein paper strip moistened with sterile saline or a topical anesthetic can be used to stain the tears on the surface of the cornea. The stain diffuses into any area of disrupted epithelium and stains it bright green. The color is enhanced with a blue light. Details of the cornea and the anterior eye are much more easily examined with magnification such as a 2- to 4-power loupe or (and preferably) with a slit lamp and microscope if one is available.

e. Anterior chambers–The anterior chambers should appear deep and clear. Hyphema (hemorrhage into the anterior chamber) is almost always a sign of significant injury. Hypopyon (purulent material in the anterior chamber) is characterized by a white or gray layer of inflammatory cells at the chamber bottom.

f. Pupils–The pupils should appear round, black, and equal in size. Pupillary reactions to light should be carefully noted. Normally, both pupils constrict and dilate equally and simultaneously when one pupil is stimulated by light. While the illuminated pupil is demonstrating the direct light response, the unilluminated pupil is showing the consensual light response. The direct light responses of the 2 eyes can be compared by moving a flashlight back and forth between the eyes and pausing a few seconds at each eye to observe the pupil. Normally, each pupil constricts when illuminated; failure of one of the pupils to constrict but to dilate instead indicates the presence of an afferent pupillary defect (Marcus Gunn pupil), which may be due to an optic nerve injury or extensive retinal damage on that side.

2. Test of ocular motility–If there are no severe

eye injuries, the ocular movements may be safely tested by comparing the excursions in all directions to make sure that they are the same in both eyes. Limitation of upward or downward gaze occurs frequently in orbital floor fractures and may be the result of accompanying edema or mechanical restriction of the ocular muscles. It can also result from direct trauma to a muscle when a penetrating injury of the orbit occurs.

3. Ophthalmoscopic examination–

a. Red reflex–A direct ophthalmoscope with a good bright light is used to observe the red reflex (the red glow reflected on the fundus). Examination should take place in a darkened room with the instrument set at 0 or +1, and the eyes should be observed at a distance of 30–60 cm (1–2 ft) so that the reflex in both of them can be seen at the same time and compared. An opacity in the cornea, anterior chamber, lens, or vitreous or a gross change in the color of the retina will appear as a dark form against a red background.

b. Optic disks–The examiner should be as close to the patient as possible to maximize the relative size of the pupil. The optic disks should be examined for the presence of papilledema (choked disk). Optic disks are usually well-vascularized and have a good pink color. When nerve fibers in the optic nerve die as the result of various injuries, the blood supply to the disks decreases in proportion to the loss of fibers. The disk will show a faint pallor if only a few fibers are missing, or it may appear completely white as a result of optic atrophy following total destruction of the nerve.

c. Optic cups–The width of each optic cup is usually one-third or less of the diameter of the whole optic disk. If it is as large as half the diameter, there is an increased risk for glaucoma. Therefore, measuring the cup size is useful for screening patients for glaucoma.

d. Retinal vessels–The vessels should be examined along the upper and lower arcades proceeding from the optic disk, and the presence of hemorrhages, exudates, and other alterations in the appearance of the retina should be noted.

e. Maculas and foveas–Each macula should be checked for alterations in its usual relatively featureless appearance. Its center, the fovea, can always be located 2n disk diameters temporal to the optic disk. Its concave center usually shows a small, bright foveal light reflex.

4. Measurement of intraocular pressure–If a lacerated or ruptured globe is suspected, intraocular pressure should not be measured. In other injuries, pressure can be measured with a Schiotz tonometer or with an applanation tonometer if one is available on a slit lamp. If a tonometer is not available, a general impression of extremely high or low intraocular pressure can be obtained by gently palpating each globe in turn with one finger of each hand through the closed upper eyelid. Comparison of the firmness of the 2 eyes is occasionally useful when the intraocular

pressure is extremely high, as in angle-closure glaucoma.

5. Test of visual acuity–Visual acuity should always be tested and the results recorded before treatment is instituted. This is important both from the point of view of good care and for medicolegal reasons, since patients do not always remember the amount of visual loss that occurred at the time of a severe injury. Visual acuity should be measured with a Snellen chart if possible or with a near-acuity card and recorded appropriately. If a near-acuity card is used, it is important to record the distance at which the measurements were made and whether they were made with or without the patient's glasses. If visual acuity is poor and a refractive error is suspected, the chart or card should be read through a pinhole to substitute for corrective lenses; an improvement in acuity will confirm the presence of a refractive error. If acuity is less than 20/200, the greatest distance at which fingers can be counted should be noted for each eye. If the patient cannot see the fingers well enough to count them, the greatest distance at which hand movements can be seen should be recorded. If vision is poorer than this, light perception can be tested with a bright flashlight held as close to the eye as possible, and the ability to perceive light in each of the 4 quadrants is recorded. If there is no light perception, it should be recorded as such.

There are 2 techniques for objectively estimating visual acuity—optokinetic nystagmus and visual evoked response—that may be useful in certain situations, particularly when the patient is unable or unwilling to respond to the usual subjective measures of visual acuity.

Optokinetic nystagmus is a visually stimulated response to relatively large targets. These eye movements are observed in the intact visual system by passing an alternating series of dark and light stripes of equal width before the patient's eyes. Involuntary nystagmus is produced—slow following movement in the direction of movement of the stripes alternating with a quick recovery movement. The stimulus is usually presented as a series of vertical stripes 1–2 cm in width on a handheld drum 10–15 cm in diameter. The drum is held 20–30 cm from the patient and turned slowly while observing the patient's eyes to see the induced nystagmus. The stripes can also be presented on a 50-cm long cloth strip with the stripes running across the 10- to 12-cm width. Normally, the nystagmus can be induced in any direction, and its rate will vary with the speed of the stimulus.

The **visually evoked response** is an electroencephalographic recording over the visual cortex (occipital lobe) in response to visual stimuli. The stimulus can be a simple light flash giving an on-off response, or an estimate of visual acuity can be made by presenting an alternating pattern of dark and light squares in a checkerboard pattern on a television screen. The squares can be made progressively smaller until the response is no longer recorded and the size of the smallest squares eliciting a cortical recording can be related to standard visual acuity measurements. The responses are involuntary and cannot be controlled by the subject; acuity measurements in the range of 20/400 to 20/20 have been recorded even in infants under 1 year of age. This technique is usually available through neuro-ophthalmologic or neurologic consultation. It can be particularly valuable when evaluating patients with compensation or forensic problems.

6. Test of visual fields–Visual fields should be tested, especially in patients with suspected head injury or a significant decrease in visual acuity. Each eye is tested separately by confrontation. The patient is asked to look at the examiner's eye while the examiner's hand moves toward the center of the visual field. The point at which the patient can accurately count fingers in each of the 4 quadrants is determined, and the results in the 2 eyes are carefully compared.

7. Tests for malingering–When a patient claims poor vision or blindness in one or both eyes, the presence of normal pupillary light responses (in the absence of an afferent pupillary defect) objectively demonstrates a functioning retina and optic nerve in each eye. The following tests will frequently help reveal the presence of normal fusion.

a. Utilizing the refractor, place a strong convex lens in front of the good eye and a weak convex lens in front of the "blind" eye. If the patient reads small letters on the test chart, the eye under consideration is not blind. This test can be more subtly done with the refractor than with the trial frame, since the strong convex lens is not visible to the patient when the refractor is used.

b. Place a 1-diopter base-out prism in front of the "blind" eye. If there is sight in the eye, diplopia will result and the eye will be seen to move inward to correct the diplopia.

c. Place a pair of red-green glasses on the patient, with the red lens in front of the right eye and the green lens in front of the left eye. If the left eye is the suspected eye and the patient can read the green letters with this eye, the eye is not blind; the green letters will not be transmitted through the lens in front of the right eye.

CHEMICAL BURNS OF THE EYE

Etiology & Pathogenesis

Strong alkalis and acids cause the most severe and damaging chemical injuries that can be sustained by the eye. Alkali burns are commonly due to sodium and potassium hydroxide used as cleaning agents, to calcium hydroxide used in mason's mortar and plaster, and to anhydrous ammonia used in fertilizer. Battery acids and the strong acids used to clean metal in the electroplating industry are also common causes of severe eye injury.

Alkalis affect the lipid in cell membranes and thereby reduce the normal barriers to diffusion. This allows the chemical to rapidly penetrate the interior of the eye. Because alkalis are not quickly neutralized by tissue, their destructive action can continue for hours if they are not diluted and removed immediately by irrigation of the eye. In contrast, acids tend to be fixed by protein in tissues, and this neutralizes them in a relatively shorter period of time and keeps them from penetrating as deeply.

The corneal endothelium, which is essential to the normal function and survival of the cornea, is particularly vulnerable to chemical insult. There is often severe damage within the anterior chamber, including the aqueous outflow pathways, and this can lead to glaucoma. Obliteration of the blood vessels of the conjunctiva and sclera can cause severe ischemia of the anterior eye, including the periphery of the cornea and the underlying ciliary body and iris.

Clinical Findings

The skin on the face and eyelids shows edema and erythema, sometimes with sloughing of the surface. Eye examination may require use of a topical anesthetic, depending on whether pain is noted or nerve damage is severe enough to cause anesthesia. The conjunctiva may be mildly hyperemic, show small hemorrhages, or be blanched and have the appearance of white marble (Fig 9–2). Testing the pH of the conjunctival surface with indicator paper will help confirm the cause of the injury. The severity of injury (Table 9–1) is usually judged by the degree of corneal opacity, using the normal clarity of the pupil as a guide. The cornea may appear gray or cloudy because of epithelial and stromal edema. If the cornea is not cloudy, the anterior chamber can be clearly seen. In some cases, the iris and pupil appear hazy and indistinct. Visual acuity is decreased in proportion to the severity of corneal damage.

Injuries of the nasopharynx and upper respiratory passages are frequently found in association with aspiration of the chemical irritant.

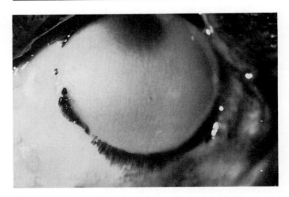

Figure 9–2. Severe alkali burn. The cornea is opaque, with the exception of a small dark area of corneal epithelium protected by the upper lid. The conjunctiva and sclera are blanched and ischemic.

Table 9–1. Classification of chemical burns of the eye.[1]

Classification	Clinical Findings
Mild	Erosion of the corneal epithelium. Faint haziness of the cornea. No ischemic necrosis of the conjunctiva or sclera.
Moderate	Corneal opacity blurring details of the iris. Minimal ischemic necrosis of the conjunctiva and sclera.
Severe	Corneal opacity blurring the pupillary outline. Severe ischemic necrosis and blanching of the conjunctiva and sclera.

[1]Modified and reproduced, with permission, from Thoft RA, Dohlman CH: Chemical and thermal burns of the eye. In: *Ocular Trauma.* Freeman HM (editor). Appleton-Century-Crofts, 1979.

Prevention

Chemical burns can be prevented by safety measures such as keeping chemicals in unbreakable containers and providing splash protection shields and eyeglasses for employees who must handle them. Workers at risk should be taught emergency treatment measures of themselves and their fellow workers.

Treatment

Emergency treatment (Table 9–2) should be started in the workplace by the patient or anyone immediately available. Any source of water (drinking fountain, hose, etc) is adequate and should be used immediately to wash the eyes with copious amounts of water until the patient can be taken to an emergency facility. At least 1 L of saline or other isotonic solution should then be used to irrigate each eye carefully, with the lids held open to thoroughly cleanse the conjunctival sac. Use of a sterile topical anesthetic may be necessary.

Moist cotton-tipped applicators should be used to sweep the conjunctival surface free of particulate matter, such as the granules found in drainpipe cleaners and plaster. The pH of the conjunctival

Table 9–2. Emergency treatment of chemical burns of the eye.

(1) **In the workplace:** Wash the eyes with copious amounts of water until the patient can be taken to an emergency facility.

(2) **In the emergency facility:**
  (a) Irrigate each eye with at least 1 L of saline or other isotonic solution, with the lids open to flush the conjunctival sac.
  (b) Use sterile topical anesthetic as necessary.
  (c) Remove particulate matter with cotton-tipped applicators.
  (d) Test the pH of the conjunctival surface, and continue irrigation until the pH approaches neutral.
  (e) Remove loose or damaged epithelium from the cornea and conjunctiva.
  (f) Dilate the pupil with cyclopentolate or scopolamine.
  (g) Give topical antibiotic drops, patch the eyes, and refer the patient to an ophthalmologist.

surface should be tested with pH test paper strips or urine pH test strips and irrigation repeated until the pH approaches the normal level of 7.0. As a general rule, there is no practical limit to the amount of irrigation that may be helpful. If there is any doubt about its efficacy, irrigation may be repeated for several hours while waiting for ophthalmologic consultation.

During irrigation, the gray color or cloudiness of the cornea may appear to clear, giving a false impression of improved clinical status. The change is usually due to sloughing of the damaged corneal epithelium, which reveals the clearer corneal stroma underneath.

After irrigation is completed, cycloplegic drops (eg, cyclopentolate or scopolamine) may be instilled to dilate the pupil and thus prevent posterior synechiae (adhesions between iris and lens). Antibiotic drops should be instilled before the eye is patched. The patch prevents blinking and should provide some comfort. The patient should be referred to an ophthalmologist.

Specific ophthalmologic treatment may include the use of topical corticosteroids and antibiotics to reduce the severe inflammatory response that occurs shortly after injury. These medications—particularly the corticosteroids—must be used with caution since they enhance the possibility of secondary infection and discourage the formation of new vessels in ischemic areas. Irrigation of the anterior chamber with saline solution may help restore the pH to more normal levels. After the initial reaction subsides and the conjunctiva and cornea have epithelialized, the severity of the injury can be judged. A scarred cornea can be replaced by a corneal transplant, and a damaged lens (cataract) can be surgically removed. Glaucoma due to scarring of aqueous outflow pathways may be medically controlled—and, if not, a surgical fistulization procedure may be done.

Prognosis

Emergency treatment of chemical burns is usually followed by a period of weeks or months of effort to rehabilitate the damaged ocular tissues. The degree of blanching or ischemia of the conjunctiva is an important factor influencing the final outcome. Ischemic damage even in the presence of apparent healing makes ultimate restoration of vision difficult. The survival of a corneal transplant depends on normal function of structures in the anterior eye. The survival of the cornea and the anterior segment of the eye are directly related to the degree of damage to the corneal endothelium, aqueous drainage pathways, and ciliary body. If the ciliary body fails to produce enough aqueous humor, the entire eye becomes soft and ultimately atrophies. In patients with severe burns, deep penetration and extensive destruction of ocular tissues can lead to perforation of the globe, infection, and loss of the eye. Milder burns in which chemical penetration is more shallow may heal with little scarring.

THERMAL BURNS OF THE EYE & EYELID

Thermal burns of the eyelids and upper face may involve the eyes. However, in cases of flash burn caused by a sudden gas explosion, most individuals forcibly close their eyes, and this reflex lid closure usually protects the ocular surface. Direct contact with molten metal or glass can cause severe injury to the lids and even to the open eye. Thermal injury occurs rapidly at the time of contact. Tissue destruction is not progressive, as is the case with some chemical burns.

Eye examination may require topical anesthesia and careful use of lid retractors. Irrigation may be necessary to remove particulate matter, especially in injuries caused by explosions.

Depending on their severity, thermal burns of the eye structures are treated in the same manner as burns occurring elsewhere on the body (see Chapter 11). Extensive loss of lid skin can lead to exposure and drying of the cornea. This can be prevented by covering the eye with a transparent plastic sheet and sealing it to the surrounding skin with a sterile antibiotic ointment, thus producing a humidity chamber over the eye. Healing of lid skin is frequently followed by scarring, contraction, and distortion of the lids, which results in some degree of exposure of the globe. Plastic surgery with skin grafting may be necessary to restore lid function.

MECHANICAL INJURIES OF THE EYE & EYELID

Mechanical injuries range from superficial abrasions to complete disruption of the globe, depending on the nature of the force striking the eye. Small, sharp, fast-moving objects can penetrate or lacerate the globe, whereas larger objects may exert enough compressive force to cause contusion injury or to rupture the eyeball.

Laceration of the Eyelid

Lid lacerations result from 2 common mechanisms: (1) contact with sharp, fast-moving objects such as glass or metal parts, which cut the skin and subcutaneous tissues (partial-thickness lacerations) or involve the posterior layers, the tarsus, and the conjunctiva (full-thickness lacerations); and (2) avulsion injuries, which are due to blunt trauma (eg, a blow to the malar eminence) and cause abrupt traction of the lid and tear it from its attachment to the medial canthal ligament. The type and extent of injury determine the method of treatment.

Partial-thickness lacerations can be closed by direct suturing with generally good results. Full-thickness lacerations require meticulous repair by an ophthalmic surgeon to accurately restore the continuity of the lid margin. If notching of the margin occurs with healing, the cornea will not be adequately protected from abrasions and other trauma. Deep stab wounds above the upper lid may sever the levator muscle of the lid. The cut end of the levator is easier to retrieve and repair if surgery is performed immediately after injury. Inadequate repair can result in chronic ptosis. Severe damage to the upper lid and blinking mechanism can also place the patient at risk for superficial corneal injuries.

In avulsion injuries, lid structures that have pulled away from the globe should be carefully examined and placed as close to their anatomic positions as possible to protect the eye while the patient is awaiting treatment by an ophthalmic surgeon. Retention of avulsed lid structures is important. They can frequently be repaired and usually heal well because of their rich blood supply. It is difficult to substitute skin grafts or skin flaps for the normal lid structures, particularly the tarsal and conjunctival structures that are essential for normal functioning of the lid. Avulsion of the medial canthal ligament sometimes disrupts the lacrimal drainage system, and failure to repair it will result in epiphora (the overflow of tears).

Injuries of the Iris

Injuries to the iris can be caused indirectly by contusion and directly by perforating or penetrating injuries of the eye.

Contusion of the globe transmits force to the iris by the rapid displacement of aqueous humor. Since water is incompressible and the eye is essentially inelastic, these forces can be very large and destructive.

Iridoplegia is caused by damage to the pupillary sphincter. The pupil may react to light either directly or consensually and only slightly or not at all. The iris root, where it attaches to the ciliary body, may be torn, producing an iridodialysis. Sometimes the ciliary body with the iris root intact is torn away from its scleral attachment, producing an angle recession that can damage the aqueous outflow, causing a form of glaucoma.

Penetrating injuries, foreign bodies, stab wounds, corneal lacerations, and ruptured globes all may perforate, tear, or disrupt the iris. Iris tissue frequently herniates through corneal or scleral wounds.

Iris injuries do not usually require treatment other than that incidental to repair of the associated major injuries. Except for an increase in the amount of light entering an eye, it may have quite useful vision without an iris or with an iris with multiple holes. An eye with more than one pupil still sees only one image.

Injuries of the Retina

Retinal injuries are caused by both blunt trauma (contusion) and penetrating wounds.

When the eye is struck in a contusion injury, the force is transmitted by the fluid contents throughout the interior of the globe. Posteriorly, the retina may become edematous in a discrete area, frequently including the macula—a condition called commotio retinae, or Berlin's edema. Vision is reduced but may improve to nearly normal when the edema clears. This process may require several weeks to a month to complete. Contusion injuries also cause forceful displacement of the vitreous, resulting in traction at its anterior attachment on the surface of the retina at the posterior edge of the ciliary body. This may disinsert the retina from the ciliary body or tear a hole in the peripheral retina. Hemorrhage may result, clouding the vitreous for a time.

Retinal tears or holes frequently cause retinal detachments, which require prompt surgical repair.

Visual prognosis depends on macular involvement. If the macula is intact, vision is usually good; if the macula is detached for even a few days, the prognosis is apt to be poor.

Penetrating injuries cause direct perforations and tears in the retina, causing hemorrhage and detachments.

Treatment of retinal detachments requires localization and closure of the tears or holes. This is done by creating an adhesion and scar between the retina and the choroid surrounding the hole. A freezing probe placed on the scleral surface over the hole will cause an inflammatory reaction in the choroid that will adhere to the retina. Sometimes it is necessary to displace the scleral surface inward to bring the choroidal and retinal surfaces together. This is usually done by placing an encircling band of silicone rubber around the entire globe.

Ruptured or Lacerated Globe

If a ruptured or lacerated globe is present or suspected, placing a metal shield or other protective covering (eg, the bottom half of a paper cup) over the injured eye will prevent external pressure from causing further damage during transport to the hospital. Patching the other eye will reduce ocular movements and thus help prevent further trauma to the injured eye.

Visual acuity should be measured and recorded. Severe injuries are almost always associated with some degree of visual loss, lid swelling, orbital swelling, exophthalmos, and hemorrhage. If lid swelling is extreme, it may be necessary to use a sterile topical anesthetic and lid retractors to lift the lids away from the globe during initial examination.

If the cornea is clear and the pupil is round and reacts to light, the globe is probably intact (Fig 9–3). Global rupture (Fig 9–4) is usually characterized by the presence of brownish or grayish tissue beneath the conjunctiva (subconjunctival hemorrhage), which is due to exposure or herniation of uveal tissue; an irregular or disrupted corneal surface; or the presence of blood or gross alteration in the appearance of the iris and pupil. Pupillary light reflexes may be abnormal. The pupil pulled or peaked toward one side of the cornea usually indicates that the iris has herniated through a laceration in that direction.

Ophthalmoscopic examination may be difficult because of corneal irregularities and hemorrhage in

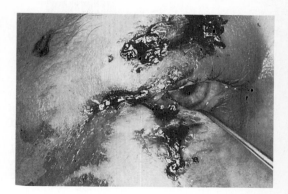

Figure 9–3. Injury in a patient with multiple facial lacerations. Eye examination with the use of a topical anesthetic and lid retractor reveals that the cornea is clear and the pupil is round and reacts to light. The globe is probably intact. (Reproduced, with permission, from Singleton BJ: *Eye Trauma and Emergencies: A Slide-Script Program.* American Academy of Ophthalmology, 1985.)

the anterior chamber and vitreous. If the fundus can be examined and the disk and vessels appear relatively normal, gross disruption of the globe is unlikely. A bright red reflex usually indicates that the interior of the globe is intact.

Intraocular pressure should not be measured if a ruptured or lacerated globe is suspected.

An x-ray for detection of any radiopaque material in the region of the globe is an essential part of the initial examination.

Definitive examination and treatment should be performed by an ophthalmic surgeon. Until a surgeon is available, both eyes should be covered again, with a sterile eye pad used on the injured eye to minimize contamination. The patient should be supported with

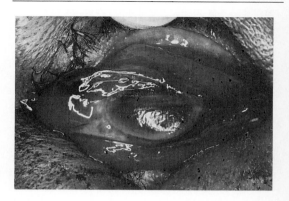

Figure 9–4. Ruptured globe, characterized by a large subconjunctival hemorrhage, grossly distorted cornea, and irregular corneal light reflection. (Reproduced, with permission, from Singleton BJ: *Eye Trauma and Emergencies: A Slide-Script Program.* American Academy of Ophthalmology, 1985.)

parenteral fluids and be considered a candidate for general anesthesia. The repair of a ruptured globe or corneal laceration is usually done under general anesthesia. A local anesthetic is not considered safe, because the distortion from its injection might cause additional damage.

The eye is safely examined under anesthesia, usually with an operating microscope, and the repair is carried out by suturing the torn sclera or lacerated cornea. Exposed intraocular structures such as the iris or ciliary body may be replaced in the eye or excised depending on their condition. When the repair is complete, the eye is filled with saline or an electrolyte solution that simulates aqueous humor. Antibiotics are injected subconjunctivally after the globe is closed and continued intravenously for 4 or 5 days to prevent infection that may have been introduced by the injury.

A ruptured globe has a grave prognosis for restoration of vision. Corneal lacerations have a better prognosis, since their surgical repair is usually easily accomplished. If scarring occurs, corneal transplant can be performed.

Contusion Injuries

Blunt trauma to the eye causes various contusion injuries ranging in severity from ecchymosis of the eyelids (black eye) to major intraocular damage.

Compression injuries of the anterior eye are characterized by corneal edema, anterior chamber hemorrhage, and increased intraocular pressure. These symptoms usually resolve without treatment. In some cases, however, return of normal intraocular pressure is followed several weeks or months later by another increase, which indicates the presence of **angle recession glaucoma.** This is caused by a tear of the attachment of the iris and ciliary body from the internal surface of the sclera at the anterior chamber angle, damaging the aqueous outflow pathway. Patients with compression injuries should always receive follow-up care at the hands of an ophthalmologist so that angle recession glaucoma can be detected and treated to prevent progressive damage to the optic nerve. Treatment usually begins with twice-daily drops of an ophthalmic beta-blocker.

Hyphema (hemorrhage into the anterior chamber) frequently clears spontaneously, but secondary hemorrhage occurs after several hours or days in up to one-third of cases as a result of lysis of the thrombus in the injured vessels of the iris or ciliary body. Secondary hemorrhage frequently continues until the anterior chamber is completely filled with blood, during which time the intraocular pressure may rise to 50–60 mm Hg (normal = 12–20 mm Hg). Lysis and reabsorption of this blood clot may take many days and cause damage to the aqueous filtration pathways and subsequent glaucoma. Breakdown products of blood can also diffuse into the cornea, stain it, and cause long-term reduction of vision. If reabsorption of the blood clot is prolonged, it can sometimes be successfully aspirated. If not, the anterior chamber is opened, and the clot is directly removed. Secondary hemorrhages may require surgical treatment. The prognosis for good vision in patients with secondary hemorrhage is poor.

The prevention of secondary hemorrhages is difficult. Bed rest with binocular patching has been a standard treatment for many years. More recent experience comparing patients treated with bed rest and others allowed normal acuity shows no significant difference in the incidence of secondary hemorrhages.

Aminocaproic acid has been used to retard fibrinolysis in the injured vessels to prevent secondary hemorrhages to the benefit of many patients. This treatment slows the lysis of the primary hyphema but when given for 5–7 days does reduce the occurrence of secondary hemorrhages. There are significant side effects, so that use of aminocaproic acid must be carefully considered and monitored.

Retinal edema, particularly in the macula, causes acute reduction of vision. Vision usually improves with clearance of edema in a few days to several weeks. Clearance is not always complete, and there may be permanent damage to the macula.

In **ruptures of the choroid,** blood spreads beneath the retina at the time of injury, and reabsorption of blood will reveal a crescent-shaped scar concentric with the optic disk. There is no treatment.

Other contusion injuries include **dislocation of the lens** (partial or complete); **traumatic cataracts;** and tears in the region of the anterior attachment of the retina to the ciliary body, which lead to vitreous hemorrhages and **detachment of the retina.**

A damaged lens—either dislocated or cataractous—may reduce vision or may be displaced anteriorly, causing increased intraocular pressure by closing the aqueous filtration angle. In either case, the lens is removed using one of the cataract surgery techniques.

Vitreous hemorrhages are removed with a suction-cutting vitrectomy instrument. Following this procedure, the retinal detachment is repaired by creating an adhesive scar between the choroid and retina, usually by freezing through the scleral surface (cryotherapy) over the area of the retinal tear or hole. The sclera may then be buckled inward to push the adhesion against the retina. This is usually done by compressing the globe with an encircling band of silicone rubber.

Intraocular Foreign Bodies

An intraocular foreign body should be suspected on the basis of the occupational history, particularly if the worker complains of an irritating sensation in the eye and no superficial foreign body is found. For example, when steel tools are used to hammer other steel objects, the hammered steel work-hardens to a glassy surface from which small, sharp chips can fly and penetrate the globe with a minimum of discomfort at the moment of impact. Vision may be nearly normal if the entry wound is small. In cases such as this, in which a radiopaque foreign body is suspected, an x-ray should be taken. Ultrasound will usually demonstrate nonradiopaque objects (eg, glass and plastic). If a foreign body is found, referral to an ophthalmologist for further evaluation and early treatment is essential.

Failure to remove iron or copper foreign bodies can cause severe impairment or loss of vision, owing to their toxic effects on ocular tissue. A retained iron or copper foreign body may dissolve away in several months to a year, but the damage done to the retina by the soluble metallic salts is irreversible, and marked visual loss—even blindness—results. The prognosis for these foreign bodies is good if they are removed before they have time to dissolve. Inert materials such as glass or plastic may cause mechanical damage to the eye, but in the absence of a local toxic reaction, the long-term prognosis is better. It is not necessary to remove every foreign body made of inert material; some of them may be left in place depending upon their position in the globe and their effect on visual function. Iron-containing magnetic foreign bodies are usually removed with an ophthalmic magnet— sometimes through the entry wound or through a surgical incision made as close as possible to the foreign body. Nonmagnetic foreign bodies are removed with grasping instruments specially designed for ophthalmic microsurgery. Penetrating wounds caused by potentially contaminated objects such as agricultural implements or by wood fragments thrown from woodworking machinery can introduce severe intraocular infections that lead to complete disruption and loss of the globe; therefore, microbiologic studies and treatment with appropriate systemic and local antibiotics are required.

Injuries to the Orbit & Optic Nerve

Orbital floor ("blowout") fractures (see Chapter 8) are frequently associated with herniation of intraorbital contents into the fracture line. There usually is severe edema within the orbit, which restricts eye movements for 7–10 days. If restriction continues, surgical repair of the fracture may be indicated to free the entrapped extraocular muscles.

Facial bone and orbital fractures that extend to the posterior orbit may involve the optic canal, with damage to the optic nerve indicated by the presence of an afferent pupillary defect. Initial and later evaluations of the patient should include documentation of visual acuity. If there is progressive loss of vision, surgical decompression of the optic nerve in the canal may preserve or, occasionally, even improve the remaining vision.

Orbital injuries may cause severe hemorrhage, marked exophthalmos of the globe, and a dramatic and abrupt increase in intraocular pressure due to compression. Although this increased pressure is usually relieved by the normal dissipation of interstitial fluid in a short period of time, it occasionally results in occlusion of the central retinal artery or vein. Pressure can sometimes be reduced by applying

gentle external massage to the globe through the closed lids. Surgical lysis of the lateral canthus of the lids may be required.

Penetrating wounds can directly damage the optic nerve by advancing through the funnel-shaped orbit to reach its apex, where the nerve and its blood supply are trapped by the optic canal. Contusion of the nerve causes severe visual impairment and is sometimes treated with large doses of systemic corticosteroids in a manner similar to treatment of spinal cord injuries.

Injuries of the Corneal Epithelium (Abrasions & Superficial Foreign Bodies)

Abrasions of the corneal epithelium can be caused by superficial mechanical trauma (eg, prolonged wearing of contact lenses), by the presence of a foreign body, or by exposure to ultraviolet radiation, chemicals, aerosols, dust, smoke, and other irritants. The occupational medical history should be taken, as described in an earlier section.

Photokeratoconjunctivitis ("welder's flash") is a specific ocular injury caused by unprotected exposure to ultraviolet radiation with wavelengths shorter than 300 nm (actinic rays). This radiation is generated by the welder's arc and damages the exposed corneal and conjunctival epithelium. Injuries are caused not only by direct observation of the arc but occur also in persons nearby who are often not wearing protective filters.

In the first few hours after exposure, there may be only mild discomfort and slight conjunctival redness. After a latent period of several hours—even as long as 6–8 hours—the injured epithelial cells slough, causing an acute onset of severe pain sometimes said to be "as though someone had thrown hot sand in my eyes." Marked tearing, photophobia, and blepharospasm (tightly closed lids) are usual.

Examination requires a sterile topical anesthetic, which may be introduced through nearly closed eyelids by placing several drops along the lid margins. When the eyes open, more anesthetic may be instilled, along with fluorescein from a sterile paper strip. The fluorescein will diffuse over the cornea where the epithelium has sloughed, staining it bright green—best observed with a blue light. Epithelial loss is confined to the area exposed in the lid opening.

Treatment consists of instillation of an antibiotic ointment and patching the eye or eyes to prevent lid movement or blinking. The epithelium will not heal rapidly and in some cases not at all if it is frequently wiped and disturbed by blinking. It will require 12–24 hours for healing to occur, and in some cases several days may be necessary. The eyes should be examined daily. Anesthetic drops and fluorescein help in following progress of reepithelialization. Continue to patch with antibiotic ointment until healing has occurred. Corneal epithelium heals without scarring.

The patient should not be given anesthetic drops or

ointment to use at home. Anesthetics slow and may even prevent epithelial healing, and when used in these circumstances they have led to severe scarring of the cornea and even the loss of an eye.

These injuries are easily prevented by wearing adequate protective filters in the face masks for the welder and goggles or UV filter glasses by visitors and workers in nearby areas where the welding flash can be seen.

Symptoms and signs of **corneal abrasions** include severe ocular pain, tearing, and blurring of vision. Inspection of the anterior eye with a flashlight usually shows irregular light reflections on the corneal surface in the area of the abraded epithelium. Use of sterile topical anesthetic and fluorescein paper strips is helpful for further examination. The fluorescein dye diffuses into the area of disrupted epithelium, stains it bright green, and can be easily observed with a blue light. If further evaluation reveals normal pupillary reactions, a bright red reflex, and no disruption of the anterior segment, the injury is usually confined to the anterior external layer of the cornea.

Small **foreign bodies** on the surface of the cornea or conjunctiva may be seen directly or detected by evidence of damaged epithelium from the fluorescein stain.

Foreign bodies can usually be removed with a cotton-tipped applicator, but a sharp instrument is occasionally helpful. The side bevel of a disposable hypodermic needle can be used to gently detach foreign bodies that are firmly attached to the corneal surface. Rust deposited in the anterior layers of the cornea frequently can be removed by the same gentle scraping maneuver. If all the foreign body or rust is not removed easily, it can usually be left to slough or absorb by itself without causing damage. After foreign bodies are removed, treatment is as for abrasions.

Abrasions are treated by applying a sterile ophthalmic antibiotic ointment effective against both gram-positive and gram-negative organisms—eg, gentamicin, tobramycin, or a mixture containing bacitracin, polymyxin, and neomycin—and covering the affected eye with a patch dressing to keep the lids closed. Corneal epithelium usually heals promptly if the surface of the cornea is allowed to rest without blinking the lid. The initial process of healing is one in which the normal epithelial cells slide from the edge of the wound over the smooth surface of the cornea to fill the gap. The eyes should be inspected in 12–24 hours to determine if healing has occurred and to rule out corneal infection, which appears as a white or gray haze in the area of the wound. If the abrasion is not completely healed, a second application of the ointment and patch dressing for an additional 12–24 hours may be required. This process should be continued until the epithelial defect is healed. Scarring usually does not occur, and vision is restored to normal.

Caution: After the initial examination with topical anesthetic, sharp pain may return until the epithelium

begins to heal. Under no circumstances should the patient be supplied with anesthetic drops or ointment to use during the healing process, since topical anesthetics will delay healing and place the patient at risk for severe corneal infection and scarring. Antibiotic mixtures containing corticosteroids should not be used for treatment, because they provide inadequate protection against bacterial infection and enhance the growth of viral and fungal pathogens.

Abrasions caused by fat-soluble petroleum products splashed into the eyes are treated initially by copious irrigation with water or saline solution to remove any remaining material. Staining with fluorescein will demonstrate the amount of epithelial loss, which may vary from a few punctate areas to complete denudation of the cornea. In either case, treatment is the same as outlined above. If the abraded area is large, the corneal stroma may appear slightly gray, owing to some degree of edema. This clears rapidly with healing of the epithelium.

Exposure to aerosols (eg, paint sprays), detergents, surfactants, dust, smoke, and vapors can produce both acute and chronic symptoms of abrasion. Acute symptoms almost invariably include marked tearing and blepharospasm, which act to protect the eyes and wash away the offending material. Treatment for acute symptoms is as for other abrasions (see above). Chronic exposure to low-level irritants causes fatigue of the lacrimal reflex and subsequent sensations of dryness and burning of the eyes. Some degree of redness is common. Irrigation with saline solution prevents most of these chronic symptoms. Adequate ventilation and avoidance of irritants in the workplace are obviously the best preventive measures.

Exposure to some chemical substances causes a delayed loss of corneal epithelium. For example, formaldehyde fumes cause diffuse damage to epithelial cells, leading to their accelerated sloughing with normal blinking. Fortunately, the abrasion will heal without scarring when the fumes are subsequently avoided. The long list of other substances that produce this effect includes butylamine, diethylamine, hydrogen sulfide, methyl silicate, mustard gas, osmium tetroxide, podophyllum resin, and sulfur.

INDIRECT INJURIES TO THE EYE

In massive crush injuries, compression of the abdominal and chest vessels can cause sudden vascular engorgement of the retina. This leads to marked edema and diffuse hemorrhages in the fundus and can result in permanent ocular damage. **Purtscher's retinopathy** is one form of this condition. There is no treatment. The prognosis for vision depends on the amount of damage done to the macula or optic nerve. Slow improvement in vision occurs as hemorrhages absorb for periods up to several months.

In fractures of the long bones, fat emboli can migrate to the retina and produce small embolic changes that have the appearance of cotton-wool spots and are sometimes associated with flame-shaped hemorrhages in the fundus. Fat emboli, thrombi from heart valve disease and endocarditis, and emboli from a variety of sources occasionally obstruct branches of the retinal artery and cause infarction of a segment of the retina. Cholesterol crystals shed from atheromatous plaques in the carotid arteries may also migrate to the retina and appear as glistening intra-arterial bodies. In intravenous drug abuse, the injected drugs frequently contain inert substances such as talc, which may be seen in the retina as small white deposits. The prognosis for each of these conditions depends entirely on their location and whether or not the macula is involved. There is no ocular treatment. Clearing of the effects of these emboli—hemorrhages and edema—requires several weeks to a month. Cholesterol crystal emboli are an indication to investigate the patency of the carotid arteries.

Rarely, a septic embolus from a distant systemic infection causes endophthalmitis. Endophthalmitis has a generally poor prognosis. Specific diagnosis requires aspiration of vitreous fluid and sometimes aqueous humor for the isolation of organisms. Periocular injection of antibiotics adjacent to the scleral surface, occasionally intravitreal injection of appropriate doses of antibiotics, and intravenous antibiotics are the usual methods of treatment. The poor prognosis is due to delay in diagnosis while the infection advances and to the unpredictable and sometimes poor ocular penetration of antibiotics.

SYMPATHETIC OPHTHALMIA

If the uveal tract (ie, the iris, ciliary body, or choroid) of one eye is injured, the uninjured (sympathizing) eye may show inflammation. This rare disorder is thought to be an autoimmune inflammatory response and can be prevented by prompt, adequate treatment of the initial injury to minimize continuing trauma to the damaged uveal tissue. Sympathetic ophthalmia can cause complete loss of vision in both eyes if unrecognized and untreated early in its course. As soon as inflammation is seen in the sympathizing eye, treatment of both eyes with local corticosteroids (topical and periocular injections) and mydriatics should be started. Large doses of systemic corticosteroids are also frequently used.

OCCLUSION OF THE CENTRAL RETINAL ARTERY

Occlusion of the central retinal artery is characterized by sudden painless loss of vision and is considered an **ocular emergency.** Permanent loss of vision will result if the retina is deprived of blood for 30–60 minutes; therefore, arterial circulation must be restored as soon as possible.

Diagnosis is based on the history and eye exami-

nation. Occlusion is usually seen in older patients with arteriosclerosis or following embolism from the great vessels. It can also be caused by pressure from an unusually tight dressing over the eye, particularly when there is orbital edema or hemorrhage. If the visual loss is incomplete, the patient may be able to detect some light. Ophthalmic examination reveals a bloodless retina with thin and thready arteries. Early findings include a faint retinal edema that appears as a grayish or white discoloration and is particularly noticeable around the macula, allowing the normal red color of the choroid in the fovea to show through as a cherry-red spot. Later, red cells in the blood column of the arteries may separate into segments and appear as "boxcars." The veins also appear thinner than normal. The optic disk retains its normal pink color for several weeks, but the retinal edema becomes more apparent.

Although central retinal artery occlusions are not usually associated with increased intraocular pressures, the most effective treatment is immediate reduction of the normal intraocular pressure in an attempt to dislodge the embolus or thrombus thought to be obstructing the artery at a restricted area of the vessel as it passes through the scleral shell just posterior to the optic disk. The pressure can be reduced by using 2 fingers to alternately massage and press the globe through the closed lids. This maneuver should be repeated 4 or 5 times over 10–15 minutes to accelerate the expression of aqueous humor and applies intermittent pressure on the artery. The patient's use of a rebreathing bag will increase the amount of carbon dioxide in the cerebral and ocular blood vessels, sometimes effecting vascular dilation.

If these maneuvers fail, paracentesis of the anterior chamber may be indicated. After a topical anesthetic is given, the conjunctiva is grasped with fine-tooth forceps. An incision is made through the clear cornea at the periphery of the anterior chamber, with the sharp scalpel blade held in the plane of the iris so as not to touch either the iris or the lens. The blade is then turned slightly to allow some of the aqueous humor to escape abruptly. This lowers the intraocular pressure and sometimes restores circulation to the retina.

OCCLUSION OF THE CENTRAL RETINAL VEIN

Occlusion of the central retinal vein produces painless visual loss and is most commonly seen in older patients with diabetes, hypertension, or other vascular occlusive diseases. Findings include a swollen optic disk, distended and tortuous retinal veins, and an edematous retina with flame-shaped hemorrhages.

There is no effective emergency treatment, although anticoagulants have occasionally been tried. Patients should be followed for specific care by an ophthalmologist.

The prognosis for improvement of vision is slightly better in patients with an occluded retinal vein than in those with an occluded retinal artery.

EYE INJURIES DUE TO RADIATION EXPOSURE

See Chapter 11 for a description of the electromagnetic spectrum and a discussion of methods to prevent occupational exposure to radiation.

Injuries Due to Ionizing Radiation

X-rays, beta rays, and other radiation sources in adequate doses can cause ocular injury. The eyelid is particularly vulnerable to x-ray damage because of the thinness of its skin. Loss of lashes and scarring can lead to inversion or eversion (entropion or ectropion) of the lid margins and prevent adequate lid closure. Scarring of the conjunctiva can impair the production of mucus and the function of the lacrimal gland ducts, thereby causing dryness of the eyes. X-ray radiation in a dose of 500–800 R directed toward the lens surface can cause cataract, sometimes with a delay of several months to a year before the opacities appear. Treatment for these injuries is the appropriate oculoplastic repair of lid deformities and scarring. Deficiencies of tears and mucus can be improved by the topical use of artificial tears and protection from evaporation by wearing protective glasses with side shields that seal to the face. Radiation cataracts can be surgically removed by the appropriate standard technique.

Injuries Due to Ultraviolet Radiation

Ultraviolet radiation of wavelengths shorter than 300 nm (actinic rays) can damage the corneal epithelium. This is most commonly the result of exposure to the sun at high altitudes and in areas where shorter wavelengths are readily reflected from bright surfaces such as snow, water, and sand. Exposure to radiation generated by a welding arc can cause welding flash burn, a form of keratitis. After a latent period of several hours, the injured epithelial cells soften and slough, causing sudden onset of pain. Treatment of these injuries consists of applying antibiotic ointment and patches until the epithelial cells have had an opportunity to heal (see Injuries of the Corneal Epithelium, above).

Wavelengths of 300–400 nm are transmitted through the cornea, and about 80% are absorbed by the lens, where they may cause cataractous changes. Accidental exposure to an inadequately shielded dental instrument used to accelerate the hardening of plastic fillings has caused significant lens opacities in dental personnel. Epidemiologic studies suggest that exposure to solar radiation in these wavelengths near the equator is correlated with an increased incidence of cataracts. They also indicate that workers exposed to bright sunlight in occupations such as farming, truck driving, and construction work appear to have a higher incidence of cataract than those who work primarily indoors. Experimental studies have shown that these wavelengths cause changes in the lens protein, which lead to cataract formation in animals.

CATARACT

Any opacity in the lens is called a cataract. Some degree of opacity is present in almost all lenses, and the significance of the changes depends solely on their effect on vision. Peripheral opacities, for example, that do not interfere with vision are of no clinical significance.

The lens is composed of lens protein arranged in an ordered pattern of cytoplasmic fibers produced by the lens epithelium. These cells continue to produce new fibers at a slow rate throughout life. The lens thus slowly increases in volume—mainly in thickness—pushing the iris forward.

Changes in the chemistry and hydration of the lens protein create various types of cataracts. These changes may be induced by a variety of agents, including near ultraviolet radiation of 300–400 nm. These wavelengths are absorbed by the central lens fibers, causing the brownish discoloration of lenticular nuclear sclerosis. Ocular inflammation and corticosteroids, both topical and systemic, produce typical posterior subcapsular cataracts.

Types of Cataracts

A. Senile Cataracts: Age-related (senile) cataract is the most common type seen. Some degree of opacity is almost universal. The progress of change and the related reduction of vision is usually quite slow. Nuclear sclerosis—an increasing density in the central mass of protein—causes a myopic change that can be corrected by changing glasses for some years—in many instances restoring vision to near normal.

B. Congenital Cataracts: These can be unilateral or bilateral, and many are thought to be of genetic origin. Some are due to maternal rubella during the first trimester of pregnancy. If the opacity prevents a clear view of the ocular fundus, surgical removal at an early age—even 2 months—is indicated to aid in the development of useful vision.

C. Traumatic Cataracts: Contusion injuries can cause opacities that may appear right away or develop slowly over weeks or even months. Penetrating wounds can tear the lens capsule, allowing aqueous humor to soften lens protein and usually creating major opacities. These cataracts almost always need to be removed acutely—in many cases at the time of wound repair.

D. Secondary Cataracts: These changes result from inflammatory processes in the eye (uveitis) and usually begin by producing opacities just inside the posterior lens capsule. Similar changes occur in association with retinitis pigmentosa, glaucoma, and, rarely, retinal detachments.

E. Cataracts Associated With Systemic Diseases: These are usually bilateral and may appear in patients with myotonia dystrophica, hypoparathyroidism, diabetes mellitus, and Down's syndrome and in many other less common conditions.

F. Toxic Cataracts: Lens opacities are reported following exposure to or ingestion of numerous chemicals. They are described at some length in Grant's Toxicology of the Eye. The most common cause at the present seems to be prolonged use of corticosteroids, either topical or systemic. At least 2 years of moderate to high doses are usually necessary to produce cataract.

Treatment

There is no effective medical treatment for cataract. Surgical removal usually results in significant improvement of vision in about 90% of patients. The results depend on whether other ocular changes are present such as macular scars or optic nerve changes. Indications for surgery depend almost entirely on the needs of the individual patient to improve vision. Of course, a rapidly swelling acute traumatic cataract needs early surgery.

There are 2 commonly used methods of cataract extraction. The lens may be removed totally in its capsule—the intracapsular technique. Extracapsular extraction removes all of the lens protein out of the lens capsular bag, leaving behind all of the capsule except for a portion of the anterior capsule removed along with the lens epithelium.

The presence of the intact posterior capsule facilitates implantation of an intraocular lens behind the iris. This lens replaces the optical power of the patient's own lens.

Complications of surgery are hemorrhage from the corneoscleral wound, infection, retinal detachment, and even damage to the macula from prolonged exposure to the light of the operating microscope.

Prognosis

The results of cataract surgery are generally excellent. Significant visual improvement is reported in nearly 90% of cases following extraction of age-related cataracts. The reduced expectations in eyes with injuries are due to unpredictable intraocular complications such as retinal scarring and macular damage.

Injuries Due to Visible Radiation (Light)

Visible light has a spectrum of 400–750 nm. If the wavelengths of this spectrum penetrate fully to the retina, they can cause thermal, mechanical, or photic injuries.

Thermal injuries are produced by light intense enough to increase the temperature in the retina by 10–20 °C. Lasers used in therapy can cause this type of injury. The light is absorbed by the retinal pigment epithelium, where its energy is converted to heat, and the heat causes photocoagulation of retinal tissue.

Mechanical injuries can be produced by exposure to laser energy from a Q-switched or mode-locked laser, which produces sonic shock waves that disrupt retinal tissue.

Photic injuries are caused by prolonged exposure to intense light, which produces varying degrees of cellular damage in the retinal macula without a significant increase in the temperature of the tissue (usually no more than 1–2 °C). Recent studies have shown photic injuries not to be burns in the literal sense but damage from the light itself. Sun gazing is the most common cause of this type of injury, but prolonged unprotected exposure to a welding arc can also damage the retinal macula. When the initial retinal edema clears, there is usually some scarring that leads to a permanent decrease in visual acuity. The intensity of light, length of exposure, and age of the exposed individual are all important factors. The older the individual, the more sensitive the retina appears to be to photic injuries. Anyone who has had cataract surgery is much more vulnerable because filtration of light by the lens is impaired. In photic injuries caused by exposure to welding sources or other excessively bright light, treatment with systemic corticosteroids may be tried. A large initial dose of 60–100 mg of prednisone is rapidly tapered over a period of 10–14 days. This may reduce the acute edema or inflammatory response, but it is not always effective.

Wavelengths of 500–750 nm are most useful for vision and appear not to cause photic damage to the retina at exposures most commonly encountered. However, repeated exposure to bright sunlight by working outdoors for 3–4 hours each day can cause prolongation of the dark adaptation response, thereby reducing night vision.

Injuries Due to Infrared Radiation

Wavelengths greater than 750 nm in the infrared spectrum can produce lens changes. Glassblower's cataract is an example of a heat injury that damages the anterior lens capsule. Denser cataractous changes can occur in unprotected workers who observe glowing masses of glass or iron for many hours a day.

EFFECTS OF VIDEO DISPLAY TERMINAL USE

In recent years, employees who spend 6–8 hours a day looking at video display terminals have complained of eyestrain, headache, and general fatigue. The brightness of the light from such terminals is not great enough to produce any ocular injury. Posture, accommodative fatigue, and the early changes of presbyopia may contribute to feelings of eyestrain and physical stress.

Measures to alleviate these problems associated with video display terminal use are discussed in Chapter 6.

REFERENCES

Deutsch TS, Feller DB: *Paton and Goldberg's Management of Ocular Injuries,* 2nd ed. Saunders, 1985.

Duane TD (editor): *Clinical Ophthalmology.* Harper & Row, 1985.

Grant WM: *Toxicology of the Eye,* 3rd ed. Thomas, 1986.

Miller D (editor): *Clinical Light Damage to the Eye.* Springer-Verlag, 1987.

Newell FW: *Ophthalmology: Principles and Concepts,* 6th ed. Mosby, 1986.

Vaughan D, Asbury T: *General Ophthalmology,* 12th ed. Appleton & Lange, 1986.

Occupational Hearing Loss

10

Robert K. Jackler, MD, & David N. Schindler, MD

Occupational hearing loss may be partial or total; unilateral or bilateral; and conductive, sensorineural, or mixed conductive and sensorineural. **Conductive hearing loss** results from dysfunction of the external or middle ear, which impairs the passage of sound vibrations to the inner ear. In the workplace, this can be caused by blunt or penetrating head injuries, explosions, and thermal injuries such as slag burns sustained when a piece of welder's slag penetrates the eardrum. **Sensory hearing loss** results from deterioration of the cochlea, usually due to loss of hair cells from the organ of Corti. Among the many common causes of sensory hearing loss are continuous exposure to noise in excess of 85 dB, blunt head injury, and exposure to ototoxic substances.

Physiology of Hearing

Sound waves consist of alternating periods of compression and rarefaction within a medium such as air. The degree of this pressure variation has a correlation in the subjective awareness of loudness. Measurement of human hearing in terms of sound pressure level (SPL) in dynes/cm^2 is cumbersome because of the differing sensitivity of the ear at the various frequencies. For this reason, a scale allowing easy comparison among frequencies and individuals has been developed. The decibel (dB) scale is a logarithmic measurement of human hearing which, through standardization, has defined normal hearing as 0 dB. The human ear has a remarkable dynamic range of roughly 0 to 120 dB (10^6 SPL), which allows for detection of sound pressure variations from the faintest noise to painful stimulation.

Frequency, or number of waves passing a point in a second, has a subjective correlate in pitch. The normal human cochlea is capable of detecting and encoding sound waves across the frequency range extending from approximately 20 Hz to 20,000 Hz. The most important range for human speech reception is between 500 and 3000 Hz. Because isolated pure tone waves seldom occur in nature, the cochlea is called upon to analyze complex wave forms.

There is considerable impedance to the passage of sound vibrations from air into the fluid-filled inner ear. To overcome this barrier, an impedance-matching mechanism known as the conducting system has evolved. This apparatus consists of the tympanic membrane and the 3 ossicles. The conducting system contributes approximately 45 dB toward normal hearing.

Evaluation of Hearing

A. Test of Spoken Words: The simplest form of hearing evaluation may be performed in a quiet room without any sophisticated equipment. The patient is asked to repeat spoken words of increasing intensity while competing noises (eg, the crumpling of paper or the sounds from a Bárány noise box) are presented to the opposite ear. Results may be expressed as the ability to hear a soft whisper, loud whisper, soft spoken voice, loud spoken voice, or shout.

B. Tuning Fork Tests: Tuning fork tests should be performed with a 512-Hz tuning fork, since frequencies below this level will elicit a tactile response.

1. Rinne test—When the patient hears air conduction (tuning fork placed by the opening of the ear canal) better than bone conduction (tuning fork placed on the mastoid bone), a sensorineural hearing loss or normal hearing is indicated. When bone conduction is louder than air conduction, a conductive hearing loss is indicated.

2. Weber test—When the tuning fork is placed on the forehead or front teeth, sound should lateralize toward a conductive loss and away from a sensorineural one.

C. Pure Tone Audiometry: Sensitivity to pure tones is measured at 250, 500, 1000, 2000, 3000, 4000, and 8000 Hz for both air conduction (headphones) and bone conduction (bone oscillator). Thresholds of hearing are expressed in decibels, with the normal range at each frequency from 0 to 20 dB. Because loud signals may stimulate the opposite ear, masking with competing sound the contralateral ear is necessary. When both air and bone conduction are decreased, a sensorineural hearing loss exists. Conductive losses are indicated by an "air-bone gap," in which the air conduction loss exceeds the bone conduction loss. Results may be presented numerically or shown graphically (Figs 10–1 to 10–5).

D. Békésy Audiometry: Pure tone thresholds may also be measured by Békésy audiometry, in which the patient uses self-directed techniques that involve pressing and releasing a signal button. This procedure is used in some occupational screening programs, but it is generally not as reliable as procedures administered by an audiologist.

E. Speech Audiometry: Two routine tests are performed to assess speech reception and comprehension, which are the most important aspects of audition.

1. Test of speech reception—The speech recep-

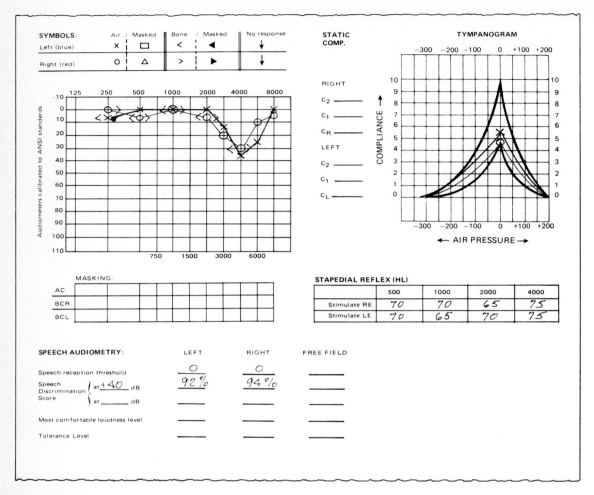

Figure 10–1. Mild noise-induced hearing loss. The audiogram shows typical bilateral high-frequency sensorineural hearing loss, which usually is most severe at 4000 Hz. Note the normal speech discrimination score.

tion threshold (SRT) is the intensity (in decibels) at which the listener is able to repeat 50% of phonetically balanced 2-syllable words (eg, baseball, playground, and airplane). The threshold is usually in close agreement with an average of the pure tone thresholds for frequencies between 500 and 3000 Hz. The normal range is between 0 and 20 dB, with losses of 20–40 dB termed "mild," 40–60 dB "moderate," 60–80 dB "severe," and greater than 80 dB "profound."

2. Test of speech discrimination—In the speech discrimination score (SDS), monosyllabic words are presented at intensities well above the threshold for speech reception (SRT plus 40 dB) in order to test speech comprehension. Results are expressed as a percentage of words correctly repeated. The normal range of SDS is 88–100%. Word lists are available for most modern languages. Significant depression of the SDS usually indicates socially significant disability.

F. Impedance Audiometry: The mechanical aspects of the middle ear sound transformer system can be assessed by tympanometry and acoustic reflex testing.

1. Tympanometry—Tympanometry employs an acoustic probe to measure the impedance of the eardrum and ossicular chain. Reduced middle ear compliance usually indicates a partial vacuum due to auditory tube dysfunction, while noncompliance suggests either a tympanic membrane perforation or middle ear effusion. An increase in compliance suggests either laxity of the tympanic membrane or disruption of the ossicular chain.

2. Acoustic reflex testing—Contraction of the middle ear muscles in response to a loud noise results in a measurable rise of middle ear impedance. Interpretation of acoustic reflex testing may yield information regarding the integrity of the auditory portion of the central nervous system. It is also an indirect

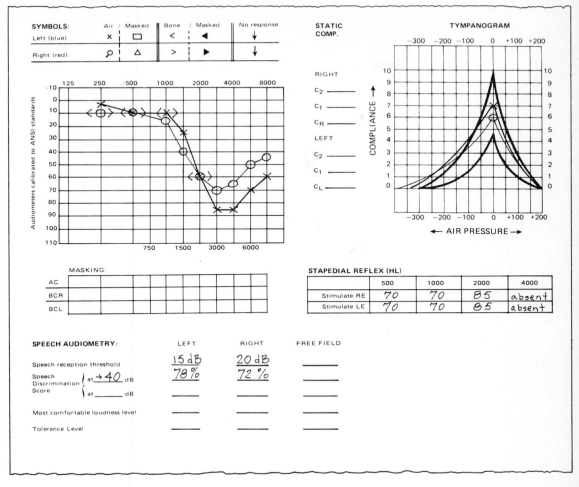

Figure 10–2. Noise-induced hearing loss. The audiogram shows moderate to severe high-frequency sensorineural hearing loss but preservation of the lower tones. Note the moderate decrease in the speech discrimination score.

measurement of recruitment (the abnormal sensitivity to loud sounds) that frequently accompanies sensorineural hearing loss.

G. Evoked Response Audiometry (Brain Stem Audiometry): In patients with unilateral or asymmetric sensorineural hearing loss, retrocochlear lesions (lesions of the eighth cranial nerve, brain stem, or cortex) must be ruled out. Evoked potentials, which are elicited in response to clicking noises and recorded via scalp electrodes, provide information about the location of lesions. In individuals with normal hearing, as well as in most patients with cochlear hearing losses, a series of 5 electroencephalographic waves may be detected, representing the central auditory system from the eighth cranial nerve (wave I) to the inferior colliculus (wave V). The significant delay or complete absence of a response may indicate a cerebellopontine angle tumor (eg, acoustic neuroma) or a lesion at the level of the brain stem. Definitive diagnosis of retrocochlear lesions

requires CT scanning or magnetic resonance imaging.

H. Stenger Test: This test is useful for detecting feigned unilateral hearing loss. The Stenger principle states that when 2 tones of the same frequency but of different loudness are presented to both ears simultaneously, only the louder tone will be heard. When the louder tone is presented to the ear with a feigned hearing loss, the patient stops responding because he or she perceives that all of the sound is coming from that side. Patients with true unilateral loss indicate that they continue to hear the sound in the opposite ear.

Differential Diagnosis of Hearing Loss

A. Occupational Hearing Loss: The following types of occupational hearing loss are discussed in separate sections below:

1. Noise-induced hearing loss (NIHL).

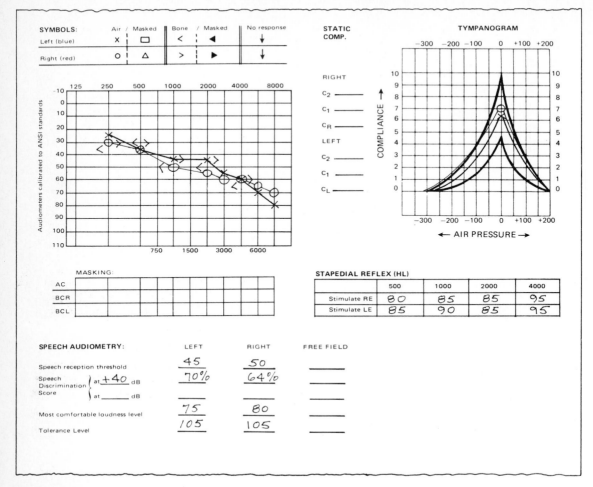

SYMBOLS:	Air / Masked	Bone / Masked	No response
Left (blue)	X □	< ◄	↓
Right (red)	O Δ	> ►	↓

STATIC COMP.

TYMPANOGRAM

RIGHT
c_2 ———
c_1 ———
c_R ———
LEFT
c_2 ———
c_1 ———
c_L ———

← AIR PRESSURE →

MASKING:

AC							
BCR							
BCL							

STAPEDIAL REFLEX (HL)

	500	1000	2000	4000
Stimulate RE	80	85	85	95
Stimulate LE	85	90	85	95

SPEECH AUDIOMETRY:

	LEFT	RIGHT	FREE FIELD
Speech reception threshold	45	50	———
Speech Discrimination Score at +40 dB	70%	64%	———
at ____ dB			
Most comfortable loudness level	75	80	———
Tolerance Level	105	105	———

Figure 10–3. Presbycusis. The audiogram shows a moderate to severe down-sloping sensorineural hearing loss. Note that the hearing threshold at 4000 Hz is better than that at 8000 Hz, a pattern suggestive but not diagnostic of an aging change rather than exposure to noise.

2. Hearing loss due to physical trauma.

3. Ototoxic hearing loss.

B. Nonoccupational Hearing Loss: The following disorders must be ruled out:

1. Presbycusis–Presbycusis is a slow and progressive deterioration of hearing that is associated with aging and not attributable to other causes. (See Fig 10–3.)

2. Hereditary sensorineural hearing loss–This is distinguished by a family history and early age at onset.

3. Metabolic disorders–Progressive hearing loss may be related to diabetes, thyroid dysfunction, renal failure, autoimmune disease, and other metabolic disorders.

4. Cochlear otosclerosis–Destruction of the otic capsule due to otosclerosis may mimic NIHL. The coexistence of conductive hearing loss with otosclerosis and the frequently positive family history help to distinguish the two.

5. Sudden sensorineural hearing loss–This is differentiated by its sudden onset in the absence of precipitating factors.

6. Vascular compromise–Sudden hearing loss may occur from vaso-occlusive disease or migraine. The role of vascular compromise in progressive hearing loss is uncertain.

7. Central nervous system disease–Cerebellopontine angle tumors, especially acoustic neuroma, may present with progressive hearing loss that is unilateral. This is in contrast to NIHL, which is usually bilateral. Patients with unilateral or asymmetric sensorineural hearing loss require further investigation to rule out these tumors. Demyelinating diseases (eg, multiple sclerosis) may present with a sudden unilateral hearing loss that typically recovers to some degree.

8. Meniere's disease–Meniere's disease and its variants generally present with unilateral hearing loss and are frequently associated with vertigo. Vertigo is not generally seen with NIHL.

9. Nonorganic hearing loss–Functional hearing

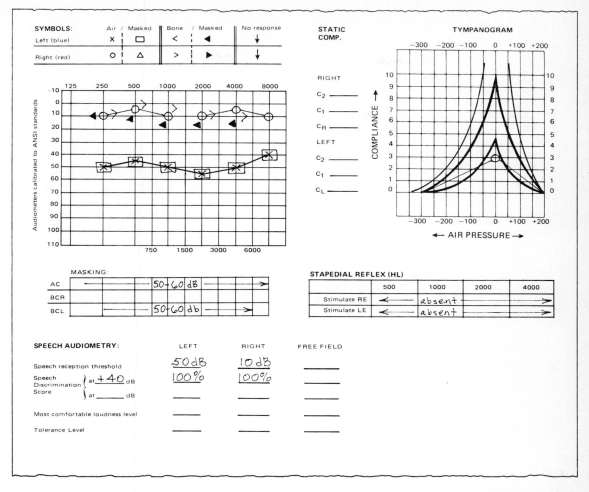

SYMBOLS:

	Air / Masked	Bone / Masked	No response
Left (blue)	x : ▢	< : ◀	↓
Right (red)	o : △	> : ▶	↓

MASKING:

AC	50-60 dB	→
BCR		
BCL	50-60 db	→

STAPEDIAL REFLEX (HL)

	500	1000	2000	4000
Stimulate RE	← absent			→
Stimulate LE	← absent			→

SPEECH AUDIOMETRY:

	LEFT	RIGHT	FREE FIELD
Speech reception threshold	50 dB	10 dB	___
Speech Discrimination Score { at +40 dB	100%	100%	___
{ at ___ dB	___	___	___
Most comfortable loudness level	___	___	___
Tolerance Level	___	___	___

Figure 10–4. The audiogram shows a disparity between the thresholds of bone conduction and air conduction. This "air-bone gap" represents the degree of hearing impairment due to dysfunction of the external or middle ear. The audiogram is typical of a left ossicular chain disruption.

loss for purposes of secondary gain is quite frequent. This may be seen in people with normal hearing or in those who embellish an existing organic hearing loss. With skillful audiometric techniques (see above), it is usually possible to distinguish organic from nonorganic hearing loss, but this may require referral to an audiologic center with considerable experience with this problem.

There are various indications of nonorganic hearing loss. Poor correlation between the speech reception thresholds and the average of the air conduction thresholds at 500, 1000, and 2000 Hz is the most common indication of functionality (Fig 10–5). The speech reception thresholds are generally within 6 dB of the average of the "speech frequencies." Test-retest variability is also suggestive. In cases of suspected unilateral functional hearing loss, the Stenger test is useful. Evoked response audiometry may also be useful for objectively establishing hear-

ing thresholds in patients unable or unwilling to cooperate with conventional testing. Although this has gained widespread use in the testing of young children, it is not yet sufficiently reliable to provide accurate thresholds in the adult with functional hearing loss. Active research is progressing in this area.

NOISE-INDUCED HEARING LOSS

Etiology & Pathogenesis

NIHL results from trauma to the sensory epithelium of the cochlea. The most obvious injury is to the stereocilia of the hair cells (the electromechanical transducers of sound energy), which may become distorted or even disrupted under acoustically generated shearing forces. Susceptibility to noise-induced hearing loss is highly variable; while some individuals are able to tolerate high noise levels for prolonged

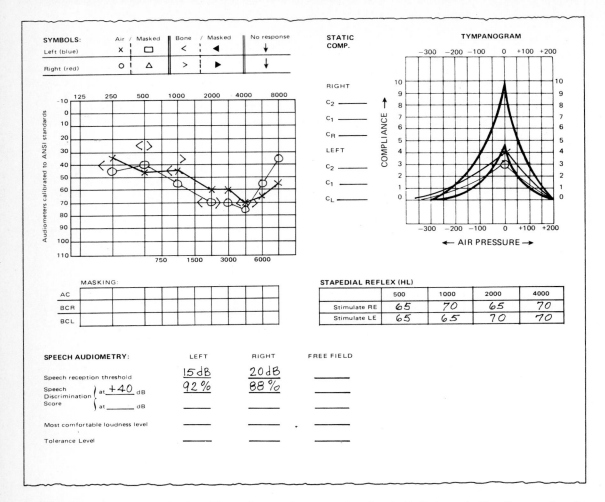

Figure 10–5. Nonorganic hearing loss. The audiogram shows pure tone thresholds that are significantly worse than the speech reception thresholds recorded on the same date.

periods of time, others who are subjected to the same environment rapidly lose hearing. Risk of permanent hearing impairment is related to the duration and intensity of exposure (see Table 10–1 and Figs 6–8, 10–1, and 10–2) as well as genetic susceptibility to noise trauma. Generally, prolonged exposure to sounds louder than 85 dB is potentially injurious. It has been estimated that 26% of production workers in the USA are exposed to noise levels of 90 dB or greater for 8 hours a day. Continuous exposure to hazardous levels of noise tends to have its maximum effect in the high-frequency regions of the cochlea. Noise-induced hearing loss is usually most severe around 4000 Hz, with downward extension toward the ''speech frequencies'' (500–3000 Hz) occurring only after prolonged or severe exposure. Interestingly, this tendency of noise-induced hearing loss to preferentially affect the high-frequency regions of the

Table 10–1. Relative intensity of common noises.

Noise Level (dB)	Environmental Source	Human Speech
140	Air raid siren	. . .
120	Jet takeoff	. . .
110	Riveting machine	. . .
100	Pneumatic hammer	Shouting in ear
90	Subway train	Shouting at a distance of 2 ft
80	Vacuum cleaner	. . .
70	Freeway traffic	Loud conversation
50	Road traffic	Normal conversation
30	Library	Soft whisper
20	Broadcasting studio	. . .
0	Threshold of hearing	. . .

cochlea remains true regardless of the frequency of the injurious noise.

The biologic effect of impulse noise is somewhat different from the effect of continuous noise. The inner ear is partially protected from the effects of continuous noise by the acoustic reflex. This reflex, which is triggered when the ear is subjected to noise louder than 90 dB, causes the middle ear muscles (the stapedius and tensor tympani) to contract and thereby stiffen the conductive system and make it more resistant to sound entry. Because this protective reflex is neurally mediated, it is delayed in onset for a period ranging from 25 to 150 ms, depending on the intensity of the sound. High-intensity impulse noises (eg, explosions) penetrate the cochlea before the acoustic reflex has been activated and thus are especially injurious. Impact noise exceeding 140 dB may cause immediate and irreversible hearing loss.

Exposure to loud noise frequently causes a slight decrease in hearing sensitivity, often associated with tinnitus. This usually lasts for several hours but may be more prolonged if the intensity of noise has been great. This phenomenon, called **temporary threshold shift (TTS),** results from reversible injury to hair cells. In contrast, **permanent threshold shift (PTS)** results from irreversible hair cell damage. PTS may be caused by a brief exposure to extremely high intensity sounds, but it is more commonly caused by prolonged repetitive exposure to lower levels of hazardous noise. The cumulative effects of long-term exposure may lead to progressive destruction of hair cell populations. Because TTS may mimic PTS, individuals should be given audiometric tests after a recovery period of 12–24 hours following exposure to hazardous levels of noise.

Clinical Findings

Patients frequently complain of gradual deterioration in hearing. The most common complaint is difficulty in comprehending speech, especially in the presence of competing background noise. Because patients with noise-induced hearing loss have a high-frequency bias to their hearing loss, they hear vowel sounds better than consonant sounds. This leads to a distortion of speech sounds that is most pronounced when they are listening to people with high-pitched voices (eg, women and children). Background noise, which is usually low-frequency in bias, masks the better-preserved portion of the hearing spectrum and further exacerbates the problems with speech comprehension.

Noise-induced hearing loss is frequently accompanied by tinnitus. Most often patients describe a high-frequency tonal sound (ringing), but the sound is sometimes lower in tone (buzzing, blowing, or hissing) or even nontonal (popping or clicking). This sensation may be intermittent or continuous and is usually exacerbated by further exposure to noise. Because tinnitus is usually most bothersome to patients when there is little ambient noise present, some of them complain of inability to fall asleep or to concentrate when in a quiet room.

On tuning fork examination, the patient hears air conduction better than bone conduction, which indicates a sensorineural hearing loss. When serial tuning forks from 512 to 4096 Hz are used, there is often a marked decrease in hearing in the higher frequencies. Formal audiometric examination usually reveals a bilateral, predominantly high-frequency sensorineural hearing loss with a maximum drop of the pure tone thresholds occurring at or around 4000 Hz on the pure tone audiogram (Figs 10–1 and 10–2). Because the most important thresholds for comprehension of human speech are between 500 and 3000 Hz, a significant decrease in speech reception threshold does not begin until frequencies below 3000 Hz are affected. The speech discrimination score is normal in the early stages of noise-induced hearing loss, but this may deteriorate as the loss becomes more severe.

Prevention

Prevention of noise-induced hearing loss requires protection of the inner ear from hazardous noise, which the Office of Workers' Compensation Programs in the US Department of Labor has defined as noise exceeding 85 dB for 8 hours a day. Although 85 dB has been characterized as the approximate biologic threshold above which permanent shifts in hearing are possible, the decision to make it the maximum acceptable level of noise in the workplace was essentially a political one representing a compromise between the need for protection of susceptible workers and the efficiency of the industrial process. Extensive noise abatement programs are under way throughout the country to attenuate noise levels to below 85 dB.

The first step in control of hazardous noise is characterization of its frequency and intensity with sound level meters and noise dosimeters. Adjustments are then made to the acceptable level of exposure based on a time-weighted average (TWA) in which the TWA formula requires halving of the permitted exposure time for each additional 5 dB above 90 dB. After all economically feasible measures to muffle offending machinery have been employed, ear protectors are provided for employees in hazardous noise areas. As shown in Fig 10–6, ear protectors vary in their ability to reduce the level of noise. In-the-ear plugs made of foam rubber or wax-impregnated cotton attenuate noise by approximately 25 dB, while over-the-ear muffs may attenuate an average of around 35 dB. When used together, earplugs and earmuffs may provide up to 45 dB of protection.

The Occupational Safety and Health Administration (OSHA) defines the steps of instituting an industrial hearing conservation program as follows: (1) Identify exposed workers. (2) Establish the extent of exposure. (3) Institute an audiometric testing program for exposed workers. (4) Obtain profes-

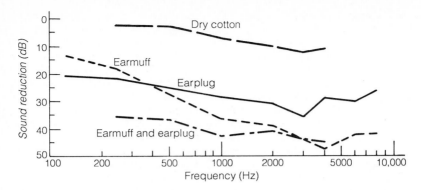

Figure 10–6. Comparison of the attentuation properties of a molded-type earplug and an earmuff protector. Note that the earplug offers greater attenuation of the lower frequencies, while the earmuff is better at the higher frequencies. (Reproduced, with permission, from Olishifski JB, Standard JJ: Industrial noise. Chapter 9 in: *Fundamentals of Industrial Hygiene*, 3rd ed. Plog BA [editor]. National Safety Council, 1989.)

sional review of audiograms and recommendations for the appropriate course of action. (5) Provide appropriate personal hearing protection. (6) Offer annual education programs for exposed employees. (7) Ensure that appropriately qualified personnel are engaged in all facets of the program. (8) Establish and maintain an effective record-keeping system encompassing all phases of the program.

Treatment

There is no medical or surgical treatment available to reverse the effects of noise-induced hearing loss. After the diagnosis has been established by otologic examination and performance of an audiometric test battery, the physician should counsel the patient on the likely consequences of continued exposure to excessive noise and should recommend techniques for avoidance of further noise-induced damage. Hearing amplification is reserved for those patients with socially impaired hearing. Hearing aids must be carefully fitted to optimally meet the needs of the individual with regard to frequency bias and gain. In bilateral hearing losses, bilateral amplification usually provides more satisfactory rehabilitation. Although whether to try hearing amplification is the patient's decision, a reasonable criterion for referral to a professional for hearing aid evaluation is a speech reception threshold below 25 dB or a speech discrimination score of less than 80%. A patient's willingness to wear a hearing aid will depend on many factors, including cosmetic considerations and concerns about the ability to insert the hearing aid and to manipulate its controls. Numerous other clever instruments known as assistive listening devices are available to enhance comprehension in small or large groups (eg, at business meetings or conventions), with telephone use, and with various audio or visual media such as television. Most of these work with wireless transmission of FM signals or infrared light

beams. Aural rehabilitation classes designed to enhance the patient's ability to comprehend speech may also be helpful and are usually available in urban areas.

There is no cure for tinnitus resulting from noise-induced hearing loss, although numerous ameliorative measures are available. In the absence of further inner ear injury, tinnitus will gradually diminish, usually over a course of weeks to months. A subtle degree of tinnitus often persists and is especially obvious when the patient is in a quiet room. For the few patients who find this to be extremely troublesome, masking the tinnitus with music or some other form of pleasant sound is often helpful. In those with significant hearing loss, the most successful treatment may be appropriate hearing amplification. Modified hearing aids designed to produce masking noises have generally been of limited success. Use of biofeedback has helped some patients suppress their tinnitus. Psychiatric referral to manage associated depression is sometimes necessary.

Prognosis

Hearing in patients with noise-induced hearing loss will generally stabilize if the patient is removed from the noxious stimulus. If not, hearing will continue to deteriorate and ultimately result in severe hearing impairment or, in extreme cases, total deafness. Although adequate noise protection is essential and should always be recommended, even with adequate hearing protection other factors may play a role in the patient's prognosis. Presbycusis can add to the noise-induced loss as the patient grows older, and preexisting noise-induced hearing loss will also cause the patient to be more susceptible to the adverse effects of ototoxic substances such as aminoglycoside antibiotics, loop diuretics, and antineoplastic agents used in the treatment of other disorders (see Ototoxic Hearing Loss, below).

HEARING LOSS DUE TO PHYSICAL TRAUMA

Etiology & Pathogenesis

A broad spectrum of injuries may cause trauma to the ears. Blunt head injury is by far the most common cause of traumatic hearing loss. A blow to the head creates a pressure wave in the skull that is transmitted through bone in a manner similar to the way a pressure wave in air is carried by the conducting mechanism of the ear. The cochlear injury observed following blunt head trauma closely resembles both histologically and audiologically that induced by high-intensity acoustic trauma. Motor vehicle accidents are the major cause of blunt head trauma and account for about 50% of temporal bone injuries. Penetrating injuries of the temporal bone are relatively rare, accounting for fewer than 10% of cases. Other occupational causes of ear injury include falls, explosions, and burns from caustic chemicals, open flames, or welder's slag that enters the ear canal.

Examination & Treatment

In the conscious patient, hearing should be assessed immediately with a 512-Hz tuning fork. Even in an ear severely traumatized and filled with blood, sound will lateralize toward a conductive hearing loss and away from a sensorineural one. Complete audiometric examinations (see Evaluation of Hearing, above) can be performed after the patient has been stabilized. Patients should also be checked for signs of vestibular injury (nystagmus) and facial nerve trauma (paralysis).

A. Injuries Causing Conductive Hearing Loss: Blunt head trauma without temporal bone fracture may cause **hematotympanum:** a collection of blood in the middle ear. If this is the sole injury, hearing usually recovers over several weeks. **Burns** sustained when a piece of welder's slag penetrates the eardrum often heal poorly, and chronic infection often results. A loud explosion with sound pressure levels exceeding 180 dB may cause **rupture of the tympanic membrane.** Traumatic membrane perforations usually heal spontaneously if secondary infection does not develop (patients should be instructed not to get the ear wet during the healing period), although hearing loss may persist. Conductive hearing loss that persists more than 3 months after injury is usually due to a tympanic membrane perforation or **disruption of the ossicular chain** (Fig 10–4). These lesions are generally suitable for surgical repair, usually on a delayed basis. Repair is by grafting the tympanic membrane or by reconstructing the ossicular chain with homograft or prosthetic materials—or both.

B. Injuries Causing Sensorineural Hearing Loss: Trauma to the inner ear most commonly results from blunt head injury. **Labyrinthine concussion** frequently occurs with transient vertigo, potentially permanent hearing loss, and tinnitus. Treatment is expectant, with vestibular suppressants such as meclizine offering symptomatic relief of vertigo. Trauma may also cause rupture of the round or oval window membranes, which can lead to leakage of inner ear fluids into the middle ear. Most perilymphatic fistulas heal spontaneously. Persistent perilymphatic leakage is difficult to diagnose and requires surgical treatment with autogenous material used to repair the defect. Most patients with surgically confirmed fistulas suffer recurrent episodes of vertigo and hearing loss, often temporally related to vigorous physical exercise.

C. Injuries Causing Mixed Conductive and Sensorineural Hearing Loss: Temporal bone injuries sometimes involve both the middle and inner ear, resulting in mixed conductive and sensorineural hearing loss. **Fractures of the temporal bone** tend to occur along lines that connect points of weakness in the skull base. Clinically, these fractures may be divided into 2 patterns: longitudinal and transverse. **Longitudinal fractures** are much more common (80% of cases) and usually result from a blow to the lateral aspect of the head. They frequently involve the structures of the middle ear but characteristically spare the inner ear. **Transverse fractures** are less common (20% of cases) and usually result from a severe occipital blow. Serious intracranial injury frequently accompanies transverse fractures. Typically, they traverse the inner ear and cause total sensorineural hearing loss and labyrinthine death. Fractures through the inner ear are often accompanied by severe vertigo that lasts for weeks or even months.

Temporal bone fractures are recognized clinically by the presence of blood, cerebrospinal fluid, or both in the ear canal or by the presence of blood in the middle ear behind an intact tympanic membrane. The ear canal should be carefully cleaned using sterile suction to assess the integrity of the tympanic membrane. Under no circumstances should a recently traumatized ear be irrigated. Battle's sign (ecchymosis over the mastoid region) is occasionally seen. Definitive diagnosis requires high-resolution CT scanning to demonstrate the fracture lines.

OTOTOXIC HEARING LOSS

Etiology & Pathogenesis

Hearing loss is frequently the result of exposure to substances that injure the cochlea. Most ototoxins injure hair cells either directly or through disruption of other cochlear homeostatic mechanisms. In the vast majority of cases, ototoxic hearing loss stems from the use of medications such as aminoglycoside antibiotics (eg, gentamicin), loop diuretics (eg, furosemide), antineoplastic agents (eg, cisplatin), and salicylates (eg, aspirin). In industries with noisy work environments, workers who are being treated with potentially ototoxic medications are at increased risk, since the combination of ototoxic drug treatment and noise trauma can lead to a greater degree of hearing loss than either of these would produce by itself.

Patients with any type of preexisting sensorineural hearing loss, including noise-induced hearing loss, are considerably more susceptible to the ototoxic effects of medications.

Hearing loss may also result from exposure to ototoxic substances in the workplace. Heavy metals, including arsenic, cobalt, lead, lithium, mercury, and thorium, have documented ototoxic potential. Other chemicals that may be ototoxic include cyanide, benzene, aniline dyes, iodine, chlorophenothane, dimethyl sulfoxide, dinitrophenol, propylene glycol, methylmercury, potassium bromate, carbon disulfide, carbon monoxide, carbon tetrachloride, and industrial solvents such as styrene and toluene.

Prevention

Audiometric evaluation is appropriate to identify and monitor ototoxic exposure. Identification of patients at heightened risk of ototoxic hearing loss is important to avoid this complication. Persons with preexisting sensory hearing loss and compromised renal or hepatic function are at substantially increased risk.

Medicinal ototoxins should be administered in the lowest dose compatible with therapeutic efficacy. Serum peak and trough levels should be monitored to reduce the risk of excessive dosages. Simultaneous administration of multiple ototoxic drugs (eg, furosemide and an aminoglycoside antibiotic) should be avoided when possible to minimize synergistic effects.

MEDICOLEGAL ISSUES

Calculation of Percentage of Hearing Loss

Several methods for calculating the percentage of hearing loss are in widespread use.

The current method recommended by the American Academy of Otolaryngology (AAO) is as follows: (1) The average hearing threshold level at 500, 1000, 2000, and 3000 Hz should be calculated for each ear. (2) The percentage of the impairment for each ear (the monaural loss) should be calculated by multiplying by 1.5 times the amount by which the above average exceeds 25 dB (low fence) up to a maximum of 100%, which is reached at 92 dB (high fence). (3) The hearing handicap (binaural assessment) should then be calculated by multiplying the smaller percentage (better ear) by 5, adding this figure to the larger percentage (poorer ear), and dividing the total by 6.

The method recommended by the National Institute for Occupational Safety and Health (NIOSH) is the same as that of the AAO except that 500 Hz is not included in the calculation. This frequently yields a higher estimate of the percentage of hearing loss. This method was used by the US Department of Labor until February of 1986, at which time the AAO method was adopted.

For the above calculations to be valid, the audiometer employed must be checked daily and periodically calibrated by an independent agency. The booth used for testing must meet the standards of background noise levels established by the American National Standards Institute (ANSI) in 1977.

A note of caution is in order regarding the calculation of percentage of hearing loss based on older audiograms. Different standards for the measurement of hearing were in use prior to establishment of the current standard by the ANSI in 1969. From 1964 to 1969, the standard of the International Organization for Standardization (ISO) was used; this is essentially the same as the current ANSI standard, and no conversion is needed. However, from 1951 to 1964, the standard of the American Standards Association (ASA) was used, and audiograms obtained in this period will require conversion for use in the above formula. To convert an audiogram from the ASA to the ANSI standard, add 14 dB at 500 Hz, 10 dB at 1000 Hz, 8.5 dB at 2000 Hz, 8.5 dB at 3000 Hz, 6 dB at 4000 Hz, and 9.5 dB at 6000 Hz. If the 3000-Hz threshold was not measured in older audiograms, a 3-tone average of 500, 1000, and 2000 Hz may be substituted.

Assessment of Disability

As previously indicated, the normal range of speech reception threshold is between 0 and 20 dB, with losses of 20–40 dB termed "mild," 40–60 dB "moderate," 60–80 dB "severe," and greater than 80 dB "profound." Of course, the extent of disability suffered by the patient depends on many psychologic, social, and work-related factors. Disability is a relative term. Assessment of the ability of an individual to do his or her job requires knowledge about the various duties performed by that individual. Some typical work-related issues for consideration include the amount of communication with coworkers and others that is required on the job, the type of communication (eg, in person or via the telephone), and the need to hear alerting signals or emergency warning alarms.

To meet the Social Security Administration's guidelines for total disability due to hearing impairment, an individual must have either (1) an average hearing threshold of 90 dB or greater for the better-hearing ear, based on both air and bone conduction at 500, 1000, and 2000 Hz; or (2) a speech discrimination score of 40% or less in the better-hearing ear. In both cases, hearing must not be restorable by hearing amplification devices.

Compensation for Occupational Hearing Loss

An example of how occupational hearing loss is compensated is provided by the statistics of the US Department of Labor. In the fiscal year 1988, there were 5100 claims. The total cost to the federal government was $23,732,164, and the average per claimant was $4654. In cases of occupational hearing loss, the Department of Labor treats aggravated or accelerated hearing losses in the same manner as losses entirely precipitated or proximally caused by the patient's employment. In other words, the amount of preemployment hearing loss is not subtracted when the percentage of loss is calculated. In contrast, local and state government regulations frequently take into account the level of preexisting hearing loss and use formulas to correct for the anticipated progression of presbycusis when calculating compensation awards.

REFERENCES

American Academy of Otolaryngology Committee on Hearing and Equilibrium: Guide for the evaluation of hearing handicap. *JAMA* 1979;**242**:2055.

Berger EH et al (editors): *Noise and Hearing Conservation Manual.* American Industrial Hygiene Association, 1986.

Feldman AS, Grimes CT: *Hearing Conservation in Industry.* Williams & Wilkins, 1985.

Hamernik RP, Henderson D, Salvi R (editors): *New Perspectives in Noise-Induced Hearing Loss.* Raven Press, 1982.

Hughes GB: *Textbook of Clinical Otology.* Thieme, 1985.

Hyde M et al: Auditory evoked potentials in audiometric assessment of compensation and medicolegal patients. *Ann Otol Rhinol Laryngol* 1986;**95**:514.

Jackler RK: Facial, auditory, and vestibular injuries associated with basal skull fractures. In: *Textbook of Neurosurgery.* Youmans JR (editor). Saunders, 1988.

Katz J (editor): *Handbook of Clinical Audiology.* Williams & Wilkins, 1985.

Kramer MB, Armbruster JM (editors): *Forensic Audiology.* University Park Press, 1982.

Kryter KD: *The Effects of Noise on Man.* Academic Press, 1985.

Lim DJ: Effects of noise and ototoxic drugs at the cellular level in the cochlea: A review. *Am J Otolaryngol* 1986;**7**:73.

Miller HM, Silverman CA: *Occupational Hearing Conservation.* Prentice-Hall, 1984.

Miller JJ: *Handbook of Ototoxicity.* CRC Press, 1985.

Occupational Noise Exposure; Hearing Conservation Amendment; Final Rule: Department of Labor, Occupational Safety and Health Administration. Fed Reg 1983; **48**:9738.

Sataloff RT, Sataloff J: *Occupational Hearing Loss.* Marcel Dekker, 1987.

Smoorenburg GF: Damage risk criteria for impulse noise. Pages 471–490 in: *New Perspectives in Noise-Induced Hearing Loss.* Hamernik RP, Henderson D, Salvi R (editors). Raven Press, 1982.

11 Injuries Due to Physical Hazards

Richard Cohen, MD, MPH

This chapter discusses injuries associated with occupational exposure to extreme temperatures (cold and heat), electricity, radiation, changes in atmospheric pressure, and vibration. Hearing loss associated with exposure to noise is covered in Chapter 10.

HYPOTHERMIA (COLD INJURY)

Cold injuries can be categorized as systemic or localized and as freezing (eg, frostbite) or nonfreezing (eg, immersion foot). Factors influencing the risk for these injuries include the atmospheric or water temperature, humidity, wind velocity, duration of exposure, type of protective equipment or clothing, type of work being performed and energy expenditure associated with it, and age and health status of the worker.

Workers at risk include both indoor and outdoor workers exposed to cold, such as meat packers and others who work with freezers, construction workers, warehouse personnel, divers, mail carriers, fire fighters, and road maintenance workers. The risk is increased if the employee is elderly; is intoxicated with drugs or alcohol; is receiving medications such as barbiturates, phenothiazines, or reserpine; or has adrenal insufficiency, diabetes, myxedema, any neurologic disease affecting hypothalamic or pituitary function or causing peripheral sensory impairment, or any cardiovascular disease causing diminished cardiac output.

SYSTEMIC HYPOTHERMIA

Pathogenesis

Systemic hypothermia is reduction of the body's core temperature below 35 °C (95 °F). Hypothermia can occur at air temperatures up to 18.3 °C (65 °F) or in water up to 22.2 °C (72 °F).

When the body is exposed to cold environments, it has 2 types of normal physiologic reactions: (1) constriction of superficial blood vessels in the skin and subcutaneous tissue, resulting in heat conservation; and (2) increase in metabolic heat production through voluntary movement and by shivering. In cases of systemic hypothermia, physiologic functions are diminished. Oxygen consumption is decreased by about 7% per degree Celsius, myocardial repolarization is slowed, and ventricular fibrillation is a major hazard. In prolonged or slowly developing hypothermia (usually accompanied by physical exhaustion), hypoglycemia is probably due to glycogen depletion (hypoglycemia inhibits shivering).

Clinical Findings

The medical history should address the circumstances under which the patient was found, the probable duration of exposure, associated injuries or frostbite, preexisting medical conditions and problems with alcohol or drug abuse, and recent changes in the state of consciousness. Because body heat is lost more quickly when a person is wet, immersed in water, or exhausted, these factors should be considered.

The onset of hypothermia is often insidious, without any specific characteristics. With profound hypothermia, there is often diminished memory, a decrease or absence of shivering, and combativeness. Initial findings may include drowsiness, slurred speech, irritability, impaired coordination, general weakness and lethargy, recent diuresis, and puffy and cool skin and face.

Physical examination often reveals diminished neurologic reflexes, slow mental and muscular reactions, weak or nonpalpable pulse, arrhythmia, low blood pressure, and increased blood viscosity. With mild hypothermia (33–35 °C), there is extensive shivering which decreases as temperature subsides to 33 °C, wherein joint and muscle stiffness become more predominant.

Core temperature should be taken with a thermometer or thermocouple capable of measuring temperatures as low as 28 °C, and esophageal or deep rectal measurement (15 cm) is best. The temperature may range from 25 to 35 °C (77–95 °F). Below 35 °C, consciousness becomes dulled, causing disorientation, irrational thinking, forgetfulness, and hallucinations. Below 30 °C, semiconsciousness and confusion may occur. Nerve conduction is slowed, although the central nervous system is protected from ischemic damage. The respiratory rate falls to 7–12 per minute, and gastrointestinal motility slows or ceases. There may be hemoconcentration due to diuresis and loss of plasma volume. The latter occurs because of subcutaneous edema, which is accompanied by an elevation in corticosteroid levels. Loss of consciousness seldom occurs at temperatures above 28 °C.

Evaluation should also include a complete blood count; measurement of blood glucose, blood urea nitrogen, electrolytes, amylase, and alcohol and drug levels; urinalysis; urine volume; coagulation screen; sputum and blood cultures; thyroid function tests; arterial blood gas measurements with pH corrected for temperature (add 0.0147 pH unit for each degree under 37 °C); chest x-ray; and ECG. There may be evidence of metabolic acidosis, hypovolemia, elevation or depression of the blood glucose level, and renal failure. The ECG may show a pathognomonic J wave at the QRS–ST junction. The level of consciousness may worsen, and death may result from ventricular fibrillation or cardiac arrest.

Prevention

Hypothermia can be prevented by wearing clothing specially designed to resist wind and rain but also to allow water vapor generated by perspiration to escape. Overheating when strenuous work is required in extreme cold can be prevented by wearing a number of thin layers of clothing that can be removed or donned as necessary. Wet garments should be replaced as soon as possible with dry ones, and constrictive garments should not be worn.

Jobs should be designed so that workers remain relatively active when exposed to cold environments and provided with dry, wind-protected, heated shelters for tasks involving stationary work positions.

Outdoor workers should have heated rest facilities and hot food and hot drinks available. Work and break schedules should take into account the expected wind velocity and temperature and should follow the recommendations of the American Conference of Governmental Industrial Hygienists (ACGIH). Under high-risk weather conditions, workers should be under constant protective observation.

Workers exposed to the cold should be physically fit, without underlying vascular, metabolic, or neurologic diseases that place them at increased risk for hypothermia. They should be cautioned to avoid smoking and drug or alcohol use. New workers should be introduced into the work schedule slowly and instructed in the use of protective clothing, recognition of impending frostbite and early signs and symptoms of hypothermia, proper warming procedures, and first-aid treatment.

Treatment & Prognosis

In cases of mild hypothermia (rectal temperatures > 32 °C), patients who are young and otherwise healthy should be treated by rewarming in a warm bed or bath or with warm packs and blankets. Mildly hypothermic elderly or debilitated patients should be treated conservatively, using an electric blanket heated to 37 °C. Patients with severe hypothermia (temperatures < 32 °C) should be treated more aggressively by experienced personnel, and cardiac rhythm and rate should be monitored. Because the risk of death due to ventricular fibrillation is high with severe hypothermia (< 32 °C), treatment methods that may trigger fibrillation (eg, central catheters, cannulas, or tubes) should be avoided unless their use is essential. If CPR is instituted, it should be continued until the patient has been rewarmed to at least 36 °C. Evaluation for and treatment of localized areas of trauma and frostbite should be undertaken.

Measures should be instituted to correct acid-base deficiencies, normalize the serum potassium and blood glucose levels, increase the blood volume, maintain cardiac output and blood pressure, and provide adequate ventilation. Adequate cardiovascular support, acid-base balance, arterial oxygenation, and intravascular volume should be established prior to rewarming to minimize the risk of organ infarction. Oxygen administration should begin prior to rewarming. Because most arrhythmias revert spontaneously to normal sinus rhythm as the patient rewarms, it is usually not necessary to give antiarrhythmic agents unless there is a preexisting cardiac condition. Ventricular arrhythmias, however, should be treated as in a euthermic patient. Blood volume expansion with dextrose-saline solution, low-molecular-weight dextran, or albumin is recommended. Potassium-containing expanders should be avoided until the serum potassium levels have stabilized. Antibiotics should be given if infection is present. If myxedema is an underlying factor or if drug intoxication is present, appropriate treatment should be given. Localized areas of frostbite should be evaluated and managed as outlined below (see Hypothermia of the Extremities).

Use of steroids or antibiotics is not recommended unless otherwise clinically indicated. Core temperature should be monitored frequently during and after initial rewarming because of the potential for delayed, repeat hypothermia.

Although controversy exists concerning active external versus active internal rewarming methods for severe hypothermia, the latter is preferred. Treatment should increase in aggressiveness with decreasing core temperature, which in severe cases may call for both selected internal and external techniques.

Peritoneal dialysis with lactated Ringer's injection or saline solution at 43 °C exchanged at a rate of 10–12 L/h until the rectal temperature reaches 35 °C has been successful. Use of inhaled warm (37 °C) oxygen and warm water enemas provides a relatively safe but slower adjunct to peritoneal dialysis. Of less usefulness and perhaps greater risk are gastric and thoracic lavage. Slow warming of administered intravenous fluids (to 45 °C) has been recommended. Hemodialysis with the dialysate warmed to 37 °C has also been used for severe hypothermia.

Active external methods include heated blankets, warm baths, hot water bottles, "piped suits" (blankets containing pipes with hot water), radiant heaters, and hot wet packs. Warm bath water should be maintained at 40–42 °C; however, warm blankets may be preferable because diagnostic and other therapeutic maneuvers may be easier outside a bathtub. Ventricular fibrillation and hypovolemic shock ("rewarming shock") have been associated with active external rewarming. This risk can be reduced by heating only the trunk and providing appropriate intravenous volume expansion.

Passive rewarming (insulation from cold) is of value only for mildly hypothermic patients or as first-aid management on the scene. Hypothermia victims without vital signs should not be pronounced dead until they have been rewarmed to a core temperature of 36 °C and are found to be unresponsive to continued cardiopulmonary resuscitation at that temperature.

The prognosis is good for otherwise healthy patients but worsens with the presence of underlying predisposing problems or a delay in treatment.

HYPOTHERMIA OF THE EXTREMITIES

The cheeks, nose, earlobes, fingers, toes, hands, and feet are the areas most likely to develop ice crystals within the tissue, resulting in localized hypothermic injury. As skin temperature falls below 25 °C, tissue metabolism slows, although oxygen demand increases if work continues. There may be tissue damage at 15 °C due to ischemia and thrombosis and at –3 °C due to actual freezing of the tissue.

Immersion foot (trench foot) is caused by a combination of cold temperature and exposure to water. This problem and chilblains are nonfreezing injuries, whereas frostbite is a freezing injury. Predisposing factors for nonfreezing injuries include inadequate clothing and constricting garments. Those for frostbite include prior cold injuries, smoking, Raynaud's phenomenon, and collagen vascular disease.

Clinical Findings

A. Chilblains: Chilblains (red, itching skin lesions) may be associated initially with edema and blistering and then progress to ulcerative or hemorrhagic lesions, which can cause scarring, fibrosis, or atrophy.

B. Immersion Foot: There are 3 clinical stages: an ischemic stage, a hyperemic stage, and a posthyperemic recovery stage.

Initially, feet are cold, numb, swollen, and waxy white or cyanotic. Two to 3 days following removal from the cold, hyperemia occurs, along with intense pain, additional swelling, redness, heat, blistering, hemorrhage, lymphangitis, ecchymoses, and in some cases sequelae such as cellulitis, gangrene, or thrombophlebitis. After 10–30 days, intense paresthesias sometimes occur and are accompanied by cold sensitivity and hyperhidrosis, which may persist for years.

Tropical immersion foot occurring at higher temperatures is similar but usually has less intense symptoms with faster recovery.

C. Frostbite: In frostbite, freezing of superficial tissues usually causes symptoms of numbness, prickling, and itching. In severe cases, there may be paresthesias and stiffness. Skin is often white and edematous.

Prevention

Prevention is the same as for systemic hypothermia (see above).

Treatment

A. Chilblains and Immersion Foot: Treatment includes elevating the extremities, gradually rewarming them by exposure to air at room temperature, and protecting pressure sites from trauma. Massage and immersion should be avoided. Antibiotics are given if infection develops.

B. Frostbite: At the site of exposure, extremities can be rewarmed by removing wet gloves, socks, and shoes; drying the extremities and covering them again with dry clothing; and either elevating them or placing them next to a warmer part of the body (eg, placing the hands in the armpits). *Caution:* Rewarming should not be attempted if refreezing is likely prior to definitive therapy.

In cases of severe frostbite, hospitalization is recommended until the extent of tissue damage has been determined. The patient should be evaluated and treated, if necessary, for systemic hypothermia (see above).

Rapid rewarming of the frostbitten parts of the body can be accomplished by placing them in water heated to 40–42 °C and leaving them there until thawing is complete but no longer (often 30 minutes). Dry heat is not recommended, and external heat should be discontinued once normal temperature has been reached. The patient should remain in bed with the affected parts elevated and uncovered at room temperature. Frostbitten parts should not be exercised, rubbed, or exposed to pressure. Dressings and bandages should not be applied.

Infection can be treated with povidone-iodine soaks, water soaks, whirlpool therapy, systemic antibiotics, or a combination of these methods. Tetanus antitoxin or a tetanus toxoid booster may be indicated. Although anticoagulants have been recommended for prevention of thrombosis, their value has not been demonstrated.

Surgery should generally be avoided and amputation not considered until it is certain that the tissue is dead. Gangrenous and necrotic tissue should be treated by specialists.

Physical therapy can be instituted as healing progresses. The patient should be instructed to avoid exposure to the cold for several months and be advised of future hypersusceptibility to frostbite.

DISORDERS DUE TO HEAT

Five medical disorders can result from excessive exposure to hot environments (in order of decreasing severity): heat stroke, heat exhaustion, heat cramps, heat syncope, and skin disorders. Among the many types of workers at risk are smelters, steel workers, blast furnace operators, glassblowers, farmers, ranchers, fishermen, and construction workers.

A stable internal body temperature requires maintenance of a balance between heat production and loss, which the hypothalamus regulates by triggering changes in muscle tone, vascular tone, and sweat gland function. Production and evaporation of sweat are a major mechanism of heat removal. The transfer of heat from the skin to surrounding gas or liquid (convection) or between 2 solids in direct contact (conduction) may also occur, but this decreases in efficiency as ambient temperature increases. The passive transfer of heat via infrared rays from a warmer to a cooler object (radiation) accounts for 65% of body heat loss under normal conditions. Radiant heat loss also decreases as temperature increases up to 37.2 °C (99 °F), at which point heat transfer reverses. At normal temperatures, evaporation accounts for about 20% of body heat loss, but at excessive temperatures it becomes the most important means for heat dissipation. It, too, is limited as humidity increases and is ineffective at 100% relative humidity.

The scheduled and regulated exposure to heated environments of increasing intensity and duration (acclimatization) allows the body to adjust to heat by beginning to sweat at lower body temperatures, increasing the quantity of sweat produced, reducing the salt content of sweat, and increasing the plasma volume, cardiac output, and stroke volume while the heart rate decreases.

Health conditions that inhibit sweat production or evaporation and increase susceptibility to heat injury include obesity; skin disease; decreased cutaneous blood flow; dehydration; hypotension; cardiac disease resulting in reduced cardiac output; use of alcohol or medications that inhibit sweating, reduce cutaneous blood flow, or cause dehydration (eg, atropine, phenothiazines, tricyclic antidepressants, diuretics, laxatives, anticholinergics, antihistamines, monoamine oxidase inhibitors, vasoconstrictors, and beta blockers); and use of drugs that increase muscle activity and thereby increase the generation of body heat (eg, phencyclidine, LSD, amphetamines, cocaine, and lithium carbonate). Infections, cancer, malnutrition, and other medical conditions characterized by debilitation and poor physical condition can reduce the effectiveness of the sweating mechanism and circulatory response to heat. Age and sex also affect susceptibility to heat injury. Older people do not acclimatize as easily because of their reduced sweating efficiency, and women generally generate more internal heat than men when performing the same task.

HEAT STROKE

Heat stroke is a life-threatening medical emergency due to thermal regulatory failure manifested by cerebral dysfunction with altered mental status, hyperpyrexia, abnormal vital signs, and, usually, hot, dry skin. Heat stroke becomes imminent as the core (rectal) temperature approaches 106 °F (41.1 °C). It is most apt to occur following excessive exposure to heat; persons at greatest risk are nonacclimatized workers performing tasks that require strenuous exertion, the elderly, the chronically infirm, or those receiving medications (eg, anticholinergic) that compromise heat dissipation mechanisms. Morbidity or mortality can result from cerebral, cardiovascular, hepatic, or renal damage.

Clinical Findings

Thermal regulatory failure is characterized by dizziness, weakness, nausea, vomiting, confusion, delirium, and visual disturbances. Convulsions, collapse, or unconsciousness may occur. The skin is hot and initially covered with perspiration; later it dries. Blood pressure may be slightly elevated but becomes hypotensive. Core temperatures usually exceed 41 °C. As with heat exhaustion, hyperventilation can occur and lead to respiratory alkalosis and compensatory metabolic acidosis. There may also be abnormal bleeding, renal failure, or arrhythmias.

Laboratory evaluation may reveal an increase in leukocytes due to dehydration; decreased serum potassium, calcium, and phosphorus levels; increased blood urea nitrogen levels; hemoconcentration; decreased blood coagulation; and concentrated urine with proteinuria, tubular casts, and myoglobinuria. Thrombocytopenia, increased bleeding and clotting times, fibrinolysis, and consumptive coagulopathy may be present. Myocardial, liver, or renal damage may be reflected in laboratory tests.

Prevention

ACGIH has developed an index of threshold limit values for exposure to heat in occupational settings. The values are based on a formula that includes the natural wet bulb temperature, shielded dry bulb temperature, and black globe temperature, which are measurements that account for effects due to solar radiant heat, air velocity, relative humidity, and ambient temperature. Exposure limits take into account the type of work-rest regimen and the work load, including body position, movement, and limb use. These determine the heat load or metabolic rate, which is then related to the index to arrive at a recommended exposure standard for workers in a particular situation. The standards are based on the assumption that workers are acclimatized and physically fit, are wearing appropriate clothing, and are supplied with adequate water and food.

For additional information on the thermal comfort zone, see Chapter 6 and Fig 6–9.

In occupations in which workers are exposed to excessive heat, medical evaluation is recommended to identify individuals at increased risk for heat disorders due to preexisting medical conditions or use of medications. Exposed workers should be trained to recognize early signs and symptoms of heat disorders and should be advised of the importance of proper attire, nutrition, and fluid intake. Employers should provide cool drinking water and make sure that there are shaded rest areas close to the work site. For workers unacclimatized to heat, balanced electrolyte solutions or 1% saline drinking water should be made available. Salt tablets are not recommended because their use may exacerbate or cause electrolyte imbalance. Organized athletic events should be managed with attention to thermoregulation; the WBGT (wet bulb globe temperature) index should be monitored, water consumption should be encouraged, and medical care should be immediately accessible.

Treatment

Treatment is aimed at rapid (within 1 hour) reduction of the core temperature and control of secondary effects. Evaporative cooling provides rapid and effective lowering of temperature and is easily accomplished in most emergency settings. Until medical care becomes available, the patient should be moved to a shady, cool place. Clothing should be removed and the entire body sprayed with cool water (15 °C); cooled or ambient air should be blown across the patient at high velocity (100 ft/min). The patient should be placed in the lateral recumbent position or supported in the hands-to-knees position to expose more skin surface to the air.

The cooling process should continue in the hospital with use of cool water or 70% isopropyl alcohol sponge baths. Other alternatives include use of cold, wet sheets accompanied by fanning.

Immersion in an ice-water bath has often been recommended but is no longer preferred both because it is often not feasible and because of its greater potential for complications of hypotension and shivering. Other treatment alternatives include ice packs and iced gastric lavage, though these are much less effective than evaporative cooling. Treatment should continue until the core temperature drops to 39 °C. Because of the risks of hypoxia and aspiration, intubation should be considered and 100% oxygen administered until the patient is cooled. The temperature should continue to be monitored, though it usually remains stable after it has returned to normal. Chlorpromazine, 25–50 mg intravenously, can be used to control shivering and thus prevent an increase in heat. Aspirin should not be used as an antipyretic because of its effects on blood coagulation.

Patients should be monitored for hypovolemic and cardiogenic shock, either or both of which may occur. Attention should be paid to maintaining a patent airway, providing oxygen, correcting fluid and electrolyte imbalances, and supporting vital processes. Central venous or pulmonary artery wedge pressure should be assessed and intravenous fluids administered if indicated. If hypovolemic shock is suspected, 500–1000 mL of 5% dextrose in saline solution may be given intravenously without overloading the circulation. Other medications appropriate for cardiovascular support should be considered. Corticosteroids have not been demonstrated to be of value.

Fluid output should be monitored through the use of an indwelling urinary catheter. Complications such as renal, hepatic, or cardiac failure, hypotension, electrolyte imbalance, or coagulopathy should be treated appropriately.

Because hypersensitivity to heat continues in some patients for prolonged periods following heat stroke, they should be advised to avoid reexposure to heat for at least 4 weeks.

HEAT EXHAUSTION

In individuals performing strenuous work, prolonged exposure to heat and inadequate salt and water intake can cause heat exhaustion, dehydration, and sodium depletion or isotonic fluid loss with accompanying cardiovascular changes.

Symptoms and signs may include intense thirst, weakness, nausea, fatigue, headache, confusion, a core (rectal) temperature exceeding 38 °C (100.4 °F), increased pulse rate, and moist skin. Symptoms associated with both heat syncope and heat cramps (see below) may also be present. Hyperventilation sometimes occurs secondary to heat exhaustion and can lead to respiratory alkalosis. Progression to heat stroke is indicated by a rise in temperature or a decrease in sweating.

Treatment consists of placing the patient in a cool and shaded environment and providing hydration and salt replenishment—orally if the patient is able to swallow. Physiologic saline solution should be administered intravenously in more severe cases. At least 24 hours' rest is recommended.

HEAT CRAMPS

Heat cramps result from sodium depletion caused by replacement of sweat losses with water alone. They are usually characterized by slow and painful muscle contractions and severe muscle spasms that last from 1 to 3 minutes and involve the muscles employed in strenuous work.

The skin is moist and cool, and involved muscle groups feel like hard, stony lumps similar to billiard balls. The temperature may be normal or slightly increased, and blood tests may show low sodium levels and hemoconcentration. Because the thirst mechanism is intact, blood volume is not significantly diminished.

The patient should be moved to a cool environment and given a balanced salt solution or an oral saline solution consisting of 4 tsp of salt per gallon of water. Salt tablets are not recommended. Rest for 1–3 days with continued salt supplementation in the diet may be necessary before returning to work.

HEAT SYNCOPE

In heat syncope, sudden unconsciousness results from cutaneous vasodilatation with consequent systemic and cerebral hypotension. Episodes commonly occur following strenuous work for at least 2 hours.

The skin is cool and moist and the pulse weak. Systolic blood pressure is usually under 100 mm Hg.

Treatment consists of recumbency, cooling, and liquids by mouth. Preexisting medical conditions should be monitored and treated if necessary.

SKIN DISORDERS DUE TO HEAT

Miliaria (heat rash) is caused by sweat retention due to obstruction of the sweat gland duct. There are 3 forms, listed here in increasing order of severity: miliaria crystallina, miliaria rubra, and miliaria profunda. As the site of duct obstruction becomes deeper in the skin, the severity increases and presentation varies (eg, vesicles, erythema, desquamation, macules).

Erythema ab igne ("from fire") is characterized by the appearance of hyperkeratotic nodules following direct contact with heat that is insufficient to cause a burn.

Intertrigo results from excessive sweating and is often seen in obese individuals. Skin in the body folds (eg, the groin and axillas) is erythematous and macerated.

Heat urticaria (cholinergic urticaria) can be localized or generalized and is characterized by the presence of wheals with surrounding erythema ("hives").

Treatment for these disorders consists of reduction or removal of heat exposure, reduction of sweating, and control of symptoms. Antihistamines may help relieve pruritus in patients with urticaria. Corticosteroids are not beneficial.

THERMAL BURNS

CLASSIFICATION

Thermal burns are classified by extent, depth, patient age, and associated illness or injury.

Extent

The "rule of nines" (Fig 11–1) is useful for rapidly assessing the extent of a burn. Therefore, it is important to view the entire patient after cleaning soot to make an accurate assessment, both initially and on subsequent examinations. Only second- and third-degree burns are included in calculating the total burn surface area (TBSA), since first-degree burns usually do not represent significant injury in terms of prognosis or fluid and electrolyte management.

Depth

Judgment of depth of injury is difficult. The **first-degree burn** may be red or gray but will demonstrate excellent capillary refill. First-degree burns are not blistered initially. If the wound is blistered, this represents a partial-thickness injury to the dermis, or a **second-degree burn.** However, a deep second-degree burn may have lost its blister and may actually appear hyperemic from fixed hemoglobin in the tissue. This redness will not have good refill and will not be as exquisitely sensitive as the hyperemia of the first-degree burn. The line between the partial- and full-thickness injury, or **third-degree burn,** may be indefinite. The initial vasoconstriction of a second-degree burn may make it appear more severe at first. Concerning healing properties of any second- or third-degree burn, the critical factors are blood supply and appendage population. In areas rich

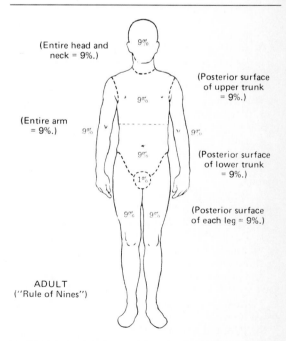

Figure 11–1. Estimation of body surface area in burns. (Reproduced, with permission, from Schroeder AS et al: *Current Medical Diagnosis & Treatment 1990.* Appleton & Lange, 1990.)

in vascularity, hair follicles, and sweat glands, the prospects for reepithelialization are good. Otherwise, even when the dermis is healthy, epithelialization may be slow and more scarring will result.

Age of the Patient

As much as extent and depth of the burn, age of the victim plays a critical part. Even a relatively small burn in an elderly patient or infant may be fatal.

Associated Injuries & Illnesses

An injury commonly associated with burns is smoke inhalation. The products of combustion, not heat, are responsible for lower airway injury. Burning plastic products produce both hydrochloric acid and hydrocyanic acid. Electrical injury that causes burns may also produce cardiac arrhythmias that require immediate attention. Premorbid physical and psychosocial disorders that complicate recovery from burn injury include cardiac or pulmonary disease, diabetes, alcoholism, drug abuse, and psychiatric illness.

Special Burn Care Units & Facilities

The American Burn Association and the American College of Surgeons have recommended that major burns be treated in specialized burn care facilities. They also advocate that even moderately severe burns be treated in a specialized facility or hospital where personnel have expertise in burn care. The American Burn Association has classified burn injuries as follows:

A. Major Burn Injuries:

1. Partial-thickness burns over more than 25% of body surface area in adults or 20% in children.

2. Full-thickness burns over more than 10% of surface area in any age group.

3. Deep burns involving the hands, face, eyes, ears, feet, or perineum.

4. Burns complicated by inhalation injury.

5. Electrical and chemical burns.

6. Burns complicated by fractures and other major trauma.

7. Burns in poor-risk patients (extremes of age or intercurrent disease).

B. Moderate Uncomplicated Burn Injuries:

1. Partial-thickness burns over 15–25% of body surface area in adults or 10–20% of body surface area in children.

2. Full-thickness burns over 2–10% of body surface area.

3. Burns not involving the specific conditions listed above.

C. Minor Burn Injuries:

1. Partial-thickness burns over less than 15% of body surface area in adults or 10% in children.

2. Full-thickness burns over less than 2% of body surface area.

INITIAL MANAGEMENT

Airway

The physician or emergency medical technician should proceed as with any other trauma. The first priority is to establish an airway, then to evaluate the cervical spine and head injuries, and then to stabilize fractures. *The burn wound itself has a lower priority.* At some point during the initial management, endotracheal intubation should be considered for most major burn cases, regardless of the area of the body involved, for as fluid resuscitation proceeds, generalized edema develops, including the soft tissues of the upper airway and perhaps the lungs as well. *Tracheostomy is rarely indicated for the burn victim,* unless dictated by other circumstances. Inhalation injuries should be followed by serial blood gas determination and bronchoscopy. The use of corticosteroids is not recommended because of the potential for immunosuppression.

Cooling the Wound

Cooling the victim for up to 20 minutes following the burn has been shown to reduce the depth of injury. Avoid prolonged application of cold water or ice packs to large surfaces, however, since they can cause systemic hypothermia and arrhythmias. Saline soaks at room temperature or cooler should be used. At the scene of an injury, a hose can be used for this purpose. Fire extinguishers and ice are not recommended, as further tissue injury may result.

History

As soon as possible, obtain a detailed history of the circumstances of the injury, including locale, substances involved, and duration of exposure; medications, mental disturbances, confusion resulting from the injury, or the presence of an endotracheal tube may later prevent the recording of an accurate history.

Vascular Access

Simultaneously with the above procedures, venous access must be sought, since the victim of a major burn is in hypovolemic shock. Ideally, a percutaneous intravenous line through nonburned skin is preferred. A peripheral line in an antecubital or subclavian vein is preferable to the femoral vein unless the femoral area is the only nonburned area. The last choice is to perform a well-secured peripheral cutdown. A burn eschar, since it has been flame-sterilized, is an acceptable location for cutdown. An arterial line may also be useful for monitoring mean arterial pressure. The line may be placed initially in the femoral artery and later changed (as peripheral resistance decreases) to a safer site such as the dorsalis pedis, temporal, or radial arteries. Swan-Ganz catheters should be used in patients with preexisting cardiopulmonary disease and in severe burn cases to determine cardiac output and peripheral resistance. Once these parameters have been established, the catheter is usually removed.

FLUID RESUSCITATION

Crystalloids

Generalized capillary leak results from burn injury over more than 25% of the total body surface area. This often necessitates replacement of a large volume of fluid. An intravenous line is recommended in the management of deep partial-thickness and full-thickness burns that cover more than 20% of total body surface area in the adult and 10% in the child.

There are many guidelines for fluid resuscitation, eg, those of Evans, Brooke, Monafo (hypertonic saline), and Parkland (Baxter). In the first 24 hours, all of these fluids deliver approximately 0.5–0.6 meq of sodium per kilogram of body weight per percent of body surface area burned. The total amount of fluid in all but the hypertonic saline formula is roughly the same but differs in distribution. The Parkland formula is currently the most widely used in the USA. It relies upon the use of lactated Ringer's injection, which is available in every emergency room. For adults and children, the fluid requirement in the first 24 hours is estimated as 3–5 mL/kg body weight per percent of body surface area burned (Fig 11–2). The smaller amounts would be used in the elderly or those with less severe burns; the larger amounts would be used in children (who have a larger relative surface-to-volume ratio) and for treatment of deep electrical burns. Four mL/kg body weight per percent of body surface area burned is begun and this amount is varied according to the patient's response. *Remember that a formula is only a guideline.*

Half the calculated fluid is given in the first 8-hour period. The remaining fluid, divided into 2 equal parts, is delivered over the next 16 hours. An extremely large volume of fluid may be required. For example, an injury over 40% of the total body surface area in a 70-kg victim may require 13 L *in the first 24 hours*. The first 8-hour period is calculated from the hour of injury.

Colloids

After 24 hours, capillary leaks have sealed in the majority of cases, and plasma volume may be restored with colloids (plasma or albumin). The Parkland formula calls for 0.3–0.5 mL/kg body weight per percent of body surface area burned to be given over the first 8-hour period of the second 24 hours. Fluids given in the following 16 hours consist of dextrose in water in quantities sufficient to maintain adequate urine output (Fig 11–3). It is hoped that during the second 24-hour period the vascular system will hold colloids and draw off edema fluid, resulting in diuresis.

Adequacy of Resuscitation

Mental alertness, urinary output, and the vital signs reflect the adequacy of fluid resuscitation. Mental alertness is important because it is the best indicator of adequate cerebral perfusion. Overmedication may cloud the sensorium during the resuscitation phase. Analgesics in the form of small doses of intravenous morphine should be used judiciously so as not to interfere with diagnosis. Renal perfusion is judged by urinary output. Adequate urinary output is 30–50 mL/h in adults and 1 mL/kg body weight/h in children. A smaller output represents inadequate renal perfusion. However, a larger output is unnecessary, and overloading results in edema in every organ.

Monitoring Fluid Resuscitation

A Foley catheter is essential for monitoring urinary output. *Diuretics have no part in this phase of patient management,* although the use of mannitol may be indicated in the resuscitation of an electrical burn

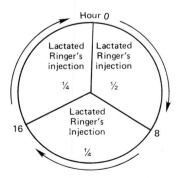

Figure 11–2. Half of the calculated crystalloid formula (lactated Ringer's injection [4 mL/kg wt/% TBSA]) is given in the first 8 hours, beginning at the time of the injury. The remainder is given evenly over the ensuing 16 hours.

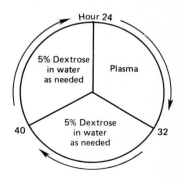

Figure 11–3. The colloid formula (aged plasma or 5% normal serum albumin, [0.3–0.5 mL/kg wt/% TBSA]) is given as calculated between hours 24 and 32. In the remaining 16-hour period, 5% dextrose in water is given as needed to maintain a urinary output of no less than 30 mL/h.

victim in whom myoglobin in the urine may precipitate in the kidneys.

Escharotomy

As edema fluid accumulates, ischemia may develop under any constricting eschar of an extremity. Similarly, an eschar of the thorax or abdomen may limit respiratory excursion. Escharotomy incisions through the anesthetic eschar can save life and limb.

THE BURN WOUND

Treatment of the burn wound is based on several principles: (1) Prevention or delay of infection. (2) Protection from desiccation and further injury of those burned areas that will spontaneously reepithelialize in 7–10 days. (3) Excision and grafting of burned areas that cannot spontaneously reepithelialize during this period.

Systemic Prophylactic Antibiotics

Regardless of the severity of the burn, prophylactic systemic antibiotics are usually not recommended. Their effectiveness is unproved, and they have the disadvantage of favoring the growth of resistant organisms.

Topical Antibiotics

Topical antibiotics delay or prevent infection. An ideal agent would readily penetrate the burn wound eschar, be effective against both gram-negative and gram-positive microorganisms as well as *Candida*, be painless and inexpensive, and have no deleterious side effects. Such an ideal agent does not currently exist. Silver sulfadiazine (Silvadene) is currently the most popular topical agent. It is painless, easy to apply, effective against most *Pseudomonas*, and a fairly good penetrator of eschar, but some microorganisms are resistant to it, and it may cause leukopenia or fever and delay epithelialization.

Mafenide (Sulfamylon) penetrates eschars better than silver sulfadiazine and is more effective against *Pseudomonas*. Mafenide inhibits carbonic anhydrase when used as a 10% solution and results in metabolic acidosis. It also delays epithelialization and may be painful. When it is diluted to a 5% solution, pain and metabolic side effects are lessened. It is useful primarily for deep burns, eg, electrical burns and burns of the ear or nose where cartilage is close to the surface, and when silver sulfadiazine is ineffective. It is best to limit the use of mafenide to no more than 10% of the total body surface area at any given time because of its metabolic effect.

Povidone-iodine is especially useful against *Candida* and both gram-positive and gram-negative microorganisms. However, it penetrates eschar poorly, is very desiccating to the wound surface, and is painful. Also, significantly high blood iodine levels have been demonstrated in patients receiving this agent.

Gentamicin and silver nitrate are no longer recommended as topical agents.

Wound Closure

The goal of therapy after fluid resuscitation is closure of the wound. Nature's own blister is the best cover to protect wounds that spontaneously epithelialize in 7–10 days (ie, superficial second-degree burns). The serum in the blister nurses the surface of the **zone of stasis** until epithelialization takes place (Fig 11–4). Where the blister has been disrupted, human amnion, porcine heterografts (preferably fresh, or frozen and meshed), or collagen composite dressings (Biobrane) can substitute. Cadaver homografts can also serve this purpose if available.

Wounds that will not heal spontaneously in 7–10 days (ie, deep second-degree or third-degree burns) are best treated by excision and autograft; otherwise, granulation and infection may develop. Granulation is nature's signal that attempts to close the wound have failed. A "skin equivalent"—a patient's own skin cells grown in culture into multilayered sheets of epithelium—is currently being tested in some burn centers.

PATIENT SUPPORT

During the wound closure phase, the patient must be supported in many ways. Most important is adequate nutrition. Enteral feedings may begin once the ileus of the resuscitation period is relieved, which usually coincides with the subsidence of edema. The

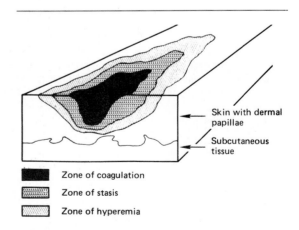

Skin with dermal papillae

Subcutaneous tissue

▉ Zone of coagulation

▨ Zone of stasis

▧ Zone of hyperemia

Figure 11–4. The burn wound has 3 general zones of tissue death. The zone of necrosis or coagulation involves irreversible skin death. The intermediate zone of capillary stasis is vulnerable to desiccation and infection that can convert potentially salvageable tissue to full-thickness destruction and irreversible skin death. There is minimal cell involvement in the outermost hyperemic zone. (Modified from Zawacki BE: Reversal of capillary stasis and prevention of necrosis in burns. *Ann Surg* 1974;**180**:98. Redrawn, with permission, from Artz CP, Moncrief JA, Pruitt BA: *A Team Approach.* Saunders, 1979.)

large nasogastric sump tube used to decompress stomach contents during resuscitation may now be replaced with a smaller, preferably soft Silastic tube. This will aid in delivering large quantities (4000–6000 kcal/d) that may be required during the wound closure period. The metabolic demands are immense. A useful guide is to provide 25 kcal/kg body weight plus 40 kcal per percent of burn surface area. Fat emulsions (Intralipid) given intravenously are useful during the resuscitation period to span the period of ileus.

Many enteral formulas are available. Eggs are a readily available source of protein and calories and are well tolerated by the patient. In many cases, more than 30 eggs per day are desirable. Early enteral feedings reduce the need for antacids and lessen the likelihood of development of Curling's ulcer, a life-threatening complication of burn injury. Gastric pH and hourly antacid delivery should be monitored during the resuscitation phase. Cimetidine may be used to reduce acid production; however, undesirable side effects such as leukopenia and confusion in the elderly may result.

Pain plays a major role during the wound closure phase. The patient is more aware of pain during dressing changes and postsurgical periods. Hydrotherapy aids in dressing removal and joint range of motion, but it can be a source of wound contamination. Analgesics are essential, but overuse or underuse may be harmful.

The Burn Team

The burn team consists of a group of highly skilled professionals—nurses, dietitians, physical therapists, occupational therapists, and counselors—who work closely with the physician in providing comprehensive services for the victim from the period of intensive care through recovery and rehabilitation. Careful attention is given to the complex problems encountered during the intensive care and recovery periods, including fluid and electrolyte abnormalities, infection, physical discomfort, malnutrition, immobility, and psychologic suffering.

The residual physical and emotional problems in burn patients, eg, body disfigurement, impaired mobility, persistent itching, decreased ability to perspire, decreased skin sensitivity, and impairment of sexual enjoyment, require long-term committed care.

ELECTRICAL INJURIES

Electrical accidents comprise up to 4% of all fatal industrial accidents. Electricians, operators of high-power electric equipment and power generators, and maintenance personnel are at greatest risk for electric shock.

Physical contact with an energized electric circuit provides a pathway for electricity to traverse the body as it seeks a ground. Conductivity to the body is affected by skin moisture as well as moisture on contacting surfaces (eg, floors). Factors influencing the severity of electrical injury include the voltage (electrical force), amperage (current intensity), current type (alternating or direct current), duration of contact, area of contact, pathway of the current through the body, and amount of tissue resistance.

Electricity from alternating currents is more dangerous than that from direct currents. The alternating currents usually cause muscle tetanization and sweating, while the direct currents cause electrolytic changes in tissue. Most tissue damage is related to the heat produced by the electric current, and tissue resistance is largely influenced by the water content of the tissue. The vascular system and muscles are good conductors of electricity, while the bones, peripheral nerves, and dry skin have higher resistance.

A sudden exposure to intense electrical energy can cause not only tissue destruction and necrosis from heat and burning but also depolarization of electrically sensitive tissues such as nerve and heart. Alternating currents with voltages and frequencies as low as domestic circuits (100 V and 60 Hz) can produce ventricular fibrillation. High voltages can cause respiratory paralysis. Most shocks involving currents exceeding 10,000 V are of such magnitude that the electrical force knocks the victim away from the power source, which minimizes the electrical injury potential but sometimes causes blunt trauma.

A tetanizing effect of voluntary muscles is greatest at frequencies between 15 and 150 cycles. Sustained grasp of the conductor does not usually occur at high voltages, because the circuit probably arcs before contact with the victim, who is thrown back instead. Current above 20 mA can cause sustained contraction of chest respiratory muscles; currents above 30–40 mA can induce ventricular fibrillation.

Clinical Findings

Exposure to electric current can cause shock, flash burns, flame burns, or direct tissue necrosis. Surface wounds covering heat-induced tissue necrosis are usually round or oval and well-demarcated, and they may have a relatively innocuous appearance. A search must be made for both the entry and the exit wound to determine the electrical pathway through the body. Depending on the contact site and the pathway, there may be damage to nerves, muscles, or major organs such as the heart, brain, eye, kidney, or gastrointestinal tract. Technetium stannous pyrophosphate scintigraphy can identify areas of significant muscle damage. In all cases, an ECG with a rhythm strip should be obtained, and the respiratory rhythm and rate should be checked. If organ, muscle, or nerve damage is suspected, appropriate diagnostic tests should be ordered such as urine myoglobin. Occult fractures may occur following muscle tetany or blunt trauma. Patients should be observed for several days, because some develop posttraumatic myositis with rhabdomyolysis.

Electrical injury causes increased vascular permeability, which may result in reduced intravascular volume and fluid extravasation in the area of internal injury. Hematocrit, plasma volume, and urine output should be monitored closely.

Acute- and delayed-onset central and peripheral nervous system complications are the most common sequelae of electrical injury. Cardiac complications usually consist of rhythm and conduction abnormalities, with rare infarction. Sepsis and psychiatric complications also occur.

Prevention

Electrical injuries can be prevented in industrial settings by making sure that electrical workers are properly qualified and trained to follow safety procedures involving the installation, grounding, and disconnection of power sources. Particular attention should be given to work requiring equipment manipulation during "live" operation. Nonconducting tools and clothing should be used whenever possible. Barricades and warning signs should be placed around high-voltage areas, and procedures to exclude other employees from these areas should be strictly enforced.

Workers should be instructed in the proper measures to free a victim from contact with the electrical current. If possible, the power should be turned off. If not, a nonconducting object such as a rope, a broom or other wooden instrument, or an article of clothing can be used to pull the victim away from the current and protect the rescuer from injury. If necessary, cardiopulmonary resuscitation should be instituted until medical help arrives. Because the victim may have suffered spinal injury, extreme care must be taken during handling or transport.

Treatment

First aid consists of freeing the victim from contact with the current. The rescuer must be protected during this procedure.

If major electrical injuries are suspected, the patient should be hospitalized and observed for secondary organ damage, impaired renal function, hemorrhage, acidosis, and myoglobinuria. A tetanus booster or antitoxin should be administered if indicated.

Superficial tissue damage should be treated conservatively and the patient observed for sepsis, which is the most common cause of death in electric shock survivors. For severe burns, a topical antibiotic (eg, mafenide or silver sulfadiazine) is applied. If major soft tissue damage is suspected, surgical exploration, fasciotomy, or both must be considered.

Lactated Ringer's injection should be administered at a rate sufficient to maintain urine output between 50 and 100 mL/h. With major muscle necrosis, mannitol can enhance hemochrome excretion. Continuous monitoring and prompt correction of acid-base or electrolyte imbalance are necessary if rhabdomyolysis occurs.

NONIONIZING RADIATION INJURIES

INJURIES DUE TO RADIOFREQUENCY & MICROWAVE RADIATION

Exposure

Injuries due to the thermal effects of acute exposure to high levels of radiofrequency and microwave radiation have been documented. Like other thermal injuries, these injuries are characterized by protein denaturation and tissue necrosis at the site of thermal exposure, with an accompanying inflammatory reaction and subsequent scar formation. Nonthermal effects of low-level exposure have been demonstrated in some laboratory studies, but their significance in humans is not clear.

Radiofrequency (RF) radiation and microwave radiation consist of energy in wave form traveling in free space at the speed of light. The radiation is defined in terms of frequency and intensity, with the frequency portion of the electromagnetic spectrum extending from 0 to 1000 GHz (1 Hz equals 1 wave or cycle per second [cps]). Microwaves occupy only a portion of the frequency spectrum, ie, the portion between 300 MHz and 300 GHz (Fig 11–5).

RF radiation has insufficient energy to cause molecular ionization, but it does cause vibration and rotation of molecules, particularly molecules that have an asymmetric charge distribution or are polar in structure. It is composed of separate electric and magnetic field vectors, each perpendicular to the other and both perpendicular to the direction of the resultant electromagnetic wave (Fig 11–6). The electric field component is measured in volts per meter, the magnetic component in amperes per meter, and the resultant power density in watts per square meter.

Absorption of radiofrequency radiation is dependent upon the orientation of the body in relation to the direction of the electromagnetic wave. Radiation at frequencies below 15 MHz and above 25 GHz is poorly absorbed and unlikely to cause significant thermally induced damage. Factors affecting conduction of radiofrequency radiation within the body include the thickness, distribution, and water content of the various tissues. As the water content increases, energy absorption and thermal effects increase. Radiofrequency radiation can be modulated according to amplitude (AM) and frequency (FM) and can be generated in pulsed or continuous form. Pulsed waves are considered more dangerous.

The risk of injury increases with higher intensities of radiation and closer proximity to the radiation

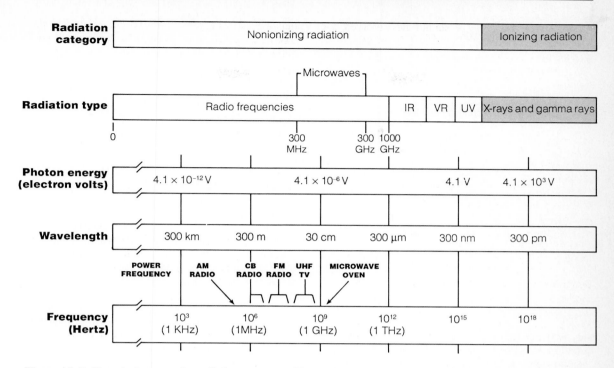

Figure 11–5. The electromagnetic radiation spectrum. IR = infrared radiation; VR = visible radiation (light); UV = ultraviolet radiation.

source. Other factors that affect human susceptibility to radiofrequency radiation injury include environmental humidity and temperature, grounding, reflecting medium, tissue vascularity, increased temperature sensitivity of tissues (eg, the testes), and lack of anatomic barriers to external radiation (eg, the eye).

Occupational exposures are likely in any workplace where employees are near equipment that generates radiofrequency radiation, particularly equipment for dielectric heating (used in sealing of plastics and drying of wood), physiotherapy, radiocommunications, radiolocation, and maintenance of aerial transmitters and high-power electrical equipment (Table 11–1). Injuries have been documented for acute exposure to energy levels exceeding 10 mW/cm^2. In most cases, the levels were greater

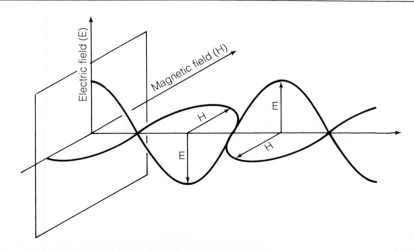

Figure 11–6. Electric field (E) and magnetic field (H) components of radiofrequency radiation.

Table 11–1. Occupational radiofrequency and microwave exposures.

Sealing and heating equipment
    Automotive trades
        Furniture and woodworking
        Glass fiber production
        Paper production
        Plastics manufacturing and fabrication
        Rubber product heating
        Textile manufacturing

Communication equipment source maintenance
    Radar
        Radio: AM, FM, CB
        Television: UHF and VHF
        Satellite
        Radio navigation

RF applications
    Microwave tube testing and aging
        RF laser
        RF welding
        Medical diathermy and healing promotion

Power transmission line workers

---

than 100 mW/cm^2. Most studies of radiofrequency radiation effects in animals and other biologic test systems have not demonstrated thermally induced effects at energy levels below 10 mW/cm^2.

Generally, acute high-level or long-term low-level exposures are not thought to cause cancer, but there is some evidence for carcinogenesis in association with exposure to extremely low frequency radiation ($<$ 200 Hz). There have been reports of increased incidence of brain tumors, malignant melanoma, and leukemia in workers exposed to extremely low-frequency electromagnetic radiation. Similarly, teratogenicity is being questioned on the basis of findings of chromosomal breaks in power station workers, an increase in the incidence of neuroblastomas found in offspring of fathers exposed to electromagnetic radiation, and an increase in the incidence of anomalies found in offspring of male physical therapists. Although concern has been expressed concerning cataract formation following long-term low-level exposure, scientific evidence is lacking.

Clinical Findings

Acute high-dose exposure is usually associated with a feeling of warmth on the exposed body part, followed by the feeling of hot or burning skin. The sensation of clicking or buzzing may also be present during the exposure. Other symptoms include irritability, headache or light-headedness, vertigo, pain at the site of exposure, watery eyes and a gritty eye sensation, dysphagia, anorexia, abdominal cramps, and nausea. Localized thermally induced masses may appear within days after exposure and consist of interstitial edema and coagulation necrosis.

The exposed skin has a sunburned appearance, with erythema and slight induration. There may be vesiculation or bullae. Blood pressure may be increased, and creatine phosphokinase levels may be elevated. Hematologic values, electroencephalographic and brain scan findings, sedimentation rate, and electrolyte values are usually within normal limits.

Beyond the immediately evident thermal injury, no further structural injury would be anticipated. In one case report, essential hypertension developed 1–3 months following exposure and then resolved with treatment. Symptoms of posttraumatic stress disorder have occurred, with emotional lability and insomnia persisting for as long as 1 year.

Differential Diagnosis

High-power equipment capable of generating radiofrequency and microwave radiation might also generate other forms of nonionizing radiation that should be considered in the differential diagnosis. Chemical reactions due to heat sources in the workplace should be investigated, because thermal decomposition products of a heated hydrocarbon can cause the acute onset of similar symptoms, although blood pressure and creatine phosphokinase levels would not be expected to rise in such circumstances. Fear and anxiety resulting from the knowledge of a possibly damaging exposure may also cause many of the functional symptoms described above, although objective evidence of thermal injury and elevated creatine phosphokinase levels would not be expected.

Prevention

Exposure assessment should include the following factors: the distance between the power source and exposed workers, the peak power density at the time of exposure, the radiofrequency and type of radiation wave (pulsed or continuous), and the duration of exposure (in minutes).

Metal barriers around the energy source can be used to contain radiofrequency radiation. Because of the rapid decrease in power density over distance, specification of a ''personnel not allowed'' area can also provide an effective barrier. Procedures to de-energize equipment are recommended when employees are working close to exposed sources. Protective clothing is generally not effective. Periodic environmental radiofrequency radiation measurements for equipment exposures are essential.

Treatment & Prognosis

Treatment is the same as for other thermal injuries and includes immediately removing the worker from exposure, cooling the wound with saline soaks, cleaning and debriding tissue if necessary, and applying a topical antibiotic (eg, mafenide or silver sulfadiazine). Future exposure to radiation should be rigorously controlled to below recommended limits.

Thermal injuries usually heal without problems. If hypertension develops, it will usually resolve following a short course of antihypertensive therapy. Posttraumatic stress disorder and other psychologic sequelae are generally responsive to short-term supportive psychotherapy.

INJURIES DUE TO INFRARED RADIATION

Infrared radiation covers the portion of the electromagnetic spectrum between visible and radiofrequency radiation (Fig 11–5). It has wavelengths between 750 and 3 million nm and is composed of 3 spectral bands—A, B, and C—which begin at 750 nm, 1400 nm, and 3000 nm, respectively. Infrared radiation is given off from any object having a temperature greater than absolute zero. Occupational exposures—in addition to sunlight—include processes in which thermal energy from infrared radiation is used, such as heating and dehydrating processes, welding, glassmaking, and the drying and baking of coatings on consumer products.

Acute, high-intensity exposure to wavelengths shorter than 2000 nm can cause thermal damage to the cornea, iris, or lens. Thermal injury to the skin can also occur, but it is usually self-limited and results in an acute skin burn with increased pigmentation. There have been reports that exposure to infrared radiation was associated with cataract formation, particularly among glassblowers and furnace workers.

Injuries can be prevented by shielding heat sources, using protective eye and skin wear, and monitoring exposure levels. Threshold limit values for exposure intensity are frequency-dependent in the biologically active wavelength spectrum of 750–2000 nm. Wavelengths in this range cause molecular excitation and vibration, resulting in heat that is absorbed by tissues and can cause thermal injury. In contrast, wavelengths exceeding 2000 nm are absorbed by water and are not biologically active because of the high water content of tissues.

INJURIES DUE TO VISIBLE RADIATION

Visible radiation (light) covers the portion of the electromagnetic spectrum between infrared and ultraviolet radiation (Fig 11–5) and the wavelengths between 400 and 750 nm. The eye is the most sensitive target organ, with damage resulting from structural, thermal, or photochemical light-induced reactions. Workers at risk are those with prolonged or repeated exposure to intense light sources, including sunlight, high-intensity lamps, lasers, flashbulbs, spotlights, and welding arcs. Extremely intense light sources such as lasers can also cause pressure-induced (mechanical) retinal damage.

The retina is the usual site of injury and is most sensitive to the wavelengths of 440–500 nm (blue light), which cause a destructive photochemical reaction. Blue light is responsible for solar retinitis (eclipse blindness) and may contribute to retinal aging and to senile macular degeneration, which can result in visual field defects. Because the lens normally filters out wavelengths between 320 and 500

nm, it provides some protection of the retina from blue light. Individuals with aphakia (absence of the lens), who are more susceptible to retinal damage, should be cautioned against looking into the midday sun and other intense light sources and urged to wear spectacle filters when working in bright environments.

Short bursts of high-intensity light can cause heat-induced flash blindness, in which the temporary visual loss and afterimage are due to bleaching of visual pigments. As the light intensity and exposure duration increase, the afterimage persists longer. With mild to moderate exposures, symptoms of flash blindness resolve quickly.

Insufficient lighting or reflected light (glare) can cause asthenopia (eyestrain), visual fatigue, headache, and eye irritation. These problems are more likely to occur in people over the age of 40 years. Symptoms are transient, and there is no indication that repeated episodes lead to ocular damage.

Contrast from surrounding light sources on areas of lesser intensity has led to complaints of asthenopia associated with video display terminal use. This can usually be corrected by decreasing surrounding light intensities, using antiglare filters, and adjusting the contrast of the light on the screen.

Treatment of eye injuries is discussed in Chapter 9. Measures to prevent injury in workers at risk include preemployment evaluations for individuals with aphakia or a history of light sensitivity and medical surveillance to detect changes in visual acuity or early signs of ocular damage; use of goggles or face shields by welders; proper illumination of the workplace to reduce glare (see Chapter 6); and use of filters on intense light sources to eliminate blue light wavelengths.

INJURIES DUE TO ULTRAVIOLET RADIATION

Ultraviolet (UV) radiation covers the portion of the electromagnetic spectrum between visible radiation and ionizing radiation (Fig 11–5) and has wavelengths between 100 and 400 nm. The wavelengths are divided into 3 bands—A, B, and C—with the A and B bands representing the longer wavelengths and producing most of the biologic effects. Wavelengths shorter than 200 nm are biologically inactive; they can exist only in a vacuum or an inert gas atmosphere and are absorbed over extremely short distances in air. Wavelengths of 200–290 nm are absorbed primarily in the stratum corneum of the skin or the cornea of the eye, while the longer wavelengths can affect the dermis, lens, iris, or retina.

Because UV radiation has relatively poor penetration, the only organs it affects are the eye and skin. Eye injury is caused by thermal action from pulsed or brief high-power exposures, and skin damage more commonly by photochemical reactions (including toxic and hypersensitivity reactions) from brief high or extended low-power exposures. The thermal effects of protein coagulation and tissue necrosis are rapid in onset. The effects of chronic exposure include accelerated aging of the skin, characterized by loss of elasticity, hyperpigmentation, wrinkling, and telangiectasia.

UV injuries occur in occupations involving drying and curing processes, arc welding, or use of lasers or germicidal UV lights (Table 11–2), but by far the greatest proportion of injuries result from occupations that expose workers to natural sunlight during the peak time of UV energy dissemination, 10 AM to 3 PM. Factors affecting the severity of injury include exposure duration, radiation intensity, distance from the radiation source, and orientation of the exposed individual relative to the source and its wave propagation plane. UV reflections from water and snow or their surrounding surfaces may increase exposure intensity.

Clinical Findings & Treatment

A. Photokeratoconjunctivitis ("Welder's Flash"): Ocular exposure to UV wavelengths shorter than 315 nm (especially wavelengths of 270 nm, to which the eye is most sensitive) can cause photokeratoconjunctivitis. Symptoms occur 6–12 hours after exposure and include severe pain, photophobia, a sensation of a foreign body or sand in the eyes, and tearing. After a latency period that varies inversely with the severity of the exposure, conjunctivitis appears, sometimes accompanied by erythema and swelling of the eyelids and facial skin. Slit lamp examination may reveal diffuse punctate staining of both corneas.

Treatment consists of providing symptomatic relief, which may include ice packs, systemic analgesics, eye patches, and mild sedation. Local anesthetics should not be used because of the risk of further injury to the anesthetized eye.

Symptoms usually resolve within 48 hours. Permanent sequelae are rare, and the eye does not develop tolerance to repeated exposure.

B. Cataracts: Cataractogenesis has been attributed to both photochemical and thermal effects of intense exposure to UV wavelengths of 295–320 nm and usually appears within 24 hours. Cataract formation following repeated exposures to UV wavelengths longer than 324 nm has been reported but is not well-documented. Treatment is by cataract extraction and, usually, intraocular lens implantation.

C. Other Eye Injuries: The lens protects the retina from the effects of UV wavelengths shorter than 300 nm, but damage to the iris and retina is possible if individuals with aphakia are exposed to these wavelengths. In others, damage is possible with exposure to longer wavelengths or to high-power UV lasers. Treatment is supportive.

Two lesions of the bulbar conjunctiva have been associated with repeated exposures to UV radiation: pterygium (a benign hyperplasia) and epidermoid carcinoma.

Table 11–2. Workers potentially exposed to ultraviolet radiation.[1]

Natural sunlight

Agricultural workers	Oil field workers
Brick masons	Open pit miners
Ranchers	Outdoor maintenance workers
Construction workers	Pipeline workers
Farmers	Police officers
Fishermen	Postal carriers
Gardeners	Railroad track workers
Greenskeepers	Road workers
Horticultural workers	Sailors
Landscapers	Ski instructors
Lifeguards	Sports professionals
Lumberjacks	Surveyors
Military personnel	

Arc welding ultraviolet
Welders
Pipeline workers
Pipecutters
Maintenance workers

Plasma torch ultraviolet
Plasma torch operators

Germicidal ultraviolet
Physicians
Nurses
Laboratory technicians
Bacteriology laboratory personnel
Barbers
Cosmetologists
Kitchen workers

Laser ultraviolet
Laboratory workers

Drying and curing processes
Printers
Lithographers
Painters
Wood curers
Plastics workers

[1]Reproduced, with permission, from Adams RM: *Occupational Skin Disease*. 2nd ed. Saunders, 1989.

D. Erythema: Absorbed UV radiation reacts with photoactive substances present in the skin and 2–24 hours later causes erythema (sunburn), the most common acute UV effect. Erythema is most severe following exposure to wavelengths of 290–320 nm and may be accompanied by edema, blistering, desquamation, chills, fever, nausea, and, rarely, circulatory collapse.

Treatment of acute sunburn and any blistering that occurs is supportive and symptomatic and may include topical and mild systemic analgesics. Most symptoms subside within 48 hours. The resulting scaling, darkening of the skin (due to increased melanin production), and thickening of the stratum corneum provide increased protection against subsequent exposures.

E. Photosensitivity Reactions: Two types of acute photosensitivity reactions of the skin can occur following exposure to UV radiation: phototoxic (nonallergic) and photoallergic reactions.

Phototoxic reactions are much more common and frequently occur in association with use of medications such as griseofulvin, tetracycline, sulfonamides, thiazides, and preparations containing coal tar or psoralens. Phototoxicity may exaggerate or aggravate the effects of some systemic diseases, including lupus erythematosus, dermatomyositis, congenital erythropoietic porphyria, porphyria cutanea tarda symptomatica, pellagra, actinic reticuloid, herpes simplex, and pemphigus foliaceus. Photosensitivity reactions may be characterized by blisters, bullae, and other skin manifestations.

Exposure to UV wavelengths above 320 nm after skin contact with furocoumarin-producing plants such as celery can cause phytophotodermatitis. A mild phototoxic reaction causes pigmentary changes along the pattern of points of contact, while bullae may result from a more severe inflammatory reaction.

Photoallergic reactions to UV radiation occur in association with bacteriostatic agents and perfume ingredients, which cause skin irritation, erythema, and blistering.

Treatment of photosensitivity reactions depends upon the particular underlying or associative cause and ranges from symptomatic care in mild cases to hospitalization and use of systemic corticosteroids in cases of severe reactions.

F. Premalignant and Malignant Skin Lesions: Premalignant lesions associated with exposure to UV radiation include actinic keratosis, keratoacanthoma, and Hutchinson's melanosis. Malignant lesions associated with exposure are basal cell carcinoma (the most common), squamous cell carcinoma, and malignant melanoma. Hazardous UV wavelengths are thought to be between 256 and 320 nm. UV radiation also promotes carcinogenesis following exposure to some chemicals, including those found in tar and pitch.

Increased risk for premalignant and malignant lesions occurs in fair-skinned individuals and in those who have repeated sunburns or tan poorly. Patients with a history of xeroderma pigmentosum are at greater risk for malignant melanoma.

Patients should be referred to a dermatologist for definitive diagnosis and treatment. Premalignant lesions may be treated by removal or use of topical medication. Treatment of malignant lesions may involve simple excision, radiation, or major surgery.

Prevention

Workplace exposure to UV radiation should be monitored on a routine basis. Fig 11–7 shows threshold limit values, based on wavelength and irradiance. Exposure intensities should be minimized if possible, and exposed individuals should be counseled concerning photosensitizing agents. Welders should be urged to wear goggles or face shields to protect their eyes.

Outdoor workers should be instructed to use sunscreen and protective clothing, and persons at increased risk due to preexisting medical conditions or excessive exposure should be examined periodically for the presence of premalignant or malignant lesions.

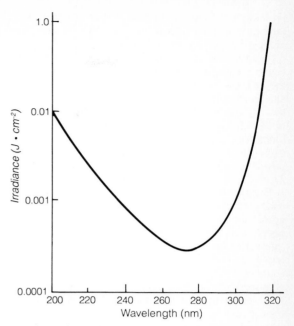

Figure 11–7. Threshold limit values for ultraviolet radiation exposure. (Redrawn and reproduced, with permission, from *TLVs: Threshold Limit Values and Biological Exposure Indices for 1988–1989.* American Conference of Governmental Industrial Hygienists, 1988.

IONIZING RADIATION INJURIES*

The 2 most significant health responses to ionizing radiation are the acute radiation syndrome that follows a brief but massive exposure and the chronic effects that are due to a brief high-dose exposure or to high cumulative exposures. Approximately 100 significant radiation incidents have occurred since 1940 as a result of exposure to radioisotopes, x-ray generators and accelerators, radar generators, and similar sources of ionizing radiation. Because of the ubiquity of ionizing radiation in our environment, the effects of long-term low-dose exposures are more difficult to pinpoint, but clusters of illnesses have been found near nuclear test sites and in association with some occupations. Workers at risk, based on their history of exposures and resulting injury, include radiologists, uranium miners, radium dial painters, nuclear power plant operators, and military personnel. Other workers at risk, based on the potential for exposure, are listed in Table 11–3.

Ionizing radiation is emitted from radioactive atomic structures as energized particles (alpha, beta,

---

*By Richard Cohen, MD, MPH, and William Vermere, PhD.

proton, and neutron particles) that impart energy through collision with other structures or as high-energy electromagnetic x-rays or gamma rays. The different forms of ionizing radiation vary in natural source, energy, frequency, and penetrability, but they all share the ability to ionize incident materials and exist at the highest energies and frequencies of the electromagnetic spectrum (Fig 11–5). Dislocation of an electron from an incident atom and the resulting biomolecular chemical reactions and instability can cause tissue damage. A summary of the clinical effects of ionizing radiation is presented in Table 11–4.

External biologic exposure to x-rays, gamma rays, and proton and neutron radiation results in high absorption, whereas beta particles penetrate skin poorly and alpha particles do not penetrate at all. Internal exposure to alpha or beta particles by inhalation, implantation, or ingestion can result in serious acute or delayed injury. If radioactive contamination is suspected, decontamination procedures should be followed scrupulously during all phases of patient management.

ACUTE RADIATION SYNDROME

Acute radiation syndrome is due to brief but heavy exposure of all or part of the body to ionizing radiation. The radiation disrupts chemical bonds, which causes molecular excitation and free radical formation. Highly reactive free radicals react with other essential molecules such as nucleic acids and enzymes, and this in turn disrupts cellular function. The clinical presentation and severity of illness are determined by the dosage, body distribution, and duration of exposure. Tissues with the most rapid cellular turnover are the most radiosensitive: reproductive, hematopoietic, and gastrointestinal tissues.

Clinical Findings

Although symptoms are unlikely with exposure to doses under 100 cGy, abnormal laboratory findings may be seen at any dose over 25 cGy. For doses of 100–400 cGy, symptoms begin within 2–6 hours and may last up to 48 hours. For doses of 600–1000 cGy, symptoms begin within 2 hours and later merge into the illness phase. For those at Chernobyl who received over 600 cGy, headache, fever, and vomiting developed within the first half hour. Within 6 days, severe lymphopenia developed, followed by severe gastroenteritis, granulocytopenia, and thrombocytopenia. For those in the lowest exposure group (80–210 cGy), slight lymphopenia occurred within a few days, followed by mild granulocytopenia and thrombocytopenia at 4 weeks.

Doses of 1000–3000 cGy can cause immediate gastrointestinal symptoms and massive fluid, blood, and electrolyte loss resulting from denudation of the gastrointestinal mucosa. Doses exceeding 3000 cGy are lethal. They cause progressive neurologic incapacitation associated with ataxia, lethargy, tremor, and convulsions. Death is almost immediate with the highest doses.

Some patients with acute radiation syndrome pass through 4 phases: prodrome, latent phase, illness, and recovery.

A. Prodrome: Symptoms and signs may include anorexia, nausea, vomiting, diarrhea, intestinal cramps, salivation, dehydration, fatigue, apathy, prostration, arrhythmia, fever, respiratory distress, hyperexcitability, ataxia, headache, and hypotension. Gastrointestinal and central nervous system findings predominate.

B. Latent Phase: The prodrome is sometimes followed by a period of relative well-being prior to the onset of illness. In cases of exposure to higher doses of radiation, the latent period is shortened or eliminated and central nervous system or gastrointestinal effects predominate.

C. Illness Phase: Symptoms and signs in this phase may include fatigue, weakness, fever, diarrhea, anorexia, weight loss, hair loss, arrhythmia, ileus, ataxia, disorientation, convulsions, coma, and shock. Effects are primarily hematopoietic and due to inhibition of hematopoietic stem cells. There may be

Table 11–3. Potential occupational exposures to ionizing radiation.

Aircraft workers
Atomic energy plant workers
Biologists
Cathode ray tube makers
Chemists
Dental Workers
Drug makers and sterilizers
Electron microscope makers and operators
Electrostatic eliminator operators
Embalmers
Fire alarm makers
Food preservers and sterilizers
Gas mantle makers
High-voltage electron, x-ray, vacuum, radar, klystron or television tube makers, users, repairmen
Industrial radiographers and fluoroscopists
Inspectors using—and workers in proximity to—sealed gamma ray sources (cesium 137, cobalt 60, iridium 192) and x-rays
Liquid level gauge painters
Luminous dial painters
Military personnel
Oil well loggers
Ore assayers
Petroleum refinery workers
Physicians and nurses
Plasma torch operators
Plastics technicians
Prospectors
Radium refinery workers
Research workers, chemists, biologists, physicists
Thickness gauge operators
Thorium ore and alloy workers
Tile glazers
Uranium workers and miners
Veterinarians
X-ray aides and technicians
X-ray diffraction apparatus operators

Table 11–4. Summary of clinical effects of ionizing radiation dosages.

	Subclinical Range	Therapeutic Range			Lethal Range	
	0–100 rem	100–200 rem (Clinical Surveillance)	200–600 rem (Therapy Effective)	600–1000 rem (Therapy Promising)	1000–5000 rem (Therapy Palliative)	>5000 rem (Therapy Palliative)
Incidence of vomiting	None	5% at 100 rem 50% at 200 rem	100% at 300 rem	100%	100%	100%
Delay time for vomiting	. . .	3 hr	2 hr	1 hr	30 min	30 min
Leading organ affected	None	Hematopoietic tissue	Hematopoietic tissue	Hematopoietic tissue	Gastrointestinal tract	Central nervous system
Characteristic signs	None	Moderate leukopenia	Severe lukopenia, purpura, hemorrhage, and infection; hair loss above 300 rem	Severe leukopenia, purpura, hemorrhage, and infection; hair loss above 300 rem	Diarrhea, fever, and disturbance of electrolyte balance	Convulsions, tremor, ataxia, and lethargy
Critical period postexposure	. . .	. . .	4–6 wk	4–6 wk	5–14 days	1–48 hr
Therapy required	Reassurance	Reassurance and hematologic surveillance	Blood transfusion and antibiotics	Consider bone marrow transplant	Maintenance of electrolyte balance	Sedatives
Prognosis	Excellent	Excellent	Good	Guarded	Hopeless	Hopeless
Convalescent period	None	Several weeks	1–12 mo	Long	. . .	. . .
Incidence of death	None	None	0–80%	80–100%	90–100%	90–100%
Time within which death occurs	. . .	. . .	2 mo	2 mo	2 wk	2 days
Cause of death	. . .	. . .	Hemorrhage and infection	Hemorrhage and infection	Circulatory collapse	Respiratory failure and brain edema

a sequential decrease in lymphocytes, granulocytes, platelets, and erythrocytes. Leukopenia and thrombocytopenia may occur with secondary infection, hemorrhagic diathesis, or anemia. Cardiovascular collapse, pericarditis, and myocarditis have been reported. With doses exceeding 200 cGy, there may be reproductive system effects, including sterility, aspermatogenesis, and cessation of menses. Fetal and embryo toxicity or death can also occur.

D. Recovery Phase: The prognosis for recovery from exposures of up to 600 cGy is good when appropriate therapy is given. For higher exposures, the prognosis worsens as the dose increases. Infection and sepsis are the major causes of morbidity and mortality in cases involving exposures below 1000 cGy, in which the major impact is hematopoietic.

Prevention

Occupational exposure to ionizing radiation should be monitored. The technology varies with the type of radiation and the target site. Personal exposure measurement devices include film badges or nuclear emulsion monitors (for x-rays, gamma rays, beta particles, and neutron radiation), thermoluminescent dosimeters, and ionization dosimeters. A scintillation counter can be used to measure some radioisotopes in urine specimens or in tissue from target organs (eg, thyroid). Environmental or area monitoring devices include the Geiger-Müller counter, ionization chamber, and scintillation detector. Where an exposure potential occurs, shielding with lead or other effective barrier can contain emissions.

To quantify risk from radiation exposure, a system of units has been created and revised many times. The International Commission on Radiological Units and Measurements (ICRU) has recommended that the older CGS units be replaced by the equivalent SI units, as shown in Table 11–5. Recommended external and internal exposure limits are shown in Tables 11–6 and 11–7. The basis for the limits is what is referred to as the "acceptable" risk. This is thought to be 1 in 10,000 per year for workers with occupational exposures and 1 in 10,000–1,000,000 per year for the general public, based on estimated radiation-induced fatal cancers and serious hereditary disorders. The upper limit of organ dose has been set to

Table 11–5. Radiation units.

Parameter	SI Units[1]	CGS Units[2]	Conversion
Activity = rate of decay (disintegration per second)	becquerel (Bq)	curie (Ci)	1 Ci = 3.7 x 10^{10} Bq. 1 Bq+ = 2.703 x 10^{-11} Ci.
Exposure (dose) = quantity of x-ray or gamma radiation at a given point	coulomb (C)/kg of air	roentgen (R)	1 C/kg of air = 3876 R. 1 R = 258 MC/kg of air.
Dose rate = dose per unit of time (counts per minute)	coulomb (C)/kg of air/hr	roentgen (R)/hr	Same as above.
Absorbed dose = quantity of radiation absorbed per unit of mass	gray (Gy) joules (J)/kg	rad erg	1 Gy = 1 J/kg. 1 Gy = 100 rads. 1 rad = 0.01 Gy. 1 rad = 100 ergs.
Dose equivalent = absorbed dose in terms of estimated biologic effect relative to an exposure of 1 roentgen of x-ray or gamma radiation	sievert (Sv)	rem	1 Sv = 100 rem. 1 rem = 0.01 Sv.

[1]SI = international system of units.
[2]CGS = centigram-gram-second system of units.

avoid the nonstochastic (threshold) effects, such as cataracts.

Treatment

The patient should be decontaminated, hospitalized, and placed under the care of hematologists, oncologists, and infectious disease specialists. Vital signs, fluid and electrolyte balance, and hematopoietic, gastrointestinal, and central nervous system functions should be monitored closely.

If the granulocyte counts fall below 1000, prophylactic use of trimethoprim, sulfamethoxazole, and nystatin has been recommended by some physicians, though this is controversial. If there is fever or suspected sepsis, antimicrobial agents by intravenous infusion should be started immediately. A combination of a semisynthetic penicillin and an aminoglycoside has been recommended, but the choice of agents

will also depend on the endemic pathogens at the particular hospital. Antimicrobial therapy should be continued until the granulocyte count exceeds 500/μL or until the patient has been afebrile for 5 consecutive days without evidence of infection. Reverse isolation should be maintained.

Granulocyte, platelet, and red cell transfusions may be necessary. Lymphocytes should be obtained immediately for HLA typing. Transfusions are recommended if the platelet count falls below 20,000/μL, the granulocyte count below 200/μL, or the hematocrit below 25%. Bone marrow transplants have been successful in combating intractable hemorrhage and infection. They should be considered for patients exposed to 600–2000 cGy, and the decision about whether to use them should be made within a week following radiation exposure.

Patients should receive supportive therapy as necessary for control of nausea, dehydration, and other symptoms.

Table 11–6. External radiation exposure limits.

Groups and Body Parts Exposed	Radiation Limit
Adults Whole body, head, trunk, arm above elbow, and leg above knee	5 rem (0.05 Sv) per year[1] **or** 3 rem (0.03 Sv) in any quarter
Hand, elbow, arm below elbow, foot, knee, and leg below knee	50 rem (0.5 Sv) per year
Lens of eye	15 rem (0.15 Sv) per year
Skin (10 cm)	50 rem (0.5 Sv) per year
Pregnant women	0.05 rem (0.5 mSv) per month while pregnant **or** 0.5 rem (5 mSv) per pregnancy
Minors	10% of annual limits for adults

[1]Includes cumulative yearly (external) deep-dose equivalent and (internal) committed effective-dose equivalent.

Table 11–7. Organ-specific internal radiation exposure limits.

Tissue	Relative Sensitivity (wt)	Risk Coefficient per Sv	Actual Dose Limit (Sv/yr)
Gonads	0.25	4 x 10^{-3}	0.2
Breast	0.15	2.5 x 10^{-3}	0.33
Red marrow	0.12	2 x 10^{-3}	0.42
Lung	0.12	2 x 10^{-3}	0.42
Thyroid	0.03	5 x 10^{-4}	0.5
Bone surfaces	0.03	5 x 10^{-4}	0.5
Each of 5 remaining organs or tissues with the largest dose	0.06	5 x 10^{-3}	0.5

ACUTE LOCALIZED RADIATION INJURIES

Exposure of isolated skin and body parts to ionizing radiation will result in hair loss (doses above 300 cGy), erythema (above 600 cGy), dry desquamation (radionecrosis) (above 1000 cGy), and wet desquamation (above 2000 cGy). Pain and itching occur shortly after exposure and are followed by erythema and blister formation. In cases of severe localized burns, there may be tissue ischemia and necrosis.

Prevention is as for acute radiation syndrome (see above).

Treatment is conservative and should not include surgery unless that is dictated by secondary complications. To conserve joint motion and prevent contractures, splinting and physical therapy may be required during convalescence. Injuries should be followed closely, because the extent of tissue damage is often not readily apparent. Subsequent fibrosis, ulceration, infection, necrosis, or gangrene may occur and require surgery or more radical medical treatment.

RADIONUCLIDE CONTAMINATION

Skin contamination with radionuclides is rarely life-threatening. Immediate decontamination measures consist of gently scrubbing the skin with soap and warm water and, if necessary, cutting the hair. Hair clippings, material removed by scrubbing, swabs of the nares and mouth, clothing, and personal effects should be saved for radioactivity analysis and dosage calculation.

For contaminated open wounds, gentle surgical debridement should be performed and wound irrigation considered. Depending on the type of radionuclide causing the injury, administration of a chelating agent may be indicated. For plutonium and alpha emitters, diethylenetriaminepentaacetic acid (DTPA) is effective and can be administered systemically as well as in the wound irrigation solution. Blocking agents may also be considered, as in the case of radioiodines. For further information, the reader is referred to Report 65 of the National Council on Radiation Protection and Measurements, which is listed in the references at the end of this chapter.

DELAYED EFFECTS OF HIGH-DOSE RADIATION

Radiodermatitis often occurs in association with ionizing radiation therapy. The skin is dry, smooth, shiny, thin, pruritic, and sensitive, and there are signs of telangiectasia, atrophy, and diffuse pigmentation. The nails are brittle and striated.

Scarring in other tissues following high-dose exposure has led to endarteritis obliterans, intestinal stenosis, pulmonary fibrosis, and cataracts.

Various cancers related to localized organ radioactivity have been described. These include bone cancer from localized radioisotopes, thyroid cancer following childhood thymus irradiation, liver cancer associated with thorium dioxide, and lung cancer associated with radon decay products (radon daughters) in uranium miners. Leukemia has been reported in patients receiving radiotherapy for ankylosing spondylitis.

Other effects of high-dose exposure include premature aging, shortening of the life span, and teratogenic and reproductive abnormalities.

EFFECTS OF LOW-DOSE RADIATION

Controversy continues over whether the risk for somatic and genetic disorders is increased by cumulative low-dose exposures. The dose-response curve in the low-dose range cannot be determined at present, so most estimates of risk continue to be based on mathematical extrapolations from experiences with higher doses. Although developmental abnormalities have been associated with doses as low as 10 cGy and cancers associated with levels below 100 cGy, the practical relevance of low-dose phenomena is extremely difficult to establish, not only because of inconsistencies in the literature but also because the cumulative average exposure for people in the USA is approximately 8–10 cGy per lifetime. In other words, the practical medical significance of these low lifetime cumulative exposures is presently unclear.

LASER INJURIES

The energy of the laser source is transformed through atomic excitation into a coherent, collimated, monochromatic beam of radiation. Lasers operate at one wavelength, usually in the ultraviolet, visible, or infrared portion of the electromagnetic spectrum. They may emit radiation in continuous or pulsed waves.

Most industrial exposures to laser radiation occur in the construction industry, where lasers are used to provide alignment and grade levels on projects such as dam construction, tunneling, dredging, floor installation, and pipe laying. In the manufacture of electronics, laser use is increasing for welding, burning, and alignment. Intense laser sources are used to cut hard metals and diamonds, and less intense thermal applications include medical treatment.

Biologic effects at low intensities are unlikely, although there is some variation with wavelength. Injuries have not been associated with repeated low-intensity exposures. At high intensities, thermal or pressure-induced damage to the skin or eyes can occur. These injuries are more likely with lasers that have a high-intensity beam outside the visible light spectrum, because the worker's proximity to the beam may not be apparent. Because of the thermal mechanism, any damage that occurs would be expected to be immediately manifested with the symptoms and signs of a corneal, retinal, or cutaneous burn. Treatment for these laser injuries is the same as that for other thermal injuries.

To prevent injuries, exposure levels should be monitored. Threshold limit values for lasers have been established by the American Conference of Governmental Industrial Hygienists (ACGIH) and are based on intensity, wavelength, and exposure time. The American National Standards Institute (ANSI) has developed a classification for lasers by degree of hazard, with class 1 representing no risk and class 4 representing a severe hazard even from diffuse reflection. Evaluation of workers following laser exposures should include an assessment of exposure intensity, wavelength, duration, viewing angle, and ANSI laser hazard classification.

Individuals working in proximity to high-power lasers should be instructed in proper operating procedures and provided with protective eye wear designed for the specific wavelength of the laser. In some cases, the eye wear may not by itself offer sufficient protection, owing to possible laser reflections. Other devices, including shields, barriers, and, where possible, remote viewing equipment, should be used. Skin protection is also important when high-power lasers are used. If feasible, systems should be designed with the beam line totally enclosed and shielded.

Preplacement examinations are recommended for individuals who will work with class 3 and 4 lasers and should consist of, as a minimum, the medical history, tests for visual acuity (near and far) and refractive errors, slit lamp examination, ophthalmoscopy, and inspection of the outer eye. Because pathologic effects have not been associated with long-term low-intensity exposures, periodic evaluation is not recommended for laser operators unless an acute high-intensity exposure occurs.

ATMOSPHERIC PRESSURE DISORDERS (DYSBARISM)

Sudden shift to an environment of lower ambient pressure, as occurs with rapid ascension to the surface from deep-sea diving or with loss of cabin pressure while flying at high altitudes, causes decompression sickness. Compression sickness can occur following movement to an environment of higher ambient pressure, but the only common example of this is barotitis.

DECOMPRESSION SICKNESS (CAISSON DISEASE)

Decompression sickness results from mechanical and physiologic effects of expanding gases and bubbles in blood and tissue. When the body is exposed to an environment of higher than atmospheric gas pressure, as in tunneling or diving, it absorbs more of the inhaled gases than it does at sea level. Nitrogen concentrations increase in tissues, particularly those of the nervous system, bone marrow, and fat. Because the blood supply is poor in bone marrow and fat, nitrogen enters and leaves these tissues more slowly than oxygen or carbon dioxide does. As the surrounding pressure decreases (decompression), nitrogen expands and will form gas bubbles if there is insufficient time for its dissolution from tissues. Because oxygen and carbon dioxide have greater fluid solubility and move more easily between tissue compartments, their tendency for bubble formation is reduced.

Most cases of decompression sickness have occurred after rapid ascension from sea depths in excess of 9 meters or after sudden pressure loss at altitudes in excess of 7000 meters.

Clinical Findings

A complete evaluation of the systems affected—as determined by the history and physical examination—should be performed with appropriate x-rays and other diagnostic procedures. Anyone exhibiting signs or symptoms of decompression sickness within 48 hours after a high-pressure exposure should be given a compression test in which 100% oxygen at 3 atm is administered for 20 minutes in a hyperbaric chamber.

There are 3 types of decompression sickness, as described below. The type and severity of symptoms will depend on the age, weight, and physical condition of the patient; the degree of physical exertion; the depth or altitude before decompression; and the rate and duration of decompression.

A. Type 1 Decompression Sickness: This type, which has the best prognosis, affects the limbs and skin. Acute pain, usually around a major joint, may be incapacitating and cause the patient to assume a stooped posture (''the bends''). Pain may begin immediately after decompression or up to 12 hours later and is sometimes accompanied by urticarial and bluish-red mottling and itching of the skin (''diver's lice'').

B. Type 2 Decompression Sickness: Type 2 is more severe than type 1. Symptoms and signs of central and peripheral nerve damage may include vertigo, ''pins and needles'' paresthesias, hypesthesia, ataxic gait, hyperreflexia, Babinski's sign, paralysis or weakness of the limbs, headache, seizures, vomiting, visual loss or visual field defects, incontinence, impaired speech, tremor, and coma. Pulmonary manifestations (''the chokes'') may include substernal pain, chest tightness, severe coughing, dyspnea, pulmonary edema, and shallow respirations. Cardiovascular findings include arrhythmia and hypertension.

Type 2 sickness, which is probably caused by gas bubbles in the central nervous system and spinal cord, may have significant sequelae, such as vascular obstruction and tissue infarction, which are sometimes accompanied by hemoconcentration, changes in osmotic pressure, or lipid emboli; hemorrhagic infarcts of the lungs; ulcers of the colon; multifocal degeneration of white matter; and hypercoagulation of blood. Massive air emboli in the circulatory system are fatal in this type of decompression sickness.

C. Type 3 Decompression Sickness: The third type is characterized by aseptic necrosis of bone (osteonecrosis), which frequently involves the head or shaft of the humerus and less often the lower end of the femur and the tibial head. Osteonecrosis usually occurs 6–60 months following decompression and is asymptomatic unless there is joint involvement, which can cause permanent impairment. X-ray examination may show bone sclerosis and mottling. Lesions are often symmetric.

Osteonecrosis may be the result of nitrogen bubbles obstructing the capillaries and has been reported in up to 50% of divers and underwater workers, although disability occurs in fewer than 3%. An increased incidence of memory deficits, retrograde amnesia, emotional instability, and other neurologic and psychiatric symptoms has been observed in divers with a history of decompression sickness.

Prevention

Divers, underwater workers, and pilots should be screened to make sure they are in good physical condition—not overweight and with no other conditions imposing an increased risk for dysbarism, such as vascular disorders, hypercoagulopathy, obstructive airway disease, dehydration, or recent bone fractures. They and their crews should receive training and education in proper compression and decompression procedures and in recognizing symptoms and signs of decompression sickness.

Treatment

A. Type 1 and Type 2 Decompression Sickness: The patient should be placed in a supine position or, if pulmonary or central nervous system symptoms are present, in Trendelenburg's position but tilted slightly to the left—theoretically, to reduce the risk of cerebral air embolism—at an angle of 10–15 degrees. For immediate first aid, 100% oxygen should be administered, and aspirin may be given for analgesia. The patient should be transported rapidly to an emergency facility that has a hyperbaric chamber for recompression and decompression. Information about the nearest facility and advice about recompression can be obtained 24 hours a day by calling the National Diving Accident Network at (919) 684-8111.

In the hyperbaric chamber, the patient is placed in an atmosphere of raised pressure. The pressure is then reduced at a slow rate, with decompression pressures and schedules determined on the basis of the duration and pressure exposure of the inciting incident. Breathing 100% oxygen by mask alternating with normal breathing should shorten the period of decompression.

Corticosteroids (dexamethasone phosphate, 10 mg intravenously followed by 4 mg intramuscularly every 6 hours for not more than 72 hours), diuretics, or both can be used for cerebral or spinal edema. Volume depletion should be corrected with oral or parenteral fluids. In severe cases, anticoagulation using heparin (7500 units intravenously followed by 500 units given as necessary) or plasma volume expansion using low-molecular-weight dextran 40 has been effective. Diazepam has been used for treatment of confusional states and oxygen toxicity if oxygen is administered during treatment.

In cases of type 2 sickness, decompression may take several days. To prevent reemergence of symptoms, the patient should breathe air for 30 minutes and then breathe oxygen for 30 minutes and continue this procedure for up to 8 hours after decompression. Careful monitoring should be maintained to guard against oxygen toxicity of the lungs and central nervous system.

B. Type 3 Decompression Sickness: Osteonecrosis and sequelae due to chronic decompression sickness are treated in the same manner as these conditions due to other causes.

COMPRESSION SICKNESS

When atmospheric pressure is increased, internal gases become compressed, usually with little effect. The only common form of compression sickness is barotitis. This can occur with descent of an aircraft from a high altitude, which causes a relative vacuum in the middle ear space if the auditory tube is already obstructed due to allergies or upper respiratory tract infection. Symptoms may include pain or a foggy feeling in the ears, dizziness, nausea, and vertigo. In more severe cases, the tympanic membrane may appear inflamed and retracted or ruptured.

Barotitis can be prevented in people at risk by avoiding high-pressure exposures or, for short exposures, by using decongestants. Barotitis is usually self-limiting but can be treated with decongestant nose drops, a nasal vasoconstrictor inhaler, or use of Valsalva's maneuver.

DISORDERS DUE TO VIBRATION

Vibration occurs when mechanical energy from an oscillating source is transmitted to another structure.

Every structure has its own natural vibration level, including the human body as a whole and each of its parts. When vibration of the same frequency is applied, resonance (amplification) of that vibration occurs, often with adverse effects. For example, at a frequency of 5 Hz, whole-body resonance occurs, and the body acts in concert with externally generated vibration and amplifies that effect.

EFFECTS OF WHOLE-BODY VIBRATION

In the USA, approximately 7 million workers operate vehicles that expose them to the back-and-forth motion of whole-body vibration and place them at risk for associated injuries. Truck and bus drivers, heavy equipment operators, miners, and others exposed to long-term whole-body vibration have been reported to have a higher incidence of musculoskeletal, neurologic, circulatory, and digestive system disorders than the general population, and European studies have found associated bony abnormalities such as intervertebral osteochondrosis and calcification of intervertebral disks. "Vibration sickness," characterized by gastrointestinal problems, decreased visual acuity, labyrinthine disorders, and intense musculoskeletal pain, has also been reported in these workers. Despite these reports, a relationship between exposure intensity or quantity and the disorders found in occupationally exposed groups has not been clearly defined. Although many questions remain unanswered regarding the effects of long-term whole-body vibration exposure, neurologic and spinal effects appear likely.

Although almost all clinical and experimental effects of whole-body vibration have occurred at frequencies less than 20 Hz, they have also been reported to occur at frequencies as high as 100 Hz, depending on other factors such as the amplitude, acceleration, duration, and direction (vertical or lateral) of the vibrating force. The International Organization for Standardization (ISO) has established guidelines for whole-body vertical vibration exposure times to various frequencies and accelerations, as shown in Fig 6–10 and discussed in Chapter 6. Not all investigators agree with existing exposure standards because of the many inconsistencies in the literature; however, prudence suggests that employers should try to minimize whole-body vibration exposures of their employees whenever possible by limiting the duration of exposure and choosing well-designed equipment that insulates workers from vibration.

VIBRATION-INDUCED WHITEFINGER DISEASE

Vibration-induced whitefinger disease is the most common example of an occupational injury due to segmental vibration of the hands. In the USA, more than 1 million workers are estimated to have significant exposure to vibration from hand tools such as power saws, grinders, sanders, pneumatic drills, jackhammers, and other equipment used in construction, foundry work, machining, and mining. Although segmental vibration injury can occur with frequencies ranging from 10 to 1500 Hz, it usually occurs with frequencies of 125–300 Hz. Other factors affecting risk include the amplitude and acceleration of the equipment used and the duration of use. Cumulative trauma most often occurs with a work history of at least 2000 hours of exposure and usually over 8000 hours.

Whitefinger disease is characterized by spasms of the digital arteries (Raynaud's phenomenon) caused by vibration-induced damage of the peripheral nerve and vascular tissue, subcutaneous tissue, bones, and joints of the hands and fingers. The pathologic process may also involve arterial muscle wall hypertrophy; demyelinating peripheral neuropathy; excess connective tissue deposition in perivascular, perineural, and subcutaneous tissues; and microvascular occlusion. Attacks of vasospasm can last for minutes to hours and are more likely to occur with exposure to the cold and with strenuous physical exertion. The worker is often standing erect, with the hand held lower than the heart and maintained in a contracted position.

Clinical Findings

Attacks in severe cases can last 15–60 minutes or as long as 2 hours. They are usually easily reversible if the individual is removed from vibration exposure. Early symptoms consist of tingling followed by numbness of the fingers. The fingers later begin to turn white in a cold environment or when cold objects are touched. Intermittent blanching often starts with the tip of one finger but progressively extends to other fingertips and eventually to the tips and bases of all fingers on the exposed hands. With increasing severity of disease, blanching or cyanosis of the fingers may extend into the summer season. Return of blood circulation (reactive hyperemia, or "red flush") following each episode is accompanied by redness and swelling, acute pain, throbbing, and paresthesias.

In more advanced cases, there may be degeneration of bone and cartilage, with resulting joint stiffness, restriction of motion, and arthralgia. Manual dexterity may decrease and clumsiness increase. With greater intensities of vibration, the period between exposure to vibration and the appearance of "whitefinger" is shorter.

There is no one specific diagnostic test, but tests of peripheral vascular function (such as arteriography or plethysmography), neurologic function (such as 2-point discrimination, sensory and motor nerve conduction velocities), cold provocation tests, skin thermography, and radiographic investigation may be helpful in defining the extent of pathology.

Differential Diagnosis

The diagnosis of vibration-induced whitefinger disease is based on the occupational history of vibration exposures, the association of these exposures with episodes of Raynaud's phenomenon (digital vasospasms), and the exclusion of idiopathic Raynaud's disease and other causes of Raynaud's phenomenon, including trauma of the fingers and hands, frostbite, occlusive vascular disease, connective tissue disorders, neurogenic disorders, drug intoxication, and exposure to vinyl chloride monomer.

Prevention

Segmental vibration can be prevented by using well-designed tools (see Chapter 6), wearing gloves to minimize vibration and keep the hands warm, and following a work-rest schedule that prevents long periods of exposure to vibration. Workers should be instructed about the early symptoms and signs of vibration-induced whitefinger disease and advised of factors that may place them at higher risk, such as the use of vasoactive drugs and cigarette smoking.

Treatment

In most cases, symptoms and signs disappear when the worker is removed from exposure to vibration. In other cases, attacks can be reduced in severity or stopped by massaging, shaking, or swinging the hands or by placing them in warm water or warm air.

For more intractable episodes, vasodilators, calcium channel blockers, or drugs for regional nerve block can be tried. Biofeedback training has also been suggested. Surgical sympathectomy may be considered for irreversible cases. For medical or surgical therapy, the patient should be referred to the appropriate vascular specialist or hand surgeon.

REFERENCES

Hypothermia (Cold Injury)

Bangs CC: Hypothermia and frostbite. *Emerg Med Clin North Am* 1984;**2**:475.

Lonning PE, Skulberg A, Abyholm F: Accidental hypothermia: Review of the literature. *Acta Anaesthesiol Scand* 1986;**30**:601.

Moss J: Accidental severe hypothermia. *Surg Gynecol Obstet* 1986;**162**:501.

Paton BC: Accidental hypothermia. *Pharmacol Ther* 1983;**22**:331.

TLVs: Threshold Limit Values and Biological Exposure Indices for 1988–1989. American Conference of Governmental Industrial Hygienists, 1988.

Disorders Due to Heat

American College of Sports Medicine: Position stand on the prevention of thermal injuries during distance running. *Med Sci Sports Exerc* 1987;**19**:529.

Criteria for Recommended Standards: Occupational Exposure to Hot Environments. US Department of Health and Human Services, National Institute for Occupational Safety and Health, 1986.

Management of heat stroke. *Lancet* 1982;**2**:910.

Olson KR, Benowitz NL: Environmental and drug-induced hyperthermia: Pathophysiology, recognition, and management. *Emerg Med Clin North Am* 1984;**2**:459.

TLVs: Threshold Limit Values and Biological Exposure Indices for 1988–1989. American Conference of Governmental Industrial Hygienists, 1988.

Tucker LE et al: Classical heat stroke: Clinical and laboratory assessment. *South Med J* 1985;**78**:20.

Thermal Burns

Demling RH: Fluid resuscitation after major burns. *JAMA* 1983;**250**:1438.

Fisher SV, Helm PA: *Comprehensive Rehabilitation of Burns.* Williams & Wilkins, 1984.

Frist W et al: Long-term functional results of selective treatment of hand burns. *Am J Surg* 1985;**149**:516.

Gallico GG III et al: Permanent coverage of large burn wounds with autologous cultured human epithelium. *N Engl J Med* 1984;**311**:448.

Goodwin CW: Major burns. In: *Principles of Trauma Care,* 3rd ed. Shires GT (editor). McGraw-Hill, 1985.

Herndon DN et al: Pulmonary injury in burned patients. *Surg Clin North Am* 1987;**67**:31.

Jones J, McMullen MJ, Dougherty J: Toxic smoke inhalation: Cyanide poisoning in fire victims. *Am J Emerg Med* 1987;**5**:317.

Kagan RJ et al: Serious wound infections in burned patients. *Surgery* 1985;**98**:640.

Monafo WW, Crabtree HJ, Galster AD: Hemodynamics and metabolic support of the severely burned patient. In: *The Society of Critical Care Medicine: Textbook of Critical Care.* Shoemaker WC, Thompson WL, Holbrook PR (editors). Saunders, 1984.

Rubin WD, Mari MM, Hiebert JM: Fluid resuscitation of the thermally injured patient: Current concepts with definition of clinical subsets and their specialized treatment. *Clin Plast Surg* 1986;**13**:9.

Shires GT (editor): Supportive therapy in burn care. *J Trauma* 1981;**21(Suppl 8)**:665. [Entire issue.]

Shires GT, Black EA (editors): Frontiers in understanding burn injury: Proceedings of the NIH Conference. *J Trauma* 1984;**24(Suppl)**:S1.

Electrical Injuries

Cooper MA: Electrical and lightning injuries. *Emerg Med Clin North Am* 1984;**2**:489.

Hammond JS et al: High voltage electrical injuries: Management and outcome of 60 cases. *South Med J* 1988;**81**:1351.

Nichter LS et al: Injuries due to commercial electric current. *JBCR* 1984;**5**:124.

Nonionizing Radiation Injuries

Adams RM: *Occupational Skin Diseases.* Saunders, 1989.

American National Standard Safety Levels With Respect to Human Exposure to Radiofrequency, Electromagnetic Fields 300 KHz to 100 GHz. ANSI No. C95.1-1982. American National Standards Institute, 1982.

Biological Effects and Exposure Criteria for Radiofrequency Electromagnetic Field. NCRP Report No. 86. National Council on Radiation Protection and Measurements, 1986.

Ham WT: Ocular hazards of light sources: Review of current knowledge. *J Occup Med* 1983;**25**:101.

Michaelson SM: Influence of power frequency electric and magnetic fields on human health. *Ann NY Acad Sci* 1987;**289**:55.

Occupational Hazards From Nonionizing Electromagnetic Radiation. Occupational Safety and Health Series No. 53. International Labour Office, Geneva, 1985.

Pitts DG: The ocular effects of ultraviolet radiation. *Am J Optom Physiol Opt* 1978;**55**:19.

Pitts DG, Cullen AP, Dayhaw-Barker P: *Determination of Ocular Threshold Levels for Infrared Cataractogenesis.* National Institute for Occupational Safety and Health Publication No. 80-121. US Department of Health and Human Services, 1980.

Polk C, Postow E: *Handbook of Biological Effects of Electromagnetic Fields.* CRC Press, 1986.

Rees RB Jr, Odom RB: Photodermatitis. In: *Current Medical Diagnosis & Treatment 1989.* Schroeder SA et al (editors). Appleton & Lange, 1989.

TLVs: Threshold Limit Values and Biological Exposure Indices for 1988–89. American Conference of Governmental Industrial Hygienists, 1988.

Ionizing Radiation Injuries

Champlin RE: Radiation accidents and nuclear energy: Medical consequences and therapy. *Ann Intern Med* 1988;**109**:730.

Gale RP: Perspective: Medical response to radiation and nuclear accidents: Lessons for the future. *JNCI* 1988;**80**:995.

Management of Persons Accidentally Contaminated With Radionuclides. NCRP Report No. 65. National Council on Radiation Protection and Measurements, 1980.

Milroy WC: Management of irradiated and contaminated casualty victims. *Emerg Med Clin North Am* 1984;**2**:667.

Ritenour ER: Health effects of low level radiation: Carcinogenesis, teratogenesis, and mutagenesis. *Semin Nucl Med* 1986;**16**:106.

Shapiro J: *Radiation Protection: A Guide for Scientists and Physicians,* 2nd ed. Harvard Univ Press, 1981.

Laser Injuries

American National Standard for the Safe Use of Lasers. ANSI No. Z136.1-1986. American National Standards Institute, 1986.

Environmental Health Criteria 23: Lasers and Optical Radiation. World Health Organization, 1982.

Atmospheric Pressure Disorders (Dysbarism)

Calder IM: Dysbarism: A review. *Forensic Sci Int* 1986;**30**:237.

Edmonds C, Lowry C, Pennefather J: *Diving and Subaquatic Medicine.* Diving Medical Center, Mosman, Australia, 1983.

Hickey DD: Outline of medical standards for divers. *Undersea Biomed Res* 1984;**11**:407.

Kizer KW: Diving medicine. *Emerg Med Clin North Am* 1984;**2**:513.

Myers RAM, Bray P: Delayed treatment of serious decompression sickness. *Ann Emerg Med* 1985;**14**:254.

Parell GJ et al: Management of inner ear barotrauma caused by SCUBA diving. *Otolaryngol Head Neck Surg* 1985;**93**:393.

US Navy Department: *US Navy Diving Manual.* NAVSEA 0994-LP-001-9010, Change 2. US Government Printing Office, 1978.

Disorders Due to Vibration

Helmkamp JC, Talbott EO, Marsh GM: Whole body vibration: A critical review. *Am Ind Hyg Assoc* 1984;**45**:162.

Seidel H, Heide R: Long-term effects of whole-body vibration: A critical survey of the literature. *Int Arch Occup Environ Health* 1986;**58**:1.

Symptomatology and diagnostic methods in the hand-arm vibration syndrome: Stockholm Workshop 1986. *Scand J Work Environ Health* 1987;**13**:271 [Entire issue.]

Taylor JS: Vibration syndrome in industry: Dermatological viewpoint. *Am J Ind Med* 1985;**8**:415.

Clinical Toxicology

12

Charles E. Becker, MD, & Jon Rosenberg, MD, MPH

Toxicology is the study of physical and chemical agents and the injury they cause to living cells. All substances are potentially toxic. One of the objectives of clinical and experimental studies in toxicology is to define the capacity of substances to produce harmful effects (ie, toxicity), measure and analyze the doses at which toxicity occurs (ie, the dose-response relationship), and assess the probability that injury or illness will occur under specified conditions of use (ie, hazard and risk assessment).

A distinction is made between toxicity and hazard. An extremely toxic chemical that is in a sealed container on a shelf has inherent toxicity but presents little or no hazard. When the chemical is removed from the shelf and used by a worker in a closed space and without appropriate protection, the hazard becomes great. Thus, the manner of use affects how hazardous the substance will be in the workplace.

TOXIC AGENTS & THEIR EFFECTS

Classification of Toxic Agents

Toxic agents can be classified or described in terms of the following:

A. Physical State of the Agent: The different physical states of toxic agents, with some examples of each, are shown in Table 12–1. A metal such as lead may be harmless in solid form, moderately toxic as a dust, and extremely toxic as a fume.

B. Chemical Structure of the Agent: Chemical structure can determine toxicity. Often one but not another isomer of a compound possesses toxicity. For example, aromatic amines are carcinogenic when substituted in other than the para- positions. The stability of a substance and the presence of impurities, contaminants, or additives can also affect toxicity.

C. Medium of the Agent: The medium in which a toxic substance is found in part determines the population exposed and thus to some extent the hazard. Some toxic substances occur in a specific medium—eg, oxides of nitrogen in air (from vehicular exhaust), trihalomethanes in water (from chlorination), and nitrosamines in food (from nitrites). In the USA, several governmental agencies, including the Environmental Protection Agency (EPA), Food and Drug Administration (FDA), and Occupational Safety and Health Administration (OSHA), have developed regulations regarding exposure to toxic substances in various media.

D. Site of Injury by the Agent: Toxic agents can be described in terms of their effects on target organs (hepatotoxins, nephrotoxins, etc).

E. Mechanism of Action of the Agent: Toxic agents are frequently categorized on the basis of their mechanism of action. Asphyxiants, for example, deprive tissues of oxygen. Simple asphyxiants (inert gases) act by diluting or displacing oxygen without causing other toxic effects. In contrast, chemical asphyxiants such as cyanide and carbon monoxide actively interfere with the delivery or utilization of oxygen—cyanide by inhibiting cytochrome oxidase and other enzymes necessary for cellular utilization of oxygen, and carbon monoxide by combining with hemoglobin to form carboxyhemoglobin, which decreases the oxygen-carrying capacity of the blood and inhibits release of oxygen to tissues.

F. Clinical Effects of the Agent:

1. Onset of effects–Toxic effects can be immediate, as occurs with some irritants that cause direct damage to tissues at the point of initial contact, usually resulting in inflammation; or delayed, as with chemical carcinogens.

2. Reversibility of effects–Whether or not the

Table 12–1. Physical states of toxic substances.

Particulates
  Dusts
    Nuisance
      Calcium carbonate
      Cellulose (paper fiber)
      Portland cement
      Silicon
    Fibrogenic
      Silica
      Coal dust
  Fibers
    Asbestos
    Mineral wool
  Fumes
    Metal
    Polymer (polytetrafluoroethylene decomposition
      products)
Gases and vapors
    Butane, methyl bromide, ethylene oxide (gas)
    Hexane, trichloroethylene, benzene (vapor)
Liquids
    Elemental mercury
Solids
    Plastics

toxic effects of a substance are reversible depends on the capacity of damaged cells to regenerate or recover. For instance, brain and other nervous system cells have little capacity to regenerate, whereas liver and muscle cells are more likely to regenerate or recover after injury.

Factors Affecting Clinical Response to a Toxic Agent

The following factors affect the dose-response relationship and the clinical response of humans to a toxic agent:

A. Duration, Frequency, and Route of Exposure: The severity of injury is usually related to the duration and frequency of exposure. The route of exposure often determines toxicity. For example, ethylene glycol is toxic when ingested but poses little threat in the workplace except when sprayed or heated.

B. Environmental Factors: Toxicity is affected by atmospheric pressure, temperature, and humidity. For example, a concentration of carbon monoxide that has little effect at sea level can cause impairment of work capacity at an altitude of 5000 ft. Chemicals are more readily absorbed through skin that is injured or wet with perspiration and has increased blood flow in response to heat and humidity.

C. Individual Factors: Individual factors that determine "susceptibility" include racial and genetic background, age and maturity, sex, body weight, nutrition, life-style, immunologic and hormonal status, and presence of disease or stress. These factors are not independent of one another. For instance, genetic factors determine many of the other factors, and poor nutrition can affect immunologic status.

While much concern about the effect of age on individual susceptibility has focused on the fetus, the elderly also metabolize many chemicals less efficiently. As the work force ages, this may become an increasing concern.

The effect of nutritional deficiency on susceptibility to toxic agents has been of concern in developed countries primarily during war or famine, but it is relevant in developing countries as they industrialize. While toxicologic studies in animals readily demonstrate the effects of nutritional deficiency on susceptibility, the results of these studies are difficult to extrapolate to humans. The role of vitamins and minerals in chemical toxicity has been much debated.

There is controversy about the role of genetic factors and the development and use of genetic screening tests to identify individuals with increased susceptibility to toxic agents in the workplace. It is questioned whether such tests are accurate and whether job discrimination could result from their use as preemployment screening. Among the many genetic traits that might increase the risk of toxicity from exposure to chemicals or radiation, the most visible have been glucose-6-phosphate dehydrogenase (G6PD) deficiency, sickle cell anemia, and α_1-antitrypsin deficiency.

G6PD deficiency is an X-linked recessive disorder that primarily affects American black males and Mediterranean Jews. Affected individuals are susceptible to hemolysis from many drugs. Although some chemicals—notably naphthalene and arsine—can cause hemolysis following overexposure, there is no evidence that workers exposed to workplace-acceptable concentrations of these chemicals are at increased risk. Screening for G6PD deficiency is thus not supported by solid evidence.

Similarly, there is no evidence that any of the 7–13% of American blacks with sickle cell trait are at increased risk of hypoxia when working as airplane pilots or of hemolysis when working with hemolytic agents, despite the fact that these "risks" have been cited to justify screening of individuals for these occupations.

Severe α_1-antitrypsin deficiency, when present in the rare homozygous condition, can lead to early emphysema in the absence of environmental agents. The more common heterozygous condition, which affects 4–9% of the US population, may in combination with other factors place affected individuals at increased risk of developing emphysema from exposure to environmental agents.

TOXICOKINETICS & TOXICODYNAMICS

Toxicokinetics is the study of the movement of toxic substances within the body (ie, their absorption, distribution, metabolism, and excretion) and the relationship between the dose that enters the body and the level of toxic substance found in the blood or other biologic sample. Toxicodynamics is the study of the relationship between the dose that enters the body and the measured response. The magnitude of a toxic response is usually related to the concentration of the toxic substance at its site of action.

Bioavailability

The bioavailability of a toxic substance indicates the extent to which the agent reaches its site of action. If it is not in a "bioavailable form," as is the case with many orally ingested toxic substances that cause vomiting or diarrhea, it will be promptly removed. In other cases, some of the agent will be inactivated before it reaches the site of action. For example, when cyanide is taken orally, it is absorbed and passes to the liver, where the enzyme rhodanese may metabolize a portion of the ingested cyanide. On the other hand, if the cyanide in the form of gaseous hydrocyanic acid (HCN) is absorbed through the pulmonary circulation, it goes directly to the brain, where it may cause damage due to hypoxia.

Cell Membrane Permeability & Cellular Barriers

Absorption, distribution, metabolism, and excretion all involve passage of toxic agents across cell membranes. Permeability is dependent upon a toxic substance's molecular size and shape, solubility at the site of absorption, degree of ionization, and relative lipid solubility.

The distribution of some toxic agents is altered by unique cellular barriers, eg, the blood-brain barrier, the blood-testis barrier, and the placenta, which may exclude toxic substances.

Many lipid-soluble toxic substances are stored in body fat. In an obese person with a fat content of 30–40%, this may form a stable reservoir for toxic substances, which may then be released slowly.

Bone is an important deep reservoir for many heavy metals (especially lead) and for radioactive materials, and the effects of these materials can persist long after they have left the circulation.

Absorption

The rate of absorption is dependent upon the concentration and solubility of the toxic agent. Agents in aqueous solution are absorbed more rapidly than those in oily suspension. Absorption is enhanced at sites that have increased blood flow or large absorptive surfaces (eg, the adult lung and gastrointestinal tract, whose surfaces are the size of a tennis court and a football field, respectively).

A. Gastrointestinal Absorption: The amount of absorption through the gastrointestinal tract is usually proportionate to the gastrointestinal surface area and its blood flow and depends on the physical state of the agent. Most toxic substances are absorbed in the small intestine. Therefore, agents that accelerate gastric emptying will increase the absorption rate, while factors that delay gastric emptying will decrease it. Some toxic substances may be affected by gastric juice; eg, the acidity of the stomach may release cyanide products and form hydrogen cyanide gas, which is even more toxic than the cyanide salt.

B. Pulmonary Absorption: The most common route of occupational exposure is pulmonary absorption. Gaseous and volatile toxic substances may be inhaled and absorbed through the pulmonary epithelium and mucous membranes in the respiratory tract. Access to the circulation is rapid because the surface area of the lungs is large and the blood flow is great. The nasal hair, the cough reflex, and the mucociliary barrier help prevent dust particles and fumes from reaching the lung.

The solubility of gases affects their absorption. Highly water-soluble gases such as ammonia and sulfuric acid are absorbed in the upper airways and cause marked irritation there. This serves as a warning and limits the injury to the lung. Noxious gases of low water solubility such as nitrogen dioxide and phosgene, which have few early warning properties, reach the lungs and cause delayed injury there.

C. Percutaneous Absorption: Many toxic substances pass through the skin, intact or broken. The amount of skin absorption is generally proportionate to the surface area of contact and to the lipid solubility of the toxic agent. The epidermis acts as a lipid barrier, and the stratum corneum provides a protective barrier against noxious agents. The dermis, however, is freely permeable to many toxic substances.

Absorption is enhanced by toxic agents that increase the blood flow to the skin. It is also enhanced by use of occlusive skin coverings (eg, permeable clothes and industrial gloves) and topical application of fat-solubilizing vehicles. Hydrated skin is more permeable than dry skin. The thick skin on the palms of the hands and the soles of the feet is more resistant to absorption than is the thin skin on the face, neck, and scrotum. Burns, abrasions, dermatitis, and other injuries to the skin may alter its protective properties and allow absorption of larger quantities of the toxic substance.

D. Ocular Absorption: The eye is also a ready site of absorption. When chemicals enter the body through the conjunctiva, they bypass hepatic elimination and may cause severe systemic toxicity. This may occur when organophosphate pesticides are splashed into the eyes.

Distribution

Toxic substances are transported via the blood to various portions of the body. Some are removed by the lymph, and some insoluble compounds are transported through tissues such as the lung via cells such as macrophages. Most toxic substances enter the bloodstream and are distributed into interstitial and cellular fluids. The pattern of distribution depends on the physiologic and physicochemical properties of the material. The initial phase of distribution usually reflects the cardiac output and regional blood flow. Lipid-soluble agents that penetrate membranes poorly are restricted in their distribution, and their potential sites of action are therefore limited. Distribution may also be limited by the binding of toxic substances to plasma proteins. Toxic agents can accumulate in higher concentration in some tissues as a result of pH gradients, binding to special cellular proteins, or partitioning into lipids. Some agents accumulate in tissue reservoirs, and this may serve to prolong the toxic action; eg, lead may be stored for years in bone and may be released later.

Metabolism

Toxic substances that are lipid-soluble may go through a series of metabolic conversions (biotransformation) to produce more polar (water-soluble) products and thereby enhance removal by urinary excretion. The most common site for biotransformation is the liver, but it can also occur in plasma, lung, or other tissue. Biotransformation may result in either a decrease (detoxification or inactivation) or an increase (activation) in the toxicity of a compound. Differences in the metabolism of toxic substances account for much of the observed differences between individuals and between animal species.

Biotransformation occurs in the liver by hydrolysis, oxidation, reduction, and conjugation. Microsomal enzymes play a key role in the process, and the activity of the microsomal enzyme system can be increased (induced) by many environmental and pharmacologic agents. Both normal individual differences in microsomal enzyme activity and susceptibility to induction are genetically determined and account for the marked variability in bioavailability of many toxic substances. Other factors that regulate key liver enzyme systems are hormones (which account for some sex-dependent differences) and disease states (eg, the presence of hepatitis, cirrhosis, or heart failure). Because the activity of many hepatic metabolizing systems is low in neonates—particularly premature neonates—they may be much more susceptible to toxic substances that are inactivated by liver metabolism. Inefficient metabolizing systems, an altered blood-brain barrier, and inadequate mechanisms of excretion combine to make the fetus and neonate sensitive to the toxic effects of many agents.

Excretion

A. Pathways and Mechanisms of Excretion: Toxic substances are excreted either unchanged or as metabolites. Excretory organs other than the lungs eliminate polar (water-soluble) compounds more efficiently than they eliminate nonpolar (lipid-soluble) compounds. As discussed above, the latter must be metabolized to more polar compounds before they can be eliminated renally. The kidney is the primary organ of elimination for most polar compounds and their metabolites. Excretion of toxic substances in the urine involves glomerular filtration, active secretion, and passive tubular reabsorption. Alkalization or acidification of the urine may dramatically change excretion of some agents. When tubular urine is more alkaline, weak acids are excreted more rapidly because they are ionized and passive tubular reabsorption is decreased. In contrast, when tubular urine is made more acid, excretion of weak acid is reduced.

Many toxic substances metabolized by the liver are excreted first in the bile and later eliminated in the stool or reabsorbed into the blood and ultimately eliminated in the urine. Toxic substances can also be excreted in sweat, saliva, and breast milk, and there may be some minor removal in hair or skin.

B. Clearance: Clearance is the rate at which a toxic agent is excreted, divided by the average concentration of the agent in the plasma. Most toxic substances are eliminated as a linear function of concentration; ie, a constant fraction of the toxic material is eliminated over time (per unit of time). If the point of saturation is reached, the body will no longer be able to eliminate a constant fraction of the material but will instead eliminate a constant amount per unit of time. Under these circumstances, the clearance becomes quite variable. Note that clearance is a measure not of how much is being removed but rather of the volume of fluid that is freed of the toxic agent per unit of time.

C. Volume of Distribution: The volume of distribution is calculated by dividing the dose of the toxic substance administered by the concentration in the blood. This volume is not necessarily a physiologic volume; it is merely an estimate of the degree of distribution of the toxic agent in tissues. The volume of distribution for most toxic agents depends largely on pH factors, protein binding, partition coefficients, and regional differences in blood flow and binding to special tissues.

D. Half-Time and Half-Life: The time it takes for the plasma concentration of a substance to be reduced by 50% is the half-time. For substances that are eliminated as a linear function (ie, independent of concentration), the time it takes to eliminate 50% of the substance is the half-life. Calculation of half-life provides a means of estimating the dose that was absorbed. For a substance eliminated in linear fashion, about 90% of the amount in the body will be eliminated in 3.5 half-lives after the end of the period of exposure.

TESTS OF TOXIC EFFECTS

Much of our information about the toxic effects of different agents comes from studying various strains and species of animals. Toxic substances frequently cause effects in animals, some immediately after administration and others after a prolonged period. Acute effects are sometimes qualitatively quite different from chronic effects. For example, the acute effect of benzene is central nervous system depression, while its chronic effects are aplastic anemia and leukemia.

Although tests in animals are the most common methods of identifying agents that cause toxicity, the results are difficult to extrapolate to humans, given the disparity among life spans (18–24 months for rodents versus 75 years for humans). In addition, different strains and species of animals may show both qualitative and quantitative differences in the pattern or intensity of response to a toxic agent. Even with the best statistical approaches and the best evidence of toxic responses in animals, there is no certain way of estimating the incidence of toxicity or determining the type of response to a toxic substance in a human population. Furthermore, there is no absolute certainty that safety factors for exposure to a toxic substance based on studies in animals would be valid for humans.

Tests for Acute, Subacute, & Chronic Toxic Effects

Tests for acute effects are usually performed when there are no data available on the potential toxicity of a single exposure or a few exposures to a specific agent. An appropriate route of administration is chosen, and a specific end point (eg, death of the laboratory animal) is selected. The signs and symptoms before death are observed, and the animal is later examined for gross and histologic damage to tissues. In some cases, topical application of an agent is used to test for skin or eye injury.

Tests for subacute or sublethal effects of a specific agent are usually performed during a period of 21–90 days in animals, with the route of administration chosen on the basis of anticipated human exposure. Two different species of rodents are usually involved in each test.

Tests for chronic effects are performed in animals when long-term human exposure to a specific agent is anticipated or a long latency period between exposure and toxicity is expected. Rats and mice are usually exposed from a few weeks of age until their premature death or their sacrifice at the end of the expected lifetime.

Tests for Teratogenesis & Toxic Effects on Reproductive Organs

Teratologic tests involve exposing pregnant female animals to a specific agent at a critical time during pregnancy and then examining their offspring for malformations. Usually 2 or 3 species are used for comparison and controls. In reproductive studies, male and female animals are exposed to an agent and subsequently observed for reproductive failure or success. In cases of successful reproduction, the first- and second-generation offspring are also observed for their ability to reproduce. In cases of unsuccessful reproduction, male animals are often tested for sperm motility, count, and morphology.

IDENTIFICATION OF THE MECHANISMS OF TOXICITY

The best approach to understanding the mechanisms of a toxic effect involves 3 essential considerations: (1) the time course of the concentration of the active forms of a toxic agent at its active sites, (2) the kinetics of interaction between the active forms of the toxic compound and its active sites, and (3) the kinetics of the sequence of events resulting from the interaction that occurs before toxicity has been manifested. These observations must then be validated against experimental evidence in animals or epidemiologic studies in humans.

A special task force on toxicologic assessment has suggested 6 questions whose answers would lead to the development of protocols that would effectively identify the mechanisms of toxicity: What is the manifestation of the toxicity? What element causes the toxicity? What factors govern the concentration of the toxic element at its active sites? What is the physical or chemical nature of the reaction of the toxic substance at its active sites? What subsequent events lead to the manifestation of toxicity? How can toxicity be modulated?

The answers to these 6 questions are not simple. For example, toxicologists are not certain about the significance of tumors in animal species in which the incidence of spontaneous liver tumor is high. It is important to understand whether toxic agents act without further biotransformation or by direct interaction with an essential cellular constituent that maintains the integrity of the cell. Even if the parent toxic substance does not cause injury, an active metabolite (eg, superoxide anion) may be detrimental to cell function.

The following types of research help identify the mechanisms of action of specific toxic agents: (1) studying the effects of a particular type of pretreatment on the toxin-metabolizing enzyme systems in various organs and tissues, (2) analyzing the effects of inhibitors or inducers on activation or detoxification pathways at potential sites of metabolism, (3) elucidating the nature of the substrate cell, (4) studying the influence of genetic and environmental factors that affect potential toxic target sites, (5) reviewing the age and sex differences in the enzymes and target systems affected by a given toxic agent, and (6) determining the manner in which a toxic effect can be modulated, eg, by alteration in diet or manipulation of hormones.

TOXICOLOGIC RISK ASSESSMENT

Steps in Risk Assessment

Risk assessment is the characterization of the potential adverse health effects of human exposure to hazardous substances. It can be divided into the following steps:

Step 1. Hazard identification—(a) Description of the population exposed to a substance (population at risk). (b) Determination of the adverse health effects that would be caused by that substance (eg, cancer and birth defects).

Step 2. Dose-response assessment—(a) Collection of epidemiologic and experimental dose-response data on the effects of the substance. (b) Identification of a "critical" dose-response relationship (discussed in detail below). (c) Quantitative expression of the dose-response relationship by mathematical extrapolation from high doses in animals to low doses in humans.

Step 3. Exposure assessment—Estimation of past, present, and future exposure levels of the population at risk and of actual doses received.

Step 4. Risk characterization—Estimation of the incidence of adverse health effects in the population predicted from the dose-response assessment (step 2) as applied to the exposure assessment (step 3).

Uncertainties Inherent in Risk Assessment

There are a number of uncertainties inherent in risk assessment for toxic substances: (1) Human data are frequently lacking or are limited due to inability to detect low-incidence effects. Epidemiologic studies do not demonstrate causation or provide quantitative dose-response data, nor do they account for mixed and multiple exposures, a sufficient latency period for effects to be expressed, and differences between the populations studied. (2) Animal data are often of uncertain relevance to humans. A rational choice of the most appropriate species may not be possible. Toxicokinetic and toxicodynamic data are usually lacking. The route, frequency, and duration of exposure may be different from those of the human population. The doses are usually much higher, and the animals studied are genetically homogeneous and free of exposure to other toxic substances. (3) The mechanisms of action for effects are poorly understood. (4) The exposure of the population at risk may not be quantified, and calculation of doses may not be possible.

Because of these uncertainties, the practice of quantitative risk assessment is sometimes criticized for being "unscientific." However, since human exposure to toxic substances may result in medical and public health risks, risk assessment often provides the only basis for decisions on how to manage potential risks.

Methods for Estimation of Risk

There are 2 basic methods for risk estimation, based on the presence or absence of a predicted threshold in the "critical" dose-response relationship identified in step 2.

A. Threshold Method: A threshold is generally assumed for all noncarcinogenic responses. Since human exposure is generally below the threshold for adverse effects in animals, estimated risk cannot be expressed as a numerical probability (eg, 1:1000). Risk is expressed instead as a safety factor. The safety factor is the ratio between the allowable daily intake (ADI) for humans and a threshold dose in animals.

An ADI is estimated by the steps outlined above. Following hazard identification (step 1), a "no-observed-adverse-effect level" (NOEL)—also called the "safe" level—is determined (step 2) from animal studies. Exposure assessment (step 3) is then performed. The NOEL in animals and the ADI in humans are converted into comparable doses (doses allowing for species differences and differences in route, frequency, and duration of exposure), and the NOEL is divided by the ADI to yield a safety factor (step 4). Calculations can also be made using the lowest dose that produced an effect, ie, the "minimum-observed-adverse-effect level" (MOEL), or "unsafe" level.

The size of the safety factor is an estimate of the probability of an effect occurring in the population, based on differences in sensitivity between an animal species and humans. A safety factor of 10 suggests human sensitivity 10 times that of animals. An additional factor of 10 (to yield 100) is used when there is human genetic variability and susceptibility due to other factors and exposures. An additional factor of 10 (to yield 1000) is used when the animal

study was faulty in design or a NOEL was not determined and a MOEL was used instead.

B. No-Threshold Method: For carcinogens, the absence of a threshold is usually assumed, and quantitative risk estimation is controversial. Following hazard identification (step 1), step 2 consists of evaluating human epidemiologic studies and selecting the most appropriate animal study for extrapolation. This includes scrutiny of dose-response data for the tumor in a particular species, extrapolation from the high doses in the animal study to low doses in humans, and selection of a particular mathematic model. Depending on the model selected, resulting estimates of risk may differ by many orders of magnitude. Exposure assessment (step 3) is then performed. The risk to the population (step 4) is estimated by applying the dose-response model from step 2 to the doses calculated from exposure data in step 3. Several assumptions must be made to arrive at a single "best estimate" of risk or—more commonly—a range of estimates of risk.

DOSE-RESPONSE CURVES

A dose-response relationship exists when changes in dose are followed by consistent changes in response, as shown in dose-response curves. A variety of toxicologic phenomena can be demonstrated by these curves. Figs 12–1A and 12–1B show the intensity of the response to various doses in an individual. Because Fig 12–1B is in a logarithmic scale, the shape of the curve is more linear. This makes it easier to determine values for specific points on the curve.

The frequency of a response in a population can be related to dose as a frequency distribution (as in Fig 12–2) or as a cumulative frequency (as in Figs 12–3 and 12–4).

In Fig 12–2, the existence of a threshold is indicated by the arrow at the point where the curve intersects the dose coordinate. Doses below this point do not produce a response. Individuals who exhibit the response at doses well below the average or the mean are considered hypersusceptible (H in Fig 12–2), while those who respond only to doses well above the average or the mean are considered resistant (R in Fig 12–2).

In Fig 12–3, cumulative frequency curves are used to compare 2 doses of the same toxic substance to the dose that is lethal to 50% of the population (LD50) and the dose that has an effect on 10% (ED10). The ED10 may, for example, represent an effect that is not harmful, such as odor. The ratio between comparable points on the curves (ie, the ratio of LD50 to ED10) will then represent the margin of safety for odor as a warning against the lethal effect.

In Fig 12–4, cumulative frequency curves are used to compare the doses at which the same toxic effect is elicited by 3 different toxic substances (A, B, and C). Substance A is clearly the most toxic, because at

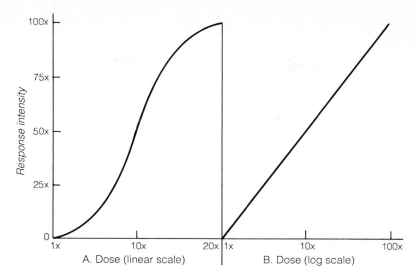

Figure 12–1. In these dose-response curves, A and B both show the intensity of the response to various doses in an individual. Because B uses a logarithmic scale, the curve is more linear.

every dose level a greater percentage of the population exhibits the response to A than to B or C. The LD50, the ED10, and the threshold for A are all lower than the corresponding values for B and C. The comparison between B and C is less clear and demonstrates the need to consider the entire dose-response curves rather than individual points when comparing toxicities. Because the LD50 of B is lower than that of C, at this dose B is more toxic than C. However, because the ED10 of C is lower than that of B, at the lower dose C is more toxic than B. The shape of a dose-response curve is important for assessing the hazard of a toxic substance. A substance that has a low threshold and shallow dose-response curve (such as C) may be more hazardous at low doses, while a substance that has a steep dose-response curve (such as B) may be more hazardous as the dose increases. Adequate assessment of the hazard of a toxic substance requires evaluation of dose-response data over a wide range of doses.

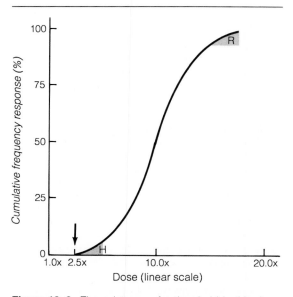

Figure 12–2. The existence of a threshold in this dose-response curve is indicated by the arrow. Doses below this point do not produce a response. Individuals who exhibit the response at doses well below the average or the mean are considered hypersusceptible (H), while those who respond only to doses well above the average or the mean are considered resistant (R).

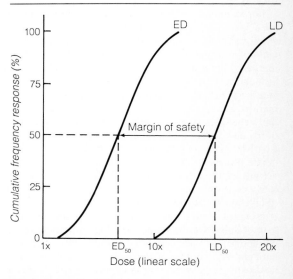

Figure 12–3. Dose-response curves comparing 2 doses of the same toxic substance. ED = effective dose; LD = lethal dose. The area between is the margin of safety.

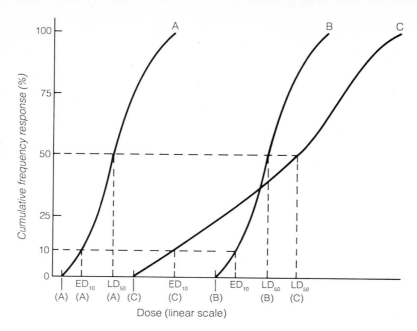

Figure 12–4. Dose-response curves comparing the doses at which the same toxic effect is elicited by 3 different toxic substances (A, B, and C).

DIAGNOSIS OF TOXIC EFFECTS

Different toxic substances often elicit similar clinical manifestations of toxicity. In some cases, the manifestations represent a response to more than one toxic agent or to a combination of toxic agents and naturally occurring causes. In general, the manifestations of acute toxicity due to high-dose exposures will be more specific than those of chronic toxicity or toxicity due to low-dose exposures.

For example, patients with acute poisoning caused by a high-dose exposure to organophosphate pesticides may present with involvement of the autonomic nervous system (nausea, vomiting, diarrhea, increased lacrimation and sweating, bronchorrhea, bronchoconstriction, blurred vision, small pupils, and bradycardia), the neuromuscular system (fasciculations, cramps, weakness, and hyporeflexia), and the central nervous system (confusion, hallucinations, and depressed consciousness). The presence of small pupils with the rest of these findings is diagnostic of organophosphate poisoning. Cholinesterase activity in blood or plasma is likely to be extremely low, confirming the diagnosis. The poisoning is likely to be accompanied by a clear history of overexposure, such as that caused by exposure to a leak or spill from pesticide spraying equipment or by deliberate or accidental ingestion. In contrast, patients with chronic or low-level exposures to organophosphate pesticides usually have poorly defined clinical manifestations, such as mild diarrhea, sweating, myalgias, and malaise (findings that are virtually indistinguishable from those of influenza), and

cholinesterase activity levels may be normal. ("Toxidromes" for other substances are discussed under Clinical Findings in subsequent chapters.)

In some cases, the manifestations of toxicity due to high-dose exposure are totally different from those due to low-dose exposure. For example, benzidine causes methemoglobinemia at high doses and bladder cancer at low doses. There are relatively few compounds that cause methemoglobinemia, and most cases can be attributed to a specific toxic substance in the workplace or the environment. However, bladder cancer has a number of known causes in addition to exposure to benzidine, and this makes it difficult to attribute bladder cancer to low-dose toxic exposure. With chronic exposure to low doses, toxic agents are more likely to cause an increase in the incidence of disorders already present in the population than they are to cause a novel disorder.

Because of this nonspecificity of clinical manifestations, a systematic approach to diagnosis is necessary and should include a greater emphasis on the history (general, occupational, and environmental), as discussed in Chapter 2. A list of possible toxic agents should be generated from the exposure history and their toxicity reviewed. The results of physical examination and laboratory tests should be grouped according to findings related to each system or organ, and the findings should then be matched with findings due to specific toxic substances. A search for causes other than exposure to toxic agents should also be made, and additional diagnostic tests should be ordered as necessary to rule out these other causes. Although biologic measurements of specific toxic substances may be helpful on occasion (see Chapter 28), they are usually not available soon enough for use in cases of acute poisoning, and it is often too late to measure them in cases of chronic exposure.

MANAGEMENT OF TOXIC EFFECTS

Management in most cases of toxicity consists of supportive care, symptomatic treatment, and removal from exposure to the toxic material. In cases of life-threatening toxicity, maintenance of cardiopulmonary function and fluid and electrolyte balance are usually indicated. Methods to enhance elimination, such as forced diuresis, hemodialysis, and hemoperfusion, have not been shown to be effective for treatment of poisoning due to most toxic agents of industrial origin.

There are only a few specific methods of treatment, or "antidotes." Chelating agents may reverse acute toxicity due to some metals (eg, lead, arsenic, and mercury), but they are less likely to affect subacute or chronic toxicity (see Chapter 25). Atropine and pralidoxime can be lifesaving in reversing the acute cholinesterase-inhibiting effects of organophosphate pesticides (see Chapter 30). In cases of acute cyanide or hydrogen sulfide poisoning, nitrites may be used to generate formation of cyanmethemoglobin or sulfmethemoglobin (see Chapter 31). Hydroxocobalamin (vitamin B_{12a}) is used in Europe and is currently being tested in the USA as an antidote for cyanide. Use of oxygen counters the effect and enhances the elimination of carbon monoxide (see Chapter 31).

REFERENCES

Clayton GD, Clayton FE (editors): *Patty's Industrial Hygiene and Toxicology: Toxicology*, 3rd ed. Vols 2A–2C. Wiley, 1981–1985.

Doull J, Klaassen CD, Amdur MO (editors): *Casarett and Doull's Toxicology: The Basic Science of Poisons*, 3rd ed. Macmillan, 1986.

Hayes AW (editor): *Principles and Methods of Toxicology*. Raven Press, 1982.

Hodgson E, Levi PE: *A Textbook of Modern Toxicology*. Elsevier, 1987.

Kamrin MA: *Toxicology*. Lewis, 1988.

National Academy of Sciences/National Research Council: *Risk Assessment in the Federal Government: Managing the Process*. National Academy Press, 1983.

Rodricks JV, Tardiff RG (editors): *Assessment and Management of Chemical Risks*. American Chemical Society, 1984.

Williams PL, Burson JL (editors): *Industrial Toxicology: Safety and Health Applications in the Workplace*. Van Nostrand/Reinhold, 1985.

13

Clinical Immunology

Donald F. German, MD

Immune hypersensitivity mechanisms play a part in many disorders of occupational medicine. In 1700, Bernardino Ramazzini, the founder of modern occupational medicine, reported that after repeated exposures to flour dust, bakers often developed respiratory problems—a disease now called baker's asthma. In the 20th century, many disorders of occupational medicine have been shown to be caused by immune reactions to environmental factors. Some of these include pigeon breeder's disease, farmer's lung, asthma induced by castor bean, nickel dermatitis, and poison oak dermatitis.

The purpose of this chapter is to review the primary immune response and the effector mechanisms, classify immune hypersensitivity disorders found in occupational medicine, list some examples of these disorders, and to comment on the controversial field of clinical ecology. The chapter concludes with a section on diagnosis of hypersensitivity diseases often seen in the practice of occupational medicine.

IMMUNE RESPONSE

The immune system serves a role that may be either protective (eg, destroying neoplastic cells, microorganisms) or damaging (eg, destroying host cells). Immune reactions generally do not occur on first exposure to foreign antigens—substances not recognized as "self." These reactions first require a period of sensitization. Lymphocyte precursors, which are derived from hematopoietic stem cells found in the mammalian yolk sac, differentiate under the influence of the thymus (T lymphocytes) or the bone marrow (B lymphocytes). Macrophages bind, process, and present antigen along with class II antigen of the major histocompatibility complex (HLA-D and HLA-DR) to CD4 (T helper-inducer) lymphocytes. CD4 lymphocytes then send a signal back to the histocompatible macrophage, stimulating the release of interleukin-1 (IL-1). IL-1 in turn acts on the CD4 lymphocytes, stimulating the release of interleukin-2 (IL-2), B cell differentiation factor (BCDF), and B cell growth factor (BCGF). The IL-2 stimulates other CD4 lymphocytes and CD8 (T suppressor) lymphocytes. The CD4 and CD8 lymphocytes modulate the immune response and B cell activity. B lymphocytes are activated by BCGF and BCDF and also IL-2 and eventually differentiate into end-stage plasma cells that produce the various immunoglobulins (Fig 13–1).

IMMUNOGLOBULINS

Immunoglobulins, the products of plasma cells, are humoral proteins that possess antibody activity. The basic immunoglobulin molecule is a monomer made up of 2 light and 2 heavy chains linked by disulfide bonds. The light chain and the N-terminal half of the heavy chain form the Fab fragment. Antigen-binding activity resides in the N-terminal portion of this fragment. The 2 Fab fragments that make up the N-terminal half of the molecule are linked at the hinge region by disulfide bonds (Fig 13–2). The C-terminal half of the immunoglobulin molecule is made up of the remainder of the heavy chains and is called the Fc fragment. The biologic function of the molecule is dependent on this fragment.

There are 5 classes of immunoglobulins, each having a different heavy chain molecule. Table 13–1 summarizes many of the properties of the immunoglobulins.

IgG is the predominant immunoglobulin in serum. It has a molecular weight of 150,000. IgG antibodies are strong precipitins, and 3 subclasses—IgG_1, IgG_2, and IgG_3—can activate complement, qualities that make it operative in serum sickness and certain types of hypersensitivity pneumonitis (eg, bird breeder's disease).

IgA is the predominant immunoglobulin on mucous membrane surfaces. It exists predominantly as a monomer (MW 160,000) in serum and as a dimer or trimer (MW 390,000–550,000) on mucous membrane surfaces. When the dimer or trimer passes through the epithelial cells to a mucous membrane surface, it acquires a smaller molecule called secretory piece (MW 70,000) that stabilizes the molecule and prevents its degradation by proteolytic enzymes. IgA antibodies protect the host from foreign antigens on mucous membrane surfaces, but they do not fix complement by the classic pathway.

IgM is a pentamer (MW 900,000) that is found almost exclusively in the intravascular compartment. IgM antibodies are potent agglutinins and fix complement. They may mediate the trimellitic anhydride pulmonary anemia syndrome. IgD is a monomeric immunoglobulin (MW 180,000). Its biologic function is unknown.

IgE is the heaviest immunoglobulin monomer (MW 190,000), with a normal concentration in serum varying from 20 to 100 IU, but the concentration may be 5 times normal or even higher in an atopic

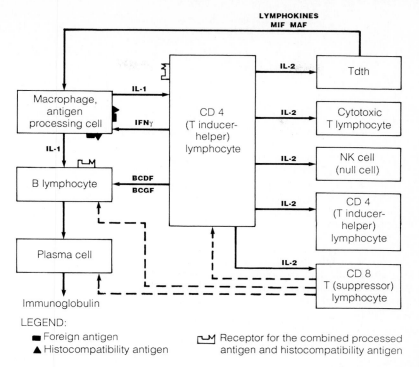

Figure 13–1. The primary immune response. MIF = macrophage inhibitory factor; MAF = macrophage-activating factor; IL-1 = interleukin-1, a product of the macrophage, which activates T4 inducer-helper cells and B cells; IL-2 = interleukin-2, which stimulates the development of Tdth (T delayed type hypersensitivity) cells, cytotoxic T cells, NK (null) cells, and T suppressor (CD8) T8 cells, which help to modulate the immune response and other (CD4) T4 cells; IFNγ = γ-interferon, a product of T4 cells that further activates the macrophage; BCDF = B cell differentiation factor and BCGF = B cell growth factor—both of them products of the CD4 cell that lead to differentiation and growth of B cells; Tdth = T delayed type hypersensitivity lymphocyte; NK cell = natural killer (null) cell, which lacks common T and B cell markers but has receptors for Fc of IgG; CD4 = an antigenic marker on T inducer-helper lymphocytes; CD8 = an antigenic marker on T suppressor lymphocytes.

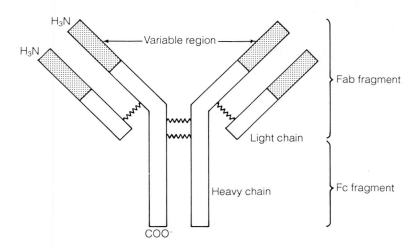

Figure 13–2. The immunoglobulin molecule is composed of 2 heavy and 2 light chains. The light chain and the amino (H₃N⁻) terminal half of the heavy chain make up Fab, the antibody-binding fragment of the molecule. The carboxyl (COO⁻) terminal halves of the heavy chains make up the Fc or crystalline half of the immunoglobulin molecule, which is responsible for the unique biologic activities of a given immunoglobulin class. Interchain disulfide bonds (∿) bind the heavy and light chains.

Table 13–1. Human immunoglobulin classes.

Class	Mean Serum Conc. mg/dL	Molecular Weight	Sed. Coef.	Half-Life in Plasma (Days)	Biologic Function
IgG	1200	150,000	7	23	Fix complement Cross placenta Strongest precipitating capacity
IgA	280	160,000 550,000	7, 10, 14	6	Secretory antibody Antiviral defense
IgM	120	900,000	19	5	Fix complement Strongest agglutinating capacity
IgD	3	180,000	7	3	B lymphocyte surface receptor in newborn
IgE	0.03	190,000	8	2.5	Reaginic antibody

individual. The Fc portion of IgE binds to receptors on the surfaces of mast cells and basophils. IgE antibodies play an important role in immediate hypersensitivity reactions such as nasal allergy and allergic bronchial asthma in veterinarians, laboratory animal handlers, and enzyme detergent industry workers.

MEDIATORS OF IMMEDIATE HYPERSENSITIVITY

Mediators of immediate hypersensitivity are chemicals generated or released by antigen-antibody reactions. They have various biologic activities and normally function in host defense, but they play a pathologic role in immune hypersensitivity. They exist in a preformed state in the granules of mast cells and basophils or are newly synthesized at the time of activation of these and some other nucleated cells (Tables 13–2 and 13–3). A number of stimuli activate mast cells and basophils, including the antigen bridging of 2 adjacent IgE molecules on the mast cell-basophil surface, anaphylatoxins (C3a, C4a, C5a), lectins (PHA, PWM), and drugs (morphine, codeine).

Preformed mediators include histamine, eosinophil chemotactic factor of anaphylaxis (ECFA), high-molecular-weight neutrophilic chemotactic factor of anaphylaxis (NCFA), proteoglycans (heparin, chondroitin sulfate), and various proteolytic enzymes. Histamine is a bioactive amine that when released binds to H_1 and H_2 receptors on adjacent cells. Binding to H_1 receptors causes smooth muscle contraction, vasodilatation, increased vascular permeability, and stimulation of nasal mucous glands. Stimulation of H_2 receptors on mast cells abrogates mediator release. Histamine is important in the pathogenesis of allergic rhinitis, allergic asthma, and anaphylaxis. ECFA and NCFA primarily stimulate eosinophil and neutrophil chemotaxis. A second peak of NCFA has been observed in late asthmatic reactions, occurring 4–6 hours after antigen challenge.

Newly generated mediators include kinins,

platelet-activating factor, and phospholipid-derived substances including leukotrienes and prostaglandins. Arachidonic acid, derived from the phospholipid bilayer of cells, is metabolized either by the lypoxygenase pathway to form leukotrienes (LT) or the cyclooxygenase pathway to form prostaglandins (PG) and thromboxanes (TXA_2 and TXB_2). Leukotrienes are generated by mast cells, granulocytes, macrophages, and basophils. LTB_4 is a potent chemoattractant for polymorphonuclear neutrophils. LTC_4, LTD_4, and LTE_4 constitute slow-reacting substance of anaphylaxis (SRS-A), which has a bronchial smooth muscle spasmogenic potency 100–1000 times that of histamine; leukotrienes are also important mediators in allergic rhinitis.

Prostaglandins are generated by almost all nucleated cells. The most important members are PGD_2, PGE_2, PGF_2, and PGI_2 (prostacyclin). Human mast cells produce large amounts of PGD_2, which causes vasodilatation, vascular permeability, and airway constriction. Activated polymorphonuclear neutro-

Table 13–2. Mediators of immediate hypersensitivity.

Preformed	Cell Source[1]
Histamine	M, B
ECFA	M
HMW NCF[2]	M
Heparin	M
Chondroitin	B
Tryptase	M
Protease	M
Lysosomal hydrolases	M, B
Newly generated	
Prostaglandins	All nucleated cells
Leukotrienes	M, (?) B, PMN, Mono
PAF	M, PMN, Eos, Mono
Kinins	M, B

[1]M = mast cells; B = basophils
[2]NCF = neutrophil chemotactic factor

Table 13–3. Action of mediators in hypersensitivity reactions.

	Bronchial Constriction	Chemotaxis PMS	Chemotaxis EOS	Platelet Activation	Increased Vascular Permeability	Mucus Production	Pruritus
Histamine	X	X	X		X	X (Nasal)	X
Leukotrienes C	X				X	X	
D	X				X	X	
E	X					X	
5-HETE		X					
PGD$_2$	X				X		
TxA$_2$	X			X			
Kallikrein					X		
PAF	X	X		X			
NCFA		X					
ECFA		X	X				

phils and macrophages generate PGF$_{2\alpha}$, a bronchoconstrictor, and PGE$_2$, a bronchodilator. PGI$_2$ causes platelet disaggregation. TxA$_2$ causes platelet aggregation, bronchial constriction, and vasoconstriction.

Platelet activating factor (PAF) is generated by macrophages, neutrophils, eosinophils, and mast cells. It causes platelet aggregation, vasodilatation, increased vascular permeability, and bronchial smooth muscle contraction. The kinins are vasoactive peptides formed in plasma when kallikrein—released by basophils and mast cells—digests plasma kininogen; they cause slow sustained contraction of bronchial and vascular smooth muscle, vascular permeability, secretion of mucus, and stimulation of pain fibers. Kinins may play a role in human anaphylaxis.

EFFECTOR CELLS

A number of effector cells participate in immune hypersensitivity reactions. These include mast cells, basophils, polymorphonuclear neutrophils, eosinophils, macrophage-monocytes, platelets, and lymphocytes. Depending on the type of immune response, many or all play a part. The effector cells have membrane receptors for various chemoattractants and mediators (Tables 13–3 and 13–4).

Mast cells are basophilic staining cells found chiefly in connective and subcutaneous tissue. They have prominent granules that are the source of many mediators of immediate hypersensitivity and have 30,000–200,000 cell surface membrane receptors for the Fc fragment of IgE. When an allergen molecule binds 2 adjacent mast cell surface-associated IgE antibodies, bridging between the 2 antibodies occurs. This perturbs the cell membrane surface, allows calcium to enter the cell, and activates enzyme systems that ultimately lead to the release of both preformed and newly generated mediators. Mast cells

also have surface receptors for anaphylatoxins C3a, C4a, and C5a.

Basophils account for approximately 1% of circulating granulocytes. They possess a segmented nucleus and granules that are larger than those of mast cells. Like mast cells, they have cell membrane surface receptors for the Fc fragment of IgE and anaphylatoxins. On exposure to antigen, activation leading to the release of mediators occurs in a manner similar to mast cells. Basophils possess some but not all of the mediators found in mast cells (Table 13–2).

Neutrophils are granulocytes that phagocytose and destroy foreign antigens and microbial organisms. They are attracted to the site of antigen by chemotactic factors, including C5a, NCFA, PAF, LTB$_4$, and ECFA. They possess receptors for the Fc fragment of IgG and IgM antibodies (specific opsonins) and for C3b (nonspecific opsonin). Neutrophils are activated when they unite with C3b or with the Fc portion of IgG or IgM antibody bound to particles or cells. Smaller antigens are phagocytosed and destroyed by lysosomal enzymes. Particles too large to be phago-

Table 13–4. Effector cell membrane receptors.

	Hist	HMW NCF	ECFA	C3a	C3b	C5a	Fc IgG	Fc IgE	Ag
MAST	X			X		X	X[1]	X	
BASO	X						X	X	
MACR					X				
MONO	X				X	X			
PMN	X	X	X	X	X	X	X		
EOS			X						
T cell	X								X
K cell							X		

[1]Fc for IgG$_4$

cytosed are destroyed by locally released lysosomal enzymes. Neutrophils contain or generate a number of antimicrobial factors, including superoxides, which produce H_2O_2; myeloperoxidase, which catalyzes the production of hypochlorite; and proteolytic enzymes, including collagenase, elastase, and cathepsin B. Some or all of these factors may play a part in a number of hypersensitivity reactions, including the type I late asthmatic response, the type II cytotoxin reaction, and type III immune complex disease (see below).

Eosinophils play both a proactive and a modulating role in inflammation. They are attracted to the site of the antigen-antibody reactions by ECFA, histamine, and LTB4. They are important in the defense against parasites. When stimulated, they release major basic protein (MBP), eosinophil peroxidase, lysosomal hydrolases, and LTC4. MBP destroys parasites, impairs ciliary beating, and causes exfoliation of respiratory epithelial cells; it may trigger histamine release from mast cells and basophils. It has been suggested that the eosinophils may play a modulating role in inflammation; they contain histaminase, which metabolizes histamine, and aryl sulfatase B, an enzyme that catabolizes various leukotrienes.

The tissue-fixed macrophages and the circulating monocytes are both phagocytes and antigen-processing cells. Monocytes are susceptible to chemoattraction by C5a. When they leave the circulation, they mature into macrophages. Both monocytes and macrophages contain receptors for C3b and the Fc portion of IgG. Activation of these cells occurs not only when these receptors are stimulated but also when they are exposed to various lymphokines and when they phagocytose antigen, silica, and asbestos. They contain aryl sulfatase, acid phosphatase, and β-glucuronidase and are able to produce H_2O_2. They produce and release SRS-A, PAF, PGE_2, PGF_2, and many complement proteins. Besides their function as effector cells of hypersensitivity, they play a vital role in the primary immune response, ingesting, processing, and presenting foreign antigen in conjunction with class 2 antigens of the major histocompatibility complex (HLA D and HLA DR) to both CD4 (T helper-inducer) lymphocytes and B lymphocytes; they generate IL-1, which stimulates CD4 cells to produce IL-2 (Fig 13–1).

Human platelets play a vital role in the clotting sequence. They contain thromboxane and vasoactive amines. Thromboxane and PAF cause platelet aggregation and initiate the clotting sequence. During antigen-induced acute airway reactions, there is evidence that platelet factor 4 (PF4) is released and stimulates mediator release from basophils.

T lymphocytes play an important role as effector cells. T delayed type hypersensitivity (Tdth) cells mediate the delayed hypersensitivity reaction. When specific antigen binds to the already sensitized Tdth cell surface receptors, the cells become activated and release mediators or lymphokines, which enhance the Tdth immune response to foreign antigen. Lympho-

kines include chemotactic factor for macrophages (CFM), migration inhibitory factor (MIF), and macrophage activation factor (MAF); these mediators—respectively—attract macrophages to the site of the T cell immune reaction, inhibit their migration away from the site, and enhance their cytolytic activity. Other lymphokines include lymphocytotoxin, leukocyte inhibition factor, colony stimulating factor, transfer factor, gamma interferon, and interleukin-2.

In addition to T and B lymphocytes, there are null cells (K [killer] cells) that lack B and most T cell markers; they do not have receptors for specific antigenic determinants but rather for the Fc fragment of cell surface antigen-bound IgG. They may play an important role in tumor immunity. CD4 lymphocytes have receptors for processed antigen presented in conjunction with class 2 major histocompatibility antigen by activated macrophages. They play a pivotal role in the immune response (Fig 13–1).

COMPLEMENT

Activation of the classic complement pathway is initiated by the union of antigen with IgE or IgM antibody. Complement-fixing sites on the Fc region of these antibody molecules are exposed, allowing binding of the first component of the complement sequence, C1q. Other components of the complement sequence are subsequently bound, activated, and cleaved, eventually leading to cell lysis (Fig 13–3). Important by-products of the classic pathway include anaphylatoxins, the potent C3a and C5a and less potent C4a; C5a is chemotactic for PMNs and monocytes and causes activation and release of mediators from mast cells and basophils. C4b and C3b opsonize target cells, thus facilitating phagocytosis. Activation of the complement sequence by the alternative pathway is initiated by a number of agents, including lipopolysaccharides, trypsinlike molecules, aggregated IgA and IgG, and cobra venom. Activation does not require the presence of antigen-antibody complexes, nor does it utilize the early components of the complement sequence, C1, C4, and C2. It requires the presence of a different series of proteins, factors B and D and properidin, which facilitate activation, and factors H and I, which act as inactivators. Just as in the classic pathway, the important molecules—C3b, C3a, and C5a—are generated. Ultimately, as a result of activation of the classic or alternative pathway, activation of the terminal complement sequence occurs, resulting in cell lysis (Fig 13–3).

CLASSIFICATION OF IMMUNE HYPERSENSITIVITY DISORDERS

Gell and Coombs have classified the various immune hypersensitivity reactions into 4 major types depending on the effector mechanisms involved.

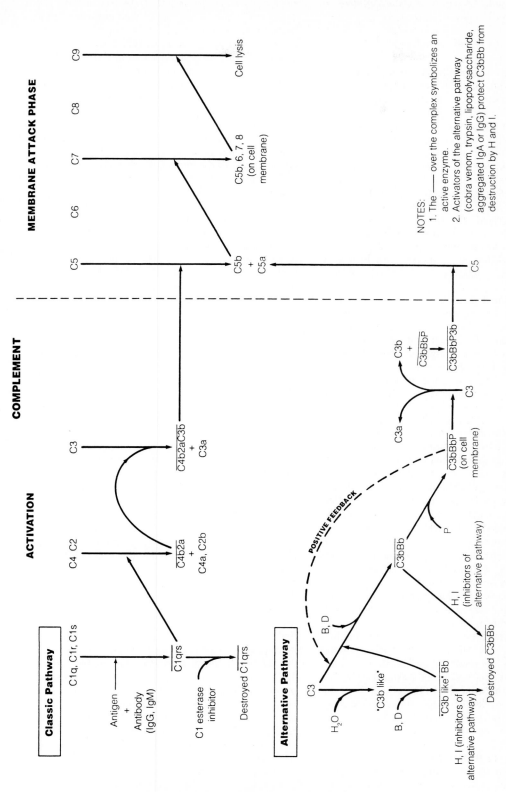

Figure 13–3. Complement. **Classic pathway:** IgG or IgM antibody binds to antigen, and C1q binds to the Fc portion of the immunoglobulin molecule. C1r and C1s bind to C1q, forming C1qrs (C1 esterase). C1qrs cleaves C4 and C2, forming C4b2a, which in turn cleaves C3. The resulting C4b2a3b cleaves C5 and activates the terminal C components (C6, C7, C8, and C9). **Alternative pathway:** Normally, some C3 is hydrolyzed by H_2O to "C3b-like molecule," which is in turn further acted on by factors B and D, leading to a "C3b-like" Bb molecule. The majority of "C3b-like"Bb is in the fluid phase and is destroyed by factors H and I. However, when C3bBb is bound to activators such as cobra venom, lipopolysaccharides, or aggregated IgG or IgA, the complex is protected from destruction. The complex is further stabilized by factor P (properdin); the resulting enzyme (C3bBbP) cleaves C3 into C3a and C3b. The C3b binds to the complex, leading to the formation of C3bBbPC3b, which cleaves C5 and activates the terminal C components (C6, C7, C8, and C9).

More than one type of reaction may be operative in many immune hypersensitivity disorders.

Type I: Immediate Hypersensitivity Reaction

The type I reaction develops in sensitized individuals immediately after contact with antigen. Patients often have a personal or family history of IgE-mediated asthma or rhinitis. The Fc portion of IgE antibody binds to surface receptors on the basophil and mast cell; each of these cells has 20,000–400,000 such receptors. When antigen bridges 2 adjacent specific IgE antibody molecules on the cell surface, perturbation of the cell occurs, eventually leading to the release of preformed and newly generated mediators. Depending on the shock organ involved, the host then may respond with rhinitis, bronchospasm, urticaria, angioedema, or hypotension. Examples of type I reactions found in occupational medicine include allergic asthma and rhinitis, seen in bakers and in animal handlers, and anaphylaxis in bee keepers.

Immediate sensitivity can be demonstrated in vivo by a scratch or intradermal skin test to specific antigen. A positive test is demonstrated by a pruritic wheal and flare reaction, which peaks at 20 minutes. When the concentration of antigen and the number of specific IgE molecules on the mast cell surface are sufficiently great, the immediate skin test after almost complete clearing is followed by the **late phase reaction (LPR),** which develops about 4 hours after the initial test. The LPR is a diffusely erythematous and edematous skin reaction with a poorly defined border. There is associated pruritus and tenderness. The LPR peaks in approximately 6 hours and may persist for 24–48 hours. IgE is the only antibody necessary to induce the LPR. Biopsy of the LPR skin site reveals perivascular hyalinization and infiltration with PMNs, mononuclear cells, and eosinophils; there is no evidence of IgG, IgA, IgM, or C3.

The IgE-mediated cutaneous LPR is thought to have its counterpart in the **late asthma reaction (LAR).** Bronchial challenge with a variety of allergens can provoke an initial brief—and then a later prolonged—increase in airway resistance lasting 12–24 hours. After such a reaction, the patient may experience recurrences of nocturnal asthma for several days or weeks. There is evidence of peribronchial inflammation. It is possible that the dual asthmatic responses seen in detergent worker's asthma, trimellitic anhydride asthma, and baker's asthma represent clinical examples of bronchial LPR. IgE antibody can be demonstrated in vitro by the radioallergosorbent test (RAST) or the enzyme-linked immunosorbent (ELISA).

Type II: Cytotoxic Reactions

In type II reactions, the antigen is a cell surface protein or antigenic substance that attaches to a cell surface protein. In transfusion reactions, the antigen is a protein on the cell membrane of the incompatible erythrocyte. In some type II hypersensitivity disorders, a low-molecular-weight substance—eg, trimellitic anhydride (TMA)—acting as a hapten attaches to a host cell surface protein that acts as a carrier. In the pulmonary disease-anemia syndrome that occurs in workers repeatedly exposed to high concentrations of volatile TMA, the chemical combines with an erythrocyte membrane protein or pulmonary basement cell membrane protein to form a complete antigen that in turn stimulates the formation of IgG or IgM antibody. On reexposure, cell surface-bound antigen-antibody union takes place, inducing a number of effects: (1) Opsonization of the target cells by IgG or IgM, which makes them more susceptible to phagocytosis by macrophages, monocytes, and polymorphonuclear leukocytes. These phagocytes are activated when their receptors for the Fc portion of IgG antibody attach to the antibody molecule on the surface of the target cell. They engulf the antigen and release lysozymal enzymes. (2) The target cell may be destroyed by killer (K) cells, which have receptors for the Fc portion of IgG. (3) The union of antigen with antibody activates the complement cascade, generating C3b, an opsonin, which facilitates phagocytosis or activation of the terminal complement sequence, leading to cell lysis. The Coombs test is helpful in demonstrating IgG antibody on the surface of red cells and leukocytes.

Type III: Immune Complex Reaction

Type III reactions depend on the union of soluble antigen with soluble IgG or IgM antibody and subsequent activation of the complement sequence. In one subtype, the Arthus reaction, an immune complex is formed locally; and in the other, serum sickness, circulating complexes are deposited in various tissues.

The **Arthus reaction** was first described in 1903 by Maurice Arthus, who intradermally injected bovine serum albumin into a previously sensitized rabbit. Induration and erythema were noted at the injection site in 2 hours, peaked at 6 hours, and resolved in 12–24 hours. In some instances, necrosis developed at the site. The type I LPR (see above) also peaks at 4–6 hours, but it is preceded by an immediate wheal and flare response and does not exhibit tissue necrosis. The Arthus reaction is the result of binding of localized but not fixed antigen to circulating antibody, forming an immune complex in situ. This reaction may be operative in hypersensitivity pneumonitis. An example is pigeon breeder's disease. The antigen, serum dried in pigeon excreta, is inhaled, sensitizing the host and leading to IgG and IgM antibody formation. On subsequent exposure to inhaled antigen, localized alveolar immune complex formation occurs. The complex activates the complement cascade, forming C4a, C3a, C5a, C4b, and C3b. C4b and C3b are opsonins, enhancing phagocytosis by polymorphonuclears, monocytes, and macrophages. C3a, C4a, and C5a are anaphylatoxins that stimulate mast cells and basophils to release histamine and other mediators which in turn cause vasodilatation and increased vascular permeability, facilitating the diffusion of other mediators and effector cells to the reaction site; C5a is also chemotactic for polymorphonuclear leukocytes and monocytes. PAF and thromboxane cause platelet aggregation and activation, leading to thrombus formation. PAF, LTB_4, and NCFA attract neutrophils, and ECFA attracts eosinophils to the site. The ingestion of immune complexes by polymorphonuclears causes activation of monocytes and macrophages and stimulates the release of lysosomal enzymes.

In **serum sickness,** or circulating immune complex disease, circulating antigen and IgG antibodies combine, forming immune complexes that in antigen excess form microprecipitates. These are filtered from the circulation at the postcapillary venule and activate the complement cascade. Just as in the Arthus reaction, the anaphylatoxins stimulate the release of mediators that induce increased vascular permeability, facilitating immune complex deposition. Examples of circulating immune complex disease include classic serum sickness, which occurs 8–13 days after injection of the foreign serum, and systemic lupus erythematosus, in which the antigen is host DNA. Clinical manifestations of serum sickness include generalized urticaria, polyserositis (arthritis, pleuritis, pericarditis), fever, and nephritis.

The presence of antibody in type III reactions may be demonstrated by the Ouchterlony gel diffusion technique (see below).

Type IV: Cellular Immunity

The type IV cellular immune or delayed reaction is initiated when antigen binds to sensitized T delayed type hypersensitivity (Tdth) lymphocytes; it does not require humoral antibody or complement. Examples include the dermatitis induced by contact with poison oak or nickel. When a low-molecular-weight sensitizer (usually less than MW 500), acting as a hapten, binds to a protein in the dermis, a hapten protein-carrier complex is formed. Langerhans' cells, which are similar to macrophages, ingest and process the antigen and present it to CD4 lymphocytes, which send a signal (IL-2) stimulating the production of sensitized Tdth lymphocytes. On subsequent challenge, Tdth cells bind to the antigen and release lymphokines. The lymphokines exert their influence in the surrounding milieu, amplifying a wide variety of biologic activities, but their main function is to attract and activate macrophages. At 24 hours after antigen challenge, there is an intense infiltration of mononuclear cells, lymphocytes and monocyte-macrophages. Erythema, induration, and pruritus and at times vesiculation and local tissue necrosis may occur.

Contact dermatitis is caused by a variety of agents, including Rhus antigens and nickel. In addition, type IV hypersensitivity may be important in the pathogenesis of hypersensitivity pneumonitis. Antigens derived from mold spores or thermophilic actinomycetes bind with sensitized Tdth lymphocytes to initiate the reaction. Patch testing with standard antigen-impregnated patches is used to demonstrate delayed type contact sensitivity.

NONIMMUNE ACTIVATION OF INFLAMMATORY REACTIONS

Inflammatory reactions can also be initiated by nonimmunologic activation of cellular and humoral effector mechanisms. Substances such as plant-derived lectins (concanavalin A from the jack bean, phytohemagglutinins from the red kidney bean, and pokeweed mitogen), gram-negative polysaccharides, pneumococcal polysaccharides, Epstein-Barr virus, trypsin, papain, silica, and asbestos act as pseudoantigens, nonimmunologically activating lymphocytes, macrophages, mast cells, basophils, and, in some cases, the complement system.

Concanavalin A (Con A) and phytohemagglutinins (PHA) selectively stimulate nonsensitized T lymphocytes, whereas gram-negative polysaccharides stimulate B lymphocytes and macrophages, leading to immunoglobulin production and macrophage activation. The intradermal injection of Con A and PHA into nonsensitized guinea pigs leads to a response resembling delayed type hypersensitivity. Inhalation of these lectins produces prominent interstitial pneumonitis in previously nonexposed rabbits. A rabbit previously sensitized and then challenged with inhaled bovine serum albumin (BSA) does not react unless Con A or PHA is simultaneously administered. Thus, these lectins enhance antigen-antibody bonding and facilitate the formation of pathologic immune complexes.

Nonimmune activation of effector cells and mechanisms can also be induced by other agents. Products derived from fungi nonimmunologically activate T cells and macrophages in the lungs, resulting in interstitial pulmonary fibrosis. These agents stimulate lymphocytes to release lymphokines, basophils and mast cells to release mediators, and macrophages to release IL-1. *Micropolyspora faeni,* a bacterium inducing farmer's lung, may activate B cells and macrophages, triggering immunelike reactions in the lung. It is possible that other pathogenic and environmental dusts induce nonimmunologic stimulation of the immune system. Silica and asbestos directly stimulate macrophages to release IL-1, which in turn stimulates fibroblast growth, collagen synthesis, and T and B cells. Patients with silicosis produce autoantibodies, immune complexes, antinuclear antibodies (ANA), and rheumatoid factor and exhibit hypergammaglobulinemia. Nonspecific activators functioning in concert with specific antigens may play an important role in the induction of immune hypersensitivity reactions observed in many occupational immune disorders.

IMMUNE HYPERSENSITIVITY OCCUPATIONAL DISORDERS

The most common immune hypersensitivity occupational disorders include allergic asthma or rhinitis, hypersensitivity pneumonitis, and contact dermatitis. The reactions are dependent on the host, the duration, the degree and type of sensitization, and the antigen.

Allergic asthma and **allergic rhinitis** occur when sensitized workers inhale specific antigen. In general, atopic patients are predisposed to sensitization to large-molecular-weight inhalants (proteins) such as animal danders, pollens, and house dust. There is no atopic predisposition to sensitization by low-molecular-weight chemicals such as toluene diisocyanate (TDA), trimellitic anhydride (TMA), or platinum salts. Allergic asthma and allergic rhinitis are type I IgE responses that occur in 3 patterns: (1) the immediate onset of symptoms after the inhalation of antigen; (2) a late-onset reaction occurring 3–6 hours after exposure—often after a worker has returned to the home environment—and lasting in some cases 12–36 hours; and (3) an immediate followed by a late onset response.

Hypersensitivity pneumonitis is a parenchymal pulmonary disease resulting from sensitization and subsequent exposure to a variety of inhalant organic dusts. Sensitization to bacterial products, small amounts of serum present in the excreta of animals, thermophilic actinomycetes (eg, *M faeni, T vulgaris,* and *Thermoactinomyces saccharii*), fungi, and vegetable proteins has produced hypersensitivity pneumonitis. Examples include pigeon breeder's disease, farmer's lung, humidifier lung, and bagassosis. The incidence varies with the type and frequency of antigen exposure and is not age-dependent. Sensitization is favored by the alveolar deposition of particulate antigen less than 5 μm in diameter.

Possible immune mechanisms operative in hypersensitivity pneumonitis include (1) a type III Arthus reaction, in which specific antibody binds to antigen, forming immune complexes that in turn activate the complement system; (2) a type IV reaction, in which sensitized Tdth cells bind to antigen and then release lymphokines; (3) nonspecific activation of immune hypersensitivity by lectins and lipopolysaccharide products of organic matter; and (4) any combination of the above.

There is evidence both to support and reject the concept that hypersensitivity pneumonitis is a type III reaction. Up to 90% of patients have antigen-specific precipitins in their serum. However, 50% of similarly exposed asymptomatic subjects also have precipitins to the same antigens, which suggests that the precipitins may merely be markers of antigen exposure. Passive transfer of serum from a rabbit with hypersensitivity pneumonitis to a nonsensitized rabbit and subsequent aerosol challenge with antigen has failed to induce the reaction, suggesting that a type III response may not be operative in this species.

Recent evidence suggests that a type IV or cell-mediated immune reaction to inhaled antigen may be important in hypersensitivity pneumonitis. Histopathologic study of the lesions reveals infiltration with neutrophils, lymphocytes, and macrophages; noncaseating granulomas, giant cells, and fibrosis may be present. Granuloma formation favors the diagnosis of cell-mediated immune reaction; CMIR; however, this may also be induced by nonphagocytosed antigen-antibody complexes. The lymphocytes of sensitized patients release lymphokines when exposed to specific antigen. Experimentally, lesions resembling alveolitis can be induced by first sensitizing rabbits using methods favoring a cell-mediated immune response and then challenging with inhaled antigen. Furthermore, when rabbits were passively sensitized by lymphocytes from sensitized rabbits and then challenged, typical lesions consistent with alveolitis developed. These studies favor a type IV response.

It is possible that nonimmune activation of effector mechanisms of hypersensitivity may be operative. Lipopolysaccharides found in the cell walls of certain bacteria and fungi may directly activate the alternative complement pathway, leading to the release of anaphylatoxins that are also chemotactic for phagocytes. Lipopolysaccharides stimulate lymphocytes to release lymphokines, including lymphocytotoxins and macrophage activators, resulting in local tissue inflammation and necrosis. Although this mechanism may play a part in hypersensitivity pneumonitis, it probably is not a primary role; studies demonstrate that sensitization must take place before a reaction occurs. It may be that hypersensitivity pneumonitis is a combination of a type III and a type IV immune response, possibly enhanced by nonimmune activation of effector mechanisms.

Contact dermatitis is a type IV reaction that usually occurs when low-molecular-weight ($<$ MW 500) sensitizers acting as haptens first bind to proteins in the dermis to form a complete antigen. The complex in turn is recognized and bound by sensitized T cells that release lymphokines, some of which activate macrophages. The most common agents are *Rhus* antigens and nickel. (See Type IV: Cellular Immunity.)

ANTIGENS INDUCING OCCUPATIONAL IMMUNE HYPERSENSITIVITY DISORDERS

Antigens inducing occupational immune hypersensitivity disorders may be of animal, vegetable, or chemical origin. Table 13–5 lists and classifies reactions caused by a number of these agents. Immune hypersensitivity reactions occur when a sensitized worker encounters antigen in the work environment.

ANIMAL PRODUCTS

Occupational exposure to animal products may cause a type I immediate response manifested by

Table 13–5. Antigens inducing occupational immune hypersensitivity disorders.

Type of Reaction	I	II	III	IV
Animal products				
Avian proteins (serum, feathers)	X		X(?)	X(?)
Danders	X			
Excreta (gerbil, rat, mouse, guinea pig, other laboratory animals)	X		X(?)	X(?)
Bacillus subtilis (alcalase) (detergent worker's lung)	X		X(?)	
Thermophilic actinomycetes (hypersensitivity pneumonitis—farmer's lung, bagassosis, malt worker's lung, humidifier fever)			X(?)	X(?)
Bee venom	X			
Vegetable products				
Western red cedar (plicatic acid)	X(?)			
Flour dust (baker's asthma)	X		X(?)	
Castor bean	X			
Green coffee dust	X			
Colophony (pine resin)	X		X(?)	
Poison oak, ivy, sumac				X
Chemical agents				
Isocyanates	X(?)		X(?)	
Trimellitic anhydride asthma	X		X(?)	
Pulmonary anemia syndrome		X		
Platinum salts	X (asthma)			
Nickel	X (asthma)			X (contact dermatitis)

symptoms of acute or chronic asthma and rhinitis. In some patients, after acute challenge, these symptoms clear only to recur in a more severe form 4–6 hours later. As previously noted, these late-onset responses may be solely IgE-mediated. Cat and dog danders and cat saliva, mouse urine, feathers, avian serum, and alcalase—an enzyme derived from *Bacillus subtilis*—have all been shown to induce IgE antibodies and type I reactions.

Avian serum has been shown to induce hypersensitivity pneumonitis in bird breeders. Depending on the type of exposure, this may take one of 2 forms: acute or chronic. With acute exposure, symptoms may develop abruptly 4–6 hours later and include chills, fever, malaise, cough, myalgia, and dyspnea that may last 24–48 hours. The chronic form occurs with insidious repeated—almost daily—exposure and is manifested by anorexia, weight loss, and progressive loss of pulmonary function secondary to pulmonary fibrosis. In addition to avian serum, thermophilic actinomycetes have been implicated in hypersensitivity pneumonitis. Hypersensitivity pneumonitis may be a type III or type IV response or a combination of the 2 types.

Alcalase, derived from *B subtilis,* is used in the manufacture of detergents in Great Britain and was at one time so used in the USA. As a result of daily exposure, atopic workers are particularly predisposed to sensitization and the development of IgE-mediated type I respiratory symptoms.

VEGETABLE PRODUCTS

Castor bean and green coffee bean dust are potent antigens for some people, inducing a type I immediate response manifested as rhinitis and asthma. There are reports of patients living near castor bean processing plants who have developed severe asthma secondary to wind shifts resulting in inhalation of minute amounts of this dust. It is estimated that 10% of workers handling green coffee beans develop IgE-mediated symptoms. The antigenic potency of the green coffee bean is destroyed by roasting. Workers who have an adverse immune response to green coffee dust are able to handle the roasted beans without difficulty.

Five percent of workers in the Western United States cedar lumber industry develop asthma after a latent period of exposure that averages about 3–4 years. They exhibit bronchospasm to inhalation challenge with plicatic acid, a low-molecular-weight derivative of red cedar. Skin testing and RAST demonstrate IgE sensitivity in approximately 50% of affected workers, but positive results are also found in unaffected workers. Atopy does not predispose workers to sensitization. It is possible that some cases are due to IgE-mediated processes.

Colophony, a pine resin by-product (rosin) used as solder flux, has been shown to cause both immediate and dual respiratory reactions in sensitized workers. The reaction is probably IgE-mediated.

In the USA, the most common agent causing occupational dermatitis is the oil from plants of the genus *Rhus* (poison oak, poison ivy, and poison sumac). Poison oak is found west of the Rocky Mountains; poison ivy and poison sumac are found to the east. The active principle is pentadecylcatechol, a low-molecular-weight substance that binds to one of the skin proteins, forming a complete antigen. Studies reveal that over 90% of subjects are sensitized on exposure to these antigens. A subject will develop a type IV allergic contact dermatitis reaction 24–72 hours after challenge.

Respiratory symptoms secondary to exposure to flour dust occur in bakers. Affected workers may exhibit (1) an immediate or (2) an immediate followed by a late-onset reaction; both are probably IgE-mediated. There is a direct relation between duration of exposure and the percentage of bakers who exhibit skin test reactivity.

CHEMICAL AGENTS

Workers in industrial plants may be exposed to a wide variety of chemical agents. Two that have been extensively studied are the isocyanates and trimellitic anhydride. Isocyanates are used in the manufacture of pesticides, polyurethane foams, and synthetic varnishes. There are many case reports of obstructive airway problems related to toluene diisocyanate (TDI). These occur with equal frequency in atopic and nonatopic workers. The mechanism of obstructive airway disease has not been elucidated, but some hypotheses to explain the pathogenesis include the following:

(1) An irritant effect: Evidence opposed to this hypothesis includes the latent period observed in many cases and the fact that all workers are not affected.

(2) Beta-adrenergic blockade: In vitro studies demonstrate that TDI acts as a weak β-adrenergic blocking agent.

(3) Immune hypersensitivity response: This is suggested by the insidious onset of symptoms after a latency period of weeks to months, peripheral eosinophilia, and the induction of symptoms in sensitized workers on reexposure to minute quantities of the material. RAST and skin testing with a conjugate of

a low-molecular-weight isocyanate with human serum albumin have demonstrated specific IgE antibodies and in some cases IgG antibodies; however, because the antibodies can be demonstrated in affected and nonaffected workers, they probably correlate with exposure and not with clinical disease.

Trimellitic anhydride (TMA) is used in the manufacture of plastics, epoxy resins, and paints. TMA dust or fumes have been associated with 4 clinical syndromes. In the **TMA immediate type reaction,** the patient may have rhinitis, conjunctivitis, or asthma. The reaction requires a latent period of exposure before the onset of symptoms. IgE antibodies to trimellityl-human serum albumin (TMHSA) conjugates have been demonstrated. Although affected workers have no atopic predisposition, this is probably a type I reaction.

The **late reacting-systemic syndrome** (''TMA flu'') is characterized by cough, occasional wheezing, dyspnea, and systemic symptoms of malaise, chills, myalgia, and arthralgia. These reactions occur 4–6 hours after exposure to TMA. This may be a type III disorder in which immune complexes of IgG antibody and TMA protein conjugates are operative. Repeated exposure and a latent period of weeks to months are required before symptoms develop. IgG antibodies to TMHSA have been demonstrated.

The **pulmonary disease-anemia syndrome** develops after exposure to TMA fumes. It occurs after repeated high-dose exposure to the volatile fumes of TMA sprayed on heated metal surfaces to prevent corrosion. A Coombs-positive hemolytic anemia and respiratory failure are evident. This is an example of a type II cytotoxic reaction in which antibodies are directed toward TMA bound to erythrocytes and pulmonary basement membrane. High titers of IgG antibody to TMHSA and to a trimellityl-erythrocyte conjugate have been demonstrated.

The **irritant respiratory syndrome** occurs with the first high-dose exposure to TMA powder and fumes. Patients develop cough and dyspnea. Immune sensitization toward TMA conjugates has not been demonstrated.

Metallic salts are an important cause of immune hypersensitivity. After poison oak, nickel is the most common cause of contact dermatitis, a type IV reaction. There are reports of asthma, probably on a type I IgE basis, secondary to exposure to fumes of nickel and platinum salts. It is thought that these salts acting as haptens binding with body proteins cause the induction of IgE immune sensitivity and, on subsequent exposure, bronchial asthma.

CLINICAL ECOLOGY

Clinical ecologists hypothesize that the total load of environmental antigens overwhelms the immune system, leading to immune aberrations, multisystem disease, and psychologic disorders. Disturbed mentation, chronic fatigue, and neurotic symptoms are reported. Noxious environmental antigens include auto exhaust fumes, tobacco smoke, perfumes, organic solvents, the off-gassing from formaldehyde products, chlorinated and fluoridated tap water, and chemical agents found in foods (synthetic fertilizers, pesticides, and food additives). The ecologists have not scientifically defined the mechanism by which such factors affect the immune system but have proposed a role for IgE, immune complex mechanisms, and other as yet undefined mechanisms.

Laboratory investigations used by proponents of these views include the use of cytotoxic tests to demonstrate damage to leukocytes by suspected agents and tests to detect alterations of the ratio and number of T and B lymphocytes and of T suppressor and T helper lymphocytes. The principal in vivo investigation employed is the **provocation-neutralization test,** which is performed in an unblinded or single-blinded manner as follows: Gradually increasing concentrations of serial dilutions of the suspected agent are administered sublingually or intradermally, and the patient is observed for various subjective symptoms; later, a "neutralizing dose" of the same agent is administered to stop the reaction.

Treatment is based on elimination of the noxious environmental and dietary factors and the subcutaneous or sublingual administration of desensitizing or neutralizing doses of agents that cannot be avoided. Elimination of noxious environmental factors may require removal of the patient from "chemical exposure" by instituting a diet of organically grown foods to avoid pesticides and chemicals found in artificial fertilizers and rotating diets in which selected safe foods are only eaten for 3–4 days in a row. The patient may be advised to move to a rural or seacoast home constructed using only natural materials.

Although there is no question of the sincerity of the proponents of clinical ecology as a field of study, to date there are no randomized double-blind placebo-controlled studies to support their position. The cytotoxic test long employed by clinical ecologists has not been scientifically substantiated. All of the double-blind studies performed to validate the efficacy of the provocation-neutralization technique have been flawed or have had a negative result.

In a recent report, Terr reviewed 50 patients who previously were diagnosed by clinical ecologists as having "environmental illness." In 41, a positive provocation-neutralization test was used to support the diagnosis. Over 80% of the patients were seen for evaluation of a workers' compensation claim of an industrial illness. The patients could be categorized into 3 groups: Eight had no disease; 11 had symptoms caused by previous nonenvironmental disease; and 31 had multiple subjective symptoms. Laboratory studies of serum immunoglobulins, total lymphocytes, lymphocyte subgroups, and helper and suppressor ratios were performed on many of the patients by the ecologists. There was no significant difference among the groups for most of the tests; there was an increase in null cells and serum IgA in the group with

physical illness. Upon review of the results of the ecology treatment, 26 had no change in symptoms, 22 were worse, and 2 had a subjective diminution of symptoms. In another study, in which 18 such patients were evaluated by 2 psychiatrists, 10 had well-recognized psychoneurotic conditions and 7 of the remainder had somatoform disorders (somatization, conversion, and hypochondriasis).

The California Medical Association Scientific Board Task Force on Clinical Ecology reviewed this subject in 1985, and their conclusion best summarizes the scientific knowledge to date: "No convincing evidence was found that patients treated by clinical ecologists have unique, recognizable syndromes, that the diagnostic tests employed are efficacious and reliable, or that the treatments used are effective."

DIAGNOSIS OF HYPERSENSITIVITY DISEASES IN OCCUPATIONAL MEDICINE

HISTORY & PHYSICAL EXAMINATION

From the standpoint of both the patient and the employer, it is important to establish an early diagnosis. Many obstructive pulmonary problems that are reversible with proper early management become fixed disabilities with prolonged exposure to offending agents. The initial work-up should include a detailed history and physical examination and, when indicated, a complete blood count, sputum smear for eosinophils, chest film, and pulmonary function evaluation.

The type of symptoms, aggravating and relieving factors, their temporal relationship with the work environment, and the effects of vacation and weekends should be noted. Late-onset respiratory reactions may not occur until a patient has returned home from work. The personal or family history of atopy (hay fever, allergic asthma, or atopic dermatitis) should be investigated. If there is bronchospasm, it is important to review medications the patient is currently receiving, including beta-blockers and nonsteroidal anti-inflammatory drugs, both of which may induce bronchial asthma; acetylcholinesterase inhibitors may cause cough. The home environment should be reviewed, including any changes that have occurred, the presence of pets and molds, any recent moves, hobbies, and the use of tobacco by the patient or others in the household. Finally, a detailed occupational history should be elicited, including information regarding present and past employment. At times it is helpful—with the permission of the employer—to visit the work site.

Physical examination should include evaluation of

the skin and the upper and lower respiratory tracts. Evidence of atopy should be sought, including the presence of allergic facies, cobblestoning of the conjunctiva, pale and boggy mucous membranes, posterior pharyngeal lymphoid plaques, expiratory wheezing, and signs of atopic dermatitis. Evidence of clubbing, increased anteroposterior diameter of the chest, and the location and quality of skin rashes should be noted. Other causes of the patient's symptoms must be ruled out.

LABORATORY INVESTIGATION

A **complete blood count** demonstrating evidence of eosinophilia may aid in the diagnosis of atopy. The presence of eosinophilia on a stained smear of **sputum** is consistent with both atopic and nonatopic asthma. **Total serum IgE** is often elevated in atopic patients.

A baseline **posteroanterior and lateral x-ray of the chest** should be obtained in patients with pulmonary problems, noting increased anteroposterior chest diameter, flattening of the diaphragms, infiltrates, evidence of bronchiectasis, hyperaeration, and diffuse micronodularity.

Pulmonary function studies before and after bronchodilator administration should be obtained in the case of pulmonary disorders; at a minimum, they should include forced expiratory volume in 1 second (FEV_1), forced vital capacity (FVC), forced expiratory flow between 25% and 75% of FVC (FEF_{25-75}), and peak expiratory flow rate (PEFR). If available, a DL_{CO} determination and measurements of blood gases may prove helpful. (See Chapter 18.)

Methacholine challenge, observing the effect of graded increasing doses of nebulized methacholine on pulmonary function, is helpful in establishing increased bronchial irritability in patients who present with an atypical history, eg, cough as a sole manifestation of bronchial involvement. Asthmatics are up to a thousand times more sensitive than normals to methacholine challenge.

IMMUNOLOGIC TESTS

Based on the initial evaluation, specific immunologic tests may be ordered. These include immediate allergy skin tests, patch tests, in vitro tests for IgE antibody, Ouchterlony gel diffusion tests, and provocative challenge with specific antigens.

Skin Tests

Scratch and intradermal skin tests are helpful in establishing sensitivity to a number of inhalant protein antigens, including molds, house dusts, animal danders, feathers, pollens, and extracts of suspected large-molecular-weight antigens in the work environment. Low-molecular-weight materials usually do not give a positive immediate skin test response unless they are linked to a protein carrier such as human serum albumin. The initial wheal and flare reaction may be followed in 4–6 hours by an IgE-mediated late phase reaction evidenced by erythema, induration, pruritus, and tenderness at the skin test site.

Patch Testing

Patch tests are useful in evaluating skin contact sensitivity. The test employs standard antigen-impregnated patches applied to the skin. They are removed after 24–48 hours. A positive reaction consists of erythema, induration, and in some cases vesiculation. In addition to antigens available in the standard antigen patch test kit obtained from the American Academy of Dermatology, suspected materials may be utilized from the work environment. (See Chapter 17.)

In Vitro Antibody Tests

The radioallergosorbent test (RAST) and the enzyme-linked immunosorbent test (ELISA) are in vitro procedures used to detect antigen-specific IgE antibody. In these tests, inert particles coated with antigen are incubated with serum. If specific antibody is present, it binds to antigen on the surface of the particles. The complex is washed, incubated with radiolabeled or enzyme-labeled anti-IgE, and then washed again. The amount of anti-IgE measured by radioactivity or enzyme activity determines the amount of specific IgE antibody attached to the antigen.

Ouchterlony Gel Diffusion Test

This test is used to demonstrate IgG precipitating antibody to antigen. Suspected antigens and the patient's serum are placed in separate wells cut into a gel-coated plate. The antigen and serum diffuse toward one another. If sufficient antibody is present, precipitin lines composed of antigen-antibody complexes form at some intermediate point. This test is helpful in type III reactions.

Inhalation Challenge Tests

These tests are conducted by exposing the worker to the suspected antigen. *Caution:* Inhalation challenge studies are not without risk. Sensitized patients are susceptible to late-onset asthmatic reactions that may develop up to 12 hours after the initial challenge. These reactions are often refractory to bronchodilator treatment.

The challenge may be performed in the work environment or in a hospital laboratory situation. The patient probably should be hospitalized and observed for 12–24 hours after a laboratory challenge.

A. Work Challenge: Probably the safest method is to remove the subject from the work environment for a few days or weeks and then, when stable, challenge with a work exposure. Baseline PEFR determinations are made on a regular basis throughout a 24-hour period for 2 or 3 days before the challenge; the worker then returns to the work environment, all the while measuring PEFR on a regular basis. In addition, pulmonary function testing is performed just before and after the work challenge. Significant falls in expected PEFR and pulmonary function test values help to confirm an adverse reaction to the work environment.

B. Laboratory Inhalation Challenge: This can be obtained in 3 ways: (1) After the worker's condition is stabilized off work, baseline tests are obtained; the worker is placed in a closed environment and asked to transfer suspected antigen dust, mixed in lactose powder, back and forth between 2 trays. (2) In another variation, the subject, in a hospital setting, is exposed to various volatile agents (eg, solder, varnish) by actually working with the materials. In each of these challenges, pulmonary function tests are obtained immediately before and for several hours after exposure. (3) Aerosol inhalation challenge involves the administration of gradually increasing amounts of aerosolized suspected material while pulmonary function tests are monitored. A 20% or greater fall in FEV_1 is considered a positive response.

REFERENCES

General

Bellanti JA (editor): *Immunology III,* 3rd ed. Saunders, 1984.

Patterson R, Goldstein RA (editors): Symposium on occupational immunologic lung disease. *J Allergy Clin Immunol* 1982;**70:**1. [Entire issue.]

Pepys J: Occupational respiratory allergy. *Clin Immunol Allergy* 1984;**4:**1.

Roitt IM et al: *Immunology.* Mosby, 1985.

Samter M et al (editors): *Immunological Diseases,* 4th ed. Little, Brown, 1988.

Stites DP, Stobo JD, Wells JV (editors): *Basic & Clinical Immunology,* 6th ed. Appleton & Lange, 1987.

Terr AI (editor): Allergy in the workplace. *Clin Rev Allergy* 1986;**4:**247. [Entire issue.]

Immune Response

Claman HN: The biology of the immune response. *JAMA* 1987;**258:**2834.

Oppenheim JJ, Ruscetti FW, Faltynek CR: Interleukins and interferons. Chap 8, pp 82–95, in: *Basic & Clinical Immunology,* 6th ed. Stites DP, Stobo JD, Wells JV (editors). Appleton & Lange, 1987.

Robb RJ: Interleukin-2: The molecule and its function. *Immunol Today* 1984;**5:**203.

Stobo JD, Levitt D, Cooper MD: Lymphocytes. Chap 7, pp 65–81, in: *Basic & Clinical Immunology,* 6th ed. Stites DP, Stobo JD, Wells JV (editors). Appleton & Lange, 1987.

Immunoglobulins

Geha RS: Human IgE. *J Allergy Clin Immunol* 1984;**74:**109.

Goodman JW: Immunoglobulins: Structure and function. Chap 4, pp 27–36, in: *Basic & Clinical Immunology,* 6th ed. Stites DP, Stobo JD, Wells JV (editors). Appleton & Lange, 1987.

Sell S: Antibodies, immunoglobulins, and receptors. Chap 5, pp 85–115, in: *Immunology, Immunopathology, and Immunity,* 4th ed. Elsevier, 1987.

Effector Cells of Immune Hypersensitivity

Katz HR, Stevens RL, Austen KF: Heterogeneity of mammalian mast cells differentiated in vivo and in vitro. *J Allergy Clin Immunol* 1985;**76:**250.

Mitchell EB, Askenase PW: Basophils in human disease. *Clin Rev Allergy* 1983;**1:**427.

Schleimer RP et al: Human mast cells and basophils: Structure, function, pharmacology, and biochemistry. *Clin Rev Allergy* 1983;**1:**327.

Weller PF: Eosinophilia. *J Allergy Clin Immunol* 1984;**73:**1.

Werb Z, Goldstein IM: Phagocytic cells: Chemotaxis and effector functions of macrophages and granulocytes. Chap 9, pp 96–113, in: *Basic & Clinical Immunology,* 6th ed. Stites DP, Stobo JD, Wells JV (editors). Appleton & Lange, 1987.

Mediators of Immediate Hypersensitivity

Marquardt DL: Histamine. *Clin Rev Allergy* 1983;**1:**343.

O'Flaherty JT, Wykle RL: Biology and biochemistry of platelet-activating factor. *Clin Rev Allergy* 1983; **1:**353.

Wasserman SI: Mediators of immediate hypersensitivity. *J Allergy Clin Immunol* 1983;**72:**101.

Complement

Cooper NR: The complement system. Chap 10, pp 114–127, in: *Basic & Clinical Immunology,* 6th ed. Stites DP, Stobo JD, Wells JV (editors). Appleton & Lange, 1987.

Fearon DT: Complement. *J Allergy Clin Immunol* 1983;**71:**520.

Muller-Eberhard H: Chemistry and function of the complement system. Chapter 12 in: *The Biology of Immunologic Disease.* Dixon FJ, Fisher DW (editors). Sinauer, 1984.

Hypersensitivity Responses to Antigens & Mitogens

Bernstein IL: Isocyanate-induced pulmonary diseases: A current perspective. *J Allergy Clin Immunol* 1982; **70:**24.

Coombs RR, Gell RG: Classification of allergic reactions responsible for clinical hypersensitivity and disease. Chap 25, pp 761–781, in: *Clinical Aspects of Immunology,* 3rd ed. Gell RG, Coombs RR, Lachmann PJ (editors). Blackwell Scientific Publications, 1975.

Bice DE, Salvaggio J, Hoffman E: Passive transfer of experimental hypersensitivity pneumonitis with lymphoid cells in the rabbit. *J Allergy Clin Immunol* 1976;**58:**250.

Emanuel DA, Kryda MJ: Farmer's lung disease. *Clin Rev Allergy* 1983;**1:**509.

Fink JN: Hypersensitivity pneumonitis. Chapter 50 in:

Allergy: Principles and Practice, 2nd ed. Middleton E Jr, Reed CE (editors). Mosby, 1983.

Gleich GJ: The late phase of the immunoglobulinE-mediated reaction: A link between anaphylaxis and common allergic disease? *J Allergy Clin Immunol* 1982;**70**:160.

Metzger WJ, Hunninghake GW, Richerson HB: Late asthmatic responses: Inquiry into mechanisms and significance. *Clin Rev Allergy* 1985;**3**:145.

Patterson R, Zeiss CR, Pruzansky JJ: Immunology and immunopathology of trimellitic anhydride pulmonary reactions. *J Allergy Clin Immunol* 1982;**70**:19.

Pepys J et al: Passive transfer in man and the monkey of type I allergy due to heat-labile and heat-stable antibody to complex salts of platinum. *Clin Allergy* 1979;**9**:99.

Richerson HB: Hypersensitivity pneumonitis: Pathology and pathogenesis. *Clin Rev Allergy* 1983;**1**:469.

Schatz M, Patterson R: Hypersensitivity pneumonitis: General considerations. *Clin Rev Allergy* 1983;**1**:451.

Willoughby WF, Willoughby JB, Gerberick GF: Polyclonal activators in pulmonary immune disease. *Clin Rev Allergy* 1985;**3**:197.

Clinical Ecology

Grieco MH: Controversial practices in allergy. *JAMA* 1982;**247**:3106.

Ramsey L: Clinical ecology: A critical appraisal. *West J Med* 1986;**144**:239.

Reisman RE: American Academy of Allergy position statements: Controversial techniques. *J Allergy Clin Immunol* 1981;**67**:333.

Stewart DE, Raskin J: Psychiatric assessment of patients with ''20th century disease'' (''total allergy syndrome''). *Can Med Assoc J* 1985;**133**:1001.

Terr AI: Environmental illness: A clinical review of 50 cases. *Arch Intern Med* 1986;**146**:145.

Terr AI: Clinical ecology in the workplace. *J Occup Med* 1989;**31**:257.

Evaluation of Diagnostic Tests

Bernstein DI, Bernstein IL: Occupational asthma. Chap 50, pp 1197–1218, in: *Allergies: Principles and Practice,* 3rd ed. Middleton E Jr et al (editors). Mosby, 1988.

Fisher AA: The role of patch testing. Chap 2, pp 9–29, in: *Contact Dermatitis,* 3rd ed. Lea & Febiger, 1986.

Fraser RG et al: Methods in clinical laboratory and functional investigation. Chap 3, pp 388–455, in: *Diagnosis of Diseases of the Chest,* 3rd ed. Saunders, 1988.

Van Arsdel PP Jr, Larson EB: Diagnostic tests for patients with suspected allergic disease: Utility and limitations. *Ann Intern Med* 1989;**110**:304.

Occupational Hematology

14

Hope S. Rugo, MD, & Lloyd E. Damon, MD

Occupationally related hematologic toxicity has occurred in cyclic fashion, historically associated with the development of the chemical industry and the advent of each World War. Common factors contributing to "epidemics" of toxicity have been the rapid introduction of many new chemicals and the exposure of large numbers of workers without adequate protection or education. As the toxicities of these agents gradually became known, regulation of their use was instituted, and exposure to some toxins such as radium has been eliminated. Hematologic toxins such as lead, benzene, arsenic, and arsine gas still exist; poisoning has still not been eliminated from the workplace; and worker education is still inadequate. As new chemicals are introduced and new products become available, it is important to be aware of potential mechanisms of toxicity so that the epidemic poisonings of the past will not be repeated.

Hematotoxicity has improved our understanding of hematologic pathophysiology, taught important pharmacologic lessons, and introduced the concept of individual susceptibility to specific toxic agents. Observation of individual variations in susceptibility to toxic agents was made by recognizing that chemicals with oxidative potential could cause cyanosis and a life-threatening hemolytic anemia in some individuals at exposure levels that had little effect on the population at large. The normal population will manifest similar toxicities, but only when exposed to much higher levels. It has therefore become important to identify workers with increased sensitivity to certain chemicals and place them in jobs with less risk of contact with these specific toxic substances.

Exposure to hematotoxins may affect blood cell survival (denaturation of hemoglobin and hemolysis), metabolism (porphyria), formation (aplasia), morphology and function (preleukemias and leukemias), or coagulation (thrombocytopenia).

DISORDERS ASSOCIATED WITH SHORTENED RED BLOOD CELL SURVIVAL

METHEMOGLOBINEMIA & HEMOLYSIS PRODUCED BY OXIDANT CHEMICALS

Methemoglobin is formed by the oxidation of ferrous (Fe^{2+}) hemoglobin to ferric (Fe^{3+}) hemoglo-

bin. It was first recognized in the 1800s when coal tars were converted into individual chemicals that served as precursors for many products ranging from explosives to synthetic dyes and perfumes. Overexposure to these chemicals—which included anilines, nitrobenzenes, and quinones—was common, and little was known about their potential toxicity. Workers in these plants came to be known as "blue workers" or suffered from "blue lip" owing to the chronic cyanosis from toxic methemoglobinemia that developed in almost all of them. Gradually it was recognized that oxidation of hemoglobin was toxic to red blood cells and could be followed by an acute and life-threatening hemolysis known as Heinz body anemia. Heinz bodies are red blood cell inclusions that represent precipitated hemoglobin and are classically seen in individuals with a deficiency of glucose-6-phosphate dehydrogenase (G6PD) after exposure to an oxidant stress. Normal individuals exposed to large amounts of oxidant chemicals will develop methemoglobinemia and occasionally Heinz body hemolytic anemia. It is not understood why some chemicals may cause methemoglobinemia, hemolysis, or both, but the disorders are certainly related to individual susceptibility. Oxidative chemicals are common in industry, and it is important to know what toxic agents have been implicated, to recognize the presenting signs and symptoms, and be able to provide appropriate treatment when it is needed.

Despite the understanding of this phenomenon which developed in the 19th century, as new compounds were developed for each World War—eg, aniline and other coal tar derivatives, new cycles of toxicity were again seen. As new chemicals continue to be synthesized, awareness of their toxicity is necessary to avoid similar outbreaks of poisoning characterized by cyanosis and hemolysis. An understanding of the pathophysiology of this phenomenon is essential to correctly handle this medical emergency; it will also help in understanding the myriad of therapeutic agents that may cause oxidative hemolysis in a susceptible individual.

Pathophysiology of Oxidant Hemolysis

Hemoglobin is unique in its ability to combine reversibly with oxygen without oxidizing its iron moiety. The small amount of oxidized hemoglobin or methemoglobin produced is readily reduced by an

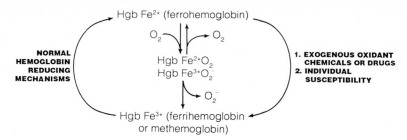

Figure 14–1. Oxidation of hemoglobin by the Embden-Meyerhof pathway.

efficient enzyme system linked to energy provided by glucose metabolism via the Embden-Meyerhof pathway (Fig 14–1).

Methemoglobin is dangerous because of its inability to bind oxygen and because it increases the oxygen affinity of the remaining heme groups in hemoglobin tetramer, thereby decreasing oxygen delivery to the tissues. Oxidation may also result in denaturation of hemoglobin with the formation of precipitated hemoglobin (Heinz bodies) within the red cell. The presence of Heinz bodies alters the surface membrane of the red cell, causing increased rigidity and leakage, with resulting hemolysis. Heinz bodies may also be formed from a second form of denatured hemoglobin, sulfhemoglobin. Unlike methemoglobin, sulfhemoglobin is irreversibly associated with the heme moiety.

The development of methemoglobinemia or oxidative hemolysis in an individual exposed to an oxidant stress is dependent on the route of exposure, the specific chemicals involved, the dose and duration of exposure, and, most importantly, individual susceptibility. Inborn structural abnormalities (unstable hemoglobins)—or, much more commonly, disorders of normal reducing capabilities such as the X-linked deficiency of the oxidation-reduction enzyme G6PD—cause some individuals to be much more susceptible to oxidant stress than others. There are many varieties of both of these abnormalities. Recognition of these high-risk individuals in the workplace is important to reduce their chance of particularly toxic exposures.

The normal individual has less than 1% circulating methemoglobin. Ninety-five percent of methemoglobin formed daily by the auto-oxidation of hemoglobin is reduced by $NADH_2$ generated by the dehydrogenation of phosphotriose by phosphotriose dehydrogenase. This reaction is catalyzed by NADH methemoglobin reductase (NADH cytochrome b_5 reductase). A rare inborn deficiency of NADH methemoglobin reductase results in congenital cyanosis due to methemoglobinemia (Fig 14–2).

An alternative methemoglobin reduction pathway exists, though it is a slow enzymatic reduction that is not physiologically functional without the presence of a redox cofactor, which may serve here as an electron carrier intermediate. In this reaction, NADPH from the first 2 steps of the hexose monophosphate shunt converts methemoglobin to reduced hemoglobin. Deficiency of the enzyme that catalyzes this reaction, NADPH methemoglobin reductase, does not result in methemoglobinemia or cyanosis. The formation of NADPH is dependent on G6PD. The presence of a redox agent such as methylene blue, which is used to treat toxic and congenital methemoglobinemia, can precipitate a hemolytic crisis in an individual with G6PD deficiency because of its own oxidative potential. In normal individuals, the administration of a redox agent may dramatically increase the rate of reduction of hemoglobin so that it greatly exceeds that of the NADH-methemoglobin reductase reaction (Fig 14–3). This is the rationale for the effectiveness of methylene blue in toxic methemoglobinemia.

Two other pathways exist, but they reduce methemoglobin only to a small extent. Glutathione is responsible for conversion of less than 7–10% of ferrihemoglobin to ferrohemoglobin, and ascorbic acid in pharmacologic amounts will reduce oxidized hemoglobin. Because of the high redox potential of ascorbic acid, however, the rate of reduction is very

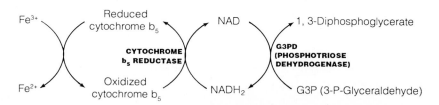

Figure 14–2. Reduction of hemoglobin by NADH methemoglobin reductase (NADH cytochrome b_5 reductase).

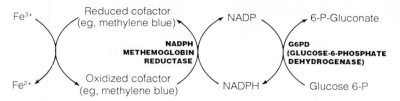

Figure 14–3. Reduction of hemoglobin by NADPH methemoglobin reductase can be accelerated by a redox agent such as methylene blue.

slow, making it less effective in therapy. In physiologic concentrations, the contribution of ascorbic acid to methemoglobin reduction is insignificant.

1. ANILINE

Historically, most work-related episodes of methemoglobinemia and hemolytic anemia have been due to exposure to aromatic nitro and amino compounds. These compounds have been used most extensively as intermediates in the synthesis of aniline dyes; they are used also as accelerators and antioxidants in the rubber industry and in the production of pesticides, plastics, paints, and varnishes. Table 14–1 lists chemicals that have been associated with methemoglobinemia and their industrial uses. Many medicinal drugs are oxidants and can cause methemoglobinemia but will not be discussed here.

The clinical presentation of methemoglobinemia is exemplified by aniline toxicity. Aniline, used in the manufacture of dyes and in the rubber industry, is the most common and best-described aromatic amine. It is fat-soluble and readily penetrates the intact skin even through clothing. The vapor form may also gain entry to the body through the lungs. Ingestion is rare in the industrial setting but causes serious toxicity when it does occur. Aniline is converted by hepatic

microsomes to phenylhydroxylamine, which behaves as a catalyst in mediating hemoglobin oxidation. Hepatic clearance of phenylhydroxylamine is slow because its oxidized form, nitrosobenzene, is rapidly converted back to phenylhydroxylamine. Another clearance pathway gradually eliminates the amine from the body.

Clinical Presentation

Acute exposure is usually associated with spills or improper usage. Symptoms will vary depending on the concentration of methemoglobin (Table 14–2). Most cases are mild and transient and present as asymptomatic blueness of the lips and nail beds. In more severe cases, the patient will appear deeply cyanotic. Freshly drawn blood appears dark maroon-brown and does not become red after exposure to air. Laboratory results reveal hypoxia and may indicate hemolysis with an elevated reticulocyte count and variable degree of anemia.

In chronic methemoglobinemia, polycythemia may be seen in response to chronic hypoxia. Hemolytic Heinz body anemia may or may not accompany methemoglobin formation, or may follow resolution of cyanosis. Heinz bodies are easily detected by examining the peripheral blood smear stained by a supravital stain but will not be evident on a smear stained with Wright's stain. Blood methemoglobin

Table 14–1. Chemicals associated with methemoglobinemia or oxidative hemolysis.

Chemical	Use
Aniline	Rubber, dyestuffs; production of MDI (methylene bisphenyl isocyanate)
Nitroaniline	Dyes
Toluidine	Dyes, organic chemicals
p-Chloroaniline	Dyes, pharmaceuticals, pesticides
o-Toluidine	Laboratory analytic reagent, production of trypan blue stain, chlorine test kits, test tapes, curing agent for urethan resins
Naphthalene	Fumigants used in clothing industry
Paradichlorobenzene	Fumigants used in clothing industry
Nitrates	Soil fertilizers
Trinitrotoluene	Explosives

levels should be followed closely. Methemoglobin is measured in the laboratory as a characteristic spectrophotometric absorption band.

Prevention

The most important safeguard in preventing oxidative hemolysis is to minimize atmospheric and cutaneous exposure to potentially oxidizing chemicals such as coal tar products. The identification of susceptible individuals such as those with G6PD deficiency may help to avoid significant toxicity in high-risk job situations. Screening for G6PD deficiency must be done before a hemolytic episode or 1–2 months after the hemolysis has resolved. Young red blood cells, particularly reticulocytes, have normal G6PD levels in most G6PD-deficient individuals. During an acute hemolytic episode, older red blood cells are destroyed and replaced by young red blood cells. The result of a G6PD deficiency screen will be normal in that acute setting. Biologic monitoring in the workplace may be done by measuring methemoglobin levels and reticulocyte counts (see Chapter 34).

Treatment

Treatment is dependent on rapid recognition of the problem. It is important to obtain as complete an exposure history as possible, since it will guide treatment. The most important aspect of therapy is to ensure removal of the offending agent. Because of the fat-soluble nature of these compounds, it is essential that clothing be removed and the patient washed thoroughly. For mild intoxication (< 20% blood methemoglobin), observation should be sufficient to watch for progression of symptoms. For moderate to severe intoxication (> 30% blood methemoglobin), 100% oxygen by mask is given to saturate the remaining hemoglobin and the antidote, methylene blue, is administered. Care must be exercised in using methylene blue to avoid increasing methemoglobin from the oxidative potential of methylene blue itself.

For initial management, methylene blue should be given intravenously as a 1% solution at a dose of 1–2 mg/kg over 10 minutes. The maximal effect should be seen within 1 hour. If no response is evident by this time, methylene blue may be repeated and exchange transfusion considered—though its role in methemoglobinemia has not been well defined. A patient who does not respond to methylene blue may have G6PD deficiency, and further administration could exacerbate hemolysis without altering hypoxia.

If the patient is better after 1 hour, methylene blue may be repeated at hourly intervals, either in intravenous form in the patient with altered consciousness or orally (50–100 mg) in an awake patient. Repeat doses should be given for symptoms, not solely on the basis of the methemoglobin level.

Ascorbic acid may be given in conjunction with the oral dose of methylene blue at a dose of 300–400 mg orally, though its role for this purpose remains

Table 14–2. Symptoms of methemoglobinemia.

% Methemoglobinemia	Symptoms
10–30	Cyanosis, mild fatigue, tachycardia
30–50	Weakness, breathlessness, headache, exercise intolerance
50–70	Altered consciousness
>70–80	Coma, death

controversial. Its onset of action is slow and its potential for urine acidification may potentiate renal toxicity in patients who are actively hemolyzing.

2. CHLORATE SALTS

Chlorate salts, used primarily in pesticides and herbicides, cause an unusual form of methemoglobinemia and hemolysis that is unresponsive to methylene blue. Hemolytic anemia has also been seen in uremic patients undergoing hemodialysis when the water supply was found to be contaminated with oxidant compounds made up of chlorine and ammonia termed chloramines. The denaturation of hemoglobin caused by chlorates is thought to be due to their direct oxidizing capacity and their ability to inhibit the hexose monophosphate shunt.

Treatment for poisoning with chlorates is supportive, since there is no specific antidote. Exchange transfusion has been advocated for severe toxicity.

HEMOLYSIS ASSOCIATED WITH EXPOSURE TO HEAVY METALS

After methemoglobinemia and oxidative hemolysis, transitional elements and heavy metals are the most important causes of work-related hemolytic anemia. These agents include arsenic, lead, mercury, copper, and others. The mechanism of hemolysis is not known, but it is thought to be related to the affinity of these directly cytolytic metals to thiol groups such as are found on the surfaces of red blood cells and in the cysteine residues of hemoglobin. When the sulfhydryl-binding metals are exposed to red cells, intravascular lysis may occur as a consequence of altered red cell membrane permeability.

1. ARSINE

The most dramatic example of acute metal-induced hemolysis is that caused by arsine. Arsine is a volatile, colorless, nonirritating gas at room temperature (boiling point –62 °C). It is usually produced accidentally by the action of acid on a metal contaminated with arsenic. However, arsine gas is now also used extensively in the growth and preparation of crystals and conducting devices in the semiconductor industry.

The toxicity of arsine may be best demonstrated by a case of 2 near fatalities reported in 1979 by Parish et al. Two workers at a chemical manufacturing plant were cleaning a floor drain that had become clogged during a clean-up operation. Although the company had discontinued production of arsenical herbicides more than 5 years previously, a steel tank used to mix the chemicals had been left on a loading platform, where it collected rainwater. In attempting to open the drain, the 2 workers emptied water from the tank onto the floor with a drain cleaner containing sodium hydroxide, sodium nitrate, and aluminum chips. They then spent 2–3 hours working to unclog the drain, noting that the drain bubbled and gave off a sewerlike odor. By the next morning, both men were hospitalized with acute hemolytic anemia.

Exposure was documented by the presence of arsenic in the drain as well as the blood and urine of both patients. Each patient required multiple-unit exchange transfusions and fluid replacement; recovery took nearly a month for both. One patient remains on chronic dialysis.

Arsine gas was formed in this incident by the action of arsenic trioxide present in the storage tank and contaminated drain with hydrogen:

$$6H_2 + A_2O_3 \longrightarrow 2AsH_3 + 3H_2O$$

(Arsenic trioxide) (Arsine)

Hydrogen was formed by the combination of sodium hydroxide and aluminum. Antimony may also be present with arsenic and under the same conditions can form stibine, a gas with toxicity similar to that of arsine. The toxicity of arsine here and in other reports is heightened by the fact that arsine is 2.5 times denser than air. This is particularly important in smelting and refinery work, where toxicity is likely to occur when workers are cleaning out large tanks containing acids and metal compounds.

The potential for arsine gas formation and exposure exists in a wide range of occupations and may be combined with exposure to stibine. Most occupational exposure occurs in the smelting, refining, and chemical industries. The respiratory tract is the most important portal of entry.

Chronic arsine poisoning has been described in workers at a zinc smelting plant and in workers engaged in the cyanide extraction of gold. These patients may be anemic, with chronic low-level hemolysis.

Clinical Presentation

A. Symptoms and Signs: Many manifestations of acute arsine poisoning are due to acute and massive intravascular hemolysis. Appearance of symptoms may be delayed for 2–24 hours after exposure. Symptoms include nausea and vomiting, abdominal cramping, headache, malaise, and dyspnea. Patients will often be alarmed by the presence of tea-colored urine not associated with pain on urination, causing them to seek medical attention. Physical examination may reveal a peculiar garlicky odor of arsine, fever, tachycardia, tachypnea, and hypotension. Later in the course of hemolysis, the patient may appear jaundiced, and there is often generalized nonspecific abdominal tenderness.

Chronic arsine poisoning has been described in workers at a zinc smelting plant and in workers engaged in the cyanide extraction of gold. These patients may be anemic, with signs of chronic low-level hemolysis.

B. Laboratory Findings: The earliest laboratory finding may be hemoglobinuria. This occurs when the amount of free plasma hemoglobin exceeds normal haptoglobin binding and renal proximal tubular reabsorption. Accordingly, plasma haptoglobin levels fall and free hemoglobin levels may be very high (> 2000 mg/dL have been reported; normal, < 1 mg/dL). The plasma may be brownish-red from the presence of methemalbumin (oxidized hemoglobin bound to albumin). Although anemia may not be present on the first blood count, evaluation of the peripheral smear will reveal red cell fragmentation with marked poikilocytosis, basophilic stippling, and polychromasia. As the hematocrit falls, reticulocytosis develops. Total bilirubin is elevated, reflecting a rise primarily in the unconjugated or indirect form. Renal function is often affected to a varying degree, with an early rise in serum creatinine. This may be due both to precipitated hemoglobin casts, causing renal tubular obstruction, and to direct toxicity of arsine on the renal tubular and interstitial cells.

Arsenic levels in blood and urine are useful as indicators of exposure rather than as guidelines for therapy.

Treatment

Initial therapy should include vigorous hydration to ensure adequate renal perfusion. For severe hemolysis with plasma hemoglobin levels greater than 400–500 mg/dL, exchange transfusion has been advocated. Repeated exchange is indicated for increasing levels of hemoglobin.

Renal function may be preserved with hydration. However, should renal failure develop, acute hemodialysis may be required. All patients must be monitored closely until all evidence of hemolysis has resolved and renal function has stabilized. Some patients may be left with renal insufficiency or chronic failure requiring dialysis or transplantation. All survivors of acute arsine poisoning must be evaluated regularly for at least 1 year to watch for residual renal dysfunction.

In chronic arsine poisoning, reduction of exposure or removal from exposure is the most important treatment.

2. LEAD

Lead will be more fully discussed with porphyria, below. In addition to the suppression of erythropoiesis and heme synthesis described there, hemolytic anemia may also be seen. Severe acute intravascular hemolysis is rare and is usually seen only with very high atmospheric exposure, as in power sanding and use of a blow torch. The anemia of chronic lead toxicity is enhanced by shortened red cell survival as well as by inhibition of hemoglobin synthesis.

It has been suggested that the pathogenesis of lead-induced hemolysis is related to its marked inhibition of pyrimidine-5' nucleotidase. The hereditary homozygous deficiency of this enzyme is marked by basophilic stippling of erythrocytes, chronic hemolysis, and intraerythrocytic accumulations of pyrimidine-containing nucleotides. These nucleotides perhaps compete with adenine nucleotides in binding to the active site of kinases in the glycolytic pathway, thereby altering red cell membrane stability. Because lead causes an acquired deficiency of this enzyme and the clinical findings are similar, severe toxicity has been likened to this hereditary disease.

3. COPPER

Copper sulfate is used in India in the whitewashing and leather industry. Toxicity is primarily due to accidental ingestion and suicide attempts and results in hemolysis, methemoglobinemia, renal failure, and often death.

Hemolysis has also been caused by hemodialysis with water contaminated by copper piping. In vitro data suggest that multiple mechanisms are involved, including inhibition of glycolysis, oxidation of NADPH, and inhibition of G6PD.

No specific treatment exists other than supportive therapy, with transfusions and hemodialysis as indicated.

THE PORPHYRIAS

The porphyrias are a group of disorders characterized by abnormalities in the heme biosynthetic pathway (Fig 14–4) that result in the abnormal accumulation of heme precursors. Although these are genetic disorders (inherited or sporadic) of enzymatic activity, acquired porphyria has been described following exposure to various toxins. Heme biosynthesis occurs chiefly in the liver and bone marrow and to a certain extent in nervous tissue. The rate-limiting step in heme biosynthesis is the synthesis of δ-aminolevulinic acid (ALA) from glycine and succinyl-CoA via δ-aminolevulinic acid synthetase. This step is under negative feedback control by heme. Clinically, symptomatic porphyria can occur either as a result of inadequate enzymatic function along any step in heme biosynthesis or as a result of inappropriate overstimulation of δ-aminolevulinic acid synthetase,

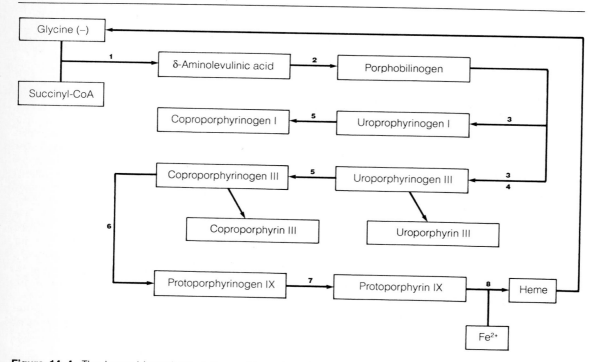

Figure 14–4. The heme biosynthetic pathway. Heme is a feedback inhibitor of enzyme (1) δ-aminolevulinic acid synthetase. Other enzymes are (2) δ-aminolevulinic acid dehydrase, (3) uroporphyrinogen I synthase, (4) uroporphyrinogen III cosynthase, (5) uroporphyrinogen decarboxylase, (6) coproporphyrinogen oxidase, (7) protoporphyrinogen oxidase, and (8) ferrochelatase.

usually in the setting of decreased heme concentration.

The clinical syndromes of porphyria are characterized by neurotoxicity or cutaneous photosensitivity (both may occur). Neurotoxicity—typically abdominal colic, constipation, autonomic dysfunction, sensorimotor neuropathy, and psychiatric problems—is considered the result of direct toxic effects of the urine-soluble heme precursors, δ-aminolevulinic acid and porphobilinogen, on nervous tissue. Neurotoxicity may also be the result of heme deficiency interrupting nervous tissue homeostasis. Cutaneous photosensitivity is manifested as repetitive vesiculation, scarring, and deformity, with hypertrichosis of sun-exposed areas of the skin. This is the result of the relatively urine-insoluble heme precursors—uroporphyrin III, coproporphyrin III, and protoporphyrin IX—fluorescing in the skin following absorption of 400-nm wavelength electromagnetic radiation. These fluorescing porphyrias can also cause discoloration of teeth and occasionally hemolysis of erythrocytes in which porphyrins accumulate.

A number of industrial and environmental toxins have induced toxic **porphyrias** similar to porphyria cutanea tarda in people heavily exposed to the agents (Table 14–3). These toxins generally cause liver injury and deranged hepatic heme synthesis. Although the exact metabolic effects of these agents are not entirely understood, unregulated stimulation of δ-aminolevulinic acid synthetase is usually demonstrable.

1. HEXACHLOROBENZENE

In an outbreak of acquired porphyria in Turkey between 1955 and 1958, over 4000 people developed a cutaneous porphyria syndrome resembling congenital erythropoietic porphyria about 6 months following ingestion of wheat containing a fungicide, hexachlorobenzene. The wheat was intended for planting and contained 2 kg of 10% hexachlorobenzene per 1000 kg of wheat to control a fungus, *Telletia tritici*. Affected people demonstrated cutaneous photosensitivity with skin hyperpigmentation, hypertrichiasis, bullae, weakness, and hepatomegaly, a condition termed kara yara, or "black sore."

Table 14–3. Toxic substances associated with acquired porphyria in humans.

Toxin	Use
Hexachlorobenzene	Fungicide
2,4-Dichlorophenol	Herbicide
2,4,5-Trichlorophenol	Herbicide
2,3,7,8-Tetrachlorodibenzo-p-dioxin	Herbicide contaminent
o-Benzyl-p-chlorophenol	Cleanser and disinfectant
2-Benzyl-4, 6-dichlorophenol	Commercial disinfectant
Vinyl chloride	Plastics
Lead	Paint compounds
Aluminum	Phosphorus binder

Porphyrinuria was nearly universal, with the urine being pigmented red or brown. The mortality rate was 10%. Breast-fed infants under 2 years of age had a 95% mortality rate when ingesting mother's milk contaminated with the fungicide. These infants developed weakness, convulsions, and cutaneous annular erythema, a condition termed pembe yara, or "pink sore." Excess porphyrins could not be detected in the urine of these infants. This is compatible with animal models of hexachlorobenzene-induced porphyria. Infant rats and mice die of neurologic toxicity from hexachlorobenzene without porphyrinuria, while adult rats and rabbits develop cutaneous photosensitivity and porphyrinuria following prolonged exposure to the chemical.

A follow-up study was done between 1977 and 1983 in which 204 patients who previously suffered from hexachlorobenzene porphyria were examined. The mean age of these individuals was 32 years, and the mean time from hexachlorobenzene exposure was 7 years. The mean duration of cutaneous porphyria symptoms was 2.4 years. At the time of study, 71% of people had hyperpigmentation and 47% had hypertrichosis. Residual scarring on sun-exposed areas of the skin was evident in 87%. Other features included perioral scarring, small hands, arthritis, short stature, weakness, paresthesias, and myotonia. Seventeen patients still had red urine and demonstrated porphyrinuria (especially uroporphyrinuria). Hexachlorobenzene was measurable in 56 samples of human milk obtained from porphyric mothers at a mean value of 0.51 ppm (versus 0.07 ppm in control).

The Hungarian experience was the first associating exposure to an industrial chemical with acquired porphyria in humans. Not only were the symptomatic attack and mortality rates significant, but the biochemical lesion persisted for decades in many survivors. The exact mechanism by which hexachlorobenzene induces porphyria remains to be elucidated. Most liver mitochondria of animals made porphyric by exposure to chlorinated benzenes, such as hexachlorobenzene, demonstrated increased activity of δ-aminolevulinic acid synthetase, the enzyme that controls the rate of porphyrin production. With the exception of mice made porphyric with diethyl-1, 4,-dihydro-2,4,6-trimethylpyridine-3,5-dicarboxylate, animal porphyric livers have demonstrated an increased production of heme. Heme normally inhibits the activity of δ-aminolevulinic acid synthetase. This suggests that porphyrinogenic compounds are somehow interfering with the repressor signal of heme on δ-aminolevulinic acid synthetase. Other theories suggest that porphyrinogenic compounds induce δ-aminolevulinic acid synthetase by altering the intracellular oxidation state through action on the electron transport chain, thus stimulating succinyl-CoA production, depressing intracellular ATP levels, or both. In any event, the net result is overproduction of porphyrins mediated by unregulated δ-aminolevulinic acid synthetase activity.

The role of iron overload in the pathogenesis of

hexachlorobenzene-induced porphyria has been examined. The suggestion that iron might be involved was based on the observation that 80% of patients with porphyria cutanea tarda—a disease associated with reduced hepatic uroporphyrinogen decarboxylase activity—have increased liver iron stores and increased levels of uroporphyrin I. Further, decreasing hepatic iron stores by phlebotomy in patients with porphyria cutanea tarda often induces disease remission and a decrease in urinary uroporphyrin I excretion. In a porcine and human liver model, ferrous iron was found to markedly inhibit uroporphyrinogen III cosynthetase activity, enhance total porphyrin production, and greatly overproduce uroporphyrin I. In rats made porphyric with hexachlorobenzene, iron overload results in decreased production of liver heme, cytochrome P-450, and cytochrome b_5 and an absence of uroporphyrinogen decarboxylase activity. In addition, the NAD: NADH ratio was over 2-fold higher in siderotic rats made porphyric with hexachlorobenzene compared to nonsiderotic rats. Furthermore, phlebotomized iron-deficient mice were protected from the porphyrinogenic effect of 2,3,7,8-tetrachlorodibenzo-p-dioxin.

Most authorities believe iron plays a permissive rather than a causative role in porphyrias. This is based on the fact that not all patients with porphyria cutanea tarda are iron-overloaded, that porphyria cutanea tarda is rare in patients with hemochromatosis, and that phlebotomy does not correct the biochemical lesion in patients with porphyria cutanea tarda. In addition, rats made porphyric by hexachlorobenzene did not require iron overload for porphyria to develop, although the porphyria was worsened by iron overload. Thus, it remains unsettled whether iron overload is permissive or etiologic in patients exposed to porphyrinogenic toxins.

2. HERBICIDES

A number of herbicides have been clearly associated with symptomatic porphyria. Bleiberg and colleagues reported on 29 patients exposed to 2,4-dichlorophenol and 2,4,5-trichlorophenol at a manufacturing plant. All 29 patients exhibited chloracne; 13 had hyperpigmentation; 11 had hirsutism; and 5 had skin fragility. Eleven patients had increased excretion of urine porphyrins (uroporphyrin and coproporphyrin). Thus, these patients had developed an acquired porphyria cutanea tarda-like syndrome after variable exposure to these herbicides. A follow-up study of 73 workers at this same herbicide plant 6 years later found no people with the porphyric syndrome and only one with persistent uroporphyrinuria. The authors of the follow-up study hypothesized that the decrease in the syndrome was due to improved personal safety habits of the workers and decreased exposure to the chemicals. An alternative explanation is that the true porphyrinogenic agent is perhaps 2,3,7,8-tetrachlorodibenzo-p-dioxin, a byproduct of 2,4,5-trichlorophenol, and that this contaminant had been effectively eliminated from the chemical stores at the factory. The contaminant was strongly implicated in an outbreak of acquired porphyria cutanea tarda, chloracne, and polyneuropathy in 80 industrial workers producing herbicides in Czechoslovakia.

3. DISINFECTANTS

The commercial disinfectants o-benzyl-p-chlorophenol and 2-benzyl-4,6-dichlorophenol have been implicated as a cause of acquired porphyria cutanea tarda in one woman exposed to these compounds.

4. ALUMINUM

A porphyria cutanea tarda-like syndrome has been described in patients with chronic renal failure being maintained on regular hemodialysis. Plasma and urine uroporphyrins are increased in these patients, whereas plasma and urine coproporphyrins are often low. Since aluminum is known to inhibit some heme synthetic enzymes and since many chronic renal failure patients on hemodialysis are aluminum-overloaded, aluminum has been implicated, but without proof, as the cause of porphyria in these patients.

5. VINYL CHLORIDE

Vinyl chloride is a known hepatotoxin used in the production of plastics. A study of 46 persons working in a polyvinyl chloride production plant revealed significantly elevated urinary coproporphyrins compared to normal controls. Exposure periods ranged from 2 to 21 years. The pathogenesis of coproporphyrinuria involves inhibition of coproporphyrinogen oxidase, inhibition of uroporphyrinogen decarboxylase, and perhaps induction of δ-aminolevulinic acid synthetase. Persons with excess urinary coproporphyrin production also manifested thrombocytopenia, splenomegaly, esophageal varices, sclerodermalike skin changes, Raynaud's syndrome, and acro-osteolysis.

6. LEAD

Lead intoxication (blood lead level > 80 mg/dL in adults; > 60 mg/dL in children) causes symptoms and signs remarkably similar to those associated with acute intermittent porphyria. The classic acute intermittent porphyria triad is abdominal pain, constipation, and vomiting—all representing the neurotoxic effects of excess δ-aminolevulinic acid and porphobilinogen. This triad is seen with equal frequency in lead intoxication. Other shared characteristics include neuromuscular pains, paresis or paralysis, paresthesias, diarrhea, and seizures. The major differences between the 2 diseases are an increase in neuropsychiatric signs in acute intermittent porphyria compared to lead intoxication and anemia, which is present in lead intoxication but virtually absent in porphyria. The anemia of lead poisoning is a characteristic microcytic anemia with basophilic stippling of erythrocytes and sideroblasts in the bone marrow.

The biochemical features of lead poisoning demonstrate why these 2 diseases are clinically so similar. Patients with lead intoxication have markedly elevated urinary δ-aminolevulinic acid levels, as in acute intermittent porphyria. Mild lead poisoning (preanemia stage) is associated with normal porphobilinogen excretion, but once anemia occurs, excess urinary porphobilinogen becomes demonstrable. Although mild elevations of urine coproporphyrins and uroporphyrin I are present, fecal uroporphyrin and coproporphyrin are normal in patients with lead poisoning. These alterations in porphyrins are present only in patients with inorganic lead intoxication, not in patients with organic lead intoxication. Excess accumulation of protoporphyrin IX has also been found in erythrocytes of lead-intoxicated patients.

Lead poisoning is associated with greatly diminished activity of δ-aminolevulinic acid dehydrase in the brain, liver, kidney, and bone marrow. Lead also blocks the incorporation of iron into protoporphyrin IX by depressing the activity of ferrochelatase, an event most closely linked with the production of anemia and elevation of free erythrocyte protoporphyrin IX levels. Coproporphyrinogen oxidase activity has also been shown to be depressed by lead. Thus, the effect of lead on heme synthesis disruption occurs at multiple steps in the synthetic pathway.

TREATMENT OF TOXIC PORPHYRIAS

Since there is often no effective means of eliminating toxic environmental or industrial substances once they are incorporated into tissues, exposure to porphyrinogenic compounds must be avoided. Although no prospective data are available to support the use of phlebotomy for this purpose, this therapy may be of benefit in patients with toxic porphyria whose disease complex resembles porphyria cutanea tarda and in whom evidence of iron overload can be demonstrated. Patients with acute intermittent porphyria occasionally respond to high-dose carbohydrate infusions (400 g/d dextrose) or hematin infusions (3 mg/kg intravenously every 12 hours for 10–12 doses). However, the use of hematin infusions in toxic porphyria may not be of benefit since, as in the case of hexachlorobenzene, the toxic agent may be interrupting the negative feedback signal by heme on δ-aminolevulinic acid synthetase.

For lead intoxication, prevention is again the best treatment. Unlike all other toxic porphyrias, specific therapy for lead intoxication is available with lead chelators (see Chapter 25).

DISORDERS ASSOCIATED WITH DECREASED OXYGEN SATURATION

CARBON MONOXIDE

Carbon monoxide is an odorless, colorless, nonirritating gas produced by the incomplete combustion of organic materials, particularly hydrocarbons. The workers at greatest risk are automobile mechanics (automobile exhaust systems), fire fighters, and chemical workers exposed to methylene chloride (converted to carbon monoxide through in vivo metabolism).

Carbon monoxide binds to hemoglobin, forming carboxyhemoglobin, which decreases hemoglobin oxygen saturation and shifts the oxygen hemoglobin dissociation curve to the left. Hemoglobin has an affinity for carbon monoxide 210 times greater than that for oxygen. Carbon monoxide also increases the stability of the hemoglobin-oxygen combination, thus inhibiting oxygen delivery to the tissues. In addition, carbon monoxide binds to the cytochrome oxidase chain, interfering with cellular respiration.

Clinical Findings

Symptoms include general malaise, headache, nausea, dyspnea, vomiting, and alteration in mental status at high levels. Severe exposure may cause coma, seizures, arrhythmias, and death. Symptoms of anoxia may be prominent without cyanosis due to the cherry-red color of carboxyhemoglobin.

Laboratory findings at low levels may show polycythemia; at higher levels, hypoxia is seen. Carboxyhemoglobin levels should be measured; a level under 6% may cause impairment in vision and time discrimination; at 40–60% alterations in mental status and death may be seen.

Treatment & Prevention

Treatment is dependent on the degree of carboxyhemoglobin. At low levels, removal from the source of exposure is sufficient. At higher levels, the treatment of choice is inspiration of 100% oxygen. Oxygen markedly decreases the half-life of carboxyhemoglobin from 5–6 hours at room air to 90 minutes at 100% inspired oxygen by dilutional displacement of the carbon monoxide. Severe toxicity, including mental status aberrations, may call for hyperbaric oxygen therapy, which decreases the half-life of carboxyhemoglobin further to 23 minutes at 3 atmospheres.

Prevention depends on adequate ventilation, with venting of combustion devices to the outside air.

DISORDERS AFFECTING BLOOD CELL FORMATION & MORPHOLOGY

Premalignant and malignant hematologic diseases have been linked to a variety of occupational exposures. Because the determination of cause and effect is very difficult to verify when the latency period is long and the exposure history is poorly documented, other methods for ascertaining this link have been explored. Cytogenetic study consists of examining the somatic chromosomes of hematologic cells in metaphase.

CYTOGENETICS

The chromosomal analysis of hematologic disorders is an important mechanism for classification and as a guide to prognosis and therapy. Cytogenetics serves 2 purposes in occupational hematology: (1) to screen populations at risk for toxic exposure so that cryptic toxic agents can be identified; and (2) in individual cases, to identify diseases that might have been caused by exposure to mutagenic agents.

Abnormalities in chromosomes can be used as a marker for exposure to noxious environmental agents. Through extensive epidemiologic study, certain abnormalities have been associated with specific diseases and prognostic categories. Toxic agents that have been shown to be associated with chromosomal abnormalities in vivo have been linked to the development of cancers and leukemias.

Cytogenetic analysis for hematologic disorders is best done by direct examination of cells obtained from bone marrow. Since these cells are continuously proliferating, it is relatively easy to examine those undergoing mitosis when the chromosomes are visible microscopically. High-resolution banding techniques are used to precisely identify deletions, translocations, inversions, and other structural chromosomal abnormalities.

Cells obtained from peripheral blood require artificial stimulation by a mitogen such as phytohemagglutinin and culture for 2–3 days to obtain enough cells in mitosis for analysis. Artifactual aberrations may be induced in cells that are manipulated after removal from the patient before fixing for analysis. The resulting risk of falsely abnormal evaluations increases the necessity and importance of well matched and multiple controls.

Screening & Prevention

Cytogenetic analysis has been used as a screening tool to monitor industrial populations for early exposure to mutagenic chemicals and to identify possible mutagens. In this way, workers at risk might be removed from potentially dangerous conditions when the effects are still reversible. Peripheral blood lymphocytes rather than bone marrow must be used for obvious reasons of worker comfort, time, and cost.

The problem with using cytogenetics for monitoring is the relative insensitivity of the method to low levels of exposure. The only known dose-response relationship for exposure and somatic chromosome aberrations has been described with ionizing radiation. In a recent study of workers exposed to low levels (below exposure limits) of chemicals in a petrochemical plant in the Netherlands, cytogenetic monitoring by chromosomal banding techniques was carried out from 1976 to 1981. Results of these studies, published in 1988, found no increase in the frequencies of chromosome aberrations in the exposed populations compared with control populations. They concluded that the examination of peripheral blood lymphocytes for chromosomal aberrations is not sufficiently sensitive for routine monitoring of cytogenetics in workers exposed to low levels of the compounds.

A second technique that has been evaluated in monitoring is sister chromatid exchange, a method of evaluating symmetric intrachromosomal rearrangements of DNA. Although this technique is faster and cheaper than cytogenetic analysis, the presence of exchanges does not necessarily correlate with the incidence of chromosomal aberrations or the development of disease.

Further progress in methods to detect induced DNA damage is needed for cytogenetic analysis to be an adequate screening tool for large populations. With the advent of molecular biologic techniques, this should be possible in the future on a population-wide scale. At present, although individual health consequences cannot be estimated by population screening methods, abnormal chromosomal or cytogenetic findings are clearly an adverse sign when correlated with specific exposure risk data.

Relationship of Cytogenetic Abnormalities to Specific Diseases

Cytogenetic study provides a means of relating chromosomal aberrations in the bone marrow of a patient with preleukemia or leukemia to exposure to mutagenic agents. The population benefited includes workers exposed to industrial agents and radiation as well as patients previously treated with chemotherapeutic agents or radiation. Many studies have suggested that this population has a much higher incidence of chromosomal abnormalities than a similar nonexposed group with the same diseases. In a summary of 3 retrospective studies of patients with de novo acute nonlymphocytic leukemia, individuals were grouped as nonexposed and exposed on the basis of occupation. Individuals who worked with insecticides, chemicals and solvents, metals or minerals, petroleum products, and ionizing radiation were considered exposed, whereas students, white-collar workers, and housewives were classified as nonexposed. Sixty-eight of 236 patients (29%) were found to be in the exposed group. Fifty-one of the 68

(75%) in the exposed group had abnormal karyotypes, versus only 60 of 168 (36%) in the nonexposed group. In addition to this generalized increase in chromosomal aberrations, abnormalities in chromosomes 5 and 7 were observed in 37% of the exposed and in 12% of the nonexposed individuals.

These specific chromosomal abnormalities have also correlated positively with the development of leukemia after exposure to therapeutic mutagens (chemotherapy or radiation) used to treat other cancers. Specifically, a loss of the entire chromosome or of part of the long arm of either or both of these chromosomes has been seen. Although these chromosome abnormalities may occur in the absence of exposure to mutagens, patients with leukemias or preleukemic conditions with deletions involving chromosomes 5 or 7 should arouse a suspicion of prior exposure to chemical carcinogens or radiation, and this history should be vigorously sought. The prognosis for patients with abnormalities of chromosomes 5 or 7—or with multiple cytogenetic abnormalities when associated with prior exposure to mutagenic agents—is poor compared to that of patients with a normal chromosome analysis.

Clearly the greatest usefulness of cytogenetics is in the area of prevention and developing better techniques to assess future pathologic consequences of exposure at a time when effects may still be reversible. As more sensitive techniques are developed, they may also serve as a guideline for determining the threshold limit values for potential mutagens.

WORK-RELATED ANEMIA AND HEMATOLOGIC MALIGNANCIES

Hematologic malignancies are discussed in detail in the chapter on occupational cancers. In this section, we will discuss only diseases not covered in that chapter: aplastic anemia, myelodysplasia, and multiple myeloma.

1. APLASTIC ANEMIA

Aplastic anemia, or medullary aplasia, is an acquired abnormality of the pluripotential hematopoietic stem cells resulting in pancytopenia. The average incidence of fatal aplastic anemia per year in the USA is about 2 per million and rises with age to an annual age-specific mortality rate of about 10 per million in people over age 65. Approximately 50% of cases of aplastic anemia in North America and Western Europe are idiopathic; most of the remainder are termed secondary aplastic anemias and may be caused by drugs, chemicals, radiation, infection, and immunologic mechanisms. A small percentage of cases are due to hereditary diseases.

The largest category of secondary aplastic anemia is due to therapeutic drugs; probably only a small fraction are due to environmental and occupational causes. The drug most commonly implicated is chloramphenicol; others include acetazolamide, phenylbutazone, phenytoin, and sulfonamides—and there are many others. This section will discuss only occupation-related cases of aplastic anemia.

Many cases of aplastic anemia develop after the occurrence of dysplastic morphologic changes in hematologic cells with associated chromosomal abnormalities. The incidence of acute nonlymphocytic leukemia in patients with aplastic anemia who survive 2 years after diagnosis is about 5–10%; in patients with preceding dysplasia, the incidence may be higher. Chemicals that are capable of inducing bone marrow damage must be assumed to be potential leukemogens. It is difficult to link specific chemicals to the development of aplastic anemia because of the absence of a specific test for exposure and the frequency of multiple or unknown exposures. Only 3 agents have been firmly established as a cause of aplastic anemia on a dose-dependent basis. These include benzene, ionizing radiation, and cytotoxic drugs such as antimetabolites and alkylating agents. Benzene and ionizing radiation are discussed at greater length in Chapter 16.

Benzene

Benzene was first described as a cause of fatal aplastic anemia in 1897. Early unregulated exposure to benzene—used widely as a solvent in the production of many products, including fabrics and pesticides—led to many cases of acute and chronic toxicity. Workers now at greatest risk of exposure are those involved in rubber manufacturing, shoemaking, petroleum and chemical production, printing, and steelworking.

Before 1950, benzene was the single most common cause of toxic aplastic anemia. With chronic doses of over 100 ppm, isolated cytopenias and aplastic anemia were common. The cytopenias usually recovered after termination of exposure; even with persistent exposure, spontaneous remissions have been described. At exposures of 100 ppm or higher, some workers will develop fatal aplastic anemia. Great variation in susceptibility to exposure has been seen, with evidence of poisoning sometimes appearing only after weeks or years. Cases of cytopenia have also been seen several years after exposure has been terminated; these cases are less likely to resolve with time and may be part of a preleukemic syndrome. In severe chronic poisoning, decreased red cell survival with hemolysis has been reported.

Toxicity is directly related to the amount and duration of exposure, although again there is individual variation in susceptibility. The diagnosis is made by examination of the bone marrow after an abnormal complete blood count is reported. The bone marrow will reveal hypocellularity with fatty replacement, though islands of hypercellularity may be seen. Although cytogenetic abnormalities have been associated with benzene exposure, specific chromosome changes have not. The initial prognosis in benzene-related aplastic anemia is better than that for idiopathic aplastic anemia; up to 40% may recover completely after removal from the source of exposure. If hypocellularity persists for more than several months, recovery is not likely to occur. Exposure has been associated with the development of acute non-lymphocytic leukemia, chronic myelogenous leukemia, and multiple myeloma—either de novo or in workers who have recovered from a bout of aplastic anemia—and in cases of irreversible aplastic anemia.

Treatment is supportive (ie, with transfusions). Drugs such as androgens to stimulate hematopoiesis have not been used extensively in benzene-induced aplastic anemia but should be tried when no other treatment option exists (such as bone marrow transplantation or colony-stimulating factors). Allogeneic bone marrow transplantation is the only known cure for irreversible aplastic anemia and is hampered by donor availability, the age of the patient, and toxicity of the transplant regimen.

Ionizing Radiation

Ionizing radiation has also been associated with aplastic anemia in a dose-dependent manner. Internal exposure to absorbed alpha particles associated with aplastic anemia was most strikingly demonstrated in the radium watch dial workers who ingested radium by wetting their paintbrushes on their tongues. External exposure to radiation is much more common and may be in the form of whole body exposure to a large dose, as in a nuclear accident or therapeutic radiation, or long-term exposure to small amounts, as may occur in the practice of radiology as a medical specialty.

Data from patients radiated for ankylosing spondylitis and from the survivors of the atomic bombing of Hiroshima and Nagasaki suggest that the risk of aplastic anemia is increased until 3–5 years after exposure, after which there is a marked decline in incidence. The most important late disturbance following irradiation of the bone marrow is leukemia. The ability to recover from a single dose of penetrating radiation is dependent on the fraction of surviving stem cells. Chromosomal aberrations are associated with exposure to ionizing radiation and rise in a linear manner as a function of the dose of radiation absorbed. The presence of these aberrations, including an increase in the number of sister chromatid exchanges, may signify excessive exposure but is not predictive of aplastic anemia or leukemia.

Strict regulation of exposure and monitoring with badges has virtually eliminated aplastic anemia due to radiation except in cases of accidental overexposure. In this case, treatment again is primarily supportive. Recovery may be seen after a prolonged period of aplastic anemia lasting 3–6 weeks and may be predicted based on the known total dose of radiation. If recovery does not occur, permanent injury to the stem cell population has resulted in chronic cellular hypoplasia or dysplasia or in leukemia. Treatment may then include bone marrow transplantation if a donor is available. Trials to study the use of hematopoietic growth factors in treating aplastic anemia are now going forward.

Other Chemicals

Aplastic anemia has been reported following exposure to a variety of other chemicals listed in Table 14–4. Toxicities often resolve completely with cessation of exposure. Again, individual susceptibility plays an important role, though it is poorly understood.

Two chemicals in particular deserve mention here. The aplastic anemia associated with **trinitrotoluene** may be accompanied by methemoglobinemia, oxidative hemolysis, liver damage, and dermatitis.

The incidence of overexposure to **arsenic** has declined with its decreasing use during the past 3 decades. Less than 10 cases of poisoning are now reported annually in the USA. If arsenic-induced aplastic anemia or pancytopenia is suspected, laboratory confirmation of the exposure (see Chapter 25) should be obtained. Complete spontaneous recovery is usually seen if the patient is removed from the source of exposure within a few days to weeks.

2. MYELODYSPLASTIC SYNDROMES

Both benzene and ionizing radiation have also been implicated in the development of myelodysplasia. Myelodysplasia or preleukemia is actually a group of 5 syndromes classified by the morphology of the bone marrow and peripheral blood. These syndromes are linked by the presence of bizarre hematopoietic morphology and the tendency to transform into acute leukemia. Most patients with myelodysplasia do not develop leukemia, though specific syndromes associated with exposure to both occupational chemicals and cytotoxic drugs have a high incidence of progression to frank leukemia. The median survival from these diseases is less than 12 months, and all patients

Table 14–4. Chemicals reported to cause aplastic anemia in an occupational setting.

Chemical	Use
Benzene	Intermediate in the synthesis of fabrics, pesticides, rubber. Solvent for glues, varnishes, inks, paints. Octane booster for gasoline.
Trinitrotoluene (TNT)	Production of explosives
Hexachloroclyclohexane (lindane) Pentachlorophenol Chlorophenothane (DDT)	Pesticide
Arsenic	Manufacture of glass, paint, enamels, weed killers, tanning agents, pesticides
Ethylene glycol monomethyl or monobutyl ether	Production of paints, lacquers, dyes, inks, cleaning agents

develop leukemias or succumb to complications related to cytopenias. These syndromes—classified as refractory anemia with excess blasts (RAEB) or RAEB in transformation—are associated with an increase in chromosomal aberrations. Exposure and treatment-related myelodysplasia is specifically associated with a high incidence of deletions involving chromosomes 5 and 7.

Myelodysplastic syndromes are more common in men than in women, and 85% of patients are over 40 years of age at the time of diagnosis. Laboratory features of RAEB include cytopenias of varying degree and often an increase in mean corpuscular volume. The marrow reveals dysplasia in all 3 cell lines and a varying degree of hypo- or hyperplasia. There may be an abnormal increase in the percentage of blast cells.

Several treatment options are available, though they are far from ideal. Allogeneic bone marrow transplantation is the only known cure and is primarily limited here by patient age, since most will not be eligible even if a donor exists. Transfusions and treatment of infections may be aided by the use of hematopoietic growth factors currently under clinical investigation.

3. MULTIPLE MYELOMA

Multiple myeloma is a clonal differentiated B cell neoplasm that accounts for 15% of all hematologic cancers. The peak incidence is between ages 55 and 65, and fewer than 2% of cases occur before the age of 40. Multiple myeloma is equally common in men and women but almost twice as common in blacks as in whites. The incidence of multiple myeloma has been increasing over the last 3 decades in North American and European men, but this rise has not been noted in the stable study populations in Minnesota and Sweden and may simply reflect an increase in our ability to diagnose the disease. The rise in incidence has aroused concern that myeloma might be associated with environmental or occupational factors.

Although no definitive link has been made between occupational exposure and the risk of multiple myeloma, many epidemiologic studies suggest an association. Exposure to petroleum products, organic solvents, heavy metals, pesticides, and asbestos has been implicated, but most studies are small and can only be used as a basis for hypotheses. Workers thought to be at risk include agricultural workers, chemicals workers, miners, smelters, and furniture workers in the early part of this century.

A study published in 1987 reviewed mortality and exposure data in a cohort of rubber manufacturers in the USA occupationally exposed to benzene. The analysis found that there was a statistically significant excess of deaths from multiple myeloma in workers exposed to low levels of benzene and that the latency period was over 20 years. A strong positive exposure-response relationship between benzene and leukemia was also found.

An important association between high-dose radiation exposure and multiple myeloma has been observed in cohorts of controls and survivors of the atomic bombings in Hiroshima and Nagasaki for the period of 1950 to 1976. The relative risk for persons with an estimated air-dose exposure of 100 cGy or more was over 4 times higher than that of controls. This excess risk became apparent about 20 years after exposure. An association has also been proposed—but not confirmed—between the risk of multiple myeloma and exposure to low-dose radiation. At present, except in the case of high-dose radiation, there are insufficient data upon which to base a firm conclusion about the relationship between exposure to ionizing radiation and the risk of developing multiple myeloma. Further large-scale incidence studies on this topic will be needed.

TOXIC THROMBOCYTOPENIA

Unlike thrombocytopenia associated with toxicant-induced aplastic anemia, isolated toxic thrombocytopenia is a rare event. A number of toxic exposures have been reported that resulted in isolated thrombocytopenia (Table 14–5). Two cases of isolated thrombocytopenia were described in 1963 in individuals exposed to the polymerizing agent **toluene diisocyanate.** Both developed thrombocytopenia 14–22 days following a significant exposure that also induced bronchospasm. These patients developed thrombocytopenic bleeding with nadir platelet counts of 6000/μL and 30,000/μL. Bone marrow samples in both cases showed increased megakaryocytes. The pathophysiologic defect was enhanced peripheral platelet destruction, presumably on an immune basis (immune thrombocytopenic purpura). One patient responded transiently to corticosteroid therapy and

Table 14–5. Toxic agents associated with isolated thrombocytopenia.

Toxic Agent	Use	Mechanism
Toluene diisocyanate	Polymerizing agent	Immune
2, 2-Dichlorovinyl dimethylphosphate Dieldrin Pyrethrin Lethane Hexachlorocyclohexane (lindane) Chlorophenothane (DDT)	Insecticide	Megakaryocyte hypoplasia
Turpentine	Organic solvent	Immune
Vinyl chloride	Plastics	Liver insufficiency with hypersplenism

then completely to splenectomy; the second patient had resolution of thrombocytopenia without any therapy.

Two more cases of toxin-induced immune thrombocytopenic purpura were described in 1969. Two children with significant **turpentine** exposure (one respiratory and cutaneous exposure, the second ingestion) developed petechiae and severe thrombocytopenia with increased bone marrow megakaryocytes. Both responded fully to corticosteroid therapy.

Insecticides can cause a selective megakaryocyte aplasia in people with significant inhalation or ingestion exposure. Isolated thrombocytopenia has been reported after exposure to 2,2-dichlorovinyl dimethyl phosphate, dieldrin, pyrethrin, lethane, hexachlorocyclohexane (lindane), and chlorophenothane (DDT). These patients demonstrated absent or decreased bone marrow megakaryocytes. Some megakaryocytes were vacuolated. Most patients received corticosteroids and responded with full platelet recovery.

A third form of toxic thrombocytopenia was described in 1984. Forty-six people exposed to **vinyl chloride** with evidence of toxic coproporphyrinuria also had thrombocytopenia. Although these patients were not described in detail, they appeared to have significant vinyl chloride liver toxicity, with esophageal varices and splenomegaly. The likely pathophysiologic mechanism of thrombocytopenia was thus enhanced peripheral platelet consumption due to hypersplenism, although there were insufficient data presented to rule out an immune or megakaryocyte toxic mechanism.

OCCUPATIONAL EXPOSURE TO ANTICANCER DRUGS

Oncology nurses and pharmacists who prepare and administer chemotherapy to patients on a regular basis are at risk for exposure to potentially mutagenic agents. Data from a variety of sources are available on the mutagenic potential of many anticancer drugs.

Epidemiologic studies have linked certain drugs (and radiation) to the development of secondary cancers; analytic in vitro methods of assessing mutagenicity have offered confirmatory evidence.

There are several obvious problems in assessing the risk to nurses. First is the low and intermittent exposure rate relative to the patients who receive these drugs therapeutically and who serve as in vivo models for the effects of heavy exposure. This limits the usefulness of epidemiologic data such as exposure rates and disease incidence when attempting to assess individual risks. Second, the methods for detecting exposure are often contradictory and may be cumbersome in time relative to work. For example, it may be difficult for nurses to obtain urine 6 hours after the end of a shift.

Methods for assessing risk include measuring blood and urine levels of drug, urine mutagenicity assays, cytogenetic monitoring and sister chromatid exchange studies, and environmental monitoring. Blood and urine levels may be difficult to interpret when drugs are rapidly metabolized. Studies evaluating oncology nurses versus control populations of other nurses or non-health care workers have been published with both positive and negative results using all of the above methods. Clearly a combination of monitoring tools is required.

In addition to the above studies, which assess potential risk, the effect on human reproduction in terms of spontaneous abortion and teratogenic effects has also been examined. Again, the results are inconclusive but suggest an increase in both effects with frequent exposure. Information on safety practices is not available.

The agents most commonly implicated in mutagenic potential are those that are also implicated as causes of secondary cancers in patients receiving therapeutic drugs such as alkylating agents. Clearly, any cytotoxic drug should be handled with great care and with the goal of absolutely minimum exposure to personnel. This can be accomplished by worker education, gloves and protective clothing, laminar hoods for preparing drugs, and proper waste disposal. Periodic atmospheric checks and biologic monitoring can improve hygienic standards, but conclusions regarding the long-term health effects based on these results are not possible.

REFERENCES

General

Jandl JH: *Blood: Textbook of Hematology.* Little, Brown, 1987.

Sauter D, Goldfrank L: Hematologic aspects of toxicology. *Hematol Oncol Clin North Am* 1987;**1**:335.

Zenz C (editor): *Occupational Medicine: Principles and Practical Applications,* 2nd ed. Year Book, 1988.

Methemoglobinemia & Oxidative Hemolysis

Bunn HF, Forget BG: *Hemoglobin: Molecular, Genetic, and Clinical Aspects.* Saunders, 1986.

Eaton JW et al: Chlorinated urban water: A cause of dialysis-induced hemolytic anemia. *Science* 1973; **181**:463.

Gordon-Smith EC: Drug-induced oxidative haemolysis. *Clin Haematol* 1980;**9**:557.

Halsted HC: Industrial methemoglobinemia. *J Occup Med* 1960;**2**:591.

Kearney TE, Manoguerra AS, Dunford JV Jr: Chemically induced methemoglobinemia from aniline poisoning. *West J Med* 1984;**140**:282.

Arsine

Fowler BA, Weissberg JB: Arsine poisoning. *N Engl J Med* 1974;**291:**1171.

Levinsky WJ et al: Arsine hemolysis. *Arch Environ Health* 1970;**20:**436.

Parish GG, Glass R, Kimbrough R: Acute arsine poisoning in 2 workers cleaning a clogged drain. *Arch Environ Health* 1979;**34:**224.

Pinto SS: Arsine poisoning: Evaluation of the acute phase. *J Occup Med* 1976;**18:**633.

Lead

Miwa S et al: A case of lead intoxication: Clinical and biochemical studies. *Am J Hematol* 1981;**11:**99.

Paglia DE, Valentine WN, Dahlgren JG: Effects of low-level lead exposure on pyrimidine 5'-nucleotidase and other erythrocyte enzymes: Possible role of pyrimidine 5'-nucleotidase in the pathogenesis of lead-induced anemia. *J Clin Invest* 1975;**56:**1164.

Valentine WN et al: Lead poisoning: Association with hemolytic anemia, basophilic stippling, erythrocyte primidine 5'-nucleotidase deficiency, and intraerythrocytic accumulation of pyrimidines. *J Clin Invest* 1976;**58:**926.

Toxic Porphyria

Bleiberg J et al: Industrially acquired porphyria. *Arch Dermatol* 1964;**89:**793.

Cripps DJ: Porphyria: Genetic and acquired. Pages 549–566 in: *Hexachlorobenzene: Proceedings of an International Symposium.* Morris CR, Cabral JR (editors). IARC Scientific Publications, 1986.

DeMatteis F: Toxic hepatic porphyrias. *Semin Hematol* 1968;**5:**409.

Doss M, Lange LE, Veltman G: Vinyl chloride-induced hepatic coproporphyrinuria with transition to chronic hepatic porphyria. *Klin Wochenschr* 1984;**62:**175.

Felsher BF, Kushner JP: Hepatic siderosis and porphyria cutanea tarda: Relation of iron excess to the metabolic defect. *Semin Hematol* 1977;**14:**243.

Gocmen A et al: Porphyria turcica: Hexachlorobenzene-induced porphyria. Pages 567–573 in: *Hexachlorobenzene: Proceedings of an International Symposium.* Morris CR, Cabral JR (editors). IARC Scientific Publications, 1986.

Goldberg A: Lead poisoning as a disorder of heme synthesis. *Semin Hematol* 1968;**5:**424.

Grossman ME, Poh-Fitzpatrick MB: Porphyria cutanea tarda: Diagnosis and management. *Med Clin North Am* 1980;**64:**807.

Hindmarsh JT: The porphyrias: Recent advances. *Clin Chem* 1986;**32:**1255.

Klein M et al: Earthenware containers as a source of fatal lead poisoning. *N Engl J Med* 1970;**283:**669.

Kushner JP, Lee GR, Nacht S: The role of iron in the pathogenesis of porphyria cutanea tarda: An in vitro model. *J Clin Invest* 1972;**51:**3044.

McColl KE, Goldberg A: Abnormal porphyrin metabolism in diseases other than porphyria. *Clin Haematol* 1980;**9:**427.

Poland AP et al: A health survey of workers in a 2,4-D and 2,4,5-T plant with special attention to chloracne, porphyria cutanea tarda, and psychologic parameters. *Arch Environ Health* 1971;**22:**316.

Toljaard JJ et al: Porphyrin metabolism in experimental hepatic siderosis in the rat. 3. Effect of iron overload and hexachlorobenzene on liver haem biosynthesis. *Br J Haematol* 1972;**23:**587.

Cytogenetics

deJong G, vanSittert NJ, Natarajan AT: Cytogenetic monitoring of industrial populations potentially exposed to genotoxic chemicals and of control populations. *Mutat Res* 1988;**204:**451.

Golomb HM et al: Correlation of occupation and karyotype in adults with acute nonlymphocytic leukemia. *Blood* 1982;**60:**404.

Mitelman F et al: Chromosome pattern, occupation, and clinical features in patients with nonlymphocytic leukemia. *Cancer Genet Cytogenet* 1981;**4:**197.

Rowley JD: Chromosome abnormalities in human leukemia as indicators of mutagenic exposure. *Carcinog Compt Surv* 1985;**10:**409.

Aplastic Anemia

Aksoy M et al: Haematological effects of chronic benzene poisoning in 217 workers. *Br J Ind Med* 1971;**28:**296.

Ichimaru M et al: Incidence of aplastic anemia in A-bomb survivors: Hiroshima and Nagasaki, 1946–1967. *Radiat Res* 1972;**49:**461.

Jandl JH: Aplastic anemias. Pages 115–127 in: *Blood: Textbook of Hematology.* Little, Brown, 1987.

Loge JP: Aplastic anemia following exposure to benzene hexachloride (Lindane). *JAMA* 1965;**193:**110.

Myelodysplasia

Koeffler HP: Myelodysplastic syndromes (preleukemia). *Semin Hematol* 1986;**23:**284.

Multiple Myeloma

Brownson RC, Reif JS: A cancer registry-based study of occupational risk for lymphoma, multiple myeloma, and leukaemia. *Int J Epidemiol* 1988;**17:**27.

Cuzick J, DeStavola B: Multiple myeloma: A case-control study. *Br J Cancer* 1988;**57:**516.

Ichimaru M et al: Multiple myeloma among atomic bomb survivors in Hiroshima and Nagasaki, 1950–1976: Relationship to radiation dose absorbed by marrow. *JNCI* 1982;**69:**323.

McLaughlin JK et al: Multiple myeloma and occupation in Sweden. *Arch Environ Health* 1988;**43:**7.

Rinsky RA et al: Benzene and leukemia: An epidemiologic risk assessment. *N Engl J Med* 1987;**316:**1044.

Toxic Thrombocytopenia

Doss M, Lange CE, Veltman G: Vinyl chloride-induced hepatic coproporphyrinuria with transition to chronic hepatic porphyria. *Klin Wochenschr* 1984;**62:**175.

Jennings GH, Gower ND: Thrombocytopenic purpura in toluene diisocyanate workers. *Lancet* 1963;**1:**406.

Kulis JC: Chemically induced, selective thrombocytopenic purpura. *Arch Intern Med* 1965;**116:**559.

Wahlberg P, Nyman D: Turpentine and thrombocytopenic purpura. *Lancet* 1969;**2:**215.

Nursing Risk

Norppa H et al: Increased sister chromatid exchange frequencies in lymphocytes of nurses handling cytostatic drugs. *Scand J Work Environ Health* 1980;**6:**299.

Sorsa M, Hemminki K, Vainio H: Occupational exposure to anticancer drugs: Potential and real hazards. *Mutat Res* 1985;**154:**135.

Occupational Infections

Richard Cohen, MD, MPH

Occupational infections are those human diseases caused by work-associated exposure to microbial agents, including bacteria, viruses, fungi, and parasites (helminths, protozoa). What distinguishes an infection as occupational is some aspect of the work that involves contact with a biologically active organism. Occupational infection can occur following contact with infected persons, as in the case of health care workers; with infected animal or human tissue, secretions, or excretions, as in laboratory workers; with asymptomatic or unknown contagious humans, as happens during business travel; or with infected animals, as in agriculture. This chapter highlights tuberculosis, hepatitis B and AIDS, travel-related infections, and brucellosis as examples of the 4 types of exposure.

The etiology, pathogenesis, clinical findings, diagnosis, and treatment of occupational and nonoccupational infections are the same except for practical differences related to identification of the source of exposure, epidemiologic control, and prevention. This chapter will focus on the occupational aspects of microbial exposures and relevant strategies for prevention.

Table 15–1 lists the more frequent occupational infections according to agent, source, exposed occupations, and preventive measures. The references at the end of the chapter are selected as those most useful for practitioners engaged in diagnosis, treatment, and prevention of occupational infectious disease.

INFECTIONS DUE TO EXPOSURE TO INFECTED HUMANS OR THEIR TISSUES

Health care and clinical laboratory workers are at increased risk of infection by organisms whose natural hosts are humans, as in the case of hepatitis, rubella, AIDS, tuberculosis, and staphylococcal disease. Some infections may be transmitted through close personal contact with infected patients. Exposure and infection due to almost any of the viruses, bacteria, fungi, and parasites pathogenic for humans can result from direct contact with the organism in culture or in human tissue. Tuberculosis is an exam-

ple of a relatively common occupational infection resulting from repeated close contact with infected patients; and type B hepatitis exemplifies a serious and relatively frequent infection resulting from manipulation of infected human blood and inoculation by infectious virus particles.

TUBERCULOSIS

Mycobacterium tuberculosis usually infects the lungs, with resulting pneumonia or granuloma formation, and may have other systemic effects also. Medical house staff have been found to have 2–3 times the tuberculosis infection rate of nonmedical personnel, and laboratory workers exposed to *M tuberculosis* have 3 times the incidence of nonexposed workers.

Tubercle bacilli may be present in gastric fluid, cerebrospinal fluid, urine, sputum, and tissue specimens harboring active lesions. Infectious patients disseminate the organism when coughing, sneezing, or talking by expelling small infectious droplets that may remain suspended in air for several hours and inhaled by susceptible persons. After an incubation period of 4–12 weeks, infection usually remains subclinical and dormant without development of active disease. However, the organism may be activated at any time, resulting in acute severe pulmonary or other systemic disease. The risk of development of clinical disease following infection is higher in selected age groups (infancy, ages 16–21), in states of undernutrition, in certain immunopathologic states (eg, AIDS), in certain genetic groups (persons with HLA-Bw15 histocompatibility antigen), and in persons with some coexisting diseases (silicosis, diabetes).

Purified protein derivative (PPD) is a chemical fractionation product of tubercle bacilli culture filtrate. Intradermal injection of 5 tuberculin units of PPD in a patient with subclinical or clinical tuberculous infection results in a delayed hypersensitivity reaction manifested by 10 mm or more of induration at the site of injection within 48–72 hours (positive or "reactive" test). The PPD test may be negative in the presence of overwhelming tuberculosis, measles, Hodgkin's disease, sarcoidosis, or immunosuppressive states. The test will usually revert to negative following elimination of viable tubercle bacilli. (However, skin testing should not be performed on

Table 15–1. Occupational infections.

Disease	Agent	Target Organ	Occupational Source	Exposed Occupations	Preventive Measures
Bacteria					
Anthrax	*Bacillus anthracis*	Skin, lung, systemic	Dust (spores) on imported wool, goat hair, hides	Weavers; goat hair, wool, or hide handlers; butchers, veterinarians, agricultural workers	Immunization
Brucellosis	*Brucella abortus, B suis, B melitensis, B canis*	Systemic	Blood, urine, vaginal discharges, milk, secretions, and tissues from cattle, swine, sheep, and caribou	Packing and slaughterhouse employees, livestock producers, veterinarians, hunters	Personal hygiene; serologic identification of infected animals.
Erysipeloid	*Erysipelothrix rhusiopathiae (insidiosa)*	Skin	Fish, shellfish, meat, poultry	Fishermen, mean and poultry workers, veterinarians	Personal hygiene, gloves
Leptospirosis	*Leptospira interrogans*	Liver, kidney, brain, systemic	Urine or tissue of domestic or wild animals or rodent excreta; contaminated water.	Field agricultural workers, abattoir workers, farmers, sewer workers, veterinarians, miners, fishermen	Personal hygiene, boots, gloves; animal immunization; identification of contaminated water supplies; doxycycline prophylaxis.
Plague	*Yersinia pestis*	Lung, systemic	Fleas from infected rats, squirrels, prairie dogs	Hunters, trappers	Immunization
Tetanus	*Clostridium tetani*	Nervous system	Soil, skin puncture by unclean sharp object	Construction workers, gardeners, farmers	Immunization
Tuberculosis	*Mycobacterium tuberculosis*	Lung, systemic	Infected patient or nonhuman primate	Patient care workers, laboratory workers, primate handlers	PPD skin testing followed by prophylaxis for positive reactors
Tularemia	*Francisella tularensis*	Ulcerating papule, systemic	Blood, tissue, secretions, or bites of infected animals or arthropods	Hunters, forestry workers, farmers, veterinarians	Personal hygiene, gloves, immunization, insect control
Fungi					
Candidiasis	*Candida albicans*	Skin	Frequent skin trauma in a wet environment	Cannery workers, dishwashers, poultry processors	Skin protection, keeping dry
Coccidioidomycosis	*Coccidioides immitis*	Lung, meninges	Soil (spores) in arid zones	Farm workers, archeologists, excavation workers, construction workers	Dust control (where practical)
Dermatophytoses, ringworm, athlete's foot	*Microsporum, Trichophyton, Epidermophyton*	Skin	Animals, hot humid environments, farmers	Animal handlers, ranchers, athletes	Personal hygiene, keeping dry
Histoplasmosis	*Histoplasma capsulatum*	Lung, systemic	Soil contaminated with fowl droppings	Farmers, poultry producers, rural demolition workers	Dust control, environmental sanitation; formaldehyde spraying of contaminated surfaces.
Protozoa and helminths					
Echinococcosis	*Echinococcus granulosus, E multilocularis*	CNS, lung, liver	Feces of infected dog, fox, other canids	Ranchers, sheepherders, veterinarians	Personal hygiene

continued

Table 15–1 (cont'd). Occupational infections.

Disease	Agent	Target Organ	Occupational Source	Exposed Occupations	Preventive Measures
Hookworm	*Ancylostoma duodenale, Necator americanus*	Small intestine	Larvae in human feces that penetrate intact skin	Barefoot farmers, excavators, sewer workers, recreation workers	Sanitary disposal of human feces; use of shoes, boots, gloves.
Toxoplasmosis	*Toxoplasma gondii*	Reticuloendothelial system, eye	Cat feces	Laboratory workers, veterinarians, cat handlers	Personal hygiene
Rickettsiae and chlamydiae Ornithosis	*Chlamydia psittaci*	Lung, systemic	Discharges or excreta of infected domestic birds (parrots, pigeons, parakeets, etc)	Bird handlers, pet shop workers, zoo attendants, poultry workers	Identification and treatment of infected birds
Q fever	*Coxiella burnetii*	Systemic, liver, lung, brain	Placental tissue, birth fluids, or excreta from infected animals (cattle, sheep, goats, wild animals)	Laboratory workers, rendering plant and slaughterhouse workers, farmers, ranchers	Personal hygiene, immunization
Rocky Mountain spotted fever	*Rickettsia rickettsii*	Systemic, skin	Ticks from infected rodents, dogs	Ranchers, farmers, foresters, rangers, lumberjacks, hunters	Tick avoidance
Viruses Encephalitis (St. Louis, equine)	Arbovirus	CNS	Laboratory virus cultures, infected arthropods	Virus laboratory workers	Adherence to biologic safety practices, immunization, insecticides
Hepatitis B	Hepatitis B virus	Liver	Accidental inoculation with infected human blood and blood products	Oral surgeons, dentists, phlebotomists, dialysis workers, clinical laboratory workers, patient care workers	Personal hygiene, immunization
Newcastle disease	Paramyxovirus	Eyes	Poultry	Poultry handlers, veterinarians, animal laboratory workers	Personal hygiene
Rabies	Rabies virus	CNS	Wild animals (skunk, fox, bat, raccoon); rarely, domestic animals.	Laboratory workers, veterinarians, trappers, hunters; persons who handle wild or unidentified animals.	Immunization of human contacts and of certain animal species (dog, cat)
Rubella	Rubella virus	Fetus, systemic	Infected humans	Health care workers	Immunization
AIDS	HIV	Immune system	Body fluids of infected humans	Health care workers	Universal body substance precautions

individuals with a history of a positive test.) PPD tests are likely to be reactive for extended periods following BCG vaccination.

PPD skin testing is an accepted method for screening high-risk populations for primary infection. Persons having a reactive test are at risk of developing active clinical infection at any time (lifelong) following the primary infection owing to reactivation of the primary infection as long as viable tubercle bacilli remain in the body.

Diagnosis and treatment of clinically active disease follows established microbiologic and antibiotic protocols, with treatment variations depending on the antibiotic resistance of the specific strain.

Prevention & Control

PPD testing can identify persons whose tests are reactive, indicating primary infection. Serial testing (biennial or more frequently) can identify recently infected individuals whose tests have become reactive ("converters") within the past 2 years. Occupational candidates for periodic PPD testing include those having contact with suspected or known infected patients, tuberculosis laboratory workers, and persons working with potentially infected primates or cattle (veterinarians, zoo keepers, primate handlers).

Recent asymptomatic "converters" or others recently discovered to be tuberculin-reactive ("reactors")—whose date of conversion is unknown and who are least likely to develop complications due to antibiotic therapy—should receive drug treatment according to protocols recommended by the Centers for Disease Control.

Isoniazid prophylaxis is recommended for persons found to have a positive PPD who fall into any of the following categories: newly infected persons, including recent converters (within 2 years); household contacts of active cases; persons with an abnormal chest film consistent with clinical tuberculosis and inadequate past antituberculous therapy or prior active disease with inadequate past therapy; persons whose reactivation may have public health consequences (eg, schoolteachers); patients with AIDS (or persons with antibodies to HIV), silicosis, insulin-dependent diabetes mellitus, hematologic or reticuloendothelial cancer, prior gastrectomy, chronic undernutrition, ileal bypass, renal failure requiring dialysis, or a history of prolonged use of glucocorticoid or immunosuppressive therapy; and all reactors under age 35 with none of the above risk factors.

Before starting isoniazid prophylaxis, a chest x-ray should be taken on all skin test reactors. Any abnormalities found should be thoroughly evaluated for evidence of clinically active disease.

If adequate prior prophylaxis or therapy for active disease has been completed or if the patient has had previous adverse reactions to isoniazid or acute liver disease due to any cause, isoniazid prophylaxis should not be given. Patients at increased risk of chronic liver disease should be identified and closely monitored for isoniazid hepatic effects.

Preventive therapy for adults is with isoniazid, 300 mg orally in a single dose daily for at least 6 months. Following completion of therapy, if no adverse reactions to isoniazid have occurred, no further follow-up or x-rays are necessary. Prophylactic management of patients suspected of having isoniazid-resistant tubercle bacilli is controversial, but rifampin with or without isoniazid has been suggested (Table 15–2).

Persons for whom prophylactic antibiotic therapy is contraindicated should receive surveillance chest x-rays if they become symptomatic. Persons having known contact with an infectious patient for whom PPD status has not been previously documented should be PPD-tested immediately and then again 8–12 weeks after the infectious contact. If conversion occurs, physical examination and chest x-ray should occur to rule out acute clinical infection.

Attenuated tubercle bacilli—particularly BCG—have been used in many countries as a vaccine. Evidence indicates that increased resistance may occur following vaccination. In the United States, use of BCG is no longer recommended.

HEPATITIS B

Hepatitis B is the most frequent laboratory-associated infection, occurring 7 times more frequently among laboratory workers than in the general population. The virus can be transmitted in blood, semen, cerebrospinal fluid, saliva, and urine. Transmission usually occurs by exposure of mucous membranes or broken skin to infected blood or blood products.

The marker for viral infection is the surface antigen (HBsAg). HBsAg is present during clinical infection in most patients for approximately 4 weeks prior to

---

Table 15–2. Prevention of tuberculosis.[1]

Tuberculosis prophylaxis consists of daily administration of isoniazid, 300 mg, for at least 6 months.

Indications
1. Household members and other close associates of newly diagnosed patients.
2. Newly infected persons (PPD "converters").
3. Significant tuberculin skin test reactors with abnormal chest x-rays.
4. Significant tuberculin skin test reactors with special clinical situations (patients receiving corticosteroids; patients with diabetes, silicosis; postgastrectomy patients, etc).
5. Other significant tuberculin skin test reactors over age 35 only in special epidemiologic situations.

Contraindications
1. Progressive tuberculosis (more than one drug needed).
2. Adequate course of isoniazid previously completed.
3. Severe adverse reaction to isoniazid previously.
4. Previous isoniazid-associated hepatic injury.
5. Acute liver disease due to any cause.

Precautions
1. Concurrent use of other medications (possible drug interactions).
2. Daily use of alcohol (possible higher incidence of isoniazid-associated liver injury).
3. Current chronic liver disease (difficulty in evaluating changes in hepatic function).
4. Pregnancy (prudent to defer until postpartum unless contact, new infection, or other urgent indication).

[1]Adapted and reproduced, with permission, from Farer LS: *Tuberculosis: What the Physician Should Know.* American Lung Association/American Thoracic Society, 1982.

the appearance of clinical disease and for approximately 8–10 weeks following the onset of clinical hepatitis. Six to 10 percent of acutely infected adults will carry the virus beyond 12 weeks and are classified as chronic carriers, remaining infectious until the surface antigen disappears.

Persons at increased risk include workers at institutions for the mentally retarded, health care workers having frequent blood contact (eg, phlebotomists, laboratory workers, surgical and emergency personnel, blood gas technicians, blood bank personnel, nurses, dialysis and oncology unit nurses, pathologists, dentists), and other workers having frequent potential for percutaneous inoculation with infected blood or saliva such as mortuary staff. The virus may remain viable in dried blood or blood components for several days, making contaminated health care equipment potentially infectious if parenteral inoculation occurs.

The incubation period is from 50 to 180 days (average, 60–90 days). The disease has an insidious onset, usually with a gradual and prolonged rise in serum alanine aminotransferase (ALT; formerly SGPT). ALT values may range between 500 and 2000 IU/L and are usually higher than serum aspartate transaminase levels (AST; formerly SGOT). Aminotransaminases may remain elevated for up to 6 months or more after clinical illness disappears. Findings on history and physical examination are indistinguishable from those associated with other forms of hepatitis. Microbial, biliary, alcoholic, drug-induced, and toxic causes of hepatitis may present with identical findings and must be ruled out.

The relatively recent commercial availability of serologic testing for the surface (s), core (c), and "e" antigens and their associated antibodies allows prompt characterization of the stage and infectivity of hepatitis B. When this is combined with serologic testing for other types of hepatitis, it assists in definitive diagnosis of type B versus non-type B hepatitis. Table 15–3 illustrates that once the patient is negative for all antigens and antibodies except for antibodies to the surface and core antigens, the disease is no longer communicable and the patient is immune to further type B infection. It also demonstrates the potential value of serologic testing as part of surveillance for asymptomatic infection and subsequent immunity.

Treatment is as for any other form of hepatitis and is for the most part supportive. Alcohol and other hepatotoxins should be avoided during convalescence.

Prevention

Because exposure to patients, patients' body fluids, contaminated glassware, and other contaminated equipment such as needles may provide an opportunity for mucous membrane or parenteral inoculation, strict "infection control" procedures should be developed for risk situations such as phlebotomy, dentistry, and hemodialysis. Splash control, rigid containment of sharp instruments (eg, contaminated needles), and use of gloves are recommended whenever contact is likely with biologic fluids such as semen, saliva, or blood, as with surgery, including dental surgery. Hygienic and safety procedures should be clearly defined and rigidly enforced. Laboratory personnel handling such fluids should consider all human specimens potentially infected with type B virus and handle them accordingly.

Workers at increased risk for hepatitis B infection should receive hepatitis B vaccine, 1 mL intramuscularly, followed by 1 mL at 1 month and again at 6

Table 15–3. Representative serologic patterns in viral hepatitis.

Serologic Markers (+, present; −, absent)					
HBsAg	HBeAg	Anti-HBc	Anti-Hbe	Anti-Hbs	Interpretation
+	−	−	−	−	Incubation period or early hepatitis B: Infective.
+	+	+	−	−	Acute hepatitis B or chronic carrier: Infective.
+	−	+	+	−	Resolving acute hepatitis or chronic carrier: Low infectivity.
−	+	+	−	−	Acute hepatitis in "window" period or low-grade chronic carrier: Infective.
−	−	+	+	−	Convalescence from acute hepatitis: Low infectivity.
−	−	+	+	+	Recent recovery from acute hepatitis: Not infective; immune.
−	−	+	−	+	Post recovery from hepatitis: Not infective; immune.
−	−	−	−	+	Past subclinical infection or active-passive immunization: Not infective; immune.

[1]Reproduced, with permission, from Mandell HN: *Laboratory Medicine in Clinical Practice.* John Wright, 1983.

months. Some recommend screening of candidates for the vaccine by testing for surface antigen antibody or core antibody; if either is present, vaccination is unnecessary. The vaccine confers immunity in 90% of vaccinees, and for this reason some experts recommend serologic testing for surface antigen antibody following vaccine administration to verify an immunologic response. The vaccine is produced by recombinant DNA technology without using human cells or plasma (Recombivax HB).

For persons not vaccinated, hepatitis B immune globulin should be administered as postexposure prophylaxis immediately following inoculation with suspected contaminated fluids. The schedule and dosage of administration may vary depending upon whether or not vaccine is administered simultaneously following exposure for previously unvaccinated individuals (Table 15–4).

Exposure surveillance as a measure of hygiene and containment practices can identify asymptomatic previously infected individuals. The combination of testing for the surface antigen, the core antibody, and the surface antigen antibody should identify all such individuals. Almost all asymptomatic cases can also be identified by testing for the surface antigen antibody alone.

Because hepatitis B is also transmitted through sexual and other intimate social contact, questions often arise about how employees in non-health care industries who develop the disease through such contact should be treated in the workplace. Other than the means of transmission mentioned above, there is no evidence that a chronic surface antigen carrier or a person acutely ill with type B hepatitis will serve as a source of infection to coworkers in the absence of parenteral contact or intimate contact. Restrictions on contact with type B hepatitis-infected workers are therefore not appropriate in most work situations.

ACQUIRED IMMUNODEFICIENCY SYNDROME (AIDS)

There is great anxiety among workers concerning potential contact with AIDS patients in the workplace. Fortunately, the virus is not transmitted through casual nonintimate workplace contact or social encounters such as eating in restaurants or using public transportation or bathroom facilities. Other than infants delivered from AIDS-infected mothers, over 98% of all new cases are in persons who are serologically positive or have the known risk factors of male homosexuality, parenteral drug abuse, medical treatment with blood or blood products, or sexual contact with an AIDS-infected person.

Transmission

Human immunodeficiency virus (HIV) has been isolated from blood, semen, saliva, tears, urine, cerebrospinal fluid, solid tissue, and cervical secretions and is likely to be present in other bodily fluids, secretions, or tissues from infected humans. Potential routes of infection include percutaneous or parenteral inoculation and direct contact of cuts, scratches, abrasions, or mucosal surfaces with material containing live virus. Possible transmission may therefore occur through parenteral inoculation, through needle sticks, broken glass, or sharps contaminated with HIV, or through spillage of infected material onto abraded skin or mucous membranes. In studies of health care and research workers who have been exposed to AIDS patients, infected secretions, concentrated virus in culture, or blood products, less than 1% have developed AIDS infection as a result of contact of infected material or virus with intact, abraded, or punctured skin. Neither ingestion nor inhalation has been shown to be a mode of transmission. The concentration of virus is higher in blood, serum, cerebrospinal fluid, and semen and much

Table 15–4. Recommendations for hepatitis B prophylaxis following percutaneous exposure. (Source: *MMWR* 1985;**34**:330.)

Source	Unvaccinated	Vaccinated
HBsAg-positive	1. HBIG once stat.[1] 2. Initiate HB vaccine[2] series.	1. Test exposed person for anti-HBs. 2. If inadequate antibody,[3] HBIG once stat plus HB vaccine booster dose.
Known source High-risk, HBsAg-positive	1. Initiate HB vaccine series. 2. Test source for HBsAg. If positive, give HBIG once.	1. Test source for HBsAg only if exposed is vaccine nonresponder; if source is HBsAg-positive, give HBIG once stat plus HB vaccine booster dose.
Low-risk, HBsAg-positive	Initiate HB vaccine series.	Nothing required.
Unknown source	Initiate HB vaccine series.	Nothing required.

[1]HBIG dose 0.06 mL/kg IM.
[2]HB vaccine dose 1 mL IM for adults, 0.5 mL IM for infants or children under 10 years of age. First dose within 1 week; second and third doses 1 and 6 months later.
[3]Less than 10 SRU by RIA, negative by EIA.

lower in AIDS patients' saliva, tears, urine, breast milk, amniotic fluid, and vaginal secretions.

It follows that transmission is most likely to occur as the result of sexual contact with an infected partner, by parenteral exposure to infected blood or blood products, and by perinatal exposure of offspring of infected mothers. Casual contact, fomites (coffee cups, drinking fountains, telephone receivers, insects, etc) have not been shown to be mechanisms or circumstances of transmission.

Risk of Occupational Infection

The following groups are at potential risk of contact with HIV-infected body fluids: blood bank technologists, dialysis technicians, emergency room personnel, morticians, dentists, medical technicians, surgeons, laboratory workers, and prostitutes. At least 6 studies involving over 1900 health care workers have been published in which the presence of antibody to HIV or evidence of clinical AIDS infection was investigated in association with needle sticks, parenteral or splash exposures to known infected material, or laboratory work with concentrated virus in culture. These and other studies consistently show that the incidence of AIDS infection following such contact with material known to be infected with HIV is consistently less than 1% and usually less than 0.5%. AIDS infection of prostitutes is occurring at increasing rates and is clearly related to both sexual activity and parenteral drug abuse.

Because the AIDS virus has been found in saliva, there has been concern that CPR and first aid activities place those providers at increased risk for AIDS. To date, the risk appears to be quite low: No cases of HIV infection have been reported as a result of mouth-to-mouth CPR or the provision of first aid services. Nevertheless, many public safety organizations (police, fire fighters, paramedics) now routinely use special patient masks for providing mouth-to-mouth CPR.

In work situations other than those described above, AIDS has not been shown to be transmitted. Workers sharing the same work environment as a coworker infected with AIDS have not been found at risk in environments such as schools, offices, factories, and construction sites. AIDS has not been transmitted via food; a food service worker infected with HIV does not place restaurant customers at increased risk of HIV infection.

Personal service workers are defined as individuals whose occupations involve close personal contact with clients: hair dressers, barbers, cosmetologists, manicurists, massage parlor personnel, or persons who perform tattooing, ear piercing, or acupuncture. There is no evidence of transmission of AIDS between personal service workers and their clients, but sensible precautions in disinfection of instruments should of course be observed.

Legal & Social Issues

Major AIDS-related issues for many workers involve fear of contagion, AIDS testing, confidentiality, civil rights, and insurance benefits.

Fear and panic among workers resulting from misinformation concerning HIV transmission can be a disruptive force in a work environment when it becomes known that a fellow worker is an AIDS victim. Other than in the few "personal service" occupations mentioned above, AIDS does not present a risk of transmission in the normal course of employment. Many people do not understand this and do not want to be near an AIDS victim. The employer, on the other hand, cannot banish the AIDS patient from the workplace in these situations, since there is no public health risk to other employees—the only basis for employment restriction would be physical or mental incapacity to perform the requirements of the job.

Coworkers who refuse to work with the AIDS victim may continue to do so until they have been educated concerning the disease and its transmission. Educational material is available from CDC and commercial sources that will provide information for employees so that the employer can then require employees, once educated, to continue their work alongside the AIDS-infected coworker.

Some employers have considered AIDS testing for prospective employees. There is no medical justification for such testing, since AIDS transmission does not occur in work activities other than those mentioned above. In some states (California is an example), statutes prohibit preemployment AIDS testing and impose restrictions on release of information concerning the diagnosis of AIDS.

As with other diseases, the employer is also bound to honor the confidentiality and privacy rights of its employees. Because there is no public health risk to coworkers in most employment situations, the employer has no obligation to release information regarding a diagnosis of AIDS in a given worker. The employer may do so only with the worker's written consent and even then would be well advised to withhold such information, since it serves no purpose and is likely to result in unnecessary disruption.

AIDS has been designated in some courts as a protected handicap, meaning that the employer cannot refuse to hire an AIDS-infected patient simply because he or she has AIDS. In order to justify denial of employment, the AIDS victim must be so debilitated as to be unable to perform the physical or mental requirements of the job.

In some states, health or life insurance contracts may be adversely affected by AIDS. Insurance carriers, employers, and subscribers should continue to evaluate their attitudes and practices.

Prevention

For occupational health professionals, employer-sponsored first aid workers, and public safety personnel who may provide medical services to HIV-infected individuals, reasonable steps should be taken to avoid skin, parenteral, or mucous membrane contact with potentially infected blood, plasma, or secretions. Hands or skin should be washed immediately and carefully if blood contact occurs. Mucous membranes—including the eyes and mouth—should be protected by eye glasses or masks during procedures that could generate splashes or aerosols of infected blood or secretions (suctioning, endoscopy). Contaminated surfaces should be disinfected using 5% sodium hypochlorite.

Personal service workers who work with needles or other instruments that can penetrate intact skin should follow precautions indicated for health care workers and practice aseptic technique and sterilization of instruments. All personal service workers should be educated concerning transmission of blood-borne infections, including AIDS and hepatitis B.

If a health care or other worker experiences parenteral or mucous membrane exposure to blood or other potentially infected bodily fluids, the likelihood of HIV infection should be determined for the source patient. If possible, the source patient should undergo serologic testing for HIV infection. If the source patient has serologic or other evidence of HIV infection or refuses to submit to testing, the exposed worker should be evaluated clinically and serologically for HIV infection as soon as possible after the event. If the result is negative, the worker should be retested 3–6 months later. If the source patient is seronegative, has no AIDS risk factors, and has no other evidence of HIV infection, the risk of infection is less than 0.01%; additional follow-up can be considered.

Pregnant health care workers should be educated regarding the possibility of transmission of HIV to newborns. Because of the increased risk of cytomegalovirus infection among AIDS patients, care of AIDS patients by pregnant women may be contraindicated.

Additional recommendations concerning general workplace exposures—including those of health care workers, precautions during invasive procedures, and precautions for laboratory workers—are updated periodically in *Morbidity and Mortality Weekly Reports*.

TRAVEL-ASSOCIATED INFECTIOUS DISEASES

International travel is a necessary part of work for many thousands of workers. It often involves travel to distant and sometimes rural locales having endemic pathogens never established or long since eradicated at the traveler's point of origin. From a workers' compensation standpoint, any illness or injury that occurs as a result of work that would not have occurred at that time due to nonoccupational activities is usually considered work-related. A manufacturing employee who develops an upper respiratory infection during the work week would have difficulty in proving that the infection was transmit-

ted from coworkers rather than from family members or casual social contacts. But salmonellosis or malaria developing following travel to an area where these disorders are endemic is clearly attributable to work-related presence in the endemic area.

Travel-related infection therefore could include the whole range of human pathogens, depending upon the agents endemic to the area being visited and opportunities by the traveler for exposure. Water purification, waste sanitation, food preparation, vector control, recreational activities during travel, and personal hygiene of the traveler influence exposure potential.

Commonly encountered travel-related diseases include traveler's diarrhea (from infection with *Salmonella, Shigella, Giardia, Entamoeba histolytica,* pathogenic *Escherichia coli,* and selected viral agents), hepatitis A, yellow fever, typhoid fever, cholera, and malaria. Other diseases that have been virtually eliminated from countries with effective childhood vaccination programs—the prime example is poliomyelitis—may be endemic in underdeveloped areas, placing the nonimmunized person at particular risk for these diseases.

Prevention

The health authorities should be consulted to determine what vaccinations are recommended or required and what diseases are endemic in areas to be visited. Standard immunizations recommended by the Immunization Practice Advisory Committee (ACIP) for persons living in the United States should be up to date (diphtheria, tetanus, measles, mumps, rubella, and poliomyelitis). Effective vaccines are available for cholera, yellow fever, typhoid fever, rabies, plague, and meningococcal meningitis. Prophylactic immunoglobulin (gamma globulin) for hepatitis A is recommended for persons visiting developing and tropical countries.

Malarial prophylaxis is strongly recommended for visits to endemic areas, particularly rural areas in tropical developing countries all over the world. Prophylaxis of chloroquine-sensitive strains of all species consists of taking 500 mg of chloroquine phosphate orally once weekly beginning 1–2 weeks before arrival and continuing for every week during travel and for 4 weeks after leaving a malaria-endemic area. In certain areas of eastern and central Africa, chloroquine-resistant strains of *Plasmodium falciparum* are prevalent. For travel to these areas, doxycycline or mefloquine (pending FDA approval) should be considered, depending upon the patient's personal medical history, drug sensitivity, length of stay, and other factors in accordance with the CDC recommendations.

As an alternative, pyrimethamine-sulfadoxine (Fansidar) can be administered, but only if febrile illness occurs when professional medical care is unavailable. The Malaria Prevention Information System (404-639-1610) can provide updated guidelines for treatment and prophylaxis.

For prophylaxis of traveler's diarrhea caused by enterotoxigenic *E coli* or viral agents such as rotaviruses, 2 regimens have been recommended. One involves administration of two 262-mg tablets of bismuth subsalicylate (Pepto-Bismol) 3 times daily. Doxycycline, 100 mg/d orally, has been used as an alternative but is contraindicated in pregnancy and for children younger than age 8 and may allow colonization by resistant salmonellae or shigellae. As an alternative, 160 mg of trimethoprim plus 800 mg of sulfamethoxazole can be taken for 3–5 days if diarrhea occurs.

Other general protective measures include insect repellents where insect vectors may transmit disease (malaria, yellow fever, dengue, filariasis, leishmaniasis, trypanosomiasis, and hemorrhagic fevers). Use of light-colored and protective clothing, mosquito netting, and avoidance of scented cosmetics may be helpful. The traveler should take care not to eat or drink contaminated food or water and should avoid uncooked foods. Swimming in contaminated waters and walking with inadequately protected feet should be avoided where possible.

Jong and Southworth have recommended items for inclusion in a traveler's personal medical kit that should be tailored to the particular destination and its endemic risks (Table 15–5).

INFECTIONS TRANSMITTED FROM ANIMALS TO HUMANS: ZOONOSES

Zoonoses are defined as diseases that infect both humans and animals. Occupations involving contact with infected animals, their infected secretions or tissues, or contact with arthropod vectors from infected animals can result in work-related zoonotic disease. Such occupations include animal laboratory workers, veterinarians, farmers, breeders, dairy workers, hunters, wildlife workers, hide and wool handlers, slaughterhouse (abattoir) workers, ranchers, rendering plant workers, pet shop workers, taxidermists, zoo attendants, agricultural workers, sewer workers, miners, military personnel, and butchers. Although these diseases are relatively rare, some of the more common occupational zoonoses in the United States include tularemia, Rocky Mountain spotted fever, brucellosis, leptospirosis, plague, psittacosis, and rabies. Brucellosis is discussed below as an example of one of the more common occupational zoonotic infections in the United States.

BRUCELLOSIS

Brucellosis in humans (undulant fever, Malta fever) is caused by several gram-negative bacteria of the genus Brucella. The species varies with the animal host, as follows: *Brucella melitensis*, goats and sheep; *Brucella suis*, swine; *Brucella abortus*, cattle; and *Brucella canis*, dogs. Over 100 reported cases of brucellosis occurred in 1985 in the United States, approximately half transmitted by occupational exposure.

Most cases occur in abattoir workers and the remainder in veterinarians, livestock industry workers, and laboratory workers. The disease is more common in animals from rural underdeveloped countries. Brucellosis is the most commonly reported laboratory-associated bacterial infection.

Pathogenesis & Clinical Findings

Occupational brucellosis occurs as a result of

Table 15–5. Traveler's personal medical kit (nonprescription items).[1]

Acetaminophen (Tylenol) or aspirin tablets: for general relief of minor aches and pains or headache.
Antibiotic ointment (bacitracin or Neosporin): topical antibiotic for minor cuts and abrasions.
Bismuth subsalicylate (Pepto-Bismol), 6 tablets per day for symptomatic treatment and for prevention of traveler's diarrhea.
Decongestant and antihistamine capsules: for nasal congestion and allergic rhinitis.
Glucose and electrolyte powdered mix (Hydra-Lyte or similar product): to be mixed in safe water for fluid replacement and rehydration during severe diarrhea.
Hydrocortisone acetate cream 0.5%: for relief of itching due to insect bites.
Insect repellent liquid (Cutter's or Jungle Juice): for topical application.
Insect repellent spray (Off): for use in unscreened rooms and other areas.
Para-aminobenzoic acid sunscreen lotion (eg, PreSun 8): for protection against sunburn.
Povidone-iodine liquid (Betadine, Isodyne): for cleansing of minor cuts and abrasions.
Water purification straw (Pocket Purifier): for purification of unsanitary water. Iodide-based; will produce purified water without the waiting period needed for water purification tablets to work; for individual use.
Water purification tablets (Potable Aqua or Coughlan's): iodine-based tablets will kill microorganisms that chlorine-based tablets will not.
Bandages: Band-Aids, 2 × 2 sterile gauze pads, roll of surgical tape.
Case or box, metal or plastic: the smallest size that will accommodate contents of the medical kit.
Dust mask for use in desert areas.
Moleskin blister protection for poorly fitting shoes.
Oral thermometer.
Safety pins.
Scissors or sterile razor blade, penknife, Swiss army knife.

[1]From Jong EC, Southworth M: Recommendations for patients traveling. *West J Med* 1983;**138**:746.

mucous membrane or skin contact with infected animal tissues. Aborted placental and fetal membrane tissues from cattle, swine, sheep, and goats are well-documented sources of human exposure. The incubation period is from 1 to 6 weeks. The onset is insidious, with fever, sweats, malaise, aches, and weakness. The fever has a characteristic pattern, often rising in the afternoon and falling during the night ("undulant fever"). The infection is systemic and may result in gastric, intestinal, neurologic, hepatic, or musculoskeletal involvement. There is usually an initial septicemic phase, following which a more chronic stage may develop characterized by low-grade fever, malaise, and in some cases psychoneurotic symptoms.

Diagnosis & Treatment

Diagnosis is aided by both culture and serologic techniques. Treatment will vary with organism sensitivity, but brucellae are often sensitive to tetracyclines or ampicillin. More resistant species may require combined therapy with streptomycin and trimethoprim-sulfamethoxazole. Prolonged treatment is often necessary.

Prevention

Identification and treatment or slaughter of infected animals combined with effective immunization of susceptible animals can eliminate disease in livestock populations. Diagnosis is by serologic testing. Personal hygiene and protective precautions should be observed in handling potentially infected animal tissues or secretions, particularly those resulting from abortion.

Immunization of humans is still experimental.

OCCUPATIONAL IMMUNIZATION, PROPHYLAXIS, & BIOLOGIC SURVEILLANCE

Recommended occupational immunizations are listed in Table 15–6. In addition, laboratory workers at risk of contact with live organisms or travelers to endemic areas should be considered for appropriate immunization, prophylaxis, or surveillance if the technology is available. Preparations are available for protection against diphtheria, tetanus, measles, mumps, rubella, smallpox, yellow fever, poliomyelitis, hepatitis B, influenza, rabies, cholera, pneumococcal pneumonia, meningococcal disease (certain serotypes), plague, typhoid fever, tuberculosis, Q fever, adenovirus infection, anthrax, pertussis, and *Haemophilus influenzae* infection. Gamma globulin has been recommended for prophylaxis of hepatitis A in travelers and the staffs of day care centers and custodial institutions where hepatitis A is endemic.

Skin testing can be useful in surveillance of tuberculosis and some mycoses (coccidioidomycosis, histoplasmosis, blastomycosis). Skin tests may also

Table 15–6. Occupational preexposure immunization and prophylaxis for susceptible (unvaccinated) adults.

	Immunization or Prophylaxis	Source or Clue to Exposure
Rubella	Vaccine, 0.5 mL SC	Indicated for those in contact with pregnant or infected patients.
Hepatitis A	Immune globulin, 0.02 mL/kg IM	Travel to endemic area
Hepatitis B	Vaccine, 1 mL IM at 0, 1, and 6 months	Frequent blood contact
Measles	Vaccine, 0.5 mL SC	Contact with infected patients
Poliomyelitis	Vaccine (Sabin), 0.5 mL at 0 and 2 months and again at 8–14 months	Contact with infected patients or laboratory culture
Smallpox	Contact CDC for vaccine and directions.	Laboratory culture
Plague	Vaccine, 1 mL at 0 month, 0.2 mL at 1 and 6 months	Laboratory culture, infected animals
Rabies	Vaccine and prophylaxis; dosage varies with vaccine type	Laboratory culture, infected animals
Tetanus	Toxoid, 0.5 mL. Give 1 dose stat and at 6–8 weeks, 1 year, and every 10 years.	Infected patients; contaminated (dirty) objects and materials.
Influenza	Vaccine (dose varies with vaccine type). If vaccine unavailable, give amantadine, 100 mg orally twice daily.	Infected patients.

detect prior infection with herpes simplex, mumps, and vaccinia.

Serologic testing for evidence of subclinical infection in selected high-risk populations should be carefully considered but may be of value for the following diseases: brucellosis, chlamydial infections, leptospirosis, plague, tularemia, salmonellosis, toxoplasmosis, some parasitic diseases (amebiasis, trichinosis), most occupational viral diseases (hepatitis A and B, herpes simplex, influenza, rabies, infectious mononucleosis), mycoplasmal pneumonia, and some rickettsioses.

As with the administration of any surveillance test or therapeutic agent, disease prevalence, occupational exposure risk, contraindications, and side effects from the prophylactic agent should all be considered before administration of any immunologic agent or use of any biologic surveillance test.

Guidelines for investigation and control of a communicable disease or common source outbreak are presented in Table 15–7.

Exposure Evaluation

Investigation of human or animal sources of infectious agents can use serologic or other clinical microbiologic techniques. Environmental exposure evaluation associated with inanimate sources such as contaminated ventilation systems or centrifuges is more esoteric. However, technologies exist for collection and measurement of airborne bacteria and viruses. A knowledgeable industrial hygienist can select the appropriate instrumentation and sampling strategy based on the presumed biologic characteristics of the organism, air velocity, sampler efficiency, anticipated concentration, "particle" size, sampler physical requirements, and the study objective.

Table 15–7. Approach to suspected communicable disease outbreak.[1]

I. Verify reported case:
   A. Review type and result of laboratory confirmation (serology, culture, etc).
   B. Review clinical presentation with patient or treating physician.
   C. If diagnosis unclear, perform laboratory determination based on clinical impression.
   D. Report suspected outbreak to public health authorities.
   E. Treat and isolate source case or material in accordance with clinical and public health guidelines.

II. If the diagnosis or etiology remains unclear, collect, analyze, and summarize:
   A. Available laboratory data.
   B. Symptoms and signs from each suspected case.
   C. Stool, blood, urine, or other appropriate fluid or tissue for further laboratory evaluation as suggested by the clinical findings.
   D. Samples for microbiologic analysis of nonhuman materials (food, animals, waste, etc) that may be sources.
   E. Epidemiologic and exposure data from a similar but clinically unaffected (control) group. Compare the case and control group for differences in rates of exposure to the various suspected microbially contaminated sources.

III. Identify susceptibles with potential exposure to source case or substance:
   A. Review usual host, period of communicability, and mode of transmission and period of communicability. (See Benenson reference.)
   B. Interview source case, family, or custodian of source material (eg, cook, farmer) to determine range of activity, travel, social interaction, or vector association during communicable period.
   C. Identify all susceptible persons or animals within source case or material's range of activity during communicable period who could have had sufficient contact with infectious case, material, or vector for disease transmission. Public agency assistance may be necessary.

IV. Identify secondary cases:
   A. Evaluate individuals identified in III, above, for evidence of infection and communicability.
   B. Continue steps III and IV.A until perimeter of outbreak is defined.

V. Institute control measures: Follow recommended actions appropriate to the suspected causal agent (see Benenson reference) for concurrent disinfection, isolation, investigation, or immunization of contacts, quarantine, hygiene, treatment, and work practices.

VI. Prevention: Institute appropriate preventive measures (eg, immunization, work practices, serologic, and other biologic surveillance).

[1]Adapted from Benenson AS (editor): *Control of Communicable Diseases in Man.* American Public Health Association, Washington, DC (updated periodically); and from Last JM (editor): *Maxcy-Rosenau's Preventive Medicine and Public Health,* 12th ed. Appleton-Century-Crofts, 1986.

REFERENCES

General

Adult immunization: Recommendations of the Immunization Practices Advisory Committee (ACIP). *MMWR* (Sept 28) 1984;**33(Suppl):**1.

Benenson AS (editor): *Communicable Diseases in Man.*

American Public Health Association, 1985.

Centers for Disease Control: *Guidelines for Isolation Precautions in Hospitals.* Department of Health and Human Services, Public Health Service, 1983.

Centers for Disease Control: *Health Information for*

International Travel. MMWR Supplement, published annually.

Centers for Disease Control: *Morbidity and Mortality Weekly Report.* Available through the Massachusetts Medical Society, CSPO Box 9120, Waltham, MA 02254-9120.

Centers for Disease Control/National Institute of Health: *Biosafety in Microbiological and Biomedical Laboratories.* US Government Printing Office, 1984.

Jawetz E et al: *Review of Medical Microbiology,* 18th ed. Appleton & Lange, 1989.

Last JM (editor): *Maxcey-Rosenau Public Health & Preventive Medicine,* 12th ed. Appleton-Century-Crofts, 1986.

The Medical Letter on Drugs and Therapeutics. Published bimonthly. The Medical Letter, Inc.

Patterson WB et al: Occupational hazards to hospital personnel. *Ann Intern Med* 1985;**102:**658.

World Health Organization: *Vaccination Certificate Requirements for International Travel.* Published annually.

World Health Organization: *Weekly Epidemiologic Record.*

Tuberculosis

American Thoracic Society: The tuberculin skin test. *Am Rev Respir Dis* 1981;**124:**356.

American Thoracic Society/Centers for Disease Control: Treatment of tuberculosis and tuberculosis infection in adults and children. *Am Rev Respir Dis* 1986;**134:**355.

Farer LS: *Tuberculosis: What the Physician Should Know.* American Lung Association/American Thoracic Society, 1982.

Hepatitis B

Collins CH: *Laboratory-Acquired Infections.* Butterworths, 1983. Mandell HN (editor): *Laboratory Medicine in Clinical Practice.* PSG Publishing Co., 1983.

Recommendations of the Immunization Practices Committee: Update on hepatitis B prevention. *MMWR* 1987; **36:**353.

Recommendations for protection against viral hepatitis. (2 parts.) *MMWR* 1985;**34:**313, 329.

AIDS

1988 Agent summary statement for human immunodeficiency virus and report on laboratory-acquired infection with human immunodeficiency virus. *MMWR* (April 1) 1988;**37(Suppl S-4):**1.

AIDS: Information on AIDS for the Practicing Physician. American Medical Association, 1987.

McCray E: Occupational risk of the acquired immunodeficiency syndrome among health care workers: Special report of the Cooperative Needlestick Surveillance Group. *N Engl J Med* 1986;**314:**1127.

Mills M, Wofsy CB, Mills J: The acquired immunodeficiency syndrome: Infection control and public health law. *N Engl J Med* 1986;**314:**931.

Recommendations for prevention of HIV transmission in health-care settings. *MMWR* (Aug 21) 1987;**36(Suppl 2S):**1.

Revision of the CDC surveillance case definition for acquired immunodeficiency syndrome. *MMWR* (Aug 14) 1987;**36(Suppl 1S):**1.

Update: Universal precautions for prevention of transmission of human immunodeficiency virus, hepatitis B virus, and other bloodborne pathogens in health care settings. *MMWR* 1988;**37:**377.

AIDS Hot Lines

Centers for Disease Control: 1-800-342-AIDS.
Public Health Service: 1-800-447-AIDS.

Travel-Related Infections

Jong EC, Southworth M: Recommendations for patients traveling. *West J Med* 1983;**138:**746.

Recommendations for the prevention of malaria in travelers. *MMWR* 1988;**37:**277.

Brucellosis

Buchanan TM, Faber LC, Feldman RA: Brucellosis in the United States 1960–1972: An abattoir-associated disease. 1. Clinical features and therapy. *Medicine* 1974; **53:**403.

Wise RI: Brucellosis in the United States: Past, present, and future. *JAMA* 1980;**244:**2318.

Immunization & Prophylaxis; Biologic Surveillance

Adult immunization: Recommendations of the Immunization Practices Advisory Committee (ACIP). *MMWR* (Sept 28) 1984;**33(Suppl):**1.Marmion BP et al: Vaccine prophylaxis of abattoir-associated Q fever. *Lancet* 1984;**2:**1411.

Exposure Evaluation

Chatigny MA: Sampling airborne microorganisms. Section E, pp E1–E10, in: *Air Sampling Instruments for Evaluation of Atmospheric Contaminants,* 5th ed. American Conference of Governmental Industrial Hygienists, 1978.

Gregory PH, Monteith JL (editors): *Airborne Microbes.* Cambridge Univ Press, 1967.

16

Occupational Cancer

Michael L. Fischman, MD, MPH, Edwin C. Cadman, MD, & Susan Desmond, MD

It is estimated that 30–40% of the population in the industrialized world will develop malignant disease during their lifetimes. Recently, various authors have attributed 70–80% of cases of cancer in humans to environmental causes.

CARCINOGENESIS: FUNDAMENTAL PROPERTIES

Evidence suggests that cancers arise from a single abnormal cell. After progressing through a number of stages, this cell may replicate itself through repeated divisions to form a large clone of tumor cells. The initial stage in development of the abnormal cell appears to result from an alteration or mutation in the genetic material, DNA. This alteration may occur spontaneously or may be caused by exogenous factors, such as exposure to carcinogenic chemicals or radiation. Whether a tumor ever develops from this altered cell may depend on a variety of factors, such as the ability of the cell to repair the damage, the presence of other endogenous or exogenous agents that foster or inhibit tumor development, and the effectiveness of the immune system.

Induction-Latency Period

Both experimental animal models of cancer and the study of human cancers with known causes have revealed the existence of a significant interval between first exposure to the responsible agent and the first manifestation of the tumor. This interval is variously referred to as the induction period, the latency period, or the induction-latency period.

For humans, the length of the induction-latency period varies from a minimum of 4–6 years for radiation-induced leukemias to perhaps 40 or more years for some cases of asbestos-induced mesotheliomas. For most tumors, however, the interval is about 12–25 years. Obviously, this long period of time may obscure the relationship between a remote exposure and a newly found tumor.

Stages in Tumor Development

Animal studies suggest that tumor development involves at least 2 distinct stages: initiation and promotion. The classic example of this phenomenon is the mouse skin tumor model. A small dose of a carcinogen, known as the initiator—typically a polycyclic aromatic hydrocarbon—is applied to the skin.

Though large doses of such substances alone can readily induce skin tumors, observation of the animals has revealed that the smaller dose alone does not result in skin tumors. However, subsequent application of certain substances, known as promoters—eg, croton oil—results in tumor development following a low dose of the aromatic hydrocarbon.

Application of the promoter alone or prior to administration of the initiator does not result in skin tumors. Similar stages have been demonstrated in the development of tumors in other organs, such as mouse liver and lung and rat trachea. For example, ingestion of a small quantity of various nitrosamines (initiators) followed by regular ingestion of polychlorinated biphenyls (promoters) results in production of liver tumors in mice.

Initiation is thought to result from an irreversible change in the genetic material (DNA) of the cell, arising from interaction with a carcinogen that is a necessary but not sufficient condition for tumor development. The mechanism by which a carcinogen-induced alteration in DNA could lead ultimately to tumor development was obscure until evidence supporting the oncogene theory was adduced. The oncogene theory states that a preexisting cellular DNA sequence, known as the proto-oncogene, is inappropriately activated during oncogenesis, conferring a malignant transforming potential on the gene and the cell containing it. It appears that there are a number of proto-oncogenes in normal human and animal cells that are responsible for normal cellular differentiation and maturation.

Though there are a number of mechanisms by which the proto-oncogene may be activated, the pathway of concern with chemical carcinogenesis involves a chemical-induced point mutation in the proto-oncogene. For example, point mutations in ras genes (so called because they were originally identified in rat sarcomas) have been observed at codons 12, 13, and 61 in human and rodent tumors. In animals, a variety of chemical initiators with mutagenic properties have been shown to activate ras and other proto-oncogenes.

Like other genes, the *ras* gene codes for a protein product, a 21,000-MW protein known as p21. It is felt that this protein product from the activated oncogene, differing by only one amino acid from the normal protein, is the direct cell-transforming agent, conferring malignant potential to the cell. It is of note that this and other abnormal proteins coded for by oncogenes can be identified in the serum and urine. It is possible that these proteins may be useful as preclinical response indicators in premalignant and early malignant lesions in occupationally exposed cohorts.

On the other hand, promotion consists of those processes subsequent to initiation that facilitate tumor development in the altered cell. The mechanisms of promotion, sometimes referred to as epigenetic as opposed to the genotoxic effects of initiators, are incompletely understood. Promotion does not result from binding to and alteration of DNA. In the case of the mouse skin tumor model, croton oil appears to interact with membrane receptors to affect cellular growth and differentiation.

Carcinogens, then, may be divided into initiating agents, known as initiators, or "early stage" carcinogens; and promoting agents, known as promoters, or "late stage" carcinogens.

The distinguishing features of initiating and promoting agents are listed in Table 16–1. Some agents (eg, cigarette smoke) that seem to possess both initiating and promoting properties are termed "complete carcinogens."

For most toxic effects, the persistence or progression of damage requires the continued presence of the offending chemical agent. For cancer initiators, however, a single exposure may induce genetic damage in the cell sufficient to result in tumor development years after exposure has ceased.

The Question of Thresholds

With most toxic effects, there are doses or exposures below which no adverse effects occur. If this threshold dose is not exceeded, there are no consequences to the health of the animal or human. With carcinogens, it is much more difficult to determine if such a threshold exists. If no threshold exists, there is no dose—other than zero—at which the risk of cancer is nil.

There is controversy about the existence of threshold doses for carcinogenic agents. An understanding of the arguments on both sides is useful, particularly in the area of policy development.

Given that a single alteration (mutation) in DNA in one cell may set the stage for tumor development, it is at least theoretically possible that exposure of the cell to only one molecule of a carcinogen will ultimately lead to tumor formation. Though the probability of tumor formation may increase with increasing frequency and magnitude of exposure to the carcinogen, a single small exposure may be sufficient. For example, in the mouse skin tumor model described above, a single exposure to a polycyclic aromatic hydrocarbon is capable of inducing a tumor.

On the other hand, a number of arguments have been advanced against the concept that there are no thresholds for carcinogens. Even if one acknowledges that a single molecule may induce a tumorigenic change in a cell, the likelihood that the molecule will reach its target cell is lowered with small doses. The agent may react with other cellular nucleophiles, such as proteins or noncritical segments of DNA. If the carcinogen is subject to rapid metabolic deactivation, as in a "first-pass" effect in the liver after ingestion, the ability of a small dose to contact the sensitive cell is reduced. DNA repair mechanisms—eg, excision of altered DNA nucleotides—may allow repair of an induced mutation before a clone of tumor cells results. There is some evidence both in humans and in animals that immunologic mechanisms may be capable of destroying transformed cells before a tumor develops. Finally, cancer induction by a number of agents appears to require a preceding pathologic effect on the tissue, eg, cellular hyperplasia or necrosis. For example, alcohol and probably some chlorinated hydrocarbon solvents, if administered in high doses, will initially induce liver damage and cirrhosis, following which a higher risk of liver tumor development exists. Since there is a threshold for the initial toxic effects below

Table 16–1. Distinctions between initiators and promoters of carcinogenesis.

Initiators	Promoters
Genotoxic.	Not genotoxic; epigenetic mechanism.
Carcinogenic alone.	Not carcinogenic alone; active only after initiator exposure.
Generally yield electrophilic compounds; highly reactive (often form free radicals).	Not electrophilic.
Covalently bind to nucleophiles (eg, DNA), leading to irreversible alteration in genetic material.	Generally do not bind to nor alter DNA; often act by induction of cellular proliferation; effects may be reversible.
Generally active in short-term tests (mutagenic).	Not active in short-term tests.
Existence of threshold dose cannot be verified.	Threshold probably exists.
Single exposure may be sufficient to induce subsequent cancer.	Repeated exposures required.

which no damage occurs, there is also a threshold for the secondary tumor formation. If any of these phenomena pertain for a given carcinogen, there will be a threshold dose below which no carcinogenic effect will occur.

Unfortunately, these arguments are not generally susceptible to experimental verification for individual carcinogens, because of limitations in the methodology and analysis of human and animal studies.

Dose-Response Relationships

Although thresholds may or may not exist, there is strong evidence for a dose-response effect for most carcinogens that have been adequately studied. In other words, larger doses result in a higher incidence and mortality rate of tumors in an exposed population than do smaller doses. Both animal experimental studies and human epidemiologic reports support this concept.

Such studies have revealed very large differences—10 million-fold or more—in the relative potency of carcinogens. For example, in animal studies, a daily dose of less than 1 μg/d of aflatoxin induced tumors in 50% of exposed animals, while an equipotent dose of trichloroethylene was greater than 1 g/d.

Although dose-response curves for some carcinogens are known, data points represent relatively high doses. We would like to know the behavior of such curves in the range of typical human exposures. We cannot predict the shape of the curve at low doses

from the high-dose data—for example, at low doses, is the curve linear, concave, or convex, or is there a threshold? Some possible models for low-dose extrapolation are illustrated in Fig 16–1.

INVESTIGATIVE METHODS IN THE ASSESSMENT OF CHEMICAL CARCINOGENICITY

Evidence to support the carcinogenicity of a chemical for humans may be derived from 4 types of studies: human epidemiologic studies, experimental studies in animals, a variety of short-term tests, and analysis of structural similarities to known carcinogens.

Epidemiologic studies potentially provide the strongest evidence for human carcinogenicity, precisely because they are conducted on human subjects. However, such studies are subject to a number of limitations that reduce their ability to detect and confirm carcinogenic effects.

Well-conducted animal bioassays can provide strong support for carcinogenicity in the animal species tested. However, the implications for humans are less clear than with epidemiologic studies.

The role of short-term assays—eg, for bacterial mutation—is not fully defined because the signifi-

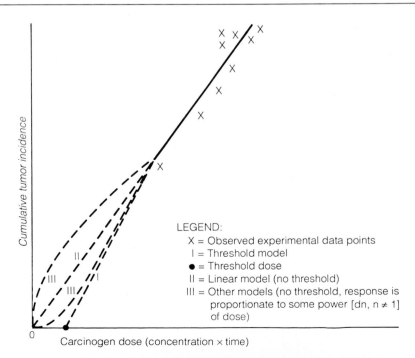

LEGEND:
X = Observed experimental data points
I = Threshold model
● = Threshold dose
II = Linear model (no threshold)
III = Other models (no threshold, response is proportionate to some power [dn, n ≠ 1] of dose)

Figure 16–1. Carcinogenesis: Possible dose-response models.

cance for human risk of positive results is unknown. Currently, at least, further study of the chemical in animal bioassays would be warranted.

Structural similarity of a chemical to known carcinogens may also suggest the need for further study in short-term or animal tests. Though the presence of such similarity has, in fact, predicted the carcinogenicity of previously untested compounds, the overall utility of structural analysis has not been established.

EPIDEMIOLOGIC STUDIES

Epidemiologic studies have the potential for providing the strongest evidence for human carcinogenicity, because the subjects studied are human. Though case reports and descriptive epidemiologic studies may provide suggestive evidence for human carcinogenicity, evidence for causality of an association can only be derived from analytic epidemiologic studies—in other words, cohort or case-control studies. The nature and design of such studies are discussed in the Appendix. When they are well-documented and yield positive results, they provide strong evidence in support of carcinogenicity.

A number of criteria have been posed to help decide whether a positive association in epidemiologic studies indicates causality. The most important are strength, consistency, biologic gradient, biologic plausibility, and temporality:

(1) The **strength** of an association is the magnitude of the relative risk in the exposed group compared to that of the control group. Strong associations are more likely to be causal because it is less likely that biases—eg, the confounding effects of smoking—would account for the association without being very obvious.

(2) **Consistency** of an association is the extent to which it is reported from multiple studies conducted under different circumstances.

(3) The **biologic gradient** of an association is its dose-response validity, ie, the observation that higher doses result in a higher frequency of adverse effects.

(4) The **biologic plausibility** of a study is based on the assessment that it makes sense in light of what is known about the mechanism of production of the adverse effect.

(5) A study's **temporality** rests on the conclusion or observation that the cause (ie, exposure) preceded the effect in time.

Despite the utility of these criteria in making assessments of causality, only one of them, temporality, is absolutely required. A weak association not consistently reported that does not exhibit a dose-response effect and does not (as yet) fully make sense may nevertheless be causal. Furthermore, fulfillment of some of the criteria may occur when in fact the association is due to chance or bias.

However, if most of the criteria are met, the likelihood of an association being causal is certainly high. The International Agency for Research on Cancer (IARC), in the preamble to its recent monographs, has established similar criteria for the designation of an agent as a carcinogen.

Limitations of Epidemiologic Studies

Failure to demonstrate a positive association in an epidemiologic study does not always indicate that there is no association between the agent and the effect studied. In some cases, a "false-negative" epidemiologic study may result because of a variety of shortcomings. Some of these limitations include difficulties in identifying exposures and effects, difficulties in choosing appropriate study (exposed) and control populations, requirements for prolonged follow-up because of long induction-latency periods, and the relative lack of sensitivity of epidemiologic methods.

The existence of all of these limitations accounts for the consensus among scientists that negative epidemiologic studies do not provide proof of non-carcinogenicity of an agent. Such negative data are generally outweighed by the finding of positive results in animal experimental studies. Greater credence may be given a negative study if the subjects studied had a sufficiently long period of exposure (an average of 15 or more years), if they were followed long enough to observe an effect (25 or more years), and if the number of exposed subjects was large enough so that an excess risk as small as 50% for the particular tumors studied could be detected.

ANIMAL BIOASSAYS

Design

Experimental studies in animals involve the administration of a test chemical to a group of animals followed by observation for the development of tumors. Procedures for such studies are now standardized and accepted by most of the sponsoring institutions, eg, the National Toxicology Program (NTP) and the International Agency for Research on Cancer (IARC). The basic requirements are listed in Table 16–2. In brief, protocols include at least 50 animals of each sex with 2 species—in each of 2

Table 16–2. IARC requirements for animal bioassays.

1. Two species of animals (generally mice and rats), both males and females.
2. Sufficient numbers of animals in each test group and concurrent control group (at least 50 per sex).
3. Duration of dose administration and observation must extend over most of the animal's life expectancy (typically 2 years for rats and mice).
4. Treated groups tested at 2 or ideally 3 different doses—at a higher dose (near the maximum tolerated dose, MTD) and at a lower dose.
5. Outcome determined from adequate pathologic examination of animals.
6. Proper statistical analysis of data.

dosage groups—and incorporate thorough pathologic examination and proper statistical analysis of results. Animals are dosed throughout their lifetimes at the maximal tolerated dose (MTD) and one-half the maximal tolerated dose.

Interpretation

Results from well-executed animal bioassays can yield clear evidence to support the carcinogenicity of a compound to the tested animal. In Supplement 4 to its Monograph series, the IARC, an independent scientific institution within the World Health Organization (WHO), has established criteria for the "assessment of evidence of carcinogenicity from studies in experimental animals." There are 4 categories, based on the following criteria: sufficient evidence, limited evidence, inadequate evidence, and no data. The first 3 are described below.

"i. *Sufficient evidence* of carcinogenicity, which indicates that there is an increased incidence of malignant tumours: (a) in multiple species or strains; or (b) in multiple experiments (preferably with different routes of administration or using different dose levels); or (c) to an unusual degree with regard to incidence, site or type of tumour, or age at onset. Additional evidence may be provided by data on dose-response effects, as well as information from short-term tests or on chemical structure.

"ii. *Limited evidence* of carcinogenicity, which means that the data suggest a carcinogenic effect but are limited because: (a) the studies involve a single species, strain or experiment; or (b) the experiments are restricted by inadequate dosage levels, inadequate duration of exposure to the agent, inadequate period of follow-up, poor survival, too few animals, or inadequate reporting; or (c) the neoplasms produced often occur spontaneously and, in the past, have been difficult to classify as malignant by histological criteria alone (eg, lung and liver tumours in mice).

"iii. *Inadequate evidence,* which indicates that because of major qualitative or quantitative limitations, the studies cannot be interpreted as showing either the presence or absence of a carcinogenic effect; or that within the limits of the tests used, the chemical is not carcinogenic . . . "

Correlation With Human Effects

In attempting to extrapolate data from animal research to conclusions about cancer risks in humans, the important issues to be considered are (1) whether all chemicals that have been shown to cause cancer in animals are also capable of causing cancer in humans, and vice versa; and (2) from a quantitative viewpoint, whether humans are equally susceptible to the carcinogenic effects of equivalent doses of known animal carcinogens.

With few exceptions, the available evidence suggests that, qualitatively, there is a good correlation between animal and human results. Until recently, it had not been possible to demonstrate in animals the carcinogenicity of arsenic, a known human skin and lung carcinogen. Arsenic was for that reason cited as an instance in which there was a discrepancy between human and animal studies, which then raised a question about the adequacy of animal bioassays to be sensitive predictors of human carcinogenicity. However, in the view of the International Agency for Research on Cancer, there is now limited evidence of carcinogenicity of arsenic compounds (arsenic trioxide, calcium arsenate) in laboratory animals, based on intratracheal instillation experiments in rats and hamsters. Thus, all known human carcinogens for which adequate animal studies have been conducted have shown at least limited evidence of carcinogenicity in some tested animals.

The issue of the specificity of animal testing as a predictor of human carcinogenicity is more difficult to resolve. Because of limitations inherent in epidemiologic studies (discussed above), it is unlikely that clear-cut evidence for human carcinogenicity can be derived for many chemicals proved to be carcinogenic in animals. Nevertheless, for the limited number of compounds for which there are adequate data in both humans and animals, most authors concur that there are no substances proved to be carcinogenic in animals that have been proved to be noncarcinogenic in humans.

Though there appears to be a good qualitative correlation between animal and human carcinogenicity, the target site at which cancers develop may be different for rodents and humans. For example, benzidine produces liver tumors in rats, hamsters, and mice but bladder tumors in humans and dogs.

The second major issue in the use of animal bioassays is the degree to which human carcinogenic effects parallel animal sensitivity. The data base that permits comparison of the sensitivity of humans relative to that of animals is quite limited. For the limited numbers of substances for which there are quantitative data in both humans and animals, it appears that the sensitivity of humans—on a total dose per body weight basis—is roughly similar to that of animals.

Limitations of Animal Bioassays

There are a number of difficult issues in the analysis of animal experimental studies that may limit their utility in human cancer risk assessment. Because of the small number of animals studied, the bioassays are relatively insensitive in detection of carcinogenicity. The agent under study must cause a 15% increase in the incidence of tumors in order for a statistically significant excess of tumors to be detected in a bioassay of standard size. A lower excess risk will not be demonstrable, particularly if there is any background rate of tumor development in untreated animals.

In an attempt to increase the sensitivity of animal experiments, high dose levels approaching the maximal tolerated dose are chosen. These doses are usually well above the human exposure levels in occupational or environmental settings. For risk quantification, the high doses add an additional difficulty, because one must make predictions based on extrapolation to the much lower doses experienced by humans. The mathematical models used for extrapolation are controversial and unproved and thus add more uncertainty to risk estimates.

Certain factors will at least theoretically affect the likelihood that the animal bioassay results will be a good predictor of the human response. The use of high doses, well above human exposures, may result in false-positive results if carcinogenicity only occurs secondary to a primary toxic pathologic alteration. If high doses overwhelm metabolic detoxifying mechanisms that normally would prevent exposure of the sensitive organ, false-positive results might occur. If metabolic processes acting in the animal studied and in humans for the particular chemical differ substantially, the possibility of both false-positives and false-negatives exists if the carcinogenic metabolite is produced only in the animal or only in humans, respectively. For most chemicals, evidence regarding comparative pharmacodynamics in humans and animals does not yet exist.

Since agents are often administered to animals by a route that is different from the one reported for human exposures, such as ingestion or intraperitoneal injection, it is at least theoretically possible that the outcome in the animal will differ from the effect in humans. However, there is no evidence to substantiate such a discrepancy in outcome based on differences in route of administration. Finally, there is some controversy about the classification of an agent as a potential carcinogen in the rare circumstance where experimental results indicate an increased frequency of benign tumors only.

SHORT-TERM TESTS

Types of Assays

A variety of assays have been designed that provide evidence of mutagenicity or the ability to induce chromosomal damage by chemicals without a long period of observation or follow-up, as is required in epidemiologic studies or animal bioassays. These short-term tests are therefore much quicker and less expensive to perform. End-points that have been assessed include gene mutation, induction of DNA damage and repair, DNA binding, chromosomal aberrations, sister chromatid exchange, or neoplastic transformation of mammalian cells. The tests ultimately rely upon the fact that most carcinogens covalently bind to DNA and thereby induce DNA damage.

The best-studied and most commonly performed short-term test is the Ames test, which utilizes a mutant strain of *Salmonella typhimurium* that is deficient in the enzymes required to synthesize histidine and will not grow unless histidine is added to the growth medium. The chemical to be tested, along with a liver microsomal enzyme fraction from rodents or humans that can metabolically activate "procar-cinogens," is added to the bacterial culture. Bacterial colonies that subsequently grow and can be counted indicate the occurrence of a reversion mutation to the wild strain, thus reflecting the mutagenic activity of the agent studied. Similar mutagenic testing is possible in cultured mammalian cells in vitro.

Tests for DNA repair can demonstrate that DNA damage has occurred following exposure to a chemical. Several tests have recently been developed that assay for the presence of chemicals covalently bound to DNA (DNA adducts). If validated, such tests may ultimately have usefulness in biologic monitoring of workers exposed to potential carcinogens.

Chromosomal aberrations in mammalian cells may be detected by cytogenetic tests that assess changes in the morphologic structure of chromosomes. Such tests can be performed on animal or human cells, including human lymphocytes. Morphologic changes that may occur include chromosomal translocations and the formation of micronuclei.

Testing for sister chromatid exchange is a more sophisticated form of cytogenetic investigation based on differential staining of sister chromatids and allowing for detection of the interchange of genetic material between chromatids. Such changes are more subtle than gross structural chromosomal aberrations. Again, tests for sister chromatid exchanges may be performed on animal or human cells.

Finally, tests for neoplastic transformation of mammalian cells in culture assess the ability of chemicals to alter growth characteristics of such cells toward neoplasia. Such altered cells can produce tumors when injected into the animal. A variety of other short-term tests are being or have been developed.

Interpretation & Limitations

The predictive value of short-term tests for the carcinogenicity of a chemical to humans is not clear. The correlation between results in short-term assays and human or animal study results is imperfect. No single short-term test is capable of detecting all chemicals positive in animal bioassays. As a result, a battery of such tests has been routinely performed on a chemical to be tested. Unfortunately, a recent study comparing the results—for a large number of chemicals—of animal bioassays and a battery of 4 commonly used short-term tests failed to demonstrate any advantage of a battery of tests over the Ames test used alone in predicting the results of the bioassays. The concordance of any of the in vitro tests with the animal bioassay results was approximately 60%. A number of compounds were identified as mutagenic in the short-term tests that were noncarcinogenic in the animal bioassays, but the explanation for these possible false-positives is unclear. While most genotoxic carcinogens are positive in short-term tests, these in vitro tests are not generally able to permit detection of chemicals that induce cancers by nongenotoxic or epigenetic mechanisms, ie, they are not sensitive to the effects of promoting agents.

Some of these tests—eg, tests for sister chromatid exchanges and measurement of DNA adducts—can be performed on cells (typically lymphocytes) taken from humans exposed occupationally or environmentally to suspect carcinogens. For example, testing for sister chromatid exchanges has been performed on ethylene oxide workers. An increased frequency of sister chromatid exchanges has been found in some of these workers. Though this merits further study, the clinical significance of these findings for the workers is unknown. The contribution of other factors such as cigarette smoking that have been shown to increase sister chromatid exchange frequency is also unclear. At this time, no predictions can be made based on results of such testing in workers. Thus, use of these tests should be limited to well-designed research studies.

Given the current state of knowledge, most authorities state that positive results in short-term tests on previously untested materials warrant further study in animal bioassays and further scrutiny in human exposure situations. Similarly, positive results on these tests provide corroboration to positive findings in animal bioassays, particularly when the animal results provide only limited or suggestive evidence of carcinogenicity. On the other hand, isolated positive short-term assay results do not constitute sufficient evidence to force immediate regulatory action.

IMPLICATIONS FOR REGULATORY ACTION & PREVENTIVE MEDICINE

When a sufficient body of evidence supporting carcinogenicity exists, corrective action to protect public and worker health must proceed, even if there is some remaining uncertainty in the conclusions. Convincingly, positive results from a well-conducted epidemiologic study merit immediate action. Sufficient evidence of carcinogenicity in animal bioassays, as defined by IARC, should also prompt immediate attempts to reduce worker exposure as much as possible. The finding of limited evidence in animal bioassays or positive results in short-term tests should at the very least serve as a stimulus for further study of the suspect chemical. When the results in different tests are contradictory, results suggesting carcinogenicity generally outweigh the negative evidence. Given the limited sensitivity of epidemiologic methods, this axiom seems particularly applicable when positive animal studies are analyzed alongside negative epidemiologic studies.

Based on analysis of epidemiologic and animal studies then available, the IARC issued, in 1987, a list of chemicals and industrial processes for which there is some evidence of human carcinogenicity. There are 28 industrial chemicals or processes in group 1 that have been shown to cause human cancer. Along with several additional carcinogenic hazards not reviewed by IARC, these are listed in Tables 16–3 and 16–4. There are 23 industrial chemicals and processes in groups 2A for which there is sufficient animal evidence but limited or inadequate human evidence of carcinogenicity, and about 70 agents in group 2B, for which there is less compelling evidence to suggest possible human carcinogenicity. Some of these agents are listed in Tables 16–5 and 16–6. There were an additional 147 substances for which there was sufficient evidence of animal carcinogenicity but for which there was either inadequate or nonexistent epidemiologic data. They conclude appropriately that, "In the absence of adequate data on humans it is reasonable, for practical purposes, to regard chemicals for which there is sufficient evidence of carcinogenicity in animals as if they presented a carcinogenic risk to humans."

The nature of the appropriate response by industry or government to evidence for carcinogenicity of a chemical is controversial. Given uncertainty about the existence of thresholds and the shape of the dose-response curve at low doses, it is not possible to establish clearly "safe" doses for carcinogens. Ideally, human exposure to known carcinogens should then be reduced to nil. In practice, political, economic, social, and technical factors constrain the power of regulators to adopt such stringent standards.

Some assistance in policy development can be derived from quantitative risk assessment methodology. Mathematical models have been designed that allow for the extrapolation from high-dose studies to lower dose exposures, providing an estimate of the excess risk or excess number of cases that might be seen in a given population as a result of these exposures. Though there is considerable uncertainty in such estimates, it can provide an approximate upper limit on the excess risk attributable to these exposures. Such risk assessments can help to place hazards from various chemicals in the occupational environment into proper perspective by allowing comparison of the risk estimate against the risk from other known hazards. These risk comparisons may allow regulators or decision-makers to prioritize exposure problems for the purpose of allocating scarce resources for clean-up or problem resolution.

Ames et al (1987) have developed an approach for such risk comparisons—the Human Exposure/Rodent Potency (HERP) percentage. The HERP compares the human exposure (daily lifetime dose in milligrams per kilogram) to the rodent TD50, the daily dose in milligrams per kilogram to halve the percentage of tumor-free animals by the end of a standard lifetime (as determined from animal bioassays). The lower the HERP percentage, the lower the possible hazard from average human exposures. Using this index, it is possible to compare the hazard of a variety of natural and synthetic carcinogens. Such comparisons frequently demonstrated a greater apparent hazard from natural carcinogens—eg, aflatoxin as a

Table 16–3. Occupational exposures associated with human cancer.

Occupational Exposure	Cancer Site
4-Aminobiphenyl	Bladder
Arsenic and arsenic compounds[1]	Lung, skin, ?liver, angiosarcoma
Asbestos	Pleura and peritoneum (mesothelioma), lung, ?larynx, gastrointestinal tract, kidney
Benzene	Leukemia (ANLL)
Benzidine	Bladder
Bis(chloromethyl) ether[2]	Lung (mainly oat cell)
Chromium compounds, hexavalent[1]	Lung
Coal tar pitches	Skin, scrotum, lung, bladder
Coal tars	Skin, scrotum, lung, ?bladder
Ionizing radiation	Leukemia, skin, other
Mineral oils, untreated and mildly treated	Skin, scrotum, ?lung
Mustard gas	Lung
β-Naphthalamine	Bladder
Nickel and nickel compounds (?oxide and sulfide)	Lung, nasal sinuses
Radium	Bone (sarcomas)
Radon	Lung
Shale oils	Skin, scrotum
Soots, tars, and oils[1]	Skin, lung, ?bladder
Talc containing asbestiform fibers	Lung, ?mesothelioma
Ultraviolet radiation	Skin
Vinyl chloride	Liver (angiosarcoma), ?brain, lung

[1]The compounds responsible for the carcinogenic effect in humans cannot be specified.
[2]And technical grade chloromethyl-methyl ether, which contains 1–8% bis(chloromethyl) ether.

Table 16–4. Industrial processes causally associated with human cancer.

Industrial Process	Possible or Probable Agent	Cancer Site
Aluminum production	Polycyclic aromatic hydrocarbons	Lung, bladder
Auramine manufacture	Auramine	Bladder
Boot and shoe manufacture and repair (certain occupations)	Benzene	Leukemia
Coal gasification	Polycyclic aromatic hydrocarbons	Lung, bladder, skin, scrotum
Coke production	Polycyclic aromatic hydrocarbons	Lung, ?kidney
Furniture manufacture	Wood dust	Nasal cavity (mainly adenocarcinoma)
Iron and steel founding	?Polycyclic aromatic hydrocarbons, silica, metal fumes	Lung
Isopropyl alcohol manufacture (strong acid process)	Diisopropyl sulfate; isopropyl oils	Paranasal sinuses, ?larynx
Magenta, manufacture of	?Magenta, ?precursors (eg, orthotoluidine)	Bladder
Nickel refining	Nickel oxides; nickel subsulfide	Nasal cavity, lung, ?larynx
Rubber industry	Aromatic amines, ?solvents	Bladder, leukemia (lymphatic), ?stomach, lung, skin, colon, prostate, lymphoma
Underground hematite mining (with exposure to radon)	?Radon	Lung

Table 16–5. Probable occupational carcinogens but limited evidence of human carcinogenicity.

Occupational Exposure	Cancer Site
Acrylonitrile	Lung
Benzo(a)pyrene	Lung, skin, bladder
Beryllium and beryllium compounds	Lung
Cadmium and certain cadmium compounds	Lung, prostate
Creosotes	Skin, scrotum
Diethyl sulfate	Larynx
Ethylene oxide	Leukemia
Formaldehyde	Nasal cavity, nasopharynx
Polychlorinated biphenyls	Liver
Silica (crystalline)	Lung

contaminant in peanut butter or hydrazines in raw mushrooms—than from better-publicized alleged hazards such as PCBs in the diet or trichloroethylene in contaminated well water. The priority setting that such an index facilitates may permit policy makers to focus attention and regulation on the most significant exposure problems.

Medical Surveillance

The proper role of medical surveillance in workers currently or previously exposed to known or suspected carcinogens is unclear. Surveillance of populations at high risk of cancer is only effective (1) if the screening test is easy to perform and sensitive, (2) if it detects premalignant abnormalities or tumors at an early stage in their development, and (3) if there is an effective intervention that reduces morbidity and mortality when applied to such ''early'' tumors. For certain tumors not associated with chemical exposures—eg, cervical cancer—screening techniques and effective therapy for early lesions have had a significant impact upon the disease. There is some evidence that a small group of workers at high risk of bladder tumors—as a result of prior exposure to aromatic amines used in dyestuff manufacture—can benefit from early detection by the use of urine cytology and cystoscopy as screening tools. For the remainder of occupational cancers, including asbestos-associated bronchogenic carcinoma, there is virtually no evidence that screening and early detection reduce mortality rates.

Table 16–6. Selected probable occupational carcinogens: Inadequate evidence of human carcinogenicity.

Occupational Exposure	Cancer Site	
	Animal	Human
Acetaldehyde	Nasal mucosa, larynx	
1,3-Butadiene	Lymphomas, lung, stomach liver	
Carbon tetrachloride	Liver	
Chloroform	Liver, kidney	
Chlorophenols and phenoxyacetic acid herbicides		?Soft tissue sarcoma and lymphoma
Chlorophenothane (DDT)	Liver, lung, lymphoma	
1,2-Dibromo-3-chloropropane (DBCP)	Nasal cavity, lung, stomach	
p-Dichlorobenzene	Liver, kidney	
Dichloromethane	Lung, liver	
1,4-Dioxane	Liver, nasal cavity	
Epichlorohydrin	Nasal cavity, forestomach	Respiratory tract
Ethylene dibromide	Forestomach, skin, lung	
Ethylene thiourea	Thyroid	
Hexachlorocyclohexanes	Liver	?Leukemia
Hydrazine	Lung, liver, mammary glands, nasal cavity	
Lead compounds, inorganic	Kidney	
4,4'-Methylenebis(2-chloroaniline) (MOCA)	Lung, liver, mammary gland	?Bladder
Polybrominated biphenyls (PBBs)	Liver	
2,3,7,8-Tetrachlorodibenzo-p-dioxin (TCDD)	Liver, lung, other	?Soft tissue sarcoma, lymphoma
Tetrachloroethylene	Liver, leukemias	

Nevertheless, properly collected medical surveillance data—particularly when combined with industrial hygiene data regarding exposure levels—may prove quite useful in future epidemiologic studies and in the refinement of our knowledge regarding human dose-response phenomena. If medical surveillance is to be performed, the protocol should be designed for each agent of concern based on the presumed target site from prior human and animal studies and the availability of screening tools. In practice, some form of medical surveillance is required by OSHA standards for asbestos, arsenic, benzene, and a variety of other carcinogens as listed in Table 16–7.

Table 16–7. Carcinogens for which medical surveillance is required.

2-Acetylaminofluorene
Acrylonitrile
4-Aminodiphenyl
Arsenic (inorganic)
Asbestos
Benzidine (and its salts)
Bis-chloromethyl ether
Coke oven emissions
1,2-Dibromo-3-chloropropane
3,3'-Dichlorobenzidine (and its salts)
4-Dimethylaminoazobenzene
Ethyleneimine
Ethylene dibromide
Ethylene oxide
4,4'-Methyelenebis (2-chloroaniline)
Methyl chloromethyl ether
α-Naphthylamine
β-Naphthylamine
4-Nitrobiphenyl
N-Nitrosodimethylamine
β-Propiolactone
Vinyl chloride

Source: Subchapter 7, General Industry Safety Orders, of title 8, Industrial Relations, California Administrative Code, 1986.

REFERENCES

Ames BN, Magaw R, Gold LS: Ranking possible carcinogenic hazards. *Science* 1987;**236:**271.

Brandt-Rauf PW: New markers for monitoring occupational cancer: the example of oncogene proteins. *Journal of Occupational Medicine* 1988;**30:**399.

Hoel DG et al: The impact of toxicity on carcinogenicity studies: implications for risk assessment. *Carcinogenesis* 1988;**9:**2045.

International Agency for Research on Cancer: *Carcinogenic Risks–Strategies for Intervention.* Davis W, Rosenfeld C (editors). IARC Scientific Publication No. 25. WHO/IARC, 1979.

International Agency for Research on Cancer: *IARC Monographs on the Evaluation of the Carcinogenic Risk of Chemicals to Humans: Chemicals, Industrial Processes and Industries Associated with Cancer in Humans, IARC Monographs, Volumes 1 to 29.* IARC Monographs Supplement 4, WHO/IARC, 1982.

International Agency for Research on Cancer: *Overall Evaluations of Carcinogenicity: An Updating of IARC Monographs Volumes 1-42* IARC Monographs Supplement 7, WHO/IARC, 1987.

Nicholson WJ: Research issues in occupational and environmental cancer. *Archives of Environmental Health* 1984;**39:**190.

Reynolds SH et al: Activated oncogenes in B6C3F1 mouse liver tumors: implications for risk assessment. *Science* 1987;**237:**1309.

Schottenfeld D: Chronic Disease in the Workplace and Environment: Cancer. *Archives of Environmental Health* 1984;**39:**150.

Schottenfeld D, Fraumeni J: *Cancer Epidemiology and Prevention.* Saunders, 1982.

Tennant RW et al: Prediction of chemical carcinogenicity in rodents from in vitro genetic toxicity assays. *Science* 1987;**236:**933.

Vainio H: Carcinogenesis and teratogenesis may have common mechanisms. *Scand J Work Environ Health* 1989;**15:**13.

Wilson R, Crouch EAC: Risk assessment and comparisons: an introduction. *Science* 1987;**236:**267.

CLINICAL PRESENTATIONS

MESOTHELIOMA

Essentials of Diagnosis

- Asbestos exposure.
- Persistent gnawing chest pain, dyspnea, dry cough, weight loss.
- Findings on examination of pleural effusion, pleural friction rub.
- Chest x-ray and CT findings of thick tumor lining chest wall.
- Diagnosis by open thoracotomy with multiple biopsies.

General Considerations

Mesothelioma was not accepted as a pathologic entity until about 50 years ago, when Klemperer and Rahn advocated general use of the term mesothelioma for primary pleural tumors originating from the surface lining cells or the mesothelium. This tumor is uncommon, accounting for only a small fraction of deaths due to cancer, but it and other asbestos-related diseases have been of great interest to occupational health physicians, public health professionals, biomedical researchers, and personal injury attorneys.

The first case reports of mesothelioma associated with asbestos were published in the 1940s, but the problem received scant attention until 1960, when Wagner reported diffuse pleural mesothelioma associated with asbestos exposure in the western Cape Province of South Africa. The incidence of mesothelioma is increasing, with an annual incidence for adults in North America of 2–3 cases per million for men and 0.7 per million for women. In Canada, England, and Italy—in areas of heavy occupational use of asbestos—rates vary from 2.3 to 21.4 cases per million.

Etiology

Diffuse mesotheliomas of the peritoneum and pleura are considered "signal tumors," pathognomonic of exposure to asbestos. Since the early report of Wagner, many additional series reports and cohort mortality studies have clearly implicated asbestos as causal in these cancers. Evidence is lacking for any relationship between asbestos exposure and the development of solitary or localized mesothelioma.

The most convincing evidence of an association between asbestos and mesothelioma was brought out in Selikoff's report that 8% of 17,800 asbestos insulation workers in the USA and Canada followed from 1967 to 1976 died from malignant mesothelioma. Selikoff and others have shown that a dose-response relationship exists between this neoplasm and asbestos exposure.

The latency period from asbestos exposure to the diagnosis of mesothelioma is 30 years or more. Quantitative asbestos fiber content of dried lung has also been shown to correlate with mesothelioma. Further evidence of the etiologic role of asbestos has been shown in experimental animals, in which intrapleural injection with asbestos fibers causes mesothelioma histologically identical to human tumors.

Epidemiologic data show that variable levels of exposure to asbestos can result in mesothelioma. In one study of 168 patients with mesothelioma in England and South Africa, one-third of cases were associated with occupational exposure intensive enough to cause asbestosis or lung cancer. Another third were asbestos-related only by trivial contact at work or in the home environment, eg, exposure of wives washing their husbands' contaminated work clothes. The remaining third had no history of contact with asbestos.

The major value of studies done to date has been in identifying a segment of the population at risk, but reports of patients with mesothelioma without a history of occupational or paraoccupational exposure to asbestos raises other questions. The proportion of patients with no exposure history ranges from nil to 87% in various studies. The long latency period from exposure to disease contributes to problems with forgotten exposures, and the variety of occupations with asbestos exposure leads to problems with overlooked exposures. Exposure occurs in the milling, mining, and transportation of raw asbestos and in the manufacture of asbestos cement pipe, friction materials, textiles, and roofing materials. Construction workers, plumbers, welders, and electricians are all exposed; and shipyard tradesmen can be "innocent bystanders" in exposure to airborne asbestos fibers. There is also evidence that nonasbestos agents can induce malignant mesotheliomas, and substances such as nickel, beryllium, silica dust, and zeolite fibers have been looked at in this regard. There is no interaction between cigarette smoking and asbestos exposure in the development of this tumor.

Pathogenesis

Asbestos is a fibrous silicate of various chemical types such as chrysotile, crocidolite, amosite, and anthophyllite; with chrysotile accounting for 90% of commercial asbestos. All types of asbestos seem to be capable of causing mesothelioma, though there is evidence that crocidolite may be the most potent. Very few mesotheliomas have been associated with the chrysotile fiber alone. The mechanisms of induction are unknown. Cancer development is apparently related not to chemical composition but to physical properties, ie, fiber size and dimension. In work done in rats, long thin fibers of a variety of types have proved carcinogenic, whereas short fibers and those with a relatively broad diameter have failed to produce mesothelioma. These findings are consistent with epidemiologic observations documenting the relatively common occurrence of tumors in populations exposed to grades of crocidolite consisting chiefly of long, thin fibers and the rarity of tumors in persons exposed to amosite and anthophyllite. The location of mesothelioma is related to the type of asbestos fiber as well. Chrysotile has been associated with pleural but not peritoneal tumors in Canadian miners, though this association may be related to tremolite, an uncommon fiber, rather than the chrysotile. Peritoneal mesothelioma has been shown to occur only in individuals exposed to amphibole asbestos, and the pathogenesis is thought to be similar to tumor in the pleural cavity. Fibers of asbestos are transported in lymphatics to the abdomen, and asbestos is also transported across the mucosa of the gut after ingestion.

The mechanism of malignant transformation of mesothelial tissue is obscure. Mesothelial cells phagocytose asbestos and proliferate when exposed to asbestos in vitro, but malignant transformation has not been documented after exposure of cultured mesothelial cells to asbestos.

Pathology

One of the major areas of difficulty in the study of mesothelioma has been the pathologic features. Many tumors metastasize and spread to the mesothelial lining of the chest and abdomen; this had led to confusion of the mesothelioma with metastatic tumors. Confusion also exists secondary to the tumor's diverse microscopic appearance.

There are 2 types: benign solitary and diffuse malignant mesothelioma. The benign solitary type remains localized, though it may become large and compress neighboring thoracic structures. This tumor has not been associated with asbestos exposure; it is a benign tumor arising from fibroblasts and other connective tissue elements in the areolar submesothelial cell layers of the pleura that is not occupational in origin. By contrast, diffuse malignant mesothelioma arises from either the pleuripotential mesenchymal cell or the primitive submesothelial mesenchymal cell, which retains the ability to form epithelial or connective tissue elements.

Malignant mesothelioma is a diffuse lesion that spreads widely in the pleural space and is usually associated with extensive pleural effusion and direct invasion of thoracic structures. On gross examination, numerous tumor nodules may be noted, and in advanced cases the tumor bulk has a hard, woody consistency. Microscopically, malignant mesotheliomas consist of a mixture of 3 histologic types: an epithelial type that may resemble metastatic disease, a mesenchymal type, and a mixed type. Histochemical techniques detecting acid mucopolysaccharide with colloidal iron or alcian blue stains can detect epithelial cells, and this staining can be removed from the tissue with hyaluronidase, a helpful technique to differentiate mesothelioma from adenocarcinoma. Studies with the electron microscope have defined certain characteristic features that are also helpful in differentiating the tumor from metastatic disease.

Clinical Findings

A. Symptoms: Symptoms in diffuse mesothelioma may be entirely absent or minimal at the time of onset of the disease. Disease progression results in the most common symptom of a persistent gnawing chest pain on the involved side, which may radiate to the shoulder and arm. In most patients, pain becomes the most incapacitating symptom. Dyspnea on exertion, dry cough (occasionally hemoptysis), and increasing weight loss are frequent accompanying symptoms. Some patients have low-grade fever, and a minority have findings such as hypertrophic pulmonary osteoarthropathy, syncopal attacks from hypoglycemia, or generalized anasarca from massive involvement of the pericardium or obstruction of the inferior and superior venae cavae.

B. Signs: Physical findings vary with the stage of disease. Most patients present with pleural effusion. Local tumor growth may depress the diaphragm and displace the liver or spleen, giving the impression of hepato- or splenomegaly. In advanced disease, there may be obvious enlargement of the affected hemithorax, with bulging of the intercostal spaces and displacement of the trachea and mediastinum to the unaffected side. After removal of pleural fluid, a pericardial or pleuropericardial rub may be heard. Advanced signs may also include fever, arthralgias, supraclavicular and axillary node enlargement, subcutaneous nodules in the chest wall, and clubbing. Encroachment on the mediastinal structures may lead to neuropathic signs such as vocal cord paralysis or Horner's syndrome. Congestion and edema may develop in the upper trunk or lower limbs secondary to compression of the superior or inferior venae cavae.

C. Laboratory Findings: Although patients may have the syndrome of inappropriate antidiuretic hormone secretion with hyponatremia, most have normal blood chemistries. Elevation of lactate dehydrogenase may occur as a nonspecific finding.

D. Imaging: X-ray studies of the chest most commonly show unilateral pleural effusion. After fluid removal, the pleura may show thickening or nodularity, seen usually at the bases. CT scanning, which is the most sensitive test for evaluating the pleural surface, may show the thickened tumor along the chest wall, and late in the disease tomograms or an overpenetrated film will show compressed lung surrounded on all sides by a tumor 2–3 cm thick. Extrapleural extension can result in soft tissue masses or radiologic evidence of rib destruction. Signs of asbestos such as interstitial pulmonary fibrosis, pleural plaques, and calcification are valuable findings when present.

E. Special Examinations:

1. Sputum cytology–Microscopic examination of sputum rarely shows malignant cells unless the tumor has invaded lung parenchyma. Asbestos bodies may be seen.

2. Thoracentesis–The considerable force necessary to enter the pleural space with a thoracentesis needle may be a clue to the presence of pleural mesothelioma. Pleural fluid is serosanguineous or hemorrhagic in 30–50% of cases but is commonly straw-colored. Cytologic examination of pleural fluid is useful in one-half to two-thirds of cases; however, distinguishing malignant mesothelioma from metastatic adenocarcinoma or benign inflammatory conditions is often difficult. The pleural fluid often contains a mixture of normal mesothelial cells, differentiated and undifferentiated malignant mesothelial cells, and a varying number of lymphocytes, histiocytes, and polymorphonuclear leukocytes. The diagnostic value of cytologic tests is limited. Mesothelial hyperplasia is not uncommon in benign pleural effusions and can easily be mistaken for malignant cells.

3. Thoracotomy and thoracoscopy–Because of the limitations of pleural fluid cytologic examination, biopsy confirmation is required. An open thoracotomy with multiple biopsies from different pleural areas is generally required for diagnosis. Thoracoscopy with biopsy of pleural masses can be an effective technique also.

Differential Diagnosis

The major disorders that must be differentiated from mesothelioma are inflammatory pleurisy, primary lung cancer, and metastatic disease. Inflammatory pleurisy is suggested by the associated clinical picture and by typical findings in the analysis of sputum and pleural fluid. In primary lung cancer, the more prominent symptoms of cough, the less common presence of severe chest pain, the presence of parenchymal tumors, and the absence of pleural abnormalities after thoracentesis help to differentiate between these 2 types of cancer. A primary tumor in the pancreas, gastrointestinal tract, and ovary should be excluded, since these tumors can metastasize to the pleural or peritoneal space and mimic mesothelioma.

Prevention

Regulations governing asbestos exposure are difficult to develop. One must use morbidity and mortality data looking retrospectively at members of occupational groups with varying exposures in the remote past or over a lifetime. The difficulties are compounded by the long latency period of asbestosis and asbestos-related cancers, especially mesothelioma. Setting permissible limits requires establishment of dose-response relationships, with subsequent determination of an acceptable level of risk. The difficulty is that all industrial processes, all fiber types, and all asbestos-related diseases have dissimilar dose-response relationships. Although it is thought that lower, shorter exposures to asbestos lead to mesothelioma than the exposures that lead to asbestosis or lung cancer, most standards are now based on preventing asbestosis.

Control of asbestos dust in industry has become progressively more rigorous during the last 40 years. It was in the 1940s that recommendations for levels of asbestos in the air of occupational settings were first established, but it was not until 1970 that federal regulations began as a result of the passage of the Occupational Safety and Health Act and the Clean Air Act. Initial standards were based on the light microscopic count of fibers of a length of 5 μm, collected by mechanical means. A concentration of 5 fibers per milliliter of air averaged over an 8-hour period was considered acceptable, with stipulation for transient excesses above that concentration. In 1986, the exposure standard of 2 fibers/mL was lowered by OSHA to 0.2 fibers/mL. Allowable exposure varies with the different mineral fibers.

Treatment

A. Surgical Measures: Surgical excision has no role in the management of peritoneal mesothelioma unless the tumor is localized; however, in spite of technical difficulties, surgery has been used with some success as a primary method of treatment in pleural mesotheliomas. Even in tumors with extensive infiltration of adjoining viscera, partial surgical resection has led to an apparent increase in longevity. Parietal pleurectomy is the accepted procedure, and more radical surgeries such as pleuropneumonectomy have been associated with an unacceptably high surgical mortality rate. Postoperative adjuvant chemotherapy and radiation therapy are rational therapy, but there are no studies to support their use. Surgical resection of all visible disease is believed to be the treatment of choice.

B. External Radiotherapy–Radiation therapy has clearly been shown to be of benefit in controlling pain and pleural effusion in mesothelioma. Although antitumor efficacy has been noted using high-dose radiation, this modality is relatively ineffective in changing the outcome of the disease.

C. Installation of Radioactive Compounds: Because colloidal gold has an affinity for serosal lining cells, instillation of radioactive colloidal gold into the pleural space has been attempted. Responses with apparent long-term survival have been reported, with no significant toxicity; but therapy must be given early in the disease, before the pleural cavity is obliterated by tumor. Radioactive phosphate in conjunction with abdominal irradiation has been used for peritoneal mesothelioma, and the small number of patients treated in this fashion have had increased lengths of survival.

D. Chemotherapy: There has been no systematic study of the role of cytotoxic drugs in mesothelioma, but there are well-documented reports of definite antitumor effects in some patients. Doxorubicin has been demonstrated to induce tumor regression and perhaps to prolong the survival of responding patients. Single-agent doxorubicin therapy has therefore become the standard therapy for patients with unresectable disease, but no patient has been cured with chemotherapy.

Other reported active antitumor agents include methotrexate and alkylating agents such as cyclophosphamide, mechlorethamine, and thiotepa. There are few studies using combination chemotherapy, but regimens containing doxorubicin appear to be most effective.

Course & Prognosis

Approximately 75% of patients are dead within 1 year after diagnosis, with average survival after diagnosis 8–10 months. Several factors correlate with improved survival in mesothelioma. Patients whose tumors are in the pleura survive twice as long as those with peritoneal tumor; survival is longer for patients with epithelial types than for those with mixed or fibrosarcomatous types; and survival is longer for patients younger than 65, those who respond well to chemotherapy, and those able to undergo surgical resection.

SKIN CANCER

Essentials of Diagnosis

● Major risk is ultraviolet radiation.

- Skin findings: crusting, ulceration, easy bleeding.
- Fair complexion at risk.

General Considerations

Neoplastic diseases of the skin are commonly divided into melanoma and nonmelanoma skin cancer, which consists mainly of basal cell and squamous cell carcinoma. Nonmelanoma skin cancer is currently the most common form of cancer in the white population of the USA. Although the dominant risk factor for nonmelanoma skin cancer (ultraviolet light) has been established, epidemiologic study of skin cancer has been limited. Skin cancer carries an excellent prognosis, with 96–99% cure rates, making death certificate reviews useless.

There is a perception that skin cancer other than melanoma is a trivial disease, and for that reason the patients are rarely hospitalized, with the result that they are commonly not included in cancer registries. Because of failure to register or record skin cancers, much of the data on incidence are from surveys conducted many years ago. The most recent surveys of nonmelanoma skin cancer conducted by the National Cancer Institute have shown an annual age-adjusted incidence rate among whites of 232.6 per 100,000 population, or an estimated 400,000 cases per year among white Americans.

Etiology

The primary causes of skin cancer in industry include ultraviolet radiation (UV), polycyclic aromatic hydrocarbons, arsenic, and ionizing radiation. Clearly, the major risk factor for skin cancer in lightly pigmented persons is radiation from the sun. The experiment of nature in which different intensities of UV radiation occur at different global latitudes has provided the opportunity for many epidemiologic studies to show an increased incidence of nonmelanoma skin cancer in Caucasians at latitudes closer to the equator. The earliest realization that excess sun exposure leads to skin cancer was made on the basis of occupation in 1890, when Unna described changes of the skin of sailors, including skin cancer that resulted from prolonged exposure to the weather.

There are approximately 4.8 million outdoor workers in the USA, with certain occupations at greater risk, such as those in agriculture and professional sports. Another estimated 300,000 workers are exposed to industrial radiation sources, eg, welding arcs, germicides, and printing processors. The carcinogenic hazard of industrial radiation—which includes wavelengths shorter than that of the sun—is not yet understood. In experimental animals, the most carcinogenic wavelength is in the 290- to 300-nm range (sunlight does not include wavelengths less than 290 nm); 254 nm is less carcinogenic, but wavelengths as low as 230 nm will still produce skin cancers.

The actual carcinogenic spectrum for humans is unknown. It is also notable that in experimental animals, a variety of foreign substances including phototoxic chemicals (eg, coal tar), chemical carcinogens (eg, benzo[a]pyrene), and nonspecific irritants (eg, xylene) under suitable conditions augment UV carcinogenesis.

Although chemical carcinogenesis of the skin does not seem to be nearly as frequent a cause of cancer as UV radiation, it was described over a century earlier. Percival Pott described the increased incidence of scrotal cancer in chimney sweeps in 1775, but not until the 1940s was a polycyclic aromatic hydrocarbon, benzo(a)pyrene, shown to be a constituent of soot. These hydrocarbons have the ability to induce skin cancers in laboratory animals, and mixtures of them are found in coal tar, pitch, asphalt, soot, creosotes, anthracenes, paraffin waxes, and lubricating and cutting oils. Exposures to mineral oil have been linked to skin and scrotal cancers among shale oil workers, jute processors, tool setters, mule spinners, wax pressmen, metal workers exposed to poorly refined cutting oils, and machine operators using lubricating oils. Latent periods between exposure to polycyclic aromatic hydrocarbons and skin cancer vary from about 20 years (coal tar) to 50 years or more (mineral oil).

Skin tumors associated with arsenic appear to occur following ingestion, injection, or inhalation rather than skin contact. Medicinal inorganic arsenicals and arsenic in drinking water are the sources most commonly implicated. Recent detailed studies in Taiwan established that use of well water with high arsenic concentrations resulted in skin cancer, with a dose-response relationship. An estimated 1.5 million workers in the USA are exposed to inorganic arsenic in such diverse trades as copper and lead smelting, the metallurgical industry, sheep dip manufacturing, and orchard growing; however, skin tumors attributed to occupational arsenic exposure are very uncommon. It is thought that many of the cases cited in the literature of agricultural workers with arsenic-induced skin cancers may be the result of other carcinogenic influences, such as sunlight and tars. Arsenic has only recently been shown to cause cancer in experimental animals.

Ionizing radiation is carcinogenic for skin as it is for many other tissues. Roentgen radiation-induced skin carcinoma was first reported in 1902, shortly after the discovery of x-rays, in those who worked the machines. There was a definite excess in skin cancer deaths among radiologists in the period from 1920 to 1939, and an excess risk has also been found for uranium miners. The latent period for radiation-induced skin cancers varies inversely with the dose, with the overall range from 7 weeks to 56 years (average, 25–30 years). Although epidemiologic studies do not give reliable data on dose-response relationships, the risk from exposures under 1000 rems appears to be small, and skin cancer may be induced by dose-equivalents of 3000 rems. There are now strict controls on industrial and occupational exposure to ionizing radiation, and currently it appears that ionizing radiation is not responsible for much cutaneous carcinogenesis.

Pathophysiology

Work by Rous in 1941 and Berenblum in 1964 elucidated the 2-stage theory of carcinogenesis. Berenblum found that a single application of a potent carcinogen such as benzo(*a*)pyrene applied in a quantity insufficient to cause tumors did allow tumor development after subsequent application of croton oil, which by itself produced no tumors at all. He theorized that the production of a tumor was initiated by the carcinogen but that its subsequent development could be promoted nonspecifically. It appears that initiation is permanent and irreversible, but promotion, up to a point, is reversible.

UV light fits into this theory of chemical carcinogenesis in that it appears to be both an initiator and a promoter for carcinoma of the skin. Two major effects of UV radiation on the skin that seem likely to be responsible for the carcinogenic effects are photochemical alteration of the DNA and alterations in immunity. Certain immunologic defects, both in skin and in lymphocytes, can be induced by UV radiation. Exposure to UV light also depletes the dermis of Langerhans cells and renders it unable to be sensitized to potent allergens. Alterations at the level of DNA are thought responsible as well for ionizing radiation-induced skin cancers.

Pathology

The histologic types of skin lesions associated with sun exposure include solar keratoses, basal cell epitheliomas, squamous cell carcinomas, keratoacanthomas, and malignant melanomas. Solar keratoses contain morphologically cancerous cells, but they are considered premalignant since invasion is limited to the most superficial part of the dermis. About 13% of all solar keratoses develop into squamous cell carcinomas, but these are rarely aggressive. The estimated incidence of metastases from all sun-induced squamous cell carcinomas is 0.5% or less. Almost all squamous cell carcinomas in Caucasians occur in highly sun-exposed areas, but 40% of basal cell epitheliomas occur on shaded areas of the head and neck.

Regardless of the source of exposure, certain features are common in all cases of arsenic-induced skin cancers. Punctate keratoses of the palms and soles and hyperpigmentation are frequently seen. The skin tumors are of several types, with squamous carcinomas arising either from normal skin or from keratoses and basal cell epitheliomas, including multiple superficial squamous cell and basal cell epitheliomas and frequently areas of intraepidermal carcinoma (Bowen's disease). Multiple tumors are the rule, most of which are found on unexposed areas, though cancer of the scrotum, which is often seen with polycyclic aromatic hydrocarbon exposure, is rare.

Early radiation workers with heavy exposure from uncalibrated machines had predominantly squamous cell carcinomas, found mainly on the hands and feet and occasionally on the face. More recently, basal cell epithelial exposures have been described following repeated occupational exposures.

Radiation-related tumors usually arise in areas of chronic radiation dermatitis, and whether they can occur on clinically normal skin is a matter of dispute. Radiation-induced malignant melanoma and sweat gland tumors have rarely been described.

Clinical Findings

Basal cell epithelioma frequently presents as a nodular or nodular-ulcerative lesion on the skin of the head and neck and only 10% of the time on the skin of the trunk. It is much less common on the upper extremities and quite uncommon on the lower extremities. The lesion is generally smooth, shiny, and translucent, with telangiectatic vessels just beneath the surface. It is usually not painful or tender, even with ulceration, except when crusting or bleeding is seen with minor trauma. Basal cell carcinomas rarely metastasize but can invade widely and deeply, extending through the subcutaneous tissue to involve neurovascular structures and occasionally eroding into bone.

Squamous cell carcinoma presents first in a premalignant stage characterized by actinic keratosis, a rough, reddened plaque on sun-exposed skin. There is then an in situ stage, which appears as a well-demarcated, slightly raised erythematous plaque with more substance and scaling than actinic keratosis. Squamous cell carcinoma usually presents as an erythematous lesion with varying degrees of scaling and crusting. Those in sun-exposed areas of the body tend to be on the most highly irradiated areas, such as the tip of the nose, the forehead, the tips of the helices of the ears, the lower lip, or the backs of the hands. Squamous cell carcinomas rarely metastasize when on the skin surface, but those on mucous membranes metastasize more frequently.

Prevention

The most important step in prevention of occupation-related skin cancers is avoidance of ultraviolet light. This is especially true for workers who are abnormally susceptible to UV light, such as those with certain hereditary diseases (eg, albinism and xeroderma pigmentosum).

Persons with fair complexions, light eye and hair color, and repeated sunburns should be discouraged from working out of doors or even indoors with ultraviolet light sources. Those who do work outdoors should wear protective clothing, such as wide-brimmed hats and long sleeves. Sunscreens should be used, but their effectiveness in preventing carcinoma is unknown even though their effectiveness for avoidance of erythema has been proved. Periodic examinations are recommended to detect the presence of malignant and premalignant skin lesions.

The incidence of scrotal cancer is now rare because

of preventive measures. If possible, a noncarcinogenic material should be substituted for a carcinogenic one. The efficacy of this approach was clearly demonstrated in Britain in 1953 when noncarcinogenic oil use became obligatory in the mule-spinning industry, with a steady fall in the number of reported cases of scrotal carcinoma. Good personal hygiene should include compulsory showering and change of clothes when entering and leaving the plant as well as washing of exposed skin after leaving contaminated areas. Isolated or closed-system operations, protective clothing, and employee education are important also in avoidance of skin cancer induced by polycyclic aromatic hydrocarbons.

Currently, the maximum allowable dose equivalent of ionizing radiation for occupational exposure to the skin is 30 rems in any year, except that forearms and hands are allowed 75 rems in any year (because there is little red marrow in the forearms and hands). These recommendations are mainly based on avoidance of hematologic disease and may need to be revised in order to prevent skin cancer.

Treatment

Biopsy is necessary in all cases of suspected skin carcinoma. For small skin cancers not located in areas where primary closure would be difficult, excisional biopsy should be done. If incisional biopsy is done, it is imperative that an adequate amount of tissue be obtained from the involved area.

Actinic keratoses may be excised or removed superficially with a scalpel followed by cautery or fulguration. One to 5 percent fluorouracil may be used topically, followed by excision of persistent lesions.

Squamous cell carcinoma should be treated with excision, but radiation is an alternative. Mohs' technique of micrographic surgery has the highest cure rate for removal of skin carcinomas. Basal cell carcinoma is treated with excision, curettage, and electrodesiccation; by irradiation; or with Mohs' technique. Cryosurgery may be used but is associated with a large number of recurrences.

THE LEUKEMIAS

Essentials of Diagnosis

- Radiation, benzene exposure.
- Weakness, malaise, anorexia, fever.
- Pallor, hepatosplenomegaly, lymph node enlargement.
- Leukocytosis; immature white cells in peripheral blood and bone marrow.
- Anemia and thrombocytopenia.

General Considerations

The 2 major forms of leukemia that have been linked to occupation are acute nonlymphocytic leukemia (ANLL) and chronic myelogenous leukemia (CML). The acute leukemias are malignant diseases of blood-forming organs characterized by a proliferation of immature blood cell progenitors in the bone marrow and other tissues. Together with replacement of the normal marrow with leukemic cells, there is a diminished production of normal erythrocytes, granulocytes, and platelets. Acute leukemias are classified morphologically by reference to the predominant cell line involved as lymphoblastic and nonlymphocytic forms. Acute leukemias, taken collectively, are relatively common diseases, with an incidence in the USA of 3.5 cases per 100,000 population per year. The annual incidence of ANLL is constant from birth throughout the first 10 years at about 10 cases per million. The incidence peaks in late adolescence, remains at 15 per million to age 55, and then rises to 50 per million at age 75. Eighty percent of all adult acute leukemias are of the nonlymphocytic variety; and unlike acute lymphoblastic leukemia, ANLL has been reported as a complication of chemical exposures and irradiation.

Chronic leukemias are classified as lymphocytic and myelogenous; only chronic myelogenous leukemia has been reported as an industrial disease. Chronic myelogenous leukemia is a neoplastic disease resulting from the development of an abnormal hematopoietic stem cell. There is excessive growth of the blood cell progenitors in the marrow, which initially can perform the functions of normal hematopoietic cells. The leukemic cells have the tendency to undergo further malignant transformation, with loss of ability to differentiate in the later stages of the disease. Large numbers of mature and immature granulocytic cells accumulate in the blood, and extramedullary hematopoiesis produces gross enlargement of the liver and spleen. Chronic myelogenous leukemia accounts for about 20% of all deaths from leukemia in the western world, with an incidence that—unlike other forms of leukemia—has not recently been increasing. Although rare cases are reported in infants, most patients with CML are aged 25–60 years, with a median age of about 45.

Etiology

The cause of human leukemia is unknown. As in the case of most other cancers, it is probable that no single factor is responsible. Most cases are thought to result from the interaction of host susceptibility factors, chemical or physical injury to chromosomes, and—in animals and presumably in humans—incorporation of genetic information of viral origin into susceptible stem cells.

A. Radiation: Radiation remains the most conclusively identified leukemogenic factor in human beings. The earliest evidence began to accumulate soon after the discovery of x-rays, which were used mainly in the medical workplace; thus, radiologists, radiation therapists, and radiation technicians were all at risk. Several studies showed an excess risk of leukemia among radiologists (approximately 9 times that of other physicians) during the years 1930–1950, with a latency period of about 18 years. With adequate shielding since that time, this excess risk has been decreasing.

The data from Hiroshima and Nagasaki atomic bomb survivors leave little doubt that the incidence of leukemia is increased following exposure to mixed gamma and neutron radiation and that the response is dependent on the dose. The risk of leukemia is increased in populations exposed to ionizing radiation at doses as low as 50–100 cGy. Between 100 cGy and 500 cGy, there is a linear correlation between dose and leukemia incidence. The data suggest that the risk of leukemia is increased at a rate of 1–2 cases per million population per year per centigray. Maximal risk occurs approximately 4–7 years after exposure, and an increased risk has been seen in Japanese people 14 years after exposure.

Whole body exposure to radiation in single doses results in suppression of marrow growth, and a single whole-body dose of 300–400 cGy is usually fatal in humans. In sublethal exposure, cytopenias may occur, and in patients who develop leukemia a delay between exposure and disease of 8–18 years may be seen. Following radiation exposure, both acute and chronic myelogenous leukemia may occur. In the atomic bomb survivors, chronic lymphocytic leukemia was not seen. The specific rates per 100,000 for people within 1500 m of the hypocenter are 8.1 for acute nonlymphocytic leukemia, 25.6 for chronic myelogenous leukemia, and 21.7 for acute lymphocytic leukemia.

Workers at risk secondary to exposure to ionizing radiation include military personnel in the vicinity of nuclear tests, uranium miners, and workers in nuclear power plants. Approximately 250,000 troops are estimated to have been present at multiple detonations of nuclear devices carried out by the USA from 1945 to 1976. In 1976, over 3000 men exposed at the 1957 nuclear test explosion ''Smoky'' were studied, and a significant excess of leukemia was discovered. A review of death certificates of former workers at the Portsmouth Naval Shipyard (where nuclear submarines are repaired and refueled) revealed an observed-to-expected ratio of leukemia deaths of 5.62 among former nuclear workers.

B. Chemicals: Certain chemicals—eg, chemotherapeutic agents—are known to be toxic to marrow cells, and many of these also possess leukemogenic potential. Occupational evidence of leukemogenicity is strongest for benzene, where recent epidemiologic studies have shown significant increases in leukemia in workers with past exposure to benzene. Benzene has been known for almost a century to be a powerful bone marrow poison, leading to aplastic or hypoplastic anemia. It is now widely believed that any chemical capable of inducing bone marrow damage must be assumed to be a potential leukemogen. Over the past few decades, evidence has been accumulating that benzene produces not only aplastic anemia but also leukemia, and that the fatal cases of leukemia outnumber those of true aplastic anemia. In 1928,

Delore and Borgomano described the first case of acute leukemia in a worker with such heavy exposure to benzene that none of his coworkers could work for more than 2 months without becoming ill. In 1932, Lignac produced several cases of leukemia in white rats given benzene in olive oil, but many subsequent animal studies were inconclusive. Only in the last few years have investigators shown benzene to systematically induce cancers in rats.

Benzene is a cyclic hydrocarbon obtained in distillation of petroleum and coal tar. It is used widely in chemical synthesis in many industries, in the manufacture of explosives, and in the production of cosmetics, soaps, perfumes, drugs, and dyes. Benzene was once used in the dry cleaning industry, but that is no longer the case. In addition, nearly 2% of unleaded gasoline is benzene.

An estimated 2 million workers in the USA have exposure to benzene. One of the most recent studies in workers exposed to benzene in the manufacture of rubber showed a nearly 6-fold greater incidence of death from leukemia than would be expected. Workers exposed for 5 years or more had a 21-fold increased risk of death from leukemia. Many other studies—including several undertaken in the shoe manufacturing industry—have shown an increase in the risk of leukemia in workers with exposure to benzene.

Chemicals other than benzene are suspected of causing leukemia, but the epidemiologic data in this area are incomplete. An increase in leukemia in chemists in Norway has been discovered, and an increase in marrow chromosome breakage has been noted in patients with leukemia who have histories suggesting occupational exposure to carcinogens. Indirect evidence of leukemogenicity of organic hydrocarbons comes from a study that showed an increased incidence of leukemia in Nebraska farmers, thought to be secondary to exposure to chemicals used on the farm.

Pathophysiology

A. Ionizing Radiation: The effects of radiation on human tissue depend on multiple factors, such as type of radiation, dose of radiation, length of exposure, body part exposed, and oxygen content of the exposed tissue. Damage secondary to radiation is greatest in rapidly dividing cells such as bone marrow stem cells, epithelial cells, and gamete-forming cells. The mechanism of radiation-induced injury at the cellular level involves direct and indirect damage to nucleic acids and proteins. DNA is a radiosensitive target, with even minor molecular damage resulting in profound effects on the cell and the organism. Radiation-induced molecular damage may be so severe that the cell no longer functions, and cell death results. Cells exposed to radiation may survive with no effects (if only a small number of nonessential molecules are affected) or may survive with altered structure and function. If the alteration is within the DNA, clinical disease may not appear until after a latency period. Cancer induction appears to depend upon an interaction of defective cellular repair and damage to the cell's regulator genes.

B. Benzene: Benzene toxicity may present as an acute illness or as a chronic disease developing up to 30 years after exposure. Chronic or recurrent exposure to concentrations of benzene exceeding 100 ppm (320 mg/m^3) leads to a very high incidence of cytopenias. When the exposure ends, there is usually spontaneous remission. Among workers who have been exposed to atmospheric concentrations of benzene in excess of 300 ppm for at least 1 year, as many as 20% will acquire pancytopenia or aplastic anemia. The chronic form of illness is related to the localization of benzene in the bone marrow, where benzene appears to exert a colchicinelike effect, blocking mitosis of the marrow proliferative cells. Mutagenic effects also occur and play a role in the occasional subsequent development of leukemia. Aplastic anemia generally occurs in subjects while they are still exposed to high concentrations of benzene; leukemia may occur at the same time or shortly after cessation of exposure. Leukemia often develops in subjects with benzene-induced hyporegenerative anemia or pancytopenia of long standing and represents the acute terminal stage of the disease. Approximately one patient in 60 with benzene-induced pancytopenia or aplastic anemia and one patient in 10 with unremitting, progressive marrow failure who survive beyond 1 year develop within the next several years one of the forms of acute nonlymphocytic leukemia. One of these—acute lymphoblastic leukemia—is disproportionately prevalent, constituting between 20% and 50% of all cases of benzene-induced ANLL.

Clinical Findings

A. Symptoms and Signs:

1. Radiation–As noted above, 300–400 cGy of whole body radiation is lethal in humans. Sublethal exposures will cause symptoms of nausea and vomiting, after which bone marrow suppression occurs. Thrombocytopenia, anemia, and neutropenia will develop, with their attendant symptoms. The development of leukemia occurs after a delay of 8–18 years after the onset of exposure. With the development of CML, the patient exhibits pallor, weakness, sternal tenderness, fever, purpura, skin nodules, or retinal hemorrhages. Gum bleeding after dental procedures or major ecchymoses after minor trauma may be seen. The symptoms of acute leukemia, which may also develop after radiation exposure, are described below.

2. Benzene–Acute exposure to benzene may result in headache, dizziness, and vertigo. Chronically, there is inhibition of marrow cell proliferation, and symptoms appear as circulating marrow progeny decrease. A decrease in hematocrit results in pallor, shortness of breath, and weakness. Thrombocytopenia leads to the appearance of petechiae and purpura. Infection and painful mouth occur secondary to decrease in numbers of neutrophils. Leukemia may

present with general complaints such as weakness, malaise, anorexia, and fever as well as enlargement of the liver, spleen, and lymph nodes.

B. Laboratory Findings:

1. Radiation–Most cases of CML present with the well-recognized hematologic characteristics of granulocytic hyperplasia in the bone marrow, peripheral myeloid leukocytosis, thrombocytosis, anemia, and basophilia. Granulocytic leukocytosis is the fundamental abnormality, averaging 200,000/μL, with a range of 15,000–600,000/μL. The bone marrow is hypercellular, with granulocytic hyperplasia and, often, increased numbers of megakaryocytes. The presence of the Philadelphia chromosome on chromosomal analysis is associated with a better prognosis.

Other patients may have findings of acute leukemia, with pancytopenia of normal blood cells and circulating leukemic cells, some of which may contain Auer rods. Their bone marrow may be either hypo- or hypercellular, with 10% or more leukemic blast cells and a decrease in megakaryocytes and granulocyte and red cell precursors.

2. Benzene–Patients with benzene toxicity usually present with pancytopenia, but any combination of anemia, thrombocytopenia, or leukopenia may occur. The anemia is usually normochromic and normocytic, with normal red cell morphology. White cell morphology is also initially normal, with a decrease in neutrophils and an increase in the percentage of mononuclear cells. There will be an inappropriately low reticulocyte count, and hemolytic parameters such as bilirubin and LDH will be normal. With the development of acute leukemia, the peripheral smear will show immature or abnormal cells. Most patients have blast cells circulating at the time of diagnosis, and some of these may contain Auer rods. Bone marrow examination will be hypocellular, with no evidence of fibrosis. With the development of leukemia, the marrow will be positive for leukemic blast cells, with massive proliferation of primitive cells in the presence of leukopenia.

Prevention

A. Radiation: X-rays were discovered by Roentgen in 1895, and by 1902 the basic principles of radiation protection had already been elaborated: to minimize dose by reducing the time of exposure and by using shielding and distance. Since 1928, the International Council on Radiation Protection (ICRP) and the National Council on Radiation Protection have defined acceptable levels of radiation exposure for workers. The concept of dose equivalent or "rem" (roentgen equivalent man) is used because the same amounts of absorbed radiation energy can produce different levels of damage, depending on the type of radiation present. Acceptable exposures for different organs vary, with maximum permissible dose ranging from 5 rems of whole body exposure to 30 rems of skin or bone exposure.

B. Benzene: Regulated standards of benzene

began in 1926, and in 1974 NIOSH published a recommended standard based on the evidence for hematologic changes: 10 ppm as an 8-hour time-weighted average (TWA), with a ceiling limit of 25 ppm. In 1977, OSHA issued an emergency standard decreasing the acceptable 8-hour TWA exposure to 1 ppm after a study showing excess deaths due to leukemia in benzene-exposed workers, but these recommendations as a permanent standard have not been upheld. This remains an area of controversy in that with current allowable levels the lifetime incidence of excess leukemia for exposed workers is estimated to be from 1.4 to 15.2%. Periodic hematologic screening is believed to be mandatory in populations exposed to increased atmospheric levels of benzene, with both removal from the work environment and further hematologic testing indicated for any aberrations found.

Treatment & Prognosis

With excess exposure or signs of toxicity in workers exposed to either radiation or benzene, removal from the offending environment is the first priority. Benzene-induced aplastic anemia is treated like any pancytopenia, ie, with supportive care in the form of transfusions, infection precautions, etc. The outcome is similar to that of other aplastic anemias, with a 5-year survival rate of 30%. Half of deaths occur in the first 6 months. Bone marrow transplantation is a promising form of therapy in some patients.

There have been major recent advances in the treatment of acute leukemias with the use of combination chemotherapy. ANLL is most successfully treated with an induction protocol consisting of daunorubicin and cytarabine, resulting in a 60% complete response in adults. The median duration of remission in responders is 1–1½ years, and 25% of all complete responders are well at 4–5 years. In chronic granulocytic leukemia, survival averages 2–3 years from the date of diagnosis, and therapy has little effect on survival. Treatment does reduce fatigue and relieves other symptoms. Treatment with alkylating agents—usually busulfan—often results in clinical remission of the disease, and repeated courses are given as the disease recurs. Terminally, many patients develop an acute leukemialike course, with survival thereafter 6 months or less.

HEPATIC ANGIOSARCOMA

Essentials of Diagnosis

- Major exposure to vinyl chloride.
- Right upper quadrant abdominal pain, weight loss.
- Hepatomegaly on physical examination.
- Diagnosis by hepatic arteriogram and open liver biopsy.

General Considerations

Angiosarcoma of the liver is a rare tumor, but its epidemiologic links to vinyl chloride, Thorotrast (thorium dioxide), and arsenic have been studied extensively and have provided valuable insights into other occupational cancers. It occurs most commonly in middle-aged men, with a male-to-female ratio of 4:1. The mean age at presentation is 53. Characteristic features of the disease include a long period of asymptomatic laboratory abnormalities, difficulty in diagnosis, and poor response to treatment.

Etiology

Vinyl chloride is the raw material with which the common plastic polyvinyl chloride is made, and—as is true of many other industrial products—was initially thought to be harmless. In 1974, several cases of angiosarcoma of the liver were reported in men in Louisville, Kentucky, who were all workers at a local industrial plant that polymerized vinyl chloride. By 1981, ten cases of hepatic angiosarcoma were identified among 1855 employees over 35 years of age, with no other cases of angiosarcoma identified in the Louisville area. In one review of 20 patients with angiosarcoma of the liver after vinyl chloride exposure, the mean time from first exposure to development of tumor was 19 years, with a range of 11–37 years. In addition to the Louisville experience, other patients with this cancer from plants elsewhere producing vinyl chloride have been noted. Similar hepatic lesions in experimental animals exposed to high concentrations of vinyl chloride have also been observed.

Although the evidence is not as striking, angiosarcoma of the liver has also been associated with arsenical pesticides, arsenic-contaminated wine, and Fowler's solution used medicinally. Methylhydrazine, urethan, diethylnitrosamine, and dimethylnitrosamine have induced angiosarcoma in laboratory animals, but there is no evidence to date that any of these have caused human angiosarcomas.

Pathophysiology

The carcinogenicity of the vinyl chloride monomer is related to the metabolic formation of reactive metabolites. There is an enhanced positive mutagenic response in certain strains of *Salmonella typhimurium* exposed to vinyl chloride monomer metabolized by microsomal enzymes or liver homogenates. Vinyl chloride is deactivated by conjugation with the hepatic nonprotein sulfhydryl compounds glutathione and cystine. It is hoped that further knowledge of metabolism and pharmacokinetics of the vinyl chloride molecule will provide a scientific basis for guidelines concerning tolerable levels of exposure.

The 2 distinctive hepatic lesions seen after exposure to vinyl chloride are a peculiar hepatic fibrosis and angiosarcoma. The hepatic fibrosis is characterized by 3 features: a nonspecific portal fibrosis, capsular and subcapsular fibrosis in a nodular form (the most characteristic lesion), and focal intralobular accumulation of connective tissue fibers. In addition to this pattern of fibrosis seen in all specimens, a focal irregular sinusoidal dilatation is seen. A spectrum of changes occurs with increasing degrees of atypia and proliferation of sinusoidal cells, culminating in progressive multicentric, infiltrative angiosarcoma. The neoplasm is hemorrhagic and cystic and replaces most of the normal tissue. Microscopic examination shows that the angiosarcoma is multicentric, with several structural patterns, including sinusoidal, papillary, and cavernous. Hepatic angiosarcomas caused by Thorotrast and inorganic arsenicals have shown many of the histologic features observed in the evolution of the hepatic angiosarcoma in the vinyl chloride workers.

Clinical Findings

A. Symptoms and Signs: The symptoms of hepatic angiosarcoma are nonspecific, and some patients may be asymptomatic. Abdominal pain is the common symptom, usually found in the right upper quadrant. Fatigue, weakness, and weight loss are seen in 25–50% of patients. The most common physical sign is hepatomegaly, with ascites, jaundice, and splenomegaly seen less often. Other less common physical findings include abdominal mass, tenderness, spider angiomas, and cachexia.

B. Laboratory Findings: A mild anemia is commonly present in these patients, and target cells and schistocytes are occasionally seen. Leukocytosis and thrombocytopenia are seen in about half of the patients. Other abnormalities include prolonged prothrombin time, elevated fibrin split products, and hypofibrinogenemia.

Almost all patients have some abnormality of liver function testing. Most common is elevation of serum alkaline phosphatase. Many patients also exhibit elevated serum AST (SGOT), total serum bilirubin, serum LDH, and serum ALT (SGPT), with decreased serum albumin. In all patients tested in series published to date, tests for alpha-fetoprotein, carcinoembryonic antigen, and hepatitis B antigen have been negative.

C. Imaging: Routine abdominal x-rays and gastrointestinal contrast studies are usually normal. Occasionally, a mass lesion can be seen pushing aside the stomach; esophageal varices are common. Chest x-rays will often show abnormalities at or near the right hemidiaphragm, including elevation of the diaphragm, a right pleural effusion, atelectasis, or pleural masses. Radionuclide liver scans are abnormal in most patients, but the abnormalities can range from distinct filling defects to nonspecific nonhomogeneous uptake (which can be confused with cirrhosis). Splenomegaly may also be seen by radionuclide scan. Hepatic arteriograms can be the most helpful, usually demonstrating normal-sized hepatic arteries that may be displaced by tumor, peripheral tumor stain and puddling during the middle of the arterial phase, and a central area of hypovascularity. Hepatic ultrasound may also demonstrate a hepatic mass.

D. Special Examinations: Definitive diagnosis of angiosarcoma is best made by open liver biopsy. Closed biopsy can be complicated by hemorrhage with this vascular tumor. Because of the difficulty in making the diagnosis and rapid clinical deterioration, over 50% of hepatic angiosarcomas are diagnosed only after death.

E. Screening Tests: Employees as risk of exposure should receive preemployment testing consisting of history and physical examination, chest x-ray, pulmonary function testing, complete blood count, urinalysis, biochemical screening (liver function tests), and liver-spleen scan. After these results are known, patients with splenomegaly are further evaluated with upper gastrointestinal x-rays, hepatic venography and transjugular liver biopsy, and portal vein catheterization. Those with abnormal liver scans or liver biochemical test abnormalities that persist on retesting at 3 weeks undergo selective hepatic arteriography and hepatic venography and transjugular biopsy.

These tests are generally accepted in high-risk populations, but of note are serious drawbacks in using biochemical screening. The principal anatomic lesion in vinyl chloride-associated liver disease is fibrosis with relative sparing of the hepatocyte, so tests of hepatocellular function can be normal. Indocyanine green hepatic uptake is discussed in Chapter 20.

Prevention

Preventive measures for angiosarcoma include new limitations for employee exposure to vinyl chloride. The current USA occupational standard is 1 ppm averaged over any 8-hour period or 5 ppm averaged over 15 minutes or less. Tighter seals on polymerization vats and protective respirators for workers cleaning the vats are also recommended.

Treatment

Partial hepatectomy with intent to cure is possible in only a very limited number of patients because of extensive fibrosis in the uninvolved liver. Hepatic radiation has not been evaluated in a controlled trial. Chemotherapy with doxorubicin, cyclophosphamide, and fluorouracil have resulted in some temporary tumor regression.

Course & Progress

Major complications occurring prior to terminal events are common in these patients and include congestive heart failure secondary to arteriovenous shunts, hemolytic anemia, peripheral platelet destruction, hepatic failure, and hemoperitoneum. The major cause of death is irreversible rapidly progressive hepatic failure. Overall survival is usually measured in months, with the median survival approximately 6 months and only a small percentage of patients surviving 2 years.

LUNG CANCER

Essentials of Diagnosis

- Asbestos, radon, chloromethyl ether exposure.

- Cough, hemoptysis, dyspnea, weight loss.
- Mass lesion, atelectasis, hilar or mediastinal adenopathy on chest x-ray.
- Cytology, bronchoscopic biopsy and brushings, transthoracic needle biopsy, or thoracotomy for diagnosis.

General Considerations

Lung cancer is the leading cause of cancer deaths in many countries, including the USA. About 99,000 men and 51,000 women were estimated to develop lung cancer in 1987. Because of the high fatality rates, the disease accounts for 25% of all cancer deaths, 34% of such deaths in men and 15% in women.

Etiology

Cigarette smoking is the most important risk factor for cancer of the lung. In 1980, cigarette smoking was thought to cause or contribute to nearly 90% of lung cancers. Its relative importance may decline if recent trends toward reduced cigarette consumption and the use of cigarettes with decreased tar and nicotine continue. The proportion of risk attributable to exposures at the workplace is thought to be small but significant, since specific occupational factors could be avoided by appropriate regulatory measures. Furthermore, the effects of some known occupational carcinogens are greatly enhanced by cigarette smoking.

A. Asbestos: Asbestos is the substance generally considered to pose the greatest carcinogenic threat in the workplace. Asbestos-related lung cancer was first reported in 1934, but perhaps the most striking data were presented in 1947 when Britain's Chief Factory Inspector reported that lung cancer was found in 31 (13.2%) of 235 men with asbestosis who died between 1924 and 1946. However, it was not until separate epidemiologic studies were published in 1955 by Doll and also by Breslow that asbestos exposure was indeed recognized as being associated with cancer of the lung. Since then, many studies have documented the increase in lung cancer in workers with prior asbestos exposure, including a landmark study by Selikoff in which he followed 17,800 asbestos workers from 1967 to 1976 and found 486 deaths due to lung cancer (against an expected 105.6 deaths). Lung cancer is a major asbestos-related disease, accounting for 20% of all deaths in asbestos-exposed cohorts. Exposures are usually to mixed forms of asbestos, and all fiber types (chrysotile, amosite, crocidolite, anthophyllite) are thought to increase the risk of lung cancer, though crocidolite may be more dangerous than chrysotile. A latency period of approximately 20 years has been noted before the majority of lung cancer cases are seen. In addition, a dose-response relationship between asbestos exposure and lung cancer has now been established. Asbestos exposure was shown in Selikoff's study to increase the risk of lung cancer 5-fold. Nearly all other investigators have found the risk not to be this high, however. For example, individuals who worked in shipyards during the 1940s are thought to have a risk of lung cancer up to 1.7 times what would have been expected. These risks should be contrasted with the 25-fold increase of lung cancer risk in persons who have been heavy smokers of cigarettes for 20 years. Several studies have also shown evidence that cigarette smokers also exposed to asbestos have an even greater increased risk of developing cancer of the lung. It is still not proved that any other cancer in an individual who has worked with asbestos is actually related to the asbestos exposure.

B. Radon: Another group with a known excess mortality rate from lung cancer is uranium miners. Excesses in pulmonary disease were noted as early as 1879 in the uranium mining towns of Europe, with some cases of tuberculosis and silicosis, but much of it lung cancer. Large-scale mining of uranium began in the USA in 1948 because of the need for uranium in building nuclear weapons. By the 1960s, 20% of deaths in uranium miners in the USA were due to lung disease. Excessive lung cancer in uranium miners is independent of cigarette smoking, though exposure to both is synergistic.

Ores containing uranium include all of its decay products, which form a series of radionuclides one of which is the inert gas radon. Radon diffuses out of the rock into the mine atmosphere, where it decays into radioisotopes of polonium, bismuth, and lead—termed "radon daughters." These radionuclides are found in the air and may be inhaled as free ions or as attachments to dust particles. Epidemiologic studies of workers in United States uranium mines have demonstrated that the risk of lung cancer is proportionate to the cumulative radon daughter exposure. Increased risk of lung cancer has also been found for fluorspar miners, iron ore (hematite) miners, and hard rock miners. In laboratory animals as well, respiratory tumors have been induced by inhaled radon daughter products.

C. Chemicals: Exposure to multiple chemical substances can cause an increase in lung cancers in exposed workers. Among the most important of these are the chloromethyl ethers, which include chloromethyl methyl ether (CMME) and bis(chloromethyl) ether (BCME). Chloromethyl ethers are produced in-house in order to chloromethylate other organic chemicals in the manufacture of ion exchange resins, bactericides, pesticides, dispersing agents, water repellents, solvents for industrial polymerization reactions, and flame-proofing agents. The potential for chloromethyl ethers to cause cancer was first suspected in humans in 1912. In Philadelphia, a cluster of 3 cases of lung cancer occurred among approximately 45 men working in a single building of a large chemical plant. Other studies have confirmed these findings, with evident dose-response relationships. A large proportion of tumors occurred in young men and nonsmokers. Inhalation studies in animals have shown that the chloromethyl ethers produce bronchial epithelial metaplasia and atypia, and both CMME and BCME are carcinogenic, BCME being the much more potent of the two.

Studies of Japanese and German workers in factories that manufactured mustard gas have shown an excess of respiratory cancers. This is consistent with the findings that mustard gas can produce lung tumors in laboratory animals. An increased incidence of lung cancer has been noted in several populations of copper smelter workers exposed to arsenic trioxide. This relationship between arsenic and lung cancer has been observed in several other occupational groups, though experimental animal studies have not been successful to date. Nickel, chromium, and polycyclic aromatic hydrocarbons have all been implicated also in the causation of occupational lung cancer, with some incomplete information available on beryllium, vinyl chloride, and acrylonitrile.

Pathology

The 4 major types of lung cancer are squamous cell (epidermoid) carcinoma, small cell (oat cell) carcinoma, adenocarcinoma, and large cell carcinoma. All histologic types of lung cancer are linked to cigarette smoking. There is no one cell type that is pathognomonic of an occupationally related lung cancer. Recently, a report on workers exposed to chloromethyl ether listed 12 of 13 cases as having small cell carcinoma. Earlier work suggested that the peripheral distribution of the fibers was associated with a higher incidence of adenocarcinomas in this region. This has not been shown to be correct in recent more thorough studies. The lung cancers in asbestos-exposed persons occur equally throughout the lung. In addition, there is no particular type of lung cancer that predominates in the asbestos-exposed individual.

Clinical Findings

A. Symptoms and Signs: The findings in patients with lung cancer may arise secondary to local tumor growth, invasion of nearby structures, regional growth of nodal metastases, or paraneoplastic syndromes. The primary tumor may cause cough, hemoptysis, wheezing, dyspnea, or pneumonitis secondary to obstruction. Tumor spread may cause tracheal obstruction or esophageal compression; and superior vena cava syndrome may result from compression of vascular structures. The peripheral nervous system may be involved, with recurrent laryngeal nerve paralysis (causing hoarseness), sympathetic nerve involvement (Horner's syndrome), or phrenic nerve paralysis. Patients may also present with nonspecific symptoms such as weight loss, anorexia, and fatigue.

B. Laboratory Findings: In approximately 60% of cases, a positive diagnosis can be made on the basis of sputum cytologic examination. Using flexible fiberoptic bronchoscopy, one can visualize approximately 65% of lesions in lung cancer patients, with biopsy and brushings true-positive in approximately 90% of these. Transthoracic fine needle aspiration biopsy with fluoroscopic guidance can also be a useful procedure. If other diagnostic procedures fail to lead to diagnosis, the patient should undergo exploratory thoracotomy.

C. Imaging: The chest x-ray currently offers the greatest possibility for early diagnosis. Findings are related to the tumor cell type, with variation as to central or peripheral location of tumor mass and whether or not regional spread has occurred. Squamous cell cancers are more often located centrally, with associated hilar adenopathy. Adenocarcinoma presents more often as a peripheral nodule with pleural and chest wall involvement, and large cell carcinoma is seen as a large peripheral mass with associated pneumonitis. A central lesion with atelectasis and both hilar and mediastinal adenopathy are common features of small cell carcinoma.

Prevention

Complete avoidance of exposure to the carcinogen is the ultimate goal, but this is not always possible. When practicable, a noncarcinogenic agent should be substituted, but if no appropriate replacement can be found the concentration of the known carcinogen should be limited in the workplace. Adequate ventilation must be assured, and a respirator may be worn. Since tobacco use is known to increase the incidence of lung cancer in occupationally exposed groups, workers should be encouraged to avoid cigarette use, and hiring only nonsmokers for especially hazardous occupations should be considered.

Attempts have been made to lessen the impact of pulmonary cancer by identifying the condition early in the course, thereby perhaps improving cure rates. Serial chest x-rays and sputum cytologic examinations are now recommended by NIOSH and OSHA in high-risk occupational groups. The main problem with this approach is that there is no evidence early detection improves the prognosis for persons with lung cancer. Thus far, serial chest x-rays have been more useful than sputum cytologic examinations in detecting lung cancer.

Treatment & Prognosis

Therapy of occupational lung cancers is no different from treatment for each of the specific cell types of lung cancer that may be seen. Surgical resection is currently the best hope for cure in non-small cell cancer. Unfortunately, most patients do not qualify for a curative surgical procedure, and these patients are treated with chemotherapy or radiotherapy in an attempt to improve palliation, since cures at this stage are rare. Survival is related to both cell type and stage of disease, with squamous cell cancers having the best prognosis. In general, even in patients with localized disease, 5-year survival is the exception rather than the rule. Small cell carcinoma has traditionally had the worst prognosis, with early and widespread metastases, although there have been some encouraging results with chemotherapy in limited disease.

OCCUPATIONAL BLADDER CANCER

Essentials of Diagnosis

- Cigarette smoking a major etiologic factor.
- Occupational links: α- and β-naphthylamine, benzidine.
- Transitional cells on histologic examination.
- Presenting complaints of hematuria and vesical irritability.

General Considerations

Bladder cancer accounts for about 2% of all malignant tumors. The American Cancer Society has estimated that there will be 40,000 new cases of bladder cancer in 1990, with an estimated 11,000 deaths. The male-to-female ratio is 3:1, but the sex incidence is probably secondary to the relationship between bladder cancer and smoking. The incidence of bladder cancer increases with age, with a peak incidence in the seventh decade. The incidence of urinary tract neoplasms is higher in industrialized countries than in the underdeveloped regions and higher in rural than in urban areas.

Etiology

Cigarette smoking appears to be the most important known preventable cause of bladder cancer, with as many as 50% of cases in men and 33% in women attributed to this common habit. The roles of coffee-drinking and the use of artificial sweeteners have also been the objects of scrutiny. Occupations have long been suspect, and it is believed that 20% of all bladder cancers are due to work exposures.

As early as 1895, a Swiss urologist described a high incidence of bladder tumors among aniline dye workers. Large-scale production of aromatic amines as dye intermediates was started in the USA during World War I, and by 1934 the first occupational bladder cancers in the USA were described. Twenty-five cases of bladder tumor were reported in workers exposed to β-naphthylamine or benzidine and 2 cases in workers exposed to α-naphthylamine. A few years later, 58 additional cases were reported from the same plant; β-naphthylamine was reported to induce urinary bladder tumors in dogs; and subcutaneous injections of benzidine induced carcinomas in rats. During the next 3 decades, several studies both in the USA and Great Britain showed an increase in urinary bladder tumors in workers exposed to these chemicals. The latency period between exposure and cancer is quite variable, ranging from 4 to over 40 years, with a mean of 20 years. The duration of exposure necessary to result in cancer may be as low as 133 days.

Occupational categories with a confirmed or strongly suspected increased risk for bladder cancer are dyestuff and chemical manufacturing, pigment and paint manufacturing, cable manufacturing, textile manufacturing (dyeing), leather working, roofing and other activities involving handling of coal tar, the coal tar industry, electrical workers, hairdressers, mechanics, metal workers, cobblers, and rubber workers. Recently, benzene-derived dyes—Direct Blue 6, Direct Black 38, and Direct Brown 95—have been reported to cause cancers resulting from occupational exposures. NIOSH concluded in 1979 that all benzidine-derived dyes should be recognized as potential human carcinogens, and since then virtually all companies in the USA have stopped their manufacture.

Pathogenesis

Most occupation-related urinary tract tumors are thought to be caused by contact with carcinogens in the urine. Because of the concentrating ability of the kidney, the bladder is exposed to higher concentrations of these materials than other body tissues. In addition, this exposure occurs over prolonged periods of time in certain areas of the urinary tract, most notably the bladder trigone area. Most of the proved urinary carcinogens are aromatic amines, which may be inhaled, ingested, or absorbed through the skin. Aromatic amines must be conjugated to sulfates or glucuronic acid in the liver before they can exert their carcinogenic effects. After transport to the kidneys, they are exposed in the urine to the enzyme β-glucuronidase and the optimal pH for its activity, with the result that there is enhanced splitting of the conjugated form and heavy exposure of urinary tract epithelium to hydroxylated carcinogens.

Pathology

Other less common work-related urologic neoplasms include tumors of the renal pelvis, ureter, and urethra—all with the same histologic and etiologic features as bladder tumors. Thus, all 4 types are usually considered together as "lower urinary tract cancers" for epidemiologic purposes. Over 90% of urothelial tumors are of the transitional cell type, approximately 6–8% squamous cell and 2% adenocarcinoma. The tumors may be papillary or flat, in situ or invasive, and are graded according to degree of cellular atypia, nuclear abnormalities, and number of mitotic figures.

Clinical Findings

Although there are no pathognomonic signs or symptoms of bladder cancer, approximately 75% of patients have hematuria, which is usually painless and gross. Thirty percent of patients have vesical irritability alone, with increased frequency, dysuria, urgency, and nocturia. In advanced cases, patients present with symptoms secondary to lymphatic or venous occlusion, such as leg edema.

Urinalysis generally shows red blood cells, and bleeding can be severe enough to cause anemia. Uremia can occur if the bladder tumor has obstructed the ureters as they enter the bladder.

The diagnosis of bladder cancer may be made on the basis of urinary cytologic examination, which has been proposed as a screening tool. Most patients undergo excretory urography, which is useful in ruling out upper tract disease, and may show a filling defect in the bladder. Definitive diagnosis relies on cystoscopy and transurethral biopsy of the suspicious areas.

Bladder carcinoma that has invaded the muscular wall is potentially lethal and may metastasize even before urinary symptoms bring the patient to a physician. Bladder cancer generally spreads by local extension, through lymphatics, or by hematogenous dissemination. Clinical sites of metastatic disease include the pelvic lymph nodes, lungs, bones, and liver (in decreasing order of occurrence). Once the diagnosis has been confirmed by biopsy, a chest x-ray, radionuclide bone scan, and liver and renal function studies should be done. CT scans are extremely useful in staging. Current staging depends on depth of involvement, nodal involvement, and the presence or absence of distant metastases.

Prevention

Prevention of exposure to known carcinogens is the most effective means of preventing occupational urinary tract cancer. On an immediate basis, personal protective equipment can be used, and ultimately the recommended means of control is by engineering methods aimed at zero exposure levels.

One appealing means of control is screening, and the use of urinary cytologic examinations has been suggested for this purpose. Estimates are of 75% sensitivity and 99.9% specificity for this test, which would be used only to screen certain occupations at risk. The gains from screening may be small, however, since there is no evidence that the survival of screen-detected cases is better.

Treatment

Therapy varies with the stage, and current series have relied heavily on operative treatment. Carcinoma in situ can be treated initially with transurethral resection of the malignant areas, followed by a course of intravesical thiotepa. Superficial disease is usually managed by transurethral resection and fulguration but is associated with a high incidence of recurrence that decreases with postoperative instillation of thiotepa. Carefully selected patients with bladder carcinoma may undergo partial cystectomy, but invasive disease usually requires radical cystectomy. The current role of preoperative radiation therapy is controversial. Chemotherapy is reserved for metastatic disease, with cisplatin and methotrexate being the most efficacious single agents. Doxorubicin and vinblastine also demonstrate antitumor activity.

Prognosis

Prognosis varies with the stage of the disease. Patients with superficial disease who are appropriately treated should have excellent 5-year survival expectations, since disease becomes invasive in only one-third of these patients. The 5-year survival rate in patients with documented muscle invasion ranges from 40% to 50%. With local spread of disease in the pelvis, 10–17% of patients survive 5 years, and there are few long-term survivors once visceral metastases have occurred.

CANCERS OF THE HEAD & NECK

Head and neck cancer cases represent 4.5% of the total new cancer cases each year in the USA. Patients present with complaints of difficulty in swallowing and hoarseness. The male-to-female ratio is 3:1 or 4:1, and the usual age at diagnosis is over age 40. There has been no major change in the incidence of head and neck cancer in males and females in the past 3 decades.

The most important etiologic agent for these tumors in general is cigarette smoking, with alcohol and cigarette smoking having additive effects. Occupational carcinogens are discussed below with the specific anatomic types of cancer.

The major forms of head and neck cancer that have been linked to occupational exposures are squamous cell cancers of the nasal cavity and sinuses and laryngeal carcinoma. Other associations include those between ultraviolet radiation exposure in outdoor workers and lip cancer and those between ionizing radiation and salivary gland tumors.

1. CANCER OF THE NASAL CAVITY & SINUSES

Cancers of the nasal cavity and sinuses are relatively rare, accounting for approximately 8 cases per million in the USA per year. This disease is very uncommon in workers under 50, and rates increase with age. Evidence suggests a fairly steady or slightly declining incidence over the years. About half of all malignant neoplasms in this anatomic area are squamous cell in type, with about 10% adenocarcinomas. Other histologic types include lymphoma, adenoid cystic carcinoma, and melanoma.

Etiology

Many different occupational exposures have been linked to cancer of the nasal cavity and paranasal sinuses. These include wood dust, nickel, chromium, mustard gas, and cutting oils. Employment in several industries has also been associated with these cancers, including furniture and shoe manufacturing and coal mining. Furnacemen in the gas, coke, and chemical industries, furnacemen in foundries, and textile workers have also been shown to be at increased risk. The process of manufacturing isopropyl alcohol has been associated with this form of cancer as well and is considered probably due to the dimethyl sulfate used during the process.

A. Wood and Other Organic Dusts: The earliest report that linked cancer of the nose to exposure to wood dust was in 1965, when a laryngologist in

England observed an unusually high incidence of cancer of the nasal cavity and sinuses among workers in the furniture industry in that area. Fifteen of the 20 reported cases were involved in the production of wooden chairs. Woodworkers without carcinoma were also examined, and many exhibited chronic hypertrophic rhinitis, dry atrophic nasal mucosa, or nasal polyps. Since this first report, many studies have shown an increased incidence of carcinoma of the sinonasal area in persons exposed to wood dust. Adenocarcinoma of the ethmoids and middle turbinates are the most frequent cell types encountered in these workers. The exact substance in wood dust responsible for carcinogenesis has not been identified.

An excess of both adenocarcinomas and squamous carcinomas of the nasal sinuses has also been observed among workers in the boot and shoe industry. As in the case of woodworkers, the specific etiologic agent in boot and shoe manufacture is unknown. Dusts involved in the textile industry and flour dusts in bakeries and flour mills have also been linked to sinonasal cancers.

B. Nickel: Both nasal cancer and lung cancer have been linked to occupational nickel exposure. Most studies have been done on nickel refinery workers exposed to complex particulates (insoluble nickel sulfide dust; nickel oxides; soluble nickel sulfate, nitrate, or chloride) and gaseous nickel carbonyl. The mean latency period between exposure and diagnosis of cancer in refinery workers is 20–30 years.

The earliest report of an increased risk of sinonasal carcinoma in nickel refinery workers was in 1932 and pertained to 10 cases occurring in Wales, where a nickel carbonyl process was employed. Studies confirming these findings have subsequently been done in Canada, Norway, Germany, Japan, and the USSR. Clearly, nickel and nickel carbonyl are carcinogenic under experimental conditions, yet epidemiologic evidence points away from the nickel carbonyl process and incriminates exposure to dust from the preliminary processes. Neoplasms in nickel workers occur most frequently in the nose and the ethmoid sinuses, usually of the squamous or anaplastic cell type.

C. Other Occupational Exposures: Tumors of the nasal epithelium and mastoid air cells have been noted in women exposed to radium used for painting dials of watches and in radon chemists. Workers involved in the manufacture of hydrocarbon gas have been noted to have excess cases of cancer of the paranasal sinuses. Chromium is known to cause ulceration and perforation of the nasal septum, and there is an excess risk of sinonasal cancer in workers involved in manufacturing chromate pigments. Mustard gas and isopropyl alcohol have also been linked to excess cancers of the nasal cavity and paranasal sinuses.

Clinical Findings

The earliest symptoms of nasal cavity neoplasms are a low-grade chronic infection, associated with discharge, obstruction, and minor intermittent bleeding. The patient often complains of "sinus trouble" and may have been inappropriately treated with antibiotics for prolonged periods before the true diagnosis was known. Subsequent symptoms depend on the pattern of local growth. Maxillary sinus tumors develop silently when they are confined to the sinus, producing symptoms only with extension outside the walls. With extension into the oral cavity, pain may be referred to the upper teeth. Nasal obstruction and bleeding are common complaints, along with "sinus pain" or "fullness" of the involved antrum. Palpation and observation of the face may show a mass. Ethmoid sinus carcinoma presents initially with mild to moderate sinus aching or pain. A painless mass may present along the inner canthus, and with invasion of the medial orbit, diplopia develops.

In all cases, the patient should have careful inspection and palpation of the facial structures, with attention to the eye and especially the extraocular movements. The nasal and orbital cavities should be examined closely, and a fiberoptic nasoscope is a useful aid in visualizing the posterior and superior nasal cavities and the nasopharynx. Sinoscopy of the maxillary antrum may also be required. Helpful radiologic studies include facial bone or sinus x-ray series and CT scan of the involved areas. Identification of the site of tumor origin is important in determining the treatment plan.

Tumor in the nasal cavity is usually biopsied with a punch forceps. Biopsy of tumor in the maxillary antrum is usually approached with a Caldwell-Luc procedure, which is an incision through the gingivobuccal sulcus opposite the premolars. Biopsy of ethmoid tumors is usually taken from the extension into the nasal cavity. An undiagnosed orbital mass may also be biopsied secondary to incomplete examination of other areas. Frontal sinuses are approached by supraorbital incision and osteotomy.

Surgical therapy is usually indicated because of the frequency of osseous involvement; it involves resection of all gross disease. Any desire for wide margins is tempered by the reluctance to mutilate, and reconstructive and cosmetic surgery using prosthetic devices is often necessary. Radiation therapy is nearly always necessary because the resection margins are often narrow and the neoplasm is frequently of high grade. Chemotherapy is reserved for advanced disease. Prognosis is best for nasal cavity cancers, because they tend to be diagnosed at an early stage. The 5-year survival rate is approximately 30–40% for tumors of the maxillary and ethmoid sinuses and dismal for frontal and sphenoid sinus carcinomas.

2. LARYNGEAL CARCINOMA

Cancer of the larynx represents about 2% of the total cancer risk in the USA. In most areas of the world, there is evidence that cancer of the larynx is increasing in men and, in more developed countries, also among women. This is primarily a disease of older workers—the median age is usually in the sixth or seventh decade. At the time of diagnosis, approximately 60% are localized, 30% show regional spread, and 10% have distant metastases. Laryngeal tumors are classified into 3 groups according to anatomic site of origin, with 40% supraglottic, 59% glottic, and 1% subglottic cancers in the USA. Nearly all are squamous cell carcinomas.

Cancer of the larynx appears to be primarily related to cigarette smoking. Alcohol is less important in the causation of laryngeal cancer than in other tumors of the head and neck. Occupational exposure to asbestos has been suggested as a risk factor for development of this disease, with one retrospective study finding asbestos to be a more important risk factor than either tobacco or alcohol. Most other studies do not support this contention, however. Epidemiologic studies have also linked laryngeal cancer to "strong acid" manufacturing of ethanol and isopropanol, as well as workplace exposures to mustard gas and nickel. The risk from these agents has not been clearly established.

Symptoms of laryngeal carcinoma vary depending on the site of involvement. Any patient who complains of persistent hoarseness, difficulty in swallowing, pain on swallowing, a "lump in the throat," or a change in voice quality should be examined promptly by indirect laryngoscopy. Any limitation of motion or rigidity should be noted, and direct laryngoscopy with biopsy of suspicious lesions is necessary. Lateral soft tissue radiographs of the neck and CT scanning are also useful, especially to delineate extent of disease.

The treatment plan must include preservation of the patient's life and voice. There has been an increasing tendency to use more limited surgical procedures plus radiation therapy, or radiation therapy alone. For failures of conservative therapy or deeply infiltrative tumors, total laryngectomy is required, necessitating tracheostomy and loss of normal voice. Because of their earlier symptoms of hoarseness, true vocal cord tumors are detected early and carry the best prognosis; localized disease in this area has a 90% five-year survival rate.

REFERENCES

General

Alderson MR: *Occupational Cancer.* Butterworths, 1986.

Casciato D (editor): *Manual of Clinical Oncology.* Little, Brown, 1988.

DeVita VT, Hellman S, Rosenberg S (editors): *Cancer: Principles and Practice of Oncology,* 3rd ed. Lippincott, 1989.

Schottenfeld D: Chronic disease in the workplace and environment: Cancer. *Arch Environ Health* 1984; **39**:150.

Mesothelioma

Aisner J, Wiernik PH: Malignant mesothelioma: Current status and future prospects. *Chest* 1978;**74**:438.

Antman K, Aisner J (editors): *Asbestos-Related Malignancy.* Grune & Stratton, 1986.

Craighead JE, Mossman BT: The pathogenesis of asbestos-associated diseases. *N Engl J Med* 1982; **306**:1446.

Rom WN, Lockey JE: Diffuse malignant mesothelioma: A review. *West J Med* 1982;**137**:548.

Selikoff IJ: Health hazards of asbestos exposure. *Ann NY Acad Sci* 1979;**330**:1.

Skin Cancer

Adams RM (editor): *Occupational Skin Disease.* Saunders, 1989.

Alderson MR (editor): *Occupational Cancer.* Butterworths, 1986.

Emmett EA: Occupational skin cancers. *State Art Rev Occup Med* 1987;**2**:165.

Leukemia

Caldwell GG, Kelley DB, Heath CW Jr: Leukemia among participants in military maneuvers at a nuclear bomb test: A preliminary report. *JAMA* 1980; **244**:1575.

Checkoway H et al: An evaluation of the associations of leukemia and rubber industry solvent exposures. *Am J Ind Med* 1984;**5**:239.

Kaplan SD: Update of a mortality study of workers in petroleum refineries. *J Occup Med* 1986;**28**:514.

Maher KV, DeFonso LR: Respiratory cancer among chloromethyl ether workers. *JNCI* 1987;**78**:839.

Rinsky RA et al: Benzene and leukemia: An epidemiologic risk assessment. *N Engl J Med* 1987;**316**:1044.

Ritenour ER: Health effects of low-level radiation: Carcinogenesis, teratogenesis, and mutagenesis. *Semin Nucl Med* 1986;**16**:106.

Upton AC: Hiroshima and Nagasaki: Forty years later. *Am J Ind Med* 1984;**6**:75.

Wongsrichanalai C, Delzell E, Cole P: Mortality from leukemia and other diseases among workers at a petroleum refinery. *J Occup Med* 1989;**31**:106.

Hepatic Angiosarcoma

Dannaher CL, Tamburro CH, Yam LT: Occupational carcinogenesis: The Louisville experience with vinyl chloride-associated hepatic angiosarcoma. *Am J Med* 1981;**70**:279.

Doll R: Effects of exposure to vinyl chloride: An assessment of the evidence. *Scand J Work Environ Health* 1988;**14**:61.

Locker GY et al: The clinical features of hepatic angiosarcoma: A report of four cases and a review of the English literature. *Medicine* 1979;**58**:48.

Lung Cancer

Alderson MR: *Occupational Cancer.* Butterworths, 1986.

Antman K, Aisner J (editors): *Asbestos-Related Malignancy.* Grune & Stratton, 1986.

Axelson O et al: Indoor radon exposure and active and passive smoking in relation to the occurrence of lung cancer. *Scand J Work Environ Health* 1988;**14**:286.

Easton DF, Peto J, Doll R: Cancers of the respiratory tract in mustard gas workers. *Br J Ind Med* 1988;**45**:652.

Morgan WK, Seaton A (editors): *Occupational Lung Disease,* 2nd ed. Saunders, 1984.

Selikoff IJ, Hammond EC, Seidman H: Mortality experience of insulation workers in the Unites States and Canada, 1943–1976. *Ann NY Acad Sci* 1979;**330**:91.

Bladder Cancer

Morrison AS: Advances in the etiology of urothelial cancer. *Urol Clin North Am* 1984;**11**:557.

Schulte PA et al: Occupational cancer of the urinary tract. *State Art Rev Occup Med* 1987;**2**:85.

Ward E et al: Bladder tumors in two young males occupationally exposed to MBOCA. *Am J Ind Med* 1988;**14**: 267.

Yamaguchi N et al: Periodic urine cytology surveillance of bladder tumor incidence in dyestuff workers. *Am J Ind Med* 1982;**3**:139.

Head & Sinuses

Doll R, Mathews JD, Morgan LG: Cancers of the lung and nasal sinuses in nickel workers: A reassessment of the period of risk. *Br J Ind Med* 1977;**34**:102.

Ellingwood KE, Million RR: Cancer of the nasal cavity and ethmoid/sphenoid sinuses. *Cancer* 1979;**43**:1517.

Kessler E, Brandt-Rauf PW: Occupational cancers of the brain and bone. *State Art Rev Occup Med* 1987;**2**:155.

Wills JH: Nasal carcinoma in woodworkers: A review. *J Occup Med* 1982;**24**:526.

Occupational Skin Disorders

Occupational Skin Disorders   17

James R. Nethercott, MD

Work-related dermatoses accounted for 20% of all cases of occupational disease in the USA in 1988 (data from US Department of Labor). The proportion varies widely among the States. Skin disease accounts for the majority of compensated occupational disease claims in some States; in California and Florida, for example, contact dermatitis due to plants is common in agricultural workers.

Contact dermatitis is the most common skin disorder reported as an occupational disease. Four-fifths of cases are associated with exposure to irritating chemicals such as solvents, cutting oils, detergents, alkalies, and acids. Ultraviolet light may react with certain chemicals (eg, coal tar, creosote) to cause irritant contact dermatitis at sites of exposure to the chemical and light. One-fifth of cases can be related to a specific contact sensitizer such as epoxy resins, chromium, plant resins, and many others.

Chemical burns due to exposure to strong irritants occur relatively frequently. Depigmentation of the skin resembling vitiligo occurs rarely and may be related to a number of specific chemicals that induce the change through skin contact. Acne and folliculitis may result from skin contact with oils and greases. A distinct entity called chloracne—different from teenage acne—may be induced by exposure to a number of chlorinated hydrocarbons (eg, polybrominated biphenyls, polychlorinated biphenyls, dioxins).

Physical injury may cause calluses at sites of repeated trauma. Such "occupation marks" are typical of a number of types of work (eg, calluses on the necks of violinists). Hand-arm vibration, as occurs in chain saw operators, grinding machine operators, and underground mine rock drillers, may result in vasospastic disease in the hands—vibration-induced white finger disease—in workers with prolonged or severe exposure.

Neoplastic skin disease may also be work-related, but the incidence is unknown since few cases are submitted to compensation authorities, the reporting of skin cancers to cancer registries is incomplete, and death from skin cancer is unusual.

Preventive measures include personal protective equipment (gloves, boots, etc), engineering controls, worker education, and administrative controls such as rotation of workers at a given task to reduce skin exposure. These measures are most helpful in preventing chemical burns, allergic contact dermatitis, vibration-induced disease, and certain work-aggravated diseases (eg, psoriasis, lichen planus, vitiligo).

Chronic irritant contact dermatitis (see below) is poorly understood, and present methods of protection are unsatisfactory.

ACUTE IRRITANT CONTACT DERMATITIS

Essentials of Diagnosis

- History of exposure to a severe cutaneous irritant such as an acid, alkali, or solvent under occlusion.
- Damage to the skin in precise sites of contact and a sharply delineated border from unaffected skin.
- Erythema or vesiculation acutely followed by sloughing of damaged skin.
- May require combination of a contactant and ultraviolet light to induce the injury: photo-irritant contact dermatitis.

General Considerations

Acid burns are characterized by immediate damage and early onset of resolution; alkali burns tend to cause injury over a number of hours subsequent to contact and thus the initial extent of the injury may underestimate the final outcome. (See fuller discussions in Chapter 26.)

Phototoxic contact dermatitis is a specific type of chemical burn in which the irritant causing the injury is capable of doing so only when it is activated by ultraviolet light. Brushing up against the plant or handling the offending phototoxic chemical results in deposition of phototoxin on the skin. Sun exposure then induces an immediate response characterized by redness and swelling, often with vesicle or bulla formation. The eruption resolves in 48–72 hours, often leaving brown discoloration (postinflammatory hyperpigmentation) that may persist for months to years. Contact phytophotodermatitis tends to occur in a linear pattern. Tar products such as creosote and plant resins containing psoralens are the most common causes. Table 17–1 outlines the causes and occupational groups that may be affected by phototoxic contact dermatitis.

Clinical Findings
A. Symptoms and Signs: Pain at the site of injury often has a burning quality. The skin becomes erythematous, and vesicles or bullae may form. In

Table 17–1. Occupational phototoxic dermatitis: Causes and workers affected.

Agent	Occupation
Tars, creosote	Construction workers, roofers, railway workers
Queen Anne's lace, wild carrot	Forestry workers, clean-up workers, utility workers
Celery, parsnips, citrus fruits	Agricultural workers, grocery clerks
Psoralens, sulfonamides	Pharmaceutical workers
Oil of bergamot	Cosmetics industry workers

severe cases, the skin may become white and non-blanching, whereupon it slowly turns black and develops a distinct border distinguishing it from surrounding normal skin.

For chemicals that are only moderately irritating, burns may occur only at sites of contact under occlusion (eg, under a rubber glove or a hat band) or only in sensitive areas (eg, eyelids, genitals). Breaks in the skin may enhance the irritant effect, and such sites may be the most severely injured or the only sites of injury. Friction enhances the irritant effect also, as does low humidity or high temperature in the work area. Table 17–2 lists possible contributing factors.

The acute injury resolves with sloughing of the damaged tissue. This may be as mild as peeling of the outer epidermis or as severe as marginating and sloughing of necrobiotic tissue down to underlying

Table 17–2. Factors contributing to the development of cutaneous irritation.*

Factors related to the substance
  Chemical class
  pH
  Solubility in water and in fats
  Detergent action
  Physical state: gas, volatile liquid, heavy liquid, semisolid, solid
  Concentration (amount, contact with skin)
Host factors
  General: age, sex, race, genetic background
  Dryness
  Sweating
  Pigmentation
  Presence of hair
  Sebaceous activity
  Concurrent and preexisting skin disease
  Pruritogenic threshold
Environmental factors
  Temperature: hot, cold
  Humidity and moisture
Other factors
  Surface area affected
  Region of skin
  Duration of exposure
  Presence or absence of occlusion
  Friction
  Pressure
  Occlusion
  Lacerations

*Adapted from Adams RM (editor): *Occupational Skin Disease.* Saunders, 1989.

soft tissue. Healing then progresses to yield either (1) no visible evidence of past injury, (2) hypo- or hyperpigmentation, or (3) varying degrees of scarring depending on the depth of injury.

B. Laboratory Findings: Skin biopsy may be called for to distinguish contact injury from some more serious chronic skin disorder. Serum calcium may be low in patients with hydrofluoric acid burns. Patch tests are dangerous and not useful and should not be performed.

Differential Diagnosis

Physical injury such as that due to heat and electrical current may cause findings similar to those associated with chemical burns, but the history of the injury allows easy differentiation. Artifactual dermatitis may be induced by this mechanism, and the location and shape (ie, square or triangular blisters) of the burn combined with the history and the histologic findings are often helpful in making this diagnosis.

Prevention

Workers must be educated about the hazards of skin contact with irritant chemicals. Signs must be placed in the workplace identifying hazards. Enclosure of hazardous processes is indicated if exposure cannot be minimized.

Personal protective equipment must be provided and its use monitored and enforced. Table 17–3 sets forth appropriate types of gloves for handling different classes of cutaneous irritants for short periods.

Treatment

A. Emergency Treatment: Remove irritant as soon as possible with copious amounts of water or saline (if water-soluble) or with mineral oil or olive oil (if hydrophobic).

B. Medical Measures:

1. Local therapy–

a. Wet dressings–Apply cool wet compresses of saline solution or 10% aluminum acetate (Burow's) solution, using sterile 4×4 compresses. The compresses should be kept wet and changed every 5–10 minutes for the first 12 hours, then less often over the next 12–24 hours. After the first day, cool soaks should be applied for 30 minutes 3 times a day and changed every 5–10 minutes during that time. This technique will remove traces of the irritant, ease discomfort, dry the site by precipitating serum on the surface, and debride the area.

b. Protective agents–In the first 48 hours, protectives such as petrolatum USP or eucerin USP should be used to cover the affected skin between soaks. After the first 24 hours, hydrocortisone 1% in petrolatum may be applied after soaks.

2. Antibiotic therapy–Bacterial culture and antibiotic sensitivity tests should be started prior to initiation of antibiotic therapy. Appropriate changes in treatment should be made based on the results of these tests.

Table 17–3. Suitability of gloves for use when handling specific irritant chemicals. (After Wilkinson.)

Irritant	Preferable Gloves	Unsuitable Gloves
Inorganic acids	Heavy rubber, neoprene, polyvinyl chloride	Light rubber
Organic acids	Heavy rubber, neoprene, nitrile	Light rubber
Aliphatic solvents	Neoprene, nitrile	Rubber
Aromatic solvents	Nitrile	Most other types
Chlorinated solvents	Nitrile	Most other types
Vegetable oils	Neoprene, nitrile, polyvinyl chloride	Light rubber
Soaps and detergents	Heavy rubber, neoprene, polyvinyl chloride	Light and medium rubber

a. Antibiotic ointments–Topical antibiotic ointments, eg, polymyxin B-bacitracin or bacitracin alone, may be indicated (in place of petrolatum, etc, above) if secondary bacterial infection is thought to be a risk.

b. Systemic antibiotics–If pyoderma develops at the burn site or if contamination of the wound strongly suggests that superimposed bacterial infection is likely, oral or intravenous antibiotics may be needed.

(1) Oral antibiotics–Give cloxacillin, 250–500 mg orally every 6 hours; cephalexin, 250–1000 mg orally every 6 hours; or clindamycin, 150–450 mg orally every 6 hours.

(2) Intravenous antibiotics–Give cloxacillin, 250–500 mg intravenously every 6 hours; cephalothin sodium, 500–1000 mg intravenously every 6 hours; or clindamycin in doses ranging from 900 mg intravenously daily in 2 doses up to 4800 mg intravenously daily in 4 doses.

3. Casting–In artifactual (ie, self-inflicted) dermatitis, protection of the affected site by application of an Unna's paste cast is useful both as treatment and for diagnosis. A cast should not be applied over an infected lesion. Resolution of lesions where access to the skin is prevented is often an important clue that dermatitis has been self-inflicted.

C. Surgical Treatment: If tissue becomes necrotic, careful debridement under local or general anesthesia is indicated to forestall secondary infection and expedite healing. Depending on the size of the tissue defect, full- or split-thickness skin grafting may be indicated. Skin grafting may be necessary even where surgical debridement has not been performed if healing is to occur in a reasonable time.

D. Pain Management: Hydrofluoric acid burns—like other severe chemical burns—are painful. After necrotic tissue and bullae have been debrided following hydrofluoric acid burns, relief can be achieved by soaking or with continuous compresses—for at least

2 hours, changed every 2 minutes—of either benzethonium chloride (Phemerol), 1.2% aqueous solution, or benzalkonium chloride (Zephiran), 0.13% aqueous solution. Gauze soaking with iced magnesium sulfate is recommended by some authorities. Treatment is discontinued after 2 hours if pain subsides but may be repeated for 2 hours if pain recurs. A total of 4–6 hours of therapy is often needed before pain is totally relieved.

If soaking or compresses are not effective, local injection of 10% aqueous solution of calcium gluconate (not calcium chloride) into, under, and around the burned area is indicated. The amount injected should not exceed 0.5 mL per square centimeter of skin surface, and a small-gauge needle (27–30 gauge) should be used. The injection should be continued until pain relief occurs as a sign of adequate infiltration.

Subungual hydrofluoric acid requires removal of the affected nail unless immersion as outlined above results in relief of pain. If the burned area is greater than 4 cm^2, the patient should be watched closely for signs of hypocalcemia. Cardiac monitoring is indicated as well as measurement of blood and urine calcium levels. Administration of calcium gluconate intravenously may be necessary to prevent toxic effects and must be titrated to the measured calcium levels.

Prognosis

The prognosis depends on the severity of the burn. Mild injury may lead to no sequelae. Severe injury may lead to marked scarring, disfigurement, and disability. Relatively limited hydrofluoric acid burns may be fatal even with immediate attention to systemic intoxication.

CHRONIC IRRITANT CONTACT DERMATITIS

Essentials of Diagnosis

- Relatively long period of exposure to a mildly irritating chemical.
- Skin response is characterized by erythema, scaling, fissuring, and pruritus. Affected skin is not clearly delineated from adjacent normal skin.
- Improvement—though often not complete remission—occurs with avoidance of exposure to the irritant(s).
- Individuals with a personal or family history of atopy (hay fever, asthma, atopic eczema) are more likely to be affected.
- Work history provides evidence of exposure to a known irritant associated with the development of contact dermatitis (eg, solvents, cutting oils).

General Considerations

Chronic irritant contact dermatitis is the most common occupational skin disease. Workers appear to experience a change in the irritability of their skin after weeks or even years of exposure to a mild irritant (eg, detergent, soap, cutting oil, solvent). The disorder often develops gradually. Once the eruption becomes severe enough for the worker to seek treatment, it tends to persist. Though many industrial workers experience desiccation or "chapping" of the skin, the disorder that leads to disability appears to be different. It is more severe and persists to a varying degree after further irritant exposure ends. Affected workers often report that manual work associated with physical—not chemical—injury will exacerbate the process. Wearing occlusive clothing (eg, gloves), friction, skin abrasion, heat, sweating, and low ambient humidity all tend to predispose to the development of irritant contact dermatitis. Some workers eventually develop relative resistance to irritant exposure and improve while continuing to work with irritants—a phenomenon called "nonspecific hardening."

Clinical Findings

A. Symptoms and Signs: The worker who has had skin irritation for weeks to years presents with complaints of pruritus and often pain due to fissures that develop in the affected areas. Erythematous scaling patches with indistinct borders develop on exposed skin, and the most sensitive skin areas are usually most affected (eg, dorsal hands more than palms). Nail growth may be affected if the eponychial skin is inflamed, resulting in transverse ridging of the nails.

B. Laboratory Findings: Skin biopsy reveals a lymphocytic perivascular infiltrate in the dermis with exocytosis of lymphocytes into the epidermis. The epidermis shows parakeratosis and spongiosis. Intraepidermal vesicles may be present. The histologic picture is similar to that of allergic contact dermatitis or endogenous forms of eczematous dermatitis.

Patch tests are helpful only in excluding allergens in the worker's environment as the cause of the process, because allergic and chronic irritant contact dermatitis may be clinically indistinguishable.

Differential Diagnosis

Differentiation from allergic contact dermatitis may not be possible on morphologic grounds or on histologic examination. Positive patch tests may point to a diagnosis of allergic contact dermatitis, but the relevance of such tests must always be carefully considered.

Atopic eczema may mimic chronic irritant dermatitis. The presence of erythematous, lichenified, scaly patches in the antecubital and popliteal fossae, lichenification of the skin of the eyelids, dry skin, and a personal or family history of atopy may help make the diagnosis of atopic eczema.

Dyshidrotic eczema is a common idiopathic dermatitis that involves the palms and soles, especially the lateral borders of the fingers and toes. It is characterized by eruption of deep-seated small vesicles on the affected skin which are not typical of chronic irritant contact dermatitis. It does not tend to involve the dorsal surfaces of the hands and feet. Often aggravated by exposure to irritants, as is atopic dermatitis, dyshidrosis may lead the worker to conclude that the problem is work-induced rather than work-aggravated. Allergic contact dermatitis due to metals (eg, chrome, nickel) may cause dermatitis that mimics dyshidrotic eczema.

Nummular dermatitis is characterized by edematous, erythematous, vesicular, round patches, 0.5–2 cm in diameter, on the extremities, usually in women. It may be exacerbated by workplace exposure to irritants.

Prevention

Workers with a personal history of atopic eczema (but not mucosal allergic disease) are at greater risk of developing chronic irritative contact dermatitis and should be so advised. Proper attention should be paid to the use of personal protective equipment and engineering controls to limit skin contact with irritants. Our lack of a clear understanding of the mechanism of this disease has meant that further modification of risk is not yet possible.

Treatment

Topical corticosteroid therapy should be chosen according to the severity of the dermatitis: (1) for mild disease, use hydrocortisone 1% cream; (2) for moderate disease, give betamethasone (Valisone) 0.1% cream or fluocinolone acetonide (Synalar) 0.025% cream; and (3) for severe disease, give betamethasone diproprionate 0.05% cream (Diprosone), halcinonide 0.1% cream (Halog), or clobetasol propionate (Temovate) 0.05% cream. These preparations should be applied 3 times daily and as necessary for pruritus. Ointments may be used if the skin is dry and fissured.

Protection of the hands as much as possible from exposure to workplace and household irritants is essential. Personal protective equipment and emollient creams to prevent desiccation and protect the skin are indicated. The use of mild soaps or soap substitutes for skin cleansing is advisable.

The practitioner must set realistic expectations for the results of therapy at the outset. The disorder is likely to improve but not fully resolve, and the worker should be told this at the first visit. Advice to leave the job should be given only if the worker is unable to continue in spite of intensive efforts on the part of the doctor to modify the process with treatment.

Prognosis

The prognosis is guarded, with many affected workers likely to continue to have dermatitis for many years after the onset of the process. Most continue to function, and in any case a change in occupation often fails to be followed by improvement.

ALLERGIC CONTACT DERMATITIS

Essentials of Diagnosis

- Often an acute vesicular dermatitis at definite sites of contact with the allergen.
- May mimic chronic irritant contact dermatitis or constitutional dermatitis (eg, dyshidrotic eczema, nummular eczema), but established exposure to the allergen and a positive patch test allows differentiation.
- Positive patch tests.
- The work history often identifies exposure to a known cause of cutaneous allergy (eg, chromium, epoxy resin, formaldehyde, *Rhus* oleoresin).
- Occurs at sites of light exposure if photoallergic in origin.
- Occurs at sites uncovered by clothing if contactant is airborne.
- Linear lesions are typical of plant dermatitis.
- A generalized maculopapular eruption (id reaction) may occur if the site of contact dermatitis is severely inflamed.

General Considerations

After a latent period of about 2 weeks following exposure to the sensitizing chemical—which binds to a protein component in the skin to become a complete antigen—the body develops a cell-mediated immune response. Subsequent reexposure leads to a lymphocyte-mediated inflammatory reaction in the skin associated with development of edema of the epidermis with collection of fluid between epidermal cells (spongiosis) and development of vesicles or even bullae. This response is specific for the given allergen, though cross-reactions to chemically similar substances occasionally occur. The immune response, once acquired, tends to be permanent. Occasionally, the individual will acquire specific immune tolerance—called "specific hardening." The immune recognition may eventually be lost if there is no further exposure. Much less exposure is required to elicit this allergic response than is usually necessary for initial induction of the immune process.

Allergic contact dermatitis accounts for approximately 20% of workers who develop occupational contact dermatitis. There are many causes, as outlined in Table 17–4.

Clinical Findings

A. Symptoms and Signs: The eruption occurs at sites of contact but may be more pronounced at sites of sensitive skin (eg, eyelids, genitals). Pruritus is characteristic. Erythematous scaling patches with indistinct borders are typical. Vesicles and bullae may occur with severe responses. Linear lesions with vesicles are characteristic of dermatitis due to plant oleoresins (eg, poison ivy).

A generalized morbilliform reaction called autosensitization dermatitis or "id" reaction may occur if the primary site of contact is severely inflamed.

Photoallergic responses occur at sites of contact combined with exposure to light. Light that passes through window glass (ie, wavelengths > 320 nm) acts synergistically with the contactant to elicit the allergic response. Sparing of the skin of the upper eyelids and under the chin—sites with less light exposure—is characteristic of photoallergic and photoirritant contact dermatitis.

If the contactant is airborne (eg, ragweed oleoresin), the dermatitis will occur at exposed sites. Lack of sparing as seen in photoallergic contact dermatitis differentiates airborne contact dermatitis from these. Once sensitized by contact, oral ingestion or even inhalation of the offending allergen may occasionally reproduce the response at sites of previous allergic contact reaction.

B. Laboratory Findings: The histopathologic changes evident are as noted in the section on chronic irritant contact dermatitis (see above). Patch tests are used to determine whether the worker is hypersensitive to a specific agent. When performed in a standard fashion as recommended by the International Contact Dermatitis Group and interpreted cautiously, the method can yield useful information about the presence of a specific immune response to a particular chemical. Industrial chemicals pose a particular problem since the worker may be exposed to a chemical for which no data exist with respect to the concentration that is appropriate for patch testing. In each instance—whether involving a commonly used chemical or an unusual one—the clinician is trying to expose the worker to the chemical in a subirritant concentration under occlusion with a standard method of skin application (eg, A1 test strip, Finn Chamber). The chemical is removed with the appli-

Table 17–4. Common causes of occupational allergic contact dermatitis and typical occupational groups affected.

Causal Agent	Occupational Group
Epoxy resins	Electronics workers, aircraft assembly workers, construction workers, electrical utility workers, painters
Formaldehyde	Embalmers, resin manufacturers, insulation workers, woodworkers
Paraphenylenediamine and related dyes	Hairdressers, rubber workers
Acrylic monomers	Dental technicians, printers, acrylic ink manufacturers
Rubber accelerators (thiurams, mercaptobenzothiazole)	Tire builders, tire repairmen, workers wearing rubber protective clothing
Metals (chromium, nickel, cobalt, platinum)	Cement workers, hairdressers, electronics assemblers
Plants (*Rhus,* chrysanthemums, tulips, exotic woods)	Outdoor workers, florists
Pharmaceuticals (penicillin, neomycin, chlorpromazine, glutaraldehyde)	Veterinarians, health care workers, pharmacists

ance after 48 hours and the site examined. If possible, the site should be examined again at least once more, usually at 96 hours or later. Because in occasional cases a positive response may not be evident for as long as 7 days, the patient should be advised to return for reassessment of the sites if a reaction develops subsequent to the second reading. Reactions developing later than this may represent acquisition of an allergic response that has been induced by the patch test procedure. The presence of an inflammatory response in the skin at the site of exposure—if it persists to 96 hours and is not sharply delineated (which would suggest an irritant reaction)—is evidence of a specific cell-mediated response to the chemical.

Care must be taken in application of the patch test and evaluation of the response. The relevance of a positive response to a workplace exposure should not be assumed but proved. Care must always be exercised in deciding whether to perform such tests as sensitization to the chemical applied even if a standard patch test chemical is used, though the frequency of this occurrence is not well documented. Patch tests should never be used as preemployment screening tests because of the risk of inducing contact allergy to a workplace chemical through the patch test procedure.

Failure to demonstrate a response on patch testing may indicate that ultraviolet (UV) light exposure is required for the suspect chemical to produce a response. Clinical findings may indicate that the process is photoallergic. In such instances, the worker is patch-tested with the suspect photoallergen at 2 sites. One patch test is removed at 24 hours, and the skin is exposed to UV light with a wavelength longer than 320 nm. This may be accomplished with the use of a Kromayer mercury quartz lamp screened with a piece of window glass 3 mm thick. The skin is exposed for approximately 10–15 minutes. The 2 sites (ie, exposed and unexposed to UV) are then examined at 48 and 96 hours. The presence of a response only at the site where UV light exposure occurred confirms the presence of photoallergic contact allergy.

Differential Diagnosis

The differentiation between chronic contact dermatitis and allergic contact dermatitis may be difficult. Positive patch test results of established relevance allow the correct diagnosis to be made.

Chemical burns and severe acute allergic contact reactions may be clinically indistinguishable. History, skin histology, and patch tests should allow differentiation. Confusion and constitutional eczema or psoriasis limited to the palms may cause diagnostic difficulty, but investigation and, in the case of psoriasis, response to specific therapy will allow appropriate diagnosis.

Prevention

Evaluation of the allergenicity of chemicals prior to their use allows implementation of control measures (eg, personal protective equipment, engineering controls).

Treatment

Therapy is similar to that of chronic irritant contact dermatitis (see above). Avoidance of exposure to the allergen may be more effective in terms than is the case with contact irritants. Realistic expectations for the results of therapy should be established early.

The worker often has allergic contact dermatitis superimposed on chronic irritant contact dermatitis or endogenous eczema. The presence of the occupational allergen in the home or the presence of a substance that cross-reacts with it may result in persistence of the dermatitis—as occurs, for example, in workers sensitized to rubber products. Avoidance of the allergen may lead to improvement in the dermatitis by eliminating the immune stimulus to skin inflammation, but it may not result in complete resolution.

Prognosis

If the worker has acute allergic contact dermatitis due to a specific allergen that can be avoided, the prognosis is excellent. If chronic dermatitis has developed, the probable outcome is less satisfactory. Often, though the condition improves, the skin does not become completely normal even with avoidance of exposure to the contactant.

CONTACT URTICARIA

Essentials of Diagnosis

- Edematous, erythematous, pruritic evanescent papules (hives) or extensive lesions (angioedema) at sites of contact.
- Onset of skin reaction within seconds to minutes after exposure.

General Considerations

The disorder may be due to a specific allergen or may result from a pharmacologic response.

A. Immunologic: The process commonly involves a specific IgE-mediated response involving liberation of histamine and other vasoactive substances from mast cells in the skin or mucous membrane. There is a latent period of weeks to years between initial exposure and subsequent response to a specific contactant. In some cases there is evidence of cell-mediated and IgE-mediated immune responses.

B. Nonimmunologic: Certain substances (eg, sodium benzoate) cause a mast cell response, liberating histamine and other vasoactive chemicals, or appear to have a direct effect on vessels in the skin. This response occurs in nearly all exposed persons if the exposure is intense enough. There is no latent period (see above)—the reaction occurs at the initial exposure.

C. Common Occupational Associations With Contact Urticaria: Handlers of small animals are reported to develop contact urticaria when exposed to danders, saliva, and urine. Food handlers have been reported to react to contact with foods, especially shellfish. Hairdressers may react to contact with ammonium persulfate. Platinum-exposed workers may manifest contact urticaria as well as respiratory symptoms on exposure to platinum salts. Pharmaceutical workers are at risk of reacting to antibiotics such as penicillin, cephalosporins, neomycin, streptomycin, and other drugs.

Clinical Findings

A. Symptoms and Signs: Within moments after contact, discrete edematous, erythematous, pruritic plaques and papules (hives) may erupt; or larger areas, such as an entire hand or cheek, may suddenly become swollen, erythematous, and pruritic (angioedema). The lesions last for minutes to hours and then resolve unless there is continuing or repeated exposure.

Skin reactivity to the contactant may be limited to only one area of the skin (eg, the hand). If the person ingests the contactant (eg, peanut oil), sudden swelling of the tongue or epiglottis may lead to a fatal outcome from asphyxiation. If given parenterally (eg, a drug), the contactant may induce anaphylaxis. Inhalation, which may occur in some circumstances (eg, pharmaceutical industry), may cause an asthmatic reaction.

B. Laboratory Findings: Skin biopsy usually is not helpful, since the changes are too subtle to be discerned in most instances. Peripheral blood eosinophilia may be evident with extensive and persistent skin lesions. A significant fall in various pulmonary function parameters (see Chapter 18) may be evident with pulmonary function testing after inhalation exposure. In a few instances, a positive radioallergosorbent test (RAST) may signify the presence of an IgE antibody to a specific allergen (eg, penicillin).

The direct application of the offending substance as an open patch test to uninvolved skin—or to the site of previous development of the urtication—may reproduce the response, thus confirming the diagnosis. Scratch, prick, or intradermal skin testing may be used with certain complex or high-molecular-weight chemicals (eg, penicillin) if development of a wheal and flare occurs, thus confirming hypersensitivity. Conventional patch tests read at 48 hours are not useful. Application of the suspect chemical under occlusion for 20 minutes may be helpful, but this test should be performed only if open patch tests are negative. Because anaphylaxis has been reported in association with skin tests in cases of contact urticaria, equipment for resuscitation must be available.

Differential Diagnosis

Urticaria and angioedema may result from exposure to physical agents such as ultraviolet light (solar urticaria, polymorphous light eruption) or thermal energy (cold urticaria, heat urticaria). Simple trauma to the skin may cause urticaria (dermographism) at the site of injury. Differentiation of contact urticaria from that due to physical agents is usually not difficult based on the lack of history of exposure to a contactant and reproduction of the response after appropriate exposure to the agent.

Prevention

Avoidance of the allergen when a specific cause has been identified prevents recurrence. Personal protective equipment (eg, gloves, aprons) designed to prevent skin exposure or engineering controls may be used to minimize exposure and avoid disease from exposure to nonspecific urticants.

Treatment

In instances of urticaria due to a specific allergen, further exposure should be avoided. For nonspecific contact urticants, exposure must be controlled. Antihistamines (diphenhydramine, 25–50 mg 3 times daily; hydroxyzine, 10–50 mg 3 times daily; terfenadine, 60 mg daily; astemizole, 10 mg daily) are all effective in controlling the process in some individuals. Epinephrine administered intradermally is indicated to control angioedema. Corticosteroid therapy is not indicated either topically or systemically.

Prognosis

The outlook is good. Patients with known hypersensitivity can usually avoid further complaints by assiduous avoidance of the offending sensitizer.

WORK-AGGRAVATED DERMATOSES

Many cutaneous diseases are exacerbated by exposure to irritants in the workplace. For example, workers with eczematous dermatitis who are exposed to irritants or physical injury in the workplace may experience flares of the disease. Similarly, because many skin diseases are aggravated by emotional stress, stressful working conditions may aggravate them.

Papulosquamous diseases such as psoriasis and lichen planus are characterized by the development of new skin lesions at sites of physical or chemical injury—the so-called isomorphic response, or Koebner's phenomenon. Individuals with psoriasis or lichen planus may develop new lesions at sites of physical injury from abrasions or burns. Vitiligo (see below) is without known cause in almost all cases, but patients with vitiligo are predisposed to develop new lesions at sites of physical or chemical injury.

Such diseases present a challenge to the physician because of the work association. Affected workers are understandably inclined to attribute disease entirely to the work exposure. Though some compensation authorities accept certain work-aggravated dermatoses for disability payment, this is certainly not consistent practice. The physician should give the fullest possible explanation so that the worker will understand the relationship between the disease and the job. Counseling with respect to avoidance of cutaneous injury so as to avoid further aggravation of the dermatosis is essential.

OCCUPATIONAL VITILIGO

Essentials of Diagnosis

- Areas of depigmentation only at sites of contact with depigmenting chemicals.

General Considerations

Depigmentation of the skin at the site of contact with a depigmenting chemical usually results from inhibition of melanin biosynthesis. In most instances, cessation of exposure results in slow repigmentation. Allergic contact sensitivity to the depigmenting chemical occasionally occurs, in which event widespread persistent depigmentation may occur outside the areas of original contact. Table 17–5 lists the industrial chemicals known to be associated with work-induced vitiligo. All are antioxidants used in the manufacture of such products as rubber, plastic, and soluble oils.

Clinical Findings

Patchy depigmentation of the skin at sites of contact with the depigmenting agent can be seen more clearly under Wood's light. Depigmentation of the hair may be present.

Differential Diagnosis

Idiopathic and occupational vitiligo may be indistinguishable. The diagnosis of work-related vitiligo is favored by a history of exposure to the agents listed in Table 17–5 followed by resolution after termination of exposure and by the presence of other similarly affected workers. Persistence of the eruption may relate to allergic sensitization to the depigmenting agent.

Other skin disorders characterized by hypopigmentation such as postinflammatory hypopigmentation, tinea versicolor, and pityriasis alba should be considered but these are hypopigmentation rather than depigmentation disorders. This difference is discernible upon examination with Wood's light. In doubtful

Table 17–5. Established causes of occupational vitiligo.

Hydroquinone
Hydroquinone monobenzyl ether
Hydroquinone monomethyl ether
p-Cresol
p-tert-Butyl phenol
p-tert-Amyl phenol
o-Phenyl phenol
o-Benzyl-p-chlorophenol
4-tert-Butyl catechol

cases, skin biopsy will determine whether vitiligo is present.

Prevention

Prevention consists of simple avoidance of exposure to known depigmenting agents.

Treatment

Removal from contact with the depigmenting agent should lead to resolution. Exposure to ultraviolet light will facilitate earlier repigmentation. Oral methoxsalen in combination with long-wave ultraviolet light (wavelengths greater than 320 nm) may be used to hasten repigmentation.

Prognosis

Repigmentation usually occurs over many months. In instances of allergic contact sensitivity to the depigmenting agent, the prognosis is somewhat guarded, and in some cases full repigmentation does not occur.

CHLORACNE

Chloracne is a rare constellation of cutaneous findings that may occur after exposure to certain chlorinated hydrocarbons (eg, chlorinated naphthalenes, azobenzenes, dibenzofurans, dioxin, polychlorinated biphenyls). Exposure is usually occupational, but outbreaks of disease in residential communities have occurred as a result of accidental environmental contamination. Occupational PCB exposure has been associated with the repair and manufacture of transformers containing PCB materials.

Clinical Findings

Affected adults develop comedones, straw-colored cysts, milia, and papules on the face, neck, ear lobes, shoulders, abdomen, genitalia, and legs. Blepharitis with a granular discharge from the eyelid margin is typical. Patches of hyperpigmentation of the skin of the face or torso have been reported in infants. Hepatotoxic changes, porphyria cutanea tarda, peripheral neuropathy, and hypertriglyceridemia may be found.

Differential Diagnosis

Work-associated acne vulgaris may occur as a result of exposure to petroleum products when soiling of the skin results in folliculitis and pustules. Acne vulgaris in a young person may be aggravated by exposure to high temperatures. Table 17–6 summarizes the differences.

Prevention

Avoidance of exposure that might lead to significant absorption of acnegenic chlorinated hydrocarbons is the sole preventive strategy.

Treatment

Resolution occurs slowly once exposure to the

Table 17–6. Differential diagnosis of chloracne. (Adapted from Adams.)

Condition	Age	Sites	Clinical Appearance
Acne vulgaris	Usually 13–26 years	Face, chest, neck, back to waist	Comedones, papules, pustules, cysts, scars
Folliculitis	Any age	Any area under oil-soaked clothing	Black comedones, papules, pustules, melanosis
Chloracne	Any age	Face, especially "crow's feet," neck, ear lobes, shoulders, abdomen, genitalia, legs	Straw-colored cysts, numerous comedones and milia, papules, often pruritic; other systemic effects

offending agent is terminated. Local measures such as use of abrasive cleansers (Pernox, Brasivol) 3 times a day may be of some value. Application of anticomedonal topical agents (benzoyl peroxide gel 2.5–20% at bedtime) may be of benefit.

Prognosis

Eventual improvement after months to years is likely, depending on the causative agent. Hydrocarbons with higher chlorination numbers tend to persist longer in the body and thus cause more persistent disease.

OCCUPATIONAL RAYNAUD'S DISEASE (Vibration-Induced Whitefinger Disease)

Essentials of Diagnosis

- History of exposure to vibratory energy for varying periods depending on the intensity of exposure (eg, chain saws, hand-held hard rock diamond drills, jack hammers).
- Reversible vasospastic change in the fingers on exposure to cold, characterized by blanching, loss of sensation, and reduction in skin temperature.
- No evidence of autoimmune disease or vascular occlusive disease that could account for the findings.

General Considerations

Damage to the microvasculature of the hand by vibration leads to alteration in the control of blood flow in the hand such that cold exposure—and occasionally emotional upset–results in a transient restriction of blood flow in the capillary bed of the fingers. The disorder is usually mild, but severe cases may lead to tissue injury with trophic changes such as ulceration of the skin or even loss of digits. Table 17–7 lists the common occupational causes and typical groups of workers affected.

Clinical Findings

A. Symptoms and Signs: The key to diagnosis is a history of vasospasm of the fingers on cold exposure that can be reproduced by cold stimulation. The worker reports that the fingertips turn white on cold exposure and feel numb. Following exposure, the fingers throb, turn red, and then bluish as blood flow returns. Painful ulceration of the fingertips may occur in severe cases, sometimes necessitating amputation. Peripheral pulses should be normal.

The changes are restricted to extremities exposed to vibration, usually one or both hands. A history of vibration exposure must be sought and carefully documented to establish that the worker has vibration-induced disease rather than idiopathic Raynaud's disease. When doubt exists, accelerometer measurements to establish the intensity and frequency of vibration generated by the suspected tool must be performed.

B. Laboratory Findings: Cold stimulation in a cold water bath will usually reproduce the clinical findings. Changes in 2-point discrimination may be used to document sensory loss with cold stimulation. Using a Doppler device, one can demonstrate reduction in blood flow in the vasculature; and plethysmography confirms a decrease in pulse pressure with cold exposure. Skin temperature measurements reveal an exaggerated fall in temperature after cold exposure which is slow to recover once the exposure ends.

Differential Diagnosis

Differentiation from systemic lupus erythematosus and rheumatoid arthritis, in either of which similar vasospastic changes without trophic skin changes may occur, is based on the lack of other clinical findings (eg, arthritis, photosensitivity, typical skin lesions) and lack of serologic abnormalities.

Scleroderma of the acrosclerotic type and the CREST syndrome are characterized by similar vasospastic findings. In these diseases, much more severe cutaneous changes (eg, telangiectatic mats of the

Table 17–7. Whitefinger disease: Occupational risks.

Equipment	Occupational Category
Chain saw	Lumberers, construction workers
Grinding wheel	Foundry workers, metal workers, auto body repair workers
Jack leg drill	Miners, surveyors
Pneumatic tools	Demolition workers, road construction workers, auto mechanics

palms, hidebinding, and loss of pulp of the fingers) as well as serologic abnormalities are present.

A cervical rib may cause vasospastic disease, but an x-ray of the thoracic outlet allows easy diagnosis.

In all of these disorders, absence of a history of vibration exposure is usually helpful to diagnosis.

Idiopathic Raynaud's disease is indistinguishable clinically from vibration-induced whitefinger disease.

Prognosis

In most instances, vibration-induced white finger disease is a nuisance but does not lead to significant functional impairment. It can interfere with leisure activities. Rarely, loss of a digit or even a hand may occur in severe cases when the worker persists with vibration exposure.

ACTINIC SKIN DAMAGE (Solar Elastosis, "Farmer's Skin," "Sailor's Skin")

Sun exposure leads to degeneration of elastin in the dermis and atrophy of the epidermis. This results in wrinkles, yellowish discoloration with relative sparing of skin immediately adjacent to hair follicles, and even comedo formation. Damage typically involves the face, the V of the neck, the nape, the arms, and the dorsal surfaces of the hands.

Injury to the pigment cell population of the skin leads to persistent patches of hyperpigmentation on sun-exposed areas, especially the face and dorsal hands, which are called solar lentigines. Elastic tissue degeneration is evident histologically. The presence of these skin findings is an indication of significant harmful sun exposure and should alert the examiner to the possibility of cutaneous malignancy (see below).

CUTANEOUS MALIGNANCY

There are 3 principal forms of malignant skin tumors. Squamous cell and basal cell carcinoma are derived from keratinocytes in the epidermis; malignant melanoma develops from the pigment-forming cells. Table 17–8 lists the recognized occupational causes of skin cancer and typical occupational groups exposed to each.

Squamous Cell Carcinoma

After many years of repeated actinic skin damage, the keratinocytes may begin to proliferate abnormally, causing warty excrescences on the skin known as actinic keratoses. These lesions in themselves are unsightly but not sinister. A small proportion of actinic keratoses undergo transformation into squamous cell carcinomas, which only rarely metastasize to regional lymph nodes or spread by hematogenous dissemination.

Squamous cancers may develop on skin not exposed to sun if there has been exposure to petroleum distillates (eg, mule spinner's disease) or tar products (scrotal cancer in chimney sweeps). Such cancers are more likely to metastasize. This association between skin cancer and occupational exposure is one of the oldest established occupational disease relationships.

Rarely, skin cancer has been reported to develop at the site of trauma to the skin. Cancer may occur also in burn scars.

Lastly, skin damaged by prolonged exposure to heat (eg, carrying bowls of hot charcoal against the body for heat as occurs in some parts of India—kangri ["fire basket"] cancer) may result in skin cancer.

Basal Cell Carcinoma

Proliferation of cells of basal layer of the epidermis results in basal cell carcinoma. This tumor may present as a solid nodule or may erode and present as an ulcer (rodent ulcer). Sun-induced basal cell carcinomas occur principally on the head and neck.

Occupational arsenic exposure (eg, gold mining) may cause multiple superficial basal cell tumors on nonexposed areas that tend to be thin, flat lesions referred to as superficial basal cell carcinomas.

Malignant Melanoma

Malignant melanoma is a rare tumor that may present as a slowly growing nodule developing in a solar lentigo (see actinic skin damage, above) or may develop de novo as a rapidly growing black nodule (nodular melanoma). Multiple melanoma may develop over a period of several years as a multicolored changing lesion called superficial spreading melanoma.

All of these tumors of pigment-forming cells,

Table 17–8. Occupational cutaneous carcinogens and occupations with significant exposure. (Adapted from Adams.)

Agent	Occupational Category
Ultraviolet light (256–320 nm)	Outdoor workers (farmers, fishermen, sailors, etc)
Polycyclic hydrocarbons (3,4-benzo[a]pyrine, 3-methylcholanthrene, dibenzanthracene, 7,12-dimethyl benzanthracene)	Roofers, petroleum workers
Ionizing radiation (x-rays, gamma rays, beta rays, gamma particles, protons, neutrons)	Radiologists, x-ray technicians, uranium miners, refiners
Inorganic arsenic	Gold miners, chemical workers
Physical injury	Construction workers, industrial workers doing heavy physical work, general laborers

which often develop in sun-exposed sites, appear to be more common following actinic damage. Workers with long exposure out of doors are at increased risk of developing malignant melanoma. There is some epidemiologic evidence that occupational exposure other than to sunlight may predispose to this tumor.

Malignant melanomas developing in lentigenes tend not to metastasize; the other types are more likely to do so.

CUTANEOUS INFECTIONS

Skin infection caused by contact with infectious agents is known to occur in many occupations (Table 17–9). Bacteria, viruses, monomorphic fungi, dermatophytic fungi, and parasites have all been reported to cause work-related disease.

Treatment is as for skin infections in the general population. It is important to investigate the circumstances and make recommendations for protection of the work force against spread of infection.

Table 17–9. Occupational cutaneous infections.[1]

Causal Agent	Occupational Association
Bacteria	
Bacillus anthracis	Wool sorters, tanners
Brucella abortus, B suis, B melitensis	Meat packers, veterinarians
Erysipelothrix insidiosa (erysipeloid)	Fishermen, meat handlers
Francisella tularensis	Farmers, meat handlers veterinarians, laboratory workers
Mycobacterium tuberculosis	Pathologists, veterinarians, farmers, meat handlers
Mycobacterium marinum	Fishermen, fish tank cleaners
Fungi	
Candida albicans and other *Candida* sp	Food workers, health professions
Trichophyton, Microsporum	Health professions
Sporothrix schenkii	Farmers, nurserymen, gardeners
Blastomyces dermatitidis	Farmers, laborers
Coccidioides immitis	Farmers, construction workers
Actinomyces, Nocardia (mycetoma)	Agricultural workers
Viruses	
Pox virus (orf)	Sheep handlers, farmers, veterinarians
Paravaccinia virus (milker's nodules)	Milkers, farmers, veterinarians
Herpes simplex virus	Health professionals
Protozoa, metazoa, helminths, and arthropods	
Ancylostoma capillaria (larva migrans)	Agricultural workers, life guards
Schistosoma sp (swimmer's itch)	Life guards at the lakes of North Central USA
Acardiae, *Glycyphagus* sp (foot mites)	Longshoremen
Pyemotes ventricosus (grain mites)	Grain handlers
Trombicula autumnalis (chiggers)	Outdoor workers
Ticks (hard or soft)	Outdoor workers
Sarcoptes scabiei (scabies)	Health professionals, teachers
Caterpillar hairs	Outdoor workers

[1]Adapted from Adams RM (editor): *Occupational Skin Disease.* Saunders, 1989.

REFERENCES

General

Adams RM (editor): *Occupational Skin Diseases.* Saunders, 1989.

Nethercott JR, Gallant C: Disability due to occupational contact dermatitis. *State Art Rev Occup Med* 1986; **1:**199.

U.S. Department of Labor: *Supplementary Data System.* Bureau of Labor Statistics, 1989.

Acute Irritant Contact Dermatitis

Edelman P: Hydrofluoric acid burns. *State Art Rev Occup Med* 1986;**1:**89.

Rook A, Wilkinson DS: Artefacts. In: *Textbook of Dermatology,* 3rd ed. Rook A, Wilkinson DS, Ebling FJ (editors). Blackwell, 1978.

Tepperman PB: Fatality due to acute systemic fluoride poisoning following a hydrofluoric acid skin burn. *J Occup Med* 1980;**22:**691.

Wilkinson DS: Protective gloves. In: *Essentials of Industrial Dermatology.* Griffin W, Wilkinson DS (editors). Blackwell, 1985.

Chronic Irritant Contact Dermatitis

Fisher AA: *Contact Dermatitis,* 2nd ed. Lea & Febiger, 1973.

Hjorth N, Fregert S: Irritant dermatitis. In: *Textbook of Dermatology,* 3rd ed. Rook A, Wilkinson DS, Ebling FJ (editors). Blackwell, 1978.

Nethercott JR, Gallant C: Disability due to occupational contact dermatitis. *State Art Rev Occup Med* 1986; **1:**199.

Allergic Contact Dermatitis

Adams RM (editor): *Occupational Skin Diseases*. Saunders, 1989.

Cronin E: *Contact Dermatitis*. Churchill Livingstone, 1980.

Fregert S: *Manual of Contact Dermatitis*. Year Book, 1975.

Hannuksela M: Epicutaneous testing. *Allergy* 1979;**34:**5.

Nethercott JR, Gallant C: Disability due to occupational contact dermatitis. *Occup Med* 1986;**1:**199.

Contact Urticaria

Adams RM (editor): *Occupational Skin Diseases*. Saunders, 1989.

Fisher A: Contact urticaria. In: *Occupational Skin Diseases*. Adams RM (editor). Saunders, 1989.

Lahti A: Non-immunologic contact urticaria. *Acta Derm Venereol [Suppl][Stockh]* 1980;**60(Suppl 91):**1.

Work-Aggravated Dermatoses

Adams RM (editor): *Occupational Skin Diseases*. Saunders, 1989.

Chloracne

Adams RM (editor): *Occupational Skin Diseases*. Saunders, 1989.

Taylor JS: Chloracne: A continuing problem. *Cutis* 1974; **13:**585.

Occupational Raynaud's Disease

Adams RM (editor): *Occupational Skin Diseases*. Saunders, 1989.

Wasserman DE, Taylor W: Occupational vibration. In: *Environmental and Occupational Medicine*. Rom WN (editor). Little, Brown, 1982.

Actinic Skin Damage

Fitzpatrick TB et al (editors): *Sunlight and Man: Normal and Abnormal Photobiologic Responses*. Univ of Tokyo Press, 1974.

Rook A, Wilkinson DS, Ebling FJ (editors): *Textbook of Dermatology,* 3rd ed. Blackwell, 1978.

Cutaneous Malignancy

Adams RM (editor): *Occupational Skin Diseases*. Saunders, 1989.

Fitzpatrick TB et al (editors): *Sunlight and Man: Normal and Abnormal Photobiologic Responses*. Univ of Tokyo Press, 1974.

Mihm MC Jr et al: Early detection of primary cutaneous malignant melanoma: A color atlas. *N Engl J Med* 1973; **289:**989.

Occupational Lung Diseases 18

Dean Sheppard, MD, William G. Hughson, MD, PhD, & Judd Shellito, MD

The lung is a common site of occupational disease. Urban dwellers inhale and retain as much as 2 mg of dust daily, and workers in dusty occupations may inhale 10–100 times that amount. What is remarkable is that most people never develop environmentally induced disease despite exposure to many potentially injurious agents. Because the lung has a limited number of ways in which to respond to injury, a wide variety of agents cause only a few familiar patterns of disease. Acute responses include upper airway obstruction, bronchoconstriction, alveolitis, and pulmonary edema; and chronic responses include asthma, parenchymal fibrosis, and cancer. Responses to agents encountered in the workplace can mimic virtually every type of pulmonary response. The specific type of response is dictated by the site of deposition of the noxious agent, the dose and duration of exposure, the susceptibility of lung cells, and the interaction between the agent and local host defense mechanisms. Because individual host factors can rarely be identified, it is essential to protect all workers from exposures that might cause disease in any of them.

This chapter will focus on pulmonary responses in asthma, hypersensitivity pneumonitis, silicosis, coal worker's pneumoconiosis, asbestos-induced diseases, and berylliosis, with emphasis on chronic effects. Acute pulmonary effects of a variety of toxic agents are discussed in other chapters.

Factors Affecting Deposition of Inhaled Materials

Deposition of inhaled materials is primarily dependent on water solubility for gases and particle size for solids. Because water-soluble gases, such as ammonia and sulfur dioxide, are almost entirely removed from inspired air by the aqueous layer lining the nose, oropharynx, and upper airways, they are most likely to cause disease in the upper respiratory tract. Water-insoluble gases, such as nitrogen dioxide and phosgene, are able to bypass the upper airways and cause injury to the distal airways and alveoli.

Though most particles are not perfect spheres, the deposition pattern of inhaled particles is similar to that of spheres and is best described in terms of aerodynamic diameter. During periods of quiet breathing through the nose, virtually all particles with aerodynamic diameters in excess of 10 μm are deposited on the nasal mucosa. During strenuous exercise, however, because of increased airflow and

mouth breathing, up to 20% of particles between 10 and 20 μm in diameter are deposited within the airways. Particles between 3 and 10 μm in diameter can be deposited throughout the tracheobronchial tree. More central deposition is favored by high rates of inspiratory flow, by airway obstruction, and by the presence of increased quantities of mucus. Particles between 0.1 and 3 μm in diameter are preferentially deposited within the alveoli. Smaller particles tend to remain in the airstream and are exhaled. A fiber (a particle whose length exceeds its width by at least 3-fold) is deposited on the basis of aerodynamic diameter rather than length—which is why fibers up to 25 μm in length are often deposited in alveoli.

Pulmonary Function Tests

Pulmonary function tests provide quantitative information about pulmonary physiology. When used in conjunction with the clinical and occupational history and chest x-rays, they can help determine the nature and severity of occupational lung disease.

Information provided by these tests is useful only if it is accurate. Lack of patient cooperation, poor testing methods, and unreliable equipment can cause misleading results. Published standards for the accuracy of testing equipment and for proper methods for administering and interpreting pulmonary function tests must be adhered to in order to obtain meaningful data.

The results of pulmonary function tests are frequently used to characterize an individual's functional capacity and ability to work. For this reason, it is important to distinguish between impairment and disability. A finding (by a physician) of respiratory **impairment** is based on decisions about whether abnormal pulmonary findings will affect respiratory function (eg, in pulmonary fibrosis), whether further occupational exposures should be proscribed (eg, in occupational asthma), and whether the prognosis is good or grave (eg, in lung cancer). **Disability** is an administrative judgment that requires the expertise of nonmedical as well as medical personnel and is based on factors such as age, level of education, earning capacity, and potential for rehabilitation.

A. Forced Spirometry Measurements: Spirometry is the measurement of expired and inspired lung volumes. The forced vital capacity (FVC) is determined by asking the patient to give a maximum expiration as rapidly as possible after a maximum inspiration. At least 3 satisfactory FVC maneuvers are recorded to ensure accuracy and reliability; the 2 highest results must agree within 5% or 100 mL of air, whichever is greater. The forced expiratory volume in 1 second (FEV_1) and the FEV_1/FVC ratio are derived from the FVC curve. The FVC, FEV_1, and FEV_1/FVC ratio are usually reduced in patients with obstructive lung diseases. Patients with restrictive lung diseases usually have a normal or increased FEV_1/FVC ratio, however, because both FEV_1 and FVC are reduced by similar amounts. These spirometry measurements are used in assessment of pulmonary impairment by comparing the patient's results with normal values derived from studies of large populations of healthy people. The American Thoracic Society criteria for pulmonary impairment are shown in Table 18–1; other rating systems are also used.

B. Static Lung Volumes: A spirometer measures only the air that enters or leaves the mouth during an FVC maneuver. Therefore, any disease process that obstructs airflow from the lungs (eg, occupational asthma) or restricts air entrance into the lungs (eg, asbestosis) reduces the FVC. Differentiation of restrictive from obstructive processes usually requires measurement of total lung capacity (TLC), functional residual capacity (FRC), and residual volume (RV) (Fig 18–1). These are measured by body plethysmography or inert gas dilution. Both methods require accurate instruments and careful attention to testing methods. Restrictive lung diseases cause a reduction in TLC and other lung volumes (Fig 18–2). Conversely, obstructive lung diseases may result in hyperinflation and an increase in TLC.

C. Diffusing Capacity for Carbon Monoxide (DL_{CO}): In this test, the patient inhales a low concentration of carbon monoxide (CO) either as a single breath or in a multiple-breath steady-state protocol. The amount of CO absorbed per unit of time is closely correlated with the capacity of the lungs to absorb oxygen, and a reduction in the DL_{CO} reflects impaired gas exchange. The DL is nonspecific; it is diminished in obstructive, restrictive, or vascular diseases that reduce the pulmonary capillary surface membrane available for gas exchange. Nevertheless, it may be used as one of the criteria in assessing pulmonary impairment (Table 18–1).

Bronchial Provocation Tests

Provocation tests are useful in the diagnosis of occupational asthma and hypersensitivity pneumonitis. Asthmatic patients have nonspecific bronchial hyperactivity and develop airflow obstruction after inhaling low concentrations of methacholine chloride or histamine. A decrease in the FEV_1 of 20% or more is considered a positive test result. Inhalation challenge testing with specific antigens can also trigger asthmatic attacks. Bronchoconstriction may occur early (in 10–20 minutes), late (in 4–8 hours), or in a combined reaction with early and late components (Fig 18–3). Most patients with hypersensitivity pneumonitis experience dyspnea and cough along with restrictive pulmonary function changes that peak 4–6 hours after exposure to the offending agent (Fig 18–4). The reaction is specific and diagnostic.

Bronchial provocation tests are expensive and may be hazardous. Patients should usually be hospitalized for testing, since late reactions can be severe and may require urgent treatment.

Exercise Tests

In exercise tests to measure the patient's ability to perform physical work, cycling and treadmill protocols are commonly used. These tests provide quantitative information about pulmonary and cardiac function, and they may be useful adjuncts to the diagnostic information provided by the chest x-rays and pulmonary function tests.

Since claimed impairment due to occupational lung disease may in fact be due to occult cardiac disease or physical deconditioning, exercise tests are used for differentiating the causes of dyspnea and fatigue. Some asthmatic patients develop bronchospasm with exercise. Results of pulmonary function tests performed before and after the exercise test can establish this diagnosis.

ASTHMA

Asthma is a pulmonary disorder characterized by widespread partial obstruction of the airways that varies in severity, is reversible either spontaneously or as a result of treatment, and is not due to cardiovascular disease. In occupational asthma, air-

Table 18–1. American Thoracic Society criteria for pulmonary impairment.[1]

Test	Normal Function	Mild Impairment	Moderate Impairment	Severe Impairment
FVC	> 80%	60–79%	51–59%	< 50%
FEV_1	> 80%	60–79%	41–59%	< 40%
$FEV_1/FVC \times 100$	> 75%	60–74%	41–59%	< 40%
DL_{CO}	> 80%	60–79%	41–59%	< 40%

[1]Modified and reproduced, with permission, from Renzetti AD et al: Evaluation of impairment disability secondary to respiratory disorders. *Am Rev Respir Dis* 1986;**133**:1205.

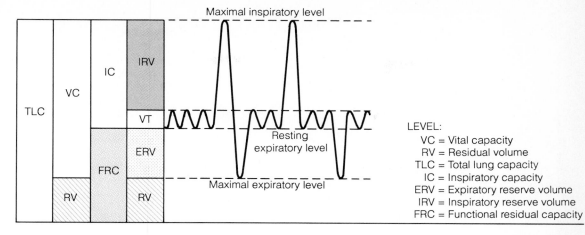

Figure 18–1. Lung capacity and static lung volumes. TLC = total lung capacity; VC = vital capacity; RV = residual volume; IC = inspiratory capacity; FRC = functional residual capacity; IRV = inspiratory reserve volume; V_T = tidal volume; ERV = expiratory reserve volume. (Redrawn and reproduced, with permission, from Comroe JH Jr et al: *The Lung: Clinical Physiology and Pulmonary Function Tests,* 2nd ed. Year Book, 1962.)

way obstruction follows workplace exposure to inhaled gases, dusts, fumes, or vapors. In the USA, asthma occurs in about 5% of the general population, and at least 2% of these cases are occupational in origin. In Japan, the proportion due to occupation is as high as 15%.

Etiology

In healthy individuals, airway smooth muscle tone is controlled by a balance of cholinergic (bronchoconstriction) and adrenergic (bronchodilation) stimulation. This bronchomotor tone is decreased by administration of atropine or β-adrenergic agonists and is increased after inhalation of various irritants. Whereas healthy individuals cannot perceive a difference in bronchomotor tone after inhalation of nonspecific irritants, asthmatic patients may show an exaggerated response. This reactivity of asthmatic airways is often manifested by a diurnal variation in the FEV_1 of 20% or more. In contrast, the diurnal variation in airways of healthy individuals is less than 10%.

The airway hyperirritability so characteristic of the asthmatic state occurs in response to specific allergens as well as to nonspecific irritants. In such cases, bronchoconstriction is augmented by immune mechanisms that cause inflammation, mucosal edema, and the accumulation of viscous secretions. The following have all been invoked in the pathogenesis of occupational asthma: type I (immediate) and type III (immune-complex-mediated) reactions due to IgE and IgG antibodies, respectively; activation of complement via the alternative pathway; and nonimmunologic release of histamine. The clinical pattern of symptoms and airflow obstruction depends on the relative contributions of these immune responses.

Pathogenesis

Pathogenetic mechanisms in occupational asthma are classified as reflex, inflammatory, pharmacologic, and allergic.

A. Reflex Bronchoconstriction: In reflex bronchoconstriction, irritant receptors in the airway wall are stimulated by agents such as cold air, inert dust particles, gases, and fumes. The reaction does not

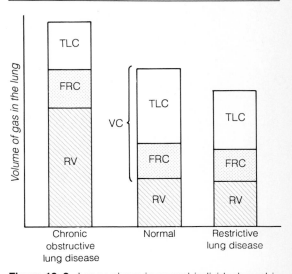

Figure 18–2. Lung volume in normal individuals and in patients with chronic obstructive lung disease and restrictive lung disease. TLC = total lung capacity; FRC = functional residual capacity; RV = residual volume; VC = vital capacity. (Redrawn and reproduced, with permission, from *Asbestos, Smoking, and Disease: The Scientific Evidence.* Commercial Union Insurance Companies, Boston, 1982.)

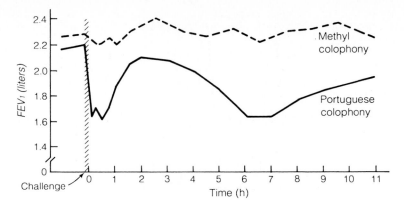

Figure 18–3. Inhalation challenge testing with 5-minute exposures to 2 forms of colophony. The Portuguese colophony triggers a dual asthmatic reaction with early and late components. (Redrawn and reproduced, with permission, from Parkes WR: *Occupational Lung Disorders,* 2nd ed. Butterworths, 1981.)

involve immune mechanisms and is nonspecific. In many cases, the patient has a history of asthma prior to occupational exposure and possesses abnormally reactive airways. For this reason, such cases are often not accepted as related to occupation.

B. Inflammatory Bronchoconstriction: This form of bronchoconstriction begins as a nonspecific reaction following the inhalation of irritant gases and vapors in high concentrations. Damage to the mucosa of airways usually consists of edema, necrosis, and intense inflammation, which cause dyspnea, wheezing, and cough. Symptoms usually resolve within several weeks, but they can then recur at a lower level of exposure. A minority of those surviving the acute event will develop chronic asthmatic attacks provoked both by specific allergens and by nonspecific irritants. The mechanisms underlying this persistent

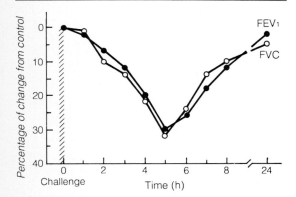

Figure 18–4. Inhalation challenge testing with pigeon serum in a patient with pigeon-breeder's lung. Restrictive pulmonary function changes peak 4–6 hours after exposure. FVC = forced vital capacity; FEV_1 = forced expiratory volume in 1 second. (Modified and reproduced, with permission, from Fink JN: Hypersensitivity pneumonitis. *J Allergy Clin Immunol* 1984;**74:**1.)

response to a single massive exposure to an irritant are unknown.

C. Pharmacologic Bronchoconstriction: This occurs when agents in the working environment exert a specific pharmacologic effect on the lung. There is a dose-response relationship between the level of exposure and the severity of bronchoconstriction. The mechanism may be the release of chemical mediators or a direct effect on the autonomic innervation of the lungs. For example, organophosphate pesticides inhibit cholinesterase, and this results in bronchoconstriction due to excessive parasympathetic stimulation.

D. Allergic Bronchoconstriction: The most common cause of occupational asthma is allergic bronchoconstriction. Susceptible workers develop IgE or IgG antibodies following exposure to workplace antigens such as animal and plant proteins. If high-molecular-weight compounds are the responsible allergens (eg, in enzyme detergent manufacturing, in industries where animals are handled, and in bakeries), atopic workers become sensitized more readily than do nonatopic workers. However, if low-molecular-weight compounds are responsible (eg, in western red cedar mills and in isocyanate manufacturing), atopy is often not a predisposing factor. In occupational asthma due to allergic bronchoconstriction, antibody production is a consequence of workplace exposure. The latency period between first exposure and onset of clinical disease varies from weeks to years, though there may be a typical latency in certain industries. The time course of symptoms and airway obstruction following exposure to a workplace antigen depends on the nature and severity of the immune response. At least 200 agents in the workplace have been shown to cause asthma. This list is growing as new materials and manufacturing processes are introduced.

Patterns of Occupational Asthma

Bronchoconstriction following nonspecific airway

irritation or the pharmacologic action of a specific exposure is usually immediate. In contrast, allergic bronchoconstriction may occur immediately after exposure, following a delay of several hours, or in a pattern with both early and late components.

Early-onset (immediate) asthma develops shortly after exposure, reaches its maximum within 10–20 minutes, and ends within about 2 hours. Sensitized workers have airway mast cells coated with IgE. Inhaled antigen reacts with the specific antibody (type I reaction), causing mast cell release of pre-formed chemical mediators such as histamine and newly formed mediators such as leukotrienes and prostaglandin D_2. This in turn causes bronchoconstriction and local inflammation with resultant dyspnea, wheezing, cough, and airflow obstruction.

Late-onset (nonimmediate) asthma begins sometime after exposure and is maximal at 4–6 hours. It usually resolves within 24 hours, though some attacks may persist for days. Recurrent nocturnal attacks of dyspnea and cough may be the only manifestation of occupational asthma, and the clinician must be aware that the onset of symptoms may not be simultaneous with workplace exposures. The mechanism for late-onset asthma is uncertain. It has been postulated that circulating IgG antibodies in plasma bind to the antigen to form complexes and stimulate a type III reaction. In most instances, however, specific IgG antibodies have not been found. Another possibility is that late-onset asthma is caused by chemical mediators released during allergic reactions involving IgE. In addition, chemotactic factors are released when mast cells degranulate, and these attract eosinophils and neutrophils. Such cellular infiltration requires 4–6 hours, coinciding with the time course of late-onset asthma. This combination of chemical and cellular inflammation probably accounts for the nonspecific bronchial hyperactivity demonstrated by many patients.

Dual-onset asthma combines the clinical features and mechanisms of early- and late-onset asthma. The initial early attack resolves, only to be followed hours later by a return of symptoms and bronchospasm (Fig 18–3).

Key elements influencing the pattern of symptoms and airflow obstruction seen in workers with occupational asthma are the recovery time and the effects of cumulative exposures. Some individuals improve rapidly after leaving work, and recovery is virtually complete before the next workday. Such workers show a similar deterioration during each shift. At the other extreme are those who need more than 2 days to recover. Repeated exposures over several weeks, even with weekends off, result in a steady deterioration of pulmonary function. Dyspnea, wheezing, cough, and other symptoms and signs may be indistinguishable from those of chronic obstructive lung disease due to nonoccupational causes. The reactive nature of the disease may be masked by a fixed reduction in expiratory flow rates seemingly unrelated to work activities. In such cases, the true relationship between the patient's occupation and asthma becomes apparent only after prolonged cessation of exposure allows sufficient time for recovery of normal pulmonary function. When return to work finally occurs, the simultaneous reappearance of symptoms and airflow obstruction makes the link obvious.

Examples of Occupational Asthma

A. Byssinosis: Dust from cotton, flax, hemp, or jute frequently causes chest tightness, cough, and dyspnea among textile workers. The exact mechanism responsible for bronchospasm in these workers is not certain. Dust extracts are capable of causing direct release of histamine and contain endotoxins from bacteria and fungi that can activate the complement system. Precipitating IgG antibodies are found in exposed workers, and a type III reaction has been postulated. A characteristic feature is that symptoms are worse on the first day at work after a weekend or vacation (''Monday fever'') and abate during the week. Progressive removal of antibody or depletion of chemical mediators may explain this pattern. Time away from work allows reconstitution of mediators, and antibody levels are highest on the first day of the workweek. Clinical disease usually does not develop until there has been 10 or more years of exposure. Symptoms vary from occasional tightness of the chest on the first day of the workweek to chronic dyspnea and permanent respiratory disability.

B. Asthma Due to Grain Dusts: Grain dust is a mixture of grain proteins and their degradation products, pollens, fungi, insects, and the excreta of birds and rodents. Immediate- and late-onset bronchospasm may follow inhalation challenge, and fever, malaise, and leukocytosis sometimes accompany late asthmatic attacks. The complex composition of grain dust makes it difficult to identify the specific component responsible for asthma. The dust is an irritant, and reflex bronchoconstriction may account for acute reversible changes following exposure. Extracts of grain dust activate complement pathways and induce direct release of histamine from mast cells. Some studies have found good correlation between a positive skin reaction to grain dust extract and bronchial reactions, but others have failed to do so.

C. Asthma Due to Wood Dusts: A wide variety of wood dusts cause asthma and rhinitis. They are nonspecific irritants and can cause reflex bronchospasm. The most extensively studied dust is from western red cedar. This contains a low-molecular-weight compound, plicatic acid, which causes release of histamine from mast cells and activation of the complement pathway. Specific IgG and IgE antibodies to plicatic acid conjugated with human serum albumin have also been demonstrated, and exposed workers may show late- or dual-onset bronchospasm. Recurrent nocturnal attacks are common, and the relationship to occupation is readily overlooked.

D. Asthma Due to Isocyanates: Isocyanates are important intermediaries in the production of polyurethane. They are formed by the reaction of amines with phosgene. Toluene diisocyanate (TDI), which is used chiefly in the manufacture of foams, is a potent irritant. Eye, nose, and throat discomfort occurs in virtually everyone exposed to TDI levels of 0.5 ppm or more, and cough is often the predominant symptom. Asthma occurs in 5–10% of workers, and exposure to extremely low concentrations of TDI (< 0.001 ppm) may cause attacks of the immediate-, late-, or dual-onset type. Recovery often takes days or even weeks. IgE and IgG antibodies to isocyanate conjugated with protein have been demonstrated in some studies, but the immunologic mechanism remains unclear.

E. Asthma Due to Metal Salts: Exposure to complex salts of platinum occurs in many industrial operations, including electroplating, jewelry manufacturing, and the production of fluorescent screens. Specific IgE antibodies to platinum salts conjugated with human serum albumin have been demonstrated in sensitized workers. Rhinitis and urticaria frequently accompany asthma, and this triad is sometimes called "platinosis." Other metals known to cause occupational asthma include nickel, chromium, cobalt, vanadium, and tungsten carbide. The mechanisms responsible for these asthmatic reactions are unknown.

Pathology

The pathologic findings in occupational asthma are identical to those in asthma due to nonoccupational causes. There is no unique tissue marker to identify the specific agent responsible for the attack. The lungs of patients dying of asthma are distended, and the bronchi and bronchioles are plugged with large amounts of viscid, tenacious mucus. This mucus contains eosinophils, bronchial epithelial cells, and Charcot-Leyden crystals. Bronchial walls are thickened and edematous, and mucous glands and smooth muscle cells are hypertrophied. About 25% of patients have evidence of local bronchiectasis. Since most knowledge concerning the morphologic characteristics of asthma comes from autopsy studies, the changes described probably represent the effects of prolonged, severe disease. Evidence from bronchial biopsies indicates that structural abnormalities may disappear between acute episodes.

Clinical Findings

A. Symptoms and Signs: Episodic dyspnea, chest tightness, and wheezing are the classic symptoms in patients with occupational asthma. For many, however, predominant complaints are recurrent attacks of "bronchitis" with cough, sputum production, and rhinitis. Symptoms may begin hours after exposure has ceased, and in some patients recurrent nocturnal attacks of dyspnea and cough may be the only complaints. It is essential to take a detailed occupational history that includes not only the work activities and exposures of the patient but also those of coworkers and the workplace in general. It is also useful to find out whether other workers have similar symptoms.

B. Laboratory Findings: Skin tests are commonly used to determine atopic status with respect to environmental antigens. Unfortunately, few purified antigens are available for the identification of workplace allergies. Examples include extracts of animal products, flour, and coffee. Serum IgE and IgG antibodies to occupational antigens can also be measured. The presence of an antibody indicates that the worker has been exposed and become sensitized. This is not sufficient to make a diagnosis of occupational asthma, however, since many workers with antibodies have no symptoms. Similarly, many patients with obvious asthma have not developed antibodies to the offending agent. Although skin tests and serologic measurements are useful if they support the clinical findings, they often lack specificity and sensitivity.

C. Pulmonary Function Tests: Many patients with occupational asthma have normal pulmonary function test results at the time of presentation. Because airflow obstruction in asthma is variable, it is essential to perform serial measurements before, during, and after work to determine whether occupational exposures are responsible. Peak expiratory flow rates (PEFR) can be determined in the workplace and at home using inexpensive meters and should be recorded at intervals each day for at least 2 weeks. Patients with prolonged recovery times may need to stop work for several weeks to ascertain whether their asthma is work-related.

D. Imaging: Fleeting infiltrates caused by mucus plugs are a common x-ray finding. Hyperinflation and flattening of the diaphragm reflect air trapping, and bronchial wall thickening due to chronic inflammation or bronchiectasis may be seen. The results of chest x-rays are often normal between symptomatic episodes.

E. Special Examinations: Measurement of nonspecific bronchial hyperreactivity is carried out by bronchial provocation tests with histamine or methacholine. Approximately 95% of asthmatic patients develop symptoms and significant airflow obstruction after inhalation of these agents. However, because test results may be normal in patients with occupational asthma—particularly during asymptomatic periods—these tests cannot be used to exclude the diagnosis of occupational asthma. The most specific diagnostic information is provided by an inhalation provocation test using the suspected industrial agent. This can be performed either by nebulized inhalation or in whole-body exposure chambers. Identifying and purifying the agent, administering it to the patient, and monitoring the concentration achieved are often technically difficult. Provocation tests are time-consuming and potentially dangerous. Hospitalization is advisable, since late reactions can only be detected with continuous monitoring, and severe bronchospasm may require urgent treatment.

Differential Diagnosis

Dyspnea, chest tightness, wheezing, and cough are common features of nonoccupational asthma, chronic obstructive pulmonary disease due to smoking, and congestive heart failure. Other causes of bronchospasm must be excluded, since issues of permanent disability and workers' compensation frequently arise. Accurate diagnosis depends on a high index of suspicion, a detailed occupational history, and an appreciation of the fact that attacks of asthma may occur hours after exposure has ceased. Monitoring of expiratory flow rates in the workplace, together with bronchial provocation testing in the laboratory, provides a definitive diagnosis.

Prevention

The most important preventive step is efficient environmental control of processes involving known sensitizers and irritants. Initial development of asthma often follows accidents in which workers are exposed to high concentrations of the offending agent. Industrial hygiene measures to ensure safe handling of materials, avoidance of spills, good housekeeping, and education of workers can prevent illness. Methods to protect workers, including respirators and extraction ventilation systems, help limit exposure when hazardous processes cannot be avoided. Substitution of a harmful material with an innocuous one should be considered whenever possible. Prophylactic use of medications such as inhaled or oral bronchodilators cannot prevent development of asthma in exposed workers.

Treatment

A. Emergency Measures: Acute asthma attacks require treatment with supplemental oxygen and inhaled and intravenous bronchodilators. Corticosteroids may be indicated. Consideration should be given to hospitalization, since the acute attack may resolve only to be followed by late-onset bronchoconstriction after the patient has left the emergency room.

B. Specific Measures: The definitive treatment of occupational asthma is elimination of the offending substance from the worker's environment. In manufacturing industries, this can sometimes be accomplished by substitution of a harmless agent for the one causing asthma. When this cannot be done, protective measures such as respirators and extraction ventilation systems may lower exposure levels to the point where bronchospasm does not occur. In cases in which immune mechanisms are responsible, however, even minute quantities of the allergen may trigger an attack; the only solution then is removal of the worker from the workplace—a solution that may be complicated by economic and legal considerations. Vocational rehabilitation and job retraining may be required, and the cooperation of the company, the affected worker, the labor union, and the workers' compensation board is necessary to return the individual to gainful employment.

Hyposensitization with certain occupational allergens (eg, platinum salts) has been attempted. A common problem with this technique is precise identification of the responsible substance and preparation of an antigen solution suitable for subcutaneous administration.

Inhaled β-adrenergic agonists are sometimes useful in early-onset bronchospasm, and corticosteroids may help control late-onset attacks. Inhalation of cromolyn sodium, which stabilizes mast cell membranes, can ameliorate both the early- and late-onset components of bronchospasm.

C. General Measures: Asthmatic patients should be advised to avoid potential allergens and irritants. It is often helpful to alter the home environment by removal of pets, frequent cleaning of carpets and furniture to minimize house dust exposure, and proper maintenance of heating and air-conditioning systems to suppress growth of fungi and bacteria. The patient and family members should be strongly encouraged to stop smoking.

Course & Prognosis

The course of occupational asthma is quite variable. Many patients recover completely, with no long-term sequelae. Others develop chronic asthma that is triggered either by specific antigens or nonspecific irritants. In some cases, bronchial hyperreactivity is so severe that the patient can never again be exposed to dusts or fumes.

Studies in which individuals who recovered completely were compared with individuals who had persistent asthma have shown that the latter had diminished expiratory flow rates, a significantly longer duration of symptoms before diagnosis, and a greater degree of bronchial hyperreactivity. Thus, early diagnosis of occupational asthma and early removal of patients from exposure are important.

HYPERSENSITIVITY PNEUMONITIS (Extrinsic Allergic Alveolitis)

In susceptible individuals of any age, repetitive inhalation of antigenic material may precipitate hypersensitivity pneumonitis, characterized by a granulomatous inflammatory reaction in the pulmonary alveolar and interstitial spaces. This condition has many common names, such as farmer's lung and detergent worker's lung, which reflect its occurrence in specific occupations.

Etiology & Pathogenesis

The antigens associated with hypersensitivity pneumonitis can be grouped into 4 major categories, as shown in Table 18–2. In some cases, causal antigens have not been defined.

The pathogenesis of hypersensitivity pneumonitis is poorly understood, but the condition is assumed to be immunologically mediated. Hypersensitivity pneumonitis usually requires repetitive exposure to a high concentration of antigen, and the inhaled antigen must be small enough to reach the lower respiratory

Table 18–2. Types of antigens causing hypersensitivity pneumonitis.

Antigen Type	Examples of Disease	Source
Animal antigens	Furrier's lung	Animal fur
	Pigeon-breeder's or bird-breeder's lung	Avian protein in bird droppings and feathers
Bacterial antigens	Detergent worker's lung	*Bacillus subtilis* enzymes in detergents
Fungal antigens	Bagassosis	Contaminated sugarcane residue
	Cheese washer's lung	Moldy cheese rind
	Farmer's lung	Thermophilic actinomycetes in moldy hay
	Humidifier fever	Contaminated furnace or air-conditioning humidifier systems
	Maple bark stripper's lung	Wood bark
	Mushroom worker's lung	Mushroom compost
Inorganic haptens	Isocyanate lung	Toluene diisocyanate
	Vineyard sprayer's lung	Copper sulfate

tract. Nondigestibility of the antigen may allow for prolonged retention in pulmonary tissue or macrophages and thereby predispose to sensitization.

The specific immune mechanisms involved in hypersensitivity pneumonitis are thought to be type III (immune complex-mediated) and type IV (cell-mediated) reactions. In the presence of excess antigen, antigen-antibody complexes may be deposited in the lungs, where they activate complement, attract neutrophils, and cause tissue damage. The fact that antibodies reactive with the offending antigen are found in the serum and bronchoalveolar lavage fluids of most patients with hypersensitivity pneumonitis and that there is a latent interval between antigen exposure and symptoms suggests that type III mechanisms are involved. The histopathologic findings of granulomatous cellular infiltrate in patients are compatible with type IV mechanisms. In addition, peripheral blood lymphocytes and lymphocytes lavaged from the lungs of patients with hypersensitivity pneumonitis will proliferate in vitro in response to the offending antigen, as is characteristic of type IV reactions. There is little evidence for type I (immediate hypersensitivity) reactions in hypersensitivity pneumonitis.

Only a small percentage of individuals exposed to an antigen develop symptoms and signs of lung disease. This cannot be explained on the basis of cumulative antigen exposure or the presence of antibodies to the specific antigen, since epidemiologic studies of antigen-exposed populations have shown

that serum antibodies are also found in a large number of healthy individuals. For example, antibodies to pigeon proteins are found in up to 50% of exposed pigeon breeders, while symptoms and signs of hypersensitivity pneumonitis are observed in only 10%. Conversely, cases of obvious hypersensitivity pneumonitis have been described in individuals without antibodies.

Studies both in animals and in humans have correlated altered suppressor T lymphocyte function with the development of lung disease after antigen exposure. This suggests that patients with hypersensitivity pneumonitis have an immunoregulatory defect that alters the immune response to inhaled antigen and eventually leads to lung damage.

Pathology

Biopsy of lung tissue in patients with hypersensitivity pneumonitis typically shows thickening of the alveolar walls with edematous fluid and a cellular infiltrate of monocytes, lymphocytes, plasma cells, and histiocytes. Characteristically, there are numerous noncaseating granulomas, usually associated with giant cells. These granulomas tend to be poorly formed in comparison with those found in sarcoidosis and tuberculosis. In cases in which granulomas are not seen, there may be nonspecific interstitial fibrosis, with varying degrees of collagenous fibrosis and honeycombing. Typically, the interstitium is involved more diffusely than in idiopathic pulmonary fibrosis.

Clinical Findings

A. Symptoms and Signs: In the acute form of hypersensitivity pneumonitis, symptoms of cough, dyspnea, fever, and chills do not develop until 4–12 hours after exposure to antigen. This latent interval may make it difficult for the patient to relate the symptoms to a particular work exposure. There is often a history of similar episodes, each resolving within a day or so. Physical examination reveals tachypnea, cyanosis, and bibasilar crackles. Wheezing is usually not present.

In the chronic form, which may result from repetitive low-level antigen exposure or from recurrent episodes of acute hypersensitivity pneumonitis, the symptoms tend to be persistent and show little worsening or resolution with changes in antigen exposure. There is insidious dyspnea, with cough, fatigue, and weight loss. Fever is uncommon. Physical examination reveals bibasilar crackles. Digital clubbing has been reported but is unusual. In advanced cases, there may be clinical evidence of cor pulmonale.

B. Laboratory Findings: Leukocytosis may be prominent, with white blood cell counts ranging from 20,000 to 30,000/μL in acute hypersensitivity pneumonitis and with counts less elevated in chronic cases. Differential cell counts show an excess of neutrophils. Eosinophilia is not common. Levels of serum immunoglobulins other than IgE tend to be elevated.

In most cases, patients have serum IgG antibodies

to the specific antigen responsible for the disease. These antibodies can be measured as precipitins by radial gel immunodiffusion, by radioimmunoassay, or by enzyme-linked immunosorbent assay. In the appropriate clinical setting, the presence of serum precipitins for an antigen related to hypersensitivity pneumonitis is helpful, but this alone is not diagnostic of disease.

C. Pulmonary Function Tests: Most patients with acute or chronic hypersensitivity pneumonitis have abnormal pulmonary function test results. The FVC is decreased, while the FEV_1/FVC ratio is normal or elevated. Total lung capacity is diminished, and there may be diffusion impairment as well. Arterial blood gases may show hypoxemia at rest, which is further exacerbated with exercise. Hypercapnia is not a feature of hypersensitivity pneumonitis. Pulmonary function tests are useful for following the progress of the patient's disease.

D. Imaging: Findings on chest x-ray in patients with hypersensitivity pneumonitis are nonspecific. They may be normal in acute cases but more often show bilateral alveolar infiltrates that have a mottled or nodular character. Both upper and lower lung fields may be involved, and serial chest x-rays sometimes show migratory infiltrates. In chronic cases, the x-ray shows a pattern of increased interstitial markings compatible with interstitial fibrosis. These abnormalities are more commonly seen in the upper lung zones, and there may also be signs of honeycombing.

E. Special Examinations:

1. Bronchial provocation tests—Inhalation challenge testing with specific antigens may be helpful in cases in which clinical and immunologic findings are equivocal. The safest way to perform these tests is to expose the patient to antigen in the suspect environment for a limited period of time and then monitor symptoms, temperature, white blood cell count, spirometry, lung volumes, and diffusing capacity. In some cases, patients are able to bring suspected antigens to the laboratory, where their responses to them can be carefully followed. In other cases, an extract of a suspected antigen can be prepared and administered to the patient in graded concentrations with a nebulizer. An example of results of inhalation challenge testing in a patient with pigeon-breeder's lung is shown in Fig 18–4. When patients with hypersensitivity pneumonitis are exposed to an offending antigen, most of them experience dyspnea and cough along with restrictive pulmonary function changes that peak 4–6 hours after exposure. These findings are antigen-specific and diagnostic. Because inhalation challenge testing may produce high fever and severe hypoxemia, it is currently done only in research centers by physicians experienced with the technique.

2. Bronchoalveolar lavage—A number of studies have sampled cells and fluid obtained by bronchoalveolar lavage from the lungs of patients with hypersensitivity pneumonitis. The fluid typically shows an increased concentration of IgG, a relative increase in the number of lymphocytes (most of which are T cells), and precipitating antibodies. Lymphocytes obtained by lavage will proliferate when exposed to the appropriate antigen in vitro. The presence of abnormalities in cells and lavage fluid does not always correlate with clinically apparent disease. For example, an increase in the number of lymphocytes has been observed in asymptomatic but antigen-exposed subjects, and the increase observed in patients with hypersensitivity pneumonitis can persist long after the clinical episode has resolved. Currently, bronchoalveolar lavage is of uncertain value in the diagnosis and management of patients with hypersensitivity pneumonitis.

3. Lung biopsy—Only when the clinical picture is atypical may lung biopsy be necessary to exclude other causes of interstitial lung disease and to justify a job change to avoid antigen exposure. In such cases, open lung biopsy is preferable to transbronchial biopsy, because it provides enough tissue for an unequivocal diagnosis.

Differential Diagnosis

It is important to identify atypical presentations of hypersensitivity pneumonitis and to differentiate related conditions.

Humidifier fever, an acute form of hypersensitivity pneumonitis reported in workers exposed to aerosolized fungal antigens from a contaminated furnace or air-conditioning humidifier system, has an atypical presentation. Cases may occur in epidemic distribution and are often first recognized as a cluster of atypical pneumonias. Diagnosis is difficult because exposed workers may not be aware of a workplace humidifier system.

Massive exposure to fungal spores, usually in workers clearing fungi from the tops of silage, may cause mycotoxicosis, which differs from hypersensitivity pneumonitis in that serum precipitating antibodies are usually not present. The pathogenesis of this condition may involve direct complement activation by inhaled fungi.

Grain fever, characterized by episodes of fever and malaise in grain workers, may or may not involve pulmonary symptoms, and the pathogenesis of the syndrome is unclear.

The differential diagnosis of acute hypersensitivity pneumonitis also includes viral pneumonia, atypical pneumonias, and toxicity from exposure to fumes.

In chronic hypersensitivity pneumonitis, the clinical presentation can mimic other forms of chronic interstitial lung disease, particularly sarcoidosis and idiopathic pulmonary fibrosis. An occupational history showing a source of antigen exposure usually serves as a reason for additional testing to differentiate these conditions from hypersensitivity pneumonitis.

Prevention

Hypersensitivity pneumonitis can be prevented by

altering work conditions to avoid antigen exposure or to decrease dust formation. For example, advice on proper hay-making techniques to decrease the risk of farmer's lung is available in many rural communities.

Treatment

Antigen avoidance is the major approach to treatment. If work practices can be altered to decrease exposure to antigen, the patient may return to work but should use a respiratory protection device and have careful follow-up. If the work environment cannot be altered, the patient should be advised to change jobs. Respiratory protection alone is of limited value, since exposure to minute quantities of antigen may provoke symptoms in a sensitized individual. In an acute attack, supplemental oxygen and short-term use of corticosteroids may hasten its resolution. There is no indication for long-term use of corticosteroids, for immunologic desensitization, or for the use of antifungal agents. In advanced cases of chronic hypersensitivity pneumonitis, therapy is supportive.

Course & Prognosis

With avoidance of the offending antigen, acute hypersensitivity pneumonitis will usually resolve completely within a few weeks. For the chronic form of the disease, long-term exposure to the offending antigen results in some degree of pulmonary fibrosis and permanent lung damage. Avoidance of the antigen may still effect some improvement in symptoms.

SILICOSIS

Etiology & Pathogenesis

Silicosis is a parenchymal lung disease caused by inhalation of crystalline silica, a component of rock and sand. Workers at risk include miners, tunnelers, quarry workers, stonecutters, sandblasters, foundry workers, glassblowers, and ceramics workers.

The 3 clinical forms of silicosis—chronic, accelerated, and acute—are determined primarily by the intensity of exposure to silica. In chronic silicosis, radiographic abnormalities appear more than 15 years after onset of exposure; in accelerated silicosis, abnormalities appear within 5–15 years and there is usually prolonged high-dose exposure; and acute silicosis can develop within a few months of massive inhalation of crystalline silica.

All 3 forms of silicosis are thought to be initiated by the toxic interaction between silica crystals and alveolar macrophages. This interaction leads to the release of mediators that can directly injure the lung parenchyma as well as mediators that are responsible for recruitment and proliferation of macrophages and fibroblasts.

In most patients with chronic silicosis, radiographic abnormalities occur without significant abnormalities in pulmonary function. In some patients, however—and especially in those with progressive massive fibrosis—pulmonary function is also abnormal, characterized primarily by lung restriction or by combined restriction and obstruction. Airway obstruction may be severe and is presumably due to distortion of the airway architecture. Occasionally, compensatory emphysema obscures the initial restrictive abnormality.

Pathology

In chronic silicosis, multiple small nodules may be diffusely distributed throughout the lung parenchyma but are often more prominent in the upper lobes. Similar nodules may be present in hilar lymph nodes. Each nodule has a relatively acellular core, which is composed of swirls of collagen, and a cellular capsule containing macrophages, fibroblasts, and plasma cells. Silica crystals can be seen within the nodules under a polarizing microscope. In a small percentage of patients, small nodules coalesce to form large masses, a phenomenon called progressive massive fibrosis. The large masses can compress normal lung structures and can cavitate. Usually, however, cavitation in silicosis is due to infection with mycobacteria.

The findings in accelerated silicosis are similar to those of chronic silicosis, except that nodules are present sooner after exposure, conglomerate nodules occur more commonly, and giant cells are occasionally seen.

In acute silicosis, findings are quite different. Alveolar spaces are flooded with eosinophilic exudates, and there is little evidence of parenchymal fibrosis. Alveolar macrophages are often loaded with silica crystals.

Clinical Findings

A. Symptoms and Signs: Most patients with chronic silicosis have no symptoms. In symptomatic patients, dyspnea is common but is usually only severe if there is progressive massive fibrosis. Cough is also common but may be due to chronic bronchitis in smokers or to superimposed infection. Since chest pain and clubbing are not features of silicosis, their presence suggests another diagnosis. Physical examination usually yields normal results.

B. Imaging: Chest x-rays usually reveal small round opacities in both lungs, especially in the upper lobes. This pattern is called simple silicosis. The terms "complicated silicosis" and "progressive massive fibrosis" denote the development of conglomerate shadows in the perihilar regions, primarily in the upper lobes. Adjacent lucent regions are sometimes seen and may be due to compensatory emphysema. Calcifications can occur in parenchymal nodules and in hilar lymph nodes, where they usually involve the rim of an enlarged node—a pattern called eggshell calcification.

Differential Diagnosis

Silicosis should be distinguished from other causes of diffuse parenchymal lung infiltration. Although a history of heavy exposure to silica is helpful, it does not exclude the possibility of other diseases associated with pulmonary infiltration, such as sarcoidosis and idiopathic interstitial pulmonary fibrosis. Since both of these diseases may respond to treatment, it is important to exclude them in symptomatic patients with impaired or rapidly decreasing pulmonary function. This usually requires transbronchial or open lung biopsy. The presence of skin or eye abnormalities and other signs of systemic involvement strongly favors an alternative diagnosis such as sarcoidosis. On the other hand, in asymptomatic patients who have nearly normal pulmonary function and would not require treatment in any case, it is difficult to justify invasive diagnostic procedures. In these patients, a history of significant exposure to silica and the presence of radiographic abnormalities are sufficient for diagnosis.

In patients with a history of exposure to several types of dust, it is often difficult to distinguish silicosis from other forms of pneumoconiosis. For example, inhalation of iron dust causes a benign pneumoconiosis with radiographic abnormalities similar to those of simple silicosis.

Complications

Patients with silicosis are at increased risk for infections with tuberculous and nontuberculous mycobacteriosis. These infections should be suspected in patients with markedly asymmetric infiltrates, progressive unilateral infiltrates, or cavitation. In severe cases of complicated silicosis, patients can develop respiratory failure and cor pulmonale. Silica exposure may also predispose to the development of lung cancer, though this association is not yet proved.

Prevention

Prevention requires care to avoid exposure of workers and bystanders to silica particles. One important strategy is replacement of sand with less toxic substitutes in abrasive blasting. Although sand blasting has been banned in many industrialized countries, sand is still widely used in the USA. Other processes that produce silica particles should be enclosed or modified (eg, by wetting procedures) to reduce airborne concentrations. Proper ventilation is necessary.

Treatment

There is no known effective treatment for established silicosis. In acute silicosis, as in alveolar proteinosis, sequential whole-lung lavage may be beneficial. The treatment of mycobacterial infections in these patients is the same as in patients without silicosis. Workers with suspected silicosis and a positive result in the tuberculin test using purified protein derivative (PPD) should receive isoniazid (300 mg once daily) for 1 year.

Course & Prognosis

Acute silicosis is usually fatal. Chronic silicosis may progress during the first few years after exposure has ceased, but thereafter it usually remains stable in the absence of mycobacterial infection. Fortunately, the prognosis for simple silicosis is excellent. In patients with complicated silicosis, the prognosis depends on the severity of impairment of pulmonary function.

COAL WORKER'S PNEUMOCONIOSIS

Etiology & Pathogenesis

Coal worker's pneumoconiosis is a parenchymal lung disease caused by inhalation of coal dust. A similar disorder occurs after heavy exposure to respirable graphite or carbon black. Coal dust inhalation also causes chronic bronchitis. Workers at risk in addition to coal miners include coal trimmers, graphite miners, and millers and workers involved in the manufacture of carbon electrodes.

Most chest x-ray abnormalities in coal miners are probably due to the large amount of radiopaque coal dust that accumulates in the lungs after long-term high-dose exposure. Much of this dust is incorporated into alveolar macrophages. The pathogenesis of parenchymal destruction in the few patients (about 1%) who develop progressive massive fibrosis is controversial, since in most patients there is little inflammatory response to coal. In these cases of massive fibrosis, tissue injury may require concomitant exposure to silica, pulmonary infection, or some underlying immunologic abnormality such as rheumatoid arthritis.

Coal dust is less fibrogenic than silica and causes severe impairment in pulmonary function only in patients who develop progressive massive fibrosis, in which case impairment may consist of lung restriction, obstruction, or both.

Pathology

The principal lesion in coal worker's pneumoconiosis is the coal macule, a small pigmented area in which macrophages are filled with dust. Coal macules are distributed within alveolar spaces and surrounding terminal bronchioles, but they provoke surprisingly little response in the adjacent parenchyma. Larger macules, called coal nodules, may contain collagen but few other cells. As in silicosis, the lesions are most prominent in the upper lobes. In progressive massive fibrosis, there are large masses that include considerably more collagen.

In coal miners with pneumoconiosis and rheumatoid arthritis (Caplan's syndrome), multiple large nodules are found in both lungs. The nodules consist of collections of inflammatory cells surrounding blood vessels, and they resemble rheumatoid nodules in other organs. Similar lesions can be seen in workers with rheumatoid arthritis who have been exposed to silica or asbestos.

Clinical Findings

A. Symptoms and Signs: In cases of simple coal

worker's pneumoconiosis, patients are usually asymptomatic. Complaints of chronic cough and sputum production typical of chronic bronchitis are due to inhalation of coal dust and are not necessarily caused by parenchymal lung disease. In cases of progressive massive fibrosis, there may be severe dyspnea or respiratory failure.

B. Imaging: Chest x-rays in simple coal worker's pneumoconiosis show small irregular opacities most prominent in the upper lobes. In progressive massive fibrosis, they show large masses that are often surrounded by lucent regions thought to be due to compensatory emphysema. Chest x-ray abnormalities correlate with the past dust burden and are primarily due to retained coal dust itself.

C. Pulmonary Function Tests: Testing usually yields normal results or shows mild airway obstruction. The mild airway obstruction can be seen in nonsmoking as well as smoking miners, but severe airway obstruction rarely occurs in nonsmokers unless they develop progressive massive fibrosis. In smokers, it is rarely possible to determine the relative contributions of coal dust and smoking to the development of airway obstruction.

Differential Diagnosis

In an asymptomatic coal miner with normal pulmonary function, small irregular opacities on chest x-ray, and no evidence of systemic disease, a presumptive diagnosis of coal worker's pneumoconiosis can be made. Abnormal pulmonary function (especially lung restriction) in the absence of progressive massive fibrosis or systemic symptoms should suggest another diagnosis, such as sarcoidosis or fibrosing alveolitis.

Prevention & Treatment

Prevention is dependent on proper ventilation and improved work practices, such as wetting the coal face before mining it and wetting the dust before removing it from the mine shaft.

There is no specific treatment for coal worker's pneumoconiosis. Affected workers should be removed from further exposure. For the rare patient who develops dyspnea or respiratory failure, supportive measures include supplemental oxygen for significant hypoxemia and a trial of bronchodilator therapy for associated airway obstruction.

Course & Prognosis

Coal worker's pneumoconiosis is usually benign and does not generally progress after exposure has ceased. However, in cases of progressive massive fibrosis, patients may develop severe respiratory impairment, cor pulmonale, and fatal respiratory failure.

ASBESTOS-INDUCED DISEASES

Asbestos is a general term for a group of mineral silicates that have in common their fibrous nature and

potential to be woven. Inhalation of asbestos can cause a variety of pulmonary disorders, including parenchymal lung disease (asbestosis) and disorders of the airways and pleura. Asbestos is considerably more potent as a stimulus to tissue injury, inflammation, and fibrosis than are coal and silica.

Worldwide utilization of asbestos in insulation, construction work, and shipbuilding increased dramatically between 1940 and 1970 and then began to decline. Nonetheless, exposure will continue to occur for many years through the use and repair of asbestos-containing ships, buildings, and other structures in industrialized countries and through the continued widespread use of asbestos in many developing countries.

1. ASBESTOSIS

The term "asbestosis" is generally reserved for the parenchymal lung disease caused by asbestos.

Etiology & Pathogenesis

Asbestos is thought to cause lung inflammation and fibrosis as a result of activation of alveolar macrophages. The precise mechanism of activation is unknown, but the shape and the relative indestructibility of fibers are thought to play a role. Asbestos fibers can persist in the lungs for many years after inhalation. Because of their long and narrow shape, they often cannot be completely engulfed by macrophages, so a single fiber may activate a series of macrophages over a long period of time. This may explain why there is often a long latency period between exposure and the development of asbestosis and why the disease can continue to progress for up to 20 years after exposure has been discontinued.

Asbestosis is more likely to be associated with restrictive lung disease than is silicosis or coal worker's pneumoconiosis. Affected workers commonly have reductions in pulmonary diffusing capacity, lung volumes, or both. Mild airflow obstruction is also common in workers exposed to asbestos.

Pathology

Pathologic findings in asbestosis are similar to those seen in other types of pulmonary fibrosis, such as idiopathic interstitial fibrosis. Alveolitis is characterized by the presence of macrophages, neutrophils, and irregular areas of increased collagen and is most prominent in the lung bases and in subpleural locations. Honeycombing is occasionally seen but is not common. The only characteristic feature is the asbestos body, which consists of an asbestos fiber coated with hemosiderin. These coated fibers account for far fewer than 1% of all retained fibers. Routine light microscopic evaluation of lung sections for asbestos bodies is neither a specific nor a sensitive indicator of asbestosis, because coated fibers are occasionally found in the lungs of healthy urban dwellers without fibrosis and because they are easily missed in patients with asbestosis. If, however, asbestos bodies are found in association with lung fibrosis, this strongly suggests asbestosis. A better assessment of exposure can be obtained by counting asbestos bodies extracted from dried lung or by electron probe analysis of lung sections.

Clinical Findings

A. Symptoms and Signs: Dyspnea, the most common symptom of asbestosis, is initially manifested as decreased tolerance for exercise. Dyspnea can slowly progress over many years even after exposure has ceased. Cough is also common and is usually nonproductive or productive of scant sputum. The most prominent findings on physical examination are bibasilar rales and clubbing. Both findings are often absent, however, even in patients with severe disease.

B. Imaging: Chest x-rays typically reveal symmetric but irregular basilar opacities with relative sparing of the upper lobes. About 10% of patients with restrictive lung disease caused by asbestos have no parenchymal infiltration apparent on standard posteroanterior and lateral chest x-rays. Pleural abnormalities are often present, but their absence does not rule out the diagnosis of asbestosis. Oblique chest x-rays can be helpful in identifying the presence or extent of parenchymal abnormalities in patients with extensive pleural disease. Thin-slice CT scans may be more sensitive than plain chest x-rays in detecting parenchymal abnormalities, but the significance of abnormal findings detected by scanning is uncertain. Thus, CT scans are not recommended for routine clinical evaluation.

C. Pulmonary Function Tests: Testing may reveal a symmetric reduction in lung volumes (lung restriction), a reduction in pulmonary diffusing capacity, or both. Mild airflow reduction, especially at low lung volumes, is common.

D. Special Examinations: Pulmonary exercise testing may be useful, especially in patients who have dyspnea and normal or nearly normal static lung function. An increased gradient between alveolar-arterial oxygen values on exercise suggests pulmonary vascular obstruction or destruction, but this finding is nonspecific.

Differential Diagnosis

The major confusion is with other causes of interstitial fibrosis. In patients with symptoms, impaired pulmonary function, or both—and especially in cases in which there is evidence of progression of disease—treatable causes must be excluded. The specific diagnosis of asbestosis requires open lung biopsy to obtain a large enough tissue sample for assessment of the asbestos burden; however, other diagnoses, such as sarcoidosis or eosinophilic granuloma, can often be established with bronchoscopic transbronchial biopsy, making this less invasive procedure the preferred initial step. In patients with a clear history of significant exposure to asbestos, the coexistence of

bilateral pleural thickening or diaphragmatic calcifications and bibasilar parenchymal fibrosis strongly favors the diagnosis of asbestosis.

Complications

The major complication of asbestosis is respiratory failure. Other asbestos-induced disorders, such as lung cancer and mesothelioma, are probably best thought of as independent consequences of asbestos exposure rather than complications of asbestosis.

Prevention & Treatment

The US Environmental Protection Agency has ordered a phased elimination of all new mining, importation, and application of asbestos. Even after this has been accomplished, however, potential exposure will continue from asbestos in existing ships, buildings, and other structures. Wherever possible, existing asbestos should be enclosed, especially if it is accessible to airflow. Removal of asbestos and renovation of buildings containing asbestos should only be done by trained individuals with respiratory protection.

There is no effective treatment for asbestosis. As with coal worker's pneumoconiosis, supportive measures should be provided for patients who develop dyspnea or respiratory failure.

Course & Prognosis

Asbestosis is usually a mild disease that either progresses slowly or is nonprogressive. However, the disease can develop or progress for many years after exposure is discontinued and can lead to respiratory failure and death. Because of the long latency period and extensive exposure between 1940 and 1970, physicians will continue to see new and progressing cases for many years.

2. ASBESTOS-INDUCED PLEURAL DISORDERS

Pleural abnormalities are frequently seen in workers with significant exposure to asbestos and include areas of pleural thickening, focal pleural plaques, and pleural and diaphragmatic calcifications. Abnormalities detected on posteroanterior chest x-rays are commonly found on the parietal pleura of the lateral chest wall and are usually bilateral. Unilateral pleural abnormalities suggest an alternative explanation such as previous trauma, infection, or pneumothorax.

Although pleural plaques may calcify, especially along the surface of the diaphragm, they do not usually cause significant pulmonary impairment—their major importance is as a marker of exposure to asbestos. However, patients with extensive pleural abnormalities occasionally develop extrapulmonary lung entrapment, which causes a decrease in total lung capacity and vital capacity and can result in severe dyspnea.

Asbestos exposure can also cause benign exudative

pleural effusions, which are sometimes bilateral and are most likely to occur within 10–20 years after onset of exposure. These effusions often recur. Because they are clinically indistinguishable from other exudative effusions, a presumptive diagnosis is reached after treatable causes and mesothelioma are excluded. Evaluation should include culture and pathologic examination of pleural fluid and of pleural tissue obtained by biopsy. Most of these benign pleural effects of asbestos exposure do not require treatment. In the rare patient who develops significant pleural restriction, decortication has been suggested. However, many of these patients also have associated subpleural fibrosis, so decortication may not always result in improvement in symptoms and lung function.

3. ASBESTOS-INDUCED MESOTHELIOMA

Mesothelioma is an extremely rare tumor that originates in the cells lining the pleural space or peritoneum. Benign mesotheliomas are usually bulky local masses and are not caused by asbestos. Malignant mesotheliomas of the pleura commonly present as diffuse pleural thickening that progressively encases the lung and generally leads to volume loss in the affected hemithorax. The tumor may eventually encroach on the other lung or extend into the chest wall, but distant metastases are uncommon. Approximately 75% of patients with mesothelioma have a history of significant occupational or environmental exposure to asbestos. The diagnosis is usually suspected on the basis of progressive pleural encasement. Chest pain is common but not universal.

A major difficulty in differential diagnosis is distinguishing mesothelioma from metastatic adenocarcinoma. This distinction can sometimes be made by electron microscopy of cells from pleural fluid, but it usually requires open pleural biopsy. An eventual definitive tissue diagnosis is important for purposes of compensation.

Treatment is generally unsatisfactory, but some reports suggest limited responses to a combination of surgical resection, radiation, and chemotherapy. Death from wasting or respiratory failure usually occurs within months after diagnosis (see Chapter 16).

4. ASBESTOS-INDUCED AIRWAY DYSFUNCTION

The most prominent initial sites of the inflammatory response to retained asbestos fibers are the terminal airways. As noted above, workers exposed to asbestos frequently have a reduction in expiratory flow at low lung volumes. However, these abnormalities are usually mild in the absence of smoking and are not a likely explanation for significant dyspnea. In smokers, it is not possible to precisely quantify the relative effects of asbestos and cigarette smoke on the airways. However, since nonsmokers exposed to asbestos generally do not develop severe airway obstruction—and smokers not exposed to asbestos commonly do—it seems reasonable to attribute severe airway obstruction in asbestos-exposed smokers primarily to the effects of cigarettes. The treatment of airway obstruction is the same as for individuals not exposed to asbestos and should include smoking cessation and a trial of bronchodilator therapy.

5. ASBESTOS-INDUCED LUNG CANCER

Asbestos is an important cause of cancer, and the lung is the most common organ affected. The effects of asbestos and cigarette smoke are synergistic. Risk estimates for lung cancer are as follows: for nonsmokers whose work exposes them to asbestos, a 5-fold increase in risk; for heavy smokers (1–2 packs a day) whose work does not expose them to asbestos, a 20- to 25-fold increase in risk; and for heavy smokers whose work exposes them to asbestos, a 50- to 90-fold increase in risk compared to nonexposed nonsmokers.

Exposure to asbestos increases the incidence of all common histologic types of lung cancer (squamous cell carcinoma, small cell carcinoma, and adenocarcinoma). As with other asbestos-induced diseases, lung cancer usually occurs after a long latency period. An increased incidence is reported about 15 years after the onset of exposure and is maximal after 30 or more years. Asbestos-induced lung cancer is thus likely to continue to be a problem long after asbestos use is diminished or eliminated. The treatment and prognosis of asbestos-induced lung cancer do not differ from those of other lung cancers and are dependent on cell type and extent of disease at the time of diagnosis.

BERYLLIUM DISEASE

Beryllium is a rare metal that can cause both acute and chronic disease. In the past, most cases were due to the use of beryllium in fluorescent lights. Since 1949, when this use was discontinued, most cases have occurred in persons engaged in manufacturing metal alloys and x-ray tubes and in the mining and milling of beryllium. The number of new cases has diminished with the improvement of industrial hygiene measures in these industries.

Acute disease is due to intense exposure to beryllium, and the resulting lung injury resembles that caused by exposure to other toxic agents. Clinical manifestations include upper airway injury, bronchiolitis, and pulmonary edema. The mortality rate may be as high as 10%. Treatment with corticosteroids has been recommended, though no controlled studies have been performed.

Chronic disease often occurs without antecedent

symptoms months to years after first exposure to beryllium. Because beryllium salts are absorbed through the respiratory tract and distributed throughout the body, exposure causes systemic disease. Noncaseating granulomas can be found in the lung, lymph nodes, liver, spleen, adrenal glands, and kidney. Granulomas in the skin are thought to be due to direct exposure.

The diagnosis of chronic beryllium disease is made on the basis of a history of exposure and demonstration of granulomas on tissue biopsy. Lung manifestations are nonspecific and indistinguishable from those seen in sarcoidosis and hypersensitivity pneumonitis. Sarcoidosis is more likely if there is involvement of the uvea, the salivary glands, and the central nervous system or if erythema nodosum is present. Demonstration of beryllium in urine confirms exposure but is not diagnostic. The disease is thought to be due to a cell-mediated immune response directed at beryllium-protein complexes, and lymphocyte transformation in response to beryllium has been demonstrated in vitro with peripheral blood lymphocytes obtained by bronchoalveolar lavage from some patients with chronic beryllium disease. However, transformation of blood lymphocytes can also be seen in exposed workers without evidence of disease, and data are presently insufficient to evaluate the sensitivity and specificity of transformation of lung lymphocytes.

The clinical course of chronic beryllium disease is quite variable. Although the disease in most cases remains stable if exposure ceases, it can remit or progress in some individuals. Treatment with corticosteroids has been recommended but has not been systematically studied.

LUNG DISEASES INDUCED BY OTHER INORGANIC DUSTS

Silicates other than asbestos can also cause pneumoconiosis. **Kaolin, mica,** and **vermiculite,** for example, cause x-ray abnormalities and lesions similar to those caused by coal dust.

Inhalation of **talc** causes pulmonary fibrosis with features of both asbestosis and silicosis and also causes granulomas. Pleural plaques have been noted in workers exposed to talc, but they may be due to contamination of talc with asbestos. Intravenous injection of talc by drug addicts can cause a severe granulomatous lung disease sometimes associated with pulmonary hypertension.

Environmental exposure to **erionite,** a fibrous silicate found in high concentration in the soil and in mud houses in some parts of Turkey, has been reported to cause mesothelioma.

Synthetic vitreous fibers such as **fiberglass** and **glass wool** are physically similar to asbestos but appear to be considerably less toxic. However, because of the long latency of fiber-induced disorders, continued close surveillance of the effects of use of these fibers is essential.

It has recently been recognized that exposure to the dust of a variety of metals, including **tungsten carbide, cobalt, titanium,** and **tantalum,** can cause acute or chronic injury to the airways and lung parenchyma. As new technologies evolve, it is likely that new reactions to inorganic dusts will be identified.

REFERENCES

Pulmonary Function Tests
American Thoracic Society: Snowbird workshop on standardization of spirometry. *Am Rev Respir Dis* 1979;**91**:831.

Crapo RO, Morris AH, Gardner RM: Reference spirometric values using techniques and equipment that meet American Thoracic Society recommendations. *Am Rev Respir Dis* 1981;**123**:659.

Miller A (editor): *Pulmonary Function Tests in Clinical and Occupational Lung Disease.* Grune & Stratton, 1986.

Renzetti AD et al: Evaluation of impairment disability secondary to respiratory disorders. *Am Rev Respir Dis* 1986;**133**:1205.

Asthma
Bernstein IL: Occupational asthma. *Clin Chest Med* 1981;**2**:255.

Chan-Yeung M, Lam S: Occupational asthma. *Am Rev Respir Dis* 1986;**133**:686.

Hypersensitivity Pneumonitis
Keller RH et al: Immunoregulation in hypersensitivity

pneumonitis: Phenotypic and functional studies of bronchoalveolar lavage lymphocytes. *Am Rev Respir Dis* 1984;**130**:766.

Leblanc P et al: Relationship among antigen contact, alveolitis, and clinical status in farmer's lung disease. *Arch Intern Med* 1986;**146**:153.

Roberts RC, Moore VL: Immunopathogenesis of hypersensitivity pneumonitis. *Am Rev Respir Dis* 1977;**116**:1075.

Stankus RP, Salvaggio JE: Hypersensitivity pneumonitis. *Clin Chest Med* 1983;**4**:55.

Silicosis
Dauber JH: Silicosis. In: *Pulmonary Diseases and Disorders: Update 1.* Fishman AP (editor). McGraw-Hill, 1982.

Goldsmith DF, Winn DM, Shy CM (editors): *Silica, Silicosis and Cancer.* Praeger, 1986.

Coal Worker's Pneumoconiosis
Merchant JA, Roger RB: Coal workers' respiratory disease. In: *Environmental and Occupational Medicine.* Rom WN (editor). Little, Brown, 1982.

Asbestos-Induced Diseases

American Thoracic Society: The diagnosis of nonmalignant diseases related to asbestos. *Am Rev Respir Dis*
1986;**134**:363.

Becklake MR: Asbestos-related diseases of the lungs and
pleura: Current clinical issues. *Am Rev Respir Dis*
1982;**126**:187.

Craighead JE et al: The pathology of asbestos-associated
diseases of the lungs and pleural cavities: Diagnostic
criteria and proposed grading schema. *Arch Pathol
Lab Med* 1982;**106**:544.

Beryllium Disease

Daniels RP: Beryllium-induced lung disease: Immunologic mechanisms and diagnostic approaches. In:
Occupational Lung Disease. Gee JB, Morgan WK
(editors). Raven Press, 1983.

Cardiovascular Toxicology

19

Neal L. Benowitz, MD

Heart disease and stroke cause the majority of deaths in the USA. The major risk factors for coronary heart disease—family history, hypertension, diabetes, lipid abnormalities, and cigarette smoking—explain only a small portion of the cases. Other factors such as stress and exposure to occupational or environmental toxic agents are believed to contribute to the development of heart disease, though the magnitude of the risk is unknown. This chapter focuses on cardiovascular disease caused by occupational toxic substances.

Causation in Toxic Cardiovascular Disease

The types and possible toxic causes of cardiovascular disease are shown in Table 19–1. Massive exposure may occur (eg, in acute carbon monoxide poisoning), but toxic cardiovascular disease is usually the result of chronic low-level exposures.

Problems in establishing the cause of cardiovascular disease include the following:

(1) Cardiovascular disease is common even in the absence of toxic exposures.

(2) There is usually nothing specific, either clinically or pathologically, to point to toxic cardiovascular disease.

(3) It is rarely possible to document high tissue levels of suspected toxic substances.

(4) It is difficult to establish occupational exposure levels over the 20 or more years it may take to develop cardiovascular disease.

(5) Cardiovascular toxic substances are likely to interact with other risk factors in causing or manifesting cardiovascular disease.

With these limitations in mind, this chapter will discuss current information concerning toxic cardiovascular disease.

Evaluation of Patients

Evaluation of patients in cases of suspected toxic cardiovascular disease should include the following steps:

(1) Take a detailed occupational history (see Chapter 2), with attention to the temporal relationship between cardiovascular symptoms and exposure to toxic substances in the workplace.

(2) Attempt to document exposure to suspected toxic substances by obtaining industrial hygiene data and, if possible, directly monitoring worker exposure.

(3) Evaluate other cardiovascular risk factors.

(4) Perform a complete physical examination.

(5) Perform appropriate diagnostic studies, such as exercise stress testing and coronary angiography to establish the presence and extent of coronary artery disease; radionuclide angiography to establish myocardial disease and the presence of cardiomyopathy; and ambulatory electrocardiographic recordings taken on workdays and at other times to document work-related arrhythmias.

CARDIOVASCULAR ABNORMALITIES CAUSED BY CARBON DISULFIDE

Chronic exposure to carbon disulfide is one of the best-documented toxic causes for accelerated atherosclerosis and coronary heart disease. Carbon disulfide is a solvent widely used, especially in the rubber and viscose rayon industries, in the manufacture of carbon tetrachloride and ammonium salts and as a degreasing solvent. Epidemiologic studies have indicated that there is a 2.5- to 5-fold increase in the risk of death from coronary heart disease in workers exposed to carbon disulfide. For a complete discus-

Table 19–1. Classification of cardiovascular diseases and possible toxic causes.

Condition	Toxic Agent
Cardiac arrhythmia	Arsenic Chlorofluorocarbon propellants Hydrocarbon solvents (eg, 1,1,1-trichloroethane and trichloroethylene) Organophosphate and carbamate insecticides
Coronary artery disease	Carbon disulfide Carbon monoxide ?Lead
Hypertension	Cadmium Carbon disulfide Lead
Myocardial injury	Antimony Arsenic Arsine Cobalt Lead
Nonatheromatous ischemic heart disease	Organic nitrates (eg, nitroglycerin and ethylene glycol dinitrate)
Peripheral arterial occlusive disease	Arsenic Lead

sion of the systemic effects of carbon disulfide, see Chapter 26.

Pathogenesis

The mechanism of accelerated atherogenesis due to carbon disulfide has not been proved. One theory is that carbon disulfide reacts with amino- and thiol-containing compounds in the body to produce thiocarbamates, which are capable of complexing trace metals and inhibiting many enzyme systems. This causes metabolic abnormalities such as disturbances of lipid metabolism and thyroid function and can lead to hypercholesterolemia and hypothyroidism, which are risk factors for atherosclerosis. Inhibition of dopamine β-hydroxylase, an enzyme that converts dopamine to norepinephrine, may be responsible for some of the neuropsychiatric effects of carbon disulfide. Aldehyde dehydrogenase may be inhibited, resulting in a disulfiram-like reaction after alcohol ingestion. Other possible contributors to accelerated atherosclerosis in workers exposed to carbon disulfide are depressed fibrinolytic activity and hypertension.

Pathology

The findings are those of accelerated atherosclerotic vascular disease involving the coronary, cerebral, and peripheral arteries. Renovascular hypertension has also been reported.

Clinical Findings

A. Symptoms and Signs: Acute intoxication may produce symptoms and signs of encephalopathy or polyneuropathy, including fatigue, headaches, dizziness, disorientation, paresthesias, psychosis, and delirium.

In cases of chronic exposure, patients may present with hypertension or manifestations of atherosclerotic vascular disease such as angina or myocardial infarction. An early sign of chronic carbon disulfide poisoning is abnormal ocular microcirculation, characterized by microaneurysms and hemorrhages resembling those of diabetic retinopathy. Presenile dementia, stroke, and sudden death have been reported in patients with chronic poisoning.

B. Laboratory Findings: Findings may include a decrease in serum thyroxine levels and an increase in serum cholesterol levels, particularly those of the beta very low density lipoproteins. There are no practical methods for measuring carbon disulfide in biologic fluids.

C. Cardiovascular Studies: Delayed filling of the retinal arteries as measured by fluorescein angiography may be an early sign of vascular disease. The ECG sometimes shows evidence of ischemia or previous myocardial infarction. The presence of coronary artery disease may be confirmed by exercise stress testing and coronary angiography.

Differential Diagnosis

The vascular findings in patients with chronic carbon disulfide poisoning are the same as those seen in any patient with atherosclerotic vascular disease. The most specific finding is abnormal ocular microcirculation in the absence of diabetes. The diagnosis is based on a clinical picture of premature vascular disease and a history of exposure to excessive levels of carbon disulfide for more than 5 or 10 years.

Prevention

Carbon disulfide exposure is primarily by inhalation. The Occupational Safety and Health Administration (OSHA) recommends that workplace exposure be limited to 4 ppm (time-weighted average for a 40-hour workweek). Periodic examination of the ocular fundi may help detect early signs of vascular disease.

Treatment

Treatment consists of removing the worker from sources of carbon disulfide exposure and medical measures for atherosclerotic vascular disease.

Course & Prognosis

The course of the disease is similar to that of any atherosclerotic vascular disease. There is evidence of reversibility—at least of ocular changes—after exposure to carbon disulfide is discontinued.

CARDIOVASCULAR ABNORMALITIES CAUSED BY CARBON MONOXIDE

Excessive carbon monoxide exposure can reduce maximal exercise capacity in healthy workers; aggravate angina pectoris, intermittent claudication, and chronic obstructive lung disease; and aggravate or induce cardiac arrhythmias. Acute intoxications can cause myocardial infarction or sudden death. Chronic high-level carbon monoxide exposure may result in congestive cardiomyopathy.

Carbon monoxide is the most widely distributed of all industrial toxic agents and accounts for the greatest number of intoxications and deaths. It is formed wherever combustion engines or other types of combustion are present. Workers at high risk include forklift operators, foundry workers, miners, mechanics, garage attendants, and fire fighters. Carbon monoxide poisoning may also occur with the use of faulty furnaces or heaters, particularly improperly vented kerosene or charcoal heaters. Cigarette smoking is an important source of carbon monoxide, and occupational sources may be additive to exposure from cigarettes. The solvent methylene chloride is metabolized within the body to carbon monoxide.

For a complete discussion of carbon monoxide, see Chapter 31.

Pathogenesis

The affinity of carbon monoxide for hemoglobin is more than 200 times that of oxygen. Binding of carbon monoxide and hemoglobin to form carboxyhemoglobin reduces delivery of oxygen to body tissues because the oxygen-carrying capacity of hemoglobin is decreased and because less oxygen is released to tissues at any given oxygen tension (ie, there is a shift in the oxygen dissociation curve). Thus, a carboxyhemoglobin concentration of 20% represents a greater reduction in oxygen delivery than a 20% reduction in erythrocyte count. Other heme-containing proteins (eg, myoglobin, cytochrome oxidase, and cytochrome P-450) bind 10–15% of the total body carbon monoxide, but the medical significance of their binding at usual levels of exposure to carbon monoxide is unclear.

In healthy individuals exposed to carbon monoxide, the decrease in delivery of oxygen to tissues causes the cardiac output and coronary blood flow to increase to meet the metabolic demands of the heart. Although these compensatory responses allow healthy individuals to perform at normal work levels, their maximal exercise capacity is decreased. If, on the other hand, compensatory responses are limited, as in patients with coronary artery disease, carbon monoxide exposure may cause angina or myocardial infarction (Fig 19–1). Reduced exercise thresholds

for the development of angina have been reported when carboxyhemoglobin concentrations are as low as 2.7% (Table 19–2). Carbon monoxide decreases the ventricular fibrillation threshold in experimental animals and may do the same in humans. This would explain why sudden death occurs in people who have coronary artery disease and are exposed to carbon monoxide, as has been reported to occur on smoggy days in large cities. Severe carbon monoxide poisoning (carboxyhemoglobin concentrations > 50%) may cause severe hypoxic injury, including cardiovascular collapse.

Chronic exposure to carbon monoxide is thought to accelerate atherogenesis. Cigarette smokers demonstrate advanced coronary and peripheral atherosclerosis, and carbon monoxide is believed to be one of the primary etiologic factors. Several studies in animals have tested the effects of chronic high-level carbon monoxide exposure combined with feeding of atherogenic diets, and the results of some of these studies showed increased severity of atherosclerosis. Possible mechanisms include abnormal vascular permeability, increased vascular uptake of lipids, and increased platelet adhesiveness. Whether atheroscle-

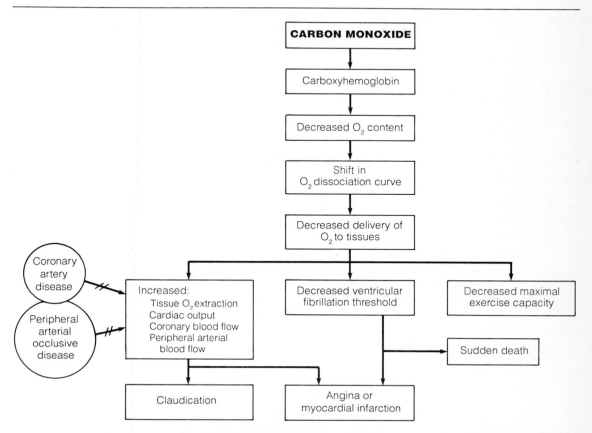

Figure 19–1. Cardiovascular consequences of exposure to carbon monoxide. The presence of coronary artery disease or peripheral arterial occlusive disease prevents (//) the usual compensatory increase in coronary or peripheral arterial blood flow, and this results in symptoms of arterial insufficiency.

Table 19–2. Effects of carbon monoxide on exercise capacity.

Group	Baseline Exercise Duration	Level of Exposure to Carbon Monoxide	Increase in Concentration of Carboxyhemoglobin	Exercise Duration After Exposure	Exercise End Point
Healthy individuals	698 sec	100 ppm for 1 h	1.7% → 4%	662 sec	Exhaustion
Patients with angina pectoris	224 sec	50 ppm for 2 h	1% → 2.7%	188 sec	Angina
Patients with intermittent claudication	174 sec	50 ppm for 2 h	1.1% → 2.8%	144 sec	Claudication
Patients with chronic lung disease	219 sec	100 ppm for 1 h	1.4% → 4.1%	147 sec	Dyspnea

rosis is accelerated at levels of carbon monoxide commonly encountered in the workplace is unclear.

Chronic exposure to carbon monoxide results in increased red blood cell mass in response to chronic tissue hypoxia and in increased blood viscosity, which could contribute to acute cardiac events.

Pathology

Cardiac necrosis is often observed in cases of fatal carbon monoxide poisoning and is presumably due to severe hypoxia. Myocardial infarction may occur in workers who have coronary artery disease and are exposed to high levels of carbon monoxide, particularly while performing strenuous work or exercise. Cardiomyopathy with cardiac enlargement and congestive heart failure has been described in workers with chronic high-level exposure to carbon monoxide (carboxyhemoglobin concentrations > 30%).

Clinical Findings

A. Symptoms and Signs: Headache is typically the first symptom of carbon monoxide poisoning and may occur at carboxyhemoglobin concentrations as low as 10%. At higher concentrations, nausea, dizziness, fatigue, and dimmed vision are commonly reported.

In patients with angina pectoris or peripheral arterial occlusive disease, carbon monoxide exposure may reduce exercise capacity to the point of angina or claudication (Table 19–2). All workers experience a reduction in maximal exercise capacity.

In neuropsychiatric tests, findings such as increased reaction time and decreased manual dexterity may be seen at carboxyhemoglobin concentrations between 5% and 10%. At concentrations of 25%, there may be decreased visual acuity and impaired cognitive function; at 35%, ataxia; at 50%, vomiting, tachypnea, tachycardia, and hypertension; and at higher levels, coma, convulsions, and cardiovascular and respiratory depression. Myocardial ischemia may be evident at any carboxyhemoglobin concentration in susceptible individuals.

B. Laboratory Findings: The only finding specific for carbon monoxide intoxication is elevation of the carboxyhemoglobin concentration. Normal carboxyhemoglobin concentrations and examples of concentrations resulting from exposure to carbon monoxide in the environment and the workplace are shown in Table 19–3.

When arterial blood gases are measured, they usually show a normal or a slightly reduced arterial oxygen tension, with substantial reductions in venous Po_2 and oxygen content. Although respiratory alkalosis due to hyperventilation is commonly observed, there is respiratory failure in the most severe poisonings. When there is marked tissue hypoxia, lactic acidosis develops.

C. Cardiovascular Studies: The ECG may show ischemic changes or myocardial infarction. Various types of arrhythmias, including atrial fibrillation and premature atrial and ventricular contractions, are observed. Abnormalities seen on ECG are usually

Table 19–3. Normal carboxyhemoglobin concentrations and examples of concentrations resulting from exposure to carbon monoxide in the environment and the workplace.

Source of Carbon Monoxide	Carboxyhemoglobin Concentration	
	Average	Range
Endogenous metabolism (normal level[1])	0.5%	. . .
Environmental exposure		
Air pollution	2%	1.5–2.5%
Cigarette smoking	6%	3–15%
Occupational exposure (nonsmokers)		
Foundry workers	4%	2–9%
Mechanics	5%	. . .
Garage attendants	7%	. . .

[1]Carbon monoxide is normally formed as a product of metabolism of hemoglobin. Endogenous levels may be higher if there is increased hemoglobin turnover.

transient, though ST–T wave abnormalities may persist for days or weeks.

Differential Diagnosis

The most important clue to carbon monoxide poisoning is the occupational or environmental exposure history. A typical symptom, such as headache, confusion, or sudden collapse, with findings of myocardial ischemia or metabolic acidosis, should suggest the diagnosis, and carboxyhemoglobin concentrations should be measured.

Prevention

Levels of carbon monoxide should be monitored if there are sources of combustion such as combustion engines or furnaces in the workplace. The current 8-hour threshold limit value is 50 ppm, which at the end of an 8-hour workday results in a carboxyhemoglobin concentration of 5%. This concentration is tolerated well by healthy individuals but not by people with cardiovascular or chronic lung disease. Workplace monitoring is easily done with a portable carbon monoxide meter. Biologic monitoring of workers involves measuring either the carboxyhemoglobin concentration in blood or the level of expired carbon monoxide, which is directly proportionate to the carboxyhemoglobin concentration. Elevated carbon monoxide levels should be anticipated in cigarette smokers.

Treatment

Carbon monoxide is eliminated from the body by respiration, and the rate of elimination depends on ventilation, pulmonary blood flow, and inspired oxygen concentration. The half-life of carbon monoxide in a sedentary adult breathing air is 4–5 hours. The half-life can be reduced to 80 minutes by giving 100% oxygen by face mask, or it can be reduced to 25 minutes by giving hyperbaric oxygen (3 atmospheres) in a hyperbaric chamber.

Course & Prognosis

Recovery is usually complete after mild to moderate carbon monoxide intoxication in the absence of a cardiac complication such as myocardial infarction. With severe carbon monoxide poisoning, particularly if coma has occurred, there may be permanent neurologic abnormalities ranging from subtle neuropsychiatric disturbances to gross motor or cognitive dysfunction to vegetative states. Abnormal findings on a CT scan of the brain (eg, lesions in the basal ganglia or the periventricular white matter) predict a poor neurologic outcome.

CARDIOVASCULAR ABNORMALITIES CAUSED BY ORGANIC NITRATES

In the 1950s, an epidemic of sudden death in young munitions workers who hand-packed cartridges was observed. It was subsequently discovered that abrupt withdrawal from excessive exposure to organic nitrates, particularly nitroglycerin and ethylene glycol dinitrate, may result in myocardial ischemia even in the absence of coronary artery disease. Occupations in which workers may be exposed to organic nitrates include explosives manufacturing, construction work involving blasting, weapons handling in the armed forces, and pharmaceutical manufacturing of nitrates.

Pathogenesis

Nitrates directly dilate blood vessels, including those of the coronary circulation. With prolonged exposure (usually 1–4 years), compensatory vasoconstriction develops that is believed to be mediated by sympathetic neural responses, activation of the renin-angiotensin system, or both. When exposure to nitrates is stopped, the compensatory vasoconstriction becomes unopposed (Fig 19–2). Coronary vasospasm with angina, myocardial infarction, or sudden

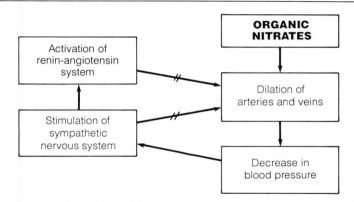

Figure 19–2. Mechanism of vasospasm after withdrawal from chronic exposure to nitrates. Vasoconstrictor forces antagonize (///) nitrate-induced vasodilation. Withdrawal of nitrates results in unopposed vasoconstriction and in coronary vasospasm.

death may result. Chest pain occurring during nitrate withdrawal has been termed "Monday morning angina" because it typically occurs 2 or 3 days after the last day of nitrate exposure. Case control studies suggest a 2.5- to 4-fold increase in the risk for cardiovascular death in workers handling explosives.

Pathology

In patients who have died following withdrawal from nitrates, there is often no or minimal coronary atherosclerosis. In one patient, coronary vasospasm was observed during angiography, and the spasm was promptly reversed by sublingual nitroglycerin.

Clinical Findings

A. Symptoms and Signs: Workers exposed to excessive levels of nitrates typically experience headaches and have hypotension, tachycardia, and warm, flushed skin. With continued exposure, the symptoms and signs become less prominent. After 1–2 days without exposure to nitrates—generally on weekends—there may be signs of acute coronary ischemia ranging from mild angina at rest to manifestations of myocardial infarction (eg, nausea, diaphoresis, pallor, and palpitations associated with severe chest pain), or sudden death may occur.

B. Laboratory Findings and Cardiovascular Studies: During episodes of pain, the ECG may show evidence of acute ischemia: either ST segment elevation or depression, with or without T wave abnormalities. At other times, the ECG may be perfectly normal. Typical findings of myocardial infarction include development of a pathologic Q wave on ECG and elevation of the MB isoenzyme creatine phosphokinase (CPK) and other cardiac enzymes. Results of exercise stress testing and coronary angiography may be normal.

Differential Diagnosis

Workers chronically exposed to nitrates may also have organic coronary artery disease, which must be identified.

Prevention

Nitrates are extremely volatile and readily absorbed through the lungs and skin. They can permeate the wrapping material of dynamite sticks, so workers who handle dynamite should be advised to wear cotton gloves. Natural rubber gloves should not be used because they tend to become permeated with nitrates and may enhance absorption.

With current automated processes in explosives manufacturing, direct handling of nitrates by employees is minimized. However, levels of nitrates in the workplace environment must be controlled by adequate ventilation and by air conditioning during periods of hot weather. The current OSHA exposure limit is 0.2 ppm for nitroglycerin, but even at lower levels (0.02 ppm or above), personal protective gear is recommended to avoid headache. Although there are no readily available biochemical measures to

detect excessive nitrate exposure, findings of progressively decreasing blood pressure and increasing heart rate during the workday are suggestive of excessive exposure. Monitoring for these signs in employees may also help prevent adverse effects of exposure to nitrates.

Treatment

Treatment of myocardial ischemia due to nitrate withdrawal includes cardiac nitrates (eg, nitroglycerin or isosorbide dinitrate) or calcium entry blocking agents. Case reports indicate that ischemic symptoms may recur, indicating a persistent tendency to coronary spasm, for weeks or months, so long-term cardiac nitrate or calcium blocker therapy may be needed. The worker should be removed from sources of organic nitrate exposure.

Course & Prognosis

In the absence of myocardial infarction or sudden death, anginal symptoms fully resolve after exposure to nitrate is stopped.

CARDIOVASCULAR ABNORMALITIES CAUSED BY HYDROCARBON SOLVENTS & CHLOROFLUOROCARBON (CFC)

Exposure to various solvents and propellants may result in cardiac arrhythmia, syncope with resultant accidents at work, or sudden death. Most serious cases of arrhythmia have been associated with abuse of or industrial exposure to halogenated hydrocarbon solvents (eg, 1,1,1-trichloroethane and trichloroethylene) or exposure to chlorofluorocarbon (freon) propellants. Nonhalogenated solvents and even ethanol present similar risks.

Exposure to solvents is widespread in industrial settings such as dry cleaning, degreasing, painting, and chemical manufacturing. Chlorofluorocarbons are used extensively as refrigerants and as propellants in a wide variety of products and processes. For example, a pathology resident developed various arrhythmias after exposure to chlorofluorocarbon aerosols used for freezing samples and cleaning slides in a surgical pathology laboratory.

Pathogenesis

Fig 19–3 illustrates 2 ways in which halogenated hydrocarbons and other solvents are thought to induce cardiac arrhythmia or sudden death: (1) At low levels of exposure, these solvents "sensitize" the heart to actions of catecholamines. For example, experimental studies have shown that the amount of epinephrine required to produce ventricular tachycardia or fibrillation is reduced after the solvents are inhaled. Catecholamine release is potentiated by euphoria and excitement due to inhalation of the

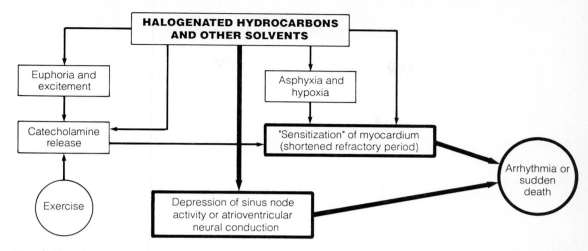

Figure 19–3. Mechanisms of arrhythmia or sudden death following low-level exposure (light arrows) or high-level exposure (heavy arrows) to halogenated hydrocarbons and other solvents.

solvent and also by exercise. This, in combination with asphyxia and hypoxia, causes arrhythmia, which can result in death. (2) At higher levels of exposure, solvents may depress sinus node activity and thereby cause sinus bradycardia or arrest, or they may depress atrioventricular neural conduction and thereby cause atrioventricular block. In some cases, they do both. Bradyarrhythmia then predisposes to escape ventricular arrhythmia or, in cases of more severe intoxication, to asystole. The arrhythmogenic action of solvents may also be enhanced by alcohol or caffeine.

Pathology

Most cardiovascular deaths following exposure to hydrocarbons are sudden deaths. Autopsies usually reveal no specific pathologic findings. The finding of a fatty liver suggests chronic exposure to high levels of halogenated solvents or to ethanol.

Clinical Findings

A. Symptoms and Signs: Symptoms of intoxication with hydrocarbon solvents or chlorofluorocarbons may include dizziness, light-headedness, headaches, nausea, drowsiness, lethargy, palpitations, or syncope. Physical examination may reveal ataxia, nystagmus, and slurred speech. The heartbeat and blood pressure are usually normal, except at the time of arrhythmias, when a rapid or irregular heartbeat is sometimes accompanied by hypotension.

Convulsions, coma, or cardiac arrest may occur in severe cases of exposure to solvents. Workers who have heart disease or chronic lung disease with hypoxemia may be more susceptible to the arrhythmogenic actions of solvents.

B. Laboratory Findings: Concentrations of some hydrocarbons can be measured in expired air or in the blood (see Chapters 27 and 34).

C. Cardiovascular Studies: Arrhythmias in-duced by solvents or chlorofluorocarbons are expected to occur only at work, while the worker is exposed to these agents. The diagnosis is based on abnormalities observed during ambulatory electrocardiographic monitoring and consist of one or more of the following: premature atrial or ventricular contractions, recurrent supraventricular tachycardia, and recurrent ventricular tachycardia. It is essential to monitor patients both on workdays and on off days and to request a log of times of exposure to solvents or chlorofluorocarbons as well as a log of symptoms of palpitations or dizzy spells. A 12-lead ECG and an exercise stress test can help determine the presence of coronary artery disease, which might increase sensitivity to hydrocarbon- or chlorofluorocarbon-induced arrhythmia.

Differential Diagnosis

The diagnosis of solvent- or chlorofluorocarbon-induced arrhythmia is based on exclusion of other causes of arrhythmias at work (eg, the presence of a cardiac disease, metabolic disturbance, or drug abuse) and demonstration of a temporal relationship between episodes of arrhythmia and exposures to the toxic agent. The diagnosis is supported by industrial hygiene measurements documenting the level of exposure in the workplace and by objective and subjective evidence that the worker was intoxicated following exposure.

Prevention

Preventive measures include proper handling of solvents and propellants, adequate ventilation in the workplace, and, in some cases, the use of protective respiratory equipment. Workers with heart disease—especially those with chronic arrhythmia—should be advised to avoid exposure to potentially arrhythmogenic chemicals.

Treatment

Beta-adrenergic blocking agents may be useful in managing solvent- or chlorofluorocarbon-induced arrhythmias. In cases of episodic arrhythmia, the worker should be removed from excessive exposure or advised to use protective respiratory equipment. If a worker collapses and resuscitation is required, use of epinephrine and other sympathomimetic drugs should be avoided if possible, since they may precipitate further arrhythmia.

Course & Prognosis

Arrhythmias are expected to fully resolve after exposure to hydrocarbons is stopped.

CARDIOVASCULAR ABNORMALITIES CAUSED BY ORGANOPHOSPHATE & CARBAMATE INSECTICIDES

Intoxication with organophosphate and carbamate insecticides can produce diverse cardiovascular disturbances, including tachycardia and hypertension, bradycardia and hypotension, heart block, and ventricular tachycardia.

Organophosphate and carbamate insecticides are widely used in agriculture and can be applied to crops by aerial spraying or by hand. Agricultural workers may thus absorb the insecticides by inhalation of mist or via cutaneous absorption. Acute insecticide poisoning affects the circulatory system and may be fatal. Chronic poisoning may cause neuropsychiatric disturbances, as described in Chapter 30.

Pathogenesis

Organophosphates and carbamates inhibit acetylcholinesterase, and this causes accumulation of acetylcholine at cholinergic synapses and myoneural junctions. The cardiovascular effects may vary over the time course of poisoning. Early in acute poisoning, acetylcholine stimulates nicotinic receptors at sympathetic ganglia and causes tachycardia and mild hypertension. Later, when acetylcholine acts at muscarinic receptors or blocks ganglionic transmission by hyperpolarization, it causes bradycardia and hypotension. As a consequence of autonomic imbalance and asynchronous repolarization of different parts of the heart, there may be QT interval prolongation and polymorphous ventricular tachycardia (torsades de pointes).

The excess of acetylcholine at the myoneural junctions initially causes muscle fasciculations and later causes muscle paralysis, including paralysis of the diaphragm, which results in respiratory failure or respiratory arrest. Other consequences are described below.

Pathology

As organophosphates act on autonomic neurotransmitters, there are no specific pathologic findings.

Clinical Findings

A. Symptoms and Signs: Typical symptoms of mild organophosphate or carbamate poisoning include weakness, headache, sweating, nausea, vomiting, abdominal cramps, and diarrhea. Moderate poisoning may be associated with chest discomfort, dyspnea, inability to walk, and blurred vision.

The signs are those of cholinergic excess and include small pupils, diaphoresis, salivation, lacrimation, an increase in bronchial secretions (which may resemble pulmonary edema), and muscle fasciculations. Early cardiovascular manifestations may include tachycardia and hypertension. Later, there may be bradycardia and hypotension. There is sometimes frank muscular weakness or, in severe poisoning, paralysis accompanied by respiratory failure, convulsions, or coma.

The failure of usual doses of atropine to reverse cholinergic signs is highly suggestive of the diagnosis of organophosphate or carbamate poisoning.

B. Laboratory Findings: The diagnosis is confirmed by the finding of markedly depressed cholinesterase activity in red blood cells. Depression to below 50% of normal is usually required for patients to have any symptoms, and depression to less than 10% of normal is usually seen in patients with severe poisoning. Plasma cholinesterase activity is usually depressed also, but this correlates less well with clinical manifestations.

Arterial blood gases may show carbon dioxide retention, hypoxia, or both.

The presence of a particular type of organophosphate may be detected in the blood or gastric fluids. Some organophosphates (eg, parathion) have metabolites that can be measured in the urine.

C. Cardiovascular Studies: Delayed repolarization with QT prolongation and episodes of ventricular tachycardia may be seen for up to 5–7 days after acute intoxication. The ECG also commonly shows nonspecific ST and T wave changes. A variety of arrhythmias, including premature ventricular contractions, ventricular tachycardia and fibrillation, and heart block with asystole, have been observed.

D. Imaging: Chest x-ray may show a pattern similar to that of pulmonary edema.

Differential Diagnosis

The signs and symptoms of cholinergic excess are fairly specific for poisoning with cholinesterase-inhibiting insecticides. However, similar findings may be seen in people treated with cholinesterase inhibitors, such as pyridostigmine for myasthenia gravis. Small pupils may also be seen following ingestion of narcotics, clonidine, phenothiazines, and sedative drugs and in patients with pontine brain infarction or hemorrhage.

Prevention

Most organophosphate and carbamate insecticides are rapidly absorbed following ingestion, inhalation, or contact with the skin or eyes. Continuing exposure may occur from contact with contaminated clothing or hair. Prevention requires use of protective clothing and respirators and monitoring of red blood cell cholinesterase levels on a regular basis.

Treatment

General measures include decontamination (removal of clothing and thorough cleaning of skin and hair), support of respiration (including mechanical ventilation in respiratory failure), and support of the circulation. Specific measures include the use of pralidoxime (2-PAM) to reverse muscular paralysis and other manifestations of excess acetylcholine and the use of atropine to reverse bronchorrhea and bradycardia.

Intensive cardiac and respiratory monitoring of patients for several days after exposure is recommended, with particular attention to the possible late development of arrhythmia or respiratory failure. Heart block and polymorphous ventricular tachycardia with a prolonged QT interval are optimally treated by cardiac pacing. Use of antiarrhythmic drugs that depress conduction (eg, quinidine, procainamide, and disopyramide) and calcium channel blockers should be avoided.

Course & Prognosis

Recovery from acute intoxication is usually complete. Chronic intoxication may be associated with neuropsychiatric consequences (see Chapters 22 and 30).

CARDIOVASCULAR ABNORMALITIES CAUSED BY HEAVY METALS

A number of metals have been associated with disturbances in cardiovascular function, but their causative role has not been fully established.

Antimony

Therapeutic use of antimonial compounds for treatment of parasitic infections produces electrocardiographic abnormalities—primarily T wave changes and QT interval prolongation—and has caused sudden death in some patients. Electrocardiographic changes have also been observed in workers exposed to antimony. Although these changes usually resolve after removal from exposure, a few studies have reported increased cardiovascular mortality rates in exposed workers. Studies in animals confirm that chronic exposure to antimony can produce myocardial disease.

Arsenic

Subacute arsenic poisoning caused by ingestion of arsenic-contaminated beer has been associated with cardiomyopathy and cardiac failure. Chronic arsenic poisoning has been reported to produce "blackfoot disease," which is characterized by claudication and gangrene presumably secondary to spasms of the large blood vessels in the extremities. Acute arsenic poisoning can cause electrocardiographic abnormalities, and in one case it was reported to cause recurrent ventricular arrhythmia of the torsades de pointes type. A recent mortality study of copper smelters exposed to arsenic indicated that these workers have an increased risk of death due to ischemic heart disease.

Arsine

Arsine gas causes red blood cell hemolysis. Massive hemolysis produces hyperkalemia, which can result in cardiac arrest. Electrocardiographic manifestations progress from high, peaked T waves to conduction disturbances and various degrees of heart block and then to asystole. Arsine may also directly affect the myocardium, causing a greater magnitude of cardiac failure than would be expected from the degree of anemia.

Cadmium

Some epidemiologic studies have linked high-level cadmium exposure with hypertension. This is supported by findings in animal studies. However, there is no evidence that exposure to cadmium levels found in the workplace increases the risk of cardiovascular disease.

Cobalt

In Quebec City, Canada, in 1965 and 1966, an epidemic of cardiomyopathy occurred in heavy drinkers of beer to which cobalt sulfate had been added as a foam stabilizer. The mortality rate in affected patients was 22%, and a major pathologic finding in those who died was myocardial necrosis with thrombi in the heart and major blood vessels. Other clinical features in affected patients included polycythemia, pericardial effusion, and thyroid hyperplasia. Cobalt is known to depress oxygen uptake by mitochondria of the heart and to interfere with energy metabolism in a manner biochemically similar to the effects of thiamine deficiency. Since individuals receiving higher doses of cobalt for therapeutic reasons have not developed cardiomyopathy, perhaps cobalt, excessive alcohol consumption, and nutritional deprivation acted synergistically to produce cardiomyopathy in this epidemic.

One case of cardiomyopathy in a worker exposed to cobalt has been reported.

Lead

Exposure to excessive levels of lead causes chronic renal diseases, and epidemiologic studies suggest that it also contributes to hypertension in the absence of renal disease. Some of the workplace studies of exposure to lead report an increased incidence of ischemic electrocardiographic changes and an increased risk of hypertensive or coronary artery disease and cerebrovascular disease in exposed workers. Nonspecific electrocardiographic changes and fatal myocarditis in the absence of hypertension have been observed in children with lead poisoning. Cardiomyopathy in moonshine drinkers has also been attributed to lead exposure. Studies in animals indicate that lead may have direct toxic effects on the myocardium.

REFERENCES

General

Goldhaber SZ: Cardiovascular effects of potential occupational hazards. *J Am Coll Cardiol* 1983;**2**:1210.

Harlan WR et al: Impact of the environment on cardiovascular disease: Report of the American Heart Association Task Force on environment and the cardiovascular system. *Circulation* 1981;**63**:243A.

Kurppa K et al: Chemical exposures at work and cardiovascular morbidity: Atherosclerosis, ischemic heart disease, hypertension, cardiomyopathy, and arrhythmias. *Scand J Work Environ Health* 1984;**10**:381.

Rosenman KD: Cardiovascular disease and environmental exposure. *Br J Ind Med* 1979;**36**:85.

Rosenman KD: Cardiovascular disease and workplace exposures. *Arch Environ Health* 1984;**39**:218.

Carbon Disulfide

MacMahon B, Monson R: Mortality in the US rayon industry. *J Occup Med* 1988;**30**:698.

Nurminen M, Hernberg S: Effects of intervention on the cardiovascular mortality of workers exposed to carbon disulphide: A 15-year follow-up. *Br J Ind Med* 1985;**42**:32.

Nurminen M et al: Quantitated effects of carbon disulfide exposure, elevated blood pressure and aging on coronary mortality. *Am J Epidemiol* 1982;**115**:107.

Tolonen M: Vascular effects of carbon disulfide: A review. *Scand J Work Environ Health* 1975;**1**:63.

Carbon Monoxide

Aronow WS, Cassidy J: Effect of carbon monoxide on maximal treadmill exercise: A study in normal persons. *Ann Intern Med* 1975;**83**:496.

Aronow WS, Isbell MW: Carbon monoxide effect on exercise-induced angina pectoris. *Ann Intern Med* 1973;**79**:392.

Hernberg S et al: Angina pectoris, ECG findings and blood pressure of foundry workers in relation to carbon monoxide exposure. *Scand J Work Environ Health* 1976;**2**(Suppl 1):54.

Olson KR: Carbon monoxide poisoning: Mechanisms, presentation, and controversies in management. *J Emerg Med* 1984;**1**:233.

Scharf SM, Thames MD, Sargent RK: Transmural myocardial infarction after exposure to carbon monoxide in coronary-artery disease: Report of a case. *N Engl J Med* 1974;**291**:85.

Stewart RD: The effect of carbon monoxide on humans. *Ann Rev Pharmacol* 1975;**15**:409.

Turino GM: Effect of carbon monoxide on the cardiorespiratory system: Carbon monoxide toxicity: Physiology and biochemistry. *Circulation* 1981;**63**:253A.

Organic Nitrates

Carmichael P, Lieben J: Sudden death in explosives workers. *Arch Environ Health* 1963;**7**:50.

Gjesdal K et al: Exposure to glyceryl trinitrate during gun powder production: Plasma glyceryl trinitrate concentration, elimination kinetics, and discomfort among production workers. *Br J Ind Med* 1985;**42**:27.

Lange RL et al: Nonatheromatous ischemic heart disease following withdrawal from chronic industrial nitroglycerin exposure. *Circulation* 1972;**46**:666.

Morton WE: Occupational habituation to aliphatic nitrates and the withdrawal hazards of coronary disease and hypertension. *J Occup Med* 1977;**19**:197.

Hydrocarbon Solvents & Chlorofluorocarbons

Bass M: Sudden sniffing death. *JAMA* 1970;**212**:2075.

Flowers NC, Horan LG: Nonanoxic aerosol arrhythmias. *JAMA* 1972;**219**:33.

Reynolds AK: Cardiac arrhythmias in sensitized hearts: Primary mechanisms involved. *Res Commun Chem Pathol Pharmacol* 1983;**40**:3.

Speizer FE, Wegman DH, Ramirez A: Palpitation rates associated with fluorocarbon exposure in a hospital setting. *N Engl J Med* 1975;**292**:624.

Organophosphate & Carbamate Insecticides

Bledsoe FH, Seymour EQ: Acute pulmonary edema associated with parathion poisoning. *Radiology* 1972;**103**:53.

Ludomirsky A et al: Q-T prolongation and polymorphous ("torsades de pointes") ventricular arrhythmias associated with organophosphorus insecticide poisoning. *Am J Cardiol* 1982;**49**:1654.

Namba T, Greenfield M, Grob D: Malathion poisoning: A fatal case with cardiac manifestations. *Arch Environ Health* 1970;**21**:533.

Namba T et al: Poisoning due to organophosphate insecticides: Acute and chronic manifestations. *Am J Med* 1971;**50**:475.

Heavy Metals

Axelson O et al: Arsenic exposure and mortality: A case-referent study from a Swedish copper smelter. *Br J Ind Med* 1978;**35**:8.

Barborik M, Dusek J: Cardiomyopathy accompanying industrial cobalt exposure. *Br Heart J* 1972;**34**:113.

Beevers DG et al: Blood-cadmium in hypertensives and normotensives. *Lancet* 1976;**2**:1222.

Borhani NO: Exposure to trace elements and cardiovascular disease. *Circulation* 1981;**63**:260A.

Glauser SC, Bello CT, Glauser EM: Blood-cadmium levels in normotensive and untreated hypertensive humans. *Lancet* 1976;**1**:717.

Goldsmith S, From AH: Arsenic-induced atypical ventricular tachycardia. *N Engl J Med* 1980;**303**:1096.

Kirkby H, Gyntelberg F: Blood pressure and other cardiovascular risk factors of long-term exposure to lead. *Scand J Work Environ Health* 1985;**11**:15.

Pirkle JL et al: The relationship between blood lead levels and blood pressure and its cardiovascular risk implications. *Am J Epidemiol* 1985;**121**:246.

Liver Toxicology

20

Robert J. Harrison, MD, MPH

The liver is the target organ of many occupational and environmental chemicals and plays a central role in their detoxification and elimination. Bacterial and viral infections and certain chemical and physical agents encountered in the workplace also involve the liver. The main causes of occupational liver disease are presented in Tables 20–1, 20–4, and 20–5.

Detection of Occupational Liver Disease

With the exception of a few chemicals that cause specific lesions (Table 20–1), hepatic injury due to industrial exposure does not differ clinically or morphologically from drug-induced damage (including damage due to ethanol). Thus, it may be difficult to differentiate occupational from nonoccupational causes on the basis of screening tests.

Occupational liver disease may be of secondary importance to damage that occurs to other organs or may occur only at high doses after accidental exposure or ingestion. While acute toxic liver injury does occur, concern is increasingly focused on chronic liver disease resulting from prolonged low-level toxic exposure. In this respect, cancer is of central concern. Because chemical studies are frequently done on animals first, the occupational health practitioner must be able to evaluate—without the assistance of adequate human studies—the results of positive carcinogenesis studies in light of actual workplace exposures (eg, methylene chloride; see Chapter 27.)

In individual cases, the clinician is usually first alerted to the presence of hepatic disease by routine enzyme tests and must then make a determination about whether the cause is occupational or nonoccupational. The occupational history and results of personal or workroom air sampling are crucial to formulation of a presumptive diagnosis. It is occasionally necessary to remove the patient from exposure to the suspected workplace toxic substance to establish the workplace relationship.

Limitations of Detection

Unfortunately, the detection of preclinical disease is made difficult by the lack of sufficiently sensitive and specific tests. It is common practice to measure liver enzymes periodically in workers exposed to a known hepatotoxin. This surveillance technique is complicated, however, by the problems of "false positives" (ie, elevated enzymes due to nonoccupational causes) and "false negatives" (normal values

in the presence of biochemical dysfunction). In addition, little is known about the effects of multiple hepatotoxic exposures common to many occupations (eg, painters, printers, laboratory technicians). (For a detailed discussion of these limitations, see Medical Surveillance and Detection of Occupational Hepatotoxicity, below.)

Epidemiologic Evidence of Liver Disease

Epidemiologic studies have been performed on many groups of workers exposed to hepatotoxic

Table 20–1. Chemical agents associated with occupational liver disease.

Compound	Type of Injury	Occupation or Use
Arsenic	Cirrhosis, hepatocellular carcinoma, angiosarcoma	Pesticides
Beryllium	Granulomatous disease	Ceramics workers
Carbon tetrachloride	Acute hepatocellular injury, cirrhosis	Dry cleaning
Dimethylformamide	Acute hepatocellular injury	Solvent, chemical mfg
Dimethylnitrosamine	Hepatocellular carcinoma	Rocket mfg
Dioxin	Porphyria cutanea tarda	Pesticides
Halothane	Acute hepatocellular injury	Anesthesiology
Hydrazine	Steatosis	Rocket mfg
Methylene dianiline	Cholestasis	MDA production workers
2-Nitropropane	Acute hepatocellular injury	Painters
Phosphorus	Acute hepatocellular injury	Munitions workers
Polychlorinated biphenyls	Subacute liver injury	Production, electrical utility
Tetrachloroethane	Acute or subacute hepatocellular injury	Aircraft mfg
Trichloroethylene	Acute hepatocellular injury	Cleaning solvent sniffing
Trinitrotoluene	Acute or subacute hepatocellular injury	Munitions workers
Vinyl chloride	Angiosarcoma	Rubber workers

agents. However, relatively few workplace hepatotoxic substances have been studied in humans. Epidemiologic studies, where available, generally provide the best evidence of toxicity; however, they may be limited by inadequate study design and other factors that make conclusions difficult.

A. Serum Aminotransferases: Cross-sectional studies that include biochemical liver tests have been conducted among many groups of workers exposed to hepatotoxic agents—though for only a few has an adequate control group been identified. Serum aminotransferase elevations have been found in workers exposed to polychlorinated and polybrominated biphenyls (PCBs, PBBs) and in painters exposed to various solvents. Exposure to commonly used aromatic and aliphatic organic solvents within permissible exposure limits is not likely to result in liver damage detectable by serum aminotransferases.

B. Microsomal Enzyme Induction: Using the noninvasive antipyrine clearance test, induction of the microsomal enzyme system has been demonstrated in workers exposed to various pesticides (chlordecone, phenoxy acids, DDT, lindane), halothane, polychlorinated biphenyls, and various solvents. Functional abnormalities of liver metabolism—measured by antipyrine clearance or other noninvasive tests of liver function—are not accompanied by other clinical or laboratory signs of toxicity and so may provide a sensitive index of biologic change.

C. Mortality Studies: Cohort mortality studies have shown an increased mortality rate from liver cirrhosis among newspaper pressmen, spray painters, and oil refinery workers and from liver cancer among vinyl chloride, rubber, dye, and shoe factory workers. Three case-control studies have shown a statistically significant association between primary liver cancer and exposure to organic solvents, particularly among laundry workers, dry cleaners, gasoline service station attendants, asphalt workers, and bartenders.

CHEMICAL AGENTS CAUSING LIVER TOXICITY

Pathogenesis & Epidemiology

Occupational hepatotoxicity caused by chemicals is most frequently part of systemic toxicity involving other organ systems of primary clinical importance (eg, central nervous system depression, following exposure to hydrocarbon solvents). Occasionally, the liver toxicity is responsible for the major clinical findings (eg, carbon tetrachloride intoxication associated with renal and central nervous system damage); rarely is liver disease the sole manifestation of toxicity.

The study of hepatotoxic potential in animals is an important first step for newly introduced chemicals. Differences among species, circumstances of exposure, and the costliness of the studies often limit extrapolation of experimental observations to the workplace. For example, while ingestion of arsenicals causes severe acute hepatic damage both in experimental animals and in humans, reports of liver disease in humans is limited to vintners exposed to arsenical pesticides.

There is no comprehensive repository of data on animal and human hepatotoxic agents. Identification of chemicals that may produce liver damage in humans has come about largely by means of clinical observation and retrospective epidemiologic studies. Some agents, such as trinitrotoluene (TNT), dimethylnitrosamine (DMA), tetrachloroethane, polychlorinated biphenyls, and vinyl chloride, led to serious industrial hepatotoxicity before their effects on experimental animals were fully investigated. In the case of chlordecone (Kepone), human hepatotoxicity was found several years after experimental animal studies demonstrated clear evidence of liver damage following exposure.

Routes of Exposure

Inhalation, ingestion, and percutaneous absorption are the routes by which toxic chemicals can gain entry to the body. Inhalation is probably the most important route for hepatotoxic material, particularly for the volatile solvents. Several chemicals are lipophilic and may be absorbed through the skin in sufficient quantities to contribute to hepatotoxicity (eg, TNT, 4,4-diaminodiphenylmethane, tetrachloroethylene, polychlorinated biphenyls, dimethylformamide). In cases of liver damage by industrial agents that are not airborne, it is often difficult to distinguish between contamination of ingested material, absorption from mucous membranes, and absorption through the skin. Oral intake of hepatotoxic agents is usually of importance only in the rare case of accidental ingestion, though mouth breathing and gum and tobacco chewing can increase the amount of gaseous substances absorbed during the work day.

Mechanisms of Toxicity

Chemical agents that cause hepatic injury may be classified into 2 major categories as shown in Table 20–2.

A. Intrinsically Toxic Agents: Agents intrinsically toxic to the liver—directly or indirectly—cause a high incidence of dose-dependent hepatic injury in exposed persons and similar lesions in experimental animals. Furthermore, the interval between exposure (under specified conditions) and onset of disease is consistent and usually short.

1. Direct hepatotoxins–Direct hepatotoxins—or their metabolic products—injure the hepatocyte and its organelles by a direct physicochemical effect, such as peroxidation of membrane lipids, denaturation of proteins, or other chemical changes that lead to destruction or distortion of cell membranes.

Table 20–2. Mechanisms of toxicity of chemicals causing hepatic injury.[1]

Category of Agent	Incidence	Experimental Reproducibility	Dose-Dependent	Example
Intrinsic toxin				
Direct	High	Yes	Yes	Carbon tetrachloride
Indirect				
Cytotoxic	High	Yes	Yes	Dimethylnitrosamine
Cholestatic	High	Yes	Yes	Methylene dianiline
Host idiosyncrasy				
Hypersensitivity	Low	No	No	Phenytoin
Metabolic abnormality	Low	No	No	Isoniazid

[1]Adapted from Zimmerman HJ: *Hepatotoxicity: Adverse Effects of Drugs and Other Chemicals on the Liver.* Appleton-Century-Crofts, 1978.

Carbon tetrachloride is the prototype and the best-studied example of the direct hepatotoxins, producing centrilobular necrosis and steatosis in humans and experimental animals. This agent appears to exert its hepatotoxic effects by the binding of reactive metabolites to a number of critical cellular molecules that interfere with vital cell function or cause lipid peroxidation of cell membranes.

Chloroform may likewise cause direct hepatic necrosis. A large number of haloalkanes (**trichloroethylene, carbon tetrabromide, tetrachloroethane**) produce hepatic injury ranging from steatosis to trivial or nondemonstrable liver damage. Their hepatotoxic potential is inversely proportionate to chain length and bond energy and directly proportionate to the number of halogen atoms in the molecule and to the atomic number of the halogen.

2. Indirect hepatotoxins–Indirect hepatotoxins are antimetabolites and related compounds that produce hepatic injury by interference with metabolic pathways. This may result in cytotoxic damage (degeneration or necrosis of hepatocytes) by interfering with pathways necessary for the structural integrity of the hepatocyte (morphologically seen as steatosis or necrosis) or may cause cholestasis (arrested bile flow) by interfering with the bile secretory process.

The cytotoxic indirect hepatotoxins include compounds of experimental interest (ethionine, galactosamine), drugs (tetracycline, asparaginase, methotrexate, mercaptopurine), and botanicals (aflatoxin, cycasin, mushroom alkaloids, tannic acid). Ethanol belongs to this category by virtue of a number of selective biochemical lesions that lead to steatosis. Only one industrial chemical, 4,4′-diaminodiphenylmethane (commonly known as methylene dianiline [MDA]), has been categorized as a cholestatic indirect hepatotoxin. Used as a plastic hardener—most commonly for epoxy resins—this agent has caused a number of epidemics (see Acute Cholestatic Jaundice, below).

B. Agents Causing Liver Injury by Virtue of Host Idiosyncrasy: Chemically induced hepatic injury may be due to some special vulnerability of the individual and not the intrinsic toxicity of the agent.

Liver damage in such cases occurs sporadically and unpredictably, has low experimental reproducibility, and is not dose-dependent. The injury may be due to allergy (hypersensitivity) or to production of hepatotoxic metabolites. A well-established example is phenytoin, which causes acute hepatitis in a small percentage of individuals with a hypersensitivity immune response.

Hepatic Metabolism of Xenobiotics

The liver is especially vulnerable to chemical injury by virtue of its role in the metabolism of foreign compounds, or xenobiotics. The metabolism of xenobiotics is thus of central clinical interest. These chemicals, taken up by the body but not incorporated into the normal metabolic economy of the cell, are metabolized chiefly by the liver. Xenobiotic lipid-soluble compounds are well-absorbed through membrane barriers and poorly excreted by the kidney, due to protein binding and tubular reabsorption. Increasing polarity of nonpolar molecules by hepatic metabolism increases water solubility and urinary excretion. In this way, hepatic metabolism prevents the accumulation of drugs and other toxic chemicals in the body.

The strategic role of the liver as the primary defense against xenobiotics depends largely on cellular enzyme systems (mixed-function oxidases; MFO). The enzyme systems responsible for the metabolism of xenobiotics are attached to the membrane layers of the smooth endoplasmic reticulum. Although enzymes that catalyze the metabolism of nonpolar xenobiotics are present in intestine, lung, kidney, and skin, the vast majority of metabolic conversions occur in the liver. Most xenobiotics that are toxic by the oral route are also hepatotoxic parenterally or by inhalation.

Xenobiotic Agents Activated by the MFO System

Many hepatotoxic agents and hepatocarcinogens must be first activated by the MFO system to a toxic or carcinogenic metabolite. Examples include carbon tetrachloride, vinyl chloride, polychlorinated biphenyls, bromobenzene, azo dyes, dimethylnitrosamine, and allyl compounds. Electrophilic intermediates react with enzymes and regulatory or structural proteins and lead to cell death.

Many drugs, insecticides, organic solvents, carcinogens, and other environmental contaminants are known experimentally to stimulate some type of microsomal activity that is associated with the metabolism of xenobiotics. The administration of ethanol concomitantly with carbon tetrachloride enhances the toxicity of the latter, presumably via induction of the MFO system. Clinically, this may explain the well-documented synergistic effect between ethanol abuse and carbon tetrachloride toxicity in humans.

Other mechanisms may be at work also, since a single dose of alcohol given to animals several hours prior to administration of carbon tetrachloride also potentiates toxicity. Experiments show that many other factors may affect the metabolism of xenobiotics: diet, age, sex, cigarette smoking, endocrine status, genetic factors, diurnal variations, underlying liver disease, and stress. There is considerable inter- and intraindividual variation in xenobiotic metabolism, and the relative importance of these factors in the occupational setting is not currently known. Enhanced microsomal enzyme function has been demonstrated in industrial workers exposed to hepatotoxins at levels below those shown to result in hepatic necrosis. Increasing attention has been directed to the use of noninvasive measurements of MFO in the preclinical detection of liver disease (see below).

DISEASE PATTERNS & MORPHOLOGY OF HEPATIC INJURY

As shown in Table 20–3, occupational exposure to xenobiotics can lead to acute, subacute, or chronic liver disease.

The clinical syndromes can be associated with several types of morphologic changes, as seen by light microscopy. Hepatic injury may be clinically overt or may be discovered only as a functional or histologic abnormality. Current concern with chronic liver disease due to subtle repeated injury has generally overshadowed the problem of acute and subacute injury caused by accidental exposure.

ACUTE HEPATIC INJURY

Acute liver disease was a cause of serious occupational liver disease in the first part of the 20th century and is still occasionally encountered. Acute hepatic injury has been reported as a result of exposure to agents listed in Table 20–4.

Table 20–3. Morphologic patterns of liver injury.[1]

Type of Injury	Examples of Causes
Acute	
Cytotoxic	
Necrosis	
Zonal	Carbon tetrachloride, chloroform
Massive	Trinitrotoluene
Steatosis	Carbon tetrachloride, chloroform, phosphorus
Cholestatic	Methylene dianiline
Subacute	Trinitrotoluene
Chronic	
Cirrhosis	Trinitrotoluene, polychlorinated biphenyls, tetrachloroethane
Sclerosis	Arsenic, vinyl chloride
Porphyria	Dioxin
Neoplasia	Arsenic, vinyl chloride

[1]Adapted from Zimmerman HJ: *Hepatotoxicity: Adverse Effects of Drugs and Other Chemicals on the Liver.* Appleton-Century-Crofts, 1978.

Clinical Findings

Occupational exposure to xenobiotics may lead to degeneration or necrosis of hepatocytes (cytotoxic injury) or to arrested bile flow (cholestatic injury). The latent period is relatively short (24–48 hours), and clinical symptoms are often of extrahepatic origin. Anorexia, nausea, vomiting, jaundice, and hepatomegaly are often present. Severely exposed individuals who have sustained massive necrosis may have coffee ground emesis, abdominal pain, clinically detectable reduction in liver size, rapid development of ascites, edema, and hemorrhagic diathesis. This is often followed within 24–28 hours by somnolence and coma.

Morphologically, hepatic necrosis may be zonal, massive, or diffuse. Centrizonal necrosis is the characteristic lesion produced by agents listed in Table 20–4 as well as by bromobenzene, halothane, the toxin of *Amanita phalloides,* and acetaminophen. Periportal or peripheral necrosis is produced by elemental phosphorus. Trinitrotoluene (TNT), polychlorinated biphenyls, and chloronaphthalenes can produce massive rather than zonal necrosis.

Varying degrees of fatty change or steatosis may also be seen morphologically in association with toxicity due to carbon tetrachloride, chloroform, tetrachloroethane, and elemental phosphorus.

Table 20–4. Agents causing acute hepatic injury.

Carbon tetrachloride
Tetrachloroethane
Trichloroethylene
Chloroform
Carbon tetrabromide
2-Nitropropane
Chlorinated naphthalenes
Dimethylnitrosamine
Elemental phosphorus
Bromobenzene
Halothane
Amanita phalloides toxin
Acetaminophen

Diagnosis & Treatment

The diagnosis and treatment of acute hepatic injuries are covered under Clinical Management of Occupational Liver Disease, below.

CARBON TETRACHLORIDE-INDUCED ACUTE HEPATIC INJURY

Carbon tetrachloride presents the classic example of an acute hepatotoxin. It was first recognized as such in the 1920s, when it was in common use as a liquid solvent, dry cleaning agent, and fire extinguisher. Since then, hundreds of poisonings and fatalities have been reported, mostly from inhalation in confined spaces.

Clinical Findings

Clinically, immediate nervous system symptoms of dizziness, headache, visual disturbances, and confusion are observed as a result of the anesthetic properties of carbon tetrachloride. This is followed by nausea, vomiting, abdominal pain, and diarrhea during the first 24 hours. Evidence of hepatic disease usually follows after 2–4 days but may appear within 24 hours. The liver and spleen become palpable and jaundice develops, accompanied by elevated serum transaminase concentrations and prolonged prothrombin time. Renal failure (see Chapter 21) may ensue a few days after the hepatic damage becomes manifest and has in fact been the cause of death in most fatal cases. Sequelae of hepatic failure such as hypoglycemia, encephalopathy, and hemorrhage may be complications. Most instances of carbon tetrachloride toxicity have occurred with accompanying ethanol intake, which may be a potentiating factor in hepatotoxicity.

ACUTE HEPATIC INJURY INDUCED BY OTHER XENOBIOTICS

Trichloroethylene has been reported to cause acute hepatotoxicity when used as a dry cleaning agent; more recently, it has been shown to cause acute centrilobular necrosis following recreational "solvent sniffing" of cleaning fluids. This may be due to contamination with dichloroacetylene rather than to trichloroethylene itself.

Carbon tetrabromide has been reported to cause a syndrome in chemists similar to acute carbon tetrachloride hepatotoxicity.

2-Nitropropane, a nitroparaffin used as a solvent in epoxy resin paints and coatings, has been reported to have caused several cases of acute fulminant hepatitis following exposure in confined spaces.

ACUTE CHOLESTATIC JAUNDICE

This is a rare manifestation of occupational toxicity. As mentioned earlier, methylene dianiline (4,4,'- diaminodiphenylmethane) was responsible for an epidemic of cholestatic jaundice observed in Epping, England ("Epping jaundice"), in 1965. This compound, used as a hardener for epoxy resin, had spilled from a plastic container onto the floor of a van that was carrying both flour and the chemical. Acute cholestatic injury was found subsequently in 84 persons who had eaten bread made from the contaminated flour. Onset was abrupt—with abdominal pain—in 60% of the cases and was insidious in one-third. Histologic evidence of bile stasis with only slight parenchymal injury was seen in most cases, and all victims recovered without evidence of persistent hepatic injury. Similar cases have subsequently been reported for industrial exposure during the manufacture and application of epoxy resins.

SUBACUTE HEPATIC NECROSIS

This form of hepatic injury is characterized by a smoldering illness, with delayed onset of jaundice. It usually follows repeated exposure to relatively small doses of a hepatotoxin. The onset of anorexia, nausea, and vomiting accompanied by hepatomegaly and jaundice may occur after several weeks to months of exposure and may lead variably to recovery or to fulminant hepatic failure. A few patients are reported to have developed macronodular cirrhosis, though clinical data are limited.

The histologic features of subacute hepatic necrosis consist of varying degrees of necrosis, fibrosis, and regeneration. In cases where the clinical course is relatively brief (2–3 weeks), necrotic features predominate. In patients with a prolonged course of several months or more, postnecrotic scarring with subacute hepatic necrosis is seen. Fortunately, subacute hepatic necrosis caused by occupational exposure is rare today.

CHRONIC HEPATIC INJURY

Several forms of chronic liver damage can result from continuing or repeated injury caused by prolonged exposure: cirrhosis and fibrosis, hepatoportal sclerosis, hepatic porphyria, and neoplasia. Acute hepatic injury due to carbon tetrachloride exposure has been anecdotally reported to lead to chronic disease.

CIRRHOSIS & FIBROSIS

The histologic pattern of progressive necrosis accompanied by regenerating nodules, fibrosis, and architectural distortion of the liver ("toxic cirrhosis'') is well described as part of the syndrome of subacute hepatic necrosis due to **trinitrotoluene, tetrachloroethane,** and the **polychlorinated biphenyls** and **chloronaphthalenes.** Additionally, some survivors of trinitrotoluene-induced injury were found to have macronodular cirrhosis.

Prolonged, repeated low-level exposure to **carbon tetrachloride** in dry cleaning plants and to **inorganic arsenical insecticides** among vintners has been reported to cause cirrhosis. Micronodular cirrhosis was described in a worker with repeated exposure to a degreasing solvent containing a mixture of trichloroethylene and **1,1,1-trichloroethane.**

Thirteen painters with no history of drug or alcohol ingestion exposed over 6–39 years to a variety of organic solvents had persistent biopsy-verified histologic changes of steatosis, focal necrosis, and enlarged portal tracts with fibrosis. Three nurses were reported to have irreversible liver injury after years of handling cystostatic drugs, with liver biopsies showing piecemeal necrosis in one and steatosis with fibrosis in the other two.

HEPATOPORTAL SCLEROSIS & HEPATIC PORPHYRIA

Portal and periportal fibrosis leading to portal hypertension (''noncirrhotic portal hypertension'') has been attributed to exposure to inorganic arsenicals and vinyl chloride. A few cases of porphyria cutanea tarda have been recorded due to occupational exposure to the herbicide **2,4,5-trichlorophenoxyacetic acid** (2,4,5-T), probably caused by contamination by dioxin. Turkish peasants developed liver disease and hepatic porphyria after ingesting wheat contaminated with the fungicide **hexachlorobenzene.**

NEOPLASIA

While many occupationally encountered chemical agents are known to cause hepatocellular carcinoma in experimental animals, only a few are demonstrated human carcinogens.

Vinyl chloride, a halogenated aliphatic compound used since the 1940s in the production of polyvinyl chloride, was known to be an animal hepatotoxin in the early 1960s. Acro-osteolysis was reported in humans in 1966 (see Chapter 26). In 1974, Creech and Johnson reported 3 cases of a rare liver tumor—angiosarcoma—in employees who had been exposed to vinyl chloride for up to 20 years. Subsequent reports and surveillance activities worldwide have recorded over 75 cases of vinyl chloride-associated hepatic angiosarcoma. Pathologically, hepatic damage in association with vinyl chloride exposure appears to progress sequentially from focal hepatocyte hyperplasia, to sinusoidal dilatation, to peliosis hepatis and sarcomatous transformation of the lining

of the cells of sinusoids and portal capillaries. Clinically, liver disease has usually not been recognized until the late stages of histologic damage and with the victim only a few months from death.

Medical surveillance of vinyl chloride-exposed workers has attempted to identify early histologic and structural abnormalities through the use of liver biopsy, ultrasonography, CT scans, and biochemical measures of liver function.

Hepatic angiosarcoma has also developed in vintners with long exposure to inorganic arsenic; in patients with psoriasis treated with inorganic potassium arsenite (Fowler's solution) in the 1940s and 1950s; and in patients injected with a colloidal suspension of thorium dioxide (Thorotrast), used for carotid angiography and liver-spleen scans from 1930 to 1955.

INFECTIOUS AGENTS CAUSING LIVER TOXICITY (Table 20–5)

Infectious hepatotoxic agents may be of importance in the pathogenesis of both acute and chronic liver disease. Occupational exposure to infectious hepatotoxic agents may occur among hospital workers, sewer workers, emergency health care personnel; animal care, slaughterhouse, and farm workers; and laboratory workers. Additional information can be found in Chapter 15.

HEPATITIS A

Exposure

Hepatitis A is an occupational risk for hospital and mental institution workers as well as for teachers and other staff of day care centers and prison personnel. While contaminated food and water are common epidemic sources, hepatitis A is primarily transmitted by person-to-person contact, generally through fecal contamination. The cause of hepatitis A is the hepatitis A virus (HAV), a 27-nm ribonucleic acid (RNA)

Table 20–5. Infectious agents associated with occupational liver disease.

Hepatitis A virus	Nursery and kindergarten staff, sewer workers
Hepatitis B virus	Health care workers with blood and body fluid contact
Cytomegalovirus	Pediatric health care workers
Coxiella burnetii	Animal care workers, farm workers, slaughterhouse workers
Leptospira icterohaemorrhagiae	Sewer workers, farm workers

[1]Adapted from Døssing M, Skinhøj P: Occupational liver injury. *Int Arch Occup Environ Health* 1985;**56:**1.

agent that is a member of the picornavirus family. Its transmission is facilitated by poor personal hygiene and intimate household or sexual contact. Transmission by blood transfusion has occurred but is rare.

In contrast with hepatitis B and with non-A, non-B hepatitis, occupational transmission of hepatitis A in the hospital is uncommon, since there is little fecal excretion of the virus after the patient develops jaundice and seeks medical attention. Nevertheless, well-documented outbreaks of hepatitis A have occurred in hospitals and institutions for the mentally retarded.

Clinical Findings & Diagnosis

The incubation period for hepatitis A is 15–50 days (average, 28–30 days). The illness caused by HAV characteristically has an abrupt onset, with fever, malaise, anorexia, nausea, abdominal discomfort, and jaundice. High concentrations of HAV (10 particles per gram) are found in stools of infected persons. Fecal virus excretion reaches its highest concentration during the incubation period and early in the prodromal phase; it diminishes rapidly once jaundice appears. Greatest infectivity is in the 2-week period immediately before the onset of jaundice.

A chronic carrier state with HAV in blood or feces has not been demonstrated. The fatality rate among reported cases is low (about 0.6%). The diagnosis of acute hepatitis A is confirmed by IgM-class anti-HAV in serum collected during the acute or early convalescent phase of the disease. IgG antibodies appear in the convalescent phase and remain positive for life, apparently conferring enduring protection against disease.

Treatment

Treatment for hepatitis A is symptomatic, with rest, analgesics, and fluid replacement where necessary.

Prevention

No vaccine is available for protection against hepatitis A virus infection.

Numerous studies have shown that a single intramuscular dose of 0.02 mL/kg of immune globulin (immune serum globulin; gamma globulin) given before exposure or during the incubation period of hepatitis A is protective against clinical illness. The prophylactic value is greatest (80–90%) when immune globulin is given early in the incubation period and declines thereafter. Since only 38% of acute hepatitis cases in the United States are caused by HAV, serologic confirmation of hepatitis A in the index case is recommended before treatment of contacts. Once the diagnosis of acute infection is made, close contacts should be promptly given immune globulin to prevent development of secondary cases. Such close contacts may include staff of day care facilities and institutions for custodial care—or hospital staff if an unsuspected patient has been fecally incontinent.

Routine immune globulin administration is not recommended under the usual office or factory conditions for persons exposed to a fellow worker with hepatitis A or to teachers with schoolroom contact. Food handlers should receive immune globulin when a common-source exposure is recognized. So should restaurant patrons when the infected person is directly involved in handling uncooked foods without gloves. This is especially the case when the patrons can be identified within 2 weeks after exposure and the food handler's hygienic practices are known to be deficient. Serologic screening of contacts for anti-HAV antibodies to the hepatitis A virus before giving immune globulin is not recommended, because screening is more costly than immune globulin and would delay administration.

An employee with symptoms and confirmed hepatitis A virus infection should be restricted from work until symptoms subside or for 1 week after the onset of jaundice.

HEPATITIS B

Exposure & Epidemiology

Hepatitis B infection (see also Chapter 15) is caused by the hepatitis B virus (HBV), a major cause of acute and chronic hepatitis, cirrhosis, and primary hepatocellular carcinoma worldwide.

High-risk health care workers with frequent blood contact include anyone having significant contact with blood, blood products, or body secretions: surgeons, oral surgeons, dental hygienists, pathologists, anesthesiologists, phlebotomists, medical technologists, respiratory therapists, emergency room personnel, and medical and surgical house staff.

The annual rate of clinically manifest hepatitis B infection in hospital workers is about 0.1%, or about 10 times that of control populations. Hospital staff with frequent blood contact have a prevalence rate of hepatitis B surface antigen (HBsAg) of 1–2% and a prevalence rate of anti-hepatitis B antibody (anti-HBs) of 15–30%, compared to healthy controls with rates of 0.3% and 3–5%, respectively. Employment in a hospital without blood exposure carries no greater risk than that for the general population.

Most hospital workers experience accidental blood contact by needlestick injuries, usually during disposal and recapping of needles, administration of parenteral injections or infusion therapy, drawing blood, and handling linens and trash containing uncapped needles. Educating hospital personnel about the risks of hepatitis B and employing methods to interrupt transmission have been successful in reducing rates of infection.

Based on serologic markers of infection, HBV is also highly prevalent in certain high-risk groups, such as immigrants from areas with high HBV endemicity, clients of institutions for the mentally retarded, parenteral drug users, homosexual men, household contacts of carriers, and hemodialysis patients.

An estimated 200,000 persons in the USA, primarily young adults, become infected yearly, and one-fourth have jaundice. More than 10,000 require hospitalization, and an average 250 die of fulminant disease. A carrier state of chronic active hepatitis develops in 3–5% of infected individuals and may result in serious complications. In the USA there are an estimated 0.5–1 million carriers who have an estimated 12- to 3000-fold higher risk than other persons of developing primary liver cancer.

Forms of Illness & Transmission

Three forms of hepatitis B are encountered in clinical practice: acute hepatitis B, inapparent sporadic episodes of unknown origin, and the chronic carrier state—detected by screening for HBsAg—in apparently healthy persons. Transmission occurs via percutaneous or permucosal routes when exposure to blood, semen, cerebrospinal fluid, saliva, or urine occurs. HBV is not transmitted via the fecal-oral route or by contamination of food or water.

Course of Illness

The onset of acute hepatitis B is generally insidious, with anorexia, malaise, nausea, vomiting, abdominal pain, and jaundice. Skin rash, arthralgia, and arthritis can also occur. The incubation period ranges from 45 to 60 days after exposure to HBV. HBsAg can be detected in serum 30–60 days after exposure to HBV and persists for variable periods. Antibody to hepatitis B surface antigen (anti-HBs) develops after a resolved infection and indicates long-term immunity. The antibody to the core antigen (anti-HBc) develops in all HBV infections and persists indefinitely. Overall fatality rates for acute infection do not exceed 2%.

The chronic carrier state is defined as the presence of HBsAg-positive serum on at least 2 occasions at least 6 months apart and is characterized by high levels of HBsAg and anti-HBc and various levels of serum transaminases, reflecting liver disease activity. The natural course of HBsAg-positive chronic active hepatitis is progressive, frequently evolving to cirrhosis, hepatocellular carcinoma, and death due to hepatic failure or bleeding esophageal varices.

Treatment

There is no known form of treatment, and corticosteroids are ineffective in the treatment of chronic active hepatitis due to HBV.

Prevention

Postexposure prophylaxis should be based on the hepatitis vaccination status of the exposed person, whether the source of blood and the HBsAg status of the source is known or unknown. Guidelines for hepatitis B prophylaxis following percutaneous exposure are given in Chapter 15. The decision to screen hospital personnel for susceptibility before vaccination depends on the cost of the screening test and the prevalence of the antibody in the group to be vacci-

nated. If screening is performed, the antibody pattern of isolated anti-hepatitis B surface antibody (anti-HBs) cannot be interpreted as reliably indicating past hepatitis B virus infection or immunity to reinfection, particularly if low titers are accepted. A higher cutoff point should be used as a criterion for a positive reaction, or both anti-HBs and anti-hepatitis B core antibody (anti-HBc) measurements should be performed.

Although the safety of hepatitis B vaccine manufactured from pooled plasma of hepatitis B antigen-positive individuals has been well demonstrated, acceptance by health care workers has been limited owing to concern about the possible presence of HIV virus (the virus of AIDS). The availability of a synthetic hepatitis B vaccine prepared with recombinant DNA techniques will probably increase the vaccination rate among susceptible hospital personnel.

Individuals at high risk should be vaccinated with hepatitis B virus vaccine. Protective immunity is conferred in over 95% of vaccines. Postexposure immune titers, periodic immune titers, and booster shots are not recommended. The employee with hepatitis B virus infection and liver disease should be advised to avoid exposure to other potentially hepatotoxic agents such as ethanol or workplace solvents.

OTHER INFECTIOUS AGENTS

Non-A, non-B viral hepatitis may develop after parenteral blood exposure among hospital personnel. The incidence and clinical spectrum of this disease after occupational exposure is not known. Chronic hepatitis following acute non-A, non-B hepatitis varies in frequency from 20% to 70%. The value of immune serum globulin for prophylaxis is not established.

Cytomegalovirus exposure is a potential risk to health care workers, particularly pediatric staff who may be pregnant and thus at risk of transmitting infection to the fetus. Cytomegalovirus may cause hepatitis, but the more serious consequence of infection for the pregnant worker may be a neonate with a congenital malformation. Convincing evidence of higher rates of seroconversion among pediatric health care workers has not been demonstrated. Nevertheless, prudent hospital policy may be to reassign seronegative employees who wish to become pregnant to jobs where there is no contact with infected patients or their biologic fluids.

Coxiella burnetii, the agent of **Q fever,** may cause acute infection among personnel exposed to infected sheep and goats. Persons at risk include animal care technicians, laboratory research personnel, abattoir workers, and farmers. Acute hepatitis occurs in up to 50% of cases and is usually self-limited.

The clinical picture of **leptospirosis** among farm and sewer workers due to exposure to *Leptospira icterohaemorrhagiae* may also be dominated by hepatic injury.

Other causes of infectious hepatitis include **yellow fever** among forest workers (arbovirus) and **schistosomiasis** among agricultural workers *(Schistosoma mansoni, Schistosoma japonicum).*

MEDICAL SURVEILLANCE & DETECTION OF OCCUPATIONAL HEPATOTOXICITY

MEDICAL SURVEILLANCE FOR OCCUPATIONAL LIVER DISEASE

The choice of a surveillance test or tests to detect chemical liver disease in a working population exposed to potential hepatotoxins is determined by its specificity, sensitivity, and positive predictive value. (See section on Diagnostic Tests for Liver Dysfunction, below.) In an occupational setting, a screening test with high sensitivity (to correctly identify all those with disease) and specificity (to correctly identify all those without disease) is needed. Indocyanine green clearance and serum alkaline phosphatase have been suggested as the initial tests of choice for the surveillance of vinyl chloride workers (to reduce the number of false positives), followed by a test of high sensitivity such as serum c-glutamyl transpeptidase (to reduce the number of false negatives). Whether this applies to other exposed groups awaits further research. In the same way, the comparative utility of other indices of liver function, such as serum bile acid measurements and noninvasive measures of microsomal enzyme activity, remains open to question.

It is currently justified to base the choice of tests on practical criteria such as noninvasiveness, simplicity of test performance, availability, and adequacy of test analysis and cost. Although serum transaminases have a relatively high sensitivity for detection of liver disease, their low specificity limits the practical utility of periodic measurement in a worker population exposed to potential hepatotoxins. Nevertheless, serum transaminases remain the test of choice for routine surveillance of such populations.

Clearance tests have been successfully used in research settings but are not recommended for daily clinical or surveillance practice until further prospective studies in well-defined groups are completed. It is not known whether reversible changes in microsomal enzyme activity in workers exposed to hepatotoxins are harmless and adaptive or potentially harmful. On the basis of current knowledge, the consequences of changes in microsomal enzyme activity cannot be accurately assessed.

So-called preemployment "baseline" measurement of serum transaminases may be helpful in establishing causality for purposes of workers' compensation where a claim is made alleging industrial liver disease.

Gray scale ultrasonography of the liver has been used in surveillance of vinyl chloride-exposed workers but has not been routinely applied in other workplace settings for surveillance of hepatic disease.

Until more specific tests are available, workplace screening for hepatotoxicity should utilize the standard serum transaminases.

DIAGNOSTIC TESTS FOR LIVER DYSFUNCTION

The ideal test for detection of liver dysfunction would be sensitive enough to detect minimal liver disease, specific enough to point to a particular derangement of liver function, and capable of reflecting the severity of the underlying pathophysiologic problem. Unfortunately, no such laboratory test is available, and "liver function tests" are used instead (Table 20–6).

Broadly speaking, these tests encompass tests of biochemical evidence of cell death and hepatic synthesis as well as actual physiologic liver dysfunction. In addition, radiologic and morphologic evaluations are often used to delineate the nature of liver disease and as such may be viewed as tests of liver function. Biochemical tests and tests of synaptic function are commonly indicated for routine use; clearance tests are not widely available and not indicated for routine use.

Biochemical Tests for Liver Disease

A. Serum Enzyme Activity: The tests most commonly used to detect liver disease are serum glutamic-oxaloacetic transaminase (SGOT), also called aspartate aminotransferase (AST); and serum glutamic-pyruvic transaminase (SGPT), also called alanine aminotransferase (ALT). Transaminase

---

Table 20–6. Tests for evaluation of liver disease.

Biochemical tests
  Serum enzyme activity
    Serum alkaline phosphatase
    Serum lactate dehydrogenase
  Serum bilirubin
  Urine bilirubin
Tests of synthetic liver function
  Serum albumin
  Prothrombin time
  Alpha-fetoprotein
  Serum ferritin
Clearance tests
  Exogenous clearance tests
    Sulfobromophthalein
    Indocyanine green
    Antipyrine test
    Aminopyrine breath test
    Caffeine breath test
  Endogenous clearance tests
    Serum bile acid

release is due to release of enzyme protein from liver cells as a result of cell injury. Elevations of serum aminotransferase may occur with minor cell injury, making such determinations useful in the early detection and monitoring of liver disease of drug or chemical origin. However, transaminases may be elevated in viral, alcoholic, or ischemic hepatitis as well as extrahepatic obstruction, limiting the specificity of these tests. In addition, significant elevations of transaminases have been noted in a few normal, healthy subjects due to diets high in sucrose, and false positives have been reported in patients receiving erythromycin and aminosalicylic acid and during diabetic ketoacidosis. Conversely, significant liver damage may be present in individuals with normal levels of transaminases.

The height of transaminase elevation in liver disease does not correlate with the extent of liver cell necrosis on biopsy and therefore has little prognostic value.

B. Alkaline Phosphatase: Serum alkaline phosphatase activity may originate from liver, bone, intestine, or placenta. Measurement of serum 5-nucleotidase may be used to determine the tissue origin of an elevated alkaline phosphatase; if elevated, it generally implies that the source of alkaline phosphatase is hepatobiliary, not bony. Toxic liver injury that results in disturbances in the transport function of the hepatocyte or of the biliary tree may cause elevation of serum alkaline phosphatase activity. Increased serum alkaline phosphatase may also be noted in the third trimester of pregnancy as well as normally in persons over age 50, in patients with osteoblastic bone disorders, and with both intra- and extrahepatic cholestatic disease.

Assay of alkaline phosphatase enzymatic activity in serum in anicteric individuals is particularly useful in detecting and monitoring suspected drug- or chemical-induced cholestasis; it is not helpful in screening individuals for toxic liver injury except when there is primary involvement of the biliary network.

C. Serum Bilirubin: Hyperbilirubinemia may be classified as conjugated or unconjugated. Conjugated hyperbilirubinemia indicates dysfunction of the liver parenchyma or bile ducts and may be found in Dubin-Johnson syndrome and Rotor's syndrome and in viral hepatitis, drug- or toxin-induced hepatitis, shock liver, and metastatic disease of the liver. Unconjugated hyperbilirubinemia may be seen in Gilbert's disease, uncomplicated hemolytic disorders, and congestive heart failure.

Serum bilirubin is of some value in detecting toxic cholestatic liver injury but is frequently normal in the presence of more common cytotoxic damage. It is probably most useful in the presence of severe acute liver damage; although patients with fulminant hepatitis may be anicteric, the level of serum bilirubin is of prognostic importance in chemical and alcoholic hepatitis, primary biliary cirrhosis, and halothane hepatitis.

D. Urine Bilirubin: Bilirubin in the urine is direct bilirubin, since indirect bilirubin is tightly bound to albumin and not filtered by the normal kidney. A positive urine bilirubin can confirm clinically suspected hyperbilirubinemia of hepatobiliary origin or may predate the appearance of overt icterus and thus serve as a useful screening test. Quantitative analysis of urine bilirubin is of no diagnostic significance.

E. Other Biochemical Tests:

1. Serum γ-glutamyl transferase (SGGT) is considered a more sensitive indicator than aminotransferases of drug-, virus-, chemical-, and alcohol-induced hepatocellular damage. Because of its lack of specificity, however, one must interpret abnormalities in conjunction with other tests.

2. Liver-specific enzymes, such as ornithine carbamyl dehydrogenase, phosphofructose aldolase, sorbitol dehydrogenase, and alcohol dehydrogenase, have been found to be less clinically useful than the aminotransferases, glutamyl transferases, or alkaline phosphatases.

3. Serum lactate dehydrogenase may originate from myocardium, liver, skeletal muscle, brain or kidney tissue, and red blood cells. Isoenzyme fractionation may determine hepatic origin (lactate dehydrogenase 5) but is generally too nonspecific for purposes of evaluating toxic chemical liver injury.

Tests of Synthetic Liver Function

Measurement of **serum albumin** concentration may be a useful index of cellular dysfunction in liver disease. It is of little value in differential diagnosis.

Because all the clotting factors are synthesized by the liver, acute liver injury can result in prolongation of the **prothrombin time,** which is dependent on the activities of factors II, V, VII, and X. Measurement of prothrombin time is useful chiefly in fulminant hepatic failure, where a markedly elevated prothrombin time has prognostic significance, or in advanced chronic liver disease. It is a relatively insensitive indicator of liver damage and of little value in differential diagnosis.

High serum concentrations of alpha-fetoprotein are present in 70% of patients with primary hepatocellular carcinoma in the USA, and serial determinations may aid in monitoring the response to therapy or detecting early recurrence. **Alpha-fetoprotein** has no utility for surveillance in the occupational setting.

Serum ferritin levels accurately reflect hepatic and total body iron stores. Serum ferritin is useful in screening for idiopathic genetic hemochromatosis as a cause of liver disease but has no utility for surveillance in the occupational setting.

Clearance Tests

Tests that measure the clearance of substances by the liver provide the most sensitive, specific, and reliable means of detecting the early phase of liver disease. Clearance tests may be used to determine the specificity of increased enzyme activity, to detect liver disease not reflected in abnormalities of serum enzymes, and to determine when recovery has occurred in reversible liver disease. This is especially the case when decreases in the functional state of the liver occur in patients with liver disease without active necrosis, including fatty liver, and inactive cirrhosis in the absence of clinical abnormalities or abnormal enzymes.

In the occupational setting, measures of hepatic functional capacity have been used epidemiologically to demonstrate liver dysfunction in the absence of clinical or serologic abnormalities. The clinical utility of clearance tests in screening for chemical liver injury—or in confirming occupational etiology of disease in workers with known liver dysfunction— has yet to be precisely determined.

A. Exogenous Clearance Tests: Exogenous clearance tests are given to detect liver function by the administration of various test substances to the individual.

1. Sulfobromophthalein (BSP)–Practical use of hepatic clearance as a diagnostic measure began with BSP. Its use has been discontinued because of side effects of phlebitis, severe local skin reactions, and occasionally fatal anaphylactic reactions.

2. Indocyanine green–Hepatic uptake of indocyanine green, a tricarbocyanine anionic dye, is an active process dependent upon sinusoidal perfusion, membrane transport, and secretory capacity. The dye is not metabolized or conjugated by the liver and is excreted directly into the bile. After a single intravenous injection of indocyanine green, clearance is calculated from serial dye levels at 3, 5, 7, 9, 12, and 14 minutes or by ear densitometry. Unlike BSP, indocyanine green causes negligible toxicity or allergic reactions.

Studies of workers exposed to vinyl chloride have shown that indocyanine green clearance after a dose of 0.5 mg/kg is the most sensitive test for subclinical liver injury and has a specificity exceeded only by serum alkaline phosphatase. A dose-response relationship has also been found between cumulative exposure to vinyl chloride and indocyanine green clearance. This has not been demonstrated in other groups of workers exposed to occupational hepatotoxins, and indocyanine green for detection of subclinical liver disease cannot yet be recommended for routine use.

3. Antipyrine test–This is the most widely used in vivo index of hepatic microsomal enzyme activity. Antipyrine is completely and rapidly absorbed from the gastrointestinal tract, distributed in total body water, and almost completely metabolized by the liver via 3 major oxidative pathways. The rate of elimination is virtually independent of hepatic blood flow, with first-order kinetics of elimination and a half-life of about 10 hours in normal subjects. Twenty-four to 48 hours after an orally administered dose of 1 g, antipyrine clearance can be calculated by serial plasma or salivary measurements. It has been shown that clearance can be calculated from a single salivary sample collected at least 18 hours after dosing, permitting a simpler, more convenient method of study. Repeat tests cannot be done less than 3 days apart, and in order to avoid the induction of antipyrine metabolism in the individual, an interval of 1 week is recommended.

The antipyrine test has undergone the most extensive study of all clearance tests in the detection of subclinical liver disease in occupational settings. It has been used to detect mean differences in hepatic enzyme activity between workers exposed to solvent mixtures and unexposed controls. Clinically, asymptomatic chlordecone-exposed workers had increased antipyrine clearance and biopsy-proved liver disease that normalized after exposure was terminated.

4. Aminopyrine breath test–The aminopyrine breath test has the advantage of being simple, noninvasive, safe, and relatively cheap. Clinical studies have documented the use of aminopyrine breath tests in patients with chronic advanced liver disease, but the sensitivity and specificity of the test for detection of subclinical chemical liver injury in asymptomatic populations have not been assessed.

After oral administration of about 2 μCi of ^{14}C-aminopyrine, the labeled methyl group will be oxidized by the microsomal enzyme system and ultimately excreted as ^{14}CO. Breath samples are collected 2 hours after administration, and the specific activity of ^{14}CO is measured in a liquid scintillation counter. The test requires physical rest from dose to breath sampling.

5. Caffeine breath test–Inhaled ^{14}caffeine, labeled at one or all 3 methyl groups, followed by exhaled breath ^{14}CO$_2$ measurement, has recently been introduced as a noninvasive means of studying hepatic microsomal enzyme function. It has not yet undergone evaluation in asymptomatic worker populations.

B. Endogenous Clearance Tests:

1. Serum bile acids–Serum bile acid measurement may be useful in further medical workup for the individual with persistent enzyme abnormalities. Bile acids are synthesized by the liver and undergo enterohepatic circulation. Serum levels of bile acids are normally low in a fasting state (< 6 μmol/L) and reflect only hepatic excretory function and not synthesis rate or volume distribution. Fasting bile acid levels are increased in relation to the degree of liver disease and impairment in excretion.

Depending on the population screened, the positive predictive value of an abnormal (> 8.4 μmol/L) serum bile acid test ranges from 10% (general population) to 94% (hospitalized population with biopsy-proved hepatobiliary disease). In a large workplace study of vinyl chloride-exposed workers, measurement of serum bile acids was found to have a sensitivity of 78%, a specificity of 93%, and a positive predictive value of 10%. Serum transaminases have higher sensitivity than serum bile acid levels in screening for liver disease, but bile acid measurement has greater specificity when used to differentiate chemical from nonchemical liver disease.

CLINICAL MANAGEMENT OF OCCUPATIONAL LIVER DISEASE

Occupational & Medical History

A careful occupational history of exposure to known human hepatotoxins should be obtained in every case of suspected occupational liver disease. The past medical history of liver disease should be noted. The review of symptoms should include those of acute central nervous system toxicity, such as headache, dizziness, and lightheadedness, since the presence of these symptoms may indicate excessive solvent exposure. Use of protective work practices (such as respiratory protection, gloves, and work clothes) should be described, as this may indicate the extent of pulmonary and skin absorption. Material Data Safety Sheets (Chapter 2) should be obtained on the relevant products used. Airborne contaminant monitoring data (Chapter 38) should be requested and reviewed for excessive exposure. Inquiry should be made of the employer about other employees with possible liver disease.

Differential Diagnosis

Other causes of occupational liver disease should be ruled out—particularly infectious and alcohol- and drug-induced hepatitis. The most common cause of elevated serum transaminase is ingestion of ethanol. If a history of excessive ethanol ingestion is elicited, the serum transaminase should be repeated after 3–4 weeks of abstinence. If serum transaminases are normal on follow-up, ethanol should be suspected as the probable cause. Persistent serum transaminase elevation may represent chronic alcoholic hepatitis or continued occupational exposure.

The onset of liver disease after exposure to a known or suspected hepatotoxin is suggestive of occupational liver disease, particularly if normal liver function tests before exposure can be documented. Even if preexposure tests are normal, liver disease may develop coincidentally without relation to workplace exposure.

Management of Acute Liver Disease

The most common clinical problem is the individual with elevated serum transaminase on routine screening who may have occupational exposure to a known hepatotoxin. Nonoccupational causes of liver disease should be carefully ruled out and the workplace inspected for the presence of hepatotoxic exposures. If an occupational cause is suspected, the individual should be immediately removed from exposure for 3–4 weeks. The serum transaminase measurement should then be repeated; with few exceptions, serum transaminase concentration will normalize following removal from exposure. A persistently elevated serum transaminase suggests a nonoccupational cause of liver disease or, rarely, chronic occupational liver disease.

Although there is little evidence that individuals with nonoccupational liver disease are more susceptible to further liver damage due to occupational exposure, it is prudent to carefully monitor them for evidence of worsening liver damage. Appropriate engineering controls and personal protective equipment should be made available to reduce potential hepatotoxic exposures. If there is evidence of worsening liver disease or if exposure cannot be satisfactorily reduced, the individual should be reassigned.

Aside from removing the individual from exposure to the offending agent, there is no specific treatment for acute occupational liver disease.

Management of Chronic Liver Disease

Persistent abnormalities in liver function tests after removal from exposure have rarely been reported, and a thorough search for other causes should always be conducted. Occasionally, chronic liver disease may follow acute chemical hepatitis or years of low-dose exposure. Liver biopsy is usually not helpful in differentiating occupational from nonoccupational liver disease and is rarely indicated.

Treatment of hepatocellular carcinoma due to occupational exposure does not differ from that of disease due to other causes.

REFERENCES

Chopra S, Griffin PH: Laboratory tests and diagnostic procedures in evaluation of liver disease. *Am J Med* 1985;**79**:221.

Doll R: Effects of exposure to vinyl chloride: An assessment of the evidence. *Scand J Work Environ Health* 1988;**14**:61.

Døssing M, Skinhøj P: Occupational liver injury: Present state of knowledge and future perspectives. *Int Arch Occup Environ Health* 1985;**56**:1.

Goodman RA: Nosocomial hepatitis A. *Ann Intern Med* 1985;**103**:452.

Immunization Practices Advisory Committee: Recommendations for protection against viral hepatitis. *MMWR* 1985;**34**:313.

Pond SM: Effects on the liver of chemicals encountered in the workplace. *West J Med* 1982;**137**:506.

Tamburro CH, Liss GM: Tests for hepatotoxicity: Usefulness in screening workers. *J Occup Med* 1986;**28**:1034.

Toftgärd R, Gustafsson JA: Biotransformation of organic solvents: A review. *Scand J Work Environ Health* 1980;**6**:1.

Wright C, Rivera JC, Baetz JH: Liver function testing in a working population: Three strategies to reduce false-positive results. *J Occup Med* 1988;**30**:693.

Zimmerman HJ: *Hepatotoxicity: The Adverse Effects of Drugs and Other Chemicals on the Liver.* Appleton-Century-Crofts. 1978.

Zuckerman AJ: Controversies in immunization against hepatitis B. *Hepatology* 1985;**5**:1227.

Renal Toxicology

21

George A. Kaysen, MD, PhD

The kidney is exposed to a number of toxic materials in the workplace that can cause acute or chronic renal dysfunction or end-stage renal disease. These materials vary in their effects and fall into 4 principal categories: heavy metals, organic chemicals, pesticides, and other xenobiotics. Renal toxicity seldom occurs as an isolated finding in occupational medicine but rather in conjunction with other systemic consequences of toxic exposure.

The kidney is commonly the target of toxic substances. Despite their relatively small size, the kidneys receive 25% of the cardiac output and thus are potentially exposed to large doses of toxic materials. Because of its function, osmotic gradients develop in the kidney—primarily in the medulla—that concentrate toxic agents to levels far in excess of those found in other organs. Because the kidney is capable of acidifying the urine, various solutes may occur in ionic forms not present in other tissues. This combination of factors may explain why the kidney is affected by a variety of toxic materials.

ACUTE RENAL DYSFUNCTION

Acute renal dysfunction may be observed within hours to a few days following relatively high-dose exposure to certain metals, organic solvents, or pesticides. With improvement in industrial hygiene practices during the past 40–50 years, such cases are rarely encountered today. Cases that do occur usually result from confined-space exposure to very high concentrations of airborne substances.

ACUTE RENAL DYSFUNCTION CAUSED BY HEAVY METALS

Significant exposure to any of the divalent metals—chromium, cadmium, mercury, and vanadium—is capable of producing acute renal failure (acute tubular necrosis). Of these metals, the only one encountered in industrial settings in high enough concentrations to produce acute tubular necrosis with notable frequency is cadmium. Exposure to cadmium in toxic amounts is usually through inhalation, and the classic history of exposure is of workers welding

cadmium-plated metals. Welders exposed to cadmium fumes present with coughing and progressive pulmonary distress leading to adult respiratory distress syndrome. Renal failure occurs rapidly in the form of acute tubular necrosis. Severe exposure is capable of producing bilateral cortical necrosis.

ACUTE RENAL DYSFUNCTION CAUSED BY ORGANIC SOLVENTS

1. HALOGENATED HYDROCARBONS

Carbon Tetrachloride

Carbon tetrachloride (CCl_4) is used as an industrial solvent and as the basis for manufacture of fluorinated hydrocarbons. It was once used as a household cleaning agent and as a component of fire extinguisher fluid under the brand name Pyrene.

Like other organic solvents, carbon tetrachloride is lipophilic and therefore distributed in highest concentration in fat, liver, bone marrow, blood, brain, and kidney. Its toxicity is enhanced if it is consumed with ethyl alcohol or other alcohols, and chronic alcoholism potentiates the toxicity of this agent as well.

After acute exposure, patients typically present with symptoms of acute central nervous system depression, such as confusion and somnolence, frequently accompanied by nausea and vomiting. Mucous membrane irritant effects, such as burning eyes, may occur, though some workers may be symptom-free for several days following exposure and then present with complaints of vomiting, abdominal pain, constipation, diarrhea, and in some cases fever. Physical findings may be compatible with the acute abdomen at this stage of illness, and many patients have been improperly subjected to laparotomy for that reason.

After 7–10 days of illness, there may be a decline in urine output even to the point of anuria. Carbon tetrachloride intoxication may show signs of prerenal azotemia as demonstrated by a low urinary sodium excretion and by improvement after volume repletion. Sinicrope (1984) postulated that in some cases of carbon tetrachloride toxicity, renal failure may result from volume depletion and may occur as an extension of prerenal azotemia.

Once renal failure develops, it is manifested by oliguria, which may last 1–2 weeks. In the case of renal failure due to poisoning with aliphatic halogenated hydrocarbons, the kidneys are large and firm and may be tender to palpation.

Urinalysis may reveal red blood cells and protein in cases of nephrotoxic acute renal failure. Red blood cell casts may be seen in the urine, though this finding has not been generally confirmed.

The diagnosis of halogenated hydrocarbon-induced acute renal failure has been confused with that of acute glomerulonephritis. The natural history of this disease is one of spontaneous recovery. However, dialysis may be necessary to support the patient until recovery occurs.

Other Aliphatic Halogenated Hydrocarbons

Other aliphatic halogenated hydrocarbons are nephrotoxic, some to a greater and some to a lesser degree than carbon tetrachloride.

Ethylene dichloride ($CH_2Cl.CH_2Cl$) is used as a solvent for oils, fats, waxes, turpentine, rubber, and some resins; as an insecticide and fumigant; and in fire extinguishers and household cleaning fluids. It is slightly less potent as a renal toxicant than carbon tetrachloride but causes far greater central nervous system toxicity. Ingestion or heavy inhalation may produce acute tubular necrosis similar to that encountered with mercury poisoning.

Chloroform (CCl_3H) is more nephrotoxic than carbon tetrachloride. Like the latter, its toxicity can be enhanced by prior exposure to alcohol or to other substances known to increase the metabolism of exogenous agents.

Trichloroethylene ($CHCl:CCl_2$) has a number of industrial uses and has been used as an anesthetic agent as well. Acute renal failure has followed inhalation of this agent and has occurred in persons using it as a solvent for cleaning. Although it is partially unsaturated, it has toxic effects comparable with those of carbon tetrachloride and chloroform.

Tetrachloroethane (1,1,2,2,-tetrachloroethane; $CCl_2H.CCl_2H$) is an excellent solvent for cellulose acetate and is by far the most toxic of the halogenated hydrocarbons.

Vinylidene chloride (1,1-dichloroethylene; $CClH:CClH$) is a monomer used in the manufacture of plastics and is not used as a solvent. Its toxicology is similar to that of carbon tetrachloride.

Ethylene chlorohydrin (2-chloroethyl alcohol; $CH_2Cl.CH_2OH$) is used as a solvent and as a chemical intermediate. It is far more toxic than any of the other aliphatic halogenated hydrocarbons. Unlike the others, it penetrates the skin readily and is absorbed through rubber gloves. Its mechanism of toxicity is not well understood.

2. NONHALOGENATED HYDROCARBONS AS A CAUSE OF ACUTE RENAL FAILURE

Dioxane

Dioxane is a cyclic diether, colorless and with only a faint odor, freely soluble in water. The vapor pressure of dioxane is quite low, so that respiratory overexposure is rare. Although dioxane is less toxic than the halogenated hydrocarbons, toxicity can be insidious, and large amounts can be inhaled without warning. Injury may become apparent hours after exposure.

Clinically, patients present with anorexia, nausea, and vomiting. Jaundice is uncommon. In fatal cases, clinical presentation may resemble acute abdominal emergency. Urine output decreases on about the third day of illness, and the urine may contain blood or albumin. The presentation is similar in this respect to that of carbon tetrachloride intoxication.

Treatment consists of removal from exposure followed by hemodialysis or hemoperfusion.

Toluene

Both acute renal failure and distal renal tubular acidosis have been reported in painters and in people sniffing glue as a form of recreational substance abuse.

Alkyl Derivatives of Ethylene Glycol

The principal derivatives of ethylene glycol used commercially are the **monoethyl ether** (cellosolve), the **monomethyl ether** (methylcellosolve), and the **butyl ether** (butylcellosolve).

The 3 compounds are similar pharmacologically, with increasing toxicity in the order listed above. All can be absorbed through the skin or lungs as well as through the gastrointestinal tract. These agents are irritants of skin and mucous membranes and act as central nervous system depressants, with resultant symptoms of headache, drowsiness, weakness, slurred speech, staggering gait, and blurred vision. The renal injury caused by these ethers is not related to the oxalic aciduria caused by the parent compounds, which are dialcohols.

Phenol

Phenol (carbolic acid) causes local burns and may be absorbed both through the lungs and transdermally.

Although phenol causes severe local burns, systemic symptoms may also occur. These include headache, vertigo, salivation, nausea and vomiting, and diarrhea. In severe intoxication, urinary albumin excretion may be increased. Red cells and casts are found in the urine. The potentially disastrous consequences of transdermal absorption should not be underestimated.

Patients may present with hypothermia, which is followed by convulsions. The urine may be dark, and oliguria may develop. Phenol is metabolized to hydroquinone, which, when excreted in the urine, may be oxidized to colored substances, causing the urine to change to green or brown (carboluria). Prolonged exposure has been reported to result in proteinuria.

Pentachlorophenol

Pentachlorophenol is used as a preservative for timber and as an insecticide, herbicide, and defoliant. It is readily absorbed through the skin.

In addition to causing acute renal failure, pentachlorophenol causes a hypermetabolic state, with hyperpyrexia and vascular collapse. Workers exposed to pentachlorophenol in clearly subtoxic doses may present with reversible decreased proximal tubular function as manifested by reduced tubular resorption of phosphorus. When these workers are reexamined after a 21-day vacation, renal function—both glomerular filtration rate and proximal tubular function—have returned to normal.

Dinitriphenols & Dinitro-o-Cresols

These agents have been used as pesticides and herbicides. After absorption, they uncouple oxidative phosphorylation. Fatal hyperpyrexia has been reported.

Although patients develop acute renal failure, it is not known whether this is a direct effect of the agents or secondary to the metabolic consequences, such as myoglobinuria.

ACUTE RENAL DYSFUNCTION CAUSED BY UNIDENTIFIED PESTICIDES

Exposure, Pathogenesis, & Clinical Findings

A reduction in glomerular filtration rate—as well as tubular reabsorption of phosphate suggestive of mild proximal tubular dysfunction—has occurred in some agricultural workers. Changes in tubular function and in glomerular filtration rate occur in conjunction with depression of serum cholinesterase, suggesting that organophosphates may be responsible for these changes in renal function.

In an ethically questionable study, prisoners in a New York State prison were fed **carbaryl.** This pesticide is similar in action to the organophosphates, and the prisoners likewise demonstrated a decrease in glomerular filtration rate and tubular resorption of phosphate. There is no evidence that structural damage occurs after exposure to any of these agents.

Organic mercurials are used as fungicides. Absorption of these agents in agricultural workers has been reported to lead to nephrotic syndrome in the case of methoxymethyl mercury silicate, and a dose-dependent increase in the urinary excretion of γ-glutamyl transpeptidase has been reported in the case of phenyl mercury, indicating a direct nephrotoxic effect of this class of compounds.

ACUTE RENAL DYSFUNCTION CAUSED BY ARSINE

Exposure

Arsine (AsH_3) is a heavy gas and the most neph-rotoxic form of arsenic. It is produced by the action of acids on arsenicals, usually during coal or metal processing operations. Exposure to arsine may be insidious, since even as simple an operation as spraying water on metal dross may liberate arsine. Arsine is also used in the semiconductor industry. It may be shipped over long distances, with potential for public health disaster, since arsine is an extremely toxic gas.

Clinical Findings

Arsine is primarily hemotoxic and is a potent hemolytic agent after acute or chronic exposure. The first signs of poisoning are malaise, abdominal cramps, nausea, and vomiting. This may take place immediately or after a delay of up to 24 hours. Renal failure results from acute tubular necrosis secondary to hemoglobinuria.

Treatment & Prognosis

Acute tubular necrosis may be delayed by treatment with mannitol and hemodialysis immediately after exposure. However, exchange transfusion is necessary to prevent further hemolysis. Recovery from acute tubular necrosis induced by arsine may not be complete, and there is evidence that residual interstitial nephritis may result.

ACUTE RENAL DYSFUNCTION CAUSED BY PHOSPHORUS

Ingestion of only a few milligrams of elemental yellow phosphorus may produce acute hepatic and acute renal necrosis. Chronic exposure may result in proteinuria, though the kidney is not the primary organ affected by phosphorus.

CHRONIC RENAL DYSFUNCTION

Relatively few industrial materials have been shown to cause chronic renal failure. This is somewhat paradoxic given the known susceptibility of the kidney to toxic agents and the widespread use of known or suspected nephrotoxins in industry. With the application of more sensitive indicators of renal damage (such as urinary enzymes) to epidemiologic studies, previously unrecognized associations of chemical exposure and chronic renal disease will undoubtedly be identified.

The current generation of tests of renal function (serum creatinine and urea nitrogen) provide little information during the developmental stages of renal disease and thus become useful only after major impairment of renal excretory function has taken place. Other tests such as creatinine clearance may be more sensitive but are impractical for use as screening tests. The development of a new generation of noninvasive tests of renal function offers the opportunity to determine renal damage early and thus institute preventive intervention. The tests thus far studied—an example is urine N-acetylglucosaminidase (NAG)—lack sufficient specificity for renal toxicity to be clinically useful.

CHRONIC RENAL DYSFUNCTION CAUSED BY LEAD

Although organic lead, which is used as an additive to gasoline, is not nephrotoxic, its combustion products are. Lead is released into the environment at a rate of approximately 60 million kg per year as inorganic lead through the combustion of gasoline. Its environmental fate is unknown. Recent findings suggest that many patients with essential hypertension—or with what is called gouty nephropathy—and with concomitant renal failure may indeed be lead-intoxicated.

Early Phase of Lead Toxicity

Early in the course of lead nephropathy, an increase in mitotic activity is seen in the proximal tubular epithelium, where formation of intranuclear inclusion bodies also occurs—a hallmark of lead toxicity. Multiple inclusion bodies may be present in a single nucleus. The bodies consist of a dense central core with an outer fibrillary zone. They are composed of lead and nuclear protein. The lead content of these bodies may be 60–100 times that of the lead concentration in the cytoplasm. The bodies are eosinophilic and acid-fast. The kidney retains the ability to form these bodies for only about 1 year.

The glomerular filtration rate is unimpaired, but evidence of tubular damage is present. Patients develop aminoaciduria, phosphaturia, and glycosuria. These are manifestations of Fanconi's syndrome, the result of nonspecific proximal tubular dysfunction. Unlike other forms of this syndrome, however, the renal clearance of uric acid is decreased rather than increased.

Mitochondrial destruction is prominent even in this early period. Ultrastructural changes seen in the mitochondria during the first phase of lead toxicity are severe. The mitochondria are swollen and distorted in shape. During this early phase, urinary lead excretion correlates roughly with blood lead concentration. Removal of the individual from exposure to lead may cause both the histologic and functional changes of lead intoxication to remit.

Second Phase of Lead Toxicity

The second phase is defined by decreased ability to form inclusion bodies. By this stage, the proximal tubular cells have decreased ability to form nuclear inclusion bodies. The renal excretion of lead is also decreased and the manifestations of Fanconi's syndrome are absent, though hyperuricemia and decreased renal uric acid excretion persist. Gross measurements of renal function, serum urea nitrogen, and serum creatinine are normal during this period. Careful measurements of renal function and of clearance of insulin and para-aminohippurate show that the glomerular filtration rate and effective renal plasma flow may already be disturbed during this period.

Final Phase of Lead Toxicity

The final stage of lead nephropathy may occur many years after initial exposure. Clinically, the disease is characterized by hypertension, hyperuricemia, and gout in about 50% of patients. Hyperkalemia may also be present. Proteinuria is below the nephrotic range. Glomerular filtration and renal blood flow are reduced, and renal failure is progressive to the end stage.

Zinc protoporphyrin is clinically useful only for the diagnosis of acute or subacute lead intoxication. The finding of a normal value in an individual patient does not rule out chronic lead intoxication as a cause of renal failure. It is also possible that the anemia of chronic renal failure might contribute to the variance in zinc protoporphyrin measurements in patients with this condition. Measurement of blood lead is not useful unless it is elevated—some workers with a history of chronic exposure have elevated blood lead concentrations years after the last exposure—in the diagnosis of lead-induced chronic renal failure.

Treatment & Prevention

Chronic lead nephropathy can be treated by intravenous or intramuscular injections of calcium disodium edetate (EDTA) (see Chapter 25 for recommended treatment). Urinary lead excretion is measured periodically. Once lead excretion has been reduced to its normal range (< 80 μg/24 h), further treatment is discontinued. This regimen has been successful in reducing the labile lead pool, and both glomerular filtration rate and renal plasma flow have improved after treatment. Renal disease has progressed, however, after transient improvement, and it is not clear whether treatment of chronic lead nephropathy with calcium disodium edetate is of clinical value. Thus, every effort must be made to prevent chronic lead nephropathy.

While it has been stated that occupational groups with blood lead levels over 60–100 μg/dL and zinc protoporphyrin levels in excess of 100 μg/dL are at definite risk of renal dysfunction, these criteria must be viewed as excessively high. While there may be no truly safe level of blood lead, a blood lead concentration in excess of 40 μg/dL—or perhaps even 30 μg/dL—must be viewed with a great deal of concern.

CHRONIC DYSFUNCTION CAUSED BY CADMIUM

Exposure

Cadmium, which is found primarily as cadmium

sulfide in ores of zinc, lead, and copper, accumulates with age, having a biologic half-life in humans in excess of 10 years. The use of cadmium has doubled in the United States every decade in the 20th century, thus causing progressive environmental contamination.

Forty to 80 percent of accumulated cadmium is stored in the liver and kidneys, with one-third in the kidneys alone. Cadmium is also a contaminant of tobacco smoke, and in the absence of occupational exposure, accumulation is substantially greater in smokers than in nonsmokers. Nonindustrial exposure is primarily via food, and only about 25% of ingested cadmium is absorbed. "Normal" daily dietary intake varies between 15 and 75 mg/d in different parts of the world, though only a small fraction of this amount (0.5–2.5 mg/d) is absorbed. The cadmium body burden of a 45-year-old nonsmoker in the USA is about 9 mg, while in Japan the total is about 21 mg. Although clinical disease has been recognized among the general population in Japan, this has not been the case in the United States, where cadmium has been generally regarded as an exclusively industrial hazard. This may represent failure to assign the correct cause to conditions commonly regarded as the result of aging.

After exposure to cadmium, blood concentration rises sharply but falls after a matter of hours as the cadmium is taken up by the liver. In the liver it stimulates synthesis of a protein, thionine, that tightly binds the cadmium into a cadmium-thionine complex, which has an extremely long half-life once distributed to the kidney.

Clinical Findings

The principal target organs for cadmium are the kidneys and lungs, though severe osteomalacia has been reported in Japan. Both low-molecular-weight and high-molecular-weight proteinuria occur in workers who have been chronically exposed to cadmium. The appearance of high-molecular-weight proteins in the urine may result from decreased renal reabsorption of the small quantity of these proteins that are normally filtered, but it may also represent glomerular dysfunction.

Serum creatinine and plasma β_2-microglobulin tend to be higher in workers exposed to cadmium than in controls, and this dysfunction is correlated with the duration of exposure to cadmium.

The absorption of cadmium is increased during consumption of a low-calcium diet. Cadmium, once absorbed, accumulates in the renal proximal tubule, where it inhibits the activity of vitamin D_1 hydroxylase, an enzyme necessary for the conversion of vitamin D to its active form, 1,25-dihydroxycholecalciferol. This may play a role in the development of osteomalacia. Patients are in negative calcium balance and exhibit hypercalciuria. Renal stone disease is common, occurring in more than 30% of patients with chronic cadmium intoxication.

The critical target organ for renal damage is the renal cortex. The renal cortical cadmium concentration at which 10% of the population will develop renal dysfunction is estimated to be between 180 and 220 $\mu g/g$. This value correlates (with significant interpatient variability) with a urinary cadmium excretion of $10\mu g/g$ creatinine.

The incidence of renal dysfunction increases in workers chronically exposed to cadmium. Urinary cadmium excretion and the excretion of protein must therefore be monitored closely. Samples of urine and blood must be obtained in cadmium-free tubes—away from the workplace—to avoid contamination.

CHRONIC RENAL DYSFUNCTION CAUSED BY MERCURY

Exposure

Occupational mercury poisoning usually results from inhalation of metal fumes or vapor—though toxicity has been reported after exposure to oxides of mercury, mercurous or mercuric chloride, phenylmercuric acetate, mercuric oxide, and mercury-containing pesticides.

Divalent mercury is quite nephrotoxic when ingested, accumulates in the proximal tubule, and can produce acute renal failure in doses as low as 1 mg/kg. Although acute tubular necrosis will result after administration of mercuric chloride ($HgCl_2$), such exposures occur either rarely or not at all as occupational hazards.

Pathogenesis

Renal disease resulting from exposure to mercury is presumably of immunologic origin, as experiments with rats would suggest. The same experiments suggest that genetic factors may also regulate the expression of mercury toxicity in humans, further confounding the diagnosis of occupation-related disease.

Renal disease induced by mercury intoxication is primarily membranous glomerulonephritis, which presents as proteinuria—often in the nephrotic range (> 3.5 g of protein per day). Proliferative glomerular nephritis, anti-glomerular basement membrane antibody deposition, and minimal change nephrotic syndrome have also been reported following exposure to mercury. These diseases generally occur after several months of exposure and are associated neither with the proximal tubular damage that may occur from mercury exposure nor with neurologic manifestations of mercurialism.

The normal route of excretion of mercury is via the kidney. Maximum renal excretion of mercury is about 0.4 mg/d. After that degree of absorption, positive mercury balance results.

Diagnosis

Mercury can be identified in phagosomes of the proximal tubular cells in patients with occupational exposure to mercury. This finding, in conjunction with proteinuria and membranous nephropathy, is strongly suggestive—but not diagnostic—of mercury-induced renal disease. Buchet et al (1980) determined that the prevalence of reduced serum albumin and orosomucoid concentrations is greater in mercury-exposed workers than in controls. Furthermore, the urinary excretion of transferrin, albumin, and β-galactosidase was significantly correlated with urine mercury concentrations. These findings did not correlate with blood mercury concentrations but did correlate with urinary mercury excretion rates. Tubular proteinuria (excretion of β_2-microglobulin) was not characteristic of exposure to mercury. Only measurement of high-molecular-weight proteins was of value.

Treatment & Prevention

Patients with occupational exposure to mercury who develop proteinuria should be removed from further exposure and treated with dimercaprol (BAL) or penicillamine. Both compounds are effective for increasing urinary excretion of organic and inorganic mercury.

CHRONIC RENAL DYSFUNCTION CAUSED BY BERYLLIUM

Exposure

Beryllium is encountered in the manufacture of electronic tubes, ceramics, and fluorescent light bulbs and in metal foundries. Its absorption through the gut is very poor, so that the principal route of entry into the body is by inhalation.

Clinical Findings

The main manifestation of berylliosis is as a systemic granulomatous disease involving primarily the lung but also the bone and bone marrow, the liver, the lymph nodes, and many other organs. Kidney damage does not occur as an isolated finding but only in conjunction with other forms of toxicity. In the kidneys, berylliosis can produce granulomas and interstitial fibrosis. Beryllium nephropathy is associated with hypercalciuria and urinary tract stones. Renal stone disease is common in berylliosis and may occur in up to 30% of patients. Parathyroid hormone levels are depressed, and the presumed mechanism of hypercalciuria is increased calcium absorption through the gut similar to that encountered in sarcoidosis. Hyperuricemia is also characteristic of beryllium nephropathy.

CHRONIC RENAL DYSFUNCTION CAUSED BY URANIUM

It is unclear at this time whether uranium is responsible for significant occupationally related renal disease in humans. Absorption of small amounts of uranium over long periods may produce chronic interstitial renal disease. Careful study of workers in a uranium refining plant revealed an increase in urinary β_2-microglobulin excretion, a form of proteinuria associated with interstitial renal disease. Uranium salts, when administered intravenously, are highly nephrotoxic, producing tubular necrosis.

CHRONIC RENAL DYSFUNCTION DUE TO SILICOSIS

Renal disease due to silicosis does not occur in the absence of pulmonary and other systemic effects.

Exposure

Silicosis is a form of pneumoconiosis associated with pulmonary exposure to silica. Extremely heavy exposure can result in a generalized systemic disease resembling collagen vascular disease, such as systemic lupus erythematosus. Inhalation of silica may trigger an autoimmune disease in sensitive individuals, though a recent report of generalized collagen vascular disease occurring in 4 exposed workmen after heavy sandblasting would remove the generalized effect of silicosis from the realm of idiosyncratic reactions to exposed agents. It has been speculated that ingested silicates may themselves be responsible for the development of interstitial renal disease in analgesic nephropathy.

Clinical Findings

Renal failure may be associated with an active urinary sediment, proteinuria, circulating autoantibodies, and circulating immune complexes. Renal histologic studies may reveal focal glomerular sclerosis, focal proliferative glomerular nephritis, and crescentic nephritis as well as severe tubular interstitial disease. This occurs in a setting of generalized vasculitis and hypertension.

The immunologically mediated glomerular nephritis of silicosis is characterized by lymphocytic and plasma cell infiltration of the kidney and has been produced in experimental animal models.

CHRONIC RENAL DYSFUNCTION CAUSED BY ORGANIC SOLVENTS

1. CHRONIC GLOMERULONEPHRITIS

Exposure History & Epidemiology

Solvent exposure may occur in many industries—including the petrochemical, aerospace, and other industries—where there is use of paints, degreasers, and fuels. Retrospective studies comparing histories of prior exposure to organic solvents among patients with biopsy-proved glomerulonephritis and patients with other forms of renal disease show up to 5 times the incidence of prior exposure to a variety of solvents in those with glomerular disease. No specific agents have been implicated.

Specific types of glomerulonephritis in patients exposed to solvents range from crescentic nephritis to membranoproliferative glomerulonephritis. Proliferative nephritis has received the most attention. While causation cannot be proved by retrospective studies, the results are strongly suggestive of a close relationship between chronic and heavy exposure to a variety of organic solvents and chronic glomerulonephritis of a variety of histologic types. Since solvent exposure is common and glomerulonephritis relatively rare, development of disease may involve a hypersensitivity reaction or may reflect some genetic or other predisposition to the development of renal injury.

2. GOODPASTURE'S DISEASE

Goodpasture's disease occurs predominantly in young men. There are case reports of prior exposure to hydrocarbons. Goodpasture's disease is a combination of rapidly progressive glomerulonephritis and pulmonary alveolar hemorrhage. It is characterized pathologically by crescent formation, endocapillary and exocapillary proliferation, and linear deposits of immunoglobulins in the glomerulus shown by immunofluorescent microscopy.

CHRONIC RENAL DISORDERS CAUSED BY CARBON DISULFIDE

Exposure History & Clinical Findings

Carbon disulfide is used in the manufacture of rayon and neoprene tires. A variety of renal disorders are reported, along with accelerated atherosclerosis. The latter may affect the renal circulation and lead to renal dysfunction, hypertension, proteinuria, and renal insufficiency. The renal effects of carbon disulfide are probably a direct result of its atherogenic effect and not related to direct nephrotoxicity.

END-STAGE RENAL DYSFUNCTION DUE TO AGENTS THAT ALTER RENAL METABOLISM (Xenobiotic Substances)

Exposure History

Certain individuals are more apt than others to develop renal damage from exposure to toxic materials. Thus, acute renal failure may develop in alcoholic patients after exposure to subtoxic doses of halogenated hydrocarbons or to the analgesic acetaminophen. Contact with occupational or environmental hazards may similarly reduce the threshold for the appearance of overt renal damage after exposure to a generally subtoxic dose of a second substance. Recent work has demonstrated that certain organic substances with variable biologic half-lives are capable of inducing aryl hydrocarbon hydrolases both in the liver and the kidney of the mouse.

Experiments suggest that response to a toxic agent may be predetermined by prior exposure to chemicals capable of inducing enzyme synthesis (eg, P-450, aryl hydrocarbon hydrolase), which results in increased metabolism of xenobiotics. These agents permanently—albeit imperceptibly—predispose the individual to react unfavorably when challenged by a second toxic chemical. Identification of the potential role of these substances in modulating the course of a renal disease—long after exposure—will be difficult both clinically and epidemiologically.

REFERENCES

General

Hook JB: Toxic responses of the kidney. Chap 11 in: *Casarett and Doull's Toxicology,* 3rd ed. Macmillan, 1986.

Landrigan PJ et al: The work-relatedness of renal disease. *Arch Env Health* 1984;**39**:225.

Lauwerys RR, Bernard A: Early detection of the nephrotoxic effects of industrial chemicals: State of the art and future prospects. *Am J Ind Med* 1987;**11**:275.

Meyer BR et al: Increased urinary enzyme excretion in workers exposed to nephrotoxic chemicals. *Am J Med* 1985;**76**:989.

Price RG: Urinary enzymes, nephrotoxicity, and renal disease. *Toxicology* 1982;**23**:99.

Thun MJ, Clarkson TW: Spectrum of tests available to evaluate occupationally induced renal disease. *J Occup Med* 1986;**28**:1026.

Viau C et al: A cross-sectional survey of kidney function in refinery employees. *Am J Ind Med* 1987;**11**:177.

Weeden PP: Occupational renal disease: In-depth review. *Am J Kidney Dis* 1984;**3**:241.

Metals: Lead

Batuman V et al: Contribution of lead to hypertension with renal impairment. *N Engl J Med* 1983;**309**:17.

Batuman V et al: The role of lead in gout nephropathy. *N Engl J Med* 1981;**304**:520.

Cullen MR, Robins JM, Eskenasi B: Adult inorganic lead intoxication: Presentation of 31 new cases and a review of recent advances in the literature. *Medicine* 1983;**62**:221.

Harlan WR et al: Blood lead and blood pressure: Relationship in the adolescent and adult US population. *JAMA* 1985;**253**:530.

Mahaffey KR et al: National estimates of blood lead levels, United States 1976-1980: Association with selected demographic and socioeconomic factors. *N Engl J Med* 1982;**307**:573.

Wedeen RP: Occupational renal disease. *Am J Kidney Dis* 1984;**3**:241.

Wedeen RP, Malik DK, Batuman V: Detection and treatment of occupational lead nephropathy. *Arch Intern Med* 1979;**139**:53.

Metals: Cadmium

Buchet JP et al: Assessment of renal function of workers exposed to inorganic lead, cadmium or mercury vapor. *J Occup Med* 1980;**22**:741.

Cousins RJ: Metallothionein synthesis and degradation: Relationship to cadmium metabolism. *Environ Health Perspect* 1979;**28**:131.

Kazantzis G: Renal tubular dysfunction and abnormalities of calcium metabolism in cadmium workers. *Environ Health Perspect* 1979;**28**:155.

Kjellstrom T: Exposure and accumulation of cadmium in populations from Japan, the United States, and Sweden. *Environ Health Perspect* 1979;**28**:169.

Lauwerys RR et al: Investigations on the lung and kidney function in workers exposed to cadmium. *Environ Health Perspect* 1979;**28**:137.

Shaikh ZA, Smith LM: Biological indicators of cadmium exposure and toxicity. *Experientia* 1984;**40**:36.

Metals: Mercury

Buchet JP et al: Assessment of renal function of worker exposed to lead, cadmium or mercury vapor. *J Occup Med* 1980;**22**:741.

Druet P, Sapin C, Hirsch F: Genetic control of mercury-induced immune response in the rat. In: *Nephrotoxic Mechanisms of Drugs and Environmental Toxins.* Porter GA (editor). Plenum Press, 1982.

Druet P et al: Immunologically mediated glomerulonephritis induced by heavy metals. *Arch Toxicol* 1982;**50**:187.

Kazantzis G: Industrial hazard to the kidney and urinary tract. In: *Sixth International Symposium on Advanced Medicine.* States JD (editor). Pitman, 1970.

Metals: Beryllium

Kelley WN, Goldfinger SE, Hardy HL: Hyperuricemia in chronic beryllium disease. *Ann Internal Med* 1969;**70**:977.

Stoeckle JD, Hardy HL, Weber AL: Chronic beryllium disease: Long-term follow-up of sixty cases and selective review of the literature. *Am J Med* 1969; **46**:545.

Stokinger HE: Beryllium. In: *Patty's Industrial Hygiene and Toxicology,* 3rd ed. Clayton GD, Clayton FE (editors). Wiley, 1981.

Metals: Uranium

Finn WF: Renal response to environmental toxins. *Environ Health Perspect* 1977;**20**:15.

Thun MJ et al: *NIOSH Health Hazard Evaluation Report.* Cotter, 1981.

Nonmetals

Bolton WK, Suratt PM, Strugill BC: Rapidly progressive silicon nephropathy. *Am J Med* 1981;**71**:823.

Hauglustaine D et al: Silicon nephropathy: A possible occupational hazard. *Nephron* 1980;**26**:219.

Hydrocarbons

Begley J et al: Association between renal function tests and pentachlorophenol exposure. *Clin Toxicol* 1977; **11**:97.

Bell GM et al: Proliferative glomerulonephritis and exposure to organic solvents. *Nephron* 1985;**40**:161.

Churchill ON et al: Association between hydrocarbon exposure and glomerulonephritis: An appraisal of the evidence. *Nephron* 1983;**33**:169.

Finn R, Fennerty AG, Ahmad R: Hydrocarbon exposure and glomerulonephritis. *Clin Nephrol* 1980;**14**:173.

Hamilton A, Hardy HL: Alcohols and glycols. In: *Industrial Toxicology.* John Wright Publishing Sciences Group, 1983.

Hunter D: The aliphatic carbon compounds. In: *The Diseases of Occupation,* 7th ed. Little, Brown, 1988.

Ravnskov U, Lundstrom S, Norden A: Hydrocarbon exposure and glomerulonephritis: Evidence from patients' occupations. *Lancet* 1983;**2**:1214.

Sinicrope RA: Carbon tetrachloride nephrotoxicity: A reassessment of pathophysiology based upon the urinary diagnostic indices. *Am J Kidney Dis* 1984;**3**:362.

Pesticides & Herbicides

Morgan DP, Roan CC: Renal function in persons occupationally exposed to pesticides. *Arch Environ Health* 1969;**19**:633.

Smith P, Heath D: Paraquat. *CRC Crit Rev Toxicology* 1976;**4**:411.

Strunge P: Nephrotic syndrome caused by a seed disinfectant. *JAMA* 1970;**212**:178.

Arsine

Fowler BA, Weissberg JB: Arsine poisoning. *N Engl J Med* 1974;**291**:1171.

Hesdorffer CS et al: Arsine gas poisoning: The importance of exchange transfusions in severe cases. *Br J Ind Med* 1986;**43**:353.

Landrigan PJ, Costello RJ, Stringer WT: Occupational exposure to arsine: An epidemiologic reappraisal of current standards. *Scand J Work Environ Health* 1982;**8**:169.

Parish GG, Glass R, Kimbrough R: Acute arsine poisoning in two workers cleaning a clogged drain. *Arch Environ Health* 1979;**34**:224.

Pinto SS: Arsine poisoning: Evaluation of the acute phase. *J Occup Med* 1976;**18**:633.

Stokinger HD: Arsine. In: *Patty's Industrial Hygiene and Toxicology,* 3rd ed. Clayton GD, Clayton FE (editors). Wiley, 1981.

Other Xenobiotics

Hook JB, Serbia VC: Potentiation of the action of nephrotoxic agents by environmental contaminants. In: *Nephrotoxic Mechanisms of Drugs and Environmental Toxins.* Porter GA (editor). Plenum Press, 1982.

Kluwe WM: Mechanisms of acute nephrotoxicity: Halogenated aliphatic hydrocarbons. In: *Nephrotoxic Mechanisms of Drugs and Environmental Toxins.* Porter GA (editor). Plenum Press, 1982.

Kluwe WM, Hook JB: Effects of environmental chemicals on kidney metabolism and function. *Kidney Int* 1980;**18**:648.

Neurotoxicology

22

William J. Estrin, MD, & Gareth J. Parry, MB, FRACP

WORKPLACE EXPOSURES & THE NERVOUS SYSTEM

Neurologic dysfunction, neuropathies, and encephalopathies can be caused by exposure to a wide variety of hazardous agents in the workplace. Among these agents are metals (eg, arsenic, lead, manganese, mercury, tellurium, thallium, and tin), solvents and other chemicals (eg, acrylamide, carbon disulfide, hexacarbons, perchloroethylene, toluene, trichloroethylene, and vinyl chloride), organophosphates, and noxious gases (eg, carbon monoxide, ethylene oxide, and nitrous oxide).

The first section of this chapter discusses the problems of establishing the causes of neurologic disorders and offers an approach to the diagnosis and treatment of occupational diseases affecting the peripheral and central nervous systems. The second part describes the effects of the neurotoxic substances most commonly encountered in the workplace.

ESTABLISHING THE CAUSES OF NEUROLOGIC DISORDERS

In workers exposed to potentially neurotoxic chemicals who show manifestations of neurotoxicity, there are many problems in trying to establish a direct cause-and-effect relationship, particularly when the central nervous system is involved. The reasons for the difficulty can be summarized briefly:

(1) In general, the nervous system does not respond to neurotoxic substances in ways that are different from other injuries or substance exposures.

(2) Alcohol and other substances of abuse are confounders with distressingly high rates of prevalence in our society.

(3) There is relatively little information about which chemicals are neurotoxic and which are not. Only a small number of the estimated 60,000 chemicals in the workplace or general environment have been evaluated for toxic effects, and about 1000–1500 new chemicals are introduced and many are brought into production for industrial and agricultural use each year. Combustion products of some industrial chemicals may be neurotoxic, although very little research has been conducted to define the problem. It is important to remember that most industrial-agricultural-environmental chemicals are not "inert" and not biologically different from pharmaceutical drugs with similar routes of absorption, metabolism, and excretion.

(4) For chemicals known to be neurotoxic, there is considerable controversy about the level and duration of exposure required to produce neurotoxic effects. Moreover, it is difficult to establish the level and duration of exposure in a given worker.

(5) Workers are generally exposed to more than one chemical in the workplace and in the environment, and the effects of a single chemical are therefore difficult to isolate.

(6) Case detection and definition are very difficult, even for the specializing occupational physician. Very few symptoms or signs of neurologic disorders are specific for neurotoxicity caused by a given chemical, and it is often difficult to rule out other (nonchemical) causes in patients with neurologic dysfunction. Furthermore, neurologic and psychologic disorders are easily confused.

(7) Reliable tests for neurologic dysfunction that can be easily administered at the worksite are currently lacking. Development of such tests will be an important step toward diagnosing neurotoxic effects in workers.

GENERAL APPROACH TO THE DIAGNOSIS OF NEUROLOGIC DISORDERS

The general principles set forth in Chapter 2 govern the approach to the diagnosis of any occupational illness. In the evaluation of a neurotoxic illness, special reliance must be placed on information about work exposure provided by the worker and the employer. Significant questions that must be answered in every case are the following:

What substances are used by the worker and in what circumstances and for what portion of the work shift?

Was the illness the result of long-term exposure or a brief exposure to a leak or spill with a high dose of neurotoxic material?

What is the toxicity of the material?

What other disease process is occurring in the patient that must be considered in the differential diagnosis?

Difficulties with neurotoxic investigations include the nonspecificity of symptoms: headaches, dizziness, weakness, difficulties concentrating, memory loss, and numbness and tingling. These symptoms occur in many neurologic and nonneurologic diseases in addition to those induced by toxic exposure. Problems in evaluating neurotoxicologic problems include the following:

(1) The need to identify diseases not induced by toxic exposure.

(2) The possibility of exposures to more than one toxic substance.

(3) The absence of systematic environmental surveillance (industrial hygiene studies) for toxic exposure.

(4) The frequency of litigation as a confounding variable in evaluation of symptoms. The adversarial relationship between litigants tends not to serve the process of objective diagnosis. Plaintiffs may feel the need to exaggerate symptoms to build their cases, and defendants may not offer important information if it is not directly demanded.

EVALUATION OF PERIPHERAL NERVE FUNCTION

The peripheral nerves are more accessible to evaluation by testing than the central nervous system. Symptom questionnaires and less subjective tests of sensation, such as the Optocon and Biothesiometer, may be useful to screen workers for neuropathic damage. Sensory and motor nerve conduction tests are more accurate and reproducible and are easily obtained and well tolerated by most workers. However, without baseline testing, it is extremely difficult to detect subtle loss of neurologic function. In individual patients who have been subjected to toxic exposures and have severe peripheral neuropathy, electromyography and even nerve biopsy may be necessary.

Peripheral neuropathy may occur as a delayed response to acute exposure to high concentrations of a neurotoxic substance, as is seen with organophosphates and acrylamide. In such cases, the neuropathy is of acute onset and runs a monophasic course, with the degree of recovery depending on the severity of the nerve damage. In other cases, neuropathy results from chronic exposure to low concentrations of neurotoxins, such as the heavy metals and organic solvents. The result is a progressive neuropathy of insidious onset with a much slower rate of recovery when exposure is stopped.

In general, most toxic peripheral neuropathies are reversible. However, a recent study demonstrated delayed (for 2–3 years) peripheral neurotoxic effects of acrylamide exposure in primates. Therefore, although in most neuropathies there is some recovery after the offending agent is removed, one cannot be certain whether a delayed onset of symptoms and dysfunctions may occur after exposure to a toxin has been terminated.

Clinical Findings

Peripheral nerve dysfunction usually results in numbness or tingling of the distal lower, then upper extremities. If exposure continues, weakness (distal > proximal) may follow, with eventual development of atrophy and fasciculation of the muscle, usually preceded by sensory symptoms.

Peripheral neuropathy is relatively easy to detect. It is likely to be present in individuals (1) with distal sensory symptoms and evidence of diminished vibration or pain sensation distally in the lower extremities who also have (2) bilaterally reduced or absent ankle reflexes.

Diagnosis

Table 22–1 sets forth the essentials of diagnosis of peripheral nerve dysfunction.

EVALUATION OF THE CENTRAL NERVOUS SYSTEM

Central nervous system dysfunction is most frequently seen following acute exposure to relatively high concentrations of a neurotoxic substance. Such exposures generally result in a nonspecific narcotic effect—in fact, almost any toxin may have this entirely nonspecific effect. The toxic source is usually easy to identify because of its acute onset, often involving many workers and causing other symptoms such as lacrimation and skin irritation. Recovery is usually rapid and complete. Occasionally, acute high-level exposure may result in permanent central nervous system damage.

Chronic low-level exposure is much more difficult to relate to central nervous system dysfunction because of the lack of specificity of symptoms, the paucity of methods of objective assessment, bias induced by litigation, and the "healthy worker effect" (see Appendix).

Clinical Findings

Although most central neurotoxic agents do not result in structural lesions that are identifiable radiologically or pathologically (carbon monoxide and toluene exposure being exceptions), the symptoms tend to be quite disabling despite their often nonspe-

Table 22-1. Essentials of diagnosis of peripheral nerve dysfunction.

Clinical
   Distal sensory loss and paresthesias
   Distal weakness and atrophy
   Reduced or absent tendon reflexes
Electrophysiologic
   Reduced nerve conduction velocity
   Low-amplitude responses on EMG (particularly sensory)
   Denervation potentials
Morphologic (nerve biopsy)
   Axonal degeneration
   Segmental demyelination

cific nature. The most common complaint in individuals with toxic exposure affecting the central nervous system is difficulty with concentration and memory. Verbal reasoning, remote and recent memory, complex concept formation, and dexterity may also be affected by central neurotoxic exposure. Vocabulary level seems to be somewhat resistant to the effects of neurotoxic exposure and predictable largely by educational background of the individual.

Additionally, patients often report headache, lightheadedness, vertigo, blurred vision, poor coordination, tremor, and diffuse weakness of the extremities. Exposed individuals may report difficulties with attention and with organizing ability as well as general depression, irritability, and fatigue. Most commonly, patients who have been exposed to a central neurotoxin report cognitive dysfunction without any other physical manifestations of neurologic dysfunction. In such cases, formal neuropsychologic evaluation is required in addition to a detailed neurologic examination. Interpretation of these tests is extremely difficult in the absence of evaluations prior to the exposure. Pre-event values are almost never available.

STEPS IN A COMPLETE NEUROLOGIC EVALUATION

Complete evaluation of a patient or group of workers with a suspected occupational neurotoxicity disorder often requires the participation of a team of specialists, including a neuropsychiatrist, neurologist, electrophysiologist, industrial hygienist, and occupational health physician. The components of the examination are outlined in the following paragraphs.

History & Physical Examination

A complete medical and occupational history should be taken, and general physical and neurologic examinations should be performed. Information should be elicited about the presence and duration of common neurologic symptoms.

Neurologic Tests

Tests for evaluation of neuropsychologic and neurologic function developed by occupational health researchers are described briefly below. In applying such tests and examinations, it is important that a representative random sample of the exposed worker population be selected and that a comparable control group of similar age, education, socioeconomic status, and sex distribution be obtained. Although many of these techniques have been developed specifically for local worksite evaluation of groups, similar analyses can be employed with individual workers who have been exposed to potentially neurotoxic substances.

One efficient approach is administration of an abbreviated subset of standardized tests such as the

WAIS (Wechsler Adult Intelligence Scale) by neuropsychologic technicians. A limited number of research studies have used computerized batteries of tests. Exposure-specific symptom and exposure questionnaires may be given. Tests include the Continuous Performance Test, Simple Reaction Time, Digit Span Forward, Digit Span Backward, Aural Digit Span, Symbol-Digit Test, Pattern Memory, Horizontal Addition, Hand-Eye Coordination, and Purdue Pegboard.

TREATMENT OF DISORDERS DUE TO NEUROTOXIC DAMAGE

With a few prominent exceptions such as chelation for heavy metal exposure, there is no specific treatment for peripheral or central nervous system dysfunction induced by toxic exposure. The passage of time brings some recovery. Psychotherapy, physical therapy, and occupational therapy should be strongly considered for individuals with continuing functional impairment. Careful neurologic follow-up of such individuals is essential.

EFFECTS OF SPECIFIC HAZARDOUS SUBSTANCES ON THE NERVOUS SYSTEM

The following descriptions present only the neurologic outcomes of each representative exposure. General descriptions of each material and its health effects and exposure limits are not included. For such information, the reader is referred to the corresponding chapters on metals (Chapter 25), chemicals (Chapter 26), solvents (Chapter 27), gases (Chapter 31), etc. Action levels (eg, blood lead) are to be found in Chapter 34 on biologic monitoring.

ACRYLAMIDE
(See also Chapter 26.)

The acrylamide *monomer* (not the polymer) is neurotoxic, and most instances of acrylamide intoxication occur by inhalation and skin absorption during its manufacture.

Acute exposure causes an encephalopathy that is usually of brief duration, though persistent cerebellar dysfunction has been seen with very large exposure. Peripheral neuropathy may develop both as a delayed manifestation of acute exposure (2–3 weeks later) and with chronic exposure. The earliest signs following acute exposure are numbness in the feet, accompanied by profuse sweating of the hands and feet and occasionally urinary retention. The sensory loss may be severe enough to produce sensory ataxia, but there is usually only mild weakness, at least in the early stages.

There is usually early and generalized loss of reflexes, which helps to distinguish this neuropathy from other toxic neuropathies. Effects of low-dose acrylamide exposure may be delayed for 2–3 years (as suggested by studies of primates). Other manifestations include skin peeling, which occasionally progresses to exfoliative dermatitis, reddening of the palms, and joint pain. After removal from exposure, there is usually slow recovery of function, but some residual sensory ataxia is not uncommon in the more severe cases.

Acrylamide neuropathy, like that caused by organic solvents, results from the accumulation of neurofilaments in axons and is characterized by distal axonal degeneration that affects both peripheral and central axonal extensions. Unlike other solvent neuropathies, acrylamide neuropathy is associated with little secondary demyelination.

ARSENIC (See Chapter 25.)

Acute arsenic exposure usually consists of accidental ingestion and produces mainly the following symptoms and signs: nausea, abdominal pain, vomiting, diarrhea, and vasomotor collapse. If an individual survives the acute syndrome, neuropathy usually appears 1–3 weeks later. Typically, numbness with intensely painful dysesthesias begins in the feet and hands and progresses proximally. Distal weakness may also occur within 1–2 weeks after acute exposure and may progress for 4–6 weeks. Arsenical neuropathy is characterized primarily by axonal degeneration with occasional demyelination.

Chronic exposure to arsenic may also lead to neuropathy, which evolves more slowly than in acute cases. Nerve conduction studies show reduced amplitude of sensory and motor compound action potentials, and there is denervation on electromyography. Occasionally, following acute exposure, there may be marked slowing of nerve conduction velocity, with dispersion of action potentials indicating demyelination. These findings, together with elevated cerebrospinal fluid protein, may suggest Guillain-Barré syndrome.

Chelation with dimercaprol or penicillamine has not been useful in the treatment of acute arsenic intoxication. However, peripheral neuropathy is not affected by chelation in any case. Slow recovery occurs if initial exposure is survived, and the residual deficit is proportionate to the severity of neuropathy.

CARBON DISULFIDE
(See also Chapter 26.)

Acute inhalation exposure to carbon disulfide concentrations above 400 ppm produces narcosis. Subacute exposure to high concentrations (> 300 ppm) produces encephalopathy manifested mainly as dramatic psychologic disturbance with mania, profound depression, and hallucinations. Attacks on relatives and coworkers and attempted suicides have been reported.

Chronic exposure to lower concentrations (50–150 ppm) is associated with a distal axonal neuropathy with sensory and motor features. The neuropathy appears 4–6 months after exposure to higher levels (150 ppm) but may take several years to develop with low-level exposure. There may also be an encephalopathy, usually characterized by organic psychosis with both extrapyramidal and pyramidal features (spastic paraparesis, pseudobulbar palsy).

CARBON MONOXIDE
(See also Chapter 31.)

Acute inhalation exposure to CO results in encephalopathy characterized by headache, confusion, and somnolence, leading to coma and death if exposure continues. Recovery following removal from exposure may be protracted owing to the affinity of hemoglobin for CO and, in severe cases, to brain edema. Recovery may be incomplete, leaving the patient with diffuse hypoxic encephalopathy or focal deficits, including mononeuropathy multiplex. These focal deficits are thought to be due to ischemia of brain or peripheral nerve.

Alternative explanations for peripheral nerve involvement include compression of nerves in comatose patients and perhaps a direct toxic effect of CO on nerve. Occasionally, following apparently good recovery, there is a delayed deterioration that can appear as early as a few days or not until 6 weeks later. Late deterioration is characterized by confusion and apathy combined with extrapyramidal features such as bradykinesia and rigidity. Most cases progress to an akinetic, mute state or death. Patients with late deterioration are usually those with severe, prolonged exposure.

The existence of chronic neurotoxicity from CO inhalation is controversial. The initial claim that fatigue, headache, and dizziness could result from chronic low-level exposure was discredited when it was found that these symptoms occurred with equal frequency in exposed and nonexposed individuals.

ETHYLENE OXIDE
(See also Chapter 26.)

There are increasing reports about the neurotoxicity of ethylene oxide, used extensively as a sterilizing agent for heat-sensitive biomedical materials.

The most prominent effect is on peripheral nerves, with distal sensory loss and some weakness. Encephalopathy may accompany the neuropathy or may occur independently. There are now several cohorts of hospital sterilizer workers who have been exposed to intermittent high inhalation doses (over 400 ppm) of ethylene oxide over many years. Neuropsychologic testing and several nerve velocity and amplitude studies strongly suggest that ethylene oxide is both a central and a peripheral neurotoxin and that central effects may be more persistent than peripheral ones.

LEAD (See also Chapter 25.)

Lead is regularly present in the blood of urban dwellers. Lead intoxication can result in encephalopathy and neuropathy.

Acute exposure to lead—occurring almost exclusively by ingestion in children with pica—causes encephalopathy with cerebral edema. Gastrointestinal, hematopoietic, and renal effects are well described. Chronic exposure—by ingestion or inhalation—results in peripheral motor neuropathy, which may affect the upper limbs more severely than the lower limbs and particularly involves muscles supplied by the radial nerve. Chronic exposure may also cause loss of anterior horn cells, to give a clinical picture indistinguishable from that of amyotrophic lateral sclerosis.

The cerebral edema of lead encephalopathy in children may require the administration of corticosteroids and osmotic agents. Recovery depends on the severity of the intoxication, and there is often incomplete resolution of the neuropathy.

MANGANESE (See also Chapter 25.)

After prolonged inhalation exposure to manganese (6 months to over 20 years), encephalopathy (manganese madness) develops, with hallucinations, emotional instability, and bizarre behavior. A few months after onset of these symptoms, generalized weakness, dysarthria, ataxia, tremor, impotence, and headache appear. Later, extrapyramidal features develop that are similar to those in Parkinson's disease; there may be dystonia or tremor alone without other findings.

MERCURY (See also Chapter 25.)

Neurologic disease may follow exposure to both organic and inorganic mercury. Occupational exposure is usually related to exposure to inorganic mercury by inhalation and possibly by ingestion (although inorganic mercury is poorly absorbed from the gut). Symptoms may develop after many years of inhalation exposure, particularly if exposure is infrequent and the dosage is low. The most characteristic feature of inorganic mercurialism is a coarse, rapid tremor that begins in the hands and may slowly spread to involve the eyelids, the tongue, the facial muscles, and the remainder of the extremities. There may also be muscular excitability, weakness, and

personality changes such as those that gave rise to the expression "mad as a hatter" among workers in the felt hat industry. Peripheral neuropathy may also occur, but it is uncommon and may be overshadowed by central nervous system dysfunction. Mercurial neuropathy is of the sensorimotor type, which may resemble Guillain-Barré syndrome—especially when the cerebrospinal fluid protein is elevated without pleocytosis.

Chronic exposure to organic mercury—not likely in the industrial setting—causes mental impairment, tremor, ataxia, dysarthria, deafness, and constriction of visual fields. An early complaint is of paresthesias, which may involve the face and tongue as well as the extremities and is probably due to involvement of the dorsal root and trigeminal ganglia.

N-HEXANE & METHYL N-BUTYL KETONE (HEXACARBONS) (See also Chapter 27.)

These hydrocarbons are metabolized to 2,5-hexanedione, which is responsible for most if not all of the neurotoxic effects. Acute exposure to hexacarbons produces euphoria, which leads to abuse of these chemicals by inhalation (glue-sniffers, gasoline-sniffers, etc). Chronic exposure causes distal axonal neuropathy. Macular degeneration without neuropathy has also been reported following chronic exposure.

N-Hexane produces neuropathy by causing a disturbance in axonal transport. Cross-bridging and secondary accumulation of axonal neurofilaments occur multifocally, with axonal degeneration occurring distally to the axonal "bulge." This distal axonal degeneration affects both the peripheral and central sensory axons. The axonal changes produce secondary demyelination, which results in marked slowing of nerve conduction velocities. Nerve biopsy is useful in obscure cases, as it may confirm the presence of segmental demyelination with axonal swellings, a combination that is essentially diagnostic of hexacarbon neuropathy.

NITROUS OXIDE

Nitrous oxide, hitherto considered harmless, has been associated with a number of cases of myeloneuropathy. Most have been the result of high level recreational inhalation exposure, though it has been suggested that chronic exposure of dentists to gas leaking into their offices may also cause the syndrome.

Acute high-level inhalation exposure causes encephalopathy, but recovery is complete even after multiple exposures. Repeated exposure on a daily basis for many months results in a myeloneuropathy closely resembling that associated with vitamin B_{12} deficiency. Paresthesias, sensory ataxia, and spastic leg weakness are most common. Sphincter disturbances suggest that the syndrome may be due to interference by nitrous oxide with vitamin B_{12} utilization.

ORGANOPHOSPHATES
(See also Chapter 30.)

The organophosphates are one of the few classes of neurotoxins in which the target enzymes are known. These compounds inhibit both acetylcholinesterase, which explains the central nervous system and neuromuscular toxicity, and neuropathy target esterase (NTE), an enzyme that is inhibited in neuropathy.

The structure of the specific anticholinesterase determines whether there is "aging" (loss of phosphate group) of the NTE-anticholinesterase complex associated with the delayed development of peripheral neuropathy. There are individual differences in the relative potencies of various organophosphates against these enzymes. Thus, nerve gases and insecticides are potent anticholinesterases and have prominent central nervous system and neuromuscular effects, though some insecticides are also NTE inhibitors (eg, leptophos, mipafox, trichlorphon). By contrast, triorthocresyl phosphate, a gasoline and mineral oil additive, is a potent inhibitor of NTE and causes neuropathy but has minimal anticholinesterase activity.

Most persons with intoxication from organophosphate compounds present with minor signs of parasympathetic nervous system stimulation. Acute poisoning by inhalation, ingestion, or skin absorption produces a cholinergic crisis characterized by encephalopathy in which convulsions, muscle twitching, weakness, lacrimation, and involuntary defecation and urination are common. In milder cases, there is nausea, vomiting, and diarrhea lasting from a few hours to days. The severity of these cholinergic features depends on the severity of exposure and the particular organophosphate.

With some organophosphates, if the acute episode is survived, a delayed neuropathy develops. There is little relationship between the severity of the acute effects and subsequent development of neuropathy, which in fact may develop in the absence of obvious acute effects.

Typically, neuropathy may develop 1–2 weeks after the episode, depending on the duration and magnitude of exposure, and is heralded by sharp cramping pains in the calves. This is quickly followed by numbness and tingling in the feet and sometimes the hands—and then weakness, which also begins in distal muscles. Sensory loss is always present, but weakness predominates and may be extreme. Autonomic signs and cranial nerve involvement are rarely seen. The symptoms evolve subacutely, the neuropathy appearing in 1–2 weeks depending on the duration and severity of exposure.

There are also signs of delayed central nervous system dysfunction, and occasionally these findings predominate. More commonly, however, they appear as the neuropathy resolves and mainly involve the pyramidal tracts, causing marked spasticity, though ataxia may also result.

There are few useful laboratory tests (see Chapter 30 for details). Following acute poisoning, erythrocyte cholinesterase levels may be depressed, especially with insecticides. However, by the time the neuropathy develops, they may be normal.

Neuropathy target esterase can be measured in lymphocytes and may be useful in predicting development of neuropathy following known organophosphate exposure. This procedure is not helpful in establishing neuropathy since by that time NTE levels have returned to normal.

Electrophysiologic testing confirms the presence of distal axonal degeneration, but there are no specific features.

SOLVENTS (See also Chapter 27.)

The solvents most commonly associated with neurotoxicity are acrylamide, carbon disulfide (CS_2), the hexacarbons (n-hexane, methyl n-butyl ketone), perchloroethylene (PCE), toluene, trichloroethylene (TCE), and vinyl chloride as well as methyl ethyl ketone, styrene, xylene, ethylene dichloride, methylene chloride, and methyl bromide.

Acute, high-level inhalation exposure to these organic solvents produces symptoms of a reversible though acute encephalopathy; respiratory depression, hypoxic coma, and death may occur. More controversial is the existence of a chronic, irreversible encephalopathy with personality change, dementia, and nonfocal neurologic signs related to chronic low-level exposure. Furthermore, very high level repeated exposure may occur in persons abusing organic solvents by inhalation (glue-sniffing), resulting in clinical and autopsy evidence of central nervous system damage and cerebellar atrophy.

Epidemiologic and neuropsychologic studies of workers chronically exposed to organic solvents in the workplace suggest that much lower levels of exposure by inhalation and skin absorption can also produce chronic progressive encephalopathy. In its mildest form, exposed individuals may have an organic affective disorder characterized by depression and irritability that is reversible over days, weeks, or months after exposure is terminated. In addition to mood changes, short-term memory loss and psychomotor difficulties occur.

Severe, irreversible toxic encephalopathy with overt dementia and nonfocal neurologic signs may be associated with chronic low-level exposure. There is considerable epidemiologic evidence that solvent workers (such as painters, who are chronically exposed to organic solvents) have a higher than normal incidence of psychiatric disorders and dementia developing later in life.

THALLIUM (See also Chapter 25.)

Acute ingestion exposure to high doses of thallium causes encephalopathy with prominent ataxia. In severe cases, this may progress to psychosis, convulsions, and coma. Other central nervous system effects include choreoathetosis, optic neuropathy, and signs of midbrain and pontine dysfunction. Severe poisoning usually results in dementia in survivors.

One of the most prominent features of acute poisoning is delayed neuropathy, which usually appears about a week after exposure. The neuropathy is heralded by the onset of paresthesias in the distal extremities, occurring first in the feet. Later, weakness may develop, but sensory symptoms and signs predominate. Occasionally, cranial nerve palsies occur, probably due to involvement of brain stem nuclei rather than of the peripheral cranial nerves. Reflexes are usually preserved. There may be prominent autonomic signs, including tachycardia, hypertension, increased salivation, and fever. Alopecia, which is so characteristic of thallatoxicosis, has also been attributed to autonomic neuropathy, but this is not established.

Diagnosis is usually established clinically by the association of a typical neurologic picture with alopecia.

TIN (See also Chapter 25.)

Tin intoxication (by inhalation) is caused only by the organic form, resulting in an encephalopathy characterized by severe headache with nausea and vomiting, progressing to vertigo, visual disturbance, papilledema, and finally convulsions. As suggested by the headache and the papilledema, there is raised intracranial pressure due to severe cranial edema. There may also be neuropathy, but it is usually trivial. There are no helpful laboratory tests.

Treatment depends on controlling the elevated intracranial pressure. Recovery is slow and often incomplete in severe cases.

TOLUENE (See also Chapter 27.)

Like n-hexane, toluene has become an abused chemical because of the euphoria that results from acute exposure. Chronic cerebral and cerebellar dysfunction occurs in toluene "sniffers." These effects are best documented in toluene abusers, and their occurrence in long-term occupational exposure is controversial. Abnormalities in cognitive functioning are most common, sometimes accompanied by pyramidal effects (weakness, spasticity, hyperreflexia) and incoordination. Visual loss from optic atrophy has also been described.

Complete functional recovery usually occurs, with permanent residua only in severe cases.

TRICHLOROETHYLENE (See also Chapter 27.)

Following inhalation exposure to concentrations above 100 ppm, trigeminal neuropathy develops that involves both the sensory and motor divisions. Sensory loss due to trichloroethylene occurs in a peculiar circumstantial distribution on the face and, less commonly, involving the optic and facial nerves.

Chronic inhalation exposure may cause an encephalopathy characterized by neuropsychologic disturbances and sometimes overt dementia, visual impairment, and tremor. In addition to trigeminal neuropathy, optic neuropathy and symptoms suggestive of distal sensorimotor neuropathy may occur. The mechanism of neuropathy is unclear, but its unusual distribution suggests a direct effect on the trigeminal nucleus.

VINYL CHLORIDE (See also Chapter 26.)

Acute inhalation exposure to vinyl chloride produces encephalopathy characterized by euphoria and, later, depression of consciousness. With repeated exposure, neuropsychologic effects may occur, such as headache, insomnia, difficulty in concentrating, and memory loss, as may overt effects on the central and peripheral nervous systems with long-term exposure over many years. Central nervous system effects include spasticity, ataxia, and occasionally extrapyramidal symptoms, all of which tend to be mild. Occasionally, trigeminal neuropathy occurs similar to that seen with trichloroethylene.

It has been suggested that some of the neurologic effects of vinyl chloride may be caused by an immune complex vasculopathy, but a direct neurotoxic effect is more likely. The neurologic effects are usually mild and resolve when exposure is discontinued.

REFERENCES

Baker EL, Letz R, Fidler A: A computer-administered neurobehavioral evaluation system for occupational and environmental epidemiology: Rationale, methodology, and pilot study results. *J Occup Med* 1985;**27**:206.

Baker EL et al: Occupational lead neurotoxicity: A behavioural and electrophysiological evaluation. Study design and year one results. *Br J Ind Med* 1984;**41**:352.

Bowler R, Thaler C, Becker C: California neuropsychological screening battery (CNS/B I & II). *J Clin Psychol* 1986;**42**:946.

Goldman RH et al: Lead poisoning in automobile radiator mechanics. *N Engl J Med* 1987;**317**:214.

Fidler AT, Baker EL, Letz RE: Neurobehavioral effects of occupational exposure to organic solvents among construction painters. *Brit J Ind Med* 1987;**44**:292.

Greenberg DB et al: Computerized assessment of human neurotoxicity: Sensitivity to nitrous oxide exposure. *Clin Pharmacol Ther* 1985;**38**:656.

Gregersen P, Klausen H, Uldal EC: Chronic toxic encephalopathy in solvent-exposed painters in Denmark (1976–1980): Clinical cases and social consequences after a 5-year follow-up. *Am J Ind Med* 1987;**11**:399.

Hartman DE: *Neuropsychological Toxicology: Identification and Assessment of Human Neurotoxic Syndromes.* Pergamon Press, 1988.

Hodgson MJ et al: Encephalopathy and vestibulopathy following short-term hydrocarbon exposure. *J Occ Med* 1989;**31**:51.

Landrigan PJ et al: Ethylene oxide: An overview of toxicologic and epidemiologic research. *Am J Ind Med* 1984;**6**:103.

Pasternak G et al: Cross-sectional neurotoxicology study of lead-exposed cohort. *Clin Tox* 1989;**27**:37.

Seppäläinen AM: Electrophysiological evaluation of central and peripheral neural effects of lead exposure. *Neurotoxicology* 1984;**5**:43.

Spencer PS, Schaumberg HH: Organic solvent neurotoxicity: Facts and research needs. *Scand J Work Environ Health* 1985;**11(Suppl 1)**:53.

Syndulko K et al: Endogenous event-related potentials: Prospective applications in neuropsychology and behavioral neurology. *Bull LA Neurol Soc* 1982;**47**:124.

Terrill JB, Montgomery RR, Reinhardt CF: Toxic gases from fires. *Science* 1978;**200**:1343.

Female Reproductive Toxicology

23

Linda Rudolph, MD, MPH, & Catherine Sonquist Forest, MD, MPH

Human reproductive dysfunction is a serious contemporary problem. One out of 6 couples is infertile. Approximately 20% of pregnancies end in detected spontaneous abortion (Table 23–1). However, studies have shown that total pregnancy loss in both the preimplantation and early postimplantation periods ranges as high as 75% of conceptions. In the United States, 7% of liveborn infants are of low birth weight, and 7% have birth defects. The vast majority of these outcomes remain unexplained (Table 23–2).

HISTORICAL PERSPECTIVE

The adverse reproductive effects of some chemicals have been known for centuries. For example, lead was recognized as a hazard in ancient Rome. Over 100 years ago, lead-exposed women in the pottery industry in Europe were found to be at increased risk of sterility, miscarriage, stillbirth, and infant death in the neonatal period. Studies of women exposed to lead on the job at the turn of the century prompted several European governments to prohibit women from working with lead. Numerous other chemicals became suspect during the 19th and early 20th centuries.

As great numbers of women entered the industrial workforce during World War II, the United States Department of Labor issued a directive entitled, "Standards for Maternity Care and Employment of Mothers in Industry." The directive recommended no exposure to "extrahazardous" toxic substances during pregnancy, no heavy lifting or heavy work during pregnancy, a minimum of 6 weeks leave before and after delivery, and other precautions.

After the war, as the majority of women returned to housework or nonindustrial jobs, interest in female occupational reproductive hazards waned.

Concern about reproductive hazards was rekindled in the 1950s, when there was an epidemic of mental retardation, cerebral palsy, and developmental delay in Japanese children whose mothers had consumed fish contaminated with methyl mercury released into Minamata Bay by a nearby plant manufacturing polyvinyl chloride. In 1968, use of PCB-contaminated cooking oil caused Yusho disease (see Chapter 39) in another Japanese community. Reproductive effects included intrauterine growth retardation and a variety of epidermal disorders typified by hyperpigmentation of the skin. In another tragic instance, women who had taken the drug thalidomide during their pregnancies in the late 1950s and early 1960s gave birth to infants with major limb malformations. These incidents provided compelling evidence of the potential for harm resulting from in utero exposure to drugs and industrial chemicals.

The need to further evaluate the relationship between work and adverse reproductive outcome has become yet more evident with the heightened awareness of occupational hazards since passage of the Occupational Safety and Health Act in 1970. Reproductive hazards in the workplace are currently the focus of a great deal of political, economic, and scientific controversy.

WOMEN WORKERS

Although the cause of most adverse outcomes is still unknown, scientific evidence implicating occupational exposures is gradually accumulating. At the same time, a marked increase in the number of women in the labor force has also increased the number of women potentially exposed to reproductive hazards on the job. Between 1947 and 1984, the

Table 23–1. Prevalence of adverse reproductive outcomes. (US, general population; approximately 3.7 million live births per year.)

Infertility	10–15%	(couples)
Recognized spontaneous abortions	15–20%	(pregnancies)
Stillbirths	2%	(pregnancies)
Low birth weight	7%	(live births)
Neonatal deaths	0.7%	(live births)
Infant deaths	1%	(live births)
Birth defects, all	7%	(live births)
Central nervous system defects	2%	
Cardiovascular defects	2.5%	
Mental retardation	0.4%	
Chromosomal abnormalities	0.2%	

Table 23–2. Causes of birth defects.

Chromosomal anomaly	5%
Genetic transmission	20%
Radiation	1%
Infection	2–3%
Maternal metabolic imbalance (eg, diabetes)	3–5%
Drugs and chemicals	2–3%
Unknown	63–67%

number of American women in the workforce nearly tripled, from 16.7 million to 46.5 million. Seventy-five percent of these women are of reproductive age (ages 16–44).

The influx of women into the workforce has included pregnant women and women with young families. Overall, fewer than 10% of employed women of reproductive age give birth in a given year. However, in 1980, more than 1.25 million live births (over 40%) were to women who had worked at some time during the year prior to delivery. It is estimated that over 300,000 of these women worked in job categories with potential exposure to substances toxic to the reproductive system, such as lead and anesthetic gases. Overall, the EEOC has estimated that as many as 20 million jobs may involve workplace exposure to suspected female reproductive hazards.

By and large, women are concentrated in low-paying, traditionally female jobs. Almost 80% of all employed women work in just 20 occupations, including health care, textiles, cosmetology, electronics, and other jobs with exposures to suspected reproductive toxic agents. Many women in these professions have inadequate access to health care, including prenatal care and information about reproductive toxicity.

FEMALE REPRODUCTIVE PHYSIOLOGY

The female reproductive cycle is a complex and poorly understood process. It is regulated by the autonomic nervous and endocrine systems, mediated by the hypothalamic-pituitary axis (Fig 23–1).

Preconception Physiology

In females—in contrast to the male, where gametogenesis occurs continuously—oogenesis and the initial stage of meiosis occur only in utero. After birth, no new oocytes are generated. From a zenith of 6 million oocytes, the number is reduced to 2 million at birth and dwindles to 400,000 at menarche by a process of atresia.

Meiosis begins during fetal life. The first mitotic and the beginning of the first meiotic divisions of the germ cells occur by the fifth or sixth month of gestation. The oocytes then remain dormant until puberty. Under hormonal stimulation, the follicles begin to mature each month. Further growth and development of a dominant follicle and preparation of the endometrial lining require delicate timing and balance of follicle-stimulating hormone (FSH), luteinizing hormone (LH), estrogen, and progester-

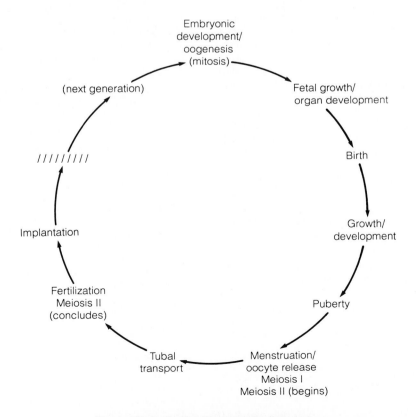

Figure 23–1. The female reproductive cycle.

interfere with cell migration or organ development to cause a serious anomaly without embryolethality; and higher doses may be embryolethal, resulting in an early (unrecognized) spontaneous abortion, which often precludes detection of other effects.

The effect of exposure to developmental toxic agents on pregnancy outcome varies markedly depending on the timing of the exposure. A substance administered early in gestation may cause irreparable damage, but, administered at a later stage in development, it may be detoxified by fetal metabolism. Interspecies differences in the development of enzyme system activity (eg, humans exhibit relatively early cytochrome P-450 enzyme activity compared to rats) may explain some of the differences in species susceptibility.

No single species has been identified as an optimal model for human susceptibility to developmental toxic agents. Because there are not yet models to predict the sensitivity of one species versus another, it is prudent to assume that humans are at least as sensitive as the most sensitive animal species. In fact, the limited available evidence indicates that humans are generally more sensitive to teratogens than are test species.

Small changes in chemical structure may radically alter the teratogenicity of an agent, making generalizations about structure-activity relationships unreliable for reproductive hazards. For example, methoxyethanol is metabolized to a potent reproductive toxin, while butoxyethanol, which is closely related (and largely substitutable in industrial processes), is considerably less toxic.

The pharmacokinetics of an agent within the fetal-maternal unit are also important. For example, some substances may accumulate in the placenta or in fetal tissue (eg, mercury accumulates in the fetal central nervous system). Similarly, although a chemical may easily cross the placenta, its more toxic metabolite may not (eg, acetaminophen).

Several recent reviews have summarized the results of animal reproductive toxicity testing (Table 23–9). For practical purposes, animal reproductive toxic agents should be considered probable human reproductive toxic agents. Regulatory agencies apply "safety factors" of 100–1000 to experimental animal data to establish arbitrary allowable levels of exposure to known reproductive toxins.

Epidemiologic Studies

When properly designed and conducted, epidemiologic studies provide the best means of evaluating whether specific exposures adversely impact the *human* reproductive system (see Appendix).

The wide range of potential adverse reproductive outcomes complicates reproductive epidemiology. Moreover, the same chemical exposure administered at a different dose or at a different gestational stage might produce different outcomes. For example, exposure before implantation may result in an early spontaneous abortion, while first-trimester exposure

to the same substance may cause a major malformation. Conversely, many different exposures may contribute to a single outcome, such as spontaneous

Table 23–9. Animal evidence for reproductive toxicity.

Altered pituitary-hypothalamic-ovarian function
  Benzene
  Carbon tetrachloride
  Kepone
  Mercury
  PCBs
Decreased fertility
  DBCP
  DDT
  Lead
  Manganese
Impaired implantation
  Cadmium
  Lead
  PCBs
Fetotoxicity or embryolethality
  Arsenic
  Benzene
  Chloroform
  2,4-D
  DDT
  Dichloromethane
  Ethylene oxide
  Lead
  Mercury (inorganic and metallic)
  Nitrogen dioxide
  Polybrominated biphenyls
  PCBs
  Selenium
  Tetrachloroethylene
  Thallium
  Vinyl chloride
  Vinylidene chloride
  Xylene
Teratogenicity
  Acrylonitrile
  Arsenic
  Bayleton
  Benlate
  Benzene
  Benzo(a)pyrene
  Cadmium
  Carbaryl
  Chlorodifluoromethane
  Chloroprene
  Chromium
  Diethylstilbestrol
  Endrin
  Glycol ethers
  Mercury
  Methacrylates (some)
  Methyl ethyl ketone
  Methyl formamide
  Phthalates (some butyl)
  Tellurium
  Thiram
  TOK (2,4-dichlorophenyl-*p*-nitrophenyl ether)
  Vinyl chloride
Transplacental carcinogens
  Arsenic
  Benzo(a)pyrene
  DES
  Vinyl chloride
Reduced reproductive capacity (in offspring)
  DES
  Kepone
  PAHs (in utero oocyte destruction)

abortion. Consistency in results between epidemiologic studies makes a cause-effect relationship appear more plausible.

Obtaining valid reproductive histories is often difficult. For example, researchers have found that nonexposed women may be less likely to recall spontaneous abortions at interview than are exposed women. This may result in an apparent increased incidence of spontaneous abortion in exposed women when in fact none may exist. Another possible bias may occur when parents overreport exposures as they strive to identify a reason for an unwanted or unexpected outcome. In addition, marked discrepancies have been observed between reports of husbands and wives in investigating adverse outcomes. For these reasons, verification of reported adverse outcomes is critical.

At the same time, many birth defects are not recorded either on birth certificates or on hospital discharge records. Inadequate reporting of occupation and malformations on birth and fetal death certificates thus impedes hypothesis-generating studies based on vital statistics.

Selection bias may occur in cross-sectional studies if women who have had successful pregnancies are more likely to terminate employment, while those with adverse outcomes remain in the work force to participate in cross-sectional surveys.

Lastly, early detection of spontaneous abortion is often difficult. Most spontaneous abortions may be dismissed as slightly abnormal menstrual periods and may not be reported. Spontaneous abortion may be the most sensitive marker for adverse reproductive effects both in terms of preconception and early postconception exposures. Since the background incidence of spontaneous abortion is much higher than that of other adverse outcomes, it does not require as large a sample size to detect small increases in incidence.

Many reproductive epidemiologic studies suffer from a lack of power because there are too few women in an industry or worksite to provide sufficient numbers per study group. Such situations probably result in frequent false-negative studies. These studies are often misinterpreted and used to state that no risk exists when in fact exposure may be associated with adverse outcome, although the study lacked sufficient power to detect an effect.

Conversely, significantly increased incidence of a given adverse outcome in a small group of women can sometimes lead to a false-positive study when the cluster is actually due only to chance. In these instances, the cluster of women is often too small to allow for valid epidemiologic study. Recently, for example, several clusters of adverse reproductive outcome were identified among VDT operators. As yet, most preliminary studies of larger groups of VDT workers have not indicated that any reproductive hazard exists, though one study did detect elevated spontaneous abortion rates. More definitive studies are still in progress.

Perhaps the most significant limitation of epidemiologic studies is that they can detect problems only after they occur in human beings. Therefore, despite the difficulties in extrapolating human risk from animal studies, good public health policy requires that one not wait for epidemiologic evidence before taking preventive actions that protect reproductive health. This is especially true in light of the paucity of epidemiologic studies on reproductive outcome in relationship to work.

Potential Human Reproductive Toxic Agents

Despite methodologic difficulties in examining female reproductive toxicity and occupational exposures, numerous studies have been conducted. Tables 23–10 through 23–15 summarize the key epidemiologic investigations to date. The studies are of variable quality, and not all have been corroborated. The tables are intended to serve as an overview of the range of occupations and chemicals that have been studied and should not be considered definitive.

Work, Exercise, & Pregnancy

A number of investigators have addressed the issue of whether working, in and of itself, influences pregnancy outcome. There have been conflicting reports regarding increases in preterm labor, low birth weight, and spontaneous abortion among working women, but most are complicated by low socioeconomic status. The current consensus is that, in the absence of clinical contraindications or specific risks, working per se during pregnancy does not increase the risk of adverse outcome.

Early studies of women engaging in intense physical activity, such as ballet dancers and Olympic athletes, have demonstrated alterations in the menstrual cycle. However, it is not appropriate to compare these women, who may have decreased percentages of body fat, diet changes, and hormonal alterations, with women experiencing more typical, though perhaps strenuous, occupational exertion.

While a shift away from splanchnic (and thus uterine) blood flow does occur during strenuous exercise, there appears to be a compensatory "flush back" phenomenon. Thus, most women can safely participate in strenuous physical activity throughout most of pregnancy. There is some evidence, however, that extremely strenuous work in the last 2 weeks of pregnancy may lead to a decline in fetal growth. Another exception may be in the case of existing uteroplacental insufficiency. Where uteroplacental insufficiency is suspected (eg, in diabetes or pre-eclampsia), clinicians should monitor fetal heart rate for bradycardia before a pregnant woman with such conditions engages in strenuous activity.

The normal woman with an uncomplicated pregnancy can continue to work until the end of pregnancy and is generally physically capable of returning to work 6–8 weeks after a normal delivery. The

Table 23–10. Effects reported in female workers: Metals.

	Menstrual Disorders	Infertility	Spontaneous Abortion	Stillbirth	Congenital Malformations	Low Birth Weight	Other
Antimony	...	...	?	...	...	...	...
Arsenic	...	...	+	...	...	...	...
Cadmium	?	?	...	?	...	+ or −	Accumulates in placenta; placental abnormalities.
Lead (H)	+	+	+	+	Varied minor malformations	+	Prematurity, neonatal death, abnormal CNS development, behavioral abnormalities.
Mercury (H)	+	?+	+	...	Cerebral palsy, intrauterine growth retardation, Minamata disease	+	Crosses placenta; accumulates in fetal CNS; psychomotor retardation.
Multiple metals	...	?+	+	...	+	...	...

(H) = Known human reproductive toxicity; + = Good evidence; + or − = Conflicting epidemiologic studies; ? = Preliminary data difficult to interpret.

American College of Obstetricians and Gynecologists has issued widely accepted *Guidelines on Pregnancy and Work*.

After the chemicals used on the job have been reviewed, exposures characterized, and scientific data interpreted, a judgment must be made about whether a reproductive hazard exists. Typically, employers, workers, and clinicians have turned to government agencies or occupational health consultants to assess occupational health risk. Ranking systems and risk assessment methodologies for reproductive hazards are currently under development. However, risk assessment is often done on a case-by-case basis. Given uncertainty regarding the level of reproductive risk present, decision-making may be based on negotiations with employers and employ-

Table 23–11. Effects reported in female workers: Solvents.

	Menstrual Disorders	Spontaneous Abortion	Congenital Malformations — Gut Atresias	Oral Clefts	CNS Defects	Cardio-vascular	All	Childhood Cancer	Other
Mixed organic solvents	?	...	+	+	+	+	...	Leukemia	Preeclampsia
Benzene	?	?	...	...	...	...	...	...	Chromosomal abnormalities in offspring
Chloroprene (rubber industry)	?	+ or −	...	...	...	...	...	...	...
Carbon disulfide	?	?	...	...	...	...	...	...	? Decreased fertility
Styrene (reinforced plastics industry)	+ or −	+ or −	...	...	...	...	+	...	? Low birth weight
Toluene	?	...	...	...	?	...	...	...	? Low birth weight
Vinyl chloride (community exposure)	...	...	...	...	+ or −	...	...	...	...
Laboratory workers	...	+ or −	+ or −	+ or −	...	...	+ or −	...	...
Printing industry	...	...	+	...	...	...	...	...	...

+ = Good evidence; + or − = Conflicting epidemiologic studies; ? = Preliminary data difficult to interpret.

Table 23–12. Effects reported in female workers: Physical agents.

	Infertility	Spontaneous Abortion	Malformations	Other	Comments
Ionizing radiation (H)	+	+	Microcephaly, mental retardation (> 20 cGy)	Childhood leukemia (1–10 cGy), intra-uterine growth retardation, premature menopause	Limit exposure to < 0.5 cGy throughout pregnancy
Heat (H)	. . .	. . .	+CNS	. . .	In cases with high maternal fever during pregnancy
Noise	+	. . .	+ or −	? ↓ Hearing in offspring	. . .
Nonionizing radiation	. . .	. . .	. . .	? Late fetal death	. . .

(H) = Known human reproductive toxicity; + = Good evidence; + or − = Conflicting epidemiologic studies; ? = Preliminary data difficult to interpret.

ees, weighing various options. These options are discussed below.

MINIMIZING THE RISK

Given the scientific uncertainty and data gaps concerning reproductive toxicity, *all* exposure to toxic chemicals and physical hazards should be minimized to the greatest extent possible. Safer chemicals should be substituted where possible. Engineering controls, such as work process enclosure and installation of effective ventilation systems to lessen ambient chemical concentrations, are also recommended. Lastly, use of personal protective equipment such as appropriate respirators, gloves, and aprons can lessen individual worker exposure. Such equipment should be used as a last resort, however, since it is often hot, bulky, and uncomfortable for workers, especially pregnant workers.

The fact that women alone bear children has led to a variety of other policies targeting female workers. One impetus for such policies is financial. Many employers fear that they will be exposed to liability in tort for fetal effects that might be attributed to

Table 23–13. Effects reported in females: Miscellaneous.

	Menstrual Disorders	Spontaneous Abortion	Malformations	Other
Aniline	?	+ or −	. . .	. . .
Carbon monoxide	. . .	. . .	CNS defect	Low birth weight
Estrogens (synthetic hormones)	?	. . .	. . .	. . .
Formaldehyde	?	+ or −	?	. . .
"Occupational fatigue" (stress, noise, work)	. . .	. . .	. . .	Low birth weight, prematurity
Diethylstilbestrol (DES) (H)	. . .	. . .	+Reproductive tract malformation	+Vaginal adenocarcinoma in offspring
DDT	?	. . .	?Polycystic ovaries	+Breast milk transfer
Polychlorinated biphenyls (PCB)	?	. . .	+Cola-staining gingival hyperplasia	+Growth retardation, low birth weight, perinatal mortality, breast milk
Polybrominated biphenyls (PBB)	?	. . .	. . .	Breast milk
Pesticides	. . .	. . .	+ or −	. . .
Vinyl chloride	. . .	. . .	+ or − (CNS)	? Low birth weight
Visual display terminals (VDT)	. . .	+ or −	. . .	. . .
Ethylene dibromide	. . .	. . .	. . .	? ↓ Fertility
Dioxins	. . .	?	?	. . .

(H) = Known human reproductive toxicity; + = Good evidence; + or − = Conflicting epidemiologic studies; ? = Preliminary data difficult to interpret.

Table 23–14. Effects reported in female workers: Occupation and industry.

	Spontaneous Abortion	Malformations					Other
		CNS	Clefts	Musculoskeletal	All		
Industry incl. construction	?	+	+	+	. . .		. . .
Chemical workers	+	. . .	. . .	. . .	. . .		. . .
Electronics (radio-TV production)	?	. . .	. . .	. . .	. . .		? Infertility
Farming (wives of farmers)	. . .	. . .	. . .	. . .	. . .		Childhood cancer
Food industry	?	. . .	. . .	. . .	. . .		. . .
Gardeners	?	. . .	. . .	?	. . .		. . .
Laboratory workers	+	. . .	. . .	. . .	. . .		. . .
Laundry workers	?	. . .	. . .	. . .	. . .		. . .
Leather industry	+ or −	. . .	. . .	. . .	. . .		. . .
Pharmaceutical manufacturing	?	. . .	. . .	. . .	. . .		. . .
Plastics industry	?	. . .	. . .	. . .	. . .		. . .
Pulp and paper industry	. . .	. . .	. . .	. . .	+ or −		. . .
Rubber industry	?	. . .	. . .	. . .	+ or −		. . .
Semiconductor industry	?	. . .	. . .	. . .	. . .		. . .
Smelter (including community exposure)	?	. . .	. . .	. . .	+		Low birth weight
Textile workers	?	. . .	. . .	. . .	. . .		Infertility
Transport and communications workers	?	. . .	?	. . .	. . .		. . .

+ = Good evidence; + or − = Conflicting epidemiologic studies; ? = Preliminary data difficult to interpret.

parental occupational exposure. The awards for such suits can be extremely large, whereas awards for other occupational illnesses and injuries are covered by the much less costly workers' compensation system. Under workers' compensation law, workers are denied the right to sue their employers, and employers are thus insulated from liability beyond the system's very limited scale of recovery.

Controversy surrounding discriminatory policies has focused attention on whether there is a biologic basis for these policies or whether they are just a reflection of societal stereotypes about women and childbearing. Several landmark judicial decisions and legislative actions have addressed the legality of "fetal protection policies" (forced maternity leaves or transfers) and "exclusionary placement policies"

Table 23–15. Effects reported in female workers: Hospital hazards.

	Spontaneous Abortion	Malformations	Other	Comments
Anesthetic gases	+	+ or −	Low birth weight	. . .
Cytotoxic (antineoplastic agents) (H)	+	+	. . .	. . .
Ethylene oxide	+	. . .	. . .	. . .
Infectious agents (H) Cytomegalovirus	. . .	Hepatosplenomegaly, microcephaly, microphthalmia	Mental retardation	Avoid contact with known CMV shedders
Hepatitis B	. . .	. . .	Chronic hepatitis (neonatal)	. . .
Herpes	+	Microcephaly, microphthalmia, retinal defects	. . .	. . .
Rubella	. . .	Heart, eye, ear, bone abnormalities	Congenital deafness	Recommend rubella vaccine
Toxoplasmosis	. . .	Microphthalmia, micro- or macrocephaly	Mental retardation	. . .
Viruses	. . .	+ or −	Late fetal death	. . .
Hexachlorophene	. . .	+ or −	. . .	. . .

(H) = Known human reproductive toxicity; + = Good evidence; + or − = Conflicting epidemiologic studies.

(excluding women of child-bearing capacity from work where exposure to toxic chemicals may occur).

Legal Rights of Fertile & Pregnant Women

Title VII of the 1964 Civil Rights Act prohibits discrimination on the basis of sex. An amendment to Title VII, the Pregnancy Discrimination Act of 1978, requires that women affected by pregnancy, childbirth, or related conditions be treated the same as any temporarily disabled worker. This law protects a woman from being fired, refused hiring, or denied promotion because she is pregnant. A woman unable to work in her usual job due to pregnancy or related reasons is entitled to the same disability benefits as any temporarily disabled worker. For example, if a man with a broken leg is entitled to job modification, light duty, job transfer, sick leave, disability leave with or without pay, or health insurance, a pregnant woman must be granted the same.

The law does not require an employer to provide any benefits to disabled workers but does prohibit reducing contracted benefits (eg, maternity leave) in order to comply with the law.

Substantial obstacles to protection of these rights include that the federal law does not apply to workplaces employing fewer than 15 people, does not affect workplaces that do not have established disability leave policies, and does not cover women who work part time. Some states have enacted legislation to overcome these obstacles.

Several exclusionary placement policies have been challenged in the courts. For instance, at a plant in West Virginia, women under 50 years of age were informed that they would be excluded from 8 out of 10 departments in the plant unless they were surgically sterilized. Only 7 of the 30 "fertile" employees could remain with the company under those conditions. Five women in the inorganic pigments department underwent sterilization in order to secure their jobs; 2 transferred to lower-paying jobs. An OSHA citation claiming violation of the general duty clause was later struck down on the basis that policies leading to "voluntary sterilization" do not constitute a "recognized hazard." The women's sex discrimination lawsuit was ultimately settled out of court, with no admission of liability by the company.

Three appellate courts have considered whether discrimination against female workers on the basis of potential fetal injury is legally permissible. In 2 cases, pregnant workers were fired from their jobs when their pregnancies became known, despite the fact that their film badges registered radiation exposure well below limits considered safe for fetuses by a nationally recognized radiation safety council. The third case, in 1978, concerned a "female employment and fetal vulnerability" policy that established "restricted" jobs. Women seeking these jobs had to provide proof of inability to bear children.

The common themes in the courts' rulings on these cases are that it is the burden of the employer instituting discriminatory policies to demonstrate (1) that the chemical or condition poses a significant (ie, not hypothetical) risk to the fetus; (2) that exposure levels hazardous to the fetus are likely to occur; (3) that at likely exposure levels, the risk exists only for female workers (ie, the male reproductive system is not vulnerable); (4) that a considerable body of expert opinion supports the conclusion that the risk is confined to the excluded group; and (5) that there exists no other alternative that would provide protection with a less discriminatory effect (eg, job transfer with rate retention).

While the scientific burden these rulings place on employers is significant, it is also consistent with current scientific knowledge. No difference in the impact of toxic substances on male versus female reproductive physiology outside of pregnancy has been demonstrated. On the contrary, NIOSH responded to proposed EEOC guidelines on reproductive hazard policies by stating that there is "no scientific basis for differential exclusion of fertile women from contact with vinyl chloride or lead . . . Reproductively active men should be equally excluded." In fact, many researchers believe that the male reproductive system may be more susceptible to reproductive toxicity than the female system. Gender-specific policies geared toward protecting the fetus also implicitly assume that the fetus is hypersusceptible to toxic insult. However, the EPA's Teratology Policy Work Group reviewed 19 pesticides and 5 industrial chemicals and concluded that when chemicals are extensively tested, other health effects besides teratogenicity are demonstrated and that "teratogenicity was never the most sensitive effect, except for one pesticide." In instances where a pregnant woman or fetus is at increased risk from workplace exposure, discriminatory policies may not be an acceptable response. Analogously, in the reverse situation, the threat to male reproductive health from DBCP was not met by policies to exclude men from work with DBCP, nor to require proof of inability to father children, nor to provide labels warning men planning to father children to avoid contact with the product—3 policies that have been instituted in response to potential female-mediated effects.

Almost invariably, scientific data are insufficient to decide whether a differential effect on women, men, or fetuses exists. Therefore, a complete evaluation of reproductive risk must be undertaken on a case-by-case basis. Careful consideration must be given to the development of nondiscriminatory policies that protect the reproductive health of men and women and the health of their offspring.

EMPLOYER-EMPLOYEE OPTIONS

Given the scientific uncertainty and data gaps concerning reproductive toxicity, exposure to *all* toxic substances should be minimized to the greatest extent possible. In general, it appears that protecting against other health effects will protect against reproductive health effects as well. However, with regard to pregnancy, employers and employees may be unwilling to accept "negligible" risk or uncertainty. If evaluation of the specific worksite reveals that a significant risk is *demonstrated* or *suspected,* the pregnant woman should be transferred to a nonexposed job with full wage and benefit retention.

In the vast majority of cases, however, the evaluation is not clear-cut. In these instances, the health professional may play a critical role in counseling workers to facilitate an arrangement acceptable to both employer and employee. Every effort should be made to advise women of the magnitude of the risk as well as their legal rights and the weaknesses in the law.

Where worksite evaluation reveals minimal exposure to known or suspected reproductive toxic agents, job transfer or job modification may be appropriate. In many cases, worksite evaluation reveals no significant risk due to exposure. Workers may be reasonably reassured in these cases.

Many employers have policies regarding transfer, and numerous others will follow a physician's recommendation. Needless to say, there are also instances where an employer is unwilling or financially unable to accommodate such temporary arrangements. It is important to keep in mind that poor access to prenatal care, low socioeconomic status, financial stress, and inadequate nutrition may substantially contribute to adverse reproductive outcomes. These factors must be considered before making recommendations that may lead to discontinuation of work and loss of benefits. If a woman does elect to leave her job, the clinician should point out her eligibility for unemployment compensation and thus protect her access to benefits.

REFERENCES

AMA Council on Scientific Affairs: Effect of physical forces on the reproductive cycle. *JAMA* 1984;**251**:247.

AMA Council on Scientific Affairs: Effects of pregnancy on work performance. *JAMA* 1984;**251**:1995.

American College of Obstetrics and Gynecology: *Guidelines on Pregnancy and Work.* US Department of Health, Education, and Welfare, 1978.

Chamberlain G (editor): *Pregnant Women at Work.* Macmillan, 1984.

Clarkson TW: The role of biomarkers in reproductive and developmental toxicology. *Environ Health Perspect* 1987;**74**:103. [Entire issue.]

Clarkson TW, Nordberg G, Sager PR (editors): *Reproductive and Developmental Toxicity of Metals.* Plenum Press, 1983.

Eskenazi B et al: Exposure to organic solvents and hypertensive disorders of pregnancy. *Am J Ind Med* 1988; **14**:177.

Goulet L, Thériault G: Association between spontaneous abortion and ergonomic factors: A literature review of the epidemiologic evidence. *Scand J Work Environ Health* 1987;**13**:399.

Hemminki K, Sorsa M, Vainio H (editors): *Occupational Hazards and Reproduction.* Hemisphere, 1985.

Johnson EM: Cross-species extrapolation and the biologic basis for safety factor determinations in developmental toxicology. *Regul Toxicol Pharmacol* 1988;**8**:22.

Karew S, Reasor M (editors): *Toxicology and the Newborn.* Elsevier, 1984.

LeMasters GK, Selevan SG: Use of exposure data in occupational reproductive studies. *Scand J Work Environ Health* 1984;**10**:1.

Lockey JE, LeMasters GK, Keye WR Jr: *Reproduction: The New Frontier in Occupational and Environmental Health Research.* Liss, 1984.

Mattison DR (editor): Reproductive toxicology. *Am J Ind Med* 1983;**4**:1.

Paul M, Himmelstein J: Reproductive hazards in the workplace: What the practitioner needs to know about chemical exposures. *Obstet Gynecol* 1988;**71**:921.

Schardein JL: *Chemically Induced Birth Defects.* Marcel Dekker, 1985.

Stein ZA, Hatch MC (editors): Reproductive problems in the workplace. *State Art Rev Occup Med* 1986;**1**:361. [Entire issue.]

US Environmental Protection Agency: *Report of the Teratology Policy Workgroup.* US Government Printing Office, 1985.

US Environmental Protection Agency: Proposed guidelines for the health assessment of suspected developmental toxicants. *Fed Reg* 1984;**49**:46324.

US Office of Technology Assessment: *Reproductive Health Hazards in the Workplace.* US Government Printing Office, 1985.

Vainio H: Carcinogenesis and teratogenesis may have common mechanisms. *Scand J Work Environ Health* 1989;**15**:13.

Wang GM, Schwetz BA: An evaluation system for ranking chemicals with teratogenic potential. *Teratogenesis Carcinog Mutagen* 1987;**7**:133.

24   Male Reproductive Toxicology

Gideon Letz, MD, MPH

Animal toxicologists have long appreciated the importance of the testis as a target organ, but only recently has male reproductive dysfunction in humans been related to exposure to chemical agents. Nitrofurantoin was the first therapeutic drug reported to cause adverse effects on the male reproductive system in humans (Heinke & Jaeschke, 1969), and during the 1970s male reproductive dysfunction was first associated with occupational exposures.

Research interest in the effects of occupational exposure on the male reproductive system has grown since then, and it is now generally recognized that assessment of male reproductive function has value in the detection and prevention of occupationally related disease.

To date, only a handful of occupational exposures have been evaluated for potential effects on the male reproductive system, and it is thus impossible to estimate the magnitude of the problem. The importance of expanding our knowledge in this area is highlighted by the finding that some reproductive toxins (notably lead, glycol ethers) cause effects in both men and women.

The dramatic event that triggered interest in this new area of occupational medicine involved the nematocide 1,2-dibromochloropropane (DBCP). The incident described below is important historically because of the severe effects observed and the attention it focused on the problem of male reproductive risk. Given the large number of chemicals currently in use, it is unlikely that DBCP is unique in its capacity to damage the male reproductive system, though it may be unique in terms of its potency and in the degree of abnormality it produces.

THE DBCP INCIDENT

In 1967, a worker at a pesticide formulation plant in California filed a workers' compensation claim contending that his infertility was related to exposure to various pesticides, including DBCP. That claim was denied, but the problem resurfaced 10 years later when similar complaints filed by other workers prompted further investigation. By that time, widespread rumor contended that workers at the Agricultural Chemicals Division (ACD) of the plant were having fertility problems.

Only 36 men worked in this area of the plant.

Though many were young and interested in having children, few had fathered children since beginning to work at the facility. A preliminary series of semen analyses in 5 men showed that all had some semen abnormality. A more systematic evaluation followed, done cooperatively with the union, plant management, and occupational health professionals from the University of California.

Exposure & Semen Analyses

Twenty-five of the 36 men employed at the ACD submitted semen samples (the rest had had vasectomies). Of the semen samples, 9 were azoospermic (no sperm seen), 3 were oligospermic (fewer than 20 million sperm/mL of seminal fluid), and 13 were normospermic (> 20 million sperm/mL). Eleven workers with counts below 1 million/mL were compared with 11 coworkers with counts above 40 million/mL, revealing a striking association between sperm count and duration of employment (Table 24–1). Those with depressed counts had an average exposure of 8 years, while those with counts in the normal range had an average exposure of less than 6 months. In addition, the workers with depressed sperm counts had elevated serum levels of LH and FSH, but as a group they had no other abnormal physical or laboratory findings.

Follow-up studies were conducted on the entire male population of the plant. The 142 men who had not had vasectomies provided semen samples. Of these, 107 had a history of exposure to DBCP, and 35 had never been exposed. A significant difference in the median sperm counts and frequency of azoospermia was noted between the 2 groups (Fig 24–1). Ten workers subsequently had testicular biopsies that showed absence of spermatogenic activity or decrease in the amount of cellularity within the seminiferous tubules. There was no inflammation and only minimal evidence of fibrosis or interstitial changes (Figs 24–2 and 24–3). Based on these

Table 24–1. Comparison of nonvasectomized DBCP workers with very low (group A) and normal (group B) sperm counts. (There were 11 subjects in each group.)

	Age (years)	Exposure (years)	Sperm Count (X 10^6/mL)
Group A	32.7 ± 1.6	8.0 ± 1.2	0.2 ± 0.1
Group B	26.7 ± 1.2	0.08 ± 0.02	93 ± 18

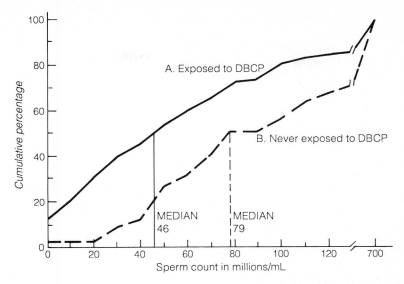

Figure 24–1. Cumulative percentage distributions for sperm counts for 2 groups: **(A)** exposed to DBCP (n = 107) and **(B)** never exposed to DBCP (n = 35). (Redrawn and reproduced, with permission, from Whorton MD et al: Testicular function in DBCP exposed pesticide workers. *J Occup Med* 1979;**21:**161.)

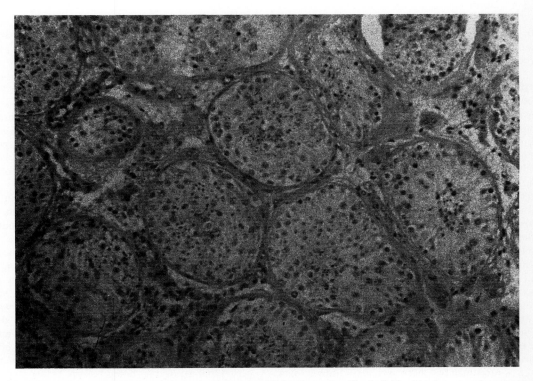

Figure 24–2. Testicular biopsy from worker exposed to DBCP for 3 months. The individual had a normal sperm count and an apparently normal biopsy. (Courtesy of Whorton MD.)

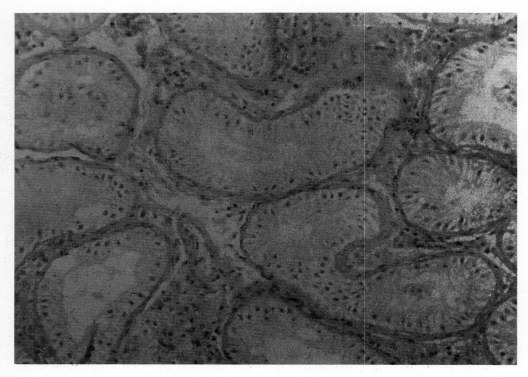

Figure 24–3. Testicular biopsy from a worker exposed to DBCP for 10 years. The individual was azoospermic and had a Sertoli cell only picture. (Courtesy of Whorton MD.)

pathologic findings and the elevated FSH levels, the presumed mechanism of action was a direct toxic effect on the primary spermatogonia.

Further Evaluations & Follow-Up

Of the 100 chemicals used in the plant, 4 had been shown to be toxic to the male reproductive system in published animal studies (epichlorohydrin, carbaryl, ethylene dibromide, and DBCP). Owing to the relative quantities of production, the suspected agent was DBCP. The confirmation of DBCP as the etiologic agent was not made until multiple studies were done at different locations. Within the next 2 years, 8 additional studies were done on 508 male DBCP-exposed workers (Whorton & Foliart, 1983). The methodologies have varied, but the findings uniformly showed that DBCP dramatically suppressed spermatogenesis: 15.7% of the men were azoospermic, and another 21.1% were oligospermic. The expected rates among workers are approximately 1% azoospermia and 8% oligospermia (Whorton & Meyer, 1984).

These statistics may underestimate the true magnitude of the DBCP effect, since not all of the men were exposed to DBCP at the time of the studies (Whorton, 1982). Unfortunately, there are very limited data available on the exposure levels in these studies. Personal air sampling results in 2 of the plants

investigated found less than 1 ppm DBCP as an 8-hour TWA concentration (Whorton et al, 1977; Egnatz et al, 1980). Since DBCP is also readily skin absorbable (Torkelson et al, 1961), it is impossible to estimate absorbed doses in the affected workers. Four follow-up evaluations have been performed on some of the affected workers 1–3 years postexposure to DBCP (for review, see Whorton & Foliart, 1983). Results are mixed, with improvement in sperm counts in most oligospermic men. Essentially, however, the azoospermic men have shown no recovery of spermatogenic function.

Agricultural use of DBCP was banned in the continental United States in 1979, and the ban was extended to Hawaii in 1985. A longitudinal study of Hawaiian pineapple workers—whose average airborne exposure to DBCP was 1 ppb or less—showed no observable effect on spermatogenic function.

A tragedy of the DBCP incident is that it was predicted by experimental data published 16 years prior to the discovery of infertility in exposed workers (Torkelson et al, 1961). This study clearly demonstrated testicular toxicity at the lowest doses tested in 3 species (rats, rabbits, guinea pigs). A no-effect level was not established, though the authors suggested that exposures should be kept below 1 ppm in air and that "close observation of the health of people exposed to this compound should be maintained."

MONITORING THE EFFECTS OF OCCUPATIONAL EXPOSURE ON MALE REPRODUCTION

The reproductive cycle is diagrammed in Fig 24–4. Under each stage are listed the parameters that could be monitored in relation to toxic exposures. In the male, end points that have been investigated include **reproductive history, blood hormone levels, testicular histology,** and **semen analyses,** all of which reflect effects of exposure prior to conception. Theoretically, any postconception event (spontaneous abortion, congenital malformation, etc) that is mediated by abnormal sperm could also be related to exposures occurring in the male prior to conception. However, to date there have been few studies of this kind, and the data are difficult to interpret.

Semen Analysis

The only unequivocal examples of occupationally related male reproductive system dysfunction have been documented using semen analyses. Research has focused on the identification of spermatotoxic agents that *directly* interfere with the normal process of gametogenesis. In most cases, the pathophysiology has not been well defined, but damage may occur by either physiologic, cytotoxic, or genetic mechanisms. In addition, there are at least 2 mechanisms by which chemicals might indirectly affect sperm cell function and reproductive outcome: (1) Exposure to toxins could produce pituitary-hypothalamic or sex hormone effects, which in turn could affect spermatogenesis or result in poor reproductive performance (decreased libido, impotence). (2) Exposure could cause abnormalities in seminal fluid, resulting in functional impairment of sperm and impaired fertility. Many drugs and xenobiotics have been found in seminal fluid. For example, semen concentrations of the anticonvulsant drug phenytoin can approach 20% of the plasma level.

Xenobiotics in semen could theoretically affect reproductive outcome in the following ways: (1) Chemical agents may directly impair sperm motility; (2) they may have a pharmacologic effect on fertilization, implantation, or placental development; or (3) they may cause systemic effects in the female by being absorbed through vaginal mucosa.

A. Methods of Assessment: Semen analysis is considered the most direct method available for clinical assessment of male infertility. It is therefore not surprising that attempts to evaluate chemical effects on male reproductive function have relied heavily on the same tests common to infertility diagnosis—sperm concentration (count), sperm motility, and sperm morphology.

1. Sperm count—The sperm count is reported as the number of sperm per milliliter of ejaculate as determined by hemocytometer. Measurement is technically easy, and automated methods are available. Interpretation of results can be confounded by a number of factors, however, such as variable periods of sexual abstinence prior to sample collection, frequency of ejaculation, and collection of an incomplete ejaculate. Multiple samples from the same individual show wide ranges in counts even in fertile men. In spite of this variability, there are many clear examples of chemically induced reductions in sperm count.

2. Sperm motility—Motility is a measure of the swimming ability of the sperm and has been reported in a number of ways, such as percentage of motile sperm or estimation on a graduated scale of 1–4. Some laboratories also distinguish between progressive and nonprogressive movement. Motility is the only assay that directly measures sperm cell function in relation to fertility. It is the most subjective assay and is sensitive to time and temperature after sample collection. Thus, it is difficult to measure in large studies, especially when samples are collected at home. Normal ranges of sperm motility are hard to define and are subject to laboratory and examiner variation. Decreased sperm motility has never been observed as an isolated change in sperm among men exposed to chemical agents.

3. Sperm morphology—Sperm head shapes and abnormalities in the midpiece and tail are noted, as well as immature forms. This assessment is quite subjective, and there has been little standardization in the definition of normal shape or in the categories of abnormal shapes. The result has been much interlaboratory and interscorer variability, but it has also been shown that quantitative approaches to visual assessment of morphology can be successful when standardized in one laboratory. The criteria for morphologic analyses must be established, and slides of concurrent controls should be analyzed in a blind fashion together with slides of semen from exposed men. To assure uniform scoring, repeated comparison should be made with a coded set of standard slides. Normal ranges have been established for several unexposed populations, and sperm morphology has been studied in men exposed to more than 40 different chemicals.

4. Double F bodies—The double F body test is a relatively new assay based on scoring the frequency of sperm with 2 fluorescent spots in smears stained with quinacrine dye. Studies in somatic cells suggest that these spots represent Y chromosomes. The double F body is thought to represent sperm with two Y chromosomes due to meiotic nondisjunction. The double F body's relationship to Y chromosome aneuploidy remains uncertain, and only a few populations of exposed men have been analyzed with it. Increases in sperm with 2 fluorescent bodies have been observed after exposure to certain chemicals (eg, DBCP and various cancer chemotherapeutic drugs), but a dose-response relationship has not been demonstrated, and validation of this assay is needed.

C. Relation of Semen Parameters to Infertility: While semen analysis is a key element in the diagnosis of male infertility, there is disagreement regarding the relative importance of the various

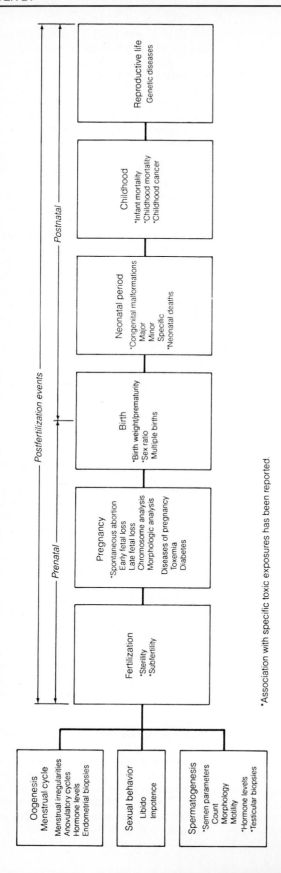

Figure 24–4. The reproductive cycle. Under each stage are listed the parameters that could be monitored in relation to toxic exposures. In the male, end points that have been investigated include reproductive history, blood hormone levels, testicular histology, and semen analyses, all of which reflect effects prior to conception. Theoretically, any postconception event (spontaneous abortion, congenital malforma-tion, etc) that is mediated by abnormal sperm could also be related to exposures occurring in the male prior to conception. The few existing studies make the available data difficult to interpret. Of the above end points, semen analysis is by far the most important in terms of medical surveillance. YFF = Double F body test (see text).

semen parameters. Several factors contribute to the uncertainties: (1) All of the parameters of semen quality and quantity show significant variation, even among fertile men; (2) each individual shows fluctuation in these end points when sampled repeatedly; (3) many measurements are subjective and qualitative, making interlaboratory comparisons difficult; and (4) variations in collection and analysis greatly influence the results.

There is more information on the relationship of fertility to sperm count than to other semen parameters. When the sperm count is less than 20 million/mL, there may be reduced fertility, but pregnancy is not absolutely precluded unless the sperm count is zero. There is no increase in fertility in men with counts above 20 million/mL. In one study, 20% of men of proved fertility had sperm counts under 20 million/mL, and plasma FSH levels were not significantly elevated until the sperm count dropped below 10 million/mL.

Reproductive History

The routine occupational history has not traditionally included questions on reproductive outcome for male workers. Since the realization that male exposures can affect reproductive outcome, such data are beginning to be routinely collected, including information about infertility, live births, spontaneous abortions, birth defects, and perinatal deaths (Fig 24–4). Questionnaires allow correlation of outcome data with exposure data and with confounding variables such as those listed in the preceding section (age, smoking, and alcohol use). Recent studies compared fertility in exposed workers to population norms. Questionnaire surveys are less sensitive indicators of male reproductive toxicity than semen analyses, but the biologic significance of positive results is clear.

Hormone Levels

Monitoring of blood levels of various hormones is useful in the clinical evaluation of patients with suspected reproductive dysfunction. LH, FSH, and testosterone are commonly measured. Leydig cell dysfunction often results in elevated LH production, while elevated FSH levels are associated with damage to the seminiferous tubules. In DBCP-exposed men, FSH levels were of little value in predicting oligospermia, though FSH was a reasonably reliable predictor of azoospermia. There is a broad range of normal testosterone levels, so that it is a poor indicator of early testicular dysfunction.

Testicular Histology

Testicular biopsy has been used in the evaluation of azoospermia or marked oligospermia. Histologic evaluation reveals specific morphologic lesions within the seminiferous tubules or Leydig cells. However, such invasive techniques must be reserved for evaluation of men with marked abnormalities in semen parameters.

RESULTS & BIOLOGIC IMPLICATIONS OF SEMEN ANALYSES

Studies of Exposure

Many studies have shown that semen parameters are reliable indicators of antispermatogenic effects. A recent survey of the literature (Wyrobek et al, 1983a) showed that human sperm assays have been used to assess the spermatogenic function in men exposed to a wide variety of agents. About 85% of the more than 100 papers reviewed concerned exposures to experimental or therapeutic drugs (many were being tested as potential male contraceptives), about 10% were to occupational or environmental exposures, and about 5% involved personal drug use (eg, ethanol, marihuana). Of the 71 chemical exposures studied, 48 were judged to have some effect on human sperm production.

Table 24–2 summarizes the available evidence in the literature on environmental or occupational exposures (excluding drugs) in relation to semen parameters. Only 18 exposure situations have been studied, and results should be considered tentative. Of the detrimental exposures listed, only the effects of DBCP have been confirmed.

Most of the studies have been on small cohorts, and negative results may be due to inadequate statistical power and do not rule out effects at higher exposure levels.

Confounding Factors in Interpreting Data

Four factors—other than chemical exposure—have been reported to affect human sperm production. These must be considered in interpreting epidemiologic data as well as by the clinician in evaluating individual patients presenting with a complaint of infertility.

A. Medical Factors: Medical conditions reported to affect sperm production in humans include viral orchitis (mumps), leprosy, urogenital tuberculosis and other genitourinary infections, renal transplantation, juvenile and adult diabetes, prostatitis, varicocele, severe allergic reactions, viral infections and other febrile illnesses, and cancer.

B. Age: The effects of age on sperm quality are generally considered insignificant. There is some suggestion, however, of small age-related effects in males from infertile marriages or in those with andrologic diseases.

C. Radiation: The spermatotoxic and mutagenic effects of radiation on animal testes are well known. Similar patterns of spermatogenic cell killing and subsequent reductions in sperm numbers have been reported for men receiving therapeutic testicular radiation.

D. Personal Habits: Some personal habits may affect human sperm production, including tobacco smoking, marihuana use, and heavy alcohol consumption. Exposure to heat and associated elevation

Table 24–2. Human sperm studies of occupational exposures.
(Adapted from Wyrobek.)

	Sperm Indicator			
	Count	Motility	Morphology	F Bodies
Detrimental effects				
Carbon disulfide	+	+	+	
Dibromochloropropane (DBCP)	+	+ ?	+ ?	+
Lead	+	+	+	
Inconclusive				
Boron	+ ?			
Cadmium	+ ?			
Carbaryl	−		+ ?	−
Ethylene dibromide	+ ?			
Kepone	+ ?	+ ?	+ ?	
Methylmercury	+ ?			
Toluenediamine and dinitrotoluene	+ ?		−	
No effects				
Anesthetic gases	−		−	
Epichlorohydrin	−		−	
Ethylene glycol monomethyl ether	−			
Formaldehyde	−	−	−	−
Glycerine production	−	+ ?	−	
p-Tertiary butyl benzoic acid	−			
Polybrominated biphenyls	−	−	−	
Waste water treatment plant	−		−	

+ = Detrimental effect observed; + ? = detrimental effect with unknown or marginal statistical significance or not clearly related to the exposure; − = no detrimental effect observed.

in scrotal temperature (eg, in hot tubs) should also be considered.

Postfertilization Effects

Another approach in investigating the reproductive effects of male exposures to industrial chemicals is to study reproductive outcomes in the wives of exposed men without reference to semen abnormalities. This is a less sensitive approach, because many pregnancies are required for analysis (Table 24–3), but if effects on reproductive outcome are observed, there is little question regarding their biologic significance. This type of study design also evaluates exposures prior to fertilization (see Fig 24–4), but the observed effects are postfertilization.

Table 24–4 summarizes all exposure situations for which there is some evidence for male-mediated postfertilization effects on reproductive outcome. Very few chemicals have been definitely associated with such adverse effects, but that may be a reflection only of the insensitivity of this epidemiologic method rather than a true absence of sperm-mediated effects. Clearly, more data are needed comparing exposure, induced sperm defects, and reproductive outcome.

Genetic Implications of Sperm Abnormalities

The biologic implications of induced changes in sperm may extend beyond the clearly defined link to testicular damage and infertility. A nonfunctional

Table 24–3. Sample size required to detect significant change in adverse reproductive outcome compared to semen parameters. (Sample size evenly divided between exposed and control.) (Adapted from Rosenberg and Kuller, 1983, and from Wyrobek, 1982.)

Reproductive outcome	Sample size[1]
Impaired fertility[2]	322 couples
Spontaneous abortion (first trimester)	322 pregnancies
Stillbirths	322 pregnancies
Low birth weight	586 live births
Major birth defects (all)	631 live births

Semen parameters	Sample size
Sperm count	70 men[3]
Abnormal morphology	8 men[4]

[1]No conception after 1 year of unprotected intercourse.
[2]To detect 2-fold increase.
[3]To detect 50% decrease in mean.
[4]To detect 50% increase in mean.

Table 24–4. Studies reported as demonstrating male-mediated postfertilization effects from occupational or environmental chemical exposures.

	Effect	Comment
Lead	Spontaneous abortion, neonatal mortality, stillbirths, and childhood cancer.	Early studies may be confounded by direct exposure to spouse from contaminated home environment.
Dibromochloropropane (DBCP)	Spontaneous abortion, altered sex ratio (based on only 17 births).	Spontaneous abortion rate 6.6% prior to exposure versus 19% postexposure.
Anesthetic gases	Spontaneous abortion.	Inconclusive results from multiple studies.
	Congenital malformations.	Inconclusive results from multiple studies.
	Altered sex ratio.	Inconclusive results from multiple studies.
Chloroprene	Spontaneous abortion.	Questionnaire study reported 3-fold elevated rate, but data not reported.
"Hydrocarbons"	Childhood cancer.	Inconclusive results; one positive, one negative study.
Vinyl chloride	Spontaneous abortion.	Inconclusive; further studies needed.
"Halogenated hydrocarbons"	Infant mortality.	Exposures not well defined.
Waste water treatment plant	Fetal loss (spontaneous abortion).	Exposures not well defined.

sperm poses no genetic hazard, whereas a genetically altered functional sperm could fertilize an egg and result in genetically defective offspring. Such sperm-mediated defects might range from spontaneous abortion to childhood cancer (see Fig 24–4).

There are a number of drugs and environmental toxins that produce fetotoxic (postfertilization) effects when administered to the male parent in experimental animal studies. Some important examples include lead, TCDD (dioxin), anesthetic gases, narcotics, and ethanol (for review see Pearn, 1983). In experimental mutagenesis, the dominant lethal assay is designed to detect such effects: Treated male rodents are mated to untreated females, and the occurrence of dominant lethality is determined by the increase of early embryonic loss as compared to control matings (Green et al, 1985). It is assumed that the exposure causes a mutation of sperm cell DNA significant enough to cause embryo lethality but not affecting the function of sperm. Sperm assays have received much attention in the assessment of chemically induced mutagenesis and carcinogenesis for several reasons:

(1) The testis contains a rapidly dividing cell population, and sperm cells are available in large numbers. Thus, the seminiferous tubules are a model tissue for the detection of in vivo DNA damage.

(2) The observed effects are at the germ cell level and therefore potentially heritable.

(3) The observed effects are of short latency (the spermatogenic cycle in humans is approximately 75 days).

(4) Chemically induced effects can be studied in human as well as experimental animal models.

Though animal assays provide several lines of evidence that induced sperm shape abnormalities may be a marker of heritable genetic abnormalities, the relevance of such assays to humans is the crucial issue. A comparison of results for 24 chemicals tested with sperm assays in at least 2 species (including humans, the mouse, and 9 other mammals) demonstrated a high degree of interspecies similarity in response.

Actual human data on the postfertilization and genetic implications of semen abnormalities are limited. With the possible exception of DBCP, there are no human data to link paternal exposure to subsequent sperm changes and to adverse postfertilization outcomes such as miscarriage, birth defects, or heritable effects in offspring fathered after exposure. One study suggests a link between poor sperm quality and embryonic failure: Fathers of 201 spontaneous abortions showed significantly higher sperm abnormalities and lower sperm counts than did fathers of 116 normal pregnancies. No data on paternal occupation or chemical exposures were given, however.

INTERPRETATION OF FUTURE STUDIES

Since the discovery of infertility in workers exposed to DBCP, many investigators have studied the effects of occupational exposures on the male reproductive system. Because such adverse effects are usually not clinically obvious, epidemiologic analyses will be required to detect previously unrecognized hazardous exposures.

Future studies will probably focus on cross-sectional comparisons of semen parameters between exposed and control groups (or longitudinal comparisons before and after exposure), since sperm studies are the most sensitive indicators of male reproductive effects.

In the planning of future studies, there should be a systematic attempt to identify high-risk populations so that another tragedy like the DBCP episode can be avoided. There is reasonable concordance between human and animal data in regard to spermatotoxic effects. Male workers may therefore be considered at risk if they are exposed to an agent—or close analogue of an agent—known to be testicular toxic in any mammal. Men exposed to agents known to be reproductive toxic agents, mutagens, or carcinogens in male animals should also be considered at risk for spermatogenic damage. Case reports may also point to potential hazardous exposures, providing caution is used not to overinterpret the data.

REFERENCES

Overstreet JW, Blazak WF: The biology of human male reproduction: An overview. *Am J Ind Med* 1983;**4**:5.

Rosenberg MJ, Kuller LH: Reproductive epidemiology. Pages 201–226, in: *Proceedings of a Symposium on Reproductive Health Policies in the Workplace*. Family Health Council of Western Pennsylvania, 1983.

Schrag SD, Dixon RL: Occupational exposures associated with male reproductive dysfunction. *Annu Rev Pharmacol Toxicol* 1985;**25**:567.

Sever LE, Hessol NF: Toxic effects of occupational and environmental chemicals on the testis. In: *Endocrine Toxicology*. Thomas JA et al (editors). Raven Press, 1985.

Steinberger E: Current status of studies concerned with evaluation of toxic effects of chemicals on the testes. *Environ Health Perspect* 1981;**38**:29.

U.S. Office of Technology Assessment: *Reproductive Health Hazards in the Workplace*. Government Printing Office, 1985.

Whorton D, Foliart D: DBCP: Eleven years later. *Repr Toxicol* 1988;**2**:155.

Whorton MD: Male occupational reproductive hazards. *West J Med* 1982;**137**:521.

Whorton MD, Foliart DE: Mutagenicity, carcinogenicity and reproductive effects of dibromochloropropane (DBCP). *Mutat Res* 1983;**123**:13.

Whorton MD et al: Testicular function in DBCP exposed pesticide workers. *J Occup Med* 1979;**21**:161.

Wyrobek AJ et al: Human sperm morphology testing: Description of a reliable method and its statistical power. Pages 527–541 in: *Bandbury Report 13: Indicators of Genotoxic Exposure*. Cold Spring Harbor Laboratories 1982.

Wyrobek AJ et al: An evaluation of human sperm as indicators of chemically induced alterations of spermatogenic function: A report of the US Environmental Protection Agency Gene-Tox Program. *Mutat Res* 1983; **115**:1.

Wyrobek AJ et al: An evaluation of the mouse sperm morphology test and other sperm tests in nonhuman animals: A report of the US Environmental Protection Agency Gene-Tox Program. *Mutat Res* 1983;**115**:73.

Metals

25

Richard Lewis, MD, MPH

The diverse and valuable physical characteristics of metals have resulted in their extensive use in industry. These materials also bring a wide array of potential health hazards into the workplace and as such are of particular importance in occupational medicine. Metals are used in the construction, automotive, aerospace, electronics, and other manufacturing industries as well as in paints, pigments, and catalysts. Because of such widespread potential exposure, familiarity with the toxicity of metals is critical for the health and safety professional.

Metals exert biologic effects chiefly through the formation of stable complexes with sulfhydryl groups and other ligands. These binding properties also form the basis for chelation therapy in the treatment of metal toxicity.

Metals are stable, which explains their wide use in structural materials. This stability also accounts for their pervasiveness in the workplace and in the environment generally. Biologic reactivity of many metals results in accumulation in selective organs and tissues and in a potential for chronic toxicity. Meticulous attention to personal and workplace hygiene is essential for the reduction of chronic exposure and the prevention of health effects.

Metals are rarely used in their pure form, usually being present in alloys. They may also be bound to organic materials, which alters their physical characteristics and toxicity. Other forms, such as hydrides and carbonyls, are highly toxic and may be formed accidentally when the parent metal reacts with acids.

Acute Metal Toxicity

Acute toxicity usually occurs after ingestion of metal-containing compounds or inhalation of high concentrations of metal fumes or gaseous metal compounds. In modern industrial operations, this type of exposure is unusual, often being due to unexpected chemical reactions or to burning or brazing in enclosed spaces. Awareness of the acute toxicity of metals, combined with a careful occupational history, will help in the detection of acute health effects that require specific treatment, such as chelation therapy. Most metals can be measured in blood or urine to confirm the diagnosis of acute poisoning.

Chronic Metal Toxicity

Research into the health effects of low-level exposure to metals continues to suggest that physiologic alterations may occur at levels that previously had been considered safe. Neurologic and neurophysiologic effects, reproductive toxicity, teratogenicity (including behavioral alterations), and carcinogenicity remain at the forefront of current research. Medical surveillance and biologic monitoring programs in industrial settings are important for determining safe levels of exposure. Prevention of chronic toxicity remains a challenge for workers exposed to metals, particularly lead.

ANTIMONY

Essentials of Diagnosis

Acute effects:
- Respiratory and mucous membrane irritation.
- Gastrointestinal distress.
- Dermatitis.
- Hemolysis and anuria (stibine gas).

Chronic effects:
- Pustular dermatitis.
- Pneumoconiosis.
- Electrocardiographic abnormalities.
- Lung cancer (antimony trioxide production).

Exposure Limits

Antimony
   ACGIH TLV: $0.5 \ mg/m^3$ TWA
   OSHA PEL: $0.5 \ mg/m^3$ TWA
   NIOSH REL: $0.5 \ mg/m^3$ TWA
Stibine
   ACGIH TLV: 0.1 ppm TWA
   OSHA PEL: 0.1 ppm TWA

General Considerations

Antimony is a soft metal found as oxides and sulfides in a variety of ores. Antimony ores often contain significant quantities of arsenic and lead.

Use

Pure antimony metal is used in the manufacture of semiconductor devices, both as a dopant compound for silicon and as a substrate material in the manufacture of intermediate crystals. Antimony alloys are used in the production of battery grids, type castings, bearings, and cable sheaths. Antimony compounds are also used in munitions, glass and pottery, fire retardants, paints and lacquers, rubber compounds, chemical catalysts, and solder. Antimonials have been used medicinally in the treatment of leishmaniasis, schistosomiasis, and filariasis.

Occupational & Environmental Exposure

Mining and smelting operations have resulted in significant worker exposure to antimony dusts and fumes. These exposures have been complicated by concomitant exposure to lead, arsenic, and sulfur dioxide. Health effects attributed to exposure to antimony during refining and extraction include respiratory tract irritation, gastrointestinal complaints, dermatitis, and pneumoconiosis. Exposure to antimony trisulfide in the manufacture of abrasive grinding wheels has been associated with an increase in electrocardiographic abnormalities and sudden death among workers. Antimony trioxide and antimony trichloride, both used in the microelectronics industry, are strongly irritating to tissues and membranes.

Stibine gas (SbH_3), a hemolytic toxin similar to arsine, may be formed when antimony alloys are processed with certain reducing acids. Stibine is also used as a grain fumigant.

Parenteral administration of antimonial compounds for medicinal purposes has been associated with electrocardiographic changes, alterations in liver function, and hemolysis. Poisoning has also occurred after storage of acidic foods and beverages in containers lined with enamels containing antimony.

Absorption, Metabolism, & Excretion

Soluble forms of antimony are readily absorbed after inhalation. Antimony is largely excreted in the urine. The trivalent form is excreted less rapidly than the pentavalent form as a result of red blood cell uptake.

Insoluble forms are excreted slowly in the urine and may be detectable years after exposure has ceased.

Clinical Findings

A. Symptoms and Signs:

1. Acute exposure–Acute exposure to antimony dusts and fumes causes intense irritation of the eyes, throat, and respiratory tract. Systemic toxicity may follow inhalation of dusts or fumes. Nausea, vomiting, abdominal pain, and bloody diarrhea may also be present. Inhalation of antimony trichloride causes headache, fatigue, abdominal pain, jaundice, and anuria due to massive hemolysis.

2. Chronic exposure–Chronic inhalation may result in dryness of the throat, dysosmia, and bronchitis as well as complaints of fatigue, headache, and anorexia. Complaints of dizziness may indicate a cardiac rhythm disturbance.

Chronic skin exposure to antimony compounds may cause pustular dermatitis. Other chronic effects include perforation of the nasal septum, bleeding gums, conjunctivitis, and laryngitis. Spontaneous abortions, menstrual disorders, and excretion of antimony in breast milk have been reported in exposed women in the Soviet Union.

Antimony is suspected of being a human carcinogen. Workers engaged in antimony trioxide production have been found to have an excess incidence of lung cancer. In addition, the high incidence of urinary bladder tumors in persons treated for schistosomiasis may be related to past treatment with antimonial agents.

B. Laboratory Findings: The red cell count may be low. Hemoglobinuria and red blood cell casts are a sign of stibine-induced hemolysis and suggest acute renal and hepatic failure. Hepatitis is a rare but serious complication of antimonial drug therapy and could occur in settings where there is acute overexposure to other antimony compounds. Electrocardiographic changes after therapeutic use or industrial exposure include T wave changes and rhythm disturbances.

Acute inhalation of antimony trichloride has resulted in acute pulmonary edema with hypoxemia and diffuse pulmonary infiltrates. Rounded opacities in the mid lung fields on chest x-ray are consistent with pneumoconiosis in workers chronically exposed to antimony ores or dusts. Pulmonary function impairment may be present on spirometry related to either acute or chronic exposure.

The presence of antimony in urine is diagnostic of past exposure but does not necessarily correlate with severity of exposure or health effects. Urine concentrations in nonexposed individuals are generally less than 0.001 mg/L. In acute exposure (such as after intravenous therapy), levels may exceed 2 mg/L. Occupational exposures generally result in levels of 0.1–0.3 mg/L.

Prevention

Personal protective devices should be worn where there is potential exposure to antimony dusts or fumes. Biologic monitoring of urinary antimony levels confirms exposure and may be useful for diagnosis if markedly elevated in acute overexposure.

Treatment

Pulmonary function and electrocardiographic monitoring are indicated when acute exposure is suspected (significant inhalation or ingestion). The occupational history will aid in the diagnosis of antimony poisoning, concentrating on acute releases of antimony fumes or vapors and work in confined spaces in patients with acute respiratory or systemic symptoms.

Irritant exposure to soluble antimony dusts or liquids is treated by removal from further exposure and cleansing exposed skin. Chelation with dimercaprol or penicillamine is indicated when significant cardiovascular, pulmonary, or hepatic impairment occurs in patients with suspected acute exposure.

Stibine-induced hemolysis requires exchange transfusion.

ARSENIC

Essentials of Diagnosis

Acute effects:
- Nausea, vomiting, diarrhea.
- Intravascular hemolysis, jaundice, oliguria (arsine).
- Cardiovascular collapse.

Chronic effects:
- Hyperkeratosis and hyperpigmentation (melanosis).
- Peripheral neuropathy.
- Anemia.
- Cardiac and peripheral vascular disease.

Exposure Limits

Arsenic
ACGIH TLV: 0.2 mg/m^3 TWA
OSHA PEL: 0.01 mg/m^3 TWA
NIOSH REL: 2 μg/m^3 ceiling (15 minutes)
Arsine
ACGIH TLV: 0.05 ppm TWA
OSHA PEL: 0.05 ppm TWA
NIOSH REL: 2 μg/m^3 ceiling (15 minutes)

General Considerations

Arsenic occurs in numerous ferrous and nonferrous ores. It is found in air, water, and food, and important industrial contributions are from smelting operations, pesticide use, and effluents from geothermal power plants. Arsenic is ubiquitous in living organisms, though it is not an essential trace element in humans.

The toxicity of arsenic varies greatly with the chemical state. Pure elemental arsenic and organic arsenic compounds (found in many seafoods) are virtually nontoxic, while trivalent arsenic trioxide and arsine gas are potent acute poisons.

Use

Metallic arsenic is used as an alloy, primarily for hardening lead in battery grids, bearings, and cable sheaths. Arsenic trioxide and arsenic pentoxide are used in the manufacture of calcium, copper, and lead arsenate pesticides. Arsenic compounds are used as pigments and refining agents in glass and as preservatives in tanning and taxidermy. Copper acetoarsenite is used as a wood preservative. Arsenic compounds are also used as herbicides and desiccants for cotton harvesting. Arsanilic acid is used in veterinary pharmaceuticals and feed additives. Arsine gas and other arsenic compounds are used in the microelectronics industry, as a source of dopant arsenic atoms, and in the manufacture of gallium arsenide substrates.

Occupational & Environmental Exposure

Exposure to arsenic compounds, primarily in the form of arsenic trioxide, occurs in the smelting of lead, copper, gold and other nonferrous metals. Readily volatilized arsenic trioxide is concentrated in flue dust and can be condensed and recovered in a cooling chamber. Furnace and flue maintenance operations carry a high risk of exposure. Pesticide manufacture and smelting operations have resulted in substantial contamination of the air and water in surrounding communities.

Metal workers may be exposed to airborne arsenic trioxide or to arsine. Workers engaged in the manufacture and application of arsenical pesticides, herbicides, and preservatives have the potential for significant arsenic exposure. Forestry and farm workers may be exposed to residual arsenic compounds after their use in the field. In the microelectronics industry, workers may be exposed to arsenic in handling source materials or finished product or in maintenance operations. Arsine exposure may also occur in this industry, but it is usually controlled through the use of closed systems. Arsine may be formed accidentally when nascent hydrogen is formed in the presence of arsenic or when water or acid reacts with metal arsenides. Pharmaceutical manufacturers may be exposed to arsanilic acid and other arsenic compounds.

Nonoccupational exposure has resulted from ingestion of contaminated well water, dried milk, soy sauce, and moonshine whiskey. Dietary intake is related to pesticide residues, feed additives, and bioaccumulation of arsenic in marine organisms. Organic arsenic compounds present in seafood are not metabolized and are excreted unchanged. Exposure may occur through burning of arsenic-treated wood and from smoking cigarettes made of tobacco sprayed with arsenical pesticides.

Absorption, Metabolism, & Excretion

Arsenic compounds are absorbed after ingestion or inhalation. Skin absorption is limited. The arsenic is readily taken up by red blood cells and then deposited in the liver, kidney, muscle, bone, skin, and hair. Trivalent arsenic (+3) avidly binds to sulfhydryl groups and interferes with numerous enzyme systems, including those involved in cellular respiration, glutathione metabolism, and DNA repair. This binding also accounts for the persistence of arsenic in the hair and nails. Pentavalent arsenic (+5) and arsine are converted to trivalent arsenic in vivo. The majority of the absorbed trivalent arsenic is metabolized to dimethylarsinic acid and monomethylarsonic acid and excreted in the urine with a half-life of 10 hours. Organic arsenic compounds are excreted unchanged in the urine.

Clinical Findings

A. Symptoms and Signs:

1. Acute exposure—Symptoms of acute arsenic poisoning may develop minutes to hours after ingestion and consist of nausea, vomiting, abdominal pain, and copious blood-tinged diarrhea. Cold, clammy skin, muscle cramps, and facial edema may be present. Seizures, coma, and circulatory collapse precede death. A dose of 120 mg of arsenic trioxide may be fatal. Liver enlargement and oliguria may also occur.

Persons who recover may develop delayed peripheral neuropathy, presenting after several weeks as symmetric distal sensory loss. The lower extremities are usually more affected than the upper. Motor involvement extending to total paralysis may also occur.

Acute exposure to arsine results in intravascular hemolysis. Other complaints include headache, nausea, and chest tightness. Exposure to 10 ppm rapidly causes delirium, coma, and death.

The triad of abdominal pain, jaundice, and oliguria should strongly suggest arsine exposure. Physical examination may reveal bronzing of the skin and hepatosplenomegaly.

2. Chronic exposure—Distal paresthesias or anesthesia indicate arsenic-induced peripheral neuropathy. In more severe cases, motor involvement may be evident as well, with weakness and reflex loss. Symptoms of sore throat, cough, and phlegm production may be due to chronic exposure to irritant arsenic dusts. Complaints of asthenia and fatigue may be due to arsenic-induced anemia. Other effects that have been reported include cardiac failure, liver disease, and renal disease. Environmental exposure in Taiwan resulted in the induction of peripheral vasospasms and gangrene, termed ''blackfoot disease.'' This has not occurred in the occupational setting.

Dermatologic manifestations of chronic exposure to arsenic compounds are common, principally after long-term ingestion of arsenic in drinking water or for medicinal purposes. Arsenical keratoses are raised punctate or verrucous lesions occurring primarily on the palms and soles. Enlarging masses or ulcerations should suggest Bowen's disease, basal cell carcinoma, and squamous cell carcinoma, which are all increased in persons with chronic arsenic exposure. In some individuals, a diffuse bronze hyperpigmentation may develop, characterized by interspersion of 10-mm macules of hypomelanosis. Alopecia may occur. Some arsenic compounds may cause an irritant dermatitis as well.

Several epidemiologic studies of smelting operations have revealed an increase in lung cancer in workers exposed to arsenic. Other cancers that have been reported in association with arsenic exposure include leukemia, lymphoma, and angiosarcoma of the liver.

Arsenic crosses the placenta and may cause fetotoxicity, decreased birth weight, or congenital malformations.

B. Laboratory Findings: Acute and chronic exposure to arsenic may cause anemia and leukopenia, and arsine-induced hemolysis results in anemia, hyperbilirubinemia, and hemoglobinuria. Hematuria and proteinuria indicate renal injury. Liver damage may result in elevation of serum enzymes and bilirubin. The ECG may reveal rhythm or conduction disturbances. Delayed sensory conduction velocities in a distal symmetric distribution may be seen on nerve conduction studies.

Total urine arsenic levels are useful in confirming recent exposure. The measurement of dimethylarsinic acid and monomethylarsonic acid eliminate confusion with dietary sources of organic arsenic compounds. Hair and nail arsenic levels may be useful in detecting systemic absorption of arsenic, primarily due to ingestion. These are also subject to external contamination and are of little use in the industrial setting.

Tissue biopsy will confirm the diagnosis of skin or respiratory cancer. Careful medical and occupational histories are necessary to determine the relationship of these common cancers to arsenic exposure.

Prevention

The use of engineering controls to contain sources of exposure to arsenic compounds will reduce exposure in smelting, metallurgy, and pesticide manufacturing operations. Personal protective equipment should be worn when performing maintenance work or during application of arsenic compounds. Medical surveillance should concentrate on skin and respiratory complaints as well as liver, hematologic, renal, and nervous system function. Biologic monitoring of arsenic in urine will complement industrial hygiene efforts to control exposure.

Treatment

Treatment following acute ingestion is by induced emesis followed by administration of activated charcoal and a cathartic. Treat shock with aggressive intravenous fluid resuscitation and pressor agents as indicated. If the diagnosis is confirmed, begin therapy with dimercaprol, 3–4 mg/kg every 4 hours for the first 2 days. Continue 3 mg/kg every 12 hours until urine arsenic is below 50 μg/d. Eliminate sources of further exposure after treatment.

Arsine poisoning requires careful monitoring of the hematocrit and renal function. Alkaline diuresis will reduce the precipitation of hemoglobin in renal tubules and the resultant renal impairment. Elevation of plasma-free hemoglobin greater than 1.5 mg/dL or oliguria is an indication for exchange transfusion. Hemodialysis is indicated if acute renal failure develops. Dimercaprol is not effective in arsine poisoning.

Prognosis

In acute arsenic poisoning, survival for more than 1 week is usually followed by complete recovery. Complete recovery from chronic arsenic poisoning may require 6 months to 1 year.

BERYLLIUM

Essentials of Diagnosis

- Tracheobronchitis, pneumonitis.
- Granulomatous pulmonary disease.

- Dermatitis (ulceration and granulomas).
- Eye, nose, and throat irritation.

Exposure Limits
ACGIH TLV: 0.002 ppm TWA
OSHA PEL: 0.002 ppm TWA, 0.005 ppm ceiling (30 minutes)
NIOSH REL: Do not exceed 0.5 μg Be/m^3

General Considerations
Beryllium is a lightweight, gray metal with high tensile strength. It is extracted from beryl ore after grinding and heating using either a sulfate or fluoride process and electrolytic reduction. Bertrandite ($4BeO.2SiO_2.H_2O$), although lower in beryllium content (0.1–3%), provides a source of acid-soluble beryllium that is more easily extracted.

Use
The unique properties of beryllium are ideally suited for the production of hard, corrosion-resistant alloys for use in the aerospace industry. Beryllium alloys (primarily copper) are used in nonsparking tools, bushings, bearings, and electronic components. Beryllium is used in nuclear reactors as a moderator to retard neutrons, a reflector to prevent neutron leakage, and a fuel source. Beryllium oxide combines high thermal conductivity with high electrical resistance for use in ceramics, microwave tubes, and semiconductors. The use of beryllium in the manufacture of fluorescent and neon lamps was discontinued in 1949 after numerous cases of beryllium toxicity were reported in that industry.

Occupational & Environmental Exposure
Exposure to beryllium in the past has occurred mainly in grinding, roasting, and milling of beryl ore, though recognition of the toxicity of beryllium has resulted in dramatic improvement in environmental conditions in these operations. Mining of beryl ore has not been associated with adverse health effects. Workers involved with the newer applications for beryllium in the aerospace, nuclear, and electronics industries may be less aware of its potential hazards. Workers engaged in the production and fabrication of beryllium alloys may be exposed to dusts and fumes. Persons residing in neighborhoods surrounding beryllium roasting operations have the potential for chronic low-level exposure to beryllium compounds, though there are strict emission standards for these operations.

Absorption, Metabolism, & Excretion
Beryllium compounds are poorly absorbed after inhalation, ingestion, or skin contact. Beryllium may be retained in the lung or deposited in bone, liver, and spleen. Renal excretion is slow and variable and serves primarily to confirm exposure, since levels are usually undetectable in nonexposed individuals. The development of chronic toxicity does not appear to be dose-dependent and may involve a hypersensitivity reaction. Pathologically, beryllium toxicity is a systemic disease, evidenced by the presence of non-caseating granulomas in numerous tissues, including lung, liver, skin, and lymph nodes.

Clinical Findings
A. Symptoms and Signs:
1. Acute or subacute exposure—Acute or subacute exposure to beryllium dusts or fumes has irritant effects on the eyes, mucous membranes, and respiratory tract. Burning eyes, sinus congestion, epistaxis, and sore throat may be presenting complaints. Affected tissues may be swollen, hyperemic, and ulcerated. Tracheobronchitis is characterized by cough, chest pain, and dyspnea. In severe cases, a chemical pneumonitis may develop, manifested by tachypnea, hemoptysis, cyanosis, and rales. Death has occurred as a result of pulmonary edema and respiratory failure.

2. Chronic exposure—Chronic berylliosis may develop after many years of exposure or following a single acute exposure. Exertional dyspnea is the usual presenting complaint, often accompanied by fatigue, weight loss, cough, and chest pain. On physical examination, there may be rales, hepatosplenomegaly, lymphadenopathy, and clubbing. In long-standing cases, there may be evidence of pulmonary hypertension such as jugular venous distention, a right ventricular heave, and an accentuated P_2 on cardiac auscultation. Exacerbations of symptoms may occur following trauma, systemic illness, or pregnancy.

After skin contact, beryllium may cause an irritant or allergic dermatitis, characterized by erythema, papules, and vesiculation. After penetration of the skin through a cut or abrasion, there may be development of a granuloma that may ulcerate through the skin surface.

Beryllium metal, beryl ore, and several beryllium alloys and compounds are proved animal carcinogens causing both lung cancers and osteogenic sarcomas in several species. Beryllium is considered a probable human carcinogen, and exposures should be reduced to the lowest feasible levels.

B. Laboratory Findings: In cases of acute pneumonitis, there is arterial hypoxemia with diffuse pulmonary infiltrates. In chronic beryllium disease, there may be hypergammaglobulinemia, anemia, elevated liver enzymes, and hyperuricemia. Pulmonary function studies may reveal a reduced FEV_1, a reduced FEV_1/FVC ratio, or both. The carbon monoxide diffusing capacity is usually impaired. In contrast to sarcoidosis, the serum angiotensin-converting enzyme levels are usually normal and the Kveim test is negative. Biopsy of affected tissues will reveal noncaseating granulomas.

Elevated urine levels of beryllium (> 0.02 mg/L) confirm exposure. Skin testing can confirm hypersensitivity to beryllium compounds but also carries the risk of sensitization and should be avoided. Lymphocyte transformation assays are a useful alternative and are effective in assessing individual reactivity to beryllium compounds. X-ray findings include diffuse bilateral nodular or linear infiltrates, often with bilateral hilar adenopathy.

Prevention

Operations that generate beryllium dusts or fumes should be enclosed and vented. Wet processes are preferred to reduce the generation of dust. Eye, skin, and respiratory protection are required during cleaning and maintenance operations. Awareness of beryllium toxicity and training and care in handling beryllium compounds will prevent inadvertent overexposure in newer industrial applications. Medical surveillance should include periodic chest x-rays and measurement of pulmonary function.

Treatment

Treatment of acute pneumonitis should include supplemental oxygen and corticosteroids. Chronic beryllium disease may also respond to steroids, starting with prednisone, 60 mg orally daily, and tapering slowly. Skin lesions should be thoroughly cleansed and treated with topical steroids.

Prognosis

Berylliosis is a chronic disease that may persist and progress even after cessation of exposure. Prevention and early detection are critical.

BORON

Essentials of Diagnosis

- Respiratory and mucous membrane irritation (boron halides, diborane, borax, boric acid).
- Central nervous system effects (boron hydrides, boric acid).
- Skin irritation (borax, borates).

Exposure Limits

Borates (anhydrous)
   ACGIH TLV: 1 mg/m^3 TWA
   OSHA PEL: 10 mg/m^3 TWA
Boron oxide
   ACGIH TLV: 10 mg/m^3 TWA
   NIOSH REL: 10 mg/m^3 TWA
Pentaborane
   ACGIH TLV: 0.005 ppm TWA
   OSHA PEL: 0.005 ppm TWA, 0.015 STEL
Diborane
   ACGIH TLV: 0.1 ppm TWA
   OSHA PEL: 0.1 ppm TWA

General Considerations

Boron is a metalloid element that occurs in bedded deposits and lake brines. Borax ($Na_2B_4O_7.10H_2O$) and kernite ($Na_2B_4O_7.4H_2O$) are important mineral sources of boron. Boron compounds are produced by the exothermic reduction of boron trioxide with magnesium. The major deposits of boron minerals are found in the United States, Turkey, and the Soviet Union.

Use

A major use for boron compounds is in the manufacture of glass, including insulating and textile fiberglass. Enamels, glazes, coatings, soaps, and cleansers also contain boron compounds. Boron compounds have been used as propellants in jet fuels and as gasoline additives. Boron is an important dopant element in the manufacture of semiconductor devices. Other diverse uses for boron are in herbicides, solar batteries, welding rods, nuclear reactors, flame retardants, abrasives, adhesives, and plastics. Boric acid has been used medicinally as a topical antiseptic.

Occupational & Environmental Exposure

Because of its many uses, workers may be exposed to boron compounds in a wide variety of settings. Workers employed in the mining and refining of boron minerals may have exposures to dusts containing boric acid. The highly toxic boron hydrides (diborane, pentaborane, and decaborane) are encountered in the production of high-energy fuels and in the rubber industry. The boron halides (boron tribromide, boron trichloride, and boron trifluoride) are used as catalysts and, along with diborane, are important sources of dopant boron atoms in the microelectronics industry. Glass workers, paint and soap manufacturers, and welders may have exposure to boron compounds.

Absorption, Metabolism, & Excretion

Boron compounds are readily absorbed after inhalation or ingestion. Some boron compounds such as boric acid are also absorbed after skin contact. Excessive absorption may lead to accumulation in the brain. Excretion is primarily renal.

Clinical Findings

A. Symptoms and Signs: The toxicity of boron is highly dependent on the source of exposure. Boron oxide, borax, and boric acid may all cause respiratory, eye, and skin irritation at high concentrations. Excessive absorption of these compounds may result in central nervous system depression, gastrointestinal distress, skin desquamation, and renal damage. Chronic exposure to boron compounds may cause alopecia. Menstrual disturbances in women have also been reported. In animal experiments, exposure to boron resulted in gonadotoxic effects, including reduction in testicular weight, sperm count, and sperm motility.

Exposure to diborane gas causes acute respiratory irritation, resulting in cough and chest tightness. Pulmonary edema may develop. Exposure to pentaborane and decaborane has been associated with severe central nervous system effects, including encephalopathy, seizures, and coma. Acute exposure may result in prolonged mental and behavioral disturbances.

Boron halides hydrolyze to the corresponding halogen acid on contact with moist surfaces. Exposure may cause eye, skin, and respiratory tract irritation as well as pulmonary edema.

B. Laboratory Findings: There may be evidence of renal failure, with proteinuria and hematuria. Liver enzymes may be elevated. The EEG may show evidence of a diffuse encephalopathy. Serum borate levels above 20 mg/L indicate excessive exposure.

Prevention

Workers should be advised to avoid skin contact with highly concentrated or irritating boron compounds through the use of gloves and protective garments. Every effort should be made to prevent worker exposure to boron halides and boron hydrides through engineering controls and process enclosure. Although borax and boric acid are upper respiratory irritants at concentrations greater than 4 mg/m^3, there is no evidence that they cause impairment of respiratory function. Medical surveillance of workers with exposure to boron hydrides should concentrate on the respiratory system and the nervous system.

Treatment

Supportive measures and anticonvulsants should be used as indicated. Careful monitoring of respiratory function is indicated after acute inhalation. Hemodialysis will remove borates from the circulation.

CADMIUM

Essentials of Diagnosis

Acute effects:
- Fever, chills, dyspnea (metal fume fever).
- Chemical pneumonitis.
- Renal failure.
- Gastrointestinal disturbance.

Chronic effects:
- Proteinuria.
- Fanconi's syndrome.
- Osteomalacia.
- Emphysema.
- Anemia.
- Anosmia.
- Lung cancer.

Exposure Limits

Cadmium oxide fume
 ACGIH TLV: 0.05 mg/m^3 TWA
 NIOSH REL: Reduce exposure to lowest feasible concentration.

General Considerations

Cadmium is a soft, silver-white, electropositive metal that is finding increasing industrial applications. Although greenockite (cadmium sulfide), the principal cadmium mineral, is rare, cadmium is commonly present in zinc, lead, and copper ores. Cadmium is a by-product of the smelting and refining of these ores and is recovered by electrolysis and distillation. Cadmium is a nonessential mineral for humans and is present in biologic tissues as a result of environmental exposure.

Use

The primary use of cadmium compounds is in electroplating. Cadmium imparts corrosion resistance to steel, iron, and a variety of other materials for use in automotive parts, aircraft, marine equipment, and industrial machinery. Cadmium alloys are used in high-speed bearings, solder, and jewelry. Cadmium sulfides and selenides are used as pigments in rubber, inks, resins, paints, textiles, and ceramics, particularly where heat stability and alkali resistance are desirable. Cadmium stearate is used as a stabilizer in plastics—primarily in polyvinyl chloride (PVC) film. Nickel-cadmium batteries are used in motor vehicles and rechargeable household appliances. Cadmium is also used in photoelectric cells and in semiconductors.

Occupational & Environmental Exposure

Workers may be exposed to cadmium in the smelting and refining of zinc, lead, and copper. The recovery and refining of cadmium compounds is associated with potential exposure to high levels of dusts and fumes. Cadmium exposure may occur in the manufacture of batteries, paints, and plastics. Welders and brazers may be exposed to cadmium oxide fumes when working with cadmium-containing solders or welding rods or when working on materials that have been coated with cadmium. Exposures may also occur at electroplating operations.

Nonoccupational exposure occurs primarily through dietary intake. Air and water contamination may be significant in areas surrounding zinc smelters. Ingestion of food that has been improperly stored in containers which have been glazed with cadmium may result in acute poisoning. Cigarette smoke is another source of chronic cadmium exposure in humans.

Absorption, Metabolism, & Excretion

Cadmium may be absorbed through inhalation or ingestion. Skin absorption is negligible under ordinary circumstances. After inhalation, 10–40% may be absorbed, depending on particle size and chemical composition. Gastrointestinal absorption is usually less than 10% but may be increased in the presence of iron, protein, calcium, or zinc deficiencies.

In the bloodstream, cadmium is bound to plasma proteins. Most is found within erythrocytes, where it is bound to hemoglobin and metallothionein, an inducible low-molecular-weight protein named for its high affinity for certain metals. Cadmium accumulates in the liver and kidneys, where binding to metallothionein protects against cellular damage.

Excretion is primarily through the kidney, with a biologic half-life of 8–30 years. Renal excretion of cadmium increases after chronic exposure due to impaired proximal tubular reabsorption, a manifestation of cadmium induced nephrotoxicity.

Clinical Findings

A. Symptoms and Signs:

1. Acute exposure–Acute inhalation of cadmium oxide fumes has accounted for several industrial fatalities. After a delay of several hours, workers complain of sore throat, headache, myalgias, nausea, and a metallic taste. Fever, cough, dyspnea, and chest tightness follow, simulating metal fume fever. In severe cases, this progresses to a fulminant chemical pneumonitis with pulmonary edema and death due to respiratory failure. Acute hepatic and renal injury may also occur. Acute exposure may result in chronic pulmonary fibrosis. Ingestion of cadmium compounds results in nausea, vomiting, headache, abdominal pain, liver injury, and acute renal failure.

2. Chronic exposure–The most frequent manifestation of chronic exposure to cadmium is proteinuria. Initially, there is increased excretion of low-molecular-weight proteins, such as β_2-microglobulin. With continued exposure, this progresses to Fanconi's syndrome, with aminoaciduria, glycosuria, hypercalciuria, and phosphaturia. Renal tubular dysfunction can result in nephrolithiasis and osteomalacia. Bone pain and pathologic fractures are related to renal calcium and phosphorus wasting and impaired synthesis of vitamin D. Chronic inhalation of cadmium dusts and fumes may also result in respiratory impairment and emphysema. Other effects that have been reported include anosmia and anemia.

Cadmium is a human carcinogen, reported as a cause of lung cancer in several studies of smelting and plating operations. An excess in genitourinary and prostate cancers has also been reported in metal workers exposed to cadmium. Cadmium persists in tissues and has been used to induce tumors (sarcomas) in laboratory animals.

Teratogenic effects and testicular effects have been observed in laboratory animals as well, though human reproductive effects have not been reported.

B. Laboratory Findings:

1. Acute inhalation–Evaluation of acute inhalations should include an arterial blood gas, a chest x-ray, spirometry, and assessment of renal and hepatic function. Hypoxemia, diffuse pulmonary infiltrates, and a reduction in FEV_1, FVC, and diffusing capacity for carbon monoxide indicate excessive exposure and impending respiratory failure. Later, the chest x-ray may reveal bronchopneumonia. Blood and urine cadmium levels are useful in acute exposure. Normal blood and urine cadmium levels are 0.004 mg/L and 0.0002 mg/L, respec-

tively. After acute cadmium fume inhalation, these may rise to 3 mg/L and 0.36 mg/L.

2. Chronic exposure–For chronic exposure, laboratory evaluation should include quantification of urine β_2-microglobulin, albumin, and total protein excretion. A complete blood count may reveal a decrease in serum hemoglobin. Evaluation of pulmonary function may reveal airway obstruction and reduction in diffusing capacity for carbon monoxide. Bone x-rays should be performed to look for abnormal mineralization and pathologic fractures.

Blood cadmium levels correlate with recent exposure but are not useful to monitor chronic exposure. Renal effects have been reported when the urine cadmium concentration exceeds 0.01 mg/g creatinine.

Prevention

Processes that result in the production of cadmium oxide fumes should be enclosed. Local exhaust ventilation and personal protective measures should be used to minimize exposure to cadmium dusts. Strict attention to workplace and personal hygiene will lessen the potential for chronic exposures. Welding on cadmium-treated metal or brazing using cadmium-containing solders should only be performed in areas that are properly ventilated. Air-supplied respirators should be used in enclosed spaces.

Biologic monitoring should focus on the early detection of proteinuria, before severe irreversible proximal renal tubular dysfunction occurs. Urine cadmium levels should be kept below 0.01 mg/g creatinine to prevent renal injury.

Treatment

Persons who have suffered acute inhalation of cadmium oxide fumes should be thoroughly evaluated for evidence of acute lung injury. Admission to the hospital for observation is indicated if excessive exposure is suspected based on the history or clinical findings. Respiratory support may be required. In severe acute poisoning, chelation with calcium disodium edetate (EDTA) may be indicated. Renal function should be closely monitored, since chelation may increase renal toxicity. Dimercaprol should not be used.

Individuals who manifest chronic toxicity (renal impairment, emphysema, bone disease) should be removed from further exposure. Supplementation with calcium and vitamin D is indicated if calcium wasting or bone disease is present.

CHROMIUM

Essentials of Diagnosis

- Sinusitis, septal perforation.
- Allergic and irritant dermatitis, ulcers.
- Respiratory irritation, bronchitis, asthma.
- Lung cancer.

Exposure Limits

Chromium metal
ACGIH TLV: 0.5 mg/m^3 TWA
OSHA PEL: 1 mg/m^3 TWA
Chromium (III) compounds
ACGIH TLV: 0.5 mg/m^3 TWA
OSHA PEL: 0.5 mg/m^3 TWA
Chromium (VI) compounds
ACGIH TLV: 0.05 mg/m^3 TWA
OSHA PEL: 0.1 ppm ceiling
NIOSH REL: 1 μg/m^3 TWA

General Considerations

Chromium is a hard, brittle gray metal. Elemental chromium does not occur naturally but is widely distributed as chromite ($FeOCr_2O_3$) or chrome iron stone. Chromite is obtained through both underground and open cast mining. Ferrochromium is produced by the reduction of chromite with carbon in an electric furnace. Chromium metal is obtained primarily through reduction of chromic oxide with aluminum powder. Chromates are produced by high-temperature roasting of chromite in an oxidizing atmosphere. The valence states that are of primary industrial interest are hexavalent (Cr [VI], chromate) and, to a lesser extent, trivalent (Cr [III], chromic) chromium. The valence state is critical for the toxicity of chromium compounds.

Use

The primary use of chromium is in plating. Numerous applications include automotive parts, household appliances, tools, and machinery, where the coating imparts corrosion resistance and a shiny, decorative finish. Chromium-iron alloys, alone or with the addition of nickel or manganese, are used to produce a variety of durable, high-strength stainless steels. Chromium alloys with nickel (nichrome) have high electrical resistance for use in electrical appliances. Chromates and dichromates are used as pigments and preservatives in paints, dyes, textiles, rubber, and inks. The radioisotope ^{56}Cr is used in nuclear medicine to label erythrocytes.

Occupational & Environmental Exposure

Exposure to chromium begins with mining and crushing operations, where there may be exposure to dusts of chromic oxide. The greatest occupational hazard historically has been in the processing of chromite ore to produce chromates, where workers were found to have a high incidence of lung cancer. Exposure to chromium fumes occurs in the production and fabrication of stainless steel. Arc welding of stainless steel also results in exposure to chromium compounds.

Electroplaters are exposed to chromic acid mists. Workers may be exposed to chromates through their use in the paint, textile, leather, glass, and rubber industries and in lithography, printing, and photography. Certain cements have a high chromium con-tent. Chromium is found in low concentrations in water, urban air, and a variety of foods.

Absorption, Metabolism, & Excretion

Chromium compounds may be absorbed through the gastrointestinal tract, the lungs, or the skin. The soluble hexavalent forms are much more readily absorbed than the insoluble trivalent forms. Intracellularly, hexavalent chromium is converted to the trivalent form, which binds avidly to proteins and nucleic acids, resulting in chromium toxicity. Chromium is an essential trace element in humans and animals, and chromium deficiency results in impaired glucose tolerance. Chromium does not generally accumulate in tissues, though inhaled insoluble forms may remain in the lung. Excretion is primarily renal, and urine levels have been found to correlate with recent airborne exposure to soluble chromium compounds.

Clinical Findings

A. Symptoms and Signs: Acute exposure to high concentrations of chromic acid or chromates will cause immediate irritation of the eye, nose, throat, and respiratory tract, resulting in burning, congestion, epistaxis, and cough. Chronic exposure may cause ulceration, bleeding, and erosion of the nasal septum. Cough, chest pain, and dyspnea may indicate exposure to irritant levels of soluble chromium compounds or the development of chromium-induced asthma. Weight loss, cough, and hemoptysis in a chromium worker should suggest the development of bronchogenic carcinoma.

Dermatologic manifestations are common in chromium workers. Penetration of the skin will cause painless erosive ulceration with delayed healing. These commonly occur on the fingers, knuckles, and forearms. Localized erythematous or vesicular lesions at points of contact or generalized eczematous dermatitis should suggest sensitization.

Ingestion of chromium compounds has caused nausea, vomiting, abdominal pain, and prostration. Death is due to uremia.

Chromium is a proven human carcinogen. Workers involved in chromate production, chrome plating, and chrome alloy work have all been found to have increased incidence of lung cancer. The chromium compounds responsible for human cancers have been identified, but hexavalent chromium compounds (chromates) are animal carcinogens and mutagenic in microbial assay systems. Trivalent chromium is not mutagenic in these same in systems.

B. Laboratory Findings: With massive exposure there will be evidence of renal and hepatic damage. Proteinuria and hematuria will precede anuria and uremia. A reduction in the FEV_1/FVC ratio on spirometry may be seen after acute irritant exposure or in workers with chromium-induced asthma. Allergy can be confirmed by patch testing.

x-ray changes consistent with pneumoconiosis may be seen in workers exposed to trivalent chromium compounds. Persistent cough, hemoptysis, or a mass lesion on chest x-ray in a chromium worker should prompt a thorough evaluation for possible lung cancer.

Prevention

Reduction of exposure to airborne soluble hexavalent chromium compounds and improved worker hygiene will reduce the respiratory and nasal complications. Avoidance of skin contact—particularly contact with damaged or inflamed skin—will reduce the risk of developing chrome ulcers or skin sensitization. Prompt evaluation for skin sensitization will prevent the development of severe or chronic dermatitis. The value of sputum cytology to screen for lung cancer is unproved.

Exposure to hexavalent chromium compounds should be reduced to the lowest feasible levels to reduce the risk of lung cancer. Chromium workers should also be encouraged to stop smoking. Biologic monitoring of urine chromium levels may be useful as an assessment of recent exposure. Workers exposed to 0.05 mg/m^3 were found to have urine levels of 40–50 μg/L at the end of an 8-hour work shift compared to 4–5 μg/L in controls.

Treatment

Persons who have suffered acute inhalation injury should be admitted to the hospital for observation. Supplemental oxygen and bronchodilators may be required. Careful attention to fluid and electrolyte balance is indicated in the setting of acute renal injury. Chromium-induced nasal and skin ulcerations should be treated with a 10% ointment of CaNa$_2$ ⁓DTA (calcium disodium edetate) and an impervious ⁓ssing with frequent application to prevent forma-⁓ of persistent, insoluble Cr (III). Persons who ⁓lop chromium respiratory or skin allergy should ⁓noved from further exposure if they cannot be ⁓tely protected.

⁓s
⁓g,
⁓an
⁓um **of Diagnosis**
⁓not *⁓cute effects:*
⁓om- ⁓ain (colic).
⁓ are ⁓y.
⁓alent ⁓re.
⁓ vitro

⁓osure, *⁓effects:*
⁓amage.
⁓uria and ⁓ias.
⁓ratio on
⁓ exposure ⁓notor).
⁓ma. Skin ⁓ces and chronic enceph-
⁓ng. Chest

- Gout and gouty nephropathy.
- Chronic renal failure.

Alkyl lead compounds:
- Fatigue and lassitude.
- Headache.
- Nausea and vomiting.
- Neuropsychiatric complaints (memory loss, difficulty in concentrating).
- Delirium, seizures, coma.

Exposure Limits

Lead, inorganic, dusts and fumes
ACGIH TLV: 0.15 mg/m^3 TWA
OSHA PEL: 0.05 mg/m^3 TWA (now under court remand)
NIOSH REL: < 100 μg Pb/m^3 TWA; air level to be maintained so that worker blood lead remains < 60 μg/100 g of whole blood
Tetraethyl lead
ACGIH TLV: 0.1 mg/m^3 TWA
OSHA PEL: 0.075 mg/m^3 TWA

General Considerations

Lead is a soft, malleable, blue-gray metal characterized by high density and corrosion resistance. Lead occurs in many ores in concentrations of 1–11%. The ores of commercial interest include the sulfide (galena), the carbonate (cerussite), and the sulfate (anglesite). Lead is concentrated through wet grinding and flotation prior to smelting. Smelting is a 3-step process, involving blending, sintering, and blast furnace reduction. Lead bullion and slag are further refined through pyrometallurgic or electrolytic processes to remove copper, arsenic, antimony, zinc, tin, bismuth, and other metal contaminants. In the USA, over one-third of the lead produced is recovered from secondary sources of lead scrap.

Lead serves no useful biologic function in humans. The release of lead into the environment from automobile emissions and the burning of coal—and its subsequent bioaccumulation in many organisms, including humans—has profound public health implications. Over the past 15 years, there has been growing concern over the health effects of low-level lead exposure and the "normal" body burden of lead. In the occupational setting, the "no effect" level for lead exposure is being scrutinized as more sensitive measures of the physiologic effects of lead are studied.

Use

The primary use of lead is in the manufacture of storage batteries. In the chemical and building industries, lead alloys (chiefly with antimony and tin) are used in pipes and cable sheathing, where they impart resistance to acids and moisture. Tin-lead alloys are used in solder for electrical applications. Lead compounds are used in paints and plastics as pigments and stabilizers. Lead glazes impart brilliance and hardness to ceramics.

Lead is used in construction for attenuation of sound and vibration and for the shielding of radioactivity. Tetraethyl and tetramethyl lead are used primarily as antiknock agents in gasoline, though this use has declined significantly to meet strict emission requirements. Other uses include ammunition (lead shot), bronze and brass, cosmetics, and jewelry.

Occupational & Environmental Exposure

Inhalation and ingestion are potential routes of lead exposure in mining, particularly the more soluble carbonate and sulfate ores. Grinding and sintering operations generate high levels of lead dust and fumes. Workers engaged in the reclamation of lead from secondary sources have potential exposure to lead as well as other metal contaminants. Exposure is a constant hazard in the manufacture of lead batteries. Paint and pigment manufacturers are exposed to lead additives. Painters may also be exposed to lead, especially during fine spray-painting operations. Torch burning to remove lead-based paints generates significant quantities of lead fumes. Welders and brazers may be exposed to lead alloys, fluxes, and coatings. Workers in munitions plants and rifle ranges may have exposure to lead dust, particularly indoors. Glass-makers, artists, and pottery workers may unknowingly be exposed to high levels of lead in pigments and glazes.

Environmental exposure may occur near lead smelters due to air, soil, and water contamination. Urban residents have exposure to lead from automobile exhausts. Children in older, low-income housing may ingest lead paint chips from decaying structures. Ingestion of moonshine whiskey is another source of acute lead poisoning. Improperly fired ceramics may release lead, especially into acidic foods and beverages.

Herbal remedies, lead cosmetics, gasoline sniffing, and retained bullets are less conventional sources of lead poisoning. Lead contamination of tap water from lead pipes is an important source of lead exposure in many older homes.

Absorption, Metabolism, & Excretion

Inhalation and ingestion are the primary routes of absorption of lead compounds. Approximately 40% of inhaled lead oxide fumes is absorbed through the respiratory tract. Absorption of particulate lead dust depends on particle size and solubility. Roughly 5–10% of ingested lead compounds are absorbed from the gastrointestinal tract. Iron and calcium deficiencies and high-fat diets may increase the gastrointestinal absorption of lead. Gastrointestinal absorption is greater in infants and children than in adults.

In the bloodstream, the majority of the absorbed lead is bound to erythrocytes. The free diffusible plasma fraction is distributed to brain, kidney, liver, skin, and skeletal muscle, where it is readily exchangeable. The concentrations in these tissues are highest with acute, high-dose exposure. Lead crosses the placenta, and fetal levels correlate with maternal levels. Bone constitutes the major site of deposition of absorbed lead, where it is incorporated into the bony matrix similar to calcium. The lead in dense bone is only slowly mobilized and gradually increases with time.

Intracellularly, lead binds to sulfhydryl groups and interferes with numerous cellular enzymes, including those involved in heme synthesis. This binding accounts for the presence of lead in hair and nails. Lead also binds to mitochondrial membranes and interferes with protein and nucleic acid synthesis.

Excretion is slow over time, primarily through the kidney. Fecal excretion, sweat, and epidermal exfoliation are other routes of excretion. The half-life of lead is long, estimated to be from 5 to 10 years. This varies with the intensity and duration of exposure and the ultimate body burden accumulated. Bone diseases (osteoporosis, fractures) may lead to increased release of stored lead and elevated blood lead levels.

Water-insoluble alkyl lead compounds are readily absorbed through intact skin. Respiratory and gastrointestinal absorption are significant as well. Tetraethyl and tetramethyl lead are converted to the trialkyl metabolites that are responsible for toxicity. The fat solubility of these compounds accounts for their accumulation in the central nervous system. Alkyl lead compounds are ultimately converted to inorganic lead and are excreted in the urine.

Clinical Findings

A. Symptoms and Signs:

1. Inorganic lead–

a. Acute exposure–After acute or subacute exposure to lead through either ingestion or inhalation, the presenting symptoms are usually gastrointestinal. Cramping, colicky abdominal pain, and constipation are often present early. Abdominal pain may be severe, suggesting biliary colic or appendicitis. Nausea, vomiting, and black, tarry stools may also accompany the acute presentation.

Neurologic manifestations of lead encephalopathy include headache, confusion, stupor, coma, and seizures and are more common in children. Funduscopic examination may reveal papilledema or optic neuritis. In severe cases, oliguria and acute renal failure may develop rapidly.

b. Chronic exposure–In the occupational setting, chronic lead intoxication is a slow, insidious disease with protean manifestations. Fatigue, apathy, irritability, and vague gastrointestinal symptoms are early signs of chronic lead intoxication. Arthralgias and myalgias may involve the extremities of axial structures. As exposure continues, central nervous system symptoms progress, with insomnia, confusion, impaired concentration, and memory problems. Long-term exposure can lead to a distal motor neuropathy presenting with wrist drop. Progression to frank lead encephalopathy with seizures and coma is rare in adults but may occur.

Other presenting symptoms include loss of libido and infertility in men and menstrual disturbances and spontaneous abortion in women. Gouty arthritis and nephropathy have also been associated with chronic lead exposure.

Physical examination may reveal pallor due to anemia. Jaundice may be present in the setting of acute hemolysis. A blue-gray pigmentation ("lead line") may be present on the gums. Neurologic examination may reveal weakness, particularly of the distal extensor muscles.

In men, there is limited evidence of altered spermatogenesis. Lead crosses the placenta, and maternal exposure prior to and during pregnancy can result in fetal exposure and toxicity.

2. Alkyl lead–The presenting symptoms of alkyl lead intoxication are neurologic. Anorexia, insomnia, fatigue, weakness, headache, depression, and irritability are early symptoms. These progress to confusion, memory impairment, excitability, dysesthesias (eg, insects crawling on the body), mania, and toxic psychosis. In severe cases, delirium, seizures, coma, and death may occur in several days.

B. Laboratory Findings: Anemia is a frequent manifestation of lead intoxication in children but is unusual in adults. The anemia is usually normochromic. Increased red cell turnover and frank hemolysis may be present, with basophilic stippling of the red blood cells and reticulocytosis. Altered heme synthesis, evidenced by an increase in protoporphyrin—measured as either free erythrocyte protoporphyrin (FEP) or zinc protoporphyrin (ZPP)—begins when blood lead levels exceed 40 μg/dL. Delta-aminolevulinic acid dehydratase (delta-ALAD), an enzyme inhibited by lead, may also be increased, though measurement of this enzyme is not readily available.

Proximal renal injury may result in Fanconi's syndrome, with aminoaciduria, glycosuria, and phosphaturia. Impaired uric acid excretion results in hyperuricemia. Elevations of BUN and serum creatinine indicate impaired renal function. Liver involvement may be suggested by mild elevations of serum aminotransferases. Nerve conduction studies may reveal delayed motor conduction velocities even without overt peripheral neuropathy. Neuropsychiatric evaluation may reveal evidence of intellectual impairment and behavioral alterations.

Blood lead levels are an indication of recent exposure (days or weeks). Whole blood lead levels in nonexposed individuals range from 5 to 15 μg/dL. While frank lead poisoning is unusual with blood lead levels below 80 μg/dL, subtle effects of lead on the central and peripheral nervous system may occur with levels between 40 and 80 μg/dL. The current OSHA standard requires that lead levels be maintained below 40 μg/dL.

In individuals with significant signs or symptoms of chronic lead intoxication but no history of significant lead exposure, measurement of chelatable lead may assist in the diagnosis. A CaNa₂EDTA (calcium disodium edetate) lead-mobilization test is indicative of the total body burden and, when abnormally high, suggests that chelation therapy should be initiated (see Treatment, below). A 24-hour urine collection for lead using with the proper acid-washed polypropylene bottles is collected before and after giving a CaNa₂EDTA dose of 30 mg/kg body weight (up to 2 g) via intravenous infusion over 1 hour in 250 mL of 5% dextrose in water (a regimen recommended by Rempel, 1989). CaNa₂EDTA may be given intramuscularly, but that route is more painful. If the urine lead in the second 24-hour sample is more than double that in the first—or if it exceeds 600 μg of lead, the test is indicative of a high body burden of lead. This will confirm past lead exposure, but the test is still only indirect evidence of lead toxicity. Chronic accumulation of lead in bone may also be measured using x-ray fluorescence and bone densitometry.

Prevention

Workplace hygiene is critical in the prevention of excessive lead exposure. Clean areas for eating should be provided. Showering and cleaning of work garments are mandatory and should be provided at the plant to prevent exposure of children in the home. For processes that have the potential for generation of airborne dusts and fumes, respiratory protection should be provided.

Medical surveillance is required under the OSHA Lead Standard for workers exposed in excess of the Action Level of 30 μg/m³ for over 30 days per year, regardless of the use of respiratory protection. The program should include the following medical and biologic monitoring procedures:

Whole blood lead levels:

(1) Every 6 months if < 40 μg/dL.

(2) Every 2 months if > 40 μg/dL until 2 consecutive determinations are < 40 μg/dL.

(3) Monthly during medical removal from exposure.

Medical examinations (Table 25–1):

(1) Yearly, if any blood lead level exceeded 40 μg/dL.

(2) Prior to assignment in an area where air lead levels are at or above the Action Level.

(3) As soon as possible, if a worker develops signs or symptoms or lead intoxication.

Removal from exposure to lead:

(1) Workers whose lead levels exceed 60 μg/dL, unless the last lead level is < 40 μg/dL.

(2) Workers whose last 3 lead levels or lead levels over the past 6 months (whichever is longer) exceed 50 μg/dL unless the last lead level is < 40 μg/dL.

(3) Workers who have an increased risk of material impairment of health from exposure to lead.

Worker removal due to elevated blood lead levels is the responsibility of the employer and should be undertaken without regard to worker health. Workers

Table 25–1. Medical examination of lead-exposed workers.

Medical and occupational history
  Focusing on lead exposure history; personal and work-place hygiene; gastrointestinal, hematologic, renal, reproductive, and neurologic problems.
Physical examination
  Focusing on the gums and on the gastrointestinal, hematologic, renal, reproductive, and neurologic systems. Pulmonary status should be evaluated in workers required to wear respiratory protective devices.
Blood pressure measurement
Blood testing
  Blood lead level.
  Zinc protoporphyrin or free erythrocyte protoporphyrin.
  Hemoglobin, hematocrit, and peripheral smear.
  Serum creatinine.
  Urinalysis, with microscopic examination.
Other tests
  As clinically indicated.

may be returned to exposure if 2 consecutive blood lead levels are less than 40 μg/dL.

Removal due to risk of substantial health impairment is a medical decision and should not be based solely on blood lead levels. Workers removed because of risk of health impairment may be returned when the final medical determination is that the worker is no longer at risk.

The occupational physician may encounter workplaces (particularly small operations) where workers have elevated blood lead and ZPP levels but are asymptomatic. In these instances, removal of an entire work force from exposure is clearly not feasible. A program of frequent medical and biologic monitoring should be instituted while industrial hygiene, engineering, and personal protective measures are instituted to reduce exposures to acceptable levels.

Treatment

In all cases of suspected lead intoxication in adults, the first step in management is removal from exposure. This may mean removal from the workplace if hygienic conditions are such that secondary exposure is significant. The decision about whether chelation therapy is needed depends on the intensity and duration of exposure and the clinical signs and symptoms. The primary indication for treatment of adults is brief, high-level exposure causing acute manifestations (encephalopathy, hemolysis, renal injury). The combined measurement of blood lead and ZPP may help in management: An elevated blood lead (> 60 μg/dL) with a normal ZPP (< 100 mg/dL) suggests a recent increase in exposure.

Much more difficult is the management of the worker with vague complaints, such as abdominal pain, fatigue, muscle aches, or irritability. In a young worker with short-term exposure and an elevated blood lead level (> 100 μg/dL), these could be considered indications for treatment both to ameliorate symptoms and reduce the body burden. In long-term lead workers, removal from exposure

remains the treatment of choice, chelation being reserved for those with severe manifestations (ie, frank encephalopathy).

While vague symptoms of ill health can occur as a result of exposure to lead, these nonspecific findings may be related to other health problems. Generally, symptoms related to lead will gradually improve after removal from exposure and reduction in blood lead levels. Symptoms that persist or worsen following removal from exposure should not be assumed to be due to lead and should prompt appropriate diagnostic evaluations.

A. Acute Poisoning: After poisoning by ingestion, induce emesis and then catharsis. Hydration is essential to reduce acute renal injury. In adults, the use of chelation therapy should be reserved for patients with significant symptoms or signs of toxicity. The patient should be hospitalized and treatment overseen by a physician who has experience with chelation therapy. The protocol recommended by Rempel (1989) is for adult patients, not for children. If the BUN and urinalysis are normal, 2 g of $CaNa_2EDTA$ in 1000 mL of 5% dextrose in water are infused intravenously over 24 hours. This is repeated daily for 5 days until a total of 10 g $CaNa_2EDTA$ has been administered. Urinalysis, BUN, and serum creatinine should be followed daily; if proteinuria, hematuria, or renal dysfunction is observed, $CaNa_2EDTA$ should be discontinued. Oral penicillamine has serious adverse reactions and should be administered only by physicians with experience in its use.

B. Chronic Poisoning: Results of the lead-mobilization test together with the presence of significant symptoms or signs of toxicity should support the decision to treat with the same hospital protocol set forth above. If acute renal failure ensues, discontinue $CaNa_2EDTA$ treatment and institute hemodialysis.

C. Lead Encephalopathy: Lead encephalopathy is extremely rare in the occupational setting. When it occurs, it is a medical emergency. Treatment with chelation therapy should be instituted as described above. Cerebral edema should be treated and seizures controlled by a physician experienced in the care of such patients. Owing to the rarity of this problem in the occupational setting, it is wise to establish a consultative relationship with a physician whose background includes medical management of lead encephalopathy cases.

D. Chronic Overexposure: For workers with mild symptoms, removal from exposure is the treatment of choice. Chelation may not be effective for workers with long-term exposure (and an excessive body burden of lead), and treatment with $CaNa_2EDTA$ may cause acute tubular necrosis. Prophylactic chelation should not be used and is prohibited by the OSHA Lead Standard.

E. Organic Level: In acute alkyl lead intoxication, chelation therapy is of no benefit. Treatment should be directed at the presenting symptoms as indicated.

Prognosis

Early diagnosis and treatment of lead toxicity will generally result in complete recovery. Once renal or neurologic impairment has occurred, only partial recovery may be expected.

MANGANESE

Essentials of Diagnosis

Acute effects:
- Fever, chills, dyspnea (metal fume fever.)

Chronic effects:
- Parkinsonlike syndrome.
- Behavioral changes, psychosis.
- Pneumonia.

Exposure Limits

Manganese dust and compounds
  ACGIH TLV: 5 mg/m^3 TWA
  OSHA PEL: 5 mg/m^3 ceiling
Manganese fume
  ACGIH TLV: 1 mg/m^3 TWA, 3 mg/m^3 STEL
  OSHA PEL: 1 mg/m^3 TWA, 3 mg/m^3 STEL
Manganese cyclopentadienyl tricarbonyl
  ACGIH TLV: 0.1 mg/m^3 TWA
  OSHA PEL: 0.1 mg/m^3 TWA
Manganese tetroxide
  OSHA PEL: 1 mg/m^3 TWA

General Considerations

Manganese is a brittle gray metal that is abundant in the earth's crust, soils, and sediments and in biologic materials. The most important source of manganese for commercial use is manganese dioxide, occurring as pyrolusite. Manganese is an essential trace element in humans and other living organisms. Manganese is present in highest concentrations in cells with high levels of metabolic activity, and several manganese-dependent enzyme systems have been identified.

Use

Ferromanganese, an iron alloy containing over 80% manganese metal, is essential in the large-scale production of steel. Manganese is also used as a depolarizer in dry cell batteries and as an oxidizing agent in the chemical industry. Manganese is used in the manufacture of matches, paints, and pesticides. The manganese carbonyls, particularly methylcyclopentadienyl manganese tricarbonyl (MMT), is finding increasing use as an antiknock agent in unleaded gasoline and in jet fuel. The manganese carbonyls are also used as a source of pure manganese metal in the electronics industry.

Occupational & Environmental Exposure

Exposure to manganese dioxide occurs in the mining, smelting, and refining of manganese ores. Manganese exposure also occurs near crushing oper-ations and reduction furnaces engaged in the production of ferrous and nonferrous alloys and in steel production. The use of manganese-containing welding rods is another source of potential worker exposure.

Exposure may also occur in the chemical industry and in the electronics industry. Workers engaged in the manufacture of fuels containing MMT may have respiratory or skin contact with this highly toxic liquid. Combustion of manganese containing fuels evolves primarily manganese oxides.

Absorption, Metabolism, & Excretion

Manganese fumes may reach the alveoli and be absorbed after inhalation. Larger particles are ingested after mucociliary clearance from the lungs. Gastrointestinal absorption is generally low (10%) but may be increased in persons who are iron-deficient. MMT may be absorbed after ingestion, inhalation, or skin contact.

Manganese is primarily excreted in the bile and may undergo enterohepatic recirculation. The biologic half-life of manganese is approximately 30 hours, though in chronically exposed workers this may be shortened to 15 hours. Blood and urine levels are elevated in exposed workers but do not correlate with toxicity. Variations in manganese homeostasis may account for individual susceptibility to the development of toxic effects.

Clinical Findings

A. Symptoms and Signs:

1. Acute exposure—Acute exposure to manganese oxide fumes may result in the development of metal fume fever, a self-limited illness characterized by fever, chills, and dyspnea. Dermal and respiratory exposure to MMT results in slight burning of the skin followed by the development of headache, a metallic taste, nausea, diarrhea, dyspnea, and chest pain. Based on animal studies, acute overexposure to MMT could cause chemical pneumonitis, hepatic toxicity, and renal toxicity.

2. Chronic exposure—Industrial exposure to manganese has more frequently resulted in chronic effects on the nervous system, usually after several years. The earliest manifestations are vague symptoms of fatigue, headache, apathy, and behavioral disturbances. Episodes of excitability, garrulousness, and sexual arousal have been termed "manganese psychosis." With continued exposure, there is development of a syndrome that closely resembles Parkinson's disease. Speech becomes slow and monotonous and the worker develops a masked facies. Tremor, bradykinesia, gait disturbance, and micrographia may all be present, comprising a syndrome identical to idiopathic parkinsonism. Excessive salivation and sweating and vasomotor disturbances may also occur. Exposure to MMT has not been associated with nervous system toxicity, though experience with this compound is limited.

Worker exposure to manganese dust has also been associated with increased susceptibility to pneumonia and respiratory infections, often refractory to treatment. An inhibitory effect of manganese dioxide on pulmonary macrophage function may be responsible for this effect.

B. Laboratory Findings: Laboratory findings are usually normal. Minor decreases in leukocyte and red blood cell counts may be seen. Liver enzyme elevations have also been reported. Elevation of protein in cerebrospinal fluid often accompanies central nervous system toxicity.

Measurement of elevated urine manganese or finding an increase in urine manganese after a dose of calcium disodium edetate, a manganese chelator, serve to confirm exposure. Levels do not correlate with degree of toxicity.

Prevention

Manganese exposure should be reduced by the use of closed systems, local exhaust ventilation, and respiratory protection. Dermal and respiratory exposure to MMT should be prevented through use of proper personal protective equipment. Medical surveillance should focus on nervous system symptoms and changes in behavior to identify affected workers while the condition is still reversible. Careful neurologic examinations should be performed routinely on all exposed workers. Workers with exposure to MMT should also have periodic assessment of respiratory, liver, and kidney function.

Treatment

Metal fume fever requires no specific treatment. Pneumonia should be treated with appropriate antibiotics as well as removal from exposure until the disease has cleared.

After skin contact with MMT, the affected areas should be cleansed immediately to reduce skin absorption. Workers who develop respiratory symptoms after inhalation of MMT should be admitted to the hospital for observation. Liver and kidney function should be monitored.

In workers with chronic exposure to manganese, the nervous system effects are reversible if they are detected early. Subjective symptoms may be the only manifestations at this stage. Once signs of parkinsonism have developed, the condition may be permanent, though progression will cease after exposure is terminated. Treatment with levodopa as for idiopathic parkinsonism is effective. Calcium disodium edetate chelation will increase urinary excretion of manganese but is ineffective in reversing the nervous system effects.

MERCURY

Essentials of Diagnosis

Inorganic mercury:
- Acute respiratory distress.

- Gingivitis.
- Tremor.
- Erethism (shyness, emotional lability).
- Proteinuria, renal failure.

Organic mercury (alkyl mercury compounds):
- Mental disturbances.
- Ataxia, spasticity.
- Paresthesias.
- Visual and auditory disturbances.

Exposure Limits

Alkyl compounds
ACGIH TLV: 0.01 mg/m^3 TWA, 0.03 mg/m^3 STEL
OSHA PEL: 0.01 mg/m^3 TWA, 0.03 mg/m^3 STEL
Vapor (all forms except alkyl)
ACGIH TLV: 0.05 mg/m^3 TWA
OSHA PEL: 0.05 mg/m^3 TWA
Aryl and inorganic compounds
ACGIH TLV: 0.1 mg/m^3
OSHA PEL: 0.1 mg/m^3 ceiling
NIOSH REL: 0.05 mg/m^3

General Considerations

Mercury is a heavy, silvery-white metal that is a liquid at room temperature. Its low vapor pressure presents the constant hazard of airborne exposure to mercury compounds. Mercury is present in numerous classes of rocks and is recovered primarily from cinnabar ore (HgS). Ore is mined using both surface and underground methods. Mercury is recovered through heating in furnaces and retorts. While mercury is ubiquitous in nature, environmental contamination and subsequent bioaccumulation—particularly in seafood—has led to strict emission controls. Mercury is not considered to be an essential element in humans.

Use

A major use of mercury is in the manufacture of control instruments, tubes, rectifiers, thermometers, barometers, batteries, and electrical devices. Mercury is used in brine cells for the electrolytic production of chlorine and caustic soda and as a catalyst in polyurethane foams. Use of alkyl mercury compounds (methyl mercury and ethyl mercury) as grain fumigants and antimildew agents has been banned in the USA—replaced by less toxic mercury compounds. Mercury is used in plating, jewelry, tanning, and taxidermy. Use in the felt industry in the 19th century led to extensive poisoning ("mad as a hatter"), and such use has been discontinued also. Mercury amalgams are used in dentistry. Mercury has been used in medicinal preparations (eg, mercurial diuretics) in the past, but these have been largely replaced by less toxic agents.

Occupational & Environmental Exposure

All workers involved in the extraction and recovery of mercury are at high risk for exposure to mercury vapor. Maintenance work on furnaces, flues, and retorts is an important potential source of exposure. Workers in chlorine plants are also at risk, though most operate using closed systems.

Workers engaged in the manufacture of electrical equipment requiring mercury may be exposed through spillage or careless handling. Metal reclaiming workers may be exposed to mercury as well as other heavy metals. In production areas where mercury is used as a catalyst, workers may be exposed through improper storing and handling or during maintenance operations. Dentists, dental technicians, and other laboratory workers may be exposed if mercury is not handled carefully. Workers may be exposed to alkyl mercury compounds during the production and application of organic mercury fungicides.

Several epidemics of organic mercury poisoning have occurred as a result of environmental contamination from industrial effluents and improper use of grain fumigants. Release of organic mercury into Minamata Bay in Japan resulted in accumulation of methyl mercury in seafood, poisoning thousands of individuals (''Minamata disease''). Similar mass poisonings have occurred after consumption of grain treated with alkyl mercury compounds. Air and water contamination with inorganic mercury from the burning of coal and from chlorine plants has had less dramatic consequences but has been a significant source of background exposure.

Absorption, Metabolism, & Excretion

Elemental mercury is absorbed after the inhalation of mercury vapor. Ingested elemental mercury forms globules that are poorly absorbed from the gastrointestinal tract. Soluble mercurial salts (Hg^{2+}) and aryl mercury compounds are also absorbed after inhalation and to a limited extent after ingestion. Alkyl mercury compounds are readily absorbed through all routes—inhalation, ingestion, or skin contact.

Inorganic and aryl mercury compounds are distributed to many tissues, primarily the brain and kidney. There they bind to sulfhydryl groups and may interfere with numerous cellular enzyme systems. Metallothionein (a low-molecular-weight protein rich in sulfhydryl groups) production is increased after mercury exposure and may exert a protective effect in the kidney. Alkyl mercury compounds have a tight carbon-mercury bond and accumulate in the central nervous system. In the bloodstream, the majority of the absorbed alkyl mercury is found in the red blood cells.

Both organic and inorganic mercury compounds readily cross the blood-brain barrier and the placenta and are secreted in breast milk. All mercury compounds are eliminated slowly in the urine, feces, saliva, and sweat. The average half-life in humans is 60 days for inorganic mercury and 70 days for alkyl

mercury compounds. Mercury also binds to thiol groups and may be measured in the hair and nails.

Clinical Findings

A. Symptoms and Signs:

1. Inorganic mercury—Inhalation of high concentrations of mercury vapor or soluble mercury salts usually is a result of work in enclosed spaces. Cough, dyspnea, inflammation of the oral cavity, and gastrointestinal complaints occur shortly after exposure. These may be followed by the development of a chemical pneumonitis with cyanosis, tachypnea, and pulmonary edema. Renal injury presents as an initial diuresis followed by proteinuria and oliguric renal failure. After recovery from the acute illness, neurologic symptoms may develop similar to those seen with chronic overexposure. Ingestion of soluble mercury compounds results in gastrointestinal complaints of nausea, vomiting, diarrhea, and abdominal pain, which may be followed by renal and neurologic sequelae.

Chronic exposure to inorganic mercury compounds results primarily in effects on the nervous system. Neuropsychiatric manifestations include changes in personality, shyness, anxiety, memory loss, and emotional lability. Tremor is an early sign of neurotoxicity. Initially, the tremor is fine and occurs at rest, progressing with further exposure to an intention tremor interrupted by coarse jerking movements. A comparison with prior handwriting may demonstrate the tremor. Head tremor and skeletal ataxia may also occur. A combination of tremor, gait ataxia, and bradykinesia may mimic parkinsonism. A sensory peripheral neuropathy is usually present with distal paresthesias. Hallucinations and dementia are late manifestations.

Other findings after excessive chronic exposure include inflammation of the oral cavity, manifested by salivation, gingivitis, and dental erosions. A bluish linear pigmentation may be present on the teeth or gums. Reddish-brown pigmentation of the lens may be apparent on slit lamp examination. Renal injury usually results in proteinuria without frank renal failure. Excessive sweating and an eczematous skin eruption may also be present.

2. Organic mercury—Exposure to alkyl mercury compounds results in the insidious onset of progressive nervous system effects. The earliest symptoms are of numbness and tingling of the extremities and lips. Loss of motor coordination follows, with gait ataxia, tremor, and loss of fine movement. Constriction of the visual fields, central hearing loss, muscular rigidity, and spasticity occur with exaggerated deep tendon reflexes. Behavioral changes, fits of laughter, and intellectual impairment may be prominent. Erythroderma, desquamation, and other skin rashes may be present. Renal disease is rare. Neurotoxicity in infants exposed in utero in the Minamata Bay epidemic resembled cerebral palsy.

B. Laboratory Findings: After acute inhalation, there may be hypoxemia (as shown by arterial blood gas measurements) and diffuse infiltrates on chest x-ray. Proteinuria indicates renal injury. The earliest manifestation of renal injury is increased excretion of low-molecular-weight proteins, including N-acetyl-β-glucosaminidase, $β_2$-microglobulin, and retinol-binding protein.

Measurement of mercury in blood and urine will confirm the diagnosis. Gross renal or neurologic manifestations are unusual unless urine mercury levels exceed 500–1000 μg/L. Subtle nervous system effects have been detected in workers with levels of 300 μg/L, and early renal effects (low-molecular-weight proteinuria with normal renal function) have been detected when urine mercury levels chronically exceed 100–150 μg/L. Normal concentrations in nonexposed individuals are less than 0.02 mg/L in whole blood and less than 10 μg/L in urine. Substantial seafood consumption may result in higher levels. A high ratio of whole blood mercury to plasma mercury suggests alkyl mercury intoxication. Hair and nail levels may be elevated in intoxication but are subject to external contamination.

Prevention

Awareness of the constant hazard of mercury vapor exposure along with proper handling of materials and meticulous attention to workplace hygiene will reduce potential exposures. Use of proper ventilation and respiratory protection is required in all operations that use mercury compounds. Special attention should focus on maintenance workers. Care in the handling and disposal of mercury compounds will prevent inadvertent contamination of the workplace. Control of industrial emissions will prevent contamination of waterways and seafood. Grain fumigation with mercury compounds should be restricted.

Medical surveillance of mercury-exposed workers should include a careful history and neurologic examination as well as periodic urinalyses. Individuals exposed to 0.05 mg/m^3 of mercury vapor in air should have urine mercury levels between 50 and 100 μg/L. Higher levels indicate excessive exposure and a decreased margin of safety in the prevention of neurologic and renal toxicity. Urine levels fluctuate, and periodic monitoring or group monitoring will be more representative of ongoing exposure. Greater accuracy may be obtained by collecting 24-hour specimens or adjusting to urine creatinine.

Treatment

After acute exposure to mercury, prompt treatment with dimercaprol (5 mg/kg intramuscularly) should be instituted. Respiratory distress and renal failure should be treated appropriately. Penicillamine is also effective for acute poisoning.

Individuals manifesting symptoms of chronic mercury toxicity should be removed from further exposure. The decision to give treatment in such cases depends on the severity of the symptoms and whether evidence of neurologic or renal toxicity is present. Recently, 2 individuals with mild chronic mercury

poisoning responded to treatment with the investigational drug 2,3-dimercaptopropane-1-sulfonate (100 mg orally 3 times daily, increasing to 4 times daily, for several weeks). The neurologic sequelae of alkyl mercury poisoning are irreversible, emphasizing the need for prevention.

NICKEL

Essentials of Diagnosis

Nickel compounds (except nickel carbonyl):
- Allergic contact dermatitis, eczema.
- Sinusitis, anosmia.
- Asthma.
- Nasal and lung cancer.

Nickel carbonyl:
- Headache, fatigue, gastrointestinal symptoms.
- Cough, dyspnea.
- Interstitial pneumonitis.
- Delirium, coma.

Exposure Limits

Nickel, metal
    ACGIH TLV: 1 mg/m^3 TWA
    OSHA PEL: 1 mg/m^3 TWA
Nickel, soluble compounds
    ACGIH TLV: 0.1 mg/m^3 TWA
    OSHA PEL: 0.1 mg/m^3 TWA
Nickel carbonyl
    ACGIH TLV: 0.1 mg/m^3 TWA
    OSHA PEL: 0.007 mg/m^3 TWA
    NIOSH REL: 0.007 mg/m^3 TWA (lowest detectable concentration)

General Considerations

Nickel is a hard, silver-white, malleable, magnetic metal that has wide industrial application. Pentlandite—$(Fe,Ni)_9S_8$—the primary commercial ore, is often deposited with other iron and copper sulfides. Nickel sulfide is concentrated by flotation and magnetic separation prior to roasting. Nickel is refined using electrolysis or the Mond process, where treatment with carbon monoxide leads to the formation of nickel carbonyl—$Ni(CO)_4$. Nickel occurs naturally in a variety of vegetables and grains.

Use

The major use of nickel is in the production of stainless steel, where it may be present in concentrations of 5–10%. Nickel alloys with other metals, such as copper (Monel metal), supply durability and fabricating properties for applications in food and dairy processing equipment, chemical synthesis, and the petroleum industry. Coins, tableware and utensils, springs, magnets, batteries (nickel-cadmium), and spark plugs also utilize nickel alloys. Soluble nickel salts are used in electroplating to impart lustrous, polishable, corrosion-resistant surfaces to parts and equipment. Nickel compounds are also used as catalysts and pigments.

Occupational & Environmental Exposure

Exposure to nickel compounds may occur during mining, milling, roasting, sintering, and refining operations. In the Mond process, workers may also be exposed to highly toxic nickel carbonyl gas. Workers engaged in the production of nickel alloys—as well as those involved in the fabrication and welding of these materials—may also be exposed to nickel dusts and fumes. In electroplating shops, workers may have respiratory and skin exposure to soluble nickel salts. Workers using nickel as a catalyst may be exposed to nickel powders. Air levels may be elevated in communities surrounding roasting and sintering plants. Nickel and (presumably) nickel carbonyl are contaminants in cigarette smoke.

Absorption, Metabolism, & Excretion

Nickel is poorly absorbed from the gastrointestinal tract. Soluble nickel compounds and nickel carbonyl are readily absorbed after inhalation.

In plasma, nickel is bound to albumin and "nickelplasmin," a metalloprotein. Absorbed nickel does not accumulate in tissues and is excreted in the urine with a half-life of approximately 1 week.

Nickel is excreted to a lesser extent in sweat and bile. Insoluble nickel compounds may accumulate in the respiratory tract—a factor that may contribute to carcinogenicity. Nickel readily crosses the placental barrier and can be measured in fetal tissue.

Clinical Findings

A. Symptoms and Signs: The most common manifestations of exposure to soluble nickel compounds are dermatologic. Nickel is a common cause of skin allergy (usually nonoccupational) and may cause erythema and vesiculation at points of contact in sensitized individuals. Chronic eczematous dermatitis involving the hands and arms may also develop in nickel workers, particularly in electroplating shops where there is exposure to liquids and aerosols. Exposure to high levels of soluble nickel aerosols may also cause rhinitis, sinusitis, anosmia, and septal perforation. Cough and wheezing should suggest the possibility of nickel-induced asthma, though this is uncommon. Nickel fumes may cause an illness resembling metal fume fever.

Exposure to nickel carbonyl causes headache, fatigue, nausea, and vomiting. These symptoms usually resolve when the affected individual is removed to fresh air. In severe cases, there is a delay of 12–36 hours before development of a diffuse interstitial pneumonitis, with fever, chills, cough, chest pain, and dyspnea. Delirium, seizures, and coma may occur prior to death.

Exposure to nickel compounds in refining and nickel subsulfide roasting operations has caused an increase in nasal and respiratory cancers in humans. Smaller studies of workers exposed to pure nickel dust, nickel oxides, and nickel alloys have not shown an excess in respiratory cancers. Nickel, nickel subsulfide, nickel carbonyl, and other nickel compounds are carcinogenic in laboratory animals. Nickel should be considered a human respiratory carcinogen, and worker exposure should be reduced to the lowest feasible levels, particularly in refining and roasting operations.

B. Laboratory Findings: The diagnosis of nickel skin allergy can be confirmed by patch testing or lymphocyte transformation testing. Nickel-induced asthma may result in an elevated eosinophil count. After exposure to nickel carbonyl, there is a moderate leukocytosis, hypoxemia, and a reduction in lung volumes and carbon monoxide diffusing capacity consistent with acute pneumonitis. Liver enzymes may be elevated. In evaluating persons who have been exposed to nickel carbonyl, urine nickel levels greater than 100 μg/L indicate moderate exposure while levels in excess of 500 μg/L indicate severe exposure.

Prevention

Skin and respiratory protection should be used where there is potential exposure to nickel dusts, fumes, or soluble nickel aerosols and liquids. Extreme caution should be employed in handling gaseous nickel carbonyl. Medical surveillance should concentrate on the skin and respiratory system, with prompt removal of those who develop dermal or respiratory allergy. A biologic threshold level of 10 μg/L in plasma is recommended for workers exposed to nickel compounds. A maximum level of 10 μg/L in the urine is recommended for workers exposed to nickel carbonyl.

Treatment

Nickel dermatitis should be treated with topical steroids and removal from further exposure. Extremely sensitive individuals may not be able to work where there is any further exposure to nickel, even with proper personal protection. Nickel sensitivity is permanent. Respiratory tract irritation will resolve after removal from exposure.

Individuals who have been exposed to nickel carbonyl should be admitted to a hospital to be monitored for the development of pulmonary complications and systemic toxicity. An 8-hour urine collection should be sent for nickel measurement. If exposure is found to be excessive (urine nickel 100 μg/L), treatment should be instituted with sodium diethyldithiocarbamate (Dithiocarb). This may be given orally in a dosage of 50 mg/kg in divided doses as follows:

50% of total dose at time 0
25% of total dose at 4 hours
15% of total dose at 8 hours
10% of total dose at 16 hours and then an additional dose equivalent to 10% of the total dose every 8 hours until symptoms have resolved or urine nickel is below 50 μg/L.

In comatose or acutely ill persons, the drug may be

given in a dose of 25 mg/kg intramuscularly every 4 hours, increasing to 100 mg/kg depending on the clinical condition.

PHOSPHORUS

Essentials of Diagnosis
- Necrosis of the jaw.
- Dermal burns.
- Respiratory irritation.
- Hepatic and renal injury.

Exposure Limits
Phosphorus (yellow)
> ACGIH TLV: 0.1 mg/m^3 TWA
> OSHA PEL: 0.1 mg/m^3 TWA

Phosphine
> ACGIH TLV: 0.4 mg/m^3 TWA, 1 mg/m^3 STEL
> OSHA PEL: 0.4 mg/m^3 TWA, 1 mg/m^3 STEL

Phosphorus oxychloride
> ACGIH TLV: 0.6 mg/m^3 TWA, 3 mg/m^3 STEL
> OSHA PEL: 0.6 mg/m^3 TWA

Phosphoric acid
> ACGIH TLV: 1 mg/m^3 TWA, 3 mg/m^3 STEL

General Considerations

Phosphorus is an essential element for energy metabolism in many biologic systems. In nature, phosphorus does not occur free but is found in rock in the mineral apatite (tricalcium phosphate). Phosphorus rock is crushed and heated, liberating elemental phosphorus, which is then condensed and submerged in water to prevent spontaneous combustion in air. Two allotropes—the highly toxic white (yellow) form and red phosphorus—are of industrial importance. Elemental phosphorus is converted to phosphoric acid, phosphine, and phosphorus chlorides and sulfides for specific industrial applications.

Use

The use of white phosphorus in matches was banned after the turn of the century after numerous workers developed severe, disabling jaw necrosis ("phossy jaw"). This has been replaced by less toxic red phosphorus and phosphorus sesquisulfide. White phosphorus is still used in explosives, fireworks, smoke bombs, and rodenticides. Phosphoric acid is used in the production of superphosphate fertilizers. In the microelectronics industry, phosphorus is used as a dopant for silicon and for substrate material in mixed crystals. Phosphorus compounds are used in the manufacture of a variety of chemicals, including organophosphate pesticides.

Occupational & Environmental Exposure

Workers may be exposed to white phosphorus during production of explosives, pesticides, or other phosphorus compounds. Production workers engaged in the manufacture of matches and fertilizers may handle large quantities of phosphorus compounds. Semiconductor manufacturers may use elemental phosphorus, phosphorus chlorides, and phosphine as sources of phosphorus atoms. Phosphine may escape during the storage of ferrosilicon. Phosphine may also be liberated through the accidental wetting of zinc phosphide rodenticides or aluminum phosphide grain fumigants or during the manufacture of acetylene from calcium carbide. Accidental or suicidal ingestion of phosphorus-containing fireworks or rodenticides has been a cause of nonoccupational poisoning.

Absorption, Metabolism, & Excretion

Phosphorus may be absorbed after inhalation, ingestion, or skin contact. Spontaneous combustion in air leads to extensive tissue destruction of the skin, eyes, and mucous membranes. In the liver, phosphorus interferes with protein and carbohydrate metabolism and inhibits glycogen storage. Fat deposition in the liver is increased. Chronic exposure to phosphorus causes subepiphyseal bone formation with impaired vascularity, leading to bone necrosis. Excretion of inorganic phosphate is primarily through the kidney.

Clinical Findings
A. Symptoms and Signs:
1. Acute exposure—Ingestion of yellow phosphorus is followed in 1–2 hours by development of nausea, vomiting, and abdominal pain owing to local tissue injury. Phosphorescent vomitus and smoking stools may be clues to the diagnosis. Systemic manifestations, including uremia, jaundice, and liver enlargement, develop after several days. Hypocalcemic tetany with carpal and pedal muscle spasms may also develop. In severe cases, cardiac arrhythmias and coma may precede death.

Phosphorus burns may result following spontaneous combustion, when contaminated skin surfaces dry. Second- and third-degree phosphorus burns with blistering are characterized by slow healing. Absorption of phosphorus in severe cases may result in systemic phosphorus toxicity.

Inhalation of phosphorus compounds may cause bronchospasm with cough, chest tightness, and wheezing. Local tissue necrosis may cause hemoptysis. In severe cases, chemical pneumonitis may develop, with respiratory failure due to pulmonary edema followed by arrhythmias and signs of systemic phosphorus poisoning.

Inhalation of phosphine gas causes headache, fatigue, nausea, vomiting, and excessive thirst as well as cough, chest tightness, and shortness of breath. Neurologic symptoms include ataxia, paresthesias, tremor, and diplopia. Death may occur in 1–2 days from respiratory failure, cardiovascular collapse, or convulsions.

2. Chronic exposure—The main hazard from chronic exposure to yellow phosphorus was the development of jaw necrosis. This usually presents as a dental affliction followed by chronic suppuration. Persistent bacterial infection imparts a fetid odor to the breath. Other forms of phosphorus have not been associated with this condition. Workers exposed to irritant phosphorus compounds may develop obstructive lung disease and chronic bronchitis.

B. Laboratory Findings: Findings in acute intoxication with phosphorus compounds include elevated liver enzymes, hyperbilirubinemia, hematuria, proteinuria, and leukopenia. Profound hypocalcemia may occur. After acute inhalation injury, arterial hypoxemia may be present. Pulmonary function tests may show obstruction or a mixed obstructive and restrictive pattern with an impaired diffusing capacity for carbon monoxide.

Perihilar infiltrates on chest x-ray suggest a chemical pneumonitis or pulmonary edema. X-ray changes in phosphorus-induced jaw necrosis include degeneration, sequestration, and necrosis.

Prevention

Phosphorus must be handled with extreme care, using wet processes to avoid accidental exposure and spontaneous combustion. Skin, eye, and respiratory protection should be worn when handling phosphorus compounds. Awareness of the potential sources of exposure to phosphine gas will prevent accidental injury. Medical surveillance should concentrate on dental hygiene and respiratory, liver, and kidney function. There is currently no method for biologic monitoring of workers exposed to phosphorus compounds.

Treatment

After ingestion, perform gastric lavage with 5–10 L of tap water and induce vomiting. Follow with mineral oil. Hypocalcemia should be treated with calcium gluconate 10%, 10 mL intravenously, with close monitoring of serum calcium. Cardiac rhythm should be closely monitored during calcium repletion. Treat skin and eye burns with copious irrigation. A topical solution of 3% copper sulfate will neutralize phosphorus on the skin; however, extensive use may result in excessive absorption of copper. Phosphorus-induced bone necrosis may respond to drainage and appropriate antibiotic therapy. Surgical excision and bone grafting may be necessary in extensive cases.

SELENIUM

Essentials of Diagnosis

Acute effects:
- Respiratory, mucous membrane, and skin irritation.
- Skin burns.

Chronic effects:
- Fatigue, lassitude.

- Gastrointestinal complaints.
- Garlic odor of breath and sweat.
- Dermatitis, paronychia, alopecia.
- Conjunctivitis.

Exposure Limits
ACGIH TLV: 0.2 mg/m^3 TWA
OSHA PEL: 0.2 mg/m^3 TWA

General Considerations

Selenium is a metalloid element that is distributed widely in igneous rock, sedimentary rock, and mineral ores, particularly in sulfur and copper deposits. Selenium for commercial use is obtained primarily through extraction from slimes produced in the electrolytic refining of copper. Selenium exists in 3 forms: a red amorphous powder, a gray hexagonal semiconducting crystal, and a red crystal. Selenium is an essential trace element in humans, serving as a cofactor for glutathione peroxidase in the prevention of oxidative damage in erythrocytes.

Selenium has also been found to be teratogenic in animals. An isolated report found 4 spontaneous abortions and one congenital malformation among 10 women exposed to sodium selenite in a laboratory.

Use

Selenium is used in the manufacture of glass and plastics to impart a red tint or to neutralize green discoloration. The photoconducting properties of selenium are useful in rectifiers and photoelectric cells. Selenium is used to alter the machinability of steel and to increase the rate of vulcanization of rubber. Selenium is also used medicinally in dandruff shampoos and topical antifungal lotions. Selenium is used in paint pigments, animal feeds, and veterinary medicines. Selenium hexafluoride is used as a gaseous insulator in transformers.

Occupational & Environmental Exposure

Workers engaged in the smelting and refining of copper may be exposed to airborne selenium fumes and selenium oxide dust. Refinery and metal workers may also be exposed to hydrogen selenide through the reaction of acid with metal selenides. Elemental selenium is encountered in the electronics, glass, ceramics, plastics, and rubber industries. Formulators may be exposed to selenium in the production of pharmaceuticals and animal feed. Selenium is available commercially in dandruff shampoos and mineral supplements. Agricultural use of sodium selenite as a pesticide and selenium contamination of phosphate fertilizers has led to soil and ground water contamination.

Absorption, Metabolism, & Excretion

Selenium compounds may be absorbed through the lungs, gastrointestinal tract, or damaged skin. Selenium is metabolized to organic forms in the liver.

Dimethylselenium is excreted through the lungs and imparts a garlic odor to the breath. Trimethylselenium is excreted in the urine. Elevated levels may be seen for several weeks following exposure.

Clinical Findings

A. Symptoms and Signs:

1. Acute exposure—Acute inhalation of selenium fumes, selenium oxide dust, selenium oxychloride vapor, hydrogen selenium, or selenium hexafluoride may cause severe respiratory irritation, resulting in cough, chest pain, and dyspnea. In severe cases, a chemical pneumonitis with pulmonary edema may develop. Neurologic, hepatic, and renal damage may occur. Selenium oxide may cause severe skin burns.

2. Chronic exposure—Chronic exposure to selenium compounds may result in nonspecific complaints of fatigue and lassitude. Gastrointestinal complaints of nausea and indigestion may be present. There is a strong garlic odor to the breath and sweat. Chronic airborne exposure may cause conjunctivitis, termed ''rose eye.'' Dermatologic manifestations include irritant or allergic dermatitis, painful paronychia, and loss of hair and nails. Reddish skin and hair discoloration may also be present.

The role of selenium in the development of cancer in humans is uncertain. A protective effect has been proposed but not confirmed. Selenium has caused liver tumors in laboratory animals.

B. Laboratory Findings: Laboratory evaluation is usually nondiagnostic. Liver enzyme elevations and anemia may be seen. Measurement of selenium in the urine will confirm overexposure, normal concentrations being less than 150 μg/L.

Prevention

Respiratory and skin protection should be used where exposure to high levels of airborne selenium compounds cannot be controlled through other means. Medical surveillance should focus on gastrointestinal and dermatologic complaints. The detection of a garlic odor in an exposed individual should suggest excessive absorption. Urine selenium should remain below 100 μg/L in individuals exposed to air levels of 0.1 mg/m^3.

Treatment

Prompt evacuation and resuscitation should be undertaken in cases of acute inhalation. Burns of the skin should be irrigated with a solution of 10% aqueous sodium thiosulfate followed by use of a 10% sodium thiosulfate cream. Administration of ascorbic acid may lessen the offensive garlic odor of exposed individuals. Chelation is contraindicated and may cause renal damage.

TELLURIUM

Essentials of Diagnosis

- Respiratory irritation.
- Garlic odor.
- Fatigue, somnolence.
- Dryness of mouth and skin.
- Anhidrosis.
- Blue-black skin discoloration.

Exposure Limits

ACGIH TLV: 0.1 mg/m^3 TWA
OSHA PEL: 0.1 mg/m^3 TWA

General Considerations

Tellurium is a bright silvery metalloid element that shares many characteristics with selenium. Its distribution in rock and ore deposits is similar to that of selenium, though tellurium is much rarer. Tellurium—like selenium—is obtained primarily by extraction from anodic slimes formed as a by-product in copper refining. Tellurium compounds are generally less toxic than the corresponding selenium compounds. Although present in varying concentrations in human tissues, tellurium is not considered an essential trace element for humans.

Use

Tellurium is used in the vulcanization of rubber to increase durability. Like selenium, tellurium is finding increasing use in electronics, primarily in the manufacture of rectifiers and semiconductors. Tellurium imparts corrosive resistance in steel and is used as a carbide stabilizer for iron. Tellurium is used in numerous alloys, catalysts, pigments, and photographic chemicals.

Occupational Exposure

Workers in the rubber industry may be exposed to tellurium compounds. Tellurium exposure may also occur in the refining of copper, silver, gold, lead, and bismuth and in foundries. Workers in the glass, ceramic, and electronics industries may also be exposed to tellurium.

Absorption, Metabolism, & Excretion

Soluble tellurium compounds are absorbed after inhalation or ingestion. Metabolism to dimethyl telluride results in the characteristic garlicky odor. Excretion is primarily through the urine and bile. Tellurium accumulates in liver and bone, and excretion may be prolonged after exposure.

Clinical Findings

A. Symptoms and Signs:

1. Acute exposure—Acute inhalation of tellurium fumes, tellurium oxide, hydrogen telluride, or tellurium hexafluoride may result in acute respiratory irritation. Acute exposure is followed by development of the characteristic garlicky odor of the breath and sweat. A blue-black discoloration of the skin may also develop. Fatigue, nausea, and other systemic complaints may be present.

2. Chronic exposure—Chronic exposure produces

garlic breath, a metallic taste, fatigue, somnolence, dryness of the mouth, and anhidrosis. Tellurium has been found to have adverse neurologic and reproductive effects in experimental animals. Demyelination, congenital hydrocephalus, and aspermatogenesis have been reported. There have been no reports of similar effects in humans.

B. Laboratory Findings: Laboratory tests are nonspecific. Hemolysis may occur after exposure to hydrogen telluride.

Prevention

Exhaust ventilation and personal protective equipment should be used where there is potential exposure to tellurium fumes. Periodic air monitoring and careful attention to workplace hygiene will reduce the chance for chronic exposure. Medical surveillance should focus on complaints of unusual odors, metallic taste, or dry or discolored skin. Urinary tellurium levels should be kept below 0.05 mg/L. Pregnant women should not work directly with tellurium compounds.

Treatment

Supportive therapy should be instituted as indicated. Pulmonary status should be monitored after acute inhalation. Severe hemolysis should be treated with exchange transfusion. Chelation is contraindicated because of its renal toxicity. Ascorbic acid reduces the garlicky odor but may also result in renal toxicity.

THALLIUM

Essentials of Diagnosis

Acute effects:
- Alopecia.
- Gastrointestinal distress.
- Ascending paralysis, coma.

Chronic effects:
- Alopecia.
- Weakness, fatigue.
- Peripheral neuropathy.

Exposure Limits

ACGIH TLV: 0.1 mg/m³ TWA
OSHA PEL: 0.1 mg/m³ TWA

General Considerations

Thallium is a heavy metal that occurs in the earth's crust as a minor constituent in iron, copper, sulfide, and selenide ores. Thallium can be recovered from flue dusts, either from pyrite (FeS_2) roasting or from lead and zinc smelting. Thallium can be prepared as both water-soluble (sulfate, acetate) and water-insoluble (halide) salts.

Use

Thallium sulfate was used as a medicinal in the treatment of syphilis, gonorrhea, gout, and tubercu-

losis in the 19th century. Abandoned because of its toxicity, it enjoyed a brief resurgence as a depilatory in the 1920s. Thallous chloride 201 is currently used in myocardial imaging for the diagnosis of cardiac ischemia.

Thallium salts have been used extensively as rodenticides in the form of impregnated grain (Thalgrain) and pastes (Zelio). Numerous accidental and suicidal poisonings led to the banning of these compounds in the USA in 1972. Currently, thallium is finding increasing uses in the manufacture of electronic components, optical lenses, imitation jewelry, dyes, and pigments.

Occupational & Environmental Exposure

At highest risk for exposure are those engaged in the production of thallium salt derivatives. In addition, workers in the electronics and optical industries have potential exposure to thallium compounds. Thallium exposure can occur at smelters, particularly in the maintenance and cleaning of ducts and flues. Thallium-containing pyrite is also used in cement production.

Environmental exposure can occur in the vicinity of smelting operations through air and water contamination. Thallium exposure in a community surrounding a cement plant in Germany was attributed to ingestion of vegetables grown in thallium-contaminated soil. Water pollution from smelters may contaminate seafood. Thallium chloride has been found in potassium chloride salt substitutes.

Metabolism & Mechanism of Action

Thallium—and especially its soluble salts—is readily absorbed through the gastrointestinal tract, skin, and respiratory system. Ingestion of 0.5–1 g may be lethal. Thallium is rapidly distributed intracellularly throughout all body tissues. Elimination is slow and occurs through intestinal and renal secretion in a ratio of 2:1. Thallium behaves much like potassium and binds avidly to several enzyme systems, including Na^+-K^+ ATPase. Thallium binds to sulfhydryl groups and interferes with cellular respiration and protein synthesis. Binding to riboflavin may contribute to its neurotoxicity.

Clinical Findings
A. Symptoms and Signs:

1. Acute exposure—Gastrointestinal symptoms predominate early and include pain, nausea, vomiting, hemorrhage, and diarrhea. Cardiac abnormalities include tachycardia and hypertension. Neurologic manifestations usually begin with pain, hyperesthesia, and hyperreflexia in the lower extremities. This may rapidly progress to areflexia, hypesthesia, and paralysis depending on the amount ingested. Ataxia, agitation, hallucinations, and coma may occur in severe cases. Alopecia, primarily of scalp and body hair, occurs at the end of the first week; however, black pigmentation of the hair root may be seen earlier. Mees' lines of nails and gingival pigmentation occur. Anhidrosis occurs early owing to destruction of sweat glands.

2. Chronic exposure—In chronic intoxication, the onset of symptoms is insidious. Alopecia and dry skin may be the only complaint. Fatigue and asthenia are frequent. Insomnia and behavioral dysfunction, cranial nerve involvement, and dementia may be presenting symptoms. Endocrine dysfunction includes impotence and amenorrhea.

B. Laboratory Findings: Findings are generally nonspecific. Hypokalemia and alkalosis may be present. Elevated liver enzymes in severe cases reflect centrilobular necrosis. Proteinuria and renal tubular necrosis can occur. The ECG may show signs of hypokalemia. The EEG reveals nonspecific slow wave activity in severe cases. Nerve conduction studies are consistent with axonal degeneration, though demyelination has been seen pathologically.

The diagnosis is confirmed by demonstrating elevated thallium levels in the urine. Normal levels range from 0 to 10 μg/L. Hair and nail levels may be elevated in chronic exposure.

Differential Diagnosis

Thallium intoxication should be considered in every case of peripheral neuropathy of unknown cause. Acute presentation may suggest lead poisoning; however, basophilic stippling of red blood cells is absent. The absence of urobilinogen in the urine distinguishes thallium poisoning from acute intermittent porphyria. In chronic intoxication from industrial exposure, the presentation may suggest depression, hypothyroidism, or organic brain syndrome.

Prevention

Proper skin and respiratory protection are essential. Eating and smoking should not be permitted in areas where thallium compounds are handled. Thallium is a cumulative toxin, and biologic monitoring of urine levels should be considered where there is chronic exposure to thallium compounds.

The banning of thallium-containing pesticides has reduced the frequency of thallium poisoning in the USA, but these compounds may still be encountered and are still available in other countries.

Treatment

In acute cases, emesis should be induced. Treatment with Prussian blue (potassium ferric cyanoferrate II) in a dose of 1 g 3 times daily will bind secreted thallium in the gut. This should be administered with a cathartic to avoid constipation. Activated charcoal should be used as an alternative. Potassium chloride will exchange with thallium in cells and increase renal excretion. This should be administered cautiously, since the rise in serum thallium may transiently worsen symptoms. Chelating agents have not been shown to be effective. In chronic intoxication, removal from exposure is the treatment of choice. Recovery is generally complete, though permanent blindness and hair loss have been reported.

TIN

Essentials of Diagnosis

Inorganic:
- Respiratory and mucous membrane irritation.
- Benign pneumoconiosis (stannosis).

Organic:
- Mild to severe skin irritation.
- Headache, visual disturbances.
- Seizures, coma.

Exposure Limits

Tin, inorganic compounds
ACGIH TLV: 2 mg/m³ TWA
OSHA PEL: 2 mg/m³ TWA
Tin, organic compounds
ACGIH TLV: 0.1 mg/m³ TWA
OSHA PEL: 0.1 mg/m³ TWA

General Considerations

Tin is a soft, pliable, silvery metal used extensively for its corrosion resistance properties. Cassiterite (SnO_2), or tinstone, is the primary commercial ore, with sulfide ores, such as stanniote (Cu_2FeSn_2) and tealite ($PbZnSnS_2$), being of lesser importance. Ores extracted by dredging are subjected to high-temperature reduction in smelting operations to obtain tin for commercial use. An increasing proportion of tin production, particularly in the USA, is through recycling of tin-plated scrap metal and tin alloys.

Use

The primary use of tin is for plating, where it imparts resistance to acids and the atmosphere. Tin-plated iron and steel are used for canning, in household utensils, and for decorative purposes. A tin-lead alloy is used for soldering electronic components. Tin alloys include bronze, babbitt metal, and pewter and are used in printing, bearings, and jewelry. Stannous fluoride is used in toothpastes. Organotin compounds are used as stabilizers in plastics and oils; as catalysts in curing silicone rubber; as preservatives in textiles and leather; and as pesticides in marine paints.

Occupational & Environmental Exposure

At smelting operations, workers may be exposed to tin oxide fumes when pouring molten tin and tin oxide dust during bagging and filter maintenance. Exposure to sulfur dioxide is a hazard in the roasting of sulfide ores of tin. Plating operations, utilizing molten tin drip tanks, may expose workers to tin oxide dust and fumes. Workers engaged in the manufacture of tin solder and other alloys are also exposed. Exposure to the highly toxic organotin compounds may occur in paint formulation and the manufacture of plastics. The use of organotin paints to protect boat hulls may result in contamination and poisoning of marine organisms in harbors. Divalent organotin compounds are used in the production of polyvinyl chloride (PVC) film, urethanes, and silicone rubber. Trivalent organotin compounds are used as biocides and may be encountered as preservatives in textiles, leathers, glass, and paper products.

Absorption, Metabolism, & Excretion

Inorganic tin is poorly absorbed from the gastrointestinal tract. Most of the ingested dose is excreted in the feces. Absorbed tin is found in many tissues, including the reticuloendothelial system in the liver and spleen. Renal excretion is minor. Inhaled compounds remain in the lung. Organic compounds may be absorbed by inhalation, ingestion, or through the skin. Excretion is dependent on chemical composition and is through both the biliary tract and the kidney.

Clinical Findings

A. Symptoms and Signs:

1. Inorganic—Workers exposed to tin dusts in high concentrations may complain of eye, throat, and respiratory irritation. Long-term exposure may result in significant chest x-ray findings, since tin is radiopaque. Changes in pulmonary function have not been associated with exposure to tin compounds. Exposure to tin fumes may cause metal fume fever (see Zinc).

2. Organic—Acute exposure to trimethyl and triethyl tin may cause severe skin irritation followed by central nervous system effects. Headache, lassitude, and visual disturbances may occur. In severe cases, nervous system toxicity may result in seizures and coma. Recovery in nonfatal cases may be delayed. Chronic exposure to organotin compounds may cause an erythematous skin rash and folliculitis, particularly over the lower abdomen and thighs.

B. Laboratory Findings: After chronic exposure to inorganic tin, the chest x-ray may reveal nodular densities throughout the lung fields. Abnormal spirometry should suggest concomitant exposure to silica or other fibrogenic agents. Acute toxicity due to organotin compounds may be manifested by evidence of abnormal renal and hepatic function as well as abnormal findings on the EEG. Elevated urinary levels or organotin compounds will confirm the diagnosis but are not readily available.

Prevention

Enclosure and ventilation of dipping and bagging operations will reduce exposure to tin oxide dusts and fumes. Respiratory protection should be used during maintenance. Organotin compounds should be handled with extreme care to avoid inhalation and skin contact. Medical surveillance should focus on the respiratory system of inorganic tin workers and the skin and nervous system in workers exposed to organic tin compounds.

Treatment

Irritant and dermatologic effects will resolve after removal from exposure. After dermal exposure to organotin compounds, the skin should be extensively cleansed with a strong detergent and water to prevent delayed absorption. Neurologic, hepatic, and renal toxicity should be treated as indicated clinically.

VANADIUM

Essentials of Diagnosis

- Respiratory irritation.
- Asthma.
- Green discoloration of the tongue.

Exposure Limits

Vanadium dust
   ACGIH TLV: 0.05 mg/m^3 TWA
   OSHA PEL: 0.05 mg/m^3 TWA
Vanadium fume
   ACGIH TLV: 0.05 mg/m^3 TWA
   OSHA PEL: 0.05 mg/m^3 TWA
Vanadium compounds
   NIOSH REL: 0.05 mg V/m^3 ceiling (15 minutes). Metallic vanadium and vanadium carbide, 1 mg V/m^3 TWA

General Considerations

Vanadium is a soft, gray metal that is nonoxidizing in acids and seawater. The principal commercial ores are vanadium sulfide and lead-zinc vanadate. Vanadium is also found in uranium-bearing sandstones in sufficient quantities for commercial extraction. Varying levels of vanadium are found in fossil fuels and contribute to environmental contamination.

Use

The primary use of vanadium is in production of ferrovanadium, in which as little as 0.05–5% vanadium imparts greater strength and elasticity. Vanadium alloys supply hardness and durability for high-speed cutting and drilling tools. Vanadium is also used as a catalyst for high-temperature polymerization, as a mordant in dyeing, and as a colorant in ceramics and glass. Organic vanadium compounds are used as catalysts and coatings.

Occupational & Environmental Exposure

Exposure to vanadium pentoxide dusts and fumes may occur during milling and roasting. Workers using vanadium compounds for alloys or additives will have contact with pure source materials. A particular inhalation hazard exists in cleaning fuel dusts from oil and coal furnaces where high levels of vanadium pentoxide may accumulate. Fossil fuel-burning power stations may emit vanadium compounds, resulting in environmental contamination and air pollution.

Absorption, Metabolism, & Excretion

Vanadium compounds may be absorbed after inhalation or ingestion. Lung content has been shown to be increased in miners and in persons living in proximity to effluents from the burning of fossil fuels. Excretion is primarily renal, with little accumulation in bone.

Clinical Findings

A. Acute Exposure: Acute exposure to high levels of vanadium pentoxide dusts or fumes results in profuse lacrimation, eye irritation, epistaxis, cough, and bronchitis. Pneumonia may follow acute exposures. Sensitivity to vanadium, resulting in cough and bronchospasm at lower levels of exposure, is consistent with allergic asthma. Skin irritation or allergy may also occur.

B. Chronic Exposure: With chronic exposure, green discoloration of the tongue may occur. Plasma cholesterol has been found to be lowered in workers exposed to vanadium. Pulmonary function tests may reveal an obstructive pattern. Patch testing may be used to confirm dermal sensitization to vanadium compounds.

Prevention

Proper respiratory protection should be worn when handling vanadium compounds and when cleaning oil and coal furnace flues. Medical surveillance should screen for respiratory and dermatologic complaints, which suggest chronic overexposure or development of respiratory or skin allergy.

Treatment

Ascorbic acid and calcium disodium edetate are protective in experimental animals, though there is no human experience with these compounds. Persons who develop respiratory or dermatologic allergy should be permanently removed from exposure.

ZINC

Essentials of Diagnosis

Zinc oxide:
- Headache, metallic taste.
- Fever, chills, myalgias.
- Cough, chest pain.

Zinc chloride:
- Severe skin and eye burns.
- Respiratory irritation.
- Pulmonary edema.

Exposure Limits

Zinc oxide fume
  ACGIH TLV: 5 mg/m^3 TWA, 10 mg/m^3 STEL
  OSHA PEL: 5 mg/m^3 TWA, 10 mg/m^3 STEL
Zinc oxide dust
  ACGIH TLV: 10 mg/m^3 TWA
  OSHA PEL: 10 mg/m^3 TWA

Zinc chloride fume
  ACGIH TLV: 1 mg/m^3 TWA, 2 mg/m^3 STEL
  OSHA PEL: 1 mg/m^3 TWA, 2 mg/m^3 STEL

General Considerations

Zinc is a silver-white metal with a blue tinge that is widely distributed in nature. Zinc deposits frequently contain cadmium, iron, lead, and arsenic. Zinc is recovered through flotation and separation followed by either smelting or electrolytic refining. Zinc is an essential element for humans and is found in all tissues. Many different enzyme systems require zinc for normal functioning. Zinc has been considered to be beneficial in wound healing and sickle cell anemia and to protect against cadmium-induced nephrotoxicity and the effects of lead on erythrocytes. Daily intake of zinc in the diet is between 10 and 15 mg.

Use

A major application of zinc is in the galvanizing of steel and other metals, where a coating is applied through dipping or electroplating. Purified zinc metal is die cast for use in automotive parts, electrical equipment, tools, machinery, and toys. Zinc oxide is used as a pigment and in the vulcanizing of rubber. Zinc chloride is used in welding and soldering fluxes, wood preservatives, dry cell batteries, oil refining, dental cement, and deodorants. Zinc forms alloys with many metals, including copper to form brass.

Occupational & Environmental Exposure

Exposure to zinc sulfide in mining and ore extraction is less significant than exposure to other heavy metal contaminants. In zinc ore roasting operations, there is potential exposure to zinc oxide dusts and fumes. Workers engaged in fabricating or welding of galvanized metal may have exposure to zinc oxide fumes. Zinc chloride exposure occurs in welding and soldering as well as with its use in manufacturing. Zinc alloy production and brass work involve exposure to zinc compounds. Ingestion of acidic foods and beverages from galvanized food containers has resulted in zinc poisoning.

Absorption, Metabolism, & Excretion

Only 20–30% of ingested zinc is absorbed from the gastrointestinal tract. Zinc may also be absorbed after inhalation of fumes. Circulating zinc is bound to plasma proteins (metallothionein and albumin) and is found in erythrocytes. Zinc is distributed widely in tissues, most of it in striated muscle. Absorbed zinc is excreted in pancreatic fluid, bile, and sweat, with only 20% excreted in the urine.

Clinical Findings

A. Symptoms and Signs:

1. Acute exposure—The most characteristic manifestation of occupational zinc toxicity is the development of metal fume fever after exposure to zinc oxide fumes. Several hours after exposure, the worker develops headache and a sweet metallic taste, followed by muscle and joint pains and fatigue. Fever, chills, profuse sweating, cough, and chest pain occur 8–12 hours after exposure, usually when the worker is at home. The symptoms resolve spontaneously after 24–48 hours, resembling an acute viral syndrome. The condition occurs more frequently early in the week, suggesting that tolerance may develop. Chronic sequelae do not occur.

Contact with zinc chloride may cause serious skin and eye burns even after brief contact.

2. Chronic exposure—Chronic skin exposure may cause an eczematous dermatitis or skin sensitization. Inhalation of zinc chloride fumes causes sinus and throat irritation, cough, hemoptysis, and dyspnea. Pulmonary edema and pneumonia may develop following excessive exposure. Ingestion of soluble zinc compounds causes nausea, vomiting, and diarrhea due to irritation of the gastrointestinal tract.

B. Laboratory Findings: The onset of symptoms of metal fume fever is accompanied by leukocytosis of $15,000-20,000/\mu L$ and a fall in FEV_1, FVC, and carbon monoxide diffusing capacity on pulmonary function testing. The chest x-ray may reveal hazy infiltrates in the mid lung fields. Nonspecific elevation of LDH and other serum enzymes may occur. Urine and plasma zinc levels may also be elevated.

After zinc chloride inhalation, findings of arterial hypoxemia and pulmonary infiltrates are consistent with acute chemical pneumonitis. Zinc chloride skin allergy can be confirmed by patch testing.

Prevention

Proper ventilation of high-temperature processes involving zinc will reduce exposure to zinc oxide dusts and fumes. Proper local exhaust ventilation should be provided when welding on galvanized metal and brazing on brass. Proper eye and skin protection should be used when handling zinc chloride. Home remedies purported to prevent metal fume fever, including milk and vitamin C, have no scientific basis. Medical monitoring for zinc exposed workers should concentrate on dermatologic and respiratory effects. Urine zinc levels have been found to range up to 0.7 mg/L in persons exposed to zinc below the current ACGIH limit.

Treatment

No specific treatment is indicated for metal fume fever, though bacterial infections of the lungs should be ruled out by sputum culture and examination. Zinc chloride skin and eye burns should be irrigated immediately with copious amounts of water. Eye irrigation with 1.7% $CaNa_2EDTA$ for 15 minutes should be instituted as soon as possible to prevent the development of corneal opacities. Persons with suspected zinc chloride inhalation should be hospitalized for observation and treated with supplemental oxygen. Persons who develop chronic dermatitis and zinc skin allergy should be removed from further exposure.

WELDING

Welding is a joining process with wide application in manufacturing and the building trades. Through the application of heat or pressure, welding joins metals with a lightweight bond, with strength and resistance approaching that of the parent metal.

Welding is a labor-intensive activity. Even though automated welding methods are finding increasing applications, manual arc welding remains the principal welding process.

Health Hazards of Welding

Welders work with a wide variety of materials under varied conditions and are exposed to many health hazards, including air contaminants (metal fumes, particulates, gases); physical agents such as radiation (infrared, ultraviolet), noise, and electricity; and ergonomic stress.

The common air contaminants of different welding processes are listed in Tables 25–2 and 25–3. **Shielded metal arc (SMA)** welding of mild steel is the most common use of welding. The main exposure is to iron oxide, and pulmonary deposition of this nonfibrogenic particulate has resulted in the development of a benign pneumoconiosis. Exposure to manganese and fluoride fumes may be considerable when certain welding rods are used.

The corrosion-resistant properties of stainless steel are due to a high concentration of chromium (18–30%). Nickel and manganese may also be present in different stainless steel alloys. Exposure to chromium (including Cr VI), nickel, and manganese may be considerable, particularly with **gas metal arc (GMA)** processes. The stainless steel surface reflects ultraviolet radiation, with formation of oxides of nitrogen and ozone. Low hydrogen welding of stainless steel generates high concentrations of fluoride fumes.

Most aluminum welding uses the **tungsten inert gas (TIG)** method. As with stainless steel, the

Table 25–2. Air contaminants of selected welding processes.

Process	Base Metal	Contaminants
Shielded metal arc	Mild steel	Dust, iron oxide, manganese
Shielded metal arc	Stainless steel	Chromium, nickel, manganese, fluorides
Gas metal arc	Stainless steel	Chromium, nickel, manganese, nitrogen oxides, ozone
Tungsten inert gas	Aluminum	Ozone, aluminum oxide
Gas	Variable	Nitrogen oxides, cadmium oxide, metal fume

Table 25–3. Potential hazards of welding processes.

Air contaminants	
Metals	
Iron oxide	Benign pneumoconiosis
Manganese	Neurotoxicity, pneumonia
Cadmium oxide	Acute lung injury
Zinc oxide	Metal fume fever
Chromium	Lung cancer, allergy
Nickel	Lung cancer, allergy
Fluoride	Skin irritation, bone deposition
Gases	
Ozone	Respiratory irritation, asthma
Nitrogen oxides	Acute lung injury
Carbon monoxide	Systemic poisoning
Physical hazards	
Radiation	
Ultraviolet	Photokeratitis, skin erythema,
Infra-red	Burns, ?cataracts
Electricity	Electric shock, electrocution
Noise	Hearing loss
Ergonomic stress	Muscle strain

gas-shielded process results in formation of ozone due to the action of ultraviolet radiation on the nascent oxygen in the atmosphere. Total dust and aluminum oxide generation are also considerable.

Brazing and **gas welding** both generate metal fume. Exposure to cadmium oxide from cadmium-containing silver solder has caused acute lung injury and death after brazing in enclosed spaces. Similar consequences have occurred from generation of the oxides of nitrogen during gas welding. In all cases, improper ventilation was the critical factor in creating the hazard.

Radiation and heat result in the most common injuries to welders: photokeratitis (welder's flash) and thermal burns. These are often related to improper use of protective goggles, gloves, and screens. Flying sparks or debris may cause burns or eye injury as well. Noise exposure may exceed 80 dB in welding processes, particularly cutting or gouging operations; in plasma welding, levels may approach 120 dB. Environmental conditions will also influence noise generation. Electrical shock is a constant hazard and requires careful grounding and shielding of cables and equipment. Most manual processes place isometric stress on the welder, particularly involving the shoulders and the upper extremities.

Coatings or contaminants may present additional hazards (Table 25–4), particularly when their presence and potential hazard are unknown or unsuspected. The formation of toxic gases, fumes, or vapors is usually due to the heating of a coated or treated metal, although phosgene exposure is related to the action of ultraviolet radiation on chlorinated hydrocarbon vapors (similar to the formation of ozone from oxygen and oxides of nitrogen from nitrogen).

Soldering is not associated with significant exposure to metal fumes because the temperatures are low. Potential contamination of the workplace with lead dust requires careful attention to hygiene. Some

fluxes, such as rosin, are skin sensitizers and may cause allergic dermatitis.

Clinical Findings
A. Acute Exposure:

1. Photokeratitis–Photokeratitis is the result of exposure of the cornea to ultraviolet radiation in the 280- to 315-nm range (UVB). The duration of exposure necessary to induce this effect varies with the distance from the arc and the light intensity. Following exposure of the unprotected eye to the welding arc for several seconds, the worker develops pain, burning, or a feeling of "sand or grit" in the eye. Physical examination shows conjunctival injection, and slit lamp examination may reveal punctate depressions over the cornea. The condition is self-limited, resolving in several hours. Careful examination for foreign bodies or evidence of thermal ocular injury is mandatory.

2. Metal fume fever–(See Zinc, above.) Metal fume fever is a benign, self-limited condition characterized by the delayed onset (8–12 hours) of fever, chills, cough, myalgias, and a metallic taste. A history of welding on galvanized metal suggests the diagnosis.

3. Upper respiratory irritation–Upper respiratory tract irritation may result from exposure to a variety of welding contaminants, including dusts, ozone, aluminum oxide, nitrogen oxides, cadmium oxide, and fluorides. Asthma may also be triggered as a result of nonspecific irritation or allergy (chromium, nickel).

4. Lung injury–While unusual, exposure to oxides of nitrogen and cadmium oxide may cause acute lung injury and delayed pulmonary edema. A history of gas welding or brazing in enclosed or poorly ventilated spaces should raise this concern and serve as an indication for careful medical evaluation and observation.

5. Musculoskeletal trauma–Injuries resulting from isometric stress on the upper extremity during welding may present as symptomatic shoulder and neck pain following prolonged activity. Asymptomatic muscle damage may result in slight increases in creatine phosphokinase levels in serum.

6. Thermal burns and electrical injuries–See Chapter 11.

Table 25–4. Coatings and contaminants encountered in welding.

Galvanized metal	Zinc oxide
Paints	Lead, cadmium, isocyanates, a!dehydes, epoxies
Biocides	Organic mercury, organic tin
Chlorinated solvents	Phosgene
Rust proofing	Phosphorus, phosphine
Alloys	Cadmium, nickel, manganese, beryllium

B. Chronic Exposure:

1. Siderosis–Siderosis (see Chapter 18) results from accumulation of nonfibrogenic iron oxide particles in the lung. While the radiographic appearance may be dramatic, with evidence of diffuse reticulonodular densities, reports of deficits of pulmonary function have been inconsistent, suggesting a mild or minimal effect. In welders who have also been exposed to crystalline silica or asbestos, radiographic differentiation of hemosiderosis from pulmonary fibrosis is difficult. Pleural thickening or calcification has not been related to welding in the absence of asbestos exposure.

2. Other chronic effects–Welders report an excess of respiratory symptoms and have increased work absences from respiratory diseases. Demonstration of clear deficits in pulmonary function attributable to welding have been inconsistent. At present, there is limited evidence that welding results in chronic respiratory impairment. In the evaluation of a welder with chronic lung disease, a careful medical and occupational history is essential, focusing on both welding exposures and other confounding factors.

Studies of lung cancer in welders have also been inconsistent, sharing the limitations of many of the respiratory studies. Some researchers attribute the small excess in lung cancer cases seen in several studies to exposure to chromium and nickel in welding of stainless steel, a small proportion of all welding exposures. Studies involving welders who worked in shipyards during the first half of this century will be confounded by significant secondary exposure to asbestos.

Prevention

Most acute injuries or poisonings related to welding processes are preventable. Strict adherence to appropriate safety procedures will prevent burns, eye injuries, and electric shock. Awareness of the potential hazards, with attention to the provision of adequate ventilation, is the best safeguard against accidental overexposure to air contaminants. In enclosed spaces, air-supplied respirators are essential, particularly with processes that result in generation of nitrogen oxides.

Carefully designed and controlled studies in the future will better assess the potential impact of welding on respiratory function and on the development of lung cancer. These effects, if present, will certainly be minimized by measures to reduce welding exposures through engineering, ventilation, and proper use of personal protection.

Treatment

Photokeratitis and metal fume fever require no specific treatment, though other diagnoses should be excluded. Welders suspected of having acute overexposure to nitrogen oxides or cadmium oxide should be hospitalized for observation. Treatment of pulmonary edema and respiratory insufficiency related to these agents is supportive. Asthmatics bothered by nonspecific irritant effects related to welding may benefit from improved ventilation and respiratory protection, though cartridge respirators will not prevent exposure to irritant gases. Frank allergic asthma to specific agents may require removal from further exposure.

Burns and radiation injuries are discussed in Chapter 11.

REFERENCES

Antimony
Cooper DA et al: Pneumoconiosis among workers in an antimony industry. *Am J Roentgenol Rad Ther Nucl Med* 1968;**103**:495.

Renes LE: Antimony poisoning in industry. *Arch Ind Hyg Occup Med* 1953;**7**:99.

Taylor PJ: Acute intoxication from antimony trichloride. *Br J Ind Med* 1966;**23**:318.

Arsenic
Blom S, Lagerkvist B, Linderholm H: Arsenic exposure to smelter workers: Clinical and neurophysiological studies. *Scand J Work Environ Health* 1985;**11**:265.

Enterline PE, Marsh GM: Cancer among workers exposed to arsenic and other substances in a copper smelter. *Am J Epidemiol* 1982;**116**:895.

Hesdorffer CS et al: Arsine gas poisoning: The importance of exchange transfusions in severe cases. *Br J Ind Med* 1986;**43**:353.

Landrigan PJ: Arsenic: State of the art. *Am J Ind Med* 1981;**2**:5.

Landrigan PJ, Costello RJ, Stringer WT: Occupational exposure to arsine: An epidemiologic reappraisal of current standards. *Scand J Work Environ Health* 1982;**8**:169.

Léonard A, Lauwerys RR: Carcinogenicity, teratogenicity and mutagenicity of arsenic. *Mutat Res* 1980;**75**:49.

Tseng WP: Effects and dose-response relationships of skin cancer and blackfoot disease with arsenic. *Environ Health Perspect* 1977;**19**:109.

Beryllium
Andrews JL, Kazemi H, Hardy HL: Patterns of lung dysfunction in chronic beryllium disease. *Am Rev Respir Dis* 1969;**100**:791.

Hasan FM, Kazemi H: Chronic beryllium disease: A continuing epidemiologic hazard. *Chest* 1974;**65**:289.

Kuschner M: The carcinogenicity of beryllium. *Environ Health Perspect* 1981;**40**:101.

National Institute for Occupational Safety and Health: *Occupational Exposure to Beryllium.* DHEW Publication No. 72-10268. US Government Printing Office, 1972.

Sprince NL, Kazemi H: Beryllium disease. In: *Environmental and Occupational Medicine*. Rom WN (editor). Little, Brown, 1983.

Sprince NL, Kazemi H: US beryllium case registry through 1977. *Environ Res* 1980;**21**:44.

Wagoner JK, Infante PF, Bayliss DL: Beryllium: An etiologic agent in the induction of lung cancer, nonneoplastic respiratory disease, and heart disease among industrially exposed workers. *Environ Res* 1980;**21**:15.

Boron

Garabrant DH et al: Respiratory effects of borax dust. *Br J Ind Med* 1985;**42**:831.

Hart RP et al: Neuropsychological function following mild exposure to pentaborane. *Am J Ind Med* 1984;**6**:37.

Mindrum G: Pentaborane intoxication. *Arch Intern Med* 1964;**114**:364.

Silverman JJ et al: Posttraumatic stress disorder from pentaborane intoxication: Neuropsychiatric evaluation and short-term follow-up. *JAMA* 1985;**254**:2603.

Stumpe AR: Toxicity of diborane in high concentrations. *Arch Ind Health* 1960;**21**:519.

Cadmium

Barnhart S, Rosenstock L: Cadmium chemical pneumonitis. *Chest* 1984;**86**:789.

Blainey JD et al: Cadmium-induced osteomalacia. *Br J Ind Med* 1980;**37**:278.

Elinder CG et al: Assessment of renal function in workers previously exposed to cadmium. *Br J Ind Med* 1985;**42**:754.

Elinder CG et al: Cancer mortality of cadmium workers. *Br J Ind Med* 1985;**42**:651.

Friberg L: Cadmium and the kidney. *Environ Health Perspect* 1984;**54**:1.

Hallenbeck WH: Human health effects of exposure to cadmium. *Experientia* 1984;**40**:136.

Lauwerys RR et al: Investigations on the lung and kidney function in workers exposed to cadmium. *Environ Health Perspect* 1979;**28**:137.

Roels H et al: Evolution of cadmium-induced renal dysfunction in workers removed from exposure. *Scand J Work Environ Health* 1982;**8**:191.

Chromium

Léonard A, Lauwerys RR: Carcinogenicity and mutagenicity of chromium. *Mutat Res* 1980;**76**:227.

Lindberg E, Vesterberg O: Monitoring exposure to chromic acid in chromeplating by measuring chromium in urine. *Scand J Work Environ Health* 1983;**9**:333.

National Academy of Sciences: *Chromium: Medical and Biologic Effects of Environmental Pollutants*. National Academy of Sciences, 1974.

Satoh K et al: Epidemiological study of workers engaged in the manufacture of chromium compounds. *J Occup Med* 1981;**23**:835.

Lead

Araki S et al: Determination of the distribution of conduction velocities in workers exposed to lead, zinc, and copper. *Br J Ind Med* 1986;**43**:321.

Baker EL et al: Occupational lead poisoning in the United States: Clinical and biochemical findings related to blood lead levels. *Br J Ind Med* 1979;**36**:314.

Cullen MR, Robins JM, Eskenazi B: Adult inorganic lead intoxication: Presentation of 31 new cases and a review of recent advances in the literature. *Medicine* 1983;**62**:221.

Grandjean P: Health significance of organolead compounds. In: *Lead Versus Health*. Rutter M, Jones RR (editors). Wiley, 1983.

Jeyaratnam J et al: Neurophysiological studies of workers exposed to lead. *Br J Ind Med* 1985;**42**:173.

Rempel D: The lead-exposed worker. *JAMA* 1989;**262**:532.

US Congress, Office of Technology Assessment: *Reproductive Health Hazards in the Workplace*. US Government Printing Office, 1985.

Williams DR, Halstead BW: Chelating agents in medicine. *J Toxicol Clin Toxicol* 1982;**19**:1081.

Manganese

Cooper WC: The health implications of increased manganese in the environment resulting from the combustion of fuel additives: A review of the literature. *J Toxicol Environ Health* 1984;**14**:23.

Saric M, Markicevic A, Hrustic O: Occupational exposure to manganese. *Br J Ind Med* 1977;**34**:114.

Smyth LT et al: Clinical manganism and exposure to manganese in the production and processing of ferromanganese alloy. *J Occup Med* 1973;**15**:101.

Mercury

Coordinating Committee for Scientific and Technical Assessments of Environmental Pollutants: *An Assessment of Mercury in the Environment*. National Academy of Sciences, 1978.

Elhassani SB: The many faces of methylmercury poisoning. *J Toxicol Clin Toxicol* 1982;**19**:875.

Joselow MM, Louria DB, Browder AA: Mercurialism: Environmental and occupational aspects. *Ann Intern Med* 1972;**76**:119.

Roels H et al: Surveillance of workers exposed to mercury vapour: Validation of a previously proposed biological threshold limit value for mercury concentration in urine. *Am J Ind Med* 1985;**7**:45.

Nickel

Barton RT, Hogetveit AC: Nickel-related cancers of the respiratory tract. *Cancer* 1980;**45**:3061.

Leonard A, Gerber GB, Jacquet P: Carcinogenicity, mutagenicity and teratogenicity of nickel. *Mutat Res* 1981;**87**:1.

Sunderman FW: The treatment of acute nickel carbonyl poisoning with sodium diethyldithiocarbamate. *Ann Clin Res* 1971;**3**:182.

Tola S, Kilpiö J, Virtamo M: Urinary and plasma concentrations of nickel as indicators of exposure to nickel in an electroplating shop. *J Occup Med* 1979;**21**:184.

Vuopala U et al: Nickel carbonyl poisoning: Report of 25 cases. *Ann Clin Res* 1970;**2**:214.

Phosphorus

Ben-Hur N et al: Phosphorus burns: A pathophysiological study. *Br J Plast Surg* 1972;**25**:238.

Harger LN, Spolyar LW: Toxicity of phosphine, with a possible fatality from this poison. *Arch Ind Health* 1958;**18**:497.

Hughes JP et al: Phosphorus necrosis of the jaw: A present-day study. *Br J Ind Med* 1961;**19**:83.

Wilson R et al: Acute phosphine poisoning aboard a grain freighter: Epidemiologic, clinical, and pathological findings. *JAMA* 1980;**244:**148.

Selenium

Derwenka EA, Cooper WC: Toxicology of selenium and tellurium and their compounds. *Arch Environ Health* 1961;**3:**71.

Diskin CJ et al: Long-term selenium exposure. *Arch Intern Med* 1979;**139:**824.

Glover JR, Chir M: Selenium and its industrial toxicology. *Ind Med Surg* 1970;**39:**26.

Selenium intoxication: New York. *MMWR* 1984;**33:**157.

Subcommittee on Selenium: *Selenium in Nutrition.* National Academy Press, 1983.

Tellurium

Derwenka EA, Cooper WC: Toxicology of selenium and tellurium and their compounds. *Arch Environ Health* 1961;**3:**71.

Lampert P, Garro F, Pentschew A: Tellurium neuropathy. *Acta Neuropathol* 1970;**15:**308.

Schroeder HA, Buckman J, Balassa JJ: Abnormal trace elements in man: Tellurium. *J Chronic Dis* 1967;**20:**147.

Thallium

Cavanagh JB et al: The effects of thallium salts, with particular reference to the nervous system changes: A report of three cases. *Q J Med* 1974;**43:**293.

Davis LE et al: Acute thallium poisoning: Toxicological and morphological studies of the nervous system. *Ann Neurol* 1981;**10:**38.

Moeschlin S: Thallium poisoning. *Clin Toxicol* 1980;**17:**133.

Saddique A, Peterson CD: Thallium poisoning: A review. *Vet Hum Toxicol* 1983;**25:**16.

Thompson DF: Management of thallium poisoning. *Clin Toxicol* 1981;**18:**979.

Tin

Fortemps E et al: Trimethyltin poisoning: Report of two cases. *Int Arch Occup Environ Health* 1978;**41:**1.

Fox AJ, Goldblatt P, Kinlen LJ: A study of the mortality of Cornish tin miners. *Br J Ind Med* 1981;**38:**378.

Krigman MR, Silverman AP: General toxicology of tin and its organic compounds. *Neurotoxicology* 1984; **5:**129.

Vanadium

Lees RE: Changes in lung function after exposure to vanadium compounds in fuel oil ash. *Br J Ind Med* 1980;**37:**253.

Levy BS, Hoffman L, Gottsegen S: Boilermakers' bronchitis: Respiratory tract irritation associated with vanadium pentoxide exposure during oil-to-coal conversion of a power plant. *J Occup Med* 1984;**26:**567.

Zinc

Brocks A, Reid H, Glazer G: Acute intravenous zinc poisoning. *Br Med J* 1977;**1:**1390.

National Institute for Occupational Safety and Health: *Criteria for a Recommended Standard: Occupational Exposure to Zinc Oxide.* DHEW Publication No. 76-104. US Government Printing Office, 1975.

Welding

Akbarkhanzadeh F: Long-term effects of welding fumes upon respiratory symptoms and pulmonary function. *J Occup Med* 1980;**22:**337.

Andersson HF, Dahlberg JA, Wettström R: Phosgene formation during welding in air contaminated with perchloroethylene. *Ann Occup Hyg* 1975;**18:**129.

Attfield MD, Ross DS: Radiological abnormalities in electric-arc welders. *Br J Ind Med* 1978;**35:**117.

Barnhart S, Rosenstock L: Cadmium chemical pneumonitis. *Chest* 1984;**86:**789.

Beaumont JJ, Weiss NS: Mortality of welders, shipfitters, and other metal trades workers in Boilmakers Local No. 104, AFL-CIO. *Am J Epidemiol* 1980; **112:**775.

Becker N, Claude J, Frentzel-Beyme R: Cancer risk of arc welders exposed to fumes containing chromium and nickel. *Scand J Work Environ Health* 1985;**11:**75.

Emmett EA et al: Skin and eye diseases among arc welders and those exposed to welding operations. *J Occup Med* 1981;**23:**85.

Fawer RF, Gardner AW, Oakes D: Absences attributed to respiratory diseases in welders. *Br J Ind Med* 1982;**39:**149.

Hagberg M, Michaelson G, Ortelius A: Serum creatine kinase as an indicator of local muscular strain in experimental and occupational work. *Int Arch Occup Environ Health* 1982;**50:**377.

Keimig DG, Pomrehn PR, Burmeister LF: Respiratory symptoms and pulmonary function in welders of mild steel: A cross-sectional study. *Am J Ind Med* 1983; **4:**489.

Keskinen H, Kalliomäki PL, Alanko K: Occupational asthma due to stainless steel welding fumes. *Clin Allergy* 1980;**10:**151.

Lunau FW: Ozone in arc welding. *Ann Occup Hyg* 1967;**10:**175.

Morgan WK, Kerr HD: Pathologic and physiologic studies of welders' siderosis. *Ann Intern Med* 1963; **58:**293.

Newhouse ML, Oakes D, Woolley AJ: Mortality of welders and other craftsmen at a shipyard in NE England. *Br J Ind Med* 1985;**42:**406.

Pabley AS, Keeney AH: Welding processes and ocular hazards and protection. *Am J Ophthalmol* 1981; **92:**77.

Sjögren B, Ulfvarson U: Respiratory symptoms and pulmonary function among welders working with aluminum, stainless steel and railroad tracks. *Scand J Work Environ Health* 1985;**11:**27.

Stern RM: Process-dependent risk of delayed health effects for welders. *Environ Health Perspect* 1981; **41:**235.

Chemicals

26

Robert J. Harrison, MD, MPH

This chapter covers selected chemicals of particular importance to the occupational health practitioner. Solvents, plastics, pesticides, and gases are covered in subsequent chapters.

ACIDS & ALKALIES

Acids and alkalies are of great importance as industrial chemicals. When ranked by volume of production, the inorganic acids and alkalies (including chlorine and ammonia) comprise 10 of the major 25 chemicals produced yearly in the USA.

1. ACIDS

Essentials of Diagnosis

Acute effects:
- Irritative dermatitis, skin burn.
- Respiratory irritation, pulmonary edema.

Chronic effects:
- Hydrofluoric acid: Osteosclerosis.
- Nitric acid (oxides of nitrogen): bronchiolitis fibrosa obliterans.
- Chromic acid: Nasal ulceration, perforation, skin ulceration.

Exposure Limits
Chromic acid (Cr VI)
    ACGIH TLV: 0.05 mg/m^3 TWA
    OSHA PEL: 1 mg/10 m^3 ceiling
    NIOSH REL: 25 μg/m^3 TWA, 50 μg/m^3 ceiling
      (15 minutes)
Hydrofluoric acid
    ACGIH TLV: 3 ppm TWA
    OSHA PEL: 3 ppm TWA, 6 ppm STEL
    NIOSH REL: 3 ppm TWA, 6 ppm ceiling (15
      minutes)
Nitric acid
    ACGIH TLV: 2 ppm TWA, 4 ppm STEL
    OSHA PEL: 2 ppm TWA, 4 ppm STEL
    NIOSH REL: 2 ppm TWA

General Considerations
An inorganic acid is a compound of hydrogen and one or more other elements (with the exception of carbon) that dissociates to produce hydrogen ions when dissolved in water or other solvents. The resultant solution has the ability to neutralize bases and turn litmus paper red. Inorganic acids of greatest industrial use are chromic, hydrochloric, hydrofluoric, nitric, phosphoric, and sulfuric acids. Inorganic acids share certain fire, explosive, and health hazards.

Organic acids and their derivatives include a broad range of substances used in nearly every type of chemical manufacture. All have primary irritant effects depending on the degree of acid dissociation and water solubility.

Use, Production, & Occupational Exposure
A. Inorganic Acids:
1. Sulfuric acid–Sulfuric acid is by far the largest chemical commodity produced; in the USA, the annual production is over 40 million tons. It is less costly than any other acid, can be easily handled, reacts with many organic compounds to produce useful products, and forms a slightly soluble salt with calcium oxide or calcium hydroxide. Most of United States sulfuric acid production is used in the manufacture of phosphate fertilizers, in which sulfuric acid is used to convert phosphate rock to phosphoric acid. Other important uses include the production of inorganic pigments, textile fibers, explosives, pulp, and paper; as a leaching agent for ores; and as a component of lead storage batteries. Workers with potential exposure to sulfuric acid include electroplaters, jewelers, metal cleaners, picklers, and storage battery makers. Occupational exposure can occur both by skin contact and by inhalation of sulfuric acid mist. A NIOSH study of lead acid battery plants found exposure to average 0.18 mg/m^3 and in some cases to be as high as 1.7 mg/m^3. NIOSH estimates that 200,000 workers are potentially exposed to sulfuric acid.

2. Phosphoric acid–The annual phosphoric acid production in the USA is over 11 million tons. Its greatest use (85%) is in the manufacture of phosphate salts for fertilizers by the digestion of phosphate rock with sulfuric acid. Other uses include the acid treatment (pickling) of sheet metal, chemical polishing of metals, as a tart flavoring agent for carbonated beverages, as a refractory bonding agent, and for boiler cleaning, textile dying, lithographic engraving, and rubber latex coagulation. Occupational exposure occurs primarily to the liquid acid by skin contact.

3. Chromic acid–Chromic acid is produced by roasting chromite ore with soda ash and treatment with sulfuric acid to form chromic acid anhydride, chromic acid (chromium trioxide), and dichromic acid. Over 90% of chromic acid is used in metal treatment procedures such as chrome plating, copper stripping, and aluminum anodizing. Without local exhaust ventilation, occupational exposure to chromic acid mist during metal plating operations can range up to several milligrams per cubic meter, but with a local exhaust system this can be markedly reduced to near undetectable limits. NIOSH estimates that 15,000 workers are potentially exposed to chromic acid mist.

4. Nitric acid–Nitric acid is produced from the oxidation of ammonia in the presence of a catalyst to yield nitric oxide, which is then further oxidized and absorbed in water to form an aqueous solution of nitric acid. Nitric acid is used for the production of fertilizers in the form of ammonium nitrate, in the manufacture of explosives, in metal etching and photoengraving, and in metal cleaning ("bright dipping") of copper and brass. Occupational exposure can occur by topical contact with the liquid acid as well as by inhalation of nitrogen oxides evolved when nitric acid reacts with reducing agents (metals, organic matter) or during the combustion of nitrogen-containing materials (welding, glassblowing, underground blasting, and decomposition of agricultural silage). Reports of occupational exposure to nitric acid are limited to measurements of nitrogen oxides that evolved by these reactions. NIOSH estimates that 27,000 workers are potentially exposed to nitric acid.

5. Hydrochloric acid–Hydrochloric acid is an aqueous solution of hydrogen chloride and is used in the production of fertilizers, dyes, paint pigments, and soap; in electroplating, leather tanning, ore refining, and pickling of metal; and in the photographic and textile industries. The United States produces over 1700 metric tons per year. Hydrochloric acid gas may also evolve from thermal degradation of polyvinyl chloride, a hazard to firefighters.

6. Hydrofluoric acid–Hydrofluoric acid (hydrogen fluoride) is a colorless liquid manufactured by reaction of sulfuric acid with calcium fluoride in heated kilns. It evolves as a gas and is then condensed as liquid anhydrous hydrogen fluoride. Major uses are for the production of cryolite for the aluminum industry; in the manufacture of chlorofluorocarbons; in steel pickling, uranium processing, enamel stripping, glass and quartz etching, and polishing; in electroplating; and in the semiconductor industry for wafer etching. Occupational exposure can occur both by direct skin contact and by inhalation of fumes. NIOSH estimates that 22,000 workers are potentially exposed, but this number is probably much higher if electronics workers are included.

7. Organic acids–Among the saturated monocarboxylic acids, **formic acid** is used mainly in the textile industry as a dye-exhausting agent, in the leather industry as a deliming agent and neutralizer, as a coagulant for rubber latex, and as a component of nickel plating baths.

Propionic acid is used in organic synthesis, as a mold inhibitor, and as a food additive.

The unsaturated monocarboxylic acid **acrylic acid** is widely used in the manufacture of resins, plasticizers, and drugs.

The aliphatic dicarboxylics **maleic, fumaric,** and **adipic acids** find use in the manufacture of synthetic resins, dyes, surface coatings, inks, and plasticizers.

The halogenated **acetic acids** are highly reactive chemical intermediates used in glycine, drug, dye, and herbicide manufacture.

Glycolic acid and **lactic acid** are widely used in the leather, textile, adhesive, and plastics industries, and **lactic acid** is also used as a food acidulant.

Metabolism & Mechanism of Action

Both inorganic and organic acids, by virtue of their water solubility and acid dissociation, will cause direct destruction of body tissue, including mucous membranes and skin. The extent of direct skin damage depends on the concentration of acid and length of exposure, while the damage to the respiratory tract by inhalation of acid mists will depend in addition on particle size. **Hydrofluoric acid,** one of the most corrosive of the inorganic acids, readily penetrates the skin and travels to deep tissue layers, causing liquefaction necrosis of soft tissues and decalcification and corrosion of bone. The intense pain that may accompany hydrogen fluoride burns is attributed to the calcium-precipitating property of the fluoride ion, which produces immobilization of tissue calcium and an excess of potassium that stimulates nerve endings. The fluoride ion may also bind body calcium, causing life-threatening systemic hypocalcemia after acute skin exposure or osteosclerotic bone changes after chronic exposure to hydrogen fluoride mist.

Clinical Findings
A. Symptoms and Signs:
1. Acute exposure–All acids act as primary irritants of the skin and mucous membranes.

a. Skin–All acids on contact with the skin cause dehydration and heat release to produce first-, second-, or third-degree burns with pain. Sensitization is rare. **Hydrofluoric acid** solutions of less than 50% may cause burns that may not become apparent for 1–24 hours; stronger solutions cause immediate pain and rapid tissue destruction, appearing reddened, pasty-white, blistered, macerated, or charred.

b. Respiratory effects–Inhalation of vapors or mists causes immediate rhinorrhea, throat burning, cough, burning eyes, and conjunctival irritation. High concentrations may cause shortness of breath, chest tightness, pulmonary edema, and death from respiratory failure. Inhalation of acid vapors or mists generally causes immediate symptoms due to high water solubility in mucous membranes, but respiratory effects may be delayed for several hours. For **nitric acid** exposure with oxides of nitrogen, overexposure tends to produce delayed symptoms 1–24 hours after inhalation, beginning with dyspnea followed by pulmonary edema and cyanosis.

c. Systemic effects–One death has been reported due to persistent hypocalcemia following exposure to **hydrofluoric acid** involving 2.5% of total body surface area.

2. Chronic exposure–

a. Skin–Chromate compounds can be allergens and can cause pulmonary as well as skin sensitization, but **chromic acid** results only in direct irritant dermatitis. Ulceration of the skin and ulceration and perforation of the nasal septum have been reported following chronic exposure to 0.1 mg/m^3 of chromic acid.

b. Dental erosion–Tooth erosion has been reported following chronic exposure to chromic, sulfuric, and phosphoric acids.

c. Respiratory effects–Bronchiolitis fibrosa obliterans—a chronic interstitial lung disease—has been described after acute pneumonitis from **nitric acid** and oxides of nitrogen. In a study of lead acid battery plant workers exposed to **sulfuric acid,** the prevalence of respiratory symptoms or changes in pulmonary function over the shift was not related to estimates of cumulative acid exposure.

d. Systemic effects–Osteosclerosis has been found in workers exposed to **hydrofluoric acid** and fluoride-containing compounds. Unlike hexavalent chromium, **chromic acid** or trivalent chromium is not considered to be carcinogenic.

One epidemiologic study has found evidence of an association between laryngeal cancer and exposure to **sulfuric acid** at a large petrochemical facility.

B. Laboratory Findings: In cases where inhalation exposure may cause more extensive mucosal irritation, the chest x-ray may show interstitial or alveolar edema, and hypoxemia may be evident by arterial blood gas analysis. Nonspecific abnormalities in liver and kidney function have been reported following massive inhalation exposures to **sulfuric acid** and **hydrofluoric acid.**

Urine fluoride levels can be used as biologic indices of exposure in **hydrofluoric acid** intoxication, with a normal mean value in urine of 0.5 mg/L (recommended occupational postshift urinary biologic standard of 7 mg/L).

Differential Diagnosis

There are many respiratory irritants (see Chapter 18), including gases such as ammonia, phosgene, halogens (chlorine, bromine), sulfur dioxide, and ozone; solvents such as glycol ethers; and dusts such as fibrous glass. The symptoms and clinical course of lung disorders due to these substances and to the acids discussed in this chapter do not differ; thus, the history is essential. Likewise, hundreds of industrial chemicals may cause direct irritant dermatitis.

Prevention

A. Work Practices: When possible, highly corrosive acids should be replaced by acids that present less hazard, and if use of corrosives is essential, only the minimum concentration should be used. Proper storage practices should include fire-resistant buildings with acid-resistant floors, retaining sills, and adequate drainage; containers should be adequately protected against impact, kept off the floor, and clearly labeled. Wherever possible, handling should be done through sealed systems or the substances transported in safety bottle carriers. Decanting should be done with special siphons or pumps. The potential for violent or dangerous reactions (ie, when water is poured into nitric acid) can be avoided by appropriate training.

Where processes produce acid mists (as in electroplating), local exhaust ventilation should be installed. Workers potentially exposed to splashes or spills must wear acid-resistant hand, arm, eye, and face protection, and respiratory protection should be available for emergency use.

Emergency showers and eyewash stations should be strategically located.

B. Medical Surveillance: Preplacement and periodic examinations should include a medical history of skin and respiratory disease and examination of the skin, teeth, and lungs. For potential hydrofluoric acid exposure near or above the permissible exposure limit, periodic postshift urinary fluoride in excess of 7 mg/L (adjusted for urine specific gravity of 1.024) may indicate poor work practices.

Treatment

Immediate onsite first aid treatment of acid burns to the eye or skin is copious flushing with running water with removal of all contaminated clothing. First-degree burns or second-degree burns involving a small area can generally be treated at the onsite medical facility with debridement and application of suitable burn dressings. All other acid burns should be treated at a hospital emergency facility.

For **hydrofluoric acid** burns, the definitive treatment is aimed at deactivation of the fluoride ion in tissue with calcium, magnesium, or quaternary ammonium solution. If the hydrogen fluoride concentration is 20% or more or if the patient has been exposed to a long delay of a lower concentration—or if a large tissue area has been affected by a lower concentration—then calcium gluconate solution should be used. The latter, prepared by mixing 10% calcium gluconate with an equal amount of saline to form a 5% solution, is infiltrated with a small needle in multiple injections (0.5 mL/cm^2 of tissue) into and 5 mm beyond the affected area. Dramatic pain relief should occur. Vesicles and bullae should be carefully debrided, with removal of necrotic tissue; if periungual or ungual tissues are involved, the nail should be split to the base. A burn dressing is then applied along with calcium gluconate 2.5% gel or magnesium sulfate paste.

If the hydrogen fluoride concentration is 20% or less and only a small surface area is involved, the burn can be flushed with water and then treated with 10% magnesium sulfate solution under a soft dressing.

The eye burned with hydrogen fluoride should be copiously irrigated and then evaluated by an ophthalmologist. One percent calcium gluconate in normal saline can be used as an irrigant.

Systemic effects from absorption should be anticipated from skin burns from hydrogen fluoride of greater than 50% concentration or from extensive burns at any concentration. Hypocalcemia can be life-threatening and should be monitored by repeated measurement of serum calcium and electrocardiography for QT interval prolongation. Ten percent calcium gluconate intravenously with adequate hydration should be used for calcium depletion.

For inhalation of acid vapors or mists, the victim should be immediately removed from the source of exposure and treated onsite with 100% oxygen. If there are symptoms of shortness of breath, chest tightness, or persistent cough, the patient should be evaluated at the hospital. Upper body or facial burns are a clue that inhalation may have occurred with possible lower airway damage. Evaluation should include a chest x-ray and arterial blood gas analysis for oxygen. Hypoxemia should be treated with 100% oxygen by mask, or by intubation in the event of severe hypoxemia, acidosis or respiratory distress. Fluid balance should be carefully monitored and intracardiac pressure measured directly if necessary. Bronchospasm may be treated with inhaled bronchodilators or intravenous aminophylline, and steroids if necessary. The benefits of steroids in the management of noncardiogenic pulmonary edema due to acid inhalation are unknown, but the drugs may be used empirically to speed recovery and prevent the subsequent development of interstitial lung disease.

2. ALKALIES

Essentials of Diagnosis

Acute effects:
- Skin and eye burns.
- Respiratory irritation.

Chronic effects:
- Corneal opacities of the eye (untreated).

Exposure Limits
Sodium hydroxide
 ACGIH TLV: 2 mg/m^3 TWA
 OSHA PEL: 2 mg/m^3 TWA
 NIOSH REL: 2 mg/m^3 ceiling (15 minutes)

General Considerations
Alkalies are caustic substances that dissolve in water to form a solution with a pH higher than 7.0. These include ammonia, ammonium hydroxide, cal-cium hydroxide, calcium oxide, potassium hydroxide, potassium carbonate, sodium hydroxide, sodium carbonate, and trisodium phosphate. The alkalies, whether in solid form or concentrated liquid form, are more destructive to tissue than most acids. They tend to liquefy tissues and allow for deeper penetration, depending on concentration, duration of contact, and area of the body involved.

Use, Production, & Occupational Exposure
In the USA, all **sodium hydroxide** (caustic soda) is produced by the electrolysis of sodium or potassium chloride in mercury cells. In this process, pure saturated brine is decomposed by electric current to liberate chlorine gas at the anode and sodium metal at the cathode. The latter reacts with water to form sodium hydroxide. Most caustic soda is produced as a 50% aqueous solution. A major use is to form sodium salts, to neutralize strong acids, and to solubilize water-insoluble chemicals. Uses include manufacture of bleaches, dyes, vitamins, plastics, pulp and paper, soaps, and detergents; petroleum treatment; food processing; and production of sodium hypochlorite. NIOSH estimates that 150,000 workers are potentially exposed to caustic soda.

Sodium carbonate (soda ash) is produced by the ammonium chloride process, by the reaction of sodium chloride and sulfuric acid, or by leaching out rock deposits. It is widely used in the manufacture of glass, sodium carbonate, aluminum, detergents, salts, and paints; the desulfurization of pig iron; and the purification of petroleum.

Potassium carbonate (potash) is produced by carbonating potassium hydroxide solutions obtained by electrolysis and is widely used in the glass industry, as potash fertilizers, in the soap industry, for wool dyeing, and in the pharmaceutical industry.

Potassium hydroxide (caustic potash) is produced by electrolysis of potassium chloride solution and is used for the manufacture of liquid soaps, as a mordant for wood, for mercerizing cotton, in paint and varnish removers, for electroplating, photoengraving, and lithography, and in printing inks. Over 248,000 tons are produced annually in the USA.

Calcium oxide (quicklime) is made by calcining limestone. Lime is used in the steel industry, in chemical pulp and paper manufacture, in potable water treatment, in sewage treatment, and in pollution control.

Occupational exposure to the alkalies is primarily by direct contact with the eyes, skin, and mucous membranes. Inhalation of caustic mists is generally limited by the irritant properties of the compound.

Metabolism & Mechanism of Action
Contact of the eyes by alkalies will cause disintegration and sloughing of corneal epithelium, corneal opacification, marked edema, and ulceration. Alkaline compounds will combine with skin tissue to form

albuminates and with natural fats to form soaps. They gelatinize tissue and result in deep and painful destruction. Accidental or intentional ingestion of alkalies may cause severe esophageal necrosis with subsequent stenosis.

Clinical Findings

A. Symptoms and Signs:

1. Acute exposure—In contrast to acids, skin contact with the alkalies may not elicit immediate pain but may start to cause immediate damage with erythema and tissue necrosis within minutes to hours. Splashes of alkali to the eyes, if not rapidly treated within minutes, may result in corneal necrosis, edema, and opacification.

2. Chronic exposure—Chronic exposure to caustic dusts for years does not significantly increase the mortality rate. Corneal opacities have resulted from untreated corneal alkali burns.

B. Laboratory Findings: No laboratory tests are of value in the diagnosis and management of problems resulting from alkali exposure.

Differential Diagnosis

Many other industrial chemicals, including acids, may cause eye and skin burns.

Prevention

A. Work Practices: Insofar as possible, solutions of caustics should be handled in closed systems that will prevent contact with or inhalation of the chemical. All persons with potential exposure to caustics should wear the proper protective clothing and equipment, such as a full-face shield, safety goggles, apron or suit, rubber gloves, and boots.

Emergency showers and eyewashes must be located where eye or skin contact may occur.

B. Medical Surveillance. Medical examination of the eyes, skin, and respiratory tract should be done for all workers with caustic exposure.

Treatment

Alkali burns of the eye and skin should be treated within minutes by copious irrigation with water and removal of all contaminated clothing. A physician or health practitioner should be consulted for eye burns and careful examination of the eye performed. If damage is suspected, follow-up with an ophthalmologist is recommended.

ACRYLAMIDE & ACRYLONITRILE

1. ACRYLAMIDE

Essentials of Diagnosis
Acute effects:
- Dermatitis.

Chronic effects:
- Peripheral neuropathy.

Exposure Limits
ACGIH TLV: 0.03 mg/m^3 TWA
OSHA PEL: 0.03 mg/m^3 TWA
NIOSH REL: 0.03 mg/m^3 TWA

General Considerations

Pure acrylamide is a white crystalline solid at room temperature and is highly soluble in water. It is a vinyl monomer with high reactivity with thiols and with hydroxy and amino groups. Commercial acrylamide is shipped in 50% aqueous form in stainless steel drums, tank trucks, and cars. Acrylamide manufacture is from the catalytic hydration of acrylonitrile.

Use

The major use of acrylamide monomer is in the production of polymers, which are useful as flocculators. Polyacrylamides are used for waste and water treatment flocculants, in products for sewage dewatering, and in a variety of products for the water treatment industry. Other uses include strengtheners for papermaking and retention aids, drilling-mud additives, textile treatment, and surface coatings. One of the more important uses is as a grouting agent, particularly in mining and tunnel construction. NIOSH estimates that approximately 20,000 workers are potentially exposed to acrylamide annually in the USA.

Occupational & Environmental Exposure

Monomer manufacturing workers are potentially exposed to acrylamide, as are papermaking workers, soil stabilization workers, textile workers, and well drillers. Intoxication has been reported in the manufacture of acrylamide monomer, in the handling of a 10% aqueous solution in a mine, in the production of flocculators, in the use of a resin mixture containing residual monomer, and in the production of polymers while manufacturing papercoating materials. One nonoccupational incident occurred in Japan where a family ingested well water containing 400 ppm acrylamide.

Metabolism & Mechanism of Action

Acrylamide is easily absorbed in animals following all routes of administration. Quantitative data on absorption or excretion in humans are not available. Following intravenous administration in rats, acrylamide is distributed throughout total body water within minutes and then excreted largely in the urine with a half-life of less than 2 hours. Protein-bound acrylamide or acrylamide metabolites have a half-life in blood and possibly in the central nervous system of about 10 days.

Clinical Findings

A. Symptoms and Signs: Acrylamide polymer may cause dermatitis but does not cause neurotoxicity. The monomer can produce numbness and tingling of hands, and weakness of the hands and legs. Acrylamide is neurotoxic in many experimental animals.

Over 60 cases of acrylamide-associated neurotoxicity have been reported in humans. Similar to the neuropathy associated with the hexacarbons *n*-hexane and methyl-*n*-butyl ketone, acrylamide neuropathy is considered a typical example of a dying-back disorder, where degeneration begins at the distal ends of the longest and largest fibers and spreads proximally. In most cases toxicity resulted from skin contact and dermal absorption, though it may be absorbed by inhalation as well. The neurologic features of acrylamide intoxication vary depending on the speed of intoxication. In the Japanese family who ingested contaminated well water, encephalopathy with confusion, disorientation, memory disturbances, hallucinations, ataxia, and peripheral neuropathy developed in approximately 1 month. Reported time to onset of symptoms in occupational cases has varied from 4 weeks to about 24 months. Clinically, acrylamide peripheral neuropathy affects both motor and sensory nerve fibers predominantly in the distal limbs. Difficulty in walking and clumsiness of the hands are usually the first symptoms, with numbness of the feet and fingers. Distal weakness is found on examination, with loss of tendon reflexes and vibration sensation. Evidence of excessive sweating affecting predominantly the extremities has been commonly reported, along with redness and exfoliation of the skin. In acute cases, central nervous system involvement may result in truncal ataxia, lethargy, and dysarthria.

Acrylamide has been found to increase the tumor yield in mice. No human epidemiologic studies of acrylamide have been reported to date.

B. Laboratory Findings: Electrophysiologic studies of workers with signs and symptoms of neurotoxicity have shown only a slight effect on maximal conduction velocity of either motor or sensory fibers. Sensory nerve action potentials are usually reduced and are the most sensitive electrophysiologic test.

Sural nerve biopsies performed on 2 patients during recovery from acrylamide neuropathy showed axonal degeneration affecting mainly large-diameter fibers.

Differential Diagnosis

The combination of truncal ataxia with peripheral neuropathy—predominantly motor—accompanied by excessive sweating and redness and peeling of the skin makes the diagnosis of acrylamide-associated neurotoxicity likely. Other occupational toxic agents associated with peripheral neuropathy must be considered (see Chapter 22), along with the presence of other underlying metabolic diseases, drug use, and endocrine disorders.

Prevention

A. Work Practices: Mechanized bag loading of polymerization reactors, closed-line transfer of liquid acrylamide, and other closed-system processes are important to minimize exposure. Where necessary, personal protective equipment designed to prevent dermal and inhalation exposure to acrylamide should be available.

B. Medical Surveillance: Preplacement and periodic examinations should exclude symptomatic peripheral neuropathies. Electrophysiologic tests may be useful in following symptomatic subjects but are not recommended for routine detection of early neuropathy. No biologic monitoring methods useful in the routine screening of exposed workers have been developed.

Treatment

Skin contaminated with acrylamide should be washed immediately with soap and water and contaminated clothing removed. There is no known treatment for acrylamide intoxication. Removal from exposure is the only effective measure that can be taken. Full recovery has been observed in most cases after 2 weeks to 2 years, though in severe cases some residual abnormalities have been noted.

2. ACRYLONITRILE

Essentials of Diagnosis

Acute effects:
- Respiratory irritation, nausea, and dizziness, irritability, followed by
- Convulsions, coma, and death.

Chronic effects:
- Nausea, dizziness, headache, apprehension, fatigue.
- Increased risk of lung cancer.

Exposure Limits

ACGIH TLV: 2 ppm TWA
OSHA PEL: 2 ppm TWA, 10 ppm ceiling (15 minutes)
NIOSH REL: 1 ppm TWA, 10 ppm ceiling (15 minutes)

General Considerations

Acrylonitrile is a volatile colorless liquid with a characteristic odor resembling that of peach seeds, discernible at 20 ppm or less. It is a highly reactive compound. Pure acrylonitrile polymerizes readily in light, and storage requires the addition of polymerization inhibitors. Its vapors are explosive and flammable in the range of 3–17% and may release hydrogen cyanide on burning.

Use

Acrylonitrile was not an important product until World War II, when it was used in the production of oil-resistant rubbers. Nearly all world production of acrylonitrile is now based on a process where propylene, ammonia, and air are reacted in the vapor phase in the presence of a catalyst. Hydrogen cyanide and acrylonitrile are the chief by-products formed; the latter undergoes a series of distillations to produce acrylonitrile.

Much of acrylonitrile monomer is used for the manufacture of acrylic fibers for the apparel, carpeting, and home furnishings industries. Acrylonitrile-containing plastics, particularly the resins acrylonitrile-butadiene-styrene (ABS) and styrene-acrylonitrile (SAN), are used in pipe and pipe fittings, automotive parts, appliances, and building components. Nitrile elastomers are used for their oil and hydrocarbon-resistant properties in the petrochemical and automobile industries. Acrylonitrile is also used to make acrylamide.

Occupational & Environmental Exposure

Potential exposure to acrylonitrile may occur in monomer-, fiber-, resin- and rubber-producing plants. Potential exposure to acrylonitrile in acrylic fiber production is greatest when the solvent is removed from newly formed fibers and during decontamination of acrylonitrile processing equipment, loading, surveillance of the processing unit, and product sampling. NIOSH estimates that 125,000 persons are potentially exposed to acrylonitrile in the workplace.

Metabolism & Mechanism of Action

Acrylonitrile is readily absorbed in animals following ingestion or inhalation. There is a biphasic half-life of 3.5 hours and 50–77 hours, with elimination predominantly in the urine. Acrylonitrile is metabolized to cyanide, and its metabolites are eliminated in the urine. In humans, absorption can occur both through inhalation and skin contact. The acute toxicity of acrylonitrile in humans is thought to be due to the action of cyanide, and thiocyanate is detected in blood and urine of workers. It has been postulated that the mutagenic effect of acrylonitrile is due to glycidonitrile, a reactive intermediate able to alkylate macromolecules.

Clinical Findings

A. Symptoms and Signs: A few deaths have been reported from acrylonitrile exposure, with respiratory distress, lethargy, convulsions, and coma at 7500 mg/m^3. Acrylonitrile was implicated in 4 cases of toxic epidermal necrosis, which developed 11–21 days after the victims returned to houses fumigated with a 2:1 mixture of carbon tetrachloride and acrylonitrile. One patient had measurable blood cyanide levels at autopsy. Symptoms of acute poisoning are described as irritability, respiratory irritation, limb weakness, respiratory distress, dizziness, nausea, cyanosis, collapse, convulsions, and cardiac arrest; these resemble cyanide poisoning.

Chronic human toxicity has been reported in rubber workers exposed to 16–100 ppm of acrylonitrile for periods of 20–45 minutes, with complaints of nasal irritation, headache, nausea, apprehension, and fatigue.

Acrylonitrile is carcinogenic in rats after 1 year of feeding and inhalation, inducing brain tumors and stomach papillomas. An excess risk of colon and lung cancers occurred among acrylonitrile polymerization workers from a textile fibers plant. Epidemiologic studies have suggested that acrylonitrile is associated with an increased lung cancer risk with a latency period of 20 years and that it should be regarded as probably carcinogenic in humans. No significant cancer excess has been observed in cohort mortality studies.

B. Laboratory Findings: Chromosomal analysis of workers exposed to acrylonitrile has not shown an increase in aberrations. Elevated serum cyanide or urine thiocyanate levels may be found in cases of acute intoxication.

Differential Diagnosis

Acute poisoning with acrylonitrile may mimic cyanide intoxication.

Prevention

A. Work Practices: Controls have proved effective in reducing employee exposure to acrylonitrile. NIOSH has recommended that acrylonitrile be handled in the workplace as a potential human carcinogen and has published detailed recommendations for adequate work practices.

B. Medical Surveillance: Preplacement and annual medical examinations should include special attention to the skin, respiratory tract, and gastrointestinal tract and to the nonspecific symptoms of headache, nausea, dizziness, and weakness that may be associated with chronic exposure.

Treatment kits for acute cyanide intoxication (see Chapter 31) should be immediately available to trained medical personnel at each area where there is a potential for release of or contact with acrylonitrile.

Biologic monitoring may be useful to reflect exposure to acrylonitrile. The relationship between the degree of exposure to acrylonitrile and the urinary excretion of thiocyanate and acrylonitrile was determined in Japanese workers from acrylic fiber factories. A mean postshift urine thiocyanate concentration of 11.4 mg/L (specific gravity 1.024) was found to correlate with an 8-hour average acrylonitrile exposure of 4.2 ppm. Normal urinary thiocyanate levels in nonsmokers does not exceed 2.5 mg/g of creatinine. Mean urinary acrylonitrile levels of 30 μg/L in Dutch plastics workers were found to correlate with a mean 8-hour TWA exposure level of 0.13 ppm and were used to monitor adequate work practices.

Treatment

Treatment of acute intoxication with acrylonitrile is similar to that of cyanide poisoning (see Chapter 31).

AROMATIC AMINES

Essentials of Diagnosis

Acute effects:
- Dermatitis.
- Asthma.
- Cholestatic jaundice.
- Methemoglobinemia.

Chronic effects:
- Bladder cancer.

Exposure Limits

Aniline
   ACGIH TLV: 2 ppm TWA
   OSHA PEL: 2 ppm TWA
p,p'-Methylene dianiline
   ACGIH TLV: 0.1 ppm TWA
   NIOSH REL: Reduce exposure to lowest feasible concentration
Naphthylamines
   OSHA PEL: Stringent workplace controls
Benzidine-based dyes
   NIOSH REL: Reduce exposure to lowest feasible concentration. Replace with less toxic material.
4,4'-Methylene-bis-(2-chloroaniline) (MBOCA).
   ACGIH TLV: 0.02 ppm TWA
   OSHA PEL: 0.02 ppm TWA
   NIOSH REL: 3 $\mu g/m^3$ (lowest detectable concentration)
o-Toluidine
   ACGIH TLV: 2 ppm TWA
   OSHA PEL: 5 ppm TWA
   NIOSH REL: 20 $\mu g/m^3$ (60 minutes)

General Considerations

The aromatic amines are a class of chemicals derived from aromatic hydrocarbons such as benzene, toluene, naphthalene, anthracene and diphenyl, etc, by the replacement of at least one hydrogen atom by an amino group. Some examples are shown below.

Aniline

o-Toluidine

Benzidine

MBOCA

Use

Aromatic amines are used mainly in the synthesis of other chemicals. The most important aromatic amines are aniline and 2,4-toluenediamine, which are used in the manufacture of isocyanates and rubber chemicals.

The principal commercial use of benzidine is in the manufacture of a wide range of dyes and pigments. At present, benzidine dihydrochloride is the only form commercially produced in the USA. At least 16 benzidine-based dyes are produced in the USA, with a total production of 1–2 million pounds. Two-thirds are used by the textile industry, 17% for the paper and pulp industry, 10% for the leather tanning industry, and about 7% for the aqueous ink and plastics industries.

Because of the demonstrated carcinogenicity of β-naphthylamine, its manufacture and use was banned in many countries. Production of β-naphthylamine ceased in the USA in 1972.

Occupational & Environmental Exposure

NIOSH estimates that about 700 people are occupationally exposed to benzidine and that 79,200 workers in 63 occupations are potentially exposed to benzidine-based dyes.

Metabolism & Mechanism of Action

The aromatic amines are nearly all lipid-soluble and are absorbed through the skin. Metabolism is largely via the formation of hydroxylamine intermediates. These metabolites are transported to the bladder as N-glucuronide conjugates and hydrolyzed by the acid pH of urine to form reactive electrophiles that bind to bladder transitional epithelial DNA. Animal studies have demonstrated that bladder epithelial prostaglandin H synthetase can activate aromatic amines that then bind to nucleic acids.

Clinical Findings

A. Symptoms and Signs:

1. Acute exposure–

a. Dermatitis–Because of their alkaline nature, certain amines constitute a direct risk of dermatitis. Many aromatic amines can cause allergic dermatitis, notably *p*-aminophenol and *p*-phenylenediamine. The latter was known for "fur dermatitis" and asthma among fur dyers.

b. Respiratory effects–Asthma due to *p*-phenylenediamine has been reported.

c. Hemorrhagic cystitis–Hemorrhagic cystitis can result from exposure to *o*- and *p*-toluidine and 5-chloro-*o*-toluidine. The hematuria is self-limited, and no increase in bladder tumors has been subsequently noted.

d. Hepatic injury–Cholestatic jaundice has resulted from industrial exposure to diaminodiphenylmethane, which also caused toxic jaundice due to contaminated baking flour ("Epping jaundice") (see

Chapter 20). The hepatitis has been reversible after cessation of exposure.

e. Methemoglobinemia–Acute poisoning by aniline and its derivatives results in the formation of methemoglobin. A significant elevation of methemoglobin levels has been demonstrated in adult volunteers after ingestion of 25 mg of aniline. The mean lethal dose has been estimated to be between 15 and 30 g, though death has followed ingestion of as little as 1 g of aniline. It has been postulated that a toxic metabolite, phenylhydroxylamine, is responsible for the methemoglobin. Peak levels of methemoglobin are observed within 1–2 hours after ingestion. Cyanosis becomes apparent at levels of methemoglobin of 10–15%, and headache, weakness, dyspnea, dizziness, and malaise occur at levels of 25–30%. Concentrations above 60–70% may cause coma and death.

f. Bladder cancer–An excess of bladder tumors was recognized in 1895 among German workers who used aromatic amines in the production of synthetic dyes. British dyestuffs workers had a high risk for the development of bladder cancer. In the USA, bladder cancer occurred in workers exposed to β-naphthylamine or benzidine in the manufacture of dyes, with a mean latency period of 20 years from onset of exposure.

Workers involved in the production of auramine and magenta from aniline and those working with 4-aminobiphenyl have an increased risk of bladder tumors. Workers exposed to 4-chloro-*o*-toluidine have been observed to have a 73-fold excess of bladder cancer. Animal studies have shown an increased risk of bladder tumors after exposure to benzidine, *o*-toluidine, *o*-dianisidine-based dyes and MBOCA and other aromatic amines.

B. Laboratory Findings: Methemoglobin levels can help in the detection of excess absorption of the single-ring aromatic compounds. Normal individuals have methemoglobin concentrations of 1–2%. A biologic threshold limit value of 5% has been proposed.

Determination of the metabolites *p*-aminophenol and *p*-nitrophenol can be useful to monitor exposure to aniline and nitrobenzene. After 6 hours of exposure to 1 ppm of nitrobenzene, the urinary concentration of *p*-aminophenol should not exceed 50 mg/L, and the recommended biologic threshold value is 10 mg/L.

Levels of free MBOCA in the urine can be used to monitor exposure to this compound. Levels of free MBOCA in urine should be minimized to the limit of detection and used as an index of the adequacy of existing work practices and engineering controls.

For workers exposed to the known or suspected carcinogenic aromatic amines, periodic screening of urine for red blood cells and evidence of dysplastic epithelium may detect early bladder cancer.

Differential Diagnosis

Aliphatic nitrates (eg, ethylene glycol dinitrate),

aliphatic nitrites, inorganic nitrites, and chlorates may also cause methemoglobinemia.

Occupation-associated bladder cancer may account for 10–15% of all cases of bladder cancer. Cigarette smoking, with inhalation of carcinogenic arylamines (eg, 2-aminonaphthalene), is also a significant risk factor.

Prevention

A. Work Practices: Every effort should be made to eliminate use of the carcinogenic aromatic amines by substitution of safer alternatives. Appropriate engineering controls for manufacturers of polyurethane products who use MBOCA—particularly the use of automated systems and local exhaust ventilation—can successfully reduce the potential for exposures. Since most cases of aniline exposure occur through skin and clothing contamination, emphasis should be given to provision of appropriate gloves and protective clothing.

For the benzidine-based dyes, worker exposure should be reduced to the lowest feasible levels through appropriate engineering controls, including the use of closed-process systems, liquid metering systems, walk-in hoods, and specific local exhaust ventilation. Dust levels can be minimized by the use of dyes in pellet, paste, or liquid form. Restricted access to areas with potential exposure and provision of suitable protective clothing and respirators should be instituted.

B. Medical Surveillance: Preemployment and periodic measurement of postshift urinary *p*-aminophenol is useful for biologic monitoring of aniline exposure. Similarly, periodic postshift urine samples for free MBOCA can be an important adjunct to industrial hygiene measures of exposure.

High-risk populations with past or current exposure to carcinogenic aromatic amines should be screened on a periodic basis with exfoliative bladder cytology. Positive findings are followed up with direct urologic examination.

Treatment

The definitive treatment of methemoglobinemia caused by aniline poisoning is administration of the reducing agent methylene blue. However, an excessive amount of methylene blue may itself provoke the formation of methemoglobin. Additionally, the ability of methylene blue to reduce methemoglobin can be impaired by hereditary G6PD deficiency and can precipitate frank hemolysis. The recommended dose of methylene blue for the initial management of methemoglobinemia is 1–2 mg/kg of body weight intravenously, equivalent to 0.1–0.2 mL of a 1% solution. Maximal response to methylene blue usually occurs within 30–60 minutes. Repeated doses should be spaced about 1 hour apart and based on methemoglobin levels; most patients, unless they are anemic, can tolerate a level of 30% or less. Methylene blue administration should be discontinued if either a negligible response or an increase in methemoglobin levels results after 2 consecutive doses or if the total dose exceeds 7 mg/kg. It is advisable to continue to monitor methemoglobin levels even after an initial response to methylene blue, since there is a potential for continued production of methemoglobin by aniline.

Treatment of bladder cancer associated with aromatic amine exposure is identical to that of nonoccupationally associated bladder tumors.

Early detection through screening programs may improve prognosis.

CARBON DISULFIDE

Essentials of Diagnosis

Acute effects:
- Irritability, manic delirium, hallucinations, paranoia.
- Respiratory irritation.

Chronic effects:
- Coronary artery disease.
- Neurobehavioral abnormalities.
- Retinal microaneurysms.
- Peripheral neuropathy with ascending symmetric paresthesias and weakness.

Exposure Limits

ACGIH TLV: 10 ppm TWA
OSHA PEL: 4 ppm TWA, 12 ppm STEL
NIOSH REL: 1 ppm TWA, 10 ppm ceiling (15 minutes)

General Considerations

Carbon disulfide is a colorless volatile solvent with a strong, sweetish aroma. The average odor threshold of 1 ppm is below the permissible exposure limit; therefore, carbon disulfide is a material with good warning properties. It evaporates at room temperature, and its vapor is 2.6 times heavier than air; it may form explosive mixtures in a range of 1–50% by volume in air.

Use

About 45% of carbon disulfide is used in the production of viscose rayon fibers and cellophane and 30% in the manufacture of carbon tetrachloride. Other uses include the manufacture of rubber vulcanizers and pesticides.

Occupational & Environmental Exposure

NIOSH estimates that approximately 20,000 employees are potentially exposed to carbon disulfide in the United States. In the production of viscose rayon, carbon disulfide is added to alkali cellulose to yield sodium cellulose xanthate. The latter is dissolved in caustic soda to yield viscose syrup, which can be spun to form textile yarn, tire yarn, or staple fiber or cast to form cellophane. Exposure to high concentrations of carbon disulfide can occur during the opening of sealed spinning machines and during cutting and drying.

Metabolism & Mechanism of Action

Inhalation is the major route of absorption in occupational exposure, and 40–50% of carbon disulfide in inhaled air is retained in the body. Excretion of carbon disulfide by the lung accounts for 10–30% of absorbed dose, and less than 1% is excreted unchanged by the kidney. The remainder is excreted in the form of various metabolites in the urine.

Carbon disulfide is metabolized by formation of dithiocarbamates and reduced glutathione conjugates as well as by oxidative transformation. Thiourea, mercapturic acids, and the glutathione conjugate 2-thiothiazolidine-4-carboxylic acid (TTCA) can be detected in urine of exposed workers. Formation of dithiocarbamate may account in part for the nervous system toxicity of carbon disulfide, while oxidation yields carbonyl sulfide, a hepatotoxic metabolite.

Clinical Findings
A. Symptoms and Signs:
1. Acute exposure–Acute carbon disulfide intoxication was described in the 1920s from the viscose rayon industry, involving exposure to concentrations of hundreds or thousands parts per million. Signs and symptoms included extreme irritability, uncontrolled anger, rapid mood changes—including manic delirium and hallucinations—paranoid ideas, and suicidal tendencies.

Exposure to 4800 ppm of carbon disulfide for 30 minutes may cause rapid coma and death. High concentrations of vapor may cause irritation of the eyes, nose, and throat; liquid carbon disulfide may cause second- or third-degree burns.

2. Chronic exposure–Chronic effects of lower level exposure to carbon disulfide include the following:

a. Eye–A high incidence of retinal microaneurysms and delayed fundal peripapillary filling by fluorescein angiography has been reported in Japanese and Yugoslavian workers exposed to carbon disulfide. Finnish studies have not confirmed these findings, and whether eye damage occurs below 20 ppm (8-hour TWA) is still unknown.

b. Ear–High-frequency hearing loss and vestibular symptoms of vertigo and nystagmus may occur.

c. Heart–Epidemiologic studies have shown a 2.5- to 5-fold increase in death from coronary artery disease as compared with control workers with exposure to carbon disulfide in the range of 10–30 parts per million. Spinners in the British rayon industry have an excess mortality rate from ischemic heart disease. In the US study, an excess of deaths from atherosclerotic heart disease was observed among the potentially most heavily exposed workers. A higher prevalence of hypertension and elevated cholesterol and lipoprotein levels can occur and may contribute to the higher incidence of atherosclerotic disease.

d. Nervous system–Scandinavian studies have shown neurobehavioral changes in psychomotor speed, motor coordination, and personality in workers exposed to low concentrations (5–30 ppm) of carbon disulfide. There is a reduction in peripheral nerve conduction upon exposure to less than 10 ppm, although clinical symptoms of polyneuropathy are not present.

e. Reproductive effects–Lower sperm counts and abnormal sperm morphology occur in chronically exposed workers. Women exposed to concentrations of less than 10 ppm may have an increased rate of menstrual abnormalities, spontaneous abortions, and premature births.

B. Laboratory Findings: Nonspecific elevations of liver enzymes and creatinine have been reported in acute intoxication. With chronic exposure, peripheral nerve conduction velocity can be decreased and neurobehavioral testing may show abnormalities in psychomotor skills and measures of personality function.

Urinary metabolites that catalyze the reaction of iodine with sodium azide can be used to detect exposure above 16 ppm (iodine-azide reaction). The concentration of end-of-shift urinary TTCA is related to exposure and can detect uptake as low as 10 ppm over the whole working shift.

Differential Diagnosis

Cardiac disease from carbon disulfide intoxication must be differentiated from atherosclerotic heart disease due to other causes. Peripheral polyneuropathy should be distinguished from that due to alcohol, drugs, diabetes, and other toxic agents. Neuropsychiatric symptoms may be due to depression, posttraumatic stress syndrome, or other toxic exposures such as organic solvents.

Prevention

A. Work Practices: Control of exposure must rely largely on engineering controls, with enclosure of processes and machines and proper use of ventilation systems. Operator rotation and respiratory protection during peak exposures should be implemented. Potential sources of ignition are prohibited in areas where carbon disulfide is stored or handled, and the substance must not be allowed to accumulate to concentrations higher than 0.1%. Impervious clothing, gloves, and face shields should be worn to prevent skin contact.

B. Medical Surveillance: Initial medical examination should include the central and peripheral nervous system, eyes, and cardiovascular system. Visual acuity should be measured and a baseline electrocardiogram obtained. Periodic medical surveillance to detect early signs or symptoms of toxicity should include questions regarding cardiac, nervous system, and reproductive function, with evaluation of blood pressure, peripheral nerve function, and mental status. Neurobehavioral testing, exercise electrocardiography, and nerve conduction velocity testing may be indicated.

Measurement of TTCA in urine collected at the end of the workshift following the first workday is the test of choice for biologic monitoring. Five milligrams per gram of creatinine corresponds to an 8-hour exposure (TWA) to the current TLV. The widely used iodine-azide test is insensitive at carbon disulfide levels of less than 16.7 ppm.

The presence of preexisting neurologic, psychiatric, or cardiac disease should be considered relative contraindications for individual exposure.

Treatment

Skin and eye contact with carbon disulfide should be treated immediately by washing with large amounts of water, and all contaminated clothing should be removed. No specific treatment is available for chronic carbon disulfide toxicity.

CHLOROMETHYL ETHERS

Essentials of Diagnosis

Acute effects:
- Respiratory irritation.
- Skin rash.

Chronic effects:
- Lung cancer.

Exposure Limits

ACGIH TLV: 0.001 ppm TWA
OSHA PEL: Stringent workplace controls

General Considerations

The haloethers bis(chloromethyl) ether (BCME) and chloromethyl methyl ether (CMME) are highly volatile colorless liquids at room temperature, miscible with many organic solvents. The haloethers are alkylating agents, which are highly reactive in vivo. Technical grade CMME contains 1–8% BCME as an impurity.

Use

BCME is formed when formaldehyde reacts with chloride ions in an acidic medium. It has been used in the past primarily for chloromethylations, eg, in the preparation of ion exchange resins, where a polystyrene resin is chloromethylated and then treated with an amine.

Occupational & Environmental Exposure

Occupational exposure to the chloromethyl ethers occurs in anion exchange resin production. Since 1948, approximately 2000 workers have been exposed to BCME in ion exchange resin manufacture where exposure levels ranged from 10 to 100 ppb. Currently, exposure to BCME in the manufacture of ion exchange resins is limited to one plant in the USA.

BCME may also be a potential hazard in the textile industry, where formaldehyde-containing reactants and resins are used in fabric finishing and as adhesives in laminating and flocking fabrics. Thermosetting emulsion polymers containing methylacrylamide as binders may liberate formaldehyde on drying and curing and then form BCME in the presence of available chloride. A NIOSH study of textile finishing plants found from 0.4 ppb to 8 ppb BCME in the workroom air. This led to the use of low-formaldehyde resins and chloride-free catalysts.

Clinical Findings

A. Symptoms and Signs:

1. Acute exposure–The chloromethyl ethers are potent skin and respiratory irritants. There are no reported cases of acute overexposure to either BCME or CMME.

2. Chronic exposure–Both BCME and CMME are carcinogenic and mutagenic in animal and cellular test systems. When rats are exposed to 0.1 ppm of BCME by inhalation for 6 hours a day, 5 days a week, for a total of 101 exposures, a high incidence of esthesioneuroblastomas and squamous cell carcinoma of the respiratory tract is observed. Both BCME and CMME produce skin papillomas and squamous tumors on direct application or subcutaneous injection. In humans, an excess of lung cancer has been suspected since 1962. An industry-wide survey of plants using chloromethyl ethers has documented a strikingly increased risk of lung cancer in exposed workers. Over 60 cases of BCME-associated lung cancer have been identified, with oat cell the principal histologic type. The historical average time-weighted exposure in these cases has been estimated to be between 10 and 100 ppm, and the latency period between exposure and lung cancer ranges from 5 to 25 years. An increasing incidence is observed with intensity and length of exposure. In addition, the risk of lung cancer is increased in smokers versus non-smokers. The mortality rate from respiratory tract cancer is significantly (almost 3 times) higher among chlormethyl ether-exposed workers, with a latency of 10–19 years. The risk of cancer among exposed workers declines after 20 years from first exposure.

B. Laboratory Findings: The lung carcinoma associated with BCME and CMME presents in similar fashion to nonoccupationally associated carcinoma. Chest radiography may show a mass that should lead to appropriate diagnostic testing. Alternatively, sputum cytology may be abnormal in the presence of a normal chest x-ray and thus may be useful as a screening technique in individual cases. Sputum cytology may be of some value in the follow-up of workers exposed to known carcinogens who remain at risk for many years following exposure.

Differential Diagnosis

Known occupational lung carcinogens include asbestos, arsenic, chromium, and uranium, and so a careful occupational history should be obtained from an individual who presents with lung carcinoma.

Prevention

A. Work Practices: Enclosed chemical processes are essential to reduce exposure below 1 ppb, and continuous monitoring has been utilized successfully to warn of excessive exposures to BCME and CMME. As the number of potentially exposed workers has markedly declined since the 1970s, medical follow-up of past exposed workers has assumed a greater role.

B. Medical Surveillance: Preplacement and annual lung examination should be included in medical surveillance of exposed workers. Periodic sputum cytology may be of value in detecting early lung cancer.

Treatment

The treatment of lung carcinoma associated with BCME/CMME exposure does not differ from that of nonoccupational cases.

DIBROMOCHLOROPROPANE

Essentials of Diagnosis

Acute effects:
- Oligospermia, azoospermia.

Exposure Limits

OSHA PEL: 1 ppb TWA
NIOSH REL: 10 ppb TWA (superseded by OSHA standard)

General Considerations

Dibromochloropropane is a brominated organochlorine nematocide which was used extensively since the 1950s on citrus fruits, grapes, peaches, pineapples, soybeans, and tomatoes. Millions of pounds were produced in the USA. In 1977, employees at a California pesticide formulation plant were found to be infertile, and further investigation documented azoospermia and oligospermia among workers exposed to dibromochloropropane. In DBCP-exposed men with both azoospermia and elevation in FSH level, follow-up evaluation has generally shown permanent destruction of germinal epithelium. In the USA, the application of dibromochloropropane to all but pineapples in Hawaii was banned in 1979 by the EPA.

DIMETHYLAMINOPROPIONITRILE

Dimethylaminopropionitrile was a component of catalysts used in manufacture of flexible polyurethane foams. In 1978, NIOSH reported urinary dysfunction and neurologic symptoms among workers at facilities which used dimethylaminopropionitrile. Workers at polyurethane manufacturing plants developed neurogenic bladder dysfunction after the introduction of a catalyst containing dimethylaminopropionitrile. Workers had urinary retention, hesitancy, and dribbling. Examination showed a pattern of decreased sensation confined to the lower sacral dermatomes, abnormal retention of contrast material on intravenous pyelogram, or abnormal cystometrograms. Nerve conduction velocity studies were normal. While the majority of workers recovered, some had prolonged effects.

Following these findings, production of catalysts containing dimethylaminopropionitrile was voluntarily discontinued.

Dimethylaminopropionitrile appears to be a unique example of a neurotoxin that produces localized autonomic dysfunction without peripheral nervous system damage. The discovery of this toxicity by an alert clinician underscores the role of the community practitioner in the discovery of new occupational diseases.

ETHYLENE OXIDE

Essentials of Diagnosis

Acute effects:
- Respiratory tract irritation.
- Skin rash.
- Headache, drowsiness, weakness.

Chronic effects:
- Increased sister chromatid exchanges in lymphocytes.
- Possible increased risk of cancer.

Exposure Limits

ACGIH TLV: 1 ppm TWA
OSHA PEL: 1 ppm TWA, 5 ppm excursion limit (15 minutes)
NIOSH REL: Less than 0.1 ppm TWA, 5 ppm ceiling (10 min/d)

General Considerations

Ethylene oxide is a colorless flammable gas with a characteristic etherlike odor. At elevated pressures, it may be a volatile liquid. It is completely miscible with water and many organic solvents. The threshold of detection in humans is about 700 ppm but quite variable, and smell cannot be relied on to warn of overexposure. To reduce the explosive hazard of ethylene oxide used as a fumigant or sterilant, it is often mixed with carbon dioxide or halocarbons (15% ethylene oxide and 85% dichlorofluoromethane).

Use

Ethylene oxide has a production volume in the USA of over 7 billion pounds a year. It is used in the manufacture of ethylene glycol (used for antifreeze and as an intermediate for polyester fibers, films, and bottles), nonionic surface-active agents (used for home laundry detergents and dishwashing formulations), glycol ethers (used for surface coatings), and ethanolamines (for soaps, detergents, and textile chemicals). It is used as a pesticide fumigant and as a sterilant in hospitals, medical products manufacture, libraries, museums, beekeeping, spice and seasoning fumigation, animal and plant quarantine, transportation vehicle fumigation, and dairy packaging.

Occupational & Environmental Exposure

Most ethylene oxide is used as a chemical intermediate in plants where closed and automated processes generally maintain exposure levels below 1 ppm. The greatest potential for worker exposure occurs during loading or unloading of transport tanks, product sampling, and equipment maintenance and repair.

Although only about 0.02% of production is used for sterilization in hospitals, NIOSH estimates that 75,000 health care workers have potential exposure to ethylene oxide. Approximately 10,000 ethylene oxide sterilization units are in use in 8100 hospitals in the USA. Field surveys of hospital gas sterilizers have generally found that 8-hour time-weighted average exposures to ethylene oxide are below 1 ppm. However, occupational exposure may be several hundred parts per million for brief periods during the opening of the sterilizer door, in the transfer of freshly sterilized items to the aeration cabinet or central supply area, during tank changes, and at the gas discharge point.

Metabolism & Mechanism of Action

Ethylene oxide is absorbed through the skin and respiratory tract. It is an alkylating agent that binds to DNA and may cause cellular mutation.

Clinical Findings

A. Symptoms and Signs:

1. Acute exposure–Ethylene oxide is irritating to the eyes, respiratory tract, and skin, and at high concentrations it can cause respiratory depression. Symptoms of upper respiratory tract irritation occur at between 200 and 400 ppm, and above 1000 ppm ethylene oxide may cause headache, nausea, dyspnea, vomiting, drowsiness, weakness, and incoordination. Direct contact of the skin or eyes with liquid ethylene oxide can result in severe irritation, burns, or contact dermatitis.

2. Chronic exposure–

a. Mutagenic and cytogenetic effects–Ethylene oxide is mutagenic in a number of short-term tests. It is a potent alkylating agent and causes an increased frequency of sister chromatid exchanges and chromosomal aberrations in both animals and humans after inhalation exposure.

b. Reproductive effects–Ethylene oxide is toxic to reproductive function in both male and female experimental animals. In humans, a retrospective study of reproductive function in Finnish hospital sterilizing staff has shown a higher rate of spontaneous abortions in women exposed to ethylene oxide.

c. Carcinogenic effects—Chronic inhalation bioassays in rats have shown that ethylene oxide results in a dose-related increase in mononuclear cell leukemia, peritoneal mesothelioma, and cerebral glioma. Intragastric administration of ethylene oxide in rats produces a dose-dependent increase of squamous cell carcinomas of the forestomach.

Retrospective cohort mortality studies have suggested an excess of leukemia and stomach cancers in ethylene oxide-exposed workers.

Based on the animal and human data regarding carcinogenicity, NIOSH lowered the 8-hour TWA to below 0.1 ppm. As exposure of hospital personnel are generally short-term peak exposures, NIOSH recommends a short-term exposure limit of 5 ppm as well.

d. Neurologic toxicity—Impairment of sensory and motor function has been observed in animals exposed to 357 ppm ethylene oxide over 48–85 days, and 4 cases of peripheral neuropathy were described among workers exposed to a leaking sterilizing chamber for 2–8 weeks. A preliminary study of sterilization workers revealed evidence of neurobehavioral dysfunction compared with controls. Further research into the chronic central nervous system effects of ethylene oxide are needed.

B. Laboratory Findings: No specific finding is characteristic of ethylene oxide exposure. Lymphocytosis has been noted after acute exposure. Where inhalation results in respiratory symptoms, the chest radiograph may show interstitial or frank alveolar edema. Where suspect, a complete blood count may be helpful in the diagnosis of leukemia. Cytogenetic analysis (ie, sister chromatid exchange) of peripheral lymphocytes cannot be used in individual cases to quantitate exposure or estimate cancer risk.

Differential Diagnosis

The mixture of chlorofluorocarbons found in sterilant cylinders may also produce upper respiratory symptoms on inhalation exposure. Many other genotoxicants, including cigarette smoke and other alkylating agents, may cause an increase in sister chromatid exchanges and chromosomal aberrations, so these findings cannot be specifically linked to ethylene oxide unless these causes are excluded.

Prevention

A. Work Practices: Proper engineering controls are essential that reduce short-term exposures to hospital sterilizer staff during procedures where ethylene oxide levels have been found to be greatest. A NIOSH survey has found that engineering controls are extremely effective in hospitals in reducing ethylene oxide exposure during sterilization. These include effective sterilization chamber ethylene oxide purging, local exhaust ventilation at the sterilizer door, adequate ventilation of floor drains, efficient handling of product carts from sterilizer to aerator,

and installation of ethylene oxide tanks in ventilated cabinets. Self-contained breathing apparatus or airline respirators are the only respirators acceptable for ethylene oxide and must be worn when concentrations of ethylene oxide are unknown, as when entering walk-in chambers or for emergency response.

B. Medical Surveillance: Preplacement and periodic examinations should include attention to the pulmonary, hematologic, neurologic, and reproductive systems. A white blood cell count should be obtained at least initially and at periodic intervals if exposure to ethylene oxide is over 0.5 ppm 8-hour TWA or if intermittent exposures exceed 5 ppm. Cytogenetic monitoring has been used by industries willing to maintain exposures below those causing any observable increase above preexposure baseline levels.

No specific biologic monitoring of blood or urine is recommended. Ethylene oxide alveolar air concentration correlates with exposure but has not been routinely used in hospital personnel.

Personnel trained in emergency response for use of self-contained breathing apparatus should be evaluated for cardiorespiratory fitness with pulmonary function or exercise testing.

Treatment

Removal from the work environment after inhalation of the gas should be immediate. If respiratory symptoms are evident, oxygen should be administered and the victim brought to the emergency ward. Any contaminated clothing should be immediately removed and, where appropriate, the skin thoroughly washed with soap and water. A chest radiograph should be obtained if warranted by respiratory symptoms, and the patient observed for several hours for the onset of pulmonary edema. No other specific treatment is indicated.

FORMALDEHYDE

Essentials of Diagnosis

Acute effects:
- Eye irritation causing lacrimation, redness, and pain.
- Cough, chest tightness, shortness of breath.
- Skin irritation, contact dermatitis.

Chronic effects:
- Bronchitis, exacerbation of asthma.

Exposure Limits

ACGIH TLV: 1 ppm TWA, 2 ppm STEL
OSHA PEL: 1 ppm TWA, 2 ppm STEL
NIOSH REL: 0.016 ppm TWA, 0.1 ppm ceiling
(15 minutes)

General Considerations

Formaldehyde is a colorless, flammable gas with a pungent, irritating odor. Known to physicians as a tissue preservative and disinfectant, formaldehyde is a basic feedstock of the modern chemical industry. It may also be encountered as formalin (37–50% formaldehyde), methyl aldehyde, methanal (methanol-formaldehyde mixture), methylene glycol, paraform, or paraformaldehyde (a linear copolymer of formaldehyde).

Use

The estimated annual capacity for formaldehyde production at 48 plants in the USA is over 8.5 billion pounds. Half of this amount is used in the manufacture of urea-formaldehyde foam and resins used as adhesives in particle board, fiberboard, and plywood; 20% is used as a chemical intermediate. Formaldehyde is used as a tissue fixative and embalming agent and as a preservative in cosmetics, glues, and shampoos. It is a byproduct of the incomplete combustion of hydrocarbons and is found in small amounts in automobile exhaust and cigarette smoke.

Occupational & Environmental Exposure

Occupational exposure to formaldehyde above 1 ppm occurs in the production of formaldehyde resin and plastics and in the manufacture of apparel, plywood particle board and wood furniture, paper, and paperboard; workers at risk include urea-formaldehyde foam insulation dealers and installers, mushroom farmers, embalmers, and laboratory workers. A survey of 23 industries and 34 job categories reported an estimated total of 1.34 million workers with formaldehyde exposure and an estimated 1.4 million medical, nursing, and biology students intermittently exposed. NIOSH industrial hygiene surveys have found formaldehyde levels up to 8 ppm in hospital autopsy rooms and up to 2.7 ppm in gross anatomy laboratories.

Residential exposure to formaldehyde up to several parts per million occurs from urea-formaldehyde foam insulation (UFFI) and particle board in mobile homes. Levels of formaldehyde are highest in new residences and decline with a half-life of 4–5 years for mobile homes and less than 1 year for UFFI homes. About 2.2 million persons are living in mobile homes less than 5 years old, and 1.3 to 1.6 million people are living in homes insulated with UFFI. Mean levels for mobile homes are about 0.5 ppm and for UFFI homes about 0.1 ppm. Diurnal and seasonal variations in exposure levels may occur.

Metabolism & Mechanism of Action

Formaldehyde is formed intracellularly as N^5,N^{10}-methylenetetrahydrofolic acid, an important metabolic intermediate. Exogenous formaldehyde can be absorbed by inhalation, ingestion, or dermal absorption. Over 95% of an inhaled dose is absorbed and rapidly metabolized to formic acid by formaldehyde dehydrogenase. Formaldehyde disappears from plasma with a half-time of 1–1.5 minutes, so that an increase cannot be detected immediately following inhalation exposure to high concentrations. Most formaldehyde is converted to CO_2 via formate, and a little is excreted in the urine as formate and other metabolites.

Formaldehyde interacts with macromolecules such as DNA, RNA, and protein. This probably accounts for its carcinogenic effect.

Clinical Findings
A. Symptoms and Signs:
1. Acute exposure–Formaldehyde vapor exposure causes direct irritation of the skin and respiratory tract. Both direct irritation (eczematous reaction) and allergic contact dermatitis (type IV delayed hypersensitivity) occur. After a few days of exposure to formaldehyde solutions or formaldehyde-containing resins, the individual may develop a sudden urticarial eczematous reaction of the skin of the eyelids, face, neck, and flexor surfaces of the arms.

Direct irritation of the eyes, nose, and throat occurs among most people exposed to 0.1–3 ppm of formaldehyde vapor. The odor threshold is 0.05–1 ppm, and some individuals may therefore note irritation of the upper respiratory tract at or just above the odor threshold. Shortness of breath, cough, and chest tightness occur at 10–20 ppm. Formaldehyde is a dose-dependent upper respiratory irritant but does not appear to cause asthma. Exposure to 50–100 ppm and above can cause pulmonary edema, pneumonitis, or death.

2. Chronic exposure–
a. Cancer–Squamous cell carcinomas of the nasal epithelium were induced in rats and mice exposed for prolonged periods (up to 2 years).

No case of nasal cancer has been reported in embalmers or chemical workers. A large case-control study of nasal cancer suggests a slightly increased risk associated with formaldehyde exposure (2 cases of nasal cancer). No other cancers have been reported in persons exposed to formaldehyde. Analysis of historical cohort mortality rates in a large United States exposed industrial workforce is controversial, with significant excess lung cancer risk found by one study but not by another. NIOSH recommends that formaldehyde be considered a potential human carcinogen and that occupational exposure be reduced to the lowest feasible limit.

b. Other health effects–Occupational asthma has occurred in nurses exposed to formaldehyde in a dialysis unit, but the cause was not confirmed by formaldehyde challenge. The direct irritant effect of formaldehyde may precipitate wheezing in those with underlying asthma or bronchial hyperreactivity.

Chronic formaldehyde exposure has been linked anecdotally to a variety of neuropsychologic problems, but there is no evidence to substantiate these reports.

There is no convincing evidence that formaldehyde causes adverse reproductive outcomes.

B. Laboratory Findings:
1. Liver and kidney–Routine tests of hepatic and

renal function are generally unremarkable. Measurement of formic acid in the urine is generally not helpful due to the short half life of formaldehyde.

2. Skin—If contact dermatitis is suspected, patch testing should be performed with appropriate concentrations of formaldehyde.

3. Respiratory system—Cough, shortness of breath, or wheezing may be associated with decreased forced expiratory volume in one second (FEV_1) by pulmonary function testing. Peak flow recordings while at work may show a decrease in maximal airflow during or after exposure to formaldehyde. After exposure to over 20–30 ppm of formaldehyde, chest x-rays may show interstitial or alveolar edema, with resultant reduction in arterial oxygen content on blood gas analysis.

Differential Diagnosis

Numerous workplace gases and vapors may produce symptoms of upper respiratory tract irritation. Symptoms of eye and throat irritation among office workers may be due to inadequate ventilation, cigarette smoke, or glues and solvents emitted from newly installed synthetic materials. Correlation of symptoms with measured levels of formaldehyde in indoor environments may be difficult.

Prevention

A. Work Practices: Safety goggles or a full-length plastic face mask should be worn where splashing is possible. At air concentrations above the permissible exposure limit, a full facepiece respirator with organic vapor cartridge is required. Protective neoprene clothing and boots and gloves impervious to formaldehyde should be worn to prevent skin contact.

B. Medical Surveillance: Biologic monitoring using urinary formate concentration is not useful with the possible exception of populations where ambient formaldehyde concentrations are greater than 1 ppm. A preplacement history of asthma or allergy should be obtained, along with a baseline FEV_1 and forced vital capacity (FVC).

Treatment

In case of eye and skin contact, immediately flush the contaminated area with water for 15 minutes and remove any contaminated clothing. Immediate removal to fresh air is required for inhalation exposure, with administration of oxygen for shortness of breath or hypoxemia. For formaldehyde exposure exceeding 20–30 ppm, emergency department observation with periodic evaluation of respiratory status is necessary for 6–8 hours.

NITRATES: NITROGLYCERIN & ETHYLENE GLYCOL DINITRATE

Essentials of Diagnosis

Acute effects:
- Headache.
- Angina.
- Fall in blood pressure.

Chronic effects:
- Sudden death.
- Increased incidence of ischemic heart disease.

Exposure Limits

Nitroglycerin
    ACGIH TLV: 0.05 ppm TWA
    OSHA PEL: 0.2 ppm ceiling
    NIOSH REL: 0.1 mg/m^3 ceiling (20 minutes)
Ethylene glycol dinitrate
    ACGIH TLV: 0.05 ppm TWA
    OSHA PEL: 1 mg/m^3 ceiling
    NIOSH REL: 0.1 mg/m^3 ceiling (20 minutes)

General Considerations

Nitroglycerin (glyceryl trinitrate, trinitropropanetriol) and ethylene glycol dinitrate (dinitroethanediol) are liquid nitric acid esters of mono- and polyhydric aliphatic alcohols. Those of the tetrahydric alcohols (erythritol tetranitrate, pentaerythritol tetranitrate) and the hexahydric alcohol (mannitol hexanitrate) are solids. They are less stable than aromatic nitro compounds.

Nitroglycerin is readily soluble in many organic solvents and acts as a solvent for many explosive ingredients, including ethylene glycol dinitrate. It is an oily liquid at room temperature with a slightly sweet odor. The sensitivity of nitroglycerin decreases with decreasing temperature, so ethylene glycol dinitrate may be added to nitroglycerin-bearing dynamites to depress the freezing point. Explosions of nitroglycerin may occur when the liquid is heated or when frozen nitroglycerin is thawed.

Ethylene glycol dinitrate is an oily colorless liquid that is more stable and less likely than nitroglycerin to explode when it burns.

Use, Production, & Occupational Exposure

Alfred Nobel first used a mixture of nitroglycerin with diatomaceous earth and later a more stable mixture of nitroglycerin, sodium nitrate, and wood pulp to form dynamite. The major application of nitroglycerin is in explosives and blasting gels, as in low-freezing dynamite in mixture with ethylene glycol dinitrate. Other explosive uses are in cordite in mixture with nitrocellulose and petroleum and in blasting gelatin with 7% nitrocellulose. Nitroglycerin also has medical therapeutic applications for the treatment of angina.

Nitroglycerin may be manufactured by a process in which glycerin is added to a mixture of nitric and sulfuric acids. Dynamite is formed by adding "dope," or mixtures of sodium nitrate, sulfur, antacids, and nitrocellulose. Ethylene glycol dinitrate is made by nitration of ethylene glycol with mixed acid.

Occupational exposures to nitroglycerin and ethylene glycol dinitrate can occur during their manufacture and during the manufacture and handling of explosives, munitions, and pharmaceuticals. Skin absorption for both nitroglycerin and ethylene glycol dinitrate has not been quantitated but is generally greater than respiratory absorption. Air sampling in dynamite plants where both nitroglycerin and ethylene glycol dinitrate are manufactured and used to produce explosives have shown that short-term higher exposures (in the range of 2 mg/m³ of ethylene glycol dinitrate) occur among mixers, cartridge fillers, and cleanup or maintenance workers.

Metabolism & Mechanism of Action

Both nitroglycerin and ethylene glycol dinitrate pass readily through the skin. Although there is an excellent correlation of blood nitrate ester levels with airborne exposures, skin absorption is more significant. Both nitroglycerin and ethylene glycol dinitrate are hydrolyzed to inorganic nitrates. The biologic half-life of both nitroglycerin and ethylene glycol dinitrate is about 30 minutes. Both act directly on arteriolar and venous smooth muscle, causing vasodilation within minutes with a consequent drop in blood pressure and an increase in regional myocardial blood flow. The headache associated with nitrate esters is secondary to cerebral vessel distention.

The tolerance that develops after 2–4 days of continuous exposure appears to be due to an increased sympathetic compensatory mechanism.

The pathogenesis of sudden death due to nitroglycerin and ethylene glycol dinitrate has been postulated to be a rebound vasoconstriction resulting in acute hypertension or myocardial ischemia.

General Considerations
A. Symptoms and Signs:

1. Acute exposure–Symptoms of acute illness include loss of consciousness, severe headache, difficulty in breathing, weak pulse, and pallor. Tolerance to these effects develops in dynamite production workers after a week of exposure, but symptoms recur upon return to work after an absence of 2 days or more. The headache associated with nitroglycerin (''powder headache'') frequently begins in the forehead and moves to the occipital region, where it can remain for hours or days. Associated symptoms include depression, restlessness, and sleeplessness. Alcohol ingestion may worsen the headache.

An acute drop in mean blood pressure of 10 mg Hg systolic and 6 mg Hg diastolic occurs on return to work after 2–3 days off. Mean blood pressure measurements increase over the week as compensatory mechanisms develop.

Blood pressure reduction has been noted after exposure to 0.5 mg/m³ for 25 minutes, and some workers develop headaches after inhalation exposure of more than 0.1 mg/m³.

2. Chronic exposure–Angina pectoris and sudden death have been described among dynamite workers handling nitroglycerin and ethylene glycol dinitrate. In affected workers, the angina usually occurs on the weekend or early in the work shift following periods away from work. The angina is relieved by reexposure to nitroglycerin or ethylene glycol dinitrate in contaminated clothes or by taking nitroglycerin sublingually. Sudden deaths without premonitory angina have also been recorded in dynamite workers. There is an excess risk of cardiac disease among nitroglycerin and ethylene glycol dinitrate workers.

Other reported chronic effects include symptoms of Raynaud's phenomenon and peripheral neuropathy. At high concentrations, the aliphatic nitrates may give rise to methemoglobinemia. A cancer study of a cohort exposed to nitrate fertilizer dust has found an excess of liver and digestive tract cancer.

B. Laboratory Findings: Coronary angiography has shown normal coronary arteries in workers with angina, and atheromatous coronary vessels have not generally been found on autopsy of workers who died suddenly. The incidence of ectopy is not increased in dynamite workers, and electrocardiograms may be normal. Abnormalities in digital plethysmography show changes in the digital wave pulse with inhalation exposures of 0.12–0.41 mg/m³.

Differential Diagnosis

An increased incidence of cardiovascular disease has been found in carbon disulfide-exposed workers. Sudden cardiac death may occur after exposure to carbon monoxide or to hydrocarbon solvents.

Prevention

A. Work Practices: Avoidance of headaches, blood pressure reduction, angina, or sudden death is best achieved by reduction of exposure through proper work practices. Control of exposure is best accomplished by closed systems, local ventilation, and the use of proper seals, joints, and access ports. The danger of detonation can be minimized by the use of nonsparking equipment, prevention of smoking and open flames, and other safety measures. Natural and synthetic rubber gloves will accelerate absorption of nitrate esters, so only cotton or cotton-lined gloves should be worn.

B. Medical Surveillance: Preplacement and periodic examination should stress a history of cardiovascular disease and physical examination of cardiac abnormalities. There is insufficient evidence concerning the efficacy of biologic monitoring for nitroglycerin or ethylene glycol dinitrate. Methemoglobin is not sensitive for routine monitoring of exposure.

Treatment

Treatment of cardiac symptoms due to nitrate ester exposure does not differ from that of symptoms of coronary insufficiency due to underlying coronary artery disease. Sublingual nitroglycerin should be used immediately for anginal symptoms. New onset angina or a change in anginal patterns should be evaluated by noninvasive cardiac imaging or angiography if indicated.

NITROSAMINES

Essentials of Diagnosis
Acute effects:
- Liver damage.

Chronic effects:
- Probable human carcinogen (selected).

Exposure Limits
OSHA PEL: Stringent workplace controls

General Considerations
N-Nitrosamines have the general structure shown below:

$$
\begin{array}{c}
R' \\
| \\
N - N = O \qquad \text{Nitrosyl group} \\
| \\
R
\end{array}
$$

where R and R' can be alkyl or aryl, eg, N-nitrosodimethylamine (NDMA), N-nitrosodiethylamine (NDEA), N-nitrosodiethanolamine (NDELA), and N-nitrosodiphenylamine (NDPhA). Derivatives of cyclic amines also occur, eg, N-nitrosomorpholine (NMOR) and N-nitrosopyrrolidine (NPyR). N-Nitrosamines are volatile solids or oils and are yellow because of their absorption of visible light by the N—N = O group.

Reactions of nitrosamines involve mainly the nitroso group and the C = H bonds adjacent to the amine nitrogen. Enzymatic reactions leading to the formation of carcinogenic metabolites is thought to occur at the alpha carbon.

$$
\begin{array}{ccc}
CH_2 & CH_2CH_2 & CH_2CH_2OH \\
| & | & | \\
N - N = O & N - N = O & N - N = O \\
| & | & | \\
CH_2 & CH_2CH_2 & CH_2CH_2OH \\
\\
\text{NDMA} & \text{NDEA} & \text{NDELA}
\end{array}
$$

NDPhA   NMOR   NPyR

Use, Production, & Exposure
Nitrosamines are formed by the reaction of a secondary or tertiary amine with nitrite ion in an acidic medium, according to the general equation shown below:

$$
NH + NO_2^- \xrightarrow{H^+} N - N = O
$$

Appreciation of the carcinogenicity of the nitrosamines has led to their characterization in many occupational and environmental circumstances. Humans may be exposed to nitrosamines in several ways: formation in the environment and subsequent absorption from food, water, air, or industrial and consumer products; formation in the body from precursors ingested separately in food, water, or air; from the consumption or smoking of tobacco; and from naturally occurring compounds.

The greatest exposure to the population as a whole occurs from cigarette smoking and the ingestion of nitrite-preserved meats.

Occupational Exposure
N-Nitrosodimethylamine was used in the USA until 1975 in the production of dimethylhydrazine, a rocket propellant. Exposures ranged up to 36 $\mu g/m^3$. In surveys, a fish meal factory was found to contain N-nitrosodimethylamine at 0.06 $\mu g/m^3$, a plant that manufactured surface-active agents contained N-nitrosodimethylamine at 0.8 $\mu g/m^3$, a chrome tannery had N-nitrosodimethylamine at 47 $\mu g/m^3$, and the rubber industry contained levels of N-nitrosomorphiline as high as 248 $\mu g/m^3$. NDMA and NEMA have occurred in foundries and leather tanneries.

Synthetic cutting fluids may contain up to 3% N-nitrosoethanolamine. Direct contact with cutting fluids and the presence of airborne mists provide the opportunity for ingestion or skin absorption.

Certain classes of pesticides have been found to contain identifiable N-nitroso contaminants formed during synthesis or as a result of interaction with nitrate fertilizers applied simultaneously to crops. EPA requires testing for nitrosamines of suspect formulation.

A. Tobacco and Tobacco Smoke: The largest nonoccupational exposure to preformed nitrosamines is derived from tobacco products and tobacco smoke, which may contain N-nitrosodimethylamine, N-nitrosodiethylamine, N-nitrosopyrrolidine, and others. Nitrosamine content is greater in sidestream smoke and from cigars.

B. Foods: Low levels of nitrosamines occur in several types of food, including cheese, processed meats, beer, and cooked bacon.

C. Cosmetics: Many cosmetics, soaps and shampoos are contaminated with N-nitrosodiethanolamine due to the nitrosation of triethanolamine by bactericides.

D. In Vivo Nitrosation: Nitrate can be reduced to nitrite in vitro and in human saliva in vivo. The reaction of ingested nitrites with amines will yield in vivo nitrosamines in the acidic medium of the stomach. Main contributors to gastric nitrite load are vegetables, cured meats, baked goods, cereals, fruits, and fruit juices.

Metabolism & Mechanism of Action

The nitrosamines are rapidly metabolized after skin or gastrointestinal absorption, with a biologic half-life for N-nitrosodimethylamine of several hours. N-Nitrosodimethylamine is enzymatically demethylated to form monomethylnitrosamine, which then yields an unstable diazohydroxide. The carcinogenic action of the nitrosamines is attributed to this electrophilic species, which can covalently react with DNA.

Clinical Findings

A. Symptoms and Signs:

1. Acute exposure—Two cases of industrial poisoning due to N-nitrosodimethylamine were reported in 1937 in chemists producing an anticorrosion agent. They developed headaches, backache, abdominal cramps, nausea, anorexia, weakness, drowsiness, and dizziness; both workers developed ascites and jaundice, and one died with diffuse hepatic necrosis. Five family members who ingested lemonade accidentally contaminated with N-nitrosodimethylamine developed nausea, vomiting, and abdominal pain within a few hours, and 2 died 4 and 5 days later with generalized bleeding. Postmortem examination showed hepatic necrosis.

2. Chronic exposure—Liver cirrhosis has been reported following chronic exposure to N-nitrosodimethylamine.

About 85% of over 200 nitrosamines tested in animals have been found to be carcinogenic, inducing tumors of the respiratory tract, esophagus, kidney, stomach, liver, and brain. N-Nitrosodimethylamine, N-nitrosodiethylamine, N-nitrosodiphenylamine, N-nitrosodiethanolamine, N-nitrosopyrrolidine, and N-nitrosomorphiline have been shown to be carcinogenic in many animal species and are transplacental carcinogens.

In humans, compelling evidence of carcinogenicity has not been found. Excess cancer deaths from stomach, large intestine, lung, brain, bladder, prostate, and hematopoietic system have been identified in rubber workers, but the studies are inconsistent and the exposures to nitrosamines not well characterized.

B. Laboratory Findings: In the few fatalities reported, elevated liver enzymes consistent with hepatic necrosis were noted.

Prevention

A. Work Practices: Nitrosamines should be handled in well-ventilated fume hoods. Nitrites should not be added to cutting fluids if amines are present. Reduction of nitrosamine exposure in the rubber industry includes the avoidance of compounds that give rise to nitrosamines. Adequate engineering controls should be instituted for working with raw polymers, elastomers, and rubber parts containing dialkylamine compounds that may emit nitrosamine when heated.

B. Medical Surveillance: Use of biologic samples for nitrosamine exposure has not been adequately evaluated. No specific medical surveillance for nitrosamines is recommended.

Treatment

There is no treatment for nitrosamine exposure.

PENTACHLOROPHENOL

Essentials of Diagnosis

Acute effects:
- Skin and respiratory tract irritation.
- Systemic collapse.

Chronic effects:
- Skin rash (chloracne secondary to chlorodibenzodioxin).

Exposure Limits

ACGIH TLV: 0.5 mg/m^3 TWA.
OSHA PEL: 0.5 mg/m^3 TWA

General Considerations

Pentachlorophenol (PCP) is a crystalline solid with low water solubility and a characteristic pungent phenolic odor. Its commercial production proceeds readily by the direct chlorination of phenol in the presence of chlorine and a catalyst or by the alkaline hydrolysis of hexachlorobenzene; both processes result in 4–12% tetrachlorophenol and less than 0.1% of trichlorophenol in the final product. In addition, the required elevated temperatures to produce PCP result in the formation of condensation products, including the toxic dimers dibenzo-*p*-dioxin and dibenzofuran. Analyses of commercial PCP have reported ranges of chlorinated dioxins and furans from 0.03 to 2510 parts per million. Tetrachlorodibenzodioxin has been found in a commercial sample of PCP, but it was not the most toxic 2,3,7,8-isomer. Thus, evaluation of the health effects of PCP must be considered separately from those of its impurities.

Use

Approximately 40 million pounds of PCP are produced each year in the USA. About 80% is used by the wood preserving industry to treat wood products such as railway ties, poles, pilings, and fence posts. Treated wood products have a useful product life 5 times that of untreated wood, resulting in significant economic savings and conservation of timber resources. PCP is usually applied to wood products as a 5% solution in mineral spirits, fuel oil, or kerosene. In the USA, commercial and industrial use of PCP as a preservative is concentrated in the south, southeast, and northwest. The remaining 20% is used in production of sodium pentachlorophenol, in plywood and fiberboard waterproofing, in termite control, and as a herbicide for use in rights-of-way and industrial sites. PCP is registered by the EPA as a termiticide, fungicide, herbicide, algicide, and disinfectant and as an ingredient in antifouling paint. It can be applied as a microbial deterrent in the preservation of wood pulp, leather, seeds, rope, glue, starch and cooling tower water.

Because of the risk of teratogenicity and fetotoxicity, the EPA since 1984 has required that PCP products in concentrations of 5% or less be used only by certified applicators and has restricted the use of PCP on products that may contact bare skin, food, water, or animals.

Occupational & Environmental Exposure

Occupational exposure to PCP occurs primarily in the gas, electric service, and wood preservative industries. Air sampling at 25 wood treatment plants using PCP showed an average exposure of 0.013 mg/m^3, and newer automated processes and closed systems at larger facilities are further reducing exposure. Acute exposure may occur with the opening of pressure vessel doors or in tank cleaning, solution preparation, and the handling of wood after treatment. Hand application of PCP may also pose a risk of overexposure. Dermal exposure is the principal route, either through direct contact with PCP or through contact with treated wood.

Nonoccupational exposure to PCP can occur after the wood has been treated and shipped, where handling may result in dermal exposure. Six months following treatment, PCP will be present on the wood surface at a concentration of about 0.5 mg per square foot. Elevated levels of PCP have been found in the blood and urine of residents of log homes where the logs have been dipped in PCP prior to construction; air samples showed an indoor air concentration of up to 0.38 $\mu g/m^3$ 5 years after construction.

Metabolism & Mechanism of Action

Absorption of PCP in the occupational setting is largely through inhalation and skin absorption. The latter is increased when PCP is dissolved in organic solvents. PCP is mainly excreted in urine as free PCP and as a conjugate with glucuronic acid. Pharmacokinetics were characterized in a single-dose oral administration study by first-order absorption, enterohepatic circulation, and first-order elimination, with 74% of the oral dose of PCP excreted unchanged within 8 days. The half-life for elimination was approximately 30 hours. However, in chronically exposed workers during 2- to 4-week vacations, the terminal half-life of elimination ranges from 30 to 60 days.

Acute intoxication with PCP is due to interference with cellular electron transport and the uncoupling of oxidative phosphorylation in mitochondria and endoplasmic reticulum. Interaction with energy-rich phosphate compounds results in hydrolysis and free energy release, leading to a hypermetabolic state with peripheral tissue hyperthermia.

Clinical Findings

A. Symptoms and Signs:

1. Acute exposure–

a. Skin–Commercial PCP can cause skin irritation after single exposures to more than a 10% concentration of the material or after prolonged or repeated contact with a 1% solution. Skin sensitization has not been demonstrated.

b. Eye, nose, and throat–Irritation can occur at levels above 0.3 mg/m^3, but higher concentrations can be tolerated by those accustomed to the compound.

c. Systemic intoxication–Systemic intoxication due to PCP became evident in the 1950s after 2 workers died following cutaneous exposure in a wood-dipping operation. Since that time, fatalities from PCP have occurred among chemical production workers, herbicide sprayers, and wood manufacturers. A unique poisoning tragedy occurred in 20 babies wearing diapers inappropriately laundered in 23% sodium pentachlorophenate; 2 babies died.

Acute intoxication is characterized by the rapid onset of profuse diaphoresis, hyperpyrexia, tachycardia, tachypnea, weakness, nausea, vomiting, abdominal pain, intense thirst, and pain in the extremities. An intense form of muscle contraction is observed before death. The minimum lethal dose of PCP in humans is estimated to be 29 mg/kg.

2. Chronic exposure–Chronic exposure to PCP is associated with conjunctivitis, chronic sinusitis, and bronchitis. Chloracne among PCP wood treatment workers is probably due to dioxin contaminants. In animal studies, pure PCP does not elicit acne.

Bone marrow aplasia has been reported after exposure to PCP. Swedish studies have reported an association between exposure to phenoxyherbicides or chlorophenols (or both) and soft tissue sarcoma, malignant lymphoma, and nasopharyngeal carcinoma, but this has not been confirmed. The EPA has concluded that the use of PCP poses a risk of oncogenicity because of the contaminants hexachlorodibenzodioxin and hexachlorobenzene.

PCP and its contaminants cause teratogenic and fetotoxic effects in test animals, but nothing is known concerning adverse reproductive outcomes in humans. Chronic exposure does not lead to peripheral nervous system effects.

B. Laboratory Findings: Acute intoxication with PCP can result in elevation of blood urea and creatinine, with metabolic acidosis and increased anion gap. Increased serum LDH activity and reduced creatinine clearance have been measured in chronically PCP-exposed workers.

Blood levels of PCP in fatal cases have ranged from 40 to 170 mg/L. Urine levels have ranged from 29 to 500 mg/L in fatal cases, and from 3 to 20 mg/L in nonfatal cases of intoxication. In PCP-exposed workers, mean urine PCP levels were 0.95–1.31 mg/L. In nonoccupationally exposed individuals in the USA, urine values of PCP average 6.3 μg/L, with a range from 1 to 193 μg/L, and an average of 15μg/L in hemodialysis patients.

Differential Diagnosis

Acute intoxication can be confused with hyperthermia from other causes, including heat stroke or sepsis. Symptoms of respiratory irritation may be due to the solvent carrier or other occupational irritants. Chloracne is associated with polychlorinated biphenyls, polychlorinated dibenzodioxins, or polychlorinated dibenzofurans.

Prevention

A. Work Practices: Appropriate respiratory protection must be worn where exposure to PCP may exceed permissible limits, particularly in higher risk operations such as formulating plants and pressure vessel and tank maintenance. Gloves of nitrile and polyvinyl chloride provide the best protection against both aqueous sodium pentachlorophenate and pentachlorophenol in diesel oil. Clothing contaminated with PCP must be removed, left at the workplace, and laundered before reuse. Washing and showering facilities should be available to prevent contamination of food, drink, and family.

B. Medical Surveillance: Preemployment urine analysis for PCP should be performed and repeated at intervals. Samples should be collected prior to the last shift of the work week and PCP measured by methods that incorporate hydrolysis. Concentrations over 2 mg/L total PCP are indicative of excessive exposure. Alternatively, plasma samples may be collected at any time during regular exposure and should not exceed 5 mg/L free PCP.

Routine medical surveillance should include attention to skin and mucous membrane irritation and skin rash. Hot weather appears to be a predisposing factor for PCP intoxication, so exposure to PCP should be minimized during those times. Significant skin absorption of pentachlorophenols may occur and can be documented by urinary pentachlorophenol monitoring.

Treatment

Solutions of PCP spilled on the skin are treated with prompt and thorough washing with soap and water. Eyes should be flushed for 15 minutes in water. All contaminated shoes and clothing should be immediately removed.

In the event of acute PCP intoxication, adequate intravenous hydration and efforts to maintain normal body temperature are essential to prevent cardiovascular collapse. Rapid onset of muscular spasms may prevent intubation and resuscitation, so careful monitoring of respiratory status is critical. Metabolic acidosis should be treated with sodium bicarbonate. Atropine sulfate is contraindicated.

POLYCHLORINATED BIPHENYLS

Essentials of Diagnosis

Acute effects:
- Skin rash (chloracne).
- Eye irritation.
- Nausea, vomiting.

Chronic effects:
- Weakness, weight loss, anorexia.
- Skin rash (chloracne).
- Numbness and tingling of extremities.
- Elevated serum triglycerides.
- Elevated liver enzymes.

Exposure Limits

ACGIH TLV: 0.5 mg/m^3 TWA (54% chlorine)
OSHA PEL: 1 mg/m^3 TWA (42% chlorine)
NIOSH REL: 1 μg/m^3

General Considerations

Polychlorinated biphenyls (PCBs) are a large family of chlorinated aromatic hydrocarbons prepared by the chlorination of biphenyl. Commercial products are a mixture of PCBs with variable chlorine content and are named according to the percentage of chlorine. In addition, all PCBs are contaminated with small but highly toxic concentrations of polychlorinated dibenzofurans, making interpretation of data regarding the health effects of PCBs difficult.

Use

Between 1930 and 1975, about 1.4 billion pounds of PCBs were produced in the USA. About half was used in capacitor and transformer dielectric fluids and the remainder as flame-resistant plasticizers, hydraulic fluids, lubricants, or ingredients in adhesives, carbonless carbon paper, and ink. In the United States, commercial PCBs were marketed under the name Aroclor. In 1977, the manufacture, processing, distribution, and use of PCBs were banned by Congress. However, as of 1980, an estimated 750 million tons were still in use (about half of all PCBs purchased by United States industries), primarily in electrical transformers, capacitors, and voltage regulators in electric light fixtures.

Occupational & Environmental Exposure

NIOSH estimates that 12,000 workers have been potentially occupationally exposed to PCBs. Much larger numbers are at risk of exposure due to accidental contamination. Leaks of PCBs from capacitors and transformers while in storage, shipment, or maintenance result in transient exposure risks for utility repair crews, railroad maintenance workers, building engineers, and custodians. Improper storage of used PCB electrical equipment may result in environmental contamination and community exposure. Electrical fires occurring in transformers containing PCBs may release polychlorinated dibenzofurans and polychlorinated dibenzodioxins formed through incomplete combustion of PCBs and chlorinated benzenes. Incidents of widespread building contamination due to PCB transformer fires have occurred in Binghamton, San Francisco, Chicago, and Miami. The EPA estimated that in 1984 approximately 107,000 transformers were in use or in storage for reuse, posing a significant risk to the general public if leakage or fire should occur.

Metabolism & Mechanism of Action

Chlorinated biphenyl compounds are readily absorbed through the respiratory tract, gastrointestinal tract and skin. Distribution is primarily into fat. Biphenyls are metabolized in the liver as the primary site of biotransformation. PCB mixtures cause induction of the hepatic microsomal monooxygenase systems. Induction is related to chlorination, and PCB mixtures containing higher percentages of chlorine are more potent than mixtures with lower levels of chlorination. More highly chlorinated isomers are also more resistant to metabolism and therefore are more persistent. Hydroxy metabolites can be detected in bile, feces, and breast milk, but urinary excretion is quite low. This leads to bioaccumulation in fat at low exposure levels and the persistence of PCBs in fatty tissue years after exposure. The formation of electrophilic arene oxide metabolites may cause DNA damage and the initiation of tumor growth.

Clinical Findings of Toxicity

A. Symptoms and Signs:

1. Acute—Acute exposure to PCBs results in mucous membrane irritation and nausea and vomiting. Transient skin irritation may result from direct handling of PCBs containing mixtures of solvents.

In the mass food poisoning incident due to rice oil contamination in western Japan in 1968 (Yusho, or rice oil disease), ingestion of PCBs resulted in chloracne. Typical chloracne presents with cystic or comedonal lesions over the face, ear lobes, retroauricular region, axillae, trunk, and external genitalia and may occur at any age. Yusho patients also showed dark pigmentation of the gingivae, oral mucosa, and nails, with conjunctival swelling. It is not clear whether all or some of these findings were due to trace contamination of the PCBs with dibenzofurans; the latter compound may have increased during cooking.

B. Chronic: In addition to the acute symptoms of upper respiratory tract irritation, chronic workplace exposure to PCBs has also resulted in chloracne. The relationship between dose of exposure and the appearance of chloracne is inconsistent, though chloracne persists for years after exposure has ceased.

Adverse reproductive effects of PCBs have been reported in many animal species; these include failure of implantation, increased number of spontaneous abortions, and low birth weight of litters. No specific birth defects have been found. Children born to Yusho mothers had skin hyperpigmentation and ocular discharge, with ectodermal dysplastic abnormalities of a wide variety becoming evident upon long-term follow-up (see Chapter 39).

PCBs fed to test animals produce hepatocellular carcinomas. However, human epidemiologic studies to date reveal no excess of deaths from cancer in workers exposed to PCBs, though the cohorts are small.

B. Laboratory Findings: Mild elevations of serum triglyceride concentrations have been found in Yusho patients and occupationally exposed individuals. Nerve conduction velocity was decreased and serum transaminase concentrations increased. These tests have limited diagnostic value.

Owing to widespread environmental contamination and bioconcentration, PCB residues are detectable in blood and fat tissue of nonoccupationally exposed individuals. Serum and plasma levels have ranged to 42 parts per billion (ppb), with means from 2.1 to 24.2 ppb. Fat levels have ranged to 6600 ppb (wet weight basis), with mean values from 800 to 1700 ppb. Levels vary with location, diet, and laboratory.

If exposure to PCB is suspected, serum or fat levels of PCBs may be measured to document absorption. In a steady state, serum is as good a reflection of body burden as fat. Results must be interpreted in light of established normals for geographic area and laboratory technique. Unfortunately, the relationship between symptoms or signs and PCB levels in serum or fat is variable. No information is available concerning long-term carcinogenic risk to the exposed individual.

Differential Diagnosis

Occupational exposure to PCBs may be accompanied by exposure to chlorinated dibenzodioxin and dibenzofuran contaminants and may be responsible for chronic toxicity. Concurrent exposure to solvents is important, because these substances may cause chronic fatigue and elevated liver enzymes. Mild chloracne should not be confused with other papular rashes. A biopsy may be necessary to establish the diagnosis.

Prevention

A. Work Practices: Work practices to avoid exposure to PCBs include the use of special PCB-resistant gloves and protective clothing. Adequate ventilation should be maintained during spill cleanup or maintenance of vessels containing PCBs; if this is not possible, approved respirators should be provided. Provision should be made for proper decontamination or disposal of contaminated clothing or equipment. Locations where PCBs are stored should be clearly posted as required by law. Environmental sampling may be necessary to ensure adequate worker protection or safety for public reentry to contaminated areas.

B. Medical Surveillance: Workers intermittently exposed to PCBs should have a baseline skin examination and liver function tests. Follow-up examination can be limited to symptomatic individuals and those exposed as a consequence of accidental contamination. Routine serum or fat PCB measurements is not recommended.

Treatment

Acute exposure should be treated by immediate decontamination of the skin with soap and water to prevent skin absorption. No specific measures are available for respiratory tract or skin absorption.

No treatment is available for chronic PCB toxicity. Chloracne is treated with topical therapy for symptomatic relief.

POLYCYCLIC AROMATIC HYDROCARBONS

Essentials of Diagnosis

Acute effects:
- Dermatitis, conjunctivitis (coal tar pitch volatiles).

Chronic effects:
- Excess cancer rates in selected occupations.

Exposure Limits

Coal tar products (volatiles)
ACGIH TLV: 0.2 mg/m³ TWA
OSHA PEL: 0.2 mg/m³ TWA
NIOSH REL: 0.1 mg/m³ TWA
Naphthalene
ACGIH TLV: 10 ppm TWA, 15 ppm STEL
OSHA PEL: 10 ppm TWA, 15 ppm STEL
Bitumens
NIOSH REL: 5 mg/m³ ceiling (15 minutes)
Carbon black
ACGIH TLV: 3.5 mg/m³ TWA
OSHA PEL: 3.5 mg/m³ TWA
NIOSH REL: 3.5 mg/m³ TWA; in presence of polycyclic aromatic hydrocarbons, 0.1 mg/m³ TWA

General Considerations

Polycyclic aromatic hydrocarbons are organic compounds consisting of 3 or more aromatic rings that contain only carbon and hydrogen and share a pair of carbon atoms. They are formed by pyrolysis or incomplete combustion of such organic matter as coke, coal tar and pitch, asphalt, and oil. The composition of the products of pyrolysis is dependent on the fuel, the temperature, and the time in the hot area. Polycyclic aromatic hydrocarbons are emitted as vapors from the zone of burning and condense immediately on soot particles or form very small particles themselves. Such processes always lead to a mixture of hundreds of polycyclic aromatic hydrocar-

bons. Compounds with 3 or 4 aromatic rings predominate. Carcinogenic polycyclic aromatic hydrocarbons are found among those with 5 or 6 rings. The simplest fused ring is naphthalene. Some important polycyclic aromatic hydrocarbons in the occupational environment are shown below.

Naphthalene   Anthracene

Benzo(*a*)pyrene

Use, Production, & Exposure

Pure polycyclic aromatic hydrocarbons have no direct use except for naphthalene and anthracene. Naphthalene is used as a raw material in the chemical, plastics, and dye industries, as a moth repellant, as an air freshener, and as a surface-active agent. Anthracene is used for the preparation of anthraquinone and dyes. Polycyclic aromatic hydrocarbons as contaminants can be found in air, water, food, and cigarette smoke as well as in the industrial environment.

Occupational Exposure

A. Coal Tars and Products: The most important source of polycyclic aromatic hydrocarbons in the air of the workplace is coal tar. Tars and pitches are black or brown, liquid or semisolid products derived from coal, petroleum, wood, shale oil, or other organic materials. Coal tars are by-products of the carbonization or coking of coal. The coke-oven plant is the principal source of coal tar. Coal tar pitch and creosote are derived from the distillation of coal tar. Numerous polycyclic aromatic hydrocarbons have been identified in coal tar, coal tar pitch, and creosote. Coal tar pitch volatiles are the volatile matter emitted into the air when coal tar, coal tar pitch, or their products are heated, and they may contain several polycyclic aromatic hydrocarbons.

The major use for coal tar pitch is as the binder for aluminum smelting electrodes; other uses include roofing material, surface coatings, pipe-coating enamels, and as a binder for briquettes and foundry cores. Creosote is used almost exclusively as a wood preservative.

Occupational exposure to polycyclic aromatic hydrocarbons in coal tar and pitches may occur in gas and coke works, aluminum reduction plants, iron and steel foundries, coal gasification facilities, and during roof and pavement tarring and the application of coal-tar paints.

NIOSH estimates that 145,000 employees are engaged in operations that involve coal tar products.

B. Carbon Black: Carbon black is derived from the partial combustion (pyrolysis) of natural gas or petroleum. It is primarily used in pigmenting and reinforcing rubber products and in inks, paints, and paper. NIOSH estimates that 35,000 employees are engaged in operations that involve direct or indirect exposure to carbon black.

C. Bitumens: Bitumens are viscous solids or liquids derived from refining processes of petroleum. They are principally used for road construction when mixed with asphalt, in roofing felt manufacture, in pipe coatings, and as binders in briquettes. Occupational exposure may occur in these operations. NIOSH estimates that 2 million US workers are exposed to bitumen and 30,000 to bitumen fumes.

D. Soots: Soots are mixtures of particulate carbon, organic tars, resins, and inorganic material produced during incomplete combustion of carbon-containing material. Occupational exposure is primarily to chimney soot; potential exposure occurs to chimney sweeps, brick masons, and heating unit service personnel.

Environmental Exposure

Polycyclic aromatic hydrocarbons occur in the air primarily due to coal burning and settle on soil, where they may leach into water. They are found in smoked fish and meats and form during the broiling and grilling of foods. They are inhaled in cigarette smoke from the burning of tobacco.

Metabolism & Mechanism of Action

Polycyclic aromatic hydrocarbons are readily absorbed by the skin, lungs, and gastrointestinal tract of experimental animals and are rapidly metabolized and excreted in the feces. In humans, they are largely absorbed from carrier particles via the respiratory route. They are activated by aryl hydrocarbon hydroxylase to a reactive epoxide intermediate, then conjugated for excretion in urine or bile. The reactive epoxide may covalently bind with DNA and probably accounts for the carcinogenic activity.

Clinical Findings

A. Symptoms and Signs:

1. Acute exposure—Acute inhalation exposure to naphthalene may cause headache, nausea, diaphoresis, and vomiting. Accidental ingestion has caused hemolytic anemia. Naphthalene may also cause erythema and dermatitis on repeated skin contact.

Exposure to coal tar products may cause phototoxicity, with skin erythema, burning, and itching (see Chapter 17), and eye burning and lacrimation.

2. Chronic exposure—Many polycyclic aromatic hydrocarbons are carcinogenic in animals. Often, benzo(*a*)pyrine (BaP) is measured to indicate the presence of polycyclic aromatic hydrocarbons where exposure to carcinogens is suspect. Anthracene and phenanthrene are noncarcinogenic, while benz(*a*)anthracene and 7,12-dimethylbenzanthracene are potent carcinogens.

Evidence for human carcinogenicity was initially described by Percivall Pott in 1775 when he associated scrotal cancer in chimney sweeps with their prolonged exposure to tar and soot. Subsequently, scrotal cancer in mulespinners exposed to shale oil and workers exposed to pitch have been reported.

Excess cancer risk associated with exposure to polycyclic aromatic hydrocarbons has been shown for workers in gas generation plants, steel plants, those engaged in aluminum reduction and roofing, and those who work near coke ovens. Tar bitumen exposure during road paving operations indicate that a significant cancer risk may occur.

B. Laboratory Findings: Photopatch testing may demonstrate photodermatitis in workers with occupational exposure to coal tar pitch and fumes.

Differential Diagnosis

Exposure to other known or potential carcinogenic exposure in the work environment should be investigated.

Prevention

A. Work Practices: Reduction of emissions from coke ovens, aluminum works, foundries, and steel works is essential. Where gaseous emissions occur during loading or transferring of heated coal tar products, fume and vapor control systems will reduce personal exposure. Skin exposure to tars, pitches, and oils containing polycyclic aromatic hydrocarbons is avoided by wearing gloves and changing contaminated work clothes.

B. Medical Surveillance: Periodic examination of workers exposed to coal tar pitch volatiles should include a history of skin or eye irritation and physical examination with attention to the skin, upper respiratory tract, and lungs. Biologic monitoring has not been adequately evaluated. Promising biologic markers for PAH exposure are urinary 1-hydroxypyrene and hydrocarbon-DNA adducts. Routine use of these is not yet recommended.

Treatment

Photodermatitis should be treated with cortisone-containing preparations, barrier creams, or removal from exposure.

STYRENE

Essentials of Diagnosis

Acute effects:
- Eye, respiratory tract, and skin irritation.

Chronic effects:
- Weakness, headache, fatigue, dizziness.
- Memory loss.

Exposure Limits

ACGIH TLV: 50 ppm TWA, 100 ppm STEL

OSHA PEL: 50 ppm TWA, 100 ppm STEL
NIOSH REL: 50 ppm TWA, 100 ppm ceiling (15 minutes)

General Considerations

Styrene, also known as vinyl benzene and phenyl-ethylene, has the chemical formula $C_6H_5CH:CH_2$. It is a colorless volatile liquid at room temperature with a sweet odor at low concentrations. The odor threshold of 1 ppm is below the permissible exposure limit, and the material has adequate warning properties. Styrene monomer must be stabilized by an inhibitor to prevent exothermic polymerization, a process that may cause explosion of its container.

Use

Commercial styrene was first produced in the 1920s and 1930s. During World War II, styrene was important in the manufacture of synthetic rubber. Over 90% of styrene is produced by the dehydrogenation of ethylbenzene. Many consumer products are made from styrene-containing compounds, including packaging and insulation, drain and vent pipes, tires and hoses, boats, and storage tanks.

Occupational & Environmental Exposure

NIOSH estimates that at least 30,000 workers in 1000 plants are potentially exposed in the United States to styrene, and more than 300,000 workers are potentially exposed to compounds containing styrene. The current use of closed systems for the production of styrene monomer and its polymers limits full-shift TWA styrene exposure to less than 10 ppm. Spills, sample collections, and maintenance operations may result in short-term higher exposures. Fabrication of articles from polystyrene or styrene copolymers also results in styrene exposures generally below 10 ppm.

The most significant exposure to styrene occurs when it is used as a solvent-reactant for unsaturated polyester products that have been reinforced with fibrous glass. Reinforced plastics/composites are used in the manufacture of boats, storage tanks, wall panels, tub and shower units, and truck camper tops. In this process, alternating layers of chopped fibers or woven mats of fibrous glass are hand-applied with catalyzed resin; up to 10% of the styrene may evaporate into the workplace air as the resin cures. Average styrene exposures in plants where the reinforced products are manufactured can range from 40 to 100 ppm, with short-term individual exposures up to 150–300 ppm. In a NIOSH study of the reinforced plastics industry, directly exposed workers engaged in the manufacture of truck parts and boats had the highest exposure to styrene, with a mean 8-hour TWA of 61 and 82 ppm, respectively.

Metabolism & Mechanism of Action

Occupational exposure occurs mainly via inhala-tion, with about 60% of inhaled styrene retained by the lungs. Percutaneous absorption is not significant. Styrene is metabolized by the liver to mandelic acid and phenylglyoxylic acid, which are excreted in the urine. After short-term exposure, the venous half-life of styrene is approximately 40 minutes. The half-times of mandelic acid and phenylglyoxylic acid are about 4 and 8 hours, respectively. In the chronically exposed worker, the half-time for mandelic acid excretion may range from 6 to 9 hours.

Clinical Findings

A. Symptoms and Signs:

1. Acute exposure—Concentrations of styrene from 100 to 200 ppm may cause eye and upper respiratory tract irritation. Styrene is a defatting agent and a primary skin irritant, resulting in dermatitis. Experimental human exposure to several hundred parts per million causes typical alcohol-organic solvent anesthetic symptoms, with listlessness, drowsiness, impaired balance, difficulty in concentrating, and decrease in reaction time. There have been no reports of fatalities due to styrene exposure.

2. Chronic exposure—Weakness, headache, fatigue, poor memory, and dizziness can occur in workers chronically exposed to styrene in concentrations of less than 100 ppm. Mean reaction time and visuomotor performance may be decreased in exposed workers. The incidence of abnormal EEGs was significantly greater as well.

An increased frequency of chromosome aberrations has been found in lymphocytes of workers employed in the reinforced plastics industry. Cancer mortality studies do not indicate an excess risk from exposure. Highly exposed women reported a slight decrease in birth weight.

B. Laboratory Findings: In one study, styrene-exposed workers had elevated γ-glutamyl transferase values. No other blood test is specific for styrene toxicity.

The most reliable indicator of styrene exposure is mandelic acid in the urine. Postshift mandelic acid levels in urine show a good correlation with average TWA styrene exposure over the range of 5–150 ppm. Levels of 500 mg of mandelic acid per liter of urine may indicate recent exposure to at least 10 ppm of styrene. A concentration of 1000 mg of mandelic acid per liter of urine corresponds to an average 8-hour TWA styrene exposure of 50 ppm.

Differential Diagnosis

Exposure to other solvents during the production of styrene and in the manufacture of reinforced plastic products may cause similar symptoms of central nervous system toxicity such as headache, fatigue, and memory loss.

Prevention

A. Work Practices: Styrene poses a significant fire hazard, and proper handling and storage are essential to prevent ignition of the liquid and vapor and a potential explosive reaction. Closed-process systems are recommended. Intensive local exhaust ventilation is the best way to reduce styrene vapor concentrations during construction of large reinforced plastic objects, though dilution ventilation is widely used to reduce styrene vapor exposure in the boat industry.

When worker exposure cannot be adequately controlled by engineering controls, protective clothing and respirators may be needed. Where workers may come into contact with liquid styrene, appropriate gloves, boots, overshoes, aprons, and face shields with goggles are recommended. Polyvinyl alcohol and polyethylene gloves and protective clothing give good protection against styrene. To prevent eye irritation at moderately low concentrations, full-facepiece respirators are recommended.

B. Medical Surveillance: Initial medical evaluation should include a history of nervous system disorders and an examination with particular attention to the nervous system, respiratory tract, and skin. Annual medical examinations should be performed on all workers with significant air exposure above the action level or with potential for significant skin exposure. Measurement of urinary mandelic acid is a useful adjunct to air monitoring. Spot urine samples should be collected at the end of the work shift and analyzed for mandelic acid concurrently with industrial hygiene monitoring of airborne styrene. If the urine mandelic acid concentration exceeds 1000 mg/ L (adjusted to a specific gravity of 1.018), the work setting should be investigated to evaluate a possible source of exposure greater than 50 ppm.

Treatment

Hands should be washed after skin exposure, and clothing saturated with styrene should be immediately removed. In the case of eye contact, flush the eye immediately with copious amounts of water for 15 minutes. No specific treatment is recommended for acute or chronic styrene exposure.

2,3,7,8-TETRACHLORODIBENZO-P-DIOXIN

Essentials of Diagnosis

Acute effects:
- Eye and respiratory tract irritation.
- Skin rash, chloracne.
- Fatigue, nervousness, irritability.

Chronic effects:
- Chloracne.

Exposure Limits

NIOSH REL: Lowest feasible concentration

General Considerations

Polychlorinated dibenzo-p-dioxins (PCDDs) and polychlorinated dibenzofurans (PCDFs) are 2 large

series of tricyclic aromatic compounds that exhibit similar physical, chemical, and biologic properties.

PCDFs

PCDDs

However, there is a pronounced difference in potency among the different PCDD and PCDF isomers. The most extensively studied is the 2,3,7,8-tetrachlorodibenzo-p-dioxin isomer (2,3,7,8-TCDD). "Dioxin" is the name used for at least 75 chlorinated aromatic isomers, including 22 isomers of the tetrachlorinated dioxin. 2,3,7,8-TCDD is the specific dioxin identified as a contaminant in the production of 2,4,5-trichlorophenol (TCP), 2-(2,4,5-trichlorophenoxy)propionic acid (silvex), and 2,4,5-trichlorophenoxyacetic acid (2,4,5-T). In its pure form, 2,3,7,8-TCDD is a colorless crystalline solid at room temperature, sparingly soluble in organic solvents and insoluble in water. The degree of toxicity of the dioxin compounds is highly dependent on the number and position of the chlorine atoms; isomers with chlorination in the 4 lateral positions (2,3,7,8) have the highest acute toxicity in animals. Under laboratory conditions, 2,3,7,8-TCDD is one of the most toxic synthetic chemicals known.

The chlorinated dibenzofurans are contaminants found in some polychlorinated biphenyl compounds (PCBs) used in transformers and capacitors, including the most toxic 2,3,7,8-tetrachlorinated dibenzofuran.

Use

2,3,7,8-TCDD is formed as a stable by-product during the production of trichlorophenol (TCP). Normally, 2,3,7,8-TCDD persists as a contaminant in TCP in amounts ranging from 0.07 to 6.2 mg/kg. Production of 2,4,5-T and silvex ceased in the United States in 1979, although stockpiles are still being distributed and used. Agent Orange, used in Vietnam as a defoliant during the 1960s, was a 50:50 mixture of esters of the herbicides 2,4-D and 2,4,5-T. Ten to twelve million gallons were sprayed over 3–4 million acres in Vietnam; the 2,3,7,8-TCDD concentration was about 2 ppm in Agent Orange available after usage was stopped.

The combustion of 2,4,5-T can result in its conversion to small amounts of 2,3,7,8-TCDD. Polychlorinated biphenyls can be converted to PCDFs. Soot from PCB transformer fires may be contaminated with more than 2000 $\mu g/g$ of PCDFs, including the most toxic 2,3,7,8- isomers. A complex mixture of PCDDs and PCDFs may occur in fly ash from municipal incinerators.

Occupational & Environmental Exposure

Occupational exposure to 2,3,7,8-TCDD can occur during the production and use of 2,4,5-T and its derivatives. Since 1949, there have been 24 accidents in chemical plants manufacturing chlorinated phenols in which workers were exposed to PCDDs. The explosion of a TCP chemical plant in 1976 in Seveso, Italy, exposed some 37,000 residents of surrounding communities to 2,3,7,8-TCDD.

Workers may be exposed to PCDDs during the production of TCP, 2,4,5-T, and pentachlorophenol. Herbicide sprayers using 2,4,5-T or silvex have been exposed to 2,3,7,8-TCDD during application. Environmental contamination occurred from spraying waste oil that contained 2,3,7,8-TCDD for dust control on the ground in Missouri. The EPA banned most uses of 2,4,5-T and silvex in 1979, though their use was allowed on sugarcane and in orchards, and miscellaneous noncrop uses were permitted. In October 1983, EPA published its intent to cancel the registration of all pesticide products containing 2,4,5-T or silvex. It is not possible to accurately estimate the number of United States workers currently exposed to 2,3,7,8-TCDD during decontamination of worksites, from waste materials contaminated with 2,3,7,8-TCDD, or from cleanup after fires in transformers containing polychlorinated biphenyls.

Metabolism & Mechanism of Action

2,3,7,8-TCDD is an extremely lipophilic substance and is readily absorbed following an oral dose in the rat. It accumulates mainly in the liver and after a single dose is largely eliminated unmetabolized in the feces with a whole body half-life of about 3 weeks. After repeated dosing in small laboratory animals, it is stored in adipose tissue. The retention in humans is not known. Dermal absorption may be important in workers exposed to phenoxy acids and chlorophenols. Exposure to 2,3,7,8-TCDD as a vapor will normally be negligible because of its low vapor pressure.

Clinical Findings

A. Signs and Symptoms:

1. Acute exposure–In some animals, 2,3,7,8-TCDD is lethal in doses of less than 1 $\mu g/kg$. Acute toxicity results in profound wasting, thymic atrophy, bone marrow suppression, hepatotoxicity, and microsomal enzyme induction.

In humans, the acute toxicity of 2,3,7,8-TCDD is known from accidental release due to runaway reactions or explosions. A process accident in Nitro, West Virginia, in 1949 was followed by acute skin, eye, and respiratory tract irritation, headache, dizziness, and nausea. These symptoms subsided within 1–2 weeks and were followed by an acneiform eruption; severe muscle pain in the extremities, thorax, and shoulders; fatigue, nervousness, and irritability; dyspnea, complaints of decreased libido, and intolerance to cold. Workers exhibited severe chloracne, hepatic enlargement, peripheral neuritis, delayed prothrombin time, and increased total serum lipid levels. A follow-up study 30 years later found persistence of chloracne in 55% but no evidence of increased risk for cardiovascular disease or for hepatic, renal, or nervous system damage.

2. Chronic exposure–In animals, 2,3,7,8-TCDD is a teratogen and is toxic to the fetus. Two-year feeding studies in rats and mice have demonstrated an excess of liver tumors; the feeding level at which no observable effects in rats occurred was 0.001 $\mu g/kg/d$.

The chronic health problems in humans have been studied in cohorts of workers exposed in accidents and during the production of TCP and 2,4,5-T contaminated with 2,3,7,8-TCDD. Because of the coincidental exposure to other herbicides, it is not possible to attribute the observed health effects solely to 2,3,7,8-TCDD exposure. Immunologic studies of dioxin-exposed individuals are inconclusive.

Chloracne can result within several weeks after exposure to 2,3,7,8-TCDD and can persist for decades. Among production workers, the severity of chloracne is related to the degree of exposure. In some workplaces, exposed persons had chloracne but no systemic illnesses; in others, workers experienced fatigue, weight loss, myalgias, insomnia, irritability, and decreased libido. The liver has become tender and enlarged, and sensory changes, particularly in the lower extremities, have been reported. Porphyria cutanea tarda has been observed. In exposed production workers systemic symptoms—except for chloracne—have not persisted after exposures ceased. Additional analysis of workers exposed to dioxin who had acne did not show excess cancer deaths.

Reproductive effects from possible human exposure to 2,3,7,8-TCDD are inconclusive. Following the Seveso explosion, an analysis of birth defect clusters was inadequate to assess reproductive risk. Case-control studies of birth defects in offspring of Vietnam veterans have shown an increased risk only for a few specific types of defects in subgroups of veterans who may have had a higher likelihood of exposure to Agent Orange.

Soft tissue sarcoma has been reported but not confirmed among workers exposed to phenoxy herbicides. There is a suggested association between exposure to phenoxyacetic herbicides contaminated with 2,3,7,8-TCDD and excess lymphoma and stomach cancer.

B. Laboratory Findings: Abnormalities reported most consistently are elevated liver enzymes, prolonged prothrombin time, and elevated cholesterol and triglycerides. Urinary porphyrins may be elevated. Following the Seveso accident, the incidence of abnormal nerve conduction tests was significantly elevated in subjects with chloracne.

Very low levels of 2,3,7,8-TCDD (4–130 parts per trillion) can be detected in adipose tissue of nonexposed populations. Concentration of polychlorinated compounds in plasma may be 1000-fold less than in adipose tissue. There is a high correlation between adipose and serum 2,3,7,8-TCDD levels; serum levels are a valid measure of body burden. The correlation between plasma and adipose tissue concentrations of 2,3,7,8-TCDD with signs and symptoms is uncertain.

Differential Diagnosis

Known causes of an acneiform eruption in the workplace include petroleum cutting oils, coal tar, and the chlorinated aromatic compounds. With systemic complaints such as weight loss, headache, myalgias, and irritability, other underlying medical illnesses should be ruled out before attributing the disorder to 2,3,7,8-TCDD.

Prevention

A. Work Practices: NIOSH recommends that 2,3,7,8-TCDD be considered a potential occupational carcinogen and that exposure in all occupational settings be controlled to the fullest extent possible. Specific guidelines for safe work practices must begin with environmental sampling to determine the presence of 2,3,7,8-TCDD contamination, including sampling of air, soil, and settled dust and wipe sampling of surfaces. For site cleanup, specific decontamination procedures should be adhered to for adequate worker protection. Protective clothing and equipment should consist of both outer and inner garments, with outer coveralls, gloves, and boots made of nonwoven polyethylene fabric. Appropriate respiratory protection must be worn, ranging from an air purifying respirator to a self-contained breathing apparatus. Follow-up sampling should be conducted after decontamination of a site to ensure adequate cleanup.

B. Medical Surveillance: Production workers exposed to compounds contaminated with 2,3,7,8-TCDD as well as site decontamination personnel should undergo baseline and periodic medical examination with special attention to the skin and nervous system. Baseline laboratory testing should include liver enzymes, cholesterol, and triglycerides, with follow-up as required.

Treatment

Skin contaminated with 2,3,7,8-TCDD should be immediately washed and any contaminated clothing removed and placed in marked containers and disposed of appropriately.

Except for symptomatic treatment of chloracne, there is no treatment for acute or chronic health effects resulting from 2,3,7,8-TCDD exposure.

VINYL CHLORIDE MONOMER & POLYVINYL CHLORIDE

Essentials of Diagnosis

Acute effects:
- Respiratory tract irritation.
- Lethargy, headache.

Chronic effects:
- Acro-osteolysis, Raynaud's phenomenon, skin thickening.
- Hepatosplenomegaly.
- Hepatic angiosarcoma.

Exposure Limits

ACGIH TLV: 5 ppm TWA

NIOSH REL: Lowest reliably detectable concentration

General Considerations

Vinyl chloride monomer (chloroethene) is a colorless, highly flammable gas at room temperature. It is usually handled as a liquid under pressure containing a polymerization inhibitor (phenol). It is soluble in ethanol and ether. The odor threshold is variable, so that odor cannot be used to prevent excess exposure.

Use

Worldwide, production capacity is over 15 billion kg annually.

NIOSH estimates that 27,000 workers in the USA are exposed to vinyl chloride, with an additional 2.2 million potentially exposed.

About 95% of vinyl chloride monomer is used for the production of polyvinyl chloride resins. Polyvinyl chloride is used primarily in the production of plastic piping and conduit, floor coverings, home furnishings, electrical applications, recreational products (records, toys), packaging (film, sheet, and bottles), and transportation materials (automobile tops, upholstery, and mats).

Occupational & Environmental Exposure

A 1977 NIOSH survey of 3 vinyl chloride monomer plants found that the 8-hour TWA ranged from 0.07 to 27 ppm. Following promulgation of the OSHA standard in 1974, exposures were reduced to less than 5 ppm. The highest exposures occur in polymerization plants, particularly during reactor vessel cleaning.

Retained unreacted monomer in polyvinyl chloride products is so low that there is little risk now to polyvinyl chloride fabrication workers.

Metabolism & Mechanism of Action

The chief route of exposure to VCM is through inhalation of the gas, though dermal absorption may be significant during manual reactor vessel cleaning. Vinyl chloride is readily absorbed through the respiratory tract. Its primary metabolite is chloroethylene oxide, which forms the reactive intermediate epoxide that can bind to RNA and DNA in vivo and may be responsible for the carcinogenicity observed in animal and human studies.

Clinical Findings
A. Symptoms and Signs:
1. Acute exposure–Vinyl chloride monomer has relatively low acute toxicity, causing respiratory irritation and central nervous system depression at high concentrations (10,000–20,000 ppm).

2. Chronic exposure–Chronic toxicity from vinyl chloride monomer exposure can result in hepatomegaly, osteolysis, Raynaud's phenomenon, and sclerodermalike skin lesions.

a. Acro-osteolysis–Symptoms of Raynaud's phenomenon, osteolysis in the terminal phalanges of some of the fingers, and thickening or raised nodules on the hands and forearms occurred rarely in workers employed in production and polymerization, especially associated with the cleaning of reactors.

Vascular changes in the digital arteries of the hand associated with acro-osteolysis have been demonstrated by arteriography, and circulating immune complexes have been identified.

b. Liver disease–Hepatic fibrosis, splenomegaly, and thrombocytopenia with portal hypertension have occurred. Pathologic changes in the liver consist of activation of hepatic sinusoidal cells and perisinusoidal fibrosis without significant parenchymal damage.

In 1974, 3 cases of hepatic angiosarcoma among polyvinyl chloride polymerization workers were reported at a plant in Louisville, Kentucky. Worldwide, 118 cases of hepatic angiosarcoma from 34 factories have been reported to a central registry. The time from first exposure to initial diagnosis for the 118 cases ranged from 10 to 35 years. Forty-three percent of the affected individuals had been employed as autoclave operators with the highest exposure to vinyl chloride monomer. An estimated 200–350 deaths from vinyl chloride-related angiosarcoma can be expected over the next 30 years.

Only 2 cases of hepatic angiosarcoma have been documented in the polyvinyl chloride processing industry, suggesting a significantly lower vinyl chloride-related neoplastic risk among fabrication workers.

c. Mortality studies–Cohort mortality studies of vinyl chloride monomer-exposed workers have documented significant mortality rates for liver cancer, particularly hepatic angiosarcoma. After cessation of exposure, the increased risk of hepatic angiosarcoma continues for at least 6 years. Other than liver cancer, no excess cancer deaths have been observed.

d. Pulmonary effects–Cases of pneumoconiosis have been reported in workers exposed to vinyl chloride monomer and polyvinyl chloride dust. Some polyvinyl chloride production and fabrication workers with high (> 10 mg/m^3) exposure to polyvinyl chloride dust have reduced pulmonary function and an increased incidence of chest x-ray abnormalities.

e. Reproductive effects–Increased fetal loss by wives of vinyl chloride monomer-exposed workers and an excess of central nervous system malformations in communities housing vinyl chloride monomer plants have suggested a relationship between vinyl chloride monomer exposure and adverse reproductive outcome.

B. Laboratory Findings: There may be an increased frequency of elevated levels of liver enzymes and alkaline phosphatase in workers with vinyl chloride exposure. Fasting levels of serum bile acids and urinary coproporphyrins have been suggested as clinically useful indicators of early chemical injury in vinyl chloride monomer-exposed worker populations with asymptomatic liver dysfunction. Gray-scale ultrasonography of the liver has been helpful in identifying early hepatic injury in asymptomatic workers.

Differential Diagnosis
Hepatic angiosarcoma has been associated with a history of arsenic exposure and thorium dioxide (Thorotrast) ingestion. The vinyl chloride monomer-associated sclerotic changes in skin, with skin nodules, Raynaud's phenomenon, and osteolysis, are clinically very similar to idiopathic scleroderma; however, sclerodactyly, calcinosis, and digital pitting scars are unusual in vinyl chloride monomer disease.

Prevention
The risk of hepatic angiosarcoma should be minimal if the 8-hour TWA is less than 1 ppm. If processing of vinyl chloride monomer production is controlled, general environmental risk is negligible.

A. Work Practices: Worker isolation is achieved in most polyvinyl chloride plants through the use of isolated process control rooms. For operators, cleaners, and utility employees, extensive engineering controls in polyvinyl chloride polymerization plants are required to reduce 8-hour TWA worker exposures to less than 1 ppm. Preventing worker exposure during routine maintenance and cleanup operation by adequate degassing of autoclaves and reaction vessels is essential. On-line gas chromatographic vinyl chloride monomer-specific detectors can identify leaks before large emissions develop.

Employees should be required to wear half-face supplied-air respirators when the concentration of vinyl chloride monomer exceeds 1 ppm. A full-face supplied-air respirator is required for reactor cleaning or other maintenance. Where skin contact is possible, protective uniforms, gloves, and head coverings and impervious boots are necessary.

Based on findings of pulmonary function changes and x-ray abnormalities, engineering controls to minimize polyvinyl chloride dust exposure should be taken.

B. Medical Surveillance: Preplacement medical examination should evaluate the presence of preexisting liver disease. Preplacement and periodic measurement of liver enzymes is recommended by NIOSH, though the specificity and sensitivity of these tests are poor. Other noninvasive measures of liver function, such as indocyanine green clearance, bile acids, and urinary uroporphyrins, may have some value in routine medical surveillance.

Treatment

The mean survival after diagnosis of hepatic angiosarcoma is several months. Chemotherapy may slightly improve the duration and quality of survival. Acro-osteolysis appears to be irreversible after cessation of exposure.

REFERENCES

Acids

Bracken WM et al: Comparative effectiveness of topical treatments for hydrofluoric acid burns. *J Occup Med* 1985;**27**:733.

National Institute for Occupational Safety and Health: *Criteria for a Recommended Standard for Occupational Exposure to Chromic Acid.* Department of Health, Education, and Welfare Publication No. (NIOSH) 73-11021. US Government Printing Office, 1974.

National Institute for Occupational Safety and Health: *Criteria for a Recommended Standard for Occupational Exposure to Hydrogen Fluoride.* Department of Health, Education, and Welfare Publication No. (NIOSH) 76-143 (1975). US Government Printing Office, 1977.

National Institute for Occupational Safety and Health: *Criteria for a Recommended Standard for Occupational Exposure to Nitric Acid.* Department of Health, Education, and Welfare Publication No. (NIOSH) 76-141. US Government Printing Office, 1977.

National Institute for Occupational Safety and Health: *Criteria for a Recommended Standard for Occupational Exposure to Sulfuric Acid.* Department of Health, Education, and Welfare Publication No. (NIOSH) 74-128 (1975). US Government Printing Office, 1975.

Steenland K et al: Incidence of laryngeal cancer and exposure to acid mists. *Br J Ind Med* 1988;**45**:766.

Alkalies

National Institute for Occupational Safety and Health: *Criteria for a Recommended Standard for Occupational Exposure to Sodium Hydroxide.* Department of Health, Education, and Welfare Publication No. (NIOSH) 76-105. US Government Printing Office, 1975.

Acrylamide

Le Quesne P: Acrylamide. In: *Neurotoxicology.* Spencer PS, Schaumberg HH (editors). Williams & Wilkins, 1980.

National Institute for Occupational Safety and Health: *Criteria for a Recommended Standard for Occupational Exposure to Acrylamide.* Department of Health, Education, and Welfare Publication No. (NIOSH) 77-112 US Government Printing Office, 1976.

World Health Organization: *Environmental Health Criteria 49:* Acrylamide. WHO, 1985.

Acrylonitrile

Chen JL et al: Cancer incidence and mortality among workers exposed to acrylonitrile. *Am J Ind Med* 1987;**11**:157.

Collins JJ et al: Mortality patterns among employees exposed to acrylonitrile. *J Occup Med* 1989;**31**:368.

Koerselman W, van der Graaf M: Acrylonitrile: A suspected human carcinogen. *Int Arch Occup Environ Health* 1984;**54**:317.

O'Berg MT et al: Epidemiologic study of workers exposed to acrylonitrile: An update. *J Occup Med* 1985;**27**:835.

Aromatic Amines

National Institute for Occupational Safety and Health: *Health Hazard Alert: Benzidine-, O-Tolidine-, and O-Dianisidine-Based Dyes.* DHHS (NIOSH) Pub. 81-106, 1981.

Stasik MJ: Carcinomas of the urinary bladder in a 4-chloro-o-toluidine cohort. *Int Arch Occup Environ Health* 1988;**60**:21.

Stern FB et al: Notification and risk assessment for bladder cancer of a cohort exposed to aromatic amines. 3. Mortality among workers exposed to aromatic amines in the last beta-naphthylamine manufacturing facility in the United States. *J Occup Med* 1985;**27**:495.

Carbon Disulfide

Beauchamp RO et al: Critical review of the literature on carbon disulfide toxicity. *CRC Crit Rev Toxicol* 1981;**11**:169.

MacMahon B, Monson RR: Mortality in the US rayon industry. *J Occup Med* 1988;**30**:698.

Sweetnam PM, Taylor SW, Elwood PC: Exposure to carbon disulphide and ischaemic heart disease in a viscose rayon factory. *Br J Ind Med* 1987;**44**:220.

Chloromethyl Ethers

Maher KV, DeFonso LR: Respiratory cancer among chloromethyl ether workers. *JNCI* 1987;**78**:839.

Travenius SZ: Formation and occurrence of bis (chloromethyl) ether and its prevention in the chemical industry. *Scand J Work Environ Health* 1982;**8 (Suppl 3)**:1.

Ward E, Smith AB, Halperin W: 4,4'-Methylene-bis (2-chloroaniline): An unregulated carcinogen. *Am J Ind Med* 1987;**12**:537.

Dibromochloropropane

Eaton M et al: Seven-year follow-up of workers exposed to 1,2-dibromo-3-chloropropane. *J Occup Med* 1986;**28**: 1145.

Whorton D, Foliart D: DBCP: Eleven years later. *Reprod Tox* 1988;**2**:155.

Dimethylaminopropionitrile

Keogh JP et al: An epidemic of urinary retention caused by dimethylaminopropionitrile. *JAMA* 1980;**243**:756.

Kreiss K et al: Neurological dysfunction of the bladder in workers exposed to dimethylaminopropionitrile. *JAMA* 1980;**243**:741.

Ethylene Oxide

Elliott L et al: Effect of engineering controls and work practices in reducing ethylene-oxide exposure during the sterilization of hospital supplies. *Scand J Work Environ Health* 1988;**14(Suppl 1)**:40.

Elliott LJ et al: Ethylene oxide exposure in hospitals. *Appl Ind Hyg* 1988;**3**:141.

Hogstedt C, Aringer L, Gustavsson A: Epidemiologic support for ethylene oxide as a cancer-causing agent. *JAMA* 1986;**255**:1575.

Landrigan PJ et al: Ethylene oxide: An overview of toxicologic and epidemiologic research. *Am J Ind Med* 1984;**6**:103.

Formaldehyde

Blair A et al: Mortality among industrial workers exposed to formaldehyde. *JNCI* 1986;**76**:1071.

Boeniger MF: Formate in urine as a biological indicator of formaldehyde exposure: A review. *Am Ind Hyg Assoc J* 1987;**48**:900.

Horvath EP Jr et al: Effects of formaldehyde on the mucous membranes and lungs: A study of an industrial population. *JAMA* 1988;**259**:701.

Landrigan PJ, Perera FP: Controversy in the regulation of formaldehyde. (Editorial.) *Am J Ind Med* 1988;**14**:375.

Roush GC et al: Nasopharyngeal cancer, sinonasal cancer, and occupations related to formaldehyde: A case-control study. *JNCI* 1987;**79**:1221.

Sterling TD, Weinkam JJ: Reanalysis of lung cancer mortality in a National Cancer Institute study on mortality among industrial workers exposed to formaldehyde. *J Occup Med* 1988;**30**:895.

Uba G et al: Prospective study of respiratory effects of formaldehyde among healthy and asthmatic medical students. *Am J Ind Med* 1989;**15**:91.

Nitrates

Daum S: Nitroglycerin and alkyl nitrates. In: *Occupational and Environmental Medicine*. Rom WR (editor). Little, Brown, 1982.

Fraser P et al: Further results from a census-based mortality study of fertiliser manufacturers. *Br J Ind Med* 1989;**46**:38.

Gjesdal K et al: Exposure to glyceryl trinitrate during gun powder production: Plasma glyceryl trinitrate concentration, elimination kinetics, and discomfort among production workers. *Br J Ind Med* 1985;**42**:27.

Nitrosamines

Ducos P et al: Occupational exposure to volatile nitrosamines in foundries using the ''Ashland'' core-making process. *Environ Res* 1988;**3**:72.

Lahiri VL et al: Nitrosamine in leather dust extracts. *Br J Ind Med* 1988;**45**:647.

National Academy of Sciences, National Research Council: *The Health Effects of Nitrate, Nitrite and N-Nitroso Compounds*. National Academy Press, 1981.

Speigelhalder B, Preussman R: Occupational nitrosamine exposure. 1. Rubber and tire industry. *Carcinogenesis* 1983;**4**:1147.

Pentachlorophenol

Exon JH: A review of chlorinated phenols. *Vet Hum Toxicol* 1984;**26**:508.

Lindroos L et al: urinary chlorophenols in sawmill workers. *Int Arch Occup Environ Health* 1987;**59**:463.

Triebig G et al: Pentachlorophenol and the peripheral nervous system: A longitudinal study in exposed workers. *Br J Ind Med* 1987;**44**:638.

Wood S et al: Pentachlorophenol poisoning. *J Occup Med* 1983;**25**:527.

Polychlorinated Biphenyls

Bertazzi PA et al: Cancer mortality of capacitor manufacturing workers. *Am J Ind Med* 1987;**11**:165.

Brown DP: Mortality of workers exposed to polychlorinated biphenyls: An update. *Arch Environ Health* 1987;**42**:333.

Emmett EA et al: Studies of transformer repair workers exposed to PCBs: 2. Results of clinical laboratory investigations. *Am J Ind Med* 1988;**14**:47.

Gustavsson P, Hogstedt C, Rappe C: Short-term mortality and cancer incidence in capacitor manufacturing workers exposed to polychlorinated biphenyls (PCBs). *Am J Ind Med* 1986;**10**:341.

Kimbrough RD: Human health effects of polychlorinated biphenyls (PCBs) and polybrominated biphenyls (PBBs). *Annu Rev Pharmacol Toxicol* 1987;**27**:87.

Polycyclic Aromatic Hydrocarbons

Heikkilä PR et al: Exposure to creosote in the impregnation and handling of impregnated wood. *Scand J Work Environ Health* 1987;**13**:431.

Jongeneelen FJ et al: 1-Hydroxypyrene in urine as a biological indicator of exposure to polycyclic aromatic hydrocarbons in several work environments. *Ann Occup Hyg* 1988;**32**:35.

Keimig DG, Slymen DJ, White O Jr: Occupational exposure to coke oven emissions from 1979–1983. *Arch Environ Health* 1986;**41**:363.

Knecht U, Woitowitz HJ: Risk of cancer from the use of tar bitumen in road works. *Br J Ind Med* 1989;**46**:24.

Perera FP et al: Detection of polycyclic aromatic hydrocarbon-DNA adducts in white blood cells of foundry workers. *Cancer Res* 1988;**48**:2288.

Styrene

Coggon D et al: Mortality of workers exposed to styrene in the manufacture of glass-reinforced plastics. *Scand J Work Environ Health* 1987;**13**:94.

Guillemin MP, Berode M: Biological monitoring of styrene: A review. *Am Ind Hyg Assoc J* 1988;**49**:497.

Lemasters GK et al: Reproductive outcomes of pregnant workers employed at 36 reinforced plastics companies. 2. Lowered birth weight. *J Occup Med* 1989;**31**:115.

Moscato G et al: Occupational asthma due to styrene: Two case reports. *J Occup Med* 1987;**29**:957.

2,3,7,8-Tetrachlorodibenzo-*p*-dioxin

American Academy of Clinical Toxicology: Commentary on 2,3,7,8-tetrachlorodibenzo-*p*-dioxin (TCDD). *Clin Toxicol* 1985;**23**:191.

Bond GG et al: Update of mortality among chemical workers with potential exposure to the higher chlorinated dioxins. *J Occup Med* 1989;**31**:121.

Evans RG et al: A medical follow-up of the health effects of long-term exposure to 2,3,7,8-tetrachlorodibenzo-*p*-dioxin. *Arch Environ Health* 1988;**43:**273.

Jennings AM et al: Immunological abnormalities 17 years after accidental exposure to 2,3,7,8-tetra-chlorodibenzo-para-dioxin. *Br J Ind Med* 1988; **45:**701.

Patterson DG et al: Correlation between serum and adipose tissue levels of 2,3,7,8-tetrachlorodibenzo-*p*-dioxin in 50 persons from Missouri. *Arch Environ Contam Toxicol* 1988;**17:**139.

Vinyl Chloride Monomer & Polyvinyl Chloride

Dahar WS et al: Update to vinyl chloride mortality study. *J Occup Med* 1988;**30:**648.

Doll R: Effects of exposure to vinyl chloride: An assessment of the evidence. *Scand J Work Environ Health* 1988;**14:**61.

Jones RD, Smith DM, Thomas PG: A mortality study of vinyl chloride monomer workers employed in the United Kingdom in 1940–1974. *Scand J Work Environ Health* 1988;**14:**153.

Wagoner JK: Toxicity of vinyl chloride and poly(vinyl chloride): A critical review. *Environ Health Perspect* 1983;**52:**61.

Wu W et al: Cohort and case-control analyses of workers exposed to vinyl chloride: An update. *J Occup Med* 1989;**31:**518.

Solvents

27

Jon Rosenberg, MD, MPH

GENERAL PROPERTIES & HEALTH EFFECTS OF SOLVENTS

A solvent is any substance—usually a liquid—that dissolves another substance, resulting in a solution (uniformly dispersed mixture). Solvents may be classified as aqueous (water-based) or organic (hydrocarbon-based). Since most of the substances that solvents are used to dissolve in industry are organic, most industrial solvents are organic chemicals. They are commonly used for cleaning, degreasing, thinning, and extraction.

Solvent chemicals are used in greatest volume as chemical intermediates in the manufacture and formulation of chemical products. However, more workers are exposed to high levels of solvents during use of the substances as cleaners, thinners, and degreasers.

Hundreds of individual chemicals are used to make over 30,000 industrial solvents. There are physical, chemical, and toxicologic properties that help to classify this large group of chemicals into families with shared or distinguishing features. These features will be discussed first, followed by a brief summary of the commonly used industrial solvents according to their chemical families.

PHYSICAL & CHEMICAL PROPERTIES OF SOLVENTS

Solubility

Lipid solubility is an important determinant of the efficiency of a substance as an industrial solvent and a major determinant of a number of health effects. The potency of solvents as general anesthetics and as defatting agents is directly proportionate to their lipid solubility.

Dermal absorption is related to both lipid solubility and water solubility (since the skin behaves like a lipid-water sandwich), so that solvents such as dimethylsulfoxide, dimethylformamide, and glycol ethers, which are highly soluble in both (amphipathic), are well absorbed through the skin. All organic solvents are lipid-soluble, but this solubility may differ to a significant degree.

Flammability & Explosiveness

Flammability and explosiveness are the properties of a substance that allow it to burn or ignite,

respectively. Some organic solvents are flammable enough to be used as fuels, whereas others (eg, halogenated hydrocarbons) are so nonflammable that they are used as fire extinguishing agents. Flash point, ignition temperature, and flammable and explosive limits are measures of flammability and explosiveness. The National Fire Prevention Association (NFPA) rates flammability hazards by a numerical code from 0 (no hazard) to 4 (severe hazard). Flash points and NFPA codes are listed in Table 27–1. These properties are important to consider when selecting a solvent or substituting one solvent for another based on undesirable health effects or efficacy.

Volatility

Volatility is the tendency of a liquid to evaporate (form a gas or vapor). Other conditions being equal, the greater the volatility of a substance, the greater the concentration of its vapors in air. Since the most common route of exposure to solvents is inhalation, exposure to a solvent is highly dependent on its volatility. Solvents as a class are all relatively volatile over a wide range. Vapor pressure and evaporation rate are 2 measures of volatility listed in Table 27–1.

Chemical Structure

Solvents can be divided into families according to chemical structure and the attached functional groups. Toxicologic properties tend to be similar within a group, such as liver toxicity from chlorinated hydrocarbons and irritation from aldehydes. The basic structures are aliphatic, alicyclic, and aromatic. The functional groups include halogens, alcohols, ketones, glycols, esters, ethers, carboxylic acids, amines, and amides.

PHARMACOKINETICS OF SOLVENTS

Absorption (Route of Exposure)

A. Pulmonary: Since organic solvents are generally volatile liquids and since the vapors are lipid-soluble and therefore well absorbed across the alveolar-capillary membrane, inhalation is the primary route for occupational exposure. The pulmonary retention or uptake (percentage of inhaled dose that is retained and absorbed) for most organic solvents ranges from 40% to 80% at rest. Because physical labor increases pulmonary ventilation and

Table 27–1. Industrial solvents: Properties, odor thresholds, and exposure limits.

	Flash Point (°F)	NFPA Flammability Code[1]	Vapor Pressure (mm Hg 25 °C)	Evaporation Rate[2]	TLV[3] (ppm)	Odor Threshold[4] (ppm)	Biologic Monitor[5]	General Hazards of Chemical Family and Unique Hazards of Specific Compounds
Aliphatic								Anesthetic > irritant.
Pentane	−40	4	500	1	600	400		
n-Hexane	−10	3	150	1.9	50	130	+	Peripheral neuropathy.
Hexane (other)	−10	3	150	1.9	500	130		Hazard relative to concentration of n-hexane.
Heptane	25	3	50	2.7	400	150		
Octane	55	3	15	5.9	300	50		
Nonane	90	0	5	2.9	200	50		
Alicyclic								Anesthetic > irritant.
Cyclohexane	10	3	95	2.6	300	25		
Aromatic								Anesthetic > irritant.
Benzene	10	3	75	2.8	10	10	+	Leukemia and aplastic anemia.
Toluene	40	3	30	4.5	100	5	+	Renal tubular acidosis, cerebellar dysfunction.
Xylenes (all)	85	3	10	9.5	100	1	+	
Ethyl benzene	60	3	5	9.4	100	1	+	
Cumene	95	2	10	14	50-S	0.1	+	
Styrene	90	3	5	12.4	50-S	0.5	+	
Petroleum distillates								Hazard relative to aliphatic and aromatic components:
Petroleum ether	~ −50	3	~ 40	~ 1.1	. . .	. . .		100% aliphatic, extremely volatile, flammable.
Rubber solvent	~ −20	3	. . .	~ 2.3	400	. . .		Mostly aliphatic, extremely volatile, flammable.
V M & P naphtha[6]	~ 30	3	~ 20	~ 7.1	300	. . .		Mostly aliphatic.
Mineral spirits I	~ 100	3	~ 5	~ 4.4	100	. . .		
Aromatic petroleum naphtha	~ 110	3	~ 5	. . .	. . .	. . .		Mostly aromatic.
Kerosene	~ 115	3	~ 5	. . .	. . .	. . .		
Alcohols								Irritant > anesthetic.
Methyl alcohol	50	3	90	5.2	200-S	100	+	Acidosis, optic neuropathy.
Ethyl alcohol	55	3	45	~ 7	1000	85		"Fetal alcohol syndrome" (ingestion).
1-Propyl alcohol	75	3	20	7.8	200-S	2		
Isopropyl alcohol	55	3	35	7.7	400	20		
n-Butyl alcohol	85	3	10	19.6	50-S	1		Auditory, vestibular nerve injury reported.
sec-Butyl alcohol	75	3	15	12.3	200	2		
tert-Butyl alcohol	50	3	15	. . .	100	50		
Iso-octyl alcohol	185	2	0.05	300	50-S	. . .		
Cyclohexanol	155	2	1	150	50-S	0.1		
Glycols								Extremely low volatility.
Ethylene glycol	230	1	0.05	. . .	50	. . .		Acidosis, seizures, renal failure (ingestion).
Phenols								Irritant > anesthetic; cytotoxic, corrosive.
Phenol	175	2	0.5	. . .	5-S	0.05	+	Dermal absorption of vapors.
Cresol	180	2	0.2	>400	5-S	. . .		
Ketones								Irritant, strong odor > anesthetic.
Acetone	−5	3	20	1.9	750	15	+	
Methyl ethyl ketone	15	3	70	2.7	200	5	+	
Methyl isobutyl ketone	70	3	5	5.6	50	1		
Diacetone alcohol	140	2	1	~ 60	50	0.1		
Mesityl oxide	90	3	10	8.4	15	0.5		
Cyclohexanone	110	2	3	22.2	25-S	1		
Esters								Irritant, strong odor > anesthetic.
Methyl formate	−2	3	475	1.6	100	600		Optic neuropathy from metabolism to formic acid.
Ethyl formate	−5	3	200	1.8	100	30		
Methyl acetate	15	3	175	2.2	200	5		Optic neuropathy from metabolism to methanol.
Ethyl acetate	25	3	75	2.7	400	5		
n-Propyl acetate	55	3	35	4.8	200	0.5		
n-Butyl acetate	75	3	10	5.2	150	0.5		
n-Amyl acetate	85	3	5	11.6	100	0.05		Odorant ("banana oil").

continued

Table 27–1 (con't). Industrial solvents: Properties, odor thresholds, and exposure limits.

	Flash Point (°F)	NFPA Flammability Code[1]	Vapor Pressure (mm Hg 25 °C)	Evaporation Rate[2]	TLV[3] (ppm)	Odor Threshold[4] (ppm)	Biologic Monitor[5]	General Hazards of Chemical Family and Unique Hazards of Specific Compounds
Ethers								
Ethyl ether	−50	4	450	1	400	10		Extremely volatile, flammable, explosive.
Dioxane	54	3	27	14	25-S	24		Carcinogenic in animals at high doses.
Glycol ethers								Skin absorption without irritation.
2-Methoxyethanol	100	2	10	21.1	5-S	2	+	Reproductive toxicity in male and female-animals.
2-Ethoxyethanol	110	2	5	28.1	5-S	3	+	Reproductive toxicity in male and female animals.
2-Butoxyethanol	340	2	1	~85	25-S	0.1		Anemia.
Propylene glycol monomethyl ether	100	3	10	. . .	100	10		
Dipropylene glycol monomethyl ether	185	2	0.5	. . .	100-S	. . .		
Glycidyl ethers								Sensitizers, genetic and reproductive toxins.
Phenyl glycidyl ether	. . .	. . .	0.01	. . .	1	. . .		
Diglycidyl ether	. . .	. . .	0.1	. . .	0.1	. . .		
Acids								Irritant > anesthetic.
Formic	. . .	. . .	. . .	45	5	0.1		
Acetic	105	2	15	11	10	0.5		
Propionic	. . .	. . .	. . .	5	10	0.2		
Amines								Irritant > anesthetic; corneal edema, visual halos.
Methylamine	. . .	. . .	gas	gas	10	3		
Dimethylamine	. . .	. . .	gas	gas	10	0.5		
Trimethylamine	. . .	. . .	gas	gas	10	0.0005		
Ethylamine	<0	4	gas	gas	10	1		
Diethylamine	−9	3	240	2.2	10	0.2		
Triethylamine	20	3	70	2.7	10	0.5		
Butylamine	10	3	70	5.1	5-S	2		
Cyclohexylamine	90	3	10	82.9	10	2.5		
Ethylenediamine	95	2	10	>5000	10	1		Allergic contact dermatitis, asthma.
Diethylene triamine	215	1	0.5	>400	1-S	. . .		
Ethanolamine	185	2	0.5	>5000	3	2.5		
Diethanolamine	280	1	0.05	>5000	3	0.5		
Chlorinated hydrocarbons								Cancer in animals; liver, kidney, cardiac effects.
Methyl chloroform (1,1,1,-trichloro-ethane)	NF	0	120	2.7	350	120	+	
Trichloroethylene	. . .	1	75	3.1	50	30	+	Alcohol intolerance, degreaser's flush.
Perchloroethylene (tetrachloroethyl-ene)	NF	0	20	6.6	50	25	+	
Methylene chloride	NF	0	420	1.8	50	250	+	Metabolized to carbon monoxide.
Carbon tetrachloride	NF	0	110	2.6	5-S	100		Cirrhosis, liver cancer.
Chloroform	NF	0	190	2.2	10	85		
1,1,2-Trichloroethane	NF	0	20	12.6	10-S	. . .		
1,1,2,2-Tetrachloro-ethane	NF	0	10	19.1	1-S	1.5		
Chlorofluorocarbons								Weak anesthetic, irritant; cardiac effects.
Trichlorofluoro-methane (F-11)	NF	0	330	1.6	1000	5		
Dichlorodifluoro-methane (F-12)	NF	0	. . .	. . .	1000	. . .		
Chlorodifluoro-methane (F-22)	NF	0	. . .	. . .	1000	. . .		
1,1,2,2-Tetrachloro-2,2-difluoro-ethane (F-112)	NF	0	. . .	. . .	500	. . .		

continued

Table 27–1 (con't). Industrial solvents: Properties, odor thresholds, and exposure limits.

	Flash Point (°F)	NFPA Flammability Code[1]	Vapor Pressure (mm Hg 25 °C)	Evaporation Rate[2]	TLV[3] (ppm)	Odor Threshold[4] (ppm)	Biologic Monitor[5]	General Hazards of Chemical Family and Unique Hazards of Specific Compounds
1,1,2-Trichloro- 1,2,2-trifluoroethane (F-113)	NF	0	325	2	1000	45		
1,2-Dichlorotetra-fluoroethane (F-114)	...	...	...	...	1000	...		
Chloropentafluoro-ethane (F-115)	...	...	...	...	1000	...		
Miscellaneous								
Turpentine	100	3	...	~ 375	100	...		Irritant > anesthetic; allergic contact dermatitis.
Dimethylsulfoxide	200	1	...	>300	...	...		Hepatotoxic > anesthetic; skin absorption.
Dimethylformamide	140	2	5	45	10-S	2		Smell in breath after exposure; skin absorption.
Tetrahydrofuran	5	3	175	2	200	2		Anesthetic, irritant.

[1]See text for explanation.
[2]Ether = 1; see text for explanation.
[3]American Conference of Governmental Industrial Hygienists (ACGIH) threshold limit value, 8-hour time-weighted average, 1988–89; S = "skin" designation.
[4]Population odor threshold determined by testing.
[5]Information available on biologic monitoring; see Chapter 34.
[6]Varnish makers' and painters' naphtha.

blood flow, the amount of solvent delivered to the alveoli and the amount absorbed are likewise increased. Levels of physical exercise commonly encountered in the workplace will increase the pulmonary uptake of many solvents by a factor of 2–3 times that at rest.

B. Percutaneous: The lipid solubility of organic solvents results in most being absorbed through the skin to some degree following direct contact. However, percutaneous absorption is also determined by water solubility and volatility. Solvents that are soluble in both lipid and water are most readily absorbed through the skin. Highly volatile substances are less well absorbed since they tend to evaporate from the skin unless evaporation is prevented by occlusion.

For a number of solvents, dermal absorption contributes to overall exposure sufficiently to result in a "skin" designation for the American Conference of Governmental Industrial Hygienists (ACGIH) Threshold Limit Values (TLVs), as set forth in Table 27–1. For a few solvents, significant absorption of vapors through the skin can also occur. This is most likely to occur when solvents with a "skin" designation and low TLV are used in a situation that results in very high airborne concentrations, such as in an enclosed space with respiratory protection.

Distribution

Since organic solvents are lipophilic, they tend to be distributed to lipid-rich tissue. In addition to adipose tissue, this includes the nervous system and liver. Since distribution occurs via the blood and since the blood-tissue membrane barriers are usually rich in lipids, solvents are also distributed to organs with large blood flows, such as cardiac and skeletal muscle. Persons with greater amounts of adipose tissue will accumulate greater amounts of a solvent over time and consequently will excrete larger amounts at a slower rate after cessation of exposure. Most solvents will cross the placenta and also enter breast milk.

Metabolism

Some solvents are extensively metabolized and some not at all. The metabolism of a number of solvents plays a key role in their toxicity and in some cases the treatment of intoxication. The role of toxic metabolites is discussed in their respective sections for n-hexane, methyl n-butyl ketone, methyl alcohol, ethylene glycol, diethylene glycol, methyl acetate, methyl formate, and glycol ethers. A number of solvents, including trichloroethylene, are metabolized in common with ethyl alcohol (ethanol) by alcohol and aldehyde dehydrogenase. Competition for these limited enzymes accounts for synergistic effects ("alcohol intolerance" and "degreaser's flush") and may result in reactions in workers exposed to these solvents while taking disulfiram (Antabuse) for alcoholism. Chronic ethanol ingestion may induce solvent-metabolizing enzymes and lower blood solvent concentrations. Other solvents may have acute and chronic interactions similar to those of ethanol.

Excretion

Excretion of solvents occurs primarily through exhalation of unchanged compound, elimination of metabolites in urine, or a combination of each. Solvents such as perchloroethylene that are poorly metabolized are excreted primarily through exhalation. The biologic half-life of parent compounds varies from a few minutes to several days, so that some solvents accumulate to some degree over the course of the work week while others do not. However, bioaccumulation beyond a few days is not an important determinant of adverse health effects for most solvents.

BIOLOGIC MONITORING

Biologic monitoring can provide a more accurate measure of exposure than environmental monitoring for some solvents (see Table 27–1 and Chapter 34). This is particularly true for substances whose pulmonary absorption is affected to a large degree by physical work and those with significant dermal exposure and absorption, ie, those with ACGIH "skin" designations (Table 27–1). Unfortunately, solvents have properties that tend to make biologic monitoring less useful or practical: (1) They tend to be rapidly absorbed and excreted, so that biologic levels change rapidly over time; and (2) exposure over very short intervals is often a more important determinant of adverse health effects than 8-hour or longer exposures. However, biologic monitoring has been investigated for a number of solvents. The ACGIH has recommended Biological Exposure Indices (BEIs) for the following solvents: n-hexane, benzene, toluene, xylenes, ethyl benzene, styrene, phenol, methyl ethyl ketone, perchloroethylene, trichloroethane (methyl chloroform), trichloroethylene, dimethylformamide, and carbon disulfide. For many solvents, significant levels may be present only in exhaled air, which is currently cumbersome to sample. A number of laboratories offer whole blood or plasma analysis of solvents. For solvents with relatively slow excretion, such as perchloroethylene and methyl chloroform, analysis of blood is a reasonable alternative to exhaled air. However, for those with relatively fast excretion (most of the rest), the timing of the sample is critical—even within minutes—and the results are therefore difficult to interpret. Most solvents distribute into several compartments in the body, so that the decline in blood levels exhibits several consecutive half-times, with the first being very short, on the order of 2–10 minutes. A blood sample taken immediately after an exposure will reflect primarily peak exposure at that time. A sample taken 15–30 minutes after termination of exposure will reflect exposure over the preceding few hours, while a sample taken 16–20 hours after exposure (prior to the next shift) will reflect mean exposure over the preceding day. The distribution of exposure over an 8-hour shift will also affect the validity of the biologic sample.

HEALTH EFFECTS OF SOLVENTS

SKIN DISORDERS

Up to 20% of cases of occupational dermatitis are caused by solvents (see Chapter 17). Almost all organic solvents are primary skin irritants as a result of defatting, or the dissolution of lipids from the skin. The potency of solvents for defatting the skin is related directly to lipid solubility and inversely to percutaneous absorptivity and volatility. In addition to concentration and duration of exposure, a critical factor in the development of solvent dermatitis is occlusion of the exposed area of skin, such as by clothes and leaking protective clothing. A few industrial solvents can also cause allergic contact dermatitis.

The most common work practice leading to solvent dermatitis is washing the hands with solvents. The occupations most commonly associated with solvent dermatitis are painting, printing, mechanics, and dry cleaning, though workers are at risk wherever solvents are used.

Clinical Findings

A. Symptoms and Signs: Diagnosis is based on the typical appearance of the skin and a history of direct contact with solvents. The typical appearance ranges from an acute irritant dermatitis manifested by erythema and edema to a chronic dry, cracked eczema. Areas of skin affected by solvent dermatitis are more permeable to chemicals than unaffected skin and are susceptible to secondary bacterial infection.

B. Laboratory Findings: Patch testing is rarely indicated since few solvents (principally turpentine and formaldehyde) cause allergic contact dermatitis. Patch testing with actual material used in the workplace may be necessary on occasion.

Differential Diagnosis

Consideration must sometimes be given to the possibility of other sources of irritant or allergic contact dermatitis. Use of waterless hand cleansers that contain alcohols and emollients that contain sensitizers may exacerbate or cause irritant or allergic dermatitis.

Treatment & Prevention

Treatment of dermatitis due to solvents is the same as for contact dermatitis from other causes: topical corticosteroids, emollients, and skin care. Prevention depends upon education of workers about proper handling of solvents, use of engineering controls to minimize direct contact with solvents, provisions for alternatives to washing with solvents, and the use of solvent-resistant barrier creams or protective clothing where appropriate.

Prognosis

The resolution of solvent dermatitis depends on elimination of direct solvent contact with involved areas of skin.

CENTRAL NERVOUS SYSTEM EFFECTS

1. ACUTE CENTRAL NERVOUS SYSTEM EFFECTS

Almost all volatile lipid-soluble organic chemicals cause general, nonspecific depression of the central nervous system, or general anesthesia. Beginning with ethyl ether, a number of industrial solvents were used historically as surgical anesthetics. There is good correlation between lipid solubility, as measured by the air:olive oil partition coefficient, and anesthetic potency. However, the mechanism of action of general anesthesia by any agent is not known. Excitable tissue is depressed at all levels of the central nervous system, both brain and spinal cord. Lipid solubility—and therefore anesthetic potency—increases with length of carbon chain, substitution with halogen or alcohol, and the presence of unsaturated (double) carbon bonds.

Clinical Findings

A. Symptoms and Signs: The symptoms of central nervous system depression from acute intoxication by organic solvents are the same as those from drinking alcoholic beverages. Indeed, there is currently no evidence that ethyl alcohol has any acute effects on the central nervous system other than general anesthesia. Symptoms range from headache, nausea and vomiting, dizziness, light-headedness, vertigo, disequilibrium, slurred speech, euphoria, fatigue, sleepiness, weakness, irritability, nervousness, depression, disorientation, and confusion to loss of consciousness and death from respiratory depression. A secondary hazard from these effects is increased risk of accidents. Excitatory manifestations of early intoxication are the result of depression of inhibitory functions and correspond to stage I anesthesia.

The acute effects are related to the concentration of the chemical in the nervous system, so resolution of symptoms correlates with the biologic half-life, which ranges from a few minutes to less than 24 hours for most industrial solvents. However, it must be kept in mind that many solvent exposures are to mixtures of solvents and that the effects of each solvent are at least additive and may be synergistic.

Tolerance to the acute effects can occur, particularly for those compounds with longer half-lives, and is generally not metabolic in nature (ie, not due to increased rates of metabolism and excretion). The development of tolerance may be accompanied by morning "hangovers" and even frank withdrawal symptoms on weekends and vacations, alleviated by ingestion of alcohol. Additive and synergistic effects have both been described for interactions between organic solvents and with drinking alcohol.

B. Laboratory Findings: Biologic monitoring may provide an accurate assessment of exposure to some solvents, but there is little information on the correlation of biologic levels with degrees of intoxication.

Differential Diagnosis

Acute solvent intoxication must be distinguished from that resulting from the use of alcohol or psychoactive drugs on the basis of exposure.

Treatment

The sole treatment for acute solvent intoxication is removal from exposure to solvents or any other anesthetic or central nervous system depressant until the signs and symptoms have completely resolved. The use of alcohol or other central nervous system depressant medication should be avoided. Analgesics for headache may be necessary, but nonnarcotic medication is usually adequate.

Prognosis

Most symptoms resolve in a time course parallel to the elimination of the solvent and any active metabolites, though headaches may persist for up to a week or more following acute exposure. Persistence of central nervous system dysfunction following severe overexposure with coma suggests hypoxic brain damage. The occurrence of persistent neurobehavioral dysfunction following acute overexposure has been reported anecdotally and in a few case series, particularly impairment of memory.

2. CHRONIC CENTRAL NERVOUS SYSTEM EFFECTS

Alcohol is now well recognized as causing neurobehavioral dysfunction in chronic alcoholics. It is reasonable to assume that sufficient chronic exposure to organic solvents could also cause chronic adverse neurobehavioral effects. A variety of terms have been applied to these effects when associated with solvent exposure: chronic toxic encephalopathy, presenile dementia, chronic solvent intoxication, painter's syndrome, psychoaffective disorder, and neurasthenic syndrome.

A number of epidemiologic studies of workers chronically exposed to organic solvents have demonstrated an increased incidence of adverse neurobehavioral effects. These effects have been best demonstrated in groups of workers with relatively high exposures, such as boat builders and spray painters, and with specific types of exposure, such as to carbon disulfide (see Chapter 26). Such effects include subjective symptoms, changes in personality or mood, and impaired intellectual function as assessed by batteries of neurobehavioral tests. The nature of these tests and uncertainty about the significance of the results are discussed in Chapter 22. Dose-response data and correlation of chronic with acute effects are generally lacking. Correlation of symptoms with test results is often lacking, so that the interpretation of neurobehavioral test results in an individual must be made with caution.

Chronic brain damage from chronic alcoholism or drug abuse is not well understood, but similar mechanisms may be present with chronic solvent exposure. Cortical atrophy may represent the underlying pathologic changes.

In addition to neuropsychologic dysfunction, there are other potential chronic central neurotoxic effects of solvents that can be considered briefly here. Acute and perhaps chronic intoxication with solvents can result in vestibulo-oculomotor disturbances presumably due to effects on the cerebellum. A syndrome called acquired intolerance to organic solvents in which dizziness, nausea, and weakness after exposure to minimal solvent vapor concentrations with normal vestibular test results was recently reported.

Clinical Findings

Symptoms commonly reported are headache, mood disturbance (depression, anxiety), fatigue, memory loss (primarily short-term), and difficulty in concentrating. Clinical examination may reveal signs of impairment in recent memory, attention span, and motor or sensory function.

Diagnosis

Test results that have been associated with solvent exposure in group studies include alteration of a variety of neurobehavioral tests; pneumoencephalography, CT scan, and cerebral blood flow studies showing evidence of diffuse cerebral cortical atrophy; and electroencephalographic abnormalities, particularly diffuse low wave patterns. These tests should not be used in the evaluation of individual patients without incorporating information from other sources.

Juntunen (1984) has proposed the following diagnostic criteria for chronic neurobehavioral toxicity from solvents:

A. Verified quantitative and qualitative exposure to organic chemicals which are known to be neurotoxic.
B. Clinical picture of organic central nervous system damage.
   1. Typical subjective symptoms.
   2. Pathologic findings in some of the following:
      a. Clinical neurologic status.
      b. Electroencephalography.
      c. Psychologic tests.
C. Other organic diseases reasonably well excluded.
D. Primary psychiatric diseases reasonably well excluded.

Differential Diagnosis

Primary psychiatric disease may be excluded by the presence of signs of organic brain dysfunction, but these signs are not always entirely objective or clear-cut. Drug or alcohol abuse may result in a clinical state identical to chronic solvent toxicity, distinguished only by history and other evidence of exposure. Diffuse organic brain disease—particularly Alzheimer's disease—must also be considered.

Treatment

Removal from exposure is recommended in all suspected cases. Alcohol and other central nervous system depressants should be avoided.

Depression may respond to antidepressants or other measures. Other neuropsychologic symptoms may respond to psychologic counseling. Treatment of chronic solvent-induced headaches involves empiric trials of medications, psychologic counseling, and biofeedback therapy.

Prognosis

The data on recovery from chronic solvent intoxication are contradictory and controversial. In one study, about half of affected workers tended to improve over 3–9 years of follow-up, but neuropsychologic testing results tended to worsen more than would be expected. A 5-year follow-up of 21 Danish painters diagnosed as having chronic toxic encephalopathy demonstrated considerable social consequences, with 10 unable to obtain or hold other jobs.

EFFECTS ON PERIPHERAL NERVOUS SYSTEM & CRANIAL NERVES

All organic solvents may be capable of causing or contributing to peripheral neuropathies (see also Chapter 22). However, only a few are specifically toxic to the peripheral nervous system, including carbon disulfide and the hexacarbons n-hexane and methyl n-butyl ketone. These 3 cause a symmetric, ascending, mixed sensorimotor neuropathy of the distal axonopathy type that can be replicated in animals. This may be referred to as a central-peripheral distal axonopathy, since the nerves in the spinal canal are also affected. Of the 3 substances, only n-hexane is currently in general use as an industrial solvent. Most industrial hexane is a mixture of isomers, and reports of neuropathy from hexane use are rare in the United States and more common in Italy and Japan, where cottage industries result in higher exposures. Methyl ethyl ketone, a common solvent, potentiates the neurotoxicity of the hexacarbons (n-hexane, methyl n-butyl ketone).

Trichloroethylene has been associated with isolated trigeminal nerve anesthesia. Other organic solvents have been associated with peripheral neurotoxicity in case reports of occupational exposure, following exposure to mixtures of solvents, or in persons exposed to extremely high levels from deliberate ''sniffing'' of solvents. Limited epidemiologic evidence and case reports of solvent abusers have associated solvent exposure with sensorineural hearing loss. Toluene caused high-frequency hearing loss in rats at levels above 1000 ppm. The effects of solvents on auditory nerve function merit additional study in the future. Toluene causes vestibular dysfunction in abusers, but whether this is specific for toluene is unclear.

An increased incidence of color vision disturbances was recently reported in solvent-exposed painters, with evidence to suggest a central rather than peripheral site of damage. Disturbances of olfactory function (hyposmia, parosmia) have been reported in cases of solvent-exposed individuals and anecdotally in a high percentage of long-term painters. Effects on olfaction could be due to local destruction of olfactory nerve endings in the nasal mucosa or to action at a central site.

Clinical Findings

Typical symptoms of solvent-induced neuropathy are slowly ascending numbness, paresthesias, and weakness. Pain and muscle cramps are occasionally present. Physical findings include diminished sensation and strength in a symmetric pattern and, in most cases, depressed distal reflexes. Trigeminal neuropathy from trichloroethylene is restricted to loss of sensory function in the distribution of the trigeminal nerve.

Diagnosis

The diagnosis of solvent-induced neuropathy is based on a history of illness and exposure, clinical examination, and neurophysiologic testing, as described in Chapter 22. Nerve conduction velocities may be normal or slightly depressed. Sensory conduction velocities and sensory action potential amplitude are the most sensitive. Electromyography may indicate denervation (fibrillations and positive sharp waves). The use of evoked potentials (visual and somatosensory) shows promise. Symptoms and other clinical findings are often found with absent or slight neurophysiologic abnormalities. A sural nerve biopsy may be helpful, and in the case of hexacarbons show accumulation of neurofilaments in the terminal axon.

Neurophysiologic testing may be helpful in screening large numbers of workers, but has not been shown to be more sensitive in early detection of clinical neuropathy than clinical examinations—though periodic monitoring of n-hexane-exposed workers with nerve conduction velocity testing has been recommended.

Odor threshold testing and other tests of olfactory function should be performed in individuals with complaints of disturbances in either smell or taste.

Differential Diagnosis

The primary differential for peripheral neuropathy is diabetes, alcoholism, drugs, familial neuropathies, and renal failure. About 25–50% of cases of peripheral neuropathy remain without etiologic diagnoses after initial evaluation excludes these causes. A chemical-related cause should be considered in all such cases.

Treatment

Treatment consists of removal of exposure to all substances toxic to the peripheral nervous system, including alcoholic beverages. Physical therapy should be encouraged for patients with weakness; this increases muscular strength to counteract loss of neuromuscular function, improves psychologic outlook, and may even improve the ability of nerves to regenerate effectively.

Careful clinical monitoring of workers exposed to substances toxic to the peripheral nervous system is important for early detection and prevention of permanent disability.

Prognosis

Symptoms may worsen initially and then improve for up to 1 year or more. The rate of recovery is related to the rate of axonal regeneration, which is approximately 1 mm/d. An axon from the tip of the toe that has died back to the cell body in the spinal cord may take a year to recover. The degree of residual disability, if any, is usually proportionate to the degree of injury at the time of diagnosis and cessation of exposure. However, permanent disability should not be judged until at least 1 year after diagnosis.

RESPIRATORY SYSTEM

All organic solvents irritate the respiratory tract to some degree. Irritation is a consequence of the defatting action of solvents, and so the same structure-activity relationships hold true for the respiratory tract as for the skin. Addition of functional groups to the hydrocarbon molecule may also increase the potency of the solvent as an irritant, as in the case of organic amine bases and organic acids, which are corrosives; and alcohols, ketones, and aldehydes, which denature proteins at high concentrations.

Respiratory tract irritation from solvents is usually confined to the upper airways, including the nose and sinuses. Solvents that are both highly soluble and potent irritants, such as formaldehyde, cannot reach the lower respiratory tract without intolerable irritation of the upper tract. However, it is possible for less potent irritants to reach the alveoli in sufficient concentrations following extremely high overexposures, such as in spills and in confined spaces, to cause acute pulmonary edema. Severe central nervous system depression is usually also a result of such exposure. Pulmonary edema without effects on the nervous system can result from exposure to phosgene gas produced by the extreme heating (as in welding) of chlorinated hydrocarbon solvents.

There are few studies of chronic pulmonary effects from exposure to organic solvents. Chronic bronchitis may occur as a result of long-term exposure to the more potent irritant compounds, such as the aldehydes.

Clinical Findings

A. Symptoms and Signs: Irritation of the upper respiratory tract is marked by sore nose and throat, cough, and possibly chest pain. If the eyes are not protected by vapor goggles, irritation of the eyes possibly accompanied by tearing may also occur. A few solvents are specific lacrimators, and induce pronounced tearing such that exposure may be sufficient to preclude inhalation and irritation of the respiratory tract. A productive cough indicates chemical bronchitis or the imposition of an infectious bronchitis. Manifestations of pulmonary edema include a productive cough, dyspnea, cyanosis, and rales.

B. Laboratory Findings: Upper airway irritation should not be associated with any laboratory abnormalities. Pulmonary edema is marked by infiltrates on chest x-ray, hypoxia and perhaps hypocapnia on arterial blood gas analysis, and impaired diffusion as shown by pulmonary function tests.

Differential Diagnosis

Infectious bronchitis may be distinguished from chemical bronchitis by sputum analysis and possibly sputum culture, although chemical bronchitis may be followed by a superimposed infection. Solvent-induced pulmonary edema must be distinguished from infectious or aspiration pneumonitis.

Treatment

Management of the acute pulmonary effects of solvents is the same as for any acute pulmonary irritant: administration of oxygen, bronchodilators, and other respiratory support as indicated.

Prognosis

Upper respiratory tract irritation should resolve quickly without sequelae in the absence of infection. Once treated appropriately, patients with acute pulmonary edema from solvent overexposure should recover completely if protected from the effects of hypoxic tissue damage.

EFFECTS ON THE HEART

The principal effect of organic solvents on the heart is "cardiac sensitization"—a state of increased myocardial sensitivity to the arrhythmogenic effects of epinephrine (see also Chapter 19). It can be demonstrated in animals—typically unanesthetized beagle dogs—by administration of epinephrine, either in fixed or multiple doses, before and after administration of a solvent and observation of the frequency of epinephrine-induced ventricular arrhythmias. Cases of sudden, otherwise unexplained death during abuse of solvents such as toluene in glue and trichloroethane in spot remover, usually associated with physical activity ("sudden sniffing deaths"), and occasional reports of sudden death in otherwise healthy workers overexposed to industrial solvents are probably due to cardiac sensitization.

From animal studies it appears that high—near-anesthetic or anesthetic—levels are required for this effect on an otherwise healthy heart and that all organic solvents may be capable of causing it, though potencies vary. Halogenated hydrocarbons, particularly 1,1,1-trichloroethane, trichloroethylene, and trichlorotrifluoroethane, were of higher potency in the dog, with thresholds to a particular dose of epinephrine at 0.5% (5000 ppm) of solvent vapors for 5 minutes, compared to approximately 5% (50,000 ppm) for heptane, hexane, toluene, and xylene; 10% (100,000 ppm) for propane; and 20% (20,000 ppm) for ethyl ether. Thresholds for these effects in humans, particularly with any condition predisposing to arrhythmias, are unknown.

Clinical Findings

A. Symptoms and Signs: Cardiac sensitization should be considered when a worker exposed to high concentrations of a solvent reports dizziness, palpitations, faintness, or loss of consciousness in conjunction with or in the absence of symptoms of central nervous system depression (see above). If the victim is examined promptly, an irregular pulse or low blood pressure may be detected.

B. Laboratory Findings: A resting ECG may be normal or abnormal and is rarely diagnostic. For workers with symptoms suggestive of cardiac sensitization, ambulatory cardiac monitoring during exposure may be helpful.

Differential Diagnosis

In the presence of high levels of exposure, the distinction between central nervous system depression alone and depression plus cardiac sensitization is difficult—and may not be important if all symptoms resolve with correction of overexposure. The need for evaluation for primary cardiac disease must be made on a case-by-case basis. The presence of cardiac disease does not preclude the possibility of solvent-related arrhythmias, which may occur at levels of solvent exposure lower than those usually associated with cardiac sensitization.

Treatment

Given the high levels of exposure usually associated with cardiac sensitization, evaluation and appropriate correction of exposure are essential. If arrhythmias appear to be related to exposure and the exposure is not excessive or cannot be controlled adequately, removal from exposure is preferable to treatment with antiarrhythmic medication and continued exposure.

Prognosis

Cases due solely to excessive exposure should resolve with correction of the workplace situation.

EFFECT ON THE LIVER

Although it is possible that any organic solvent may cause hepatocellular damage in sufficient doses for a sufficient duration, some solvents, particularly those substituted with halogen or nitro groups, are particularly hepatotoxic. Others, such as the aliphatic hydrocarbons (cycloparaffins, ethers, esters, aldehydes, and ketones), are only weakly if at all hepatotoxic. The aromatic hydrocarbons (benzene, toluene, and xylene) appear to be weakly hepatotoxic, with only a few reports of possible liver toxicity in exposed workers. A few solvents such as acetone with little direct hepatotoxicity themselves have been reported to potentiate the effects of alcohol on the liver.

Acute hepatic injury was frequently reported in the past from acute overexposure to carbon tetrachloride. More recently, acute hepatic necrosis and death from liver failure have been reported from exposure to 2-nitropropane used as a solvent in specialty paint products. Subacute liver disease has been rarely reported in modern times, while chronic liver disease including cirrhosis has been occasionally reported in workers exposed to carbon tetrachloride.

Clinical Findings

A. Symptoms and Signs: Liver injury may be symptomless or associated with right upper quadrant pain, nausea, and vomiting. Hepatic tenderness, jaundice, dark urine, and light stool may be present.

B. Laboratory Findings: Diagnosis of acute hepatic injury is based on the presence of abnormal liver function tests in a pattern consistent with hepatocellular dysfunction and a history consistent with exposure to a hepatotoxic solvent in the absence of exposure to any other known hepatotoxin. A pattern of liver enzyme abnormality different from alcohol hepatitis has been reported anecdotally for a few solvents. Serum bilirubin may be elevated. Evaluation of liver injury due to occupational exposure to solvents has been hampered by the lack of sensitivity and specificity of liver function tests and their often high incidence of abnormalities in working populations. The use of serum bile acid measurements has been proposed as a sensitive screening method for solvent-related liver dysfunction. Occasionally, liver biopsy may be necessary to distinguish solvent-induced hepatitis from chronic active hepatitis. Routine monitoring of liver function tests is not recommended unless there is potential exposure to a hepatotoxic dose of a solvent. Monitoring a patient after abstinence from alcohol may be necessary to evaluate the possible role of drinking. Removal of exposure with monitoring of liver function tests may be helpful in making a diagnosis.

Differential Diagnosis

The major entity that must be differentiated is alcohol-induced liver injury; if excessive use of alcohol cannot be ruled out, a diagnosis of solvent-induced liver injury often cannot be made with confidence. Viral and other infectious forms of hepatitis must also be considered.

Treatment

Treatment consists of removal from exposure and correction of any workplace situation that can be identified as having caused or contributed to the condition.

EFFECT ON THE KIDNEYS

Although many organic solvents, particularly halogenated aliphatic hydrocarbons, show evidence of nephrotoxicity to animals in relatively high doses, there are few reports of renal effects in exposed workers—perhaps in part due to the lack of sensitivity and specificity of renal function tests. Acute renal failure from acute tubular necrosis has been observed in workers with acute intoxication from halogenated hydrocarbons such as carbon tetrachloride. Animal studies indicate that halogenated aliphatic hydrocarbons damage primarily the proximal renal tubular cells. Renal tubular dysfunction—particularly renal tubular acidosis of the distal type—has been reported in solvent abusers using mainly toluene but has not been associated with occupational exposure. Acute renal failure from intrarenal deposition of oxalic acid can result from ingestion of ethylene glycol but has not been reported from other routes of exposure.

There are few studies of chronic renal effects in solvent-exposed workers. One cross-sectional study suggested that chronic exposure to a number of solvents or solvent mixtures may result in mild tubular dysfunction evidenced by proteinuria, and enzymuria (increased excretion of muramidase and β-glucuronidase). Another cross-sectional study found increases in urinary excretion of N-acetyl-β-glucosaminidase but normal urinalyses in some workers exposed to a variety of solvents. Case-control studies have suggested an association between solvent exposure and primary glomerulonephritis, particularly rapidly progressive glomerulonephritis associated with anti-glomerular basement membrane antibodies (the renal component of Goodpasture's syndrome).

Clinical Findings

A. Symptoms and Signs: Solvent abusers with renal tubular acidosis have presented with weakness and fatigue, probably as a result of electrolyte abnormalities. Signs of acute intoxication (central nervous system depression) have often been present. If it occurs, chronic renal tubular dysfunction as a result of chronic solvent exposure would usually be subclinical.

B. Laboratory Findings: Renal tubular dysfunction from solvents may be manifested by polyuria, glycosuria, proteinuria, acidosis, and electrolyte disorders. Hypokalemia, hypophosphatemia, hyperchloremia, and hypocarbonatemia have been seen as manifestations of renal tubular acidosis in toluene abusers. Acute renal failure from halogenated solvents is similar to that from any other cause. Routine monitoring of renal function is not generally recommended for workers exposed to solvents. However, the measurement of urinary excretion of low-molecular-weight enzymes such as N-acetyl-β-glucosaminidase, β-glucuronidase, and muramidase appears to offer promise as a monitor for evidence of early tubular dysfunction.

Differential Diagnosis

Renal tubular dysfunction, including acidosis, can be a primary disease that first manifests itself in early adulthood or may occur secondary to a variety of metabolic and hyperglobulinemic states and exposure to toxic agents, including antibiotics and heavy metals.

Treatment

If renal tubular dysfunction is found in a worker with a high level of exposure to a solvent, observation of renal tubular function during cessation and then reinstitution of exposure may be helpful in both establishing a diagnosis and in determining the effectiveness of removal from exposure.

EFFECTS ON BLOOD

Hematologic effects from solvents are not common. Benzene causes a dose-related aplastic anemia after months to years of exposure that may be a precursor to leukemia. Chlorinated hydrocarbons have been associated with a number of reported cases of aplastic anemia, which may be idiosyncratic or simply a spurious association. Some glycol ethers can cause either a hemolytic anemia due to increased osmotic fragility or hypoplastic anemia due to bone marrow depression.

Clinical Findings

A. Symptoms and Signs: Workers with anemia from solvents have generally presented with weakness and fatigue. Aplastic anemia can present with bleeding from thrombocytopenia or infections due to neutropenia.

B. Laboratory Findings: Aplastic anemia from benzene may be manifested by reductions in any or all of the 3 cell lines, which may occur suddenly without preceding changes. The bone marrow may be hyperplastic or hypoplastic and does not always correlate with abnormalities in the peripheral blood. Hemolytic anemia from glycol ethers or other hemolytic agents is indicated by low red blood cell concentration and reticulocytosis. Monitoring of blood counts is recommended only for exposure to benzene and perhaps for the hematotoxic glycol ethers, but the results may not be predictive of anemia even for these agents.

Differential Diagnosis

The usual causes of anemia, particularly hypoplastic anemia, must be considered.

Treatment

The treatment of solvent-induced anemia is removal from exposure, transfusion if needed, and correction of the workplace situation if appropriate. Workers with aplastic anemia from benzene should not be reexposed to benzene.

Prognosis

A significant percentage of workers with aplastic anemia from benzene will subsequently develop leukemia, which is frequently fatal. Other solvent-induced hematologic effects should resolve with cessation of exposure.

CANCER POTENTIAL

Benzene is the only commonly used solvent for which there is sufficient evidence of carcinogenicity in humans. It has been associated with all types of acute and chronic leukemia. Investigation of many of the halogenated hydrocarbons has produced limited to sufficient evidence of carcinogenicity in animals, particularly hepatocellular carcinomas in mice. Most have not been adequately studied in humans.

EFFECTS ON REPRODUCTIVE SYSTEM

Most organic solvents easily cross the lipid barrier of the placenta and, to a lesser degree, the testes. There is concern for their potential to cause reproductive toxicity. Few studies have been conducted in humans. One case-control study suggested an association between maternal exposure to organic solvents and central nervous system birth defects. Other studies have indicated adverse reproductive outcomes in workers such as female chemists but have not been able to identify specific exposures as causal.

With the exception of the glycol ethers and ethyl alcohol, available animal studies have generally not revealed evidence of significant teratogenicity. Ethyl alcohol causes both structural and behavioral teratogenic effects (fetal alcohol syndrome) in both animals and women drinking over 3–4 glasses of alcoholic beverages per day. Controversy exists over whether pregnant women should be advised not to drink alcoholic beverages at all during pregnancy. Since all organic solvents readily cross the placenta and reach the fetal nervous system and affect the nervous system in similar ways to alcohol, the possibility of a "fetal solvent syndrome" has been discussed. Standard teratogenicity studies would not necessarily reveal such effects, and behavioral teratogenicity studies in animals have been performed only to a limited extent. If a "fetal solvent syndrome" exists, important questions about dose-response relationships need to be addressed. For instance, what would the relationship be between effects on the mother and on the offspring? Would effects occur in offspring only at levels that produced acute intoxication in the mother, or at lower levels? And are short, high exposures worse than lower, longer exposures?

Decisions regarding exposure of pregnant workers to solvents must currently be made in the absence of definitive toxicologic data (see Chapter 23). Many solvents show evidence of fetotoxicity in animals at or near maternally toxic levels. Exposure that produces acute reversible effects on the mature maternal nervous system may produce irreversible effects on the developing fetal nervous system. Therefore, it is prudent to ensure that women who may be pregnant not be overexposed to any organic solvent. In addition, because of distribution to a possibly vulnerable fetal nervous system and the possibility of behavioral teratogenicity, exposure to organic solvents should be kept as low as possible throughout pregnancy.

There is potential for solvent exposure to males to affect reproduction directly by affecting male reproductive capacity or indirectly via damaged sperm, but no definitive data have been accumulated in humans (see Chapter 24).

PREVENTION OF SOLVENT TOXICITY

SELECTION & SUBSTITUTION OF SOLVENT

Selection of an initial solvent—or substitution of a less hazardous for a more hazardous solvent—must take into account both the desirable and undesirable properties of the solvents. This involves not only comparing toxicity but also volatility, flammability, explosiveness, reactivity, compatibility, stability, odor properties, and environmental fates. For example, carbon tetrachloride, perchloroethylene, trichlorotrifluoroethane, and mineral spirits are all used to some extent at the present time as dry-cleaning agents, though to different degrees than in the past. Carbon tetrachloride is by far the most toxic and for that reason is used chiefly as a spot removal agent. Perchloroethylene is less toxic than carbon tetrachloride and has replaced it for that reason. Perchloroethylene replaced mineral spirits because of the flammability of the latter; perchloroethylene and carbon tetrachloride are virtually nonflammable. However, perchloroethylene is moderately toxic and was recently found to be carcinogenic in laboratory animals. Trichlorotrifluoroethane is the least toxic, but it is expensive and may contribute to depletion of the ozone layer. It is used in closed systems to decrease cost and environmental pollution by recycling, but this requires an initial capital outlay for equipment.

Obviously, the choice of solvent is complicated when advantages and disadvantages exist in different categories.

ENGINEERING CONTROLS

The volatility of organic solvents makes engineering ingenuity to control vapors of paramount importance in many situations. Process enclosure, such as the closed system use of trichlorotrifluoroethane for dry cleaning, is common in chemical manufacturing but not in other circumstances. Spray painting and other spray operations create aerosols and vapors, so that engineering controls are particularly critical and may not be sufficient to reduce exposure adequately. The substitution of water-based for solvent-based paints has been the most effective means of reducing solvent exposure from painting. Auto body repair represents the last major use of solvent-based paints that has not been replaced with water-based paints.

PERSONAL PROTECTION

Respiratory protection should be used only when appropriate and as part of a comprehensive respiratory protection program conducted by the employer. The improper use of respirators by self-employed workers when using solvents is a major problem. Knowledge of the odor threshold of a substance (Table 27–1) is necessary before using a respirator for levels above the TLV for that substance. If the average odor threshold is well below the TLV—eg, at least 10-fold—the odor will serve as an adequate warning to signal breakthrough or other failure of the respirator to provide adequate protection. A decrease in the ability to detect odors (hyposmia) has been reported from chronic exposure to solvents, and a history of hyposmia should be sought as part of the initial medical evaluation for ability to use a respirator.

Protective clothing made of the proper material should be selected on the basis of studies that show the rate of penetration of materials by the solvent used. *Guidelines for the Selection of Chemical Protective Clothing*, published by ACGIH, is a good source of this information. Protective (barrier) creams can correct or prevent loss of oils from the skin and may provide some protection against percutaneous absorption of solvents.

Some workers, such as mechanics, may be unable to use gloves and adequately perform their work. Barrier creams are not recommended as substitutes for gloves.

SPECIFIC SOLVENTS & THEIR EFFECTS

ALIPHATIC HYDROCARBONS
Essentials of Diagnosis
Acute effects:
● Anesthesia: dizziness, headache, nausea, vomit-

ing, sleepiness, fatigue, "drunkenness," slurred speech, disequilibrium, disorientation, depression, loss of consciousness.
- Respiratory tract irritation: sore nose, throat, cough.

Chronic effects:
- Dermatitis: dry, cracked, erythematous skin.
- Neurobehavioral dysfunction: headache, mood lability, fatigue, short-term memory loss, difficulty concentrating; decreased attention span, neurobehavioral test abnormalities, CT scan (cerebral atrophy), EEG (diffuse slow waves).
- Peripheral neuropathy (n-hexane): slowly ascending numbness, paresthesias, weakness; normal or slightly depressed nerve conduction velocity, electromyography (denervation).

General Considerations

Aliphatic hydrocarbons consist of carbon and hydrogen molecules in straight or branched chains. They are further divided into alkanes, alkenes, and alkynes.

1. ALKANES (PARAFFINS)

Alkanes are aliphatic hydrocarbons with single-bonded (saturated) carbons:

$$
\begin{array}{ccc}
\text{H} & \text{H} & \text{H} \\
| & | & | \\
-\text{C}- & \text{C}- & \text{C}- \\
| & | & | \\
\text{H} & \text{H} & \text{H}
\end{array}
$$

with the empirical formula C_nH_{2n+2}

The physical state of an alkane depends on its number of carbons:

Carbons	State	Name
1–4	Gas	Methane, ethane, propane, butane
5–16	Liquid	Pentane, hexane, heptane, octane, nonane. . .
> 16	Solid	Paraffin wax

The gases are essentially odorless, while the vapors of the liquids have a slight "hydrocarbon" odor.

Use

A number of liquid alkanes are used in relatively pure form as solvents and also are the major constituents of a number of petroleum distillate solvents (see below). The liquid alkanes are important ingredients in gasoline, which accounts for most of the pentane and hexane used in the USA. Hexane is an inexpensive general use solvent in solvent glues, quick-drying rubber cements, varnishes, inks, and extraction of oils from seeds. The alkane gases are used as fuels, while paraffin wax is used for candles and other wax products.

Occupational & Environmental Exposure

NIOSH estimates that approximately 10,000 US workers are potentially exposed to pentane and heptane, 300,000 to octane, and 2.5 million to hexane annually. Many more individuals may be exposed to these and other alkanes in gasoline and other petroleum products. They are common contaminants of ambient air, with levels of methane reported from 1.2–1.5 ppm in rural areas and 2–3 ppm in urban air, while other alkanes are generally detected at more than 10-fold lower concentrations.

Pharmacokinetics

The alkanes are well absorbed by inhalation and to a lesser but still significant extent through the skin. None have skin TLV designations. Approximately 75% of most inhaled alkanes will be absorbed at rest, decreasing to 50% with moderate physical labor. Unbranched hydrocarbons such as n-hexane and n-heptane are metabolized by microsomal cytochrome P-450 enzymes to alcohols, diols, ketones, and diketones, which are further metabolized to carbon monoxide or conjugated with glucuronic acid and excreted in urine.

Health Effects

The alkanes are generally of low toxicity. The first 3 gases (methane, ethane, and propane) are simple inert asphyxiants whose toxicity is related only to the amount of available oxygen remaining in the environment and to their flammability and explosiveness. The vapors of the lighter, more volatile liquids, pentane through nonane, are irritants and anesthetics, while the heavier liquids, known as liquid paraffins, are primarily defatting agents. Hexane and heptane are most commonly used as general purpose solvents. They cause anesthesia, respiratory tract irritation, and dermatitis and are associated with neurobehavioral dysfunction; and the associated clinical findings, differential diagnosis, treatment, and prognosis are not different from those of other solvents (see above).

One isomer of hexane, n-hexane, causes peripheral neuropathy. A number of outbreaks of peripheral neuropathy have been described, particularly in cottage industries such as shoe and sandal making, where glues have been used containing n-hexane as a solvent. The proximate neurotoxin is the metabolite 2,5-hexanedione. Other diketones with the same spacing between ketone (carbonyl) groups, such as 3,6-hexanedione, can also cause peripheral neuropathy. A metabolite of n-heptane, 2,5-heptanedione, causes peripheral neuropathy in laboratory animal studies, but n-heptane has not been implicated in human peripheral neuropathy in the absence of concomitant exposure to n-hexane. The clinical and neurophysiologic findings of n-hexane-induced peripheral neuropathy is typical of distal axonopathies (see above and Chapter 22). Nerve biopsies are notable for swollen axons that contain increased numbers of neurofilaments. Methyl ethyl ketone and possibly methyl isobutyl ketone potentiate the neurotoxicity of n-hexane.

Exposure to n-hexane can be assessed by measuring 2,5-hexanedione in the urine or n-hexane in end-exhaled air. Concentrations of 2,5-hexanedione in urine of 5 mg/L measured at the end of a work shift and n-hexane in end-exhaled air of 40 ppm measured during a work shift correspond to exposure to a TWA of 50 ppm.

2. ALKENES (OLEFINS) & ALKYNES

Alkenes are aliphatic hydrocarbons with double (unsaturated) carbon bonds:

$$
\begin{array}{c}
\overset{\displaystyle H}{|}\quad \overset{\displaystyle H}{|}\quad \overset{\displaystyle H}{|} \\
-C=C-C- \\
|\\
H
\end{array}
\quad
\begin{array}{l}
\text{with the empirical formula} \\
C_nH_{2n}
\end{array}
$$

Dienes are alkenes with 2 double bonds. Alkynes are aliphatic hydrocarbons with triple carbon bonds. The physical state of alkenes and alkynes is determined by the number of carbons, as for alkanes.

Use

The liquid alkenes are not widely used as solvents but are common chemical intermediates. The alkenes are more reactive than alkanes, a property that leads to their use as monomers in the production of polymers, such as polyethylenes from ethylene, polypropylene from propylene, and synthetic rubber and resin copolymers from 1,3-butadiene.

Occupational & Environmental Exposure

Occupational exposure estimates are not available for most alkenes and alkynes. Occupational exposure to ethylene, propylene, and 1,3-butadiene occurs primarily through inhalation during polymer production. NIOSH estimates that 62,000 US workers are potentially exposed to 1,3-butadiene. Propylene is a common air pollutant as a result of engine exhaust emissions and industrial activity, with urban atmospheric concentrations ranging from 2.6 to 23.3 ppb in the USA and Europe. Butadiene has been detected in urban atmospheres in the USA at concentrations ranging from 1 to 5 ppb, while other alkenes and alkynes have been detected at comparable concentrations.

Pharmacokinetics

There is little information on absorption or metabolism of alkenes and alkynes. Absorption of these compounds should be similar to their corresponding alkanes. None have skin TLV designations.

Health Effects

The alkenes are similar in toxicity to the alkanes.

The unsaturated carbon bonds increase lipid solubility to some extent and therefore irritant and anesthetic potencies, compared to corresponding alkanes. n-Hexene does not cause peripheral neuropathy, as does n-hexane.

The presence of double bonds makes the alkenes more reactive than alkanes and dienes more reactive than alkenes. This reactivity is utilized in the production of polymers but may in some cases result also in additional health hazards. 1,3-Butadiene was recently found to be carcinogenic in animals, while propylene and ethylene were not.

ALICYCLIC HYDROCARBONS (Cyclic Hydrocarbons, Cycloparaffins, Naphthenes)

Essentials of Diagnosis

Acute effects:

- Anesthesia: dizziness, headache, nausea, vomiting, sleepiness, fatigue, "drunkenness," slurred speech, disequilibrium, disorientation, depression, loss of consciousness.
- Respiratory tract irritation: sore nose, throat, cough.

Chronic effects:

- Dermatitis: dry, cracked, erythematous skin.
- Neurobehavioral dysfunction: headache, mood lability, fatigue, short-term memory loss, difficulty concentrating; decreased attention span, neurobehavioral test abnormalities, CT scan (cerebral atrophy), EEG (diffuse slow waves).

General Considerations

Alicyclic hydrocarbons consist of alkanes or alkenes arranged into cyclic or ring structures:

$$
\begin{array}{c}
H\quad\quad\ H \\
\diagdown\ \ \ \diagup \\
C \\
\diagup\ \diagdown \\
H-C\quad C-H \\
|\quad\ \ | \\
H\quad\ H
\end{array}
$$

They have a slight "hydrocarbon" odor.

Use

Cyclohexane is the only alicyclic hydrocarbon that is widely used as an industrial solvent. Most of the US production is used in the synthesis of nylon. Cyclopropane is used as a general anesthetic, but this is limited by its flammability and explosiveness.

Occupational & Environmental Exposure

The use of cyclohexane in nylon production results in only limited occupational exposure. The alicyclic hydrocarbons are not reported as common environmental contaminants.

Pharmacokinetics

Similar to their corresponding alkanes and alkenes, the alicyclic hydrocarbons are well absorbed by inhalation, while percutaneous absorption is less important. Approximately 70% of cyclohexane that is inhaled is absorbed and excreted unchanged in urine and exhaled air and as cyclohexanol in urine.

Health Effects

The alicyclic hydrocarbons are similar in toxicity to their alkane or alkene counterparts in causing irritation and central nervous system depression. They cause anesthesia, respiratory tract irritation, and dermatitis and are associated with neurobehavioral dysfunction; and the associated clinical findings, differential diagnosis, treatment, and prognosis are not different from those of other solvents (see above). Cyclohexane does not cause peripheral neuropathy.

AROMATIC HYDROCARBONS

Essentials of Diagnosis

Acute effects:
- Anesthesia: dizziness, headache, nausea, vomiting, sleepiness, fatigue, "drunkenness," slurred speech, disequilibrium, disorientation, depression, loss of consciousness.
- Respiratory tract irritation: sore nose, throat, cough.

Chronic effects:
- Dermatitis: dry, cracked, erythematous skin.
- Neurobehavioral dysfunction: headache, mood lability, fatigue, short-term memory loss, difficulty concentrating; decreased attention span, neurobehavioral test abnormalities, CT scan (cerebral atrophy), EEG (diffuse slow waves).

General Considerations

Aromatic hydrocarbons are compounds that contain one or more benzene rings:

They are produced—directly or indirectly—chiefly from crude petroleum and to a lesser extent from coal tar. Aromatics used as solvents include benzene and the alkylbenzenes: toluene (methyl benzene), xylenes (*o-*, *m-*, and *p-* isomers of dimethyl benzenes), ethyl benzene, cumene (isopropyl benzene), and styrene (vinyl benzene). They have a characteristic "aromatic" sweet odor.

Use

Although benzene currently has only limited use as a general industrial solvent, it is still widely used in manufacturing, for extraction in chemical analyses, and as a specialty solvent. Approximately half the benzene produced is used to synthesize ethyl benzene for the production of styrene. In the USA, gasoline contains approximately 2–3% benzene and 30–50% other aromatics. Aromatics constitute a significant percentage of a number of petroleum distillate solvents (see below). Toluene and xylenes are 2 of the most widely used industrial solvents—principally in paints, adhesives, and the formulation of pesticides—though about a third of the toluene used goes to produce benzene and only about one-sixth is used as a solvent. The solvent uses of toluene and xylenes have been decreasing owing to environmental regulations because of their photochemical reactivity. Ethyl benzene is used chiefly as an intermediate in the manufacture of styrene and to a lesser extent as a solvent. Styrene is used chiefly as a monomer in the manufacture of plastics and rubber (see Chapters 28 and 29). Most of the cumene produced is used to manufacture phenol and acetone. Other aromatic compounds have a wide variety of uses but are not commonly used as solvents and so will not be discussed here.

Occupational & Environmental Exposure

NIOSH estimates that 4.8 million workers are potentially exposed to toluene, the fourth largest number for an individual chemical. The NIOSH estimate for xylene exposure is 140,000 workers. Aromatic hydrocarbons are common environmental contaminants from engine exhaust and other industrial sources. Levels in urban air have been reported to be as high as 130 ppb toluene, 100 ppb xylenes, 60 ppm benzene, 20 ppb ethyl benzene, < 1 ppb styrene, and 330 ppb total aromatics.

Pharmacokinetics

The pulmonary absorption values for aromatic hydrocarbons do not vary significantly as a group, ranging from approximately 50% to 70% at rest and decreasing to 40–60% with light to moderate work and 30–50% with moderate to heavy work. Percutaneous absorption of aromatic hydrocarbons can be significant, but only styrene and cumene currently have TLVs with skin designations.

All the aromatic hydrocarbons are extensively metabolized, their metabolic profiles varying with the substituents on the benzene ring. Benzene is metabolized mainly to phenol and excreted in urine as conjugated phenol and dihydroxyphenols, with a slow elimination phase half-time of about 28 hours. About 10% of benzene is excreted unchanged in exhaled air. Toluene is primarily metabolized to benzoic acid and excreted in urine as the glycine conjugate hippuric acid, with a half-time of about 1–2 hours. Approximately 15–20% of toluene is excreted unchanged in expired air. Xylenes are almost entirely metabolized to the *o-*, *m-*, and *p-*methylbenzoic acids and excreted in urine as the glycine conjugates, *o*-, *m*-, and *p*-methylhippuric acids, with a slow elimination phase half-time of about 30 hours. About 64% of absorbed ethyl benzene is excreted in urine as mandelic acid and about 25% as phenylglyoxylic acid. The principal metabolites of the aromatic hydrocarbons are used for biologic monitoring as indicated below.

Health Effects

The aromatic hydrocarbons are generally stronger irritants and anesthetics than the aliphatics. Substitution on benzene (toluene, xylene, ethyl benzene, and styrene) increases lipid solubility and these toxicities slightly. Aromatic hydrocarbons cause acute anesthetic effects, respiratory tract irritation, and dermatitis and are associated with neurobehavioral dysfunction; and the associated clinical findings, differential diagnosis, treatment, and prognosis are not different from those of other solvents (see above).

Benzene is notable for its effects on the bone marrow: reversible pancytopenia, aplastic anemia that may itself be fatal or progress to leukemia, and all types of leukemia, but predominantly acute non-lymphocytic leukemia. There is no evidence that the substituted benzenes have any of these myelotoxic effects. Earlier reports of effects of these substances on the bone marrow were probably due to their contamination with benzene.

There have been a few anecdotal reports of liver function abnormalities in workers exposed to aromatic hydrocarbons. Renal tubular acidosis of the distal type, with serious but reversible electrolyte abnormalities, has been reported in solvent abusers exposed primarily to toluene. A syndrome of persistent cerebellar ataxia has been reported after exposure to toluene, chiefly in solvent abusers but also occasionally in workers. Toluene and xylenes have been reported to raise auditory thresholds in laboratory animals at relatively low levels of exposure.

Exposure to benzene, ethyl benzene, toluene, xylenes, and styrene can be assessed by a variety of biologic monitoring techniques. These are summarized in Chapter 34. Although extensive research has been conducted on the use of these techniques, given the short half-lives and acute effects of these compounds, the utility of biologic monitoring for the routine assessment of exposure is limited. Little information is available on the use of biologic levels in the diagnosis of acute intoxication from aromatic hydrocarbons.

PETROLEUM DISTILLATES (Refined Petroleum Solvents)

Essentials of Diagnosis

Acute effects:
- Anesthesia: dizziness, headache, nausea, vomiting, sleepiness, fatigue, "drunkenness," slurred speech, disequilibrium, disorientation, depression, loss of consciousness.

- Respiratory tract irritation: sore nose, throat, cough.

Chronic effects:
- Dermatitis: dry, cracked, erythematous skin.
- Neurobehavioral dysfunction: headache, mood lability, fatigue, short-term memory loss, difficulty concentrating; decreased attention span, neurobehavioral test abnormalities, CT scan (cerebral atrophy), EEG (diffuse slow waves).

General Considerations

Petroleum distillate solvents are mixtures of petroleum derivatives distilled from crude petroleum at a particular range of boiling points. Each is a mixture of aliphatic (primarily alkane), alicyclic, and aromatic hydrocarbons, the relative concentration of each depending on the particular petroleum distillate fraction. They have a "hydrocarbon" or "aromatic" odor depending on the relative concentrations of aliphatic or aromatic hydrocarbons.

The major petroleum distillate solvents are shown in Table 27–2, with the number of carbon atoms, typical percentages of components, and range of boiling points of each.

Use

Petroleum distillates are among the most common general use solvents, since they are available at low cost in large quantities. Petroleum ether (petroleum naphtha) represents an estimated 60% of the total industrial solvent usage. Approximately 1.4 billion gallons of petroleum solvents (Table 27–2) were produced in the USA. Kerosene is used as a fuel as well as a cleaning and thinning agent; about 2.3 billion gallons are produced in the USA every year.

Occupational & Environmental Exposure

NIOSH estimates that 600,000 workers are potentially exposed to the petroleum solvents (Table 27–2) (naphtha solvents), 136,000 to the mineral spirits and 310,000 to kerosene.

Pharmacokinetics

The pharmacokinetics of petroleum distillate solvents are those of the individual aliphatic, alicyclic, and aromatic constituents.

Health Effects

The hazard of a particular petroleum distillate fraction is related to concentrations of the various classes of hydrocarbons it contains. As the fraction becomes heavier (higher boiling point, increasing number of carbons), the percentage of aromatic hydrocarbons and therefore the toxicity increases. However, this increase in toxicity is offset by a decrease in volatility. Petroleum distillate solvents cause anesthetic effects, respiratory tract irritation, and dermatitis, and have been associated with neurobehavioral dysfunction; the clinical findings, differ-

Table 27–2. Petroleum distillate solvents.

	Synonyms	Carbon Number	Class Components	Percentage (%)	Boiling Point (°C)
Petroleum ether	Petroleum, naphtha, ligroin, benzene	C_{5-6}	Alkanes (pentanes, hexanes)	100	30–60
Rubber solvent	Naphtha	C_{5-7}	Aliphatic Alicyclic Aromatic	60 35 5	45–125
Petroleum ether, high-boiling point	Light aliphatic solvent naphtha	C_{7-8}	. . .	. . .	80–130
V M & P naphtha[1]	. . .	C_{5-11}	Aliphatic Aromatic	>80 <20	95–100
Mineral spirits I	Stoddard solvent I, white spirits, petroleum distillate	C_{7-12}	Aliphatic Alicyclic Aromatic	30–50 30–40 10–20	150–200
Mineral spirits II	Stoddard solvent II, high-flash naphtha, 140-flash naphtha	C_{5-13}	Aliphatic Alicyclic Aromatic	40–60 30–40 5–15	175–200
Aromatic petroleum naphtha	Coal tar naphtha	C_{8-13}	Aliphatic Aromatic	<10 >90	95–315
Kerosene	Kerosine, stove oil	C_{10-16}	Aliphatic Alicyclic Aromatic	. . .	163–288

[1]Varnish makers' and painters' naphtha.

ential diagnosis, treatment, and prognosis are not different from those of other solvents (above).

Most of the aliphatic fractions are alkanes, including n-hexane. Therefore, the risk of peripheral neuropathy must be considered, particularly with exposure to petroleum ether, which may contain a significant percentage of n-hexane. The benzene content of petroleum distillates should be below 1%.

ALCOHOLS

Essentials of Diagnosis
Acute effects:
- Respiratory tract irritation: sore nose, sore throat, cough.
- Anesthesia: dizziness, headache, nausea, vomiting, sleepiness, fatigue, "drunkenness," slurred speech, disequilibrium, disorientation, depression, loss of consciousness.

Chronic effects:
- Dermatitis: dry, cracked, erythematous skin.
- Optic neuropathy (methyl alcohol): blurred vision, blindness, hyperemic optic disk, dilated pupil.

General Considerations
Alcohols are hydrocarbons substituted with a single hydroxyl group:

$$— C — C — OH$$

They have a characteristic pungent odor. Examples of alcohols used as solvents are ethyl alcohol, methyl alcohol, and isopropyl alcohol (Table 27–1).

Use
Alcohols are widely used as cleaning agents, thinners, and diluents; as vehicles for paints, pesticides, and pharmaceuticals; as extracting agents; and as chemical intermediates. Methyl alcohol is widely used as an industrial solvent—one-fourth of its production—and as an adulterant to denature ethanol to prevent its abuse when used as an industrial solvent. Approximately one-third of methyl alcohol used is in the production of formaldehyde. Over half of isopropyl alcohol produced is used to manufacture acetone, and the rest in a variety of solvent and chemical formulation uses. About 90% of cyclohexanol is used to produce adipic acid for nylon, the rest for esters for plasticizers. Allyl alcohol is used solely as a chemical intermediate. The higher alcohols (>5 carbons) are divided into the plasticizer range (6–11 carbons) and the detergent range (> 12 carbons). About 500 kilotons of plasticizer-range alcohols are produced annually in the USA to make esters for plasticizers and lubricants, and about 260 kilotons of detergent-range alcohols are produced to make sulfate deionizers for detergents.

Occupational & Environmental Exposure
NIOSH estimates that approximately 175,000 workers are potentially exposed to methyl alcohol and 141,000 workers to isopropyl alcohol in the USA. Exposure to isopropyl alcohol in the home is common in the form of cleaners, cosmetics, and rubbing alcohol.

Pharmacokinetics
The pharmacokinetics of the simple (primary) alcohols are similar. About 50% of inhaled alcohol is absorbed at rest, decreasing to 40% with light to moderate work loads. Methyl alcohol, n-butyl alco-

hol, isopropyl alcohol, and isooctyl alcohol are sufficiently absorbed percutaneously to be given skin TLV designations.

The primary alcohols are metabolized by hepatic alcohol dehydrogenase to aldehydes and by aldehyde dehydrogenase to carboxylic acids. The metabolic acidosis and optic neuropathy caused by methyl alcohol have been attributed to its metabolism to formic acid. Metabolic interactions of ethanol with other organic solvents, such as "degreaser's flush" in workers exposed to trichloroethylene and other chlorinated hydrocarbons, are frequently due to competition for alcohol and aldehyde dehydrogenases, with subsequent accumulation of the alcohol and aldehyde and resulting reaction. Secondary alcohols are primarily metabolized to ketones.

Health Effects

The alcohols are more potent central nervous system depressants and irritants than the corresponding aliphatic hydrocarbons, but they are weaker skin and respiratory tract irritants than aldehydes or ketones. Respiratory tract and eye irritation usually occurs at lower concentrations than central nervous system depression and thus serves as a useful warning property. This may explain why occupational exposure to alcohols has not been implicated as causing chronic neurobehavioral effects. The TLVs for most alcohols are based on prevention of irritation.

Methyl alcohol is toxicologically distinct owing to its toxicity to the optic nerve, which can result in blindness. An extensive literature is available on this effect, which occurs primarily as a result of ingestion of methanol as an ethanol substitute or adulterant. A few poorly documented cases of blindness have been reported as a result of occupational inhalation exposure in confined spaces. The minimum oral dose causing blindness to an adult male has been estimated to be about 8–10 g; the minimum lethal dose is estimated to be 75–100 g. These amounts correspond to 8-hour exposure concentrations in air of approximately 1600–2000 ppm and 15,000–20,000 ppm respectively. Blurred vision and other visual disturbances have been reported occasionally as a result of exposures to levels slightly above the TLV of 200 ppm.

Inhalation exposure to ethanol and propanols result in simple irritation and central nervous system depression, though propanols may be significantly absorbed through the skin. There are a few reports of auditory and vestibular nerve injury in workers exposed to n-butyl alcohol. Isooctyl alcohol is the most industrially important of the higher alcohols, but little toxicologic information about it is available.

GLYCOLS (DIOLS)

Essentials of Diagnosis

Acute effects:
• Anesthesia (unusual due to low vapor pressure):

dizziness, headache, nausea, vomiting, sleepiness, fatigue, "drunkenness," slurred speech, disequilibrium, disorientation, depression, loss of consciousness.

Chronic effects:
• Dermatitis: dry, cracked, erythematous skin.

General Considerations

Glycols are hydrocarbons with 2 hydroxyl (alcohol) groups attached to separate carbon atoms in an aliphatic chain:

$$\begin{array}{c} | \quad\quad | \\ -C - C - \\ \diagup \quad\quad \diagdown \\ HO \quad\quad OH \end{array}$$

Examples include ethylene glycol, diethylene glycol, triethylene glycol, and propylene glycol (Table 27–1). They have a slightly sweet odor.

Use

Glycols are used as antifreezing agents and as solvent carriers and vehicles in a variety of chemical formulations. Only ethylene glycol is in common general industrial use as a solvent, but large volumes of the others are used as vehicles and chemical intermediates. Approximately 40% of ethylene glycol is used as antifreeze, 35% to make polyesters, and 25% as solvent carriers.

Occupational & Environmental Exposure

NIOSH estimates that nearly 2 million workers are potentially exposed to ethylene glycol, 660,000 to diethylene glycol, and 226,000 to triethylene glycol, primarily as a result of their being directly handled, heated, or sprayed.

Pharmacokinetics

The glycols have such low vapor pressures that inhalation is only of moderate concern unless heated or aerosolized. Ethylene glycol does not have a skin TLV designation. Ethylene glycol and diethylene glycol are metabolized to glycol aldehyde, glycolic acid, glyoxylic acid, oxalic acid, formic acid, glycine, and carbon dioxide. Oxalic acid is the cause of the acute renal failure and metabolic acidosis that occur following ingestion of ethylene glycol. The first 2 steps in this metabolism use alcohol and aldehyde dehydrogenase and may be competitively blocked by administration of ethyl alcohol.

Health Effects

The low vapor pressures of the glycols result in little hazard in their customary industrial use. They are not significantly irritating to the skin or respiratory tract but can produce a chronic dermatitis from defatting of the skin. The systemic toxicity of ethylene glycol commonly seen after ingestion of commercial antifreeze compounds as an alcohol substitute—

seizures, central nervous system depression, metabolic acidosis, and acute renal failure—have not been reported as a result of occupational exposure.

PHENOLS

Essentials of Diagnosis

Acute effects:
- Respiratory tract irritation: sore nose, sore throat, cough.
- Tissue destruction: eg, hepatic necrosis with abdominal pain, jaundice, abnormal liver function tests; kidney necrosis with acute renal failure; skin necrosis with blisters, burns.
- Anesthesia: dizziness, headache, nausea, vomiting, sleepiness, fatigue, "drunkenness," slurred speech, disequilibrium, disorientation, depression, loss of consciousness.

Chronic effects:
- Dermatitis: dry, cracked, erythematous skin.

General Considerations

Phenols are aromatic alcohols:

Examples include phenol, cresol (methyl phenol), catechol (1,2,-benzenediol, 1,2-dihydroxybenzene), resorcinol (1,3-benzenediol, 1,3-dihydroxybenzene), and hydroquinone (1,4-benzenediol, 1,4-hydroxybenzene).

Use

The industrial use of phenols as solvents is limited due to their acute toxicity. Phenol is used as a cleaning agent, paint stripper, and disinfectant, but its chief use is as a chemical intermediate for phenolic resins, bisphenol A for epoxy resins, and other chemicals and drugs. Cresol is used as a disinfectant and chemical intermediate. Catechol is used in photography, fur dyeing, and leather tanning and as a chemical intermediate. Resorcinol is used as a chemical intermediate for adhesives, dyes, and pharmaceuticals. Hydroquinone is used in photography, as a polymerization inhibitor, and as an antioxidant.

Occupational & Environmental Exposure

NIOSH estimates that more than 10,000 workers are potentially exposed to phenol.

Pharmacokinetics

Phenol is well absorbed both by inhalation of vapors and by dermal penetration of vapors and liquids. Phenol and cresols have skin TLV designa-

tions. Phenol is rapidly eliminated within 16 hours, almost entirely as conjugated phenol in urine.

Health Effects

Phenol and related compounds are potent irritants that can be corrosive at high concentrations. As a result of their ability to complex with, denature, and precipitate proteins, they can be cytotoxic to all cells at sufficient concentrations. Direct contact with concentrated phenol can result in burns, local tissue necrosis, systemic absorption, and tissue necrosis in the liver, kidneys, urinary tract, and heart. Central nervous system depression occurs, as it does with all volatile organic solvents.

KETONES

Essentials of Diagnosis

Acute effects:
- Respiratory tract irritation: sore nose, sore throat, cough.
- Anesthesia: Dizziness, headache, nausea, vomiting, sleepiness, fatigue, "drunkenness," slurred speech, disequilibrium, disorientation, depression, loss of consciousness.

Chronic effects:
- Dermatitis: dry, cracked, erythematous skin.

General Considerations

Ketones are hydrocarbons with a carbonyl group that is attached to 2 hydrocarbon groups (the carbonyl is nonterminal):

They are produced by the dehydroxylation or oxidation of alcohols. A great many ketones are in use—some used as industrial solvents are listed in Table 27–1. Acetone and methyl ethyl ketone (2-butanone) are in most common use. The ketones have a characteristic minty odor that some people find pleasant and others offensive.

Use

Ketones are widely used as solvents for surface coatings with natural and synthetic resins; in the formulation of inks, adhesives, and dyes; in chemical extraction and manufacture; and, to a lesser extent, as cleaning agents. About one-fourth of the acetone produced is used in the manufacture of methacrylates and one-third as solvent. Almost all cyclohexanone is used to make caprolactam for nylon, but small amounts are used as solvents.

Occupational & Environmental Exposure

The wide use of ketones is reflected in the large numbers of potentially exposed workers estimated by

NIOSH: acetone, 2,816,000; methyl ethyl ketone, 3,031,000; methyl isobutyl ketone, 1,853,000; cyclohexanone, 1,190,000; isophorone, 1,507,000; and diacetone alcohol, 1,350,000. The use of many ketones has decreased owing to their regulation as photochemical reactants. Consumer exposure to acetone is common in the form of nail polish remover and general use solvent.

Pharmacokinetics

Ketones are well absorbed by inhalation of vapors and to a lesser extent after skin contact with liquid. Only cyclohexanone has a skin TLV designation. The pulmonary retention of acetone at rest has been estimated to be about 45%. Most ketones are rapidly eliminated unchanged in urine and exhaled air and by reduction to their respective alcohols, which are conjugated and excreted or further metabolized to a variety of compounds, including carbon monoxide.

Health Effects

Ketones have good warning properties in that irritation or a strong odor usually occurs at levels below those that cause central nervous system depression. Headaches and nausea as a result of the odor have been mistaken for central nervous system depression. The TLVs for most ketones are set to prevent irritation.

Methyl n-butyl ketone causes the same type of peripheral neuropathy as n-hexane. It is metabolized to the neurotoxic diketone 2,5-hexanedione to an even greater extent than n-hexane and therefore poses an even greater hazard. The neurotoxic potential of methyl n-butyl ketone was discovered following the occurrence of a large number of cases of peripheral neuropathy in a plastics manufacturing plant in Ohio in 1974. A large volume of research has been published since, from animal neurotoxicity and metabolism studies to cell culture and mechanistic studies. However, human exposure to this substance no longer occurs, since the sole manufacturer ceased production a number of years ago. Other ketones used as solvents have not been shown to cause peripheral neuropathy, but methyl ethyl ketone (MEK) potentiates the neurotoxicity of n-hexane and methyl n-butyl ketone, probably through a metabolic interaction.

ESTERS

Essentials of Diagnosis

Acute effects:
- Anesthesia: dizziness headache, nausea, vomiting, sleepiness, fatigue, "drunkenness," slurred speech, disequilibrium, disorientation, depression, loss of consciousness.
- Respiratory tract irritation: sore nose, sore throat, cough.

Chronic effects:
- Dermatitis: dry, cracked, erythematous skin.

General Considerations

Esters are hydrocarbons that are derivatives of an organic acid and an alcohol:

$$-\underset{\underset{O-C-}{\overset{\diagdown}{}}}{C}=O$$

They are named after their parent alcohols and acids, respectively, eg, methyl acetate for the ester of methyl alcohol and acetic acid. Examples of some of the many esters used as solvents are listed in Table 27–1. They have characteristic odors that range from sweet to pungent.

Use

Esters—particularly the lower esters—are commonly used as solvents for surface coatings. Vinyl acetate is used primarily in the production of polyvinyl acetate and polyvinyl alcohol. Other lower esters are used to make polymeric acrylates and methacrylates. Higher esters are used as plasticizers.

Occupational & Environmental Exposure

NIOSH estimates that 70,000 workers are potentially exposed to vinyl acetate in polymer production in the USA. Large numbers of workers are potentially exposed to other esters used as industrial solvents, particularly in surface coatings.

Pharmacokinetics

Esters are very rapidly metabolized by plasma esterases to their parent organic acids and alcohols.

Health Effects

Many esters have extremely low odor thresholds, their distinctive sweet smells serving as good warning properties. Because of this property, n-amyl acetate (banana oil) is used as an odorant for qualitative fit testing of respirators. Esters are more potent anesthetics than corresponding alcohols, aldehydes, or ketones but are also strong irritants. Odor and irritation usually occur at levels below central nervous system depression. Their systemic toxicity is determined to a large extent by the toxicity of the corresponding alcohol. There is one report of optic nerve damage from exposure to methyl acetate as a result of metabolism to methanol and hence to formic acid (see Alcohols, above). Similarly, methyl formate may cause optic neuropathy following metabolism directly to formic acid.

ETHERS

Essentials of Diagnosis

Acute effects:
- Anesthesia: dizziness, headache, nausea, vomiting, sleepiness, fatigue, "drunkenness," slurred speech, disequilibrium, disorientation, depression, loss of consciousness.

- Respiratory tract irritation: sore nose, sore throat, cough.

  Chronic effects:
- Dermatitis: dry, cracked, erythematous skin.

General Considerations

Ethers consist of 2 hydrocarbon groups joined by an oxygen linkage:

$$-C-O-C-$$

Examples include ethyl ether and dioxane (Table 27–1). They have a characteristic sweet odor often described as "ethereal."

Use

Ethyl ether was used extensively in the past as an anesthetic but has been replaced by agents less flammable and explosive. It is too volatile for most solvent uses except analytic extraction. It is used as a solvent for waxes, fats, oils, and gums. Dioxane (1,4-diethylene dioxide) is used as a solvent for a wide range of organic products, including cellulose esters, rubber, and coatings; in the preparation of histologic slides; and as a stabilizer in chlorinated solvents.

Occupational & Environmental Exposure

Occupational exposure to ethyl ether is largely confined to analytic laboratories. NIOSH estimates that 2500 workers are exposed to dioxane in its use as a solvent, and many more may be exposed through its use as a stabilizer in chlorinated solvents.

Pharmacokinetics

Ethyl ether is well absorbed by inhalation of vapors; its volatility limits percutaneous absorption. Over 90% of absorbed ethyl ether is excreted unchanged in exhaled air; the rest may be metabolized by enzymatic cleavage of the ether link to acetaldehyde and acetic acid. Dioxane is well absorbed by inhalation of vapors and through skin contact with liquid and has a skin TLV designation. It is metabolized almost entirely to β-hydroxyethoxyacetic acid and excreted in urine with a half-life of about 1 hour.

Health Effects

Ethyl ether is a potent anesthetic and a less potent irritant. Higher ethers are relatively more potent irritants. Dioxane is also an anesthetic and irritant but has also caused acute kidney and liver necrosis in workers exposed to uncertain amounts. Animal cancer studies have indicated an increased incidence of tumors at about 10,000 ppm in the diet but not at about 100 ppm by inhalation. Studies in exposed workers have been inadequate. The issue of carcinogenic risk from exposure to dioxane is controversial.

GLYCOL ETHERS

Essentials of Diagnosis

Acute effects:
- Anesthesia: dizziness, headache, nausea, vomiting, sleepiness, fatigue, "drunkenness," slurred speech, disequilibrium, disorientation, depression, loss of consciousness.

  Chronic effects:
- Dermatitis: dry, cracked, erythematous skin.
- Anemia: low erythrocyte count or pancytopenia, evidence of hemolysis or bone marrow suppression.
- Encephalopathy: confusion, disorientation.
- Reproductive toxicity (laboratory animals): major malformations with maternal exposure, low sperm count, testicular atrophy, infertility with male exposure.

General Considerations

The glycol ethers are alkyl ether derivatives of ethylene, diethylene, triethylene, and propylene glycol (an alkyl group linked to the glycol by an oxygen). The acetate derivatives of glycol ethers are included and are considered toxicologically identical to their precursors. They are known by formal chemical names, eg, ethylene glycol monomethyl ether (EGME); common chemical names (2-methoxyethanol, 2-ME), used here; and trade names (Methyl Cellosolve).

Use

The glycol ethers are widely used solvents because of their solubility or miscibility in water and most organic liquids. They are used as diluents in paints, lacquers, enamels, inks, and dyes; as cleaning agents in liquid soaps, dry cleaning fluids, and glass cleaners; as surfactants, fixatives, desiccants, antifreeze compounds, and deicers; and in extraction and chemical synthesis. Since the first 2 members of this family, 2-methoxyethanol and 2-ethoxyethanol, were found to be potent reproductive toxins in laboratory animals and their TLVs lowered on this basis, there has been a shift in use to 2-butoxyethanol and other longer-chained ethylene glycol ethers and to diethylene and propylene glycol ethers.

Occupational & Environmental Exposure

Over 1 million workers are potentially exposed to each of the most commonly used glycol ethers and their acetates. Accurate estimates are not available owing to the recent shifts in their use patterns. Because of their low volatility, the most important exposures occur as a result of direct contact with liquids, inhalation of vapors in enclosed spaces, and spraying or heating of the liquids to generate aerosols or vapors. These exposures can exceed the doses of 2-methoxyethanol and 2-ethoxyethanol that cause reproductive toxicity in laboratory animals. Environmental exposure occurs because of the presence of some glycol ethers in consumer products, such as glass cleaners, but there are no estimates of exposure levels from these uses.

Pharmacokinetics

The glycol ethers are well absorbed by all routes of exposure owing to their universal solubility. They have relatively low vapor pressures, so that dermal exposure is often of primary importance. The acetate derivatives are rapidly hydrolyzed by plasma esterases to their corresponding monoalkyl ethers. The ethylene glycol monoalkyl ethers maintain their ether linkages and are metabolized by hepatic alcohol and aldehyde dehydrogenases to their respective aldehyde and acid metabolites. The acid metabolites 2-methoxyacetic acid and 2-ethoxyacetic acid are responsible for the reproductive toxicities of 2-methoxyethanol and 2-ethoxyethanol. These metabolites are excreted in urine unchanged or conjugated to glycine and may be used as biologic indicators of exposure.

Health Effects

Acute central nervous system depression has not been reported as an effect of occupational exposure. However, a number of cases of encephalopathy have been reported in workers exposed to 2-methoxyethanol over periods of weeks to months. Manifestations have included personality changes, memory loss, difficulty in concentrating, lethargy, fatigue, loss of appetite, weight loss, tremor, gait disturbances, and slurred speech.

Bone marrow toxicity usually manifested as pancytopenia has been reported in workers and laboratory animals exposed to 2-methoxyethanol and 2-ethoxyethanol. The longer-chain ethylene glycol monoalkyl ethers cause hemolysis by increasing osmotic fragility in laboratory animals, an effect that has not been reported to date in humans.

Male reproductive toxicity was recently demonstrated in experimental animals for 2-methoxyethanol, 2-ethoxyethanol, and their acetate derivatives. Acute or chronic exposure of mice, rats, and rabbits to low levels of these compounds by inhalation, dermal, or oral routes resulted in reductions in sperm count, impaired sperm motility, increased numbers of abnormal forms, and infertility. These effects began about 4 weeks after the onset of exposure and—in the absence of testicular atrophy— were reversible following cessation of exposure.

The testicular toxicity of the glycol ethers decreases sharply with lengthening of the alkyl group, such that beginning with butyl and proceeding through n-propyl and isopropyl they are nearly or completely inactive. The acetic acid derivatives (alkoxy acids) appear to be the active testicular toxins. In limited testing, the dimethyl ethers of ethylene glycol and diethylene glycol—but not the monomethyl ether of diethylene glycol—show some evidence of causing testicular toxicity, though the latter has not been tested at the high doses that have been shown to be teratogenic. Ethylene glycol hexyl ether, ethylene glycol phenyl ether, and the propylene glycol ethers do not appear to be toxic to either the male or female reproductive systems.

The same glycol ethers that are testicular toxins have been shown to be teratogenic in the same species of laboratory animals at comparable doses. The structure-activity relationships also appear to be similar, the alkoxy acid metabolites are apparently the proximate teratogens. Major defects of the skeleton, kidneys, and cardiovascular system have been observed, with some variation in their nature and severity with species, dose, and route of administration. The ethylene glycol monoalkyl ethers with longer alkyl chains and other glycol (propylene, diethylene, and dipropylene) ethers have not been shown to be teratogenic with the exception of diethylene glycol monomethyl ether, which produced typical malformations at relatively high doses.

There have not been adequate studies of reproductive effects of the glycol ethers in humans to date. Since these effects have been consistently produced in all species tested and their metabolism and other health effects appear to be similar in humans and laboratory animals, those compounds with reproductive effects in animals should be assumed to be potential testicular toxins and teratogens in humans. In 1982, ACGIH lowered the TLVs for 2-methoxyethanol and 2-ethoxyethanol and their acetates to 5 ppm (with skin designations) based on their reproductive toxicity. Whenever possible, the risk of reproductive toxicity from these compounds should be reduced by substitution of other glycol ethers or other solvents.

GLYCIDYL ETHERS

Essentials of Diagnosis

Acute effects:
- Dermatitis (primary irritant): irritation, erythema, first and second degree burns of skin.

Chronic effects:
- Dermatitis (allergic contact): itching, erythema, vesicles.

General Considerations

The glycidyl ethers consist of a 2,3-epoxypropyl group with an ether linkage to another hydrocarbon group:

$$H-\underset{\underset{O}{\diagdown\diagup}}{C}-\underset{\underset{O}{\diagdown\diagup}}{\overset{\overset{H}{|}}{C}}-\overset{\overset{H}{|}}{\underset{\underset{H}{|}}{C}}-O-\overset{\overset{H}{|}}{\underset{|}{C}}-$$

They are synthesized from epichlorohydrin and an alcohol. Only the monoglycidyl ethers are in common use and will be discussed here.

Use

The epoxide or oxirane ring of glycidyl ethers makes these compounds very reactive, so their use is confined to processes that utilize this property, such as reactive diluents in epoxy resin systems. Epoxy resins have a wide range of applications in industry and consumer use (see Chapter 28).

Occupational & Environmental Exposure

The primary exposure of workers and consumers is in the application of uncured epoxy resins. The epoxide groups of the ethers react to form cross-linkages within epoxy resins, so that glycidyl ethers no longer exist in a completely cured resin. However, workers may be exposed to the ethers in their manufacture and in the formulation and application of the resin system. NIOSH estimates that 118,000 workers in the USA are potentially exposed to glycidyl ethers and an additional 1 million to epoxy resins.

Pharmacokinetics

The glycidyl ethers have low vapor pressures, so that inhalation at normal air temperatures is not usually a concern. However, the curing of epoxy resins often generates heat, which may vaporize some glycidyl ether. A number of uses such as epoxy paint require spraying and the generation of an aerosol. Although quantitative data are lacking, the glycidyl ethers should be well absorbed by all routes. They have a short biologic half-life owing to their reactivity. Three metabolic reactions have been proposed: reduction to diols by epoxide hydrase, conjugation with glutathione, and covalent bonding with proteins, RNA, and DNA.

Health Effects

Reported effects of glycidyl ethers from occupational exposure have been confined to dermatitis of both the primary irritant and allergic contact type. Dermatitis can be severe and may result in second-degree burns. Asthma in workers exposed to epoxy resins may be due to exposure to glycidyl ethers.

Glycidyl ethers are positive in a number of short-term tests of genotoxicity, including mutagenicity, but none have been adequately tested for carcinogenicity. They are testicular toxins in laboratory animals, but few have been tested for teratogenicity.

ORGANIC ACIDS

Essentials of Diagnosis
Acute effects:
- Respiratory tract irritation: sore nose, sore throat, cough.

Chronic effects:
- Dermatitis: dry, cracked, erythematous skin.

General Considerations

Organic acids are derivatives of carboxylic acid:

$$-C=O$$
$$\diagdown OH$$

Acetic acid (vinegar) is used in a variety of industrial settings, including photographic development. Other organic acids are used to a lesser extent. Most organic acids are such strong irritants that they can be considered as primary irritants and not anesthetics.

ALIPHATIC AMINES

Essentials of Diagnosis
Acute effects:
- Eye irritation, corneal edema, visual halos.
- Respiratory tract irritation: sore nose, sore throat, cough.
- Dermatitis (irritant): erythema, irritation of skin.

Chronic effects:
- Dermatitis (allergic contact): erythema, vesicles, itching of skin.
- Asthma (ethyleneamines): cough, wheezing, shortness of breath, dyspnea on exertion, decreased FVC on pulmonary function testing with response to bronchodilators.

General Considerations

Aliphatic amines are derivatives of ammonia in which one or more hydrogen atoms are replaced by an alkyl or alkanol group:

$$-C-C-NH_2 \qquad -C-\overset{\overset{\displaystyle OH}{|}}{C}-NH_2$$

(primary amine)   (alkanolamine)

They can be classified as primary, secondary, and tertiary monoamines according to the number of substitutions on the nitrogen atom; as polyamines if more than one amine group is present; and as alkanolamines if a hydroxyl group is present on the alkyl group (an alcohol). They have a characteristic odor like that of fish and are strongly alkaline.

Use

There are a large number of aliphatic amines that have a number of uses. They are used to some extent as solvents but to a greater degree as chemical intermediates. They are also used as catalysts for polymerization reactions, preservatives (bactericides), corrosion inhibitors, drugs, and herbicides.

Occupational & Environmental Exposure

Given the diversity of their uses, accurate estimates of the number of workers exposed to aliphatic amines are not possible. They are not common environmental pollutants.

Pharmacokinetics

Little is known of the pharmacokinetics of the aliphatic amines in industrial use. They are well absorbed by inhalation, and some have skin designations as a result of their percutaneous absorption (Table 27–1). Metabolism is probably primarily deamination to ammonia by monoamine oxidase and diamine oxidase.

Health Effects

The vapors of the volatile amines cause eye irritation and a characteristic corneal edema, with visual changes of halos around lights, that is reversible. Irritation will occur wherever contact with the vapors occurs, including the respiratory tract and skin. Direct contact with the liquid can produce serious eye or skin burns. Allergic contact dermatitis has been reported primarily from ethyleneamines, as has asthma.

CHLORINATED HYDROCARBONS

Essentials of Diagnosis

Acute effects:
- Anesthesia: Dizziness, headache, nausea, vomiting, sleepiness, fatigue, "drunkenness," slurred speech, disequilibrium, disorientation, depression, loss of consciousness.
- Respiratory tract irritation: sore nose, sore throat, cough.

Chronic effects:
- Dermatitis: dry, cracked, erythematous skin.
- Neurobehavioral dysfunction: headache, mood lability, fatigue, short-term memory loss, difficulty in concentrating; decreased attention span, neurobehavioral test abnormalities, CT scan (cerebral atrophy), EEG (diffuse slow waves).
- Hepatocellular injury: abdominal pain, nausea, jaundice, abnormal liver function tests.
- Renal tubular dysfunction: weakness, fatigue, polyuria, glycosuria, electrolyte abnormalities (acidosis, hypokalemia, hypophosphatemia, hypochloremia, hypocarbonatemia), glycosuria, proteinuria.

General Considerations

The addition of chlorine to carbon and hydrogen

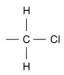

increases the stability and decreases the flammability of the resulting compounds. They have characteristic

slightly pungent odors. Six chlorinated aliphatic hydrocarbons are commonly used as solvents: trichloroethylene, perchloroethylene (tetrachloroethylene), 1,1,1-trichloroethane (methyl chloroform), methylene chloride (dichloromethane), carbon tetrachloride, and chloroform. Other chlorinated aliphatic hydrocarbons such as ethylene dichloride and chlorinated aromatics such as chlorobenzenes are rarely used as general industrial solvents and will not be discussed here. Abbreviations such as TCE and TCA will not be used since they are not standardized and can lead to errors in identification.

Use

The chlorinated hydrocarbons are used extensively as cleaning, degreasing, and thinning agents and less so as chemical intermediates. Historically, trichloroethylene was the principal solvent used in vapor degreasers, and while 80% of trichloroethylene is still used for this purpose it is being replaced by 1,1,1-trichloroethane and chlorofluorocarbons, which are somewhat safer. Perchloroethylene has replaced mineral spirits and carbon tetrachloride as the primary dry-cleaning solvent in two-thirds of facilities because of the flammability of the former and the toxicity of the latter. Methylene chloride is used as a paint stripper and extraction agent. Chloroform is used for extraction and spot cleaning. Carbon tetrachloride is used primarily as a chemical intermediate and in small quantities as a spot cleaning agent. 1,1,1-Trichloroethane is used in vapor degreasers and increasingly as a general cleaning and thinning agent.

Occupational & Environmental Exposure

Table 27–3 shows the estimated number of workers exposed and typical air and contaminated drinking water level for the common chlorinated hydrocarbon solvents. Chloroform is present in drinking water as

Table 27–3. Chlorinated hydrocarbon solvents: Occupational and environmental exposure data.

Solvent	Number of Workers Exposed[1]	Ambient Air[2]	Drinking Water[3]
Trichloroethylene	100,000 full-time 3.5 million part-time	1 ppb	1–30 ppb
Perchloroethylene	27,000 full-time 550,000 part-time	1–10 ppb	1–2 ppb
1,1,1-Trichloroethane	100,000	1 ppb	1–10 ppb
Methylene chloride	70,000	0.5–5 ppb	< 1 ppb
Carbon tetrachloride	160,000	0.1 ppb	< 1 ppb
Chloroform	80,000	< 1 ppb	<100 ppb

[1]NIOSH estimates.
[2]EPA-reported average urban concentrations.
[3]EPA-reported range in contaminated drinking water.

one of the trihalogenated methanes produced as a result of chlorination. EPA recently proposed a 100-ppb limit for total trihalogenated methanes, including chloroform, in drinking water.

Pharmacokinetics

The chlorinated hydrocarbon solvents are all relatively volatile and moderately well absorbed by inhalation. Pulmonary uptake ranges from 60% to 80% at rest and decreases to 40–50% during activity. Percutaneous absorption of vapors is usually insignificant, but dermal absorption following prolonged or extensive contact of the skin with liquid can be significant.

Biologic monitoring of the chlorinated hydrocarbons is based on their pattern of metabolism and excretion, which varies with their structure. 1,1,1-Trichloroethane and perchloroethylene are excreted mainly unchanged in exhaled air and metabolized and excreted only slightly as trichloroethanol and trichloroacetic acid. Therefore, biologic monitoring has been conducted chiefly with exhaled air and to a lesser extent with the parent compound in blood and metabolites in urine. Accumulation of both compounds occurs to some degree with daily exposure.

In contrast, less than 10% of trichloroethylene is excreted unchanged in exhaled air. The remainder is rapidly metabolized by alcohol and aldehyde dehydrogenases via chloral hydrate to trichloroethanol and trichloroacetic acid, or to unidentified metabolites. Although the biologic half-life of the parent compound is very short, trichloroethanol is an active anesthetic, and with a half-life of 10–15 hours accumulates to some extent over the course of a work week. Trichloroacetic acid, though inactive, has a much longer half-life of 50–100 hours and has been recommended for use in biologic monitoring. A value of 100 mg/L in urine voided at the end of the work week corresponds to exposure to a TWA of 50 ppm trichloroethylene. However, because of large individual variability, this value can only be used to assess groups of workers and not individuals.

Methylene chloride is both excreted unchanged in exhaled air and metabolized to carbon monoxide in a dose-dependent fashion. An 8-hour exposure to methylene chloride at its prior TLV of 100 ppm results in a carboxyhemoglobin level of about 3–5% in a nonsmoker, while exposure at its current (proposed) TLV carboxyhemoglobin levels are indistinguishable from background (1–2%). Methylene chloride in blood and exhaled air can also be used as biologic indicators of exposure.

Chloroform and carbon tetrachloride are each approximately 50% excreted unchanged in exhaled air and 50% metabolized. Both can be measured in blood and exhaled air, but little information is available on biologic monitoring for either.

Health Effects

As a class, the chlorinated hydrocarbons are more potent anesthetics, hepatotoxins, and nephrotoxins than other organic solvents. Most have been found to cause hepatocarcinomas in laboratory mice following oral administration. Evidence for carcinogenicity following inhalation has been recently demonstrated for methylene chloride and perchloroethylene, while adequate inhalation bioassays of the remainder have not been completed. Due to their common industrial use, the issue of carcinogenic risk to humans from exposure to these compounds is one of the most controversial topics in regulatory toxicology. There are surprisingly few animal studies examining their potential for reproductive toxicity, and almost none in male animals. Pertinent aspects of the toxicity of each compound will be briefly discussed.

1. TRICHLOROETHYLENE

The TLV of 50 ppm is based on prevention of central nervous system depression, which occurs at levels below those causing evidence of hepatic dysfunction. A recent National Toxicology Program (NTP) cancer bioassay in multiple rat strains conducted in an attempt to address the uncertainty over results in mice was unfortunately inadequate due to insufficient survival in dosed animals, so that the carcinogenicity of trichloroethylene remains unresolved. Limited evidence from animal studies suggests that trichloroethylene is not teratogenic or spermatotoxic.

2. PERCHLOROETHYLENE

Perchloroethylene is approximately equipotent to trichloroethylene as an anesthetic and more potent an irritant. Its TLV of 50 ppm is set to prevent both effects. A recent NTP inhalation bioassay provided clear evidence of carcinogenicity in mice and male rats and some evidence in female rats. Limited studies of the effects of perchloroethylene on reproduction in animals are not adequate for evaluation but suggest that perchloroethylene may be spermatotoxic. One case has been reported of obstructive jaundice in a newborn who was nursed in a dry-cleaning shop where perchloroethylene was used and was found in the mother's breast milk.

3. TRICHLOROETHANE

1,1,1-Trichloroethane is only weakly hepatotoxic, with minor injury reported following massive overexposure. It is the weakest anesthetic of this group; its TLV of 350 ppm is established to prevent this effect. Sudden deaths in situations indicative of acute overexposure have been attributed to cardiac arrhythmias as a result of cardiac sensitization. The compound is weakly positive for mutagenicity in *Salmonella*, but it has not been adequately tested for carcinogenicity or reproductive toxicity.

4. CARBON TETRACHLORIDE

Carbon tetrachloride is a potent anesthetic. Both acute and chronic effects on the liver and kidneys have been reported at levels not much higher than those causing central nervous system depression. The TLV of 5 ppm (skin) was established to prevent fatty infiltration of the liver demonstrated in animals at 10 ppm and potentiated by alcohol ingestion. Deaths have occurred from both hepatic and renal necrosis, and liver cancer has been reported in workers following acute liver damage from acute overexposure. The TLV has an A2 (suspected human carcinogen) designation. There is evidence that carbon tetrachloride is fetotoxic but not teratogenic, and it causes testicular and ovarian damage in animals at toxic doses—but there is no evidence about effects at nontoxic doses.

5. CHLOROFORM

Chloroform is only slightly less potent than carbon tetrachloride as an anesthetic and liver toxin. Its TLV was lowered to 10 ppm (A2) by ACGIH because of its carcinogenicity to rats (epithelial tumors of the kidney) and mice (hepatocarcinoma) and embryotoxicity to the rat at 30–300 ppm by inhalation.

6. METHYLENE CHLORIDE

Methylene chloride is similar to perchloroethylene and trichloroethylene in potency as an anesthetic and liver toxin. It is unique in that it is metabolized to carbon monoxide, with formation of carboxyhemoglobin. At exposure levels above 100 ppm, carboxyhemoglobin levels can exceed 10%, so that the presence of anoxia in addition to anesthesia must be considered. The TLV was recently lowered from 100 ppm to 50 ppm to provide a wider margin of safety in preventing liver injury and lowering carboxyhemoglobin to near background levels—and in recognition of evidence for carcinogenicity in animals. Methylenechloride was fetotoxic but not teratogenic to rats and mice exposed to 1225 ppm.

CHLOROFLUOROCARBONS (CFCs)

Essentials of Diagnosis

Acute effects:
- Respiratory tract irritation: sore nose, sore throat, cough.
- Anesthesia: dizziness, headache, nausea, vomiting, sleepiness, fatigue, "drunkenness," slurred speech, disequilibrium, disorientation, depression, loss of consciousness.
- Cardiac sensitization: dizziness, palpitations, faintness, loss of consciousness, arrhythmia on ambulatory cardiac monitoring.

Chronic effects:
- Dermatitis: dry, cracked, erythematous skin.

General Considerations

Chlorofluorocarbon solvents are aliphatic hydrocarbons (methane or ethane) that contain one or more atoms each of chlorine and fluorine. Table 27–1 lists the commonly used chlorofluorocarbon solvents.* CFCs are often referred to as Freons, which is the trade name of CFCs manufactured by Dupont. A CFC may be formulated with another organic solvent, such as methanol or methylene chloride, in a proprietary solvent mixture.

Use

The main solvent uses of CFCs are as cleaning and degreasing agents. CFC-113 has been used increasingly in dry cleaning in closed systems ("dry-to-dry") as a replacement for open systems ("wet-to-dry") using perchloroethylene. Other uses include refrigeration and air-conditioning fluids, propellants, foam blowing agents, vehicles for pesticides, paints, and other materials, and intermediates in the manufacture of plastics and resins. Restrictions have been placed on CFC use for propellants because of their role in depletion of stratospheric ozone. The completely halogenated CFCs are those implicated in this effect. Bromine-containing compounds are widely used as fire extinguishing agents (see Chapter 28).

Five CFCs account for almost 99% of all US chlorofluorocarbon production. The most common uses for these compounds are shown in Table 27–4.

Occupational & Environmental Exposures

The widespread use of CFCs in industry and in consumer products has resulted in exposure of large numbers of workers and consumers and in global contamination of the environment. In homes where aerosols are used, ambient air concentrations of CFCs can be significantly higher than that outside.

Table 27–4. Uses of chlorofluorocarbons.

Use	Chlorofluorocarbon
Cleaning and degreasing	CFC-113, CFC-11
Refrigeration and air conditioning	CFC-22, CFC-12, CFC-11
Foam blowing	CFC-11
Aerosol propellant	CFC-12, CFC-11, CFC-114
Plastics manufacturing	CFC-12, CFC-22

---

*The numbering system for chlorofluorocarbons offers a convenient method of determining their chemical formulas. The "units" digit is the number of fluorine atoms (with CFC-113, this would be 3); the "tens" digit is the number of hydrogen atoms plus 1; and the "hundreds" digit is the number of carbon atoms minus 1. (Thus, CFC 113 would contain 3 fluorine atoms, no hydrogen atoms, and 2 carbon atoms, thereby requiring 3 chlorine atoms to make trichlorotrifluoroethane.)

Pharmacokinetics

Very little information is available on the pharmacokinetics of CFCs. Most are probably resistant to metabolism and are excreted rapidly unchanged in exhaled air. Correlations undoubtedly exist between exposure and concentrations in exhaled air, but information is too limited to recommend biologic monitoring.

Health Effects

The CFCs are of relatively low toxicity. All are anesthetics but require exposure to concentrations above 500–1000 ppm before this effect is manifested. Such levels most commonly are encountered in enclosed spaces (eg, cleaning out a degreasing tank) or when the CFC is heated (eg, using a heated vapor degreaser) or sprayed (eg, when used as propellant). They have not been associated with chronic neurobehavioral effects. They are not strong irritants. Prolonged or frequent skin contact can cause a typical solvent dermatitis. Cardiac sensitization was first demonstrated for CFCs after a number of cases of sudden death of persons abusing CFC-11 and CFC-12 beginning in the late 1960s. An NCI bioassay of CFC-11 was negative for mice and inconclusive for rats, while CFC-22 may have caused a slight increase in salivary gland tumors in male rats. Two rarely used chlorofluorocarbons, CFC-31 and CFC-133a, were carcinogenic in a limited gavage assay in rats. CFC-22, CFC-31, CFC-142b, CFC-143, and CFC-143a are positive in one or more short-term genotoxicity tests. CFC-22, the only one of the genotoxic CFCs in common use, is a weak bacterial mutagen. A number of CFCs have been tested for teratogenicity, including CFC-11, CFC-12, CFC-21, CFC-22, CFC-31, CFC-114, CFC-123b, and CFC-142b, but either because of inadequate design or inadequate reporting no conclusions about effects can be reached. Unpublished studies have reported that CFC-22 is teratogenic in rats but not rabbits, producing microphthalmia and anophthalmia at inhalation levels of 50,000 ppm.

ALDEHYDES

Essentials of Diagnosis

Acute effects:
- Respiratory tract irritation: sore nose, sore throat, cough.

Chronic effects:
- Dermatitis: dry, cracked, erythematous skin.
- Asthma: cough, wheezing, shortness of breath, dyspnea on exertion, decreased FVC on pulmonary function testing reversible with bronchodilators.

General Considerations

The aldehydes are used primarily as preservatives, disinfectants, and chemical intermediates rather than as solvents. Glutaraldehyde is commonly used in hospitals as a disinfectant. The prototype aldehyde, formaldehyde, is discussed in Chapter 26. Most aldehydes are such strong irritants that at levels that would produce anesthetic effects irritation would be intolerable. Asthma has been associated with exposure to formaldehyde but not other aldehydes to date.

MISCELLANEOUS SOLVENTS

Turpentine

Turpentine is a mixture of substances called terpenes, primarily pinene. Gum turpentine is extracted from pine pitch, wood turpentine from wood chips. It has had greater home than industrial use as a solvent. It is irritating and anesthetic and is one of the few solvents that causes allergic contact dermatitis. The incidence of sensitization varies with the type of pine, being generally higher with European than American pines. Owing to the frequency of allergic dermatitis, the availability of turpentine is now extremely limited. Limonene is a terpene used as a solvent for art paints that also causes allergic contact dermatitis.

Dimethylformamide

Dimethylformamide is a useful solvent because of its solubility in both aqueous and lipid media. However, these properties also result in its being well absorbed by all routes of exposure. It is a potent hepatotoxin and has been associated with both hepatitis and pancreatitis following occupational exposure. This hazard precludes most general industrial solvent uses. Two recent case series have associated dimethylformamide exposure with testicular cancer. Exposure can be monitored biologically by measuring monomethylformamide and related metabolites in urine.

Dimethylsulfoxide

Like dimethylformamide, dimethylsulfoxide is soluble in a variety of media and is well absorbed by all routes of exposure. It appears to potentiate the absorption of other substances through the skin. Its use has not been associated with significant toxicity, but it has been subjected to little scientific study. It has a characteristic garliclike or oysterlike odor that is present in exhaled air of exposed persons. Its use as a dermally applied anti-inflammatory agent is not approved by the Federal Drug Administration, though it is used in that way in veterinary medicine.

REFERENCES

Andrews LS, Snyder R: Toxic effects of solvents and vapors. In: *Casarett and Doull's Toxicology: The Basic Science of Poisons,* 3rd ed. Klaassen CO, Amdur NW, Doull J (editors). Macmillan, 1986.

Baker EL Jr, Smith TJ, Landrigan PJ: The neurotoxicity of industrial solvents: A review of the literature. *Am J Ind Med* 1985;**8:**207.

Clayton GD, Clayton FE (editors): *Patty's Industrial Hygiene and Toxicology.* Wiley, 1981.

Collings AJ, Luxon SG (editors): *Safe Use of Solvents.* Academic Press, 1982.

Craft BF: Solvents and related compounds. In: *Environmental and Occupational Medicine.* Rom WN (editor). Little, Brown, 1983.

Daniell WE, Couser WG, Rosenstock L: Occupational solvent exposure and glomerulonephritis: A case report and review of the literature. *JAMA* 1988;**259:**2280.

Englund A, Ringen K, Mehlman MA (editors): *Occupational Health Hazards of Solvents.* Princeton Scientific, 1982.

Grayson M (editor): *Kirk-Othner Encyclopedia of Chemical Technology,* 3rd ed. Wiley, 1985.

James RC: The toxic effects of organic solvents. In: *Industrial Toxicology: Safety and Health Applications in the Workplace.* Williams PL, Burson JL (editors). Van Nostrand Reinhold, 1985.

Juntunen J: Organic solvent intoxications in occupational neurology. *Acta Neurol Scand [Suppl]* 1984;**98:**105.

Lilis R: Diseases associated with exposure to chemical substances: Organic solvents. In: *Maxcy-Rosenau Public Health and Preventive Medicine,* 12th ed. Last JM (editor). Appleton-Century-Crofts, 1986.

Lundberg P (editor): Proceedings of the international conference on organic solvent toxicity, Stockholm, 15–17 October 1984. *Scand J Work Environ Health* 1985; **11(Suppl 1):**6.

National Institute for Occupational Safety and Health: *Current Intelligence Bulletin #48: Organic Solvent Neurotoxicity.* NIOSH, 1987.

Riihimäaki V, Ulfvarson U (editors): *Safety and Health Aspects of Organic Solvents.* Proceedings of the international course on safety and health aspects of organic solvents, held in Espso, Finland, April 22–26, 1985. Alan R. Liss, 1986.

Plastics

28

Richard Lewis, MD, MPH

The emergence of the plastics industry during the past 30 years has had a major impact on many other industries, including manufacturing, construction, and transportation. Articles made from plastics are ubiquitous in industrialized societies, being found in appliances, automobiles, toys, home furnishings, clothing, insulation, food and beverage containers, and countless other applications. Advances in plastics technology have resulted in the development of materials with properties that match or surpass in quality and utility those of traditional materials such as metal, wood, and glass.

Plastics are divided into 2 main classes (Table 28–1). **Thermoplastics** are linear or branched polymers that can be repeatedly softened and reshaped with the application of heat or pressure. These materials are recyclable, though variations in formulations and additives limit the recycling of products after they have reached the consumer. **Thermoset** plastics undergo a chemical reaction during processing that results in permanent cross-linking. The finished materials are resistant to heat and cannot be re-formed. Table 28–1 lists the major thermoplastic and thermoset polymers in current use.

HEALTH HAZARDS IN THE MANUFACTURE OF PLASTICS

As the plastics industry has grown over the last several decades, health hazards in its manufacturing processes have become an important concern to the occupational health practitioner. These hazards reflect 3 principal aspects of the manufacture of plastics: resin manufacture, plastic processing, and combustion.

Resin Manufacture

Raw materials for the production of polymers from which plastics are formed are derived chiefly from crude oil and gas. The chemical processes involved in the formation of plastics include crude oil distillation followed by catalytic cracking and reformation. Other chemical reactions, such as the addition of halogen, may take place prior to polymerization.

Most of the polymerization processes take place in closed systems, and the health hazards of resin manufacture are similar to those of the petrochemical industry. Workers may have exposure to vapors and dusts containing chemical intermediates, polymers, and additives during loading, mixing, pelletizing, and maintenance operations. Proper storage and handling of chemicals and additives is mandatory. Reactions must be carefully controlled to avoid chemical release or explosion. Dry mixing and pelletizing operations may generate high concentrations of airborne dusts of combustible plastic materials, presenting an explosion hazard. The use of heavy machinery requires proper safety measures to avoid worker injury.

Plastic Processing

The plastic processing industry converts the resins into finished products. Granules and powders may be compounded with additives prior to processing, and workers in these operations may have exposures similar to those of the resin manufacturers. Thermoset and partially polymerized materials may be supplied in solid or liquid form, and workers handling these materials may have exposure to unreacted intermediates and catalysts.

Plastic processing equipment uses high temperatures and pressures and must be equipped with guards and safety rails to avoid serious burns, amputations, and crush injuries. Plastic grinding may generate polymer dust, resulting in inhalation and possible combustion hazard. The overheating of plastic materials during processing, cleaning, and maintenance may expose workers to the thermal decomposition products of the polymer materials. Finishing operations may expose workers to a variety of other

Table 28–1. Principal plastic materials.

Thermoplastics
  Polyethylene
  Polyvinyl chloride
  Polypropylene
  Polystyrene
  Polyester
  ABS (acrylonitrile-butadiene-styrene)
  Acrylics
  Nylon
  Fluoropolymers
Thermosets
  Phenolics
  Polyurethane
  Urea and melamine
  Epoxies
  Cellulosics

chemical compounds, such as solvents and adhesives. In addition, cutting of plastics may result in repetitive motion injuries, such as tendinitis, sprains, and carpal tunnel syndrome.

COMBUSTION PRODUCT HAZARDS

Thermoplastic materials must be heated during processing. The temperatures required to achieve proper fluidity vary with the composition of the polymer and the additives. Overheating of plastics results in thermal decomposition and the release of oligomers, monomers, and other combustion products. The composition of the mixture of gases and vapors that are evolved is extremely complex and depends not only on the chemical constituents of the polymer but also on the temperature. Workers may be exposed to the thermal decomposition products of plastics through accidental overheating during processing or during clean-out and maintenance operations. In addition, the burning of plastic materials during fires may present a health hazard to fire fighters and the public.

The main combustion hazards that have been identified for the major classes of plastic materials are listed in Table 28–2. This list is far from complete, and new degradation products will be identified as research progresses. It is important to note that while combustion hazards are primarily respiratory irritants (hydrochloric acid, aldehydes), significant pulmonary injury (oxides of nitrogen) and systemic poisoning (carbon monoxide, cyanides) may occur. The long-term health effects of exposure to combustion products are unknown.

THERMOPLASTICS

POLYETHYLENE

Essentials of Diagnosis
- Asphyxia (ethylene).
- Respiratory irritation (thermal decomposition products).

Exposure Limits
ACGIH TLV: Asphyxiant

General Considerations & Production
Polyethylene is a semicrystalline, lightweight thermoplastic, first produced in 1942. High- and low-density polyethylene resins account for almost one-third of the current production of plastic materials in the United States. Over 100 different brands of polyethylene are available.

Polyethylene is produced by the polymerization of ethylene in either continuous-flow or tubular reactors. Catalysts include chromic oxide, aluminum alkyls, titanium chloride, and t-butyl esters. Density can be altered by addition of other olefins, such as butene, hexene, octene, and vinyl acetate. Liquid polymer is then cooled and pelletized.

Use
A primary use of high-density polyethylene is in the production of containers (milk bottles, drums, fuel tanks), using blow molding. Other uses include the production of trash bags, pipe and wire covering by extrusion, and the production of containers, toys, and housewares by injection molding. Low-density polyethylene has higher clarity and is used for films, coating, shrink-wrapping, and food packaging and is primarily formed by extrusion.

Exposure
The principal hazard of exposure to ethylene is asphyxia. Catalysts used are potent irritants of the eyes, skin, and respiratory system.

When burned at 230 °C (450 °F), polyethylene gives off primarily carbon monoxide, though the respiratory irritants acrolein and formaldehyde may also be formed. Occupational asthma was attributed to exposure to acrolein in wrappers cutting polyethylene with a hot wire.

The induction of tumors (primarily sarcomas) in laboratory animals by implants of polyethylene has been attributed to solid state carcinogenesis rather than an effect of the polymer or monomer. Intrauterine devices made of polyethylene have been associated with endometrial metaplasia, perhaps by a similar process.

Prevention
The use of enclosed processes will prevent exposure to ethylene gas. Proper respiratory protection

Table 28–2. Thermal degradation products of some plastics.

Polymer	Degradation Products	Hazard
Polyethylene	Carbon monoxide	S
Polyvinyl chloride	Vinyl chloride	S, C
	Hydrochloric acid, phosgene	I, R
Polystyrene	Styrene	S
	Benzene	S, C
Fluoropolymers	Carbonyl fluoride	I, R
	Perfluoroisobutylene	I, R
	Hydrogen fluoride	I, R
Polyurethane	Aldehydes, ammonia	I, R
	Cyanide	S
	Isocyanates	I, R
	Nitrogen dioxide	R
Phenolics	Formaldehyde	I, R, S
	Aldehydes, ammonia	I, R
	Cyanide	S
	Nitrogen dioxide	R

A = asphyxiant; C = carcinogen; I = mucous membrane irritant; R = respiratory irritant; S = systemic poison.

should be worn by persons cleaning machinery or reaction vessels. Avoiding overheating or burning polyethylene will prevent exposure to irritant aldehydes and other decomposition products. Medical surveillance of workers should focus on the respiratory system.

Treatment

Workers overcome by ethylene in an oxygen-deficient atmosphere should be rescued by persons equipped with air-supplied respirators. Once the victim has been removed to a fresh air environment, treatment consists of cardiopulmonary resuscitation and 100% oxygen. Exposure to respiratory irritants usually results in self-limited symptoms that resolve after removal from exposure. Treat asthma with inhaled bronchodilators.

POLYPROPYLENE

Essentials of Diagnosis
- Asphyxia (propylene).
- Respiratory irritation (thermal combustion products).

Exposure Limits
ACGIH TLV: Asphyxiant

General Considerations & Production

Polypropylene was first brought into production in 1957. It is characterized by high heat resistance, strength, and resistance to corrosion by chemicals such as detergents and alcohols. Production of polypropylene generally occurs in a slurry with a hydrocarbon diluent and the addition of an organometallic catalyst. High-activity catalysts have been developed that improve the quality of the finished polymer. Solvent vapors are generated during drying and grinding.

Use

Through extrusion, a major application of polypropylene is in the production of fibers for carpeting and clothing. Blow and injection molding are used to produce medical containers, syringes, battery casings, dashboards, packing materials, and components for appliances.

Exposure

Polypropylene is an asphyxiant. As in the case of polyethylene, the main hazards are respiratory irritation due to exposure to thermal decomposition products. This may occur during the welding of pipe made from polypropylene, particularly in poorly ventilated spaces.

Prevention

Awareness of the hazards from release of propylene into enclosed spaces will prevent asphyxia during maintenance and cleaning operations. Polypropy-

lene should not be burned or heated without proper ventilation or respiratory protection.

Treatment

Treatment is the same as that for polyethylene, above.

POLYVINYL CHLORIDE

Essentials of Diagnosis
- Asthma and pneumoconiosis: wheezing, dyspnea, cough, chest tightness.
- Hepatitis and angiosarcoma: nausea, vomiting, jaundice, hepatomegaly.
- Acro-osteolysis (vinyl chloride monomer): loss of bone structure at ends of phalanges.

Exposure Limits
ACGIH TLV: 5 ppm TWA
OSHA PEL: 1 ppm TWA, 5 ppm ceiling (15 minutes)
NIOSH REL: Lowest reliable detectable concentration

General Considerations & Production

Though polyvinyl production began in 1927, it was not until the 1970s that the toxicity and carcinogenicity of vinyl chloride monomer became widely recognized as a result of worker exposure during the manufacture of polyvinyl chloride resins. Vinyl chloride is a gas at room temperature, and polymerization reactions take place in pressure vessels. Whereas in recent years worker exposure to vinyl chloride has been reduced significantly, many current workers in the industry may have had heavy exposure to this substance in the past. A full discussion of the occupational health hazards of vinyl chloride is found in Chapter 26.

Use

The commercial value of polyvinyl chloride is related to its processing versatility, strength, corrosion resistance, and cost. Rigid and flexible resins have diverse applications and are processed by a variety of molding methods. Sheet, pipe, wire and cable coating, and conduits formed by extrusion have major applications in the building and construction industries. Flexible polyvinyl chloride is used to form garden hoses; automobile upholstery, floor mats, and trim; baby pants, medical tubing, and intravenous solution bags. Compression molding is used to produce phonograph records. Polyvinyl chloride can be blow-molded into bottles and is also used to coat flooring, furnishings, and clothing.

Exposure

The potential exposure to unreacted vinyl chloride monomer was great in polyvinyl chloride production facilities prior to 1960, a time when exposures have been estimated to routinely exceed 1000 ppm. Workers often were lowered into reaction vessels during cleaning, resulting in significant exposure. Loading, drying, and bagging operations also resulted in significant exposure. Between 1970 and 1974, exposures were estimated to range between 100 and 200 ppm.

There were further reductions following the promulgation of the OSHA standard of 1 ppm in 1974. Industrial hygiene surveys by NIOSH revealed a continued reduction in exposure in the production of polyvinyl chloride resins between 1974 and 1977, with most exposures being less than 5 ppm. The workers with greatest potential exposure included reactor operators, baggers, and maintenance workers, while exposures in polyvinyl chloride fabrication were generally less than 1 ppm. Since 1977, routine worker exposures in the polyvinyl chloride manufacturing industry are assumed not to have exceeded the current standard, but intermittent peak exposures may still occur if proper work practices are not observed.

Clinical Findings

The main hazards in the production and processing of polyvinyl chloride are exposure to vinyl chloride monomer, polyvinyl chloride dust, and thermal decomposition products.

A. Acute Effects: The effects of acute massive exposure to vinyl chloride (10,000 ppm) include narcosis and chemical hepatitis.

B. Chronic Effects: Chronic excessive exposure can result in cirrhosis, with portal hypertension or development of hepatic angiosarcoma. Other chronic effects include acro-osteolysis—an immunologic disorder manifested by Raynaud's phenomenon—and clubbing and lytic lesions of the fingers and toes. Hematologic cancers and brain tumors are also increased in workers with chronic exposure to vinyl chloride.

Exposure to polyvinyl chloride dust during production of resins and fabrication has been associated with the development of mild pneumoconiosis in some workers, with slight impairment of pulmonary function. This is thought to be a granulomatous reaction, characterized by x-ray findings of small rounded opacities of low profusion. One study has found an association of exposure to polyvinyl chloride and lung cancer.

The main thermal decomposition product of polyvinyl chloride is hydrochloric acid, a respiratory irritant. In certain cases, other irritants, such as phosgene, may be formed. "Meat wrapper's asthma" was attributed to the cutting of polyvinyl chloride wrap with a hot wire and was attributed to exposure to both hydrochloric acid and an additive.

Prevention

Protection of workers in the polyvinyl chloride industry from exposure to vinyl chloride monomer will result in the reduction or elimination of the corresponding health effects, both acute and chronic. Workers should also avoid exposure to polyvinyl

chloride dust generated during grinding, drying, or cleaning operations. Medical surveillance should be directed toward the detection of abnormal liver function in workers with potential exposure to high levels of vinyl chloride. For workers exposed to polyvinyl chloride, periodic chest x-rays and assessment of respiratory function are indicated.

Treatment

Workers who have evidence of liver injury after exposure to vinyl chloride should be removed from further exposure. Biopsy may assist in the diagnosis. Acro-osteolysis is usually irreversible. Symptomatic vasospasm (Raynaud's phenomenon) may respond to use of gloves and cautious use of vasodilators. Respiratory irritation resulting in asthma should be treated with inhaled bronchodilators.

POLYSTYRENE & COPOLYMERS

Essentials of Diagnosis

- Lightheadedness and incoordination (styrene monomer).
- Altered liver function (styrene monomer): nausea and vomiting, jaundice, hepatomegaly.
- Mucous membrane and respiratory irritation: wheezing, cough.
- Acrylonitrile and butadiene: ?cancer.

Exposure Limits

Styrene
  ACGIH TLV: 50 ppm TWA
  OSHA PEL: 50 ppm TWA, 100 ppm STEL
Acrylonitrile
  ACGIH TLV: 2 ppm TWA
  OSHA PEL: 2 ppm TWA, 10 ppm ceiling
  NIOSH REL: 1 ppm TWA, 10 ppm ceiling (15 minutes)
1,3-Butatiene
  ACGIH TLV: 10 ppm TWA
  NIOSH REL: Reduce exposure to lowest feasible concentration.

General Considerations

Styrene-based polymers were widely used in the 1940s because of the demand for synthetic rubber. This group of polymers now ranks third in total production, after polyethylene and polyvinyl chloride. The major classes of styrene-based polymers are polystyrene, acrylonitrile-butadiene-styrene (ABS), and styrene-acrylonitrile (SAN).

Production

Styrene is produced by the catalytic dehydrogenation of ethylbenzene. Over 90% of styrene produced is used for polymers, primarily polystyrene and to a lesser extent ABS, SAN, and synthetic rubbers. Polystyrene resins are produced by the bulk polymerization process at low temperatures 48.8–93 °C (120–200 °F). The rate of polymerization increases at higher temperatures, and careful temperature monitoring is required to prevent uncontrolled reactions. A bead polymerization process in suspension is used to produce polystyrene foams. SAN resins are random, amorphous copolymers produced by suspension or emulsion. ABS resins are manufactured using a graft polymerization process in which styrene-acrylonitrile copolymers are added to polybutadiene rubber.

Use

The major applications of polystyrene are in packaging, disposables, toys, and building materials. Foam polystyrene is used to form egg cartons, plates, cups, and food containers through extrusion. ABS copolymers combine the chemical resistance of acrylonitrile, the impact resistance of butadiene, and the rigidity and gloss of styrene for diverse applications in business machinery housings, telecommunications equipment, automobile grills, pipe fittings, and appliances. SAN copolymers are used for appliances, battery casings, and packaging.

Exposure

Workers engaged in the production of polystyrene resins may have exposure to unreacted styrene monomer during loading and maintenance operations. The potential for runaway reactions may result in intermittent releases of high concentrations of styrene into the workroom air if conditions are not carefully controlled. The residual monomer content of polystyrene resins is low—usually less than 0.5%—but residual monomer may be released during the heating of polystyrene. Exposure to acrylonitrile and butadiene may also occur during the production of copolymers. Inhalation is the main route of exposure, but both styrene and acrylonitrile are absorbed through the skin.

Health Hazards

Polystyrene is biologically inert, and the main hazard is exposure to styrene monomer. High concentrations (over 100 ppm) of styrene cause irritation of the eyes and mucous membranes. Prolonged skin contact may cause dermatitis and defatting of the skin and may lead to skin absorption. Exposure to the styrene in the production of polymer resins may cause lightheadedness, dizziness, and incoordination. Workers with chronic exposure to styrene have been found to manifest changes in electroencephalograms, slowed nerve conduction velocities, and impaired performance on neuropsychologic tests, suggesting both central and peripheral nervous system effects. Most of these findings were subclinical. Changes in hepatic function, including increases in serum enzymes and serum bile acids, have suggested possible hepatotoxicity. Styrene is mutagenic and has been associated with the induction of chromosomal aberrations in humans.

Acrylonitrile is a potent eye, mucous membrane, and skin irritant. Excessive exposure may result in vague symptoms of headache, fatigue, and nausea. Acrylonitrile is a chemical asphyxiant equivalent to cyanide, and acute exposure may be fatal. Acrylonitrile is an animal carcinogen and a probable human carcinogen, exposure being associated with an excess of both lung and colon cancers in exposed workers.

Butadiene is a gas at room temperature and an irritant of the eyes and mucous membranes and a central nervous system depressant at high concentrations. Recently, 1,3-butadiene has been found to be an animal carcinogen and is suspected of being a human carcinogen.

The main combustion products of thermal decomposition of polystyrene are styrene, benzene, and carbon monoxide. With acrylonitrile copolymers, the major hazard is the production of hydrogen cyanide, ammonia, and the oxides of nitrogen.

Prevention

Awareness of the potential neurotoxicity of styrene and concern over possible carcinogenicity of acrylonitrile and butadiene has resulted in stricter control of worker exposures to these compounds. Both respiratory and skin protection are required during loading and maintenance operations, which carry a high risk of exposure to unreacted monomers. Styrene polymers should not be welded or burned—particularly those containing acrylonitrile. Medical surveillance of styrene-exposed workers in resin manufacture should include assessment of nervous system symptoms and careful neurologic and mental status examinations. Blood testing should include liver enzyme determinations. Biologic monitoring of workers exposed to styrene can include urine metabolites (phenylglyoxylic acid and mandelic acid) or the measurement of styrene in blood or exhaled air. Urinary thiocyanate levels can be used in the biologic monitoring of workers exposed to acrylonitrile.

Treatment

Workers who develop acute or chronic nervous system symptoms related to exposure to styrene should be removed from further exposure. Skin irritation should be treated with local care and topical steroids.

Overexposure to acrylonitrile is a medical emergency. After resuscitation of the worker, contaminated clothing should be removed and the skin cleansed to eliminate further absorption. Treatment with amyl nitrite should be given as for cyanide poisoning. Alternatively, sodium nitrite and sodium thiosulfate may be given. Persons with suspected serious poisoning should be hospitalized for observation for 24–48 hours.

Skin, eye, and mucous membrane irritation due to exposure to butadiene should be treated by cleansing the affected area followed by local care.

ACRYLICS

Essentials of Diagnosis

- Respiratory and mucous membrane irritation: cough, wheezing.

- Allergic contact dermatitis: swelling, redness, pruritus.
- Headache, fatigue, irritability (methyl methacrylate monomer).

Exposure Limits

Methylmethacrylate
   ACGIH TLV: 100 ppm TWA
   OSHA PEL: 100 ppm TWA
Methyl acrylate
   ACGIH TLV: 10 ppm TWA
   OSHA PEL: 10 ppm TWA
Ethyl acrylate
   ACGIH TLV: 5 ppm TWA, 25 ppm STEL
   OSHA PEL: 5 ppm TWA, 25 ppm STEL

General Considerations

The acrylics are a broad group of plastics of which the main classes of monomers are the acrylate or methacrylate esters. Polyacrylonitrile and other copolymers are also included in this class.

Production

Methyl methacrylate, the major monomer used in acrylic production, is formed through the reaction of acetone and hydrogen cyanide. This is then heated with methanol in the presence of sulfuric acid to liberate the monomer. Bulk polymerization is initiated by peroxide catalysts and liberates heat, which must be dissipated. Resins are supplied as clear sheets, pellets, or syrups.

Use

Acrylics combine the properties of crystal clarity, environmental and chemical resistance, and pigment compatibility for use as lightweight substitutes for glass. Extruded sheet is used in lighting fixtures, signs, displays, windows, and face shields. Acrylics are also used as coatings and laminates for other plastics, metal, and wood.

Health Hazards

Acrylic monomers are upper respiratory and mucous membrane irritants. Skin sensitization may occur, resulting in contact dermatitis after exposure to unreacted acrylic monomers. Methyl methacrylate exposure has caused symptoms of headache. Fatigue and irritability in exposed workers and central nervous system effects have been demonstrated in experimental animals. Hypotension and cardiac arrest were reported in elderly persons in whom methyl methacrylate was used as an adhesive for hip prosthesis.

Prevention

Skin contact with acrylic monomers should be avoided. In persons who develop dermatitis, patch testing should be performed to differentiate allergic from irritant effects. Once allergy has been demonstrated, workers should be removed from further exposure. Medical surveillance should include exam-ination of the skin and respiratory system and assessment of nervous system symptoms.

Treatment

Central nervous system effects related to exposure to acrylic monomers resolve with removal from exposure. Allergic dermatitis should be treated with topical steroids.

FLUOROPOLYMERS

Essentials of Diagnosis
- Polymer fume fever (fever, chills, respiratory impairment).
- Chronic lung disease: wheezing, cough, dyspnea.

Exposure Limits

ACGIH TLV: There is no TLV for polytetrafluoroethylene decomposition products. Exposure should be minimized.

General Considerations

Fluoropolymers are a class of plastics that combine properties of high resistance with low friction for application in electronics, coatings, and cable sheaths. These compounds were introduced in the 1960s and comprise a small but growing class of materials.

Production

The fluorinated monomers are produced through the fluorination of aliphatic and chlorinated hydrocarbons using hydrogen fluoride. Polytetrafluoroethylene—the main fluoropolymer resin—is polymerized in the presence of water with a peroxide catalyst. The fluoropolymers have high melt viscosity, which requires special processing and extrusion equipment capable of generating high pressures.

Use

The fluoropolymers are resistant to solvents and used in linings and components of chemical processing equipment. The low-friction and resistance properties are used in coatings and sheathing for wire and cables. Fluoropolymers are also used for nonstick coating applications on home cookware, food processing equipment, and production line conveyer parts.

Health Hazards

A variety of fluorinated and chlorinated hydrocarbons may be used in the production of fluoropolymer resins. Although these are usually reacted in closed systems, worker exposure during loading or maintenance operations may result in symptoms of solvent narcosis (lightheadedness, headache and incoordination).

Exposure to the thermal decomposition of polytetrafluoroethylene has resulted in a syndrome known as "polymer fume fever" characterized by fever, chills, malaise, cough, and dyspnea several hours after exposure, with spontaneous resolution after 12–24 hours. The cause of this syndrome has not been identified, but several respiratory irritants may be evolved during the thermal decomposition of fluoropolymers, including carbonyl fluoride, perfluoroisobutylene, and hydrogen fluoride. The syndrome has been associated with the accidental or intentional overheating of fluoropolymers during processing or maintenance operations. This has also been associated with smoking cigarettes that may have been contaminated with fluoropolymer resins. In some cases, chronic respiratory impairment has occurred in workers who have experienced episodes of polymer fume fever, indicating that the condition may not necessarily be benign and self-limited.

Prevention

Solvent compounds should be properly stored and handled to avoid excess worker exposure. Care should be taken to avoid overheating of fluoropolymers. Workers should not smoke in areas where fluoropolymers are being handled and processed. Medical surveillance should include careful questioning regarding symptoms of polymer fume fever as well as periodic assessment of pulmonary function. Industrial hygiene and engineering measures should be instituted to prevent worker exposures that result in symptoms of polymer fume fever.

Treatment

Polymer fume fever is a self-limited condition that does not require specific treatment. If bronchospasm is evident after exposure to thermal decomposition products, bronchodilators by inhalation should be provided.

THERMOSETS

PHENOLICS

Essentials of Diagnosis
- Respiratory irritation and bronchospasm: wheezing, cough, dyspnea.
- Irritant or allergic dermatitis: swelling, redness, pruritus.
- Possible pneumoconiosis: wheezing, cough, dyspnea, chest tightness.

Exposure Limits
Formaldehyde
  ACGIH TLV: 1 ppm TWA, 2 ppm STEL
  OSHA PEL: 1 ppm TWA, 2 ppm STEL
  NIOSH REL: 0.016 ppm TWA, 0.1 ppm ceiling
    (15 minutes)
Phenol
  ACGIH TLV: 5 ppm TWA
  OSHA PEL: 5 ppm TWA
  NIOSH REL: 5.2 ppm TWA, 15.6 ppm ceiling
    (15 minutes)
Cresol
  ACGIH TLV: 5 ppm TWA
  OSHA PEL: 5 ppm TWA
  NIOSH REL: 2.3 ppm TWA

General Considerations
The phenolics are hard crystalline resins formed by the reaction of a phenol and an aldehyde—most frequently formaldehyde. These were the first synthetic resins produced.

Production
Phenolic resins are of 2 main types. Single-stage resins, or resoles, contain phenol, formaldehyde, and an alkaline catalyst. The condensation process in a charged reaction vessel is interrupted while the material is still thermoplastic, and the resin is supplied as a flake, powder, or liquid that requires heating for final curing.

The 2-stage resins, or novalacs, contain excess phenol and an acid catalyst. Hexamethylene tetramine is added to the resin molding powder prior to processing to complete the cure.

Use
Most phenolic resins produced in the United States are used for the production of plywood and other building materials, adhesives, and bonding agents and insulation. Molded products are used in the automotive industry to replace metals in transmissions, brake components, and electric motors. The electrical resistance properties of resoles are used in electrical components and for laminating surfaces. Phenolics are also used to crease resistant fabrics.

Health Hazards
The main hazards in the production and handling of phenolic resins are skin irritation or allergic sensitization due to phenol or formaldehyde. Contact dermatitis may result from handling raw materials, resins, or finished products due to exposure to uncured resin. Phenol, formaldehyde, and hexamethylene tetramine are respiratory and mucous membrane irritants and may induce symptoms of eye irritation, cough, and congestion in sensitive individuals at concentrations near the current exposure limits. Phenol is absorbed through the skin, and chronic exposure has resulted in symptoms of fatigue, weight loss, and hepatic dysfunction. Hexamethylene tetramine is metabolized to formaldehyde, and both compounds can also cause systemic symptoms of headache, malaise, and fatigue. Exposure to powdered resins has been associated with chronic respiratory impairment and possible pneumoconiosis. Thermal decomposition products include phenol, formaldehyde, acrolein, and carbon monoxide. Formaldehyde is a suspect human carcinogen and is capable of inducing nasal cancers in experimental animals.

Prevention
Skin protection is mandatory in the production and

processing of phenolics. Respiratory protection should be used during loading and maintenance operations and when handling resin powders. Workers who develop skin problems should be patch-tested for sensitivity to both resin materials and finished polymers. Those who develop true allergy may need to be removed from further exposure. Medical surveillance should include a careful history to elicit irritant and systemic symptoms and periodic assessment of respiratory function. Urinary phenol levels may be of value in following workers with the greatest potential exposure to this compound.

Treatment

Allergic or irritant dermatitis should be treated by application of topical steroids. Respiratory irritation resulting in bronchospasm should be treated with inhaled bronchodilators. Persons suspected of overexposure to phenol should be removed from exposure until symptoms have resolved.

POLYURETHANE

Essentials of Diagnosis
- Corneal burns.
- Allergic or irritant dermatitis: swelling, redness, pruritus.
- Asthma.

Exposure Limits
Toluene
   ACGIH TLV: 0.005 ppm TWA, 0.02 ppm STEL
   OSHA PEL: 0.005 TWA, 0.02 ppm STEL
   NIOSH REL: 0.005 ppm TWA, 0.02 ppm ceiling (10 minutes)
Methylene bisphenyl isocyanate (MDI)
   ACGIH TLV: 0.005 ppm TWA
   OSHA PEL: 0.02 ppm ceiling
Methylene bis(4-cyclohexylisocyanate)
   ACGIH TLV: 0.005 ppm TWA
   OSHA PEL: 0.01 ppm (ceiling)

General Considerations

Polyurethanes were first developed in the 1940s as synthetic fibers, but the main current use is in the form of flexible and rigid foams. The main health hazards are related to the use of isocyanates.

Production

Polyurethanes are complex cellular polymers based on the reaction of isocyanates with alcohol groups (polyols) from either polyesters or polyethers. The reactions take place in the presence of a catalyst (usually an organotin compound), a blowing agent (fluorocarbon), and water. TDI is used for the production of flexible foams, while MDI is used for rigid foam. For some applications, tertiary amines such as triethylenediamine are used as cross-linking agents.

Use

Flexible foams are used in furniture, mattresses, automobile seats, and carpet pads. Rigid foams are used for building insulation and packaging. Urethanes are also used for surface coatings to impart resistance to abrasion and chemical corrosion.

Health Hazards

The main health hazard in the production of polyurethanes is exposure to isocyanates. These compounds can cause severe eye and skin burns. Isocyanates are potent skin sensitizers, as are tertiary amine compounds. Dermal allergy can be confirmed by patch testing. Respiratory sensitization may also occur, resulting in symptoms of chest tightness and cough. Workers who develop either dermal or respiratory sensitization may have symptoms at very low exposure levels. Thermal decomposition products include isocyanates, hydrogen cyanide, oxides of nitrogen, and carbon monoxide.

Prevention

Eye, skin, and respiratory protection is mandatory when working with isocyanates. Exposure to uncured isocyanates may occur during loading, processing, or maintenance operations. Residual isocyanates may also be released from finished foam products. Medical surveillance should concentrate on respiratory symptoms and skin problems and should include periodic assessment of pulmonary function.

Treatment

Eye contact with isocyanates should be treated with copious irrigation with water and referral to an eye specialist. Allergic dermatitis should be treated with topical steroids. Bronchospasm should be treated with inhaled bronchodilators.

AMINO RESINS

Essentials of Diagnosis
- Eye irritation.
- Respiratory irritation: wheezing, cough, dyspnea.
- Allergic sensitization.

Exposure Limits
Formaldehyde
   ACGIH TLV: 1 ppm TWA, 2 ppm STEL
   OSHA PEL: 1 ppm TWA, 2 ppm STEL
   NIOSH REL: 0.016 ppm TWA, 0.1 ppm ceiling (15 minutes)

General Considerations

The amino resins were first developed in the 1920s for use as resins and adhesives in glues, wood, paper, and textiles. Approximately 40% of commercial formaldehyde production is used in the production of amino resins.

Production

The amino resins are thermoset materials, formed by the reaction of formaldehyde with an amino group, usually urea or melamine. The controlled polymerization reaction occurs in the presence of an acid catalyst and heat, with the evolution of water and formaldehyde. Amino resins are supplied as liquids, air-dried solids, or powders.

Use

Liquid resins are used as adhesives and bonding agents in plywood and particle board or are impregnated into textiles to impart crease resistance. Molding applications include electrical devices, dinnerware, knobs, handles, and industrial laminates, where they display hardness and surface resistance properties. Urea-formaldehyde foam was used extensively in home insulation during the energy crisis of the 1970s until this use was banned in 1982.

Health Hazards

The main health hazard in the production and use of amino resins is exposure to formaldehyde. Formaldehyde is a respiratory and mucous membrane irritant to which there appears to be great variability in individual susceptibility. Dermal sensitization may occur.

Dermal sensitization to the amino resins may also occur without evidence of sensitivity to formaldehyde. Systemic symptoms such as headache, fatigue, and nausea and irritant symptoms have been associated with the use of urea-formaldehyde insulation.

Formaldehyde is an animal carcinogen and a suspected human carcinogen. Thermal decomposition products include carbon monoxide, formaldehyde, ammonia, and cyanide.

Prevention

Workers should avoid extensive skin contact with amino resins to prevent skin irritation or cutaneous sensitization. Materials should be kept in well-ventilated areas after production to avoid accumulation of unreacted formaldehyde vapor. Medical surveillance should focus on the skin and respiratory system. Individuals who demonstrate intolerance to exposure to formaldehyde or amino resins—manifested by respiratory, skin, or systemic symptoms—should be removed from exposure if adequate ventilation or personal protection cannot be provided.

Treatment

Respiratory irritation related to formaldehyde is usually self-limited. If bronchospasm is present, administer inhaled bronchodilators. Treat dermatitis with topical steroids.

OTHER POLYMERS

POLYESTERS

Polyesters are formed through a polycondensation reaction of an acid (phthalic or maleic anhydride) and an alcohol (ethylene or propylene glycol). Thermoplastic polyesters are used primarily to form soft drink containers and films. Reinforced unsaturated polyesters are used to make boat hulls, paneling, shower stalls, and automotive bodies. The unsaturated polyester is mixed with styrene and an inhibitor (hydroquinone). A catalyst is added at the time of application to promote cross-linking and curing. The material is reinforced with a filler, usually fibrous glass, and shaped by spraying, molding, or hand application.

Exposure to polyesters does not generally result in dermatologic or respiratory irritation or sensitization. A major hazard in the reinforced plastics industry is exposure to styrene vapor during the application and curing process (see Styrene, Polystyrene).

EPOXIES

Epoxy resins are formed by the reaction of epichlorohydrin and a diglycidyl ether of the bisphenol A type. Epoxies are used primarily for protective coatings and laminates for metals, woods, and other plastics. Other uses include adhesives and bonding agents, flooring, and reinforced plastics for electrical and tooling applications. The main health hazard of exposure to epoxies is allergic dermal or respiratory sensitization, usually to low-molecular-weight oligomers of the cured resin (MW 340). Hardeners include aliphatic and cyclo-aliphatic amines, which are strong irritants as well as sensitizers. Epichlorohydrin reacts with nucleic acids and has been shown to induce chromosomal aberrations in lymphocytes of exposed workers.

NYLON

Nylon polymers are polyamides formed either by the polymerization of a lactam (ϵ-caprolactam) or by the reaction of an amine and a dibasic acid. A major use of nylon is in the production of fibers and filaments for textiles and furnishings. Molded compounds are used in automotive products, housewares, and appliances. The raw materials are respiratory and skin irritants. Most reactions take place in closed systems. Nylon compounds are a rare cause of allergic sensitization.

CELLULOSICS

Cellulosics are formed by the chemical modification of naturally occurring polymers from wood and cotton. They are used for films, sheeting, tools, and personal items (brushes, pens). Exposure to organic raw wood and cotton fibers may cause allergic respiratory problems. A major hazard with the use of cellulose nitrate films was the formation of high levels of nitrogen oxides with thermal decomposition.

ADDITIVES

A large number of organic and inorganic compounds are added to plastic materials to alter their physical and chemical properties. During the evaluation of workers for potential health effects in the plastics industry, the health professional needs to consider the toxicities of the additives in addition to the hazards of monomers or polymers. The occurrence of new health effects in a long-standing polymer operation should suggest a change in additives. The following is a brief discussion of a few of the major plastic additives.

PLASTICIZERS

Plasticizers are added to polymers to increase flexibility, softness, and processability. Polyvinyl chloride polymers are particularly well suited to modification by the addition of plasticizers.

The major class of plasticizers is the phthalate esters. Di(2-ethylhexyl)phthalate is used extensively. This compound has been shown to have hepatotoxic effects and may be released in potentially toxic quantities from treated materials. It has recently been shown to be an animal carcinogen as well.

COLORANTS

Inorganic and organic pigments and dyes are used to color plastics. Titanium dioxide and iron oxides are most common, but lead, cadmium, and chrome pigments are also used. Exposure to pigment dusts may occur during compounding and maintenance operations.

FILLERS

Fillers include silica, silicates (asbestos), fibrous glass, metal oxides and powders, and polymer fibers. The main hazards are respiratory exposure to fibrogenic dusts or metal dusts or skin contact with irritant fibers.

FOAMING AGENTS

Foaming or blowing agents are used to introduce a gas or vapor into a polymer to impart a cellular structure of low density. Azodicarbonamide is most commonly used. Occupational asthma has been related to exposure to this compound in several reports. Organic solvents may also be used.

FLAME RETARDANTS

Flame retardants include polychlorinated and polybrominated compounds, phosphate esters, and inorganic compounds. These are added to materials with construction and electrical applications. Triorthocresyl phosphate, a flame retardant, causes peripheral neuropathy after ingestion, though this effect has not been seen after industrial exposure.

STABILIZERS

Heat stabilizers to prevent thermal decomposition are used extensively in polyvinyl chloride. These include organotin compounds, metal salts (lead, barium, cadmium, zinc), and epoxies.

REFERENCES

Autian J: Plastics. In: *Toxicology: The Basic Science of Poisons*, 3rd ed. Casaret LJ, Doull J (editors). Macmillan, 1986.

Eckardt RE, Hindin R: The health hazards of plastics. *J Occup Med* 1973;**15**:808.

Forman D et al: Exposure to vinyl chloride and angiosarcoma of the liver: A report of the register cases. *Br J Ind Med* 1985;**42**:750.

IARC Monographs on the Evaluation of the Carcinogenic Risk of Chemicals to Humans, vol 19, 1979.

Innes DL, Tansy MF: Central nervous system effects of methyl methacrylate vapor. *Neurotoxicology* 1981; **2**:515.

L'Abbe KA, Hoey J: Review of the health effects of urea-formaldehyde foam insulation. *Environ Res* 1984; **35**:246.

Lucier GW, Hook GER (editors): *Environmental Health Perspectives.* U.S. Dept of Health and Human Services, vol 41, 1981.

Malten KE: Old and new, mainly occupational dermatological problems in the production and processing of plastics. In: *Occupational and Industrial Dermatology,* 2nd ed. Maibach HI (editor). Year Book, 1987.

NIOSH: *Criteria for a Recommended Standard Occupational Exposure to Decomposition Products of Fluorocarbon Polymers.* U.S. Dept of Health, Education, and Welfare, 1977.

Slovak AJM: Occupational asthma caused by a plastic agent, azodicarbonamide. *Thorax* 1981;**36**:906.

Tossavainen A: Styrene use and occupational exposure in the plastics industry. *Scand J Work Environ Health* 1978;**2**:7.

Vainio H et al: Chemical hazards in the plastics industry. *J Toxicol Environ Health* 1980;**6**:259.

Williams PL, Burson JL: *Industrial Toxicology: Safety and Health Application in the Workplace.* Van Nostrand Reinhold, 1985.

The Rubber Industry

29

Richard Lewis, MD, MPH

As early as the sixth century AD, objects made from rubber were considered magical by the Aztecs and Mayas and used in religious ceremonies. In the Amazon, natives fashioned footwear from natural rubber using wood smoke (which killed bacteria) to increase strength and durability. But it was not until the early part of the 19th century that the development of waterproof footwear and garments—and tremendous public demand—resulted in the birth of the rubber industry in Great Britain and the USA.

Several historical developments served to shape the modern rubber industry. Invention of the vulcanization process by Charles Goodyear in 1839—using sulfur and heat to cross-link natural rubber molecules—as well as the use of additives to improve processing led to a demand for rubber products that exceeded the natural supplies at the time. By the end of the 19th century, rubber plants had been exported from Brazil to plantations in southeast Asia, Sri Lanka, Indonesia, Liberia, and Zaire, which remain the primary producers of natural rubber today.

Development of the pneumatic tire and its application in the automobile industry after the turn of the century led to vast increases in rubber production along with continuing improvements in rubber processing. The growth of the petrochemical industry and advances in polymer technology, coupled with significant shortages in the supply of natural rubber during the Second World War, led to the rapid expansion of the synthetic rubber industry in the 1940s. Since that time, the use of synthetic rubber has exceeded that of natural rubber for most applications.

Tire manufacturing remains the leading sector of the rubber industry today, consuming nearly half of all natural and synthetic rubber produced annually. This industry employs over one-half million workers in nearly 400 plants around the world. Other uses of rubber include automotive components, wiring and cable, hoses, clothing and footwear, medical supplies, building materials, and sports and leisure equipment.

Potential exposures in the rubber industry are diverse. A single tire may require the use of 275 raw materials. Workers' exposures will vary not only with different jobs within the industry but also with changes in production techniques and material use over time. This chapter will review the basic processes involved in rubber production, focusing on the tire industry, and will highlight the occupational health issues of the industry as a whole. Specific exposures relevant to the rubber industry are discussed elsewhere in this book.

PRODUCTION OF NATURAL RUBBER

Natural rubber is obtained primarily from a variety of trees and plants, especially the tree Hevea brasiliensis. Latex is harvested manually from trees by field workers. Preliminary processing involves filtering to remove dirt and debris and coagulation with acids (formic acid and acetic acid). The rubber is then rolled into sheets, cut, and cured with either smoke or sodium bisulfite bleach. It is then formed into bales for shipping.

The production of natural rubber shares many of the occupational health hazards of other agricultural industries. These include use of sharp cutting implements, exposure to pesticides (including sodium arsenite), and risk of tropical diseases in endemic areas. The acids and caustics used in processing are potential respiratory and skin irritants. Increasing use of processing equipment requires careful attention to safety practices to prevent worker injuries.

PRODUCTION OF SYNTHETIC RUBBER

Synthetic rubber is a general term for elastomers—polymeric materials similar to plastic resins. The distinction is based on the elastomer's ability to be stretched (extensibility) at room temperature and return to its original shape. Synthetic rubber in its crude state is thermoplastic but lacks strength and resiliency. Cross-linking using sulfur or other atoms during vulcanization creates a durable thermoset material of variable strength and pliability.

As in resin production for plastics, the manufacturing of synthetic rubber involves use of large volumes of raw materials. Polymerization reactions take place in enclosed vessels, limiting worker exposure to unreacted chemical intermediates. Workers may be exposed to chemical feedstocks during receiving and loading or with leaks and spills. Maintenance operations, such as the cleaning of reaction vessels, have been major sources of exposure in the past, prior to the implementation of proper venting and respiratory protection measures.

The most widely used synthetic rubber is a copolymer of **styrene and butadiene (SBR)** used extensively in tire manufacturing. This substance is produced through an emulsion polymerization reaction of aqueous styrene and butadiene. Unreacted monomers are captured and recycled. The latex polymer is coagulated with sulfuric acid and dried prior to shipping. Other chemicals may be added, such as carbon black, antioxidants, and curing agents depending on the intended use of the product.

Overexposure to unreacted styrene monomer can result in effects on the nervous system (giddiness, loss of coordination) and the liver. Worker exposure to 1,3-butadiene results primarily in mucous membrane and respiratory tract irritation at high concentrations. This compound is an animal carcinogen, however, and limited studies of this industry have reported excess deaths from lymphoproliferative disorders (leukemias, lymphomas) in production workers.

Neoprene (polychloroprene) combines the mechanical properties of natural rubber with increased resistance to aging, oils, and chemicals. This is used in belts, hoses, footwear, and low-voltage insulation. **Chloroprene (2-chloro-1,3-butadiene)** is flammable, and exposure to high concentrations of unreacted monomer and other chemical intermediates has caused narcosis, respiratory tract and skin irritation, alopecia, and liver and kidney damage. Studies of workers exposed to low concentrations of chloroprene in a manufacturing and polymerization plant showed no evidence of biochemical or hematologic abnormalities.

Other synthetics include **butyl rubber** (isobutylene-isoprene polymers), **nitriles** (NBR [nitrile butadiene rubber], copolymers of acrylonitrile and butadiene), and **polyurethane** elastomers (see Chapter 28). Acrylonitrile is a respiratory and mucous membrane irritant, and overexposure may mimic cyanide poisoning. Acrylonitrile is also a suspect human carcinogen.

MANUFACTURING OF TIRES & OTHER RUBBER PRODUCTS

The manufacturing of rubber products varies from relatively simple operations, such as the production of gloves and balloons by dipping into liquid latex concentrates, to the complex 40-step process involved in tire manufacturing. The basic processes and potential environmental exposures described below in tire manufacturing are relevant to many other rubber manufacturing operations.

Compounding & Mixing

Thousands of different chemicals may be used as rubber additives. The major **reinforcement and filler materials** are carbon black and amorphous silica, though asbestos-containing materials have been used in the past. **Vulcanizing agents** include sulfur, zinc oxide, stearic acid, and other sulfide compounds. Thiurams, thiocarbamates, and various amine-aldehyde compounds are used as **accelerators** to increase the rate of curing. Additional additives include **activators** (soaps and fatty acids), **extenders** (mineral oils), **plasticizers** (phthalates), **antioxidants** (amines, quinones), and **pigments.**

The initial step in fabrication involves the weighing and mixing of various additives with natural and synthetic rubbers—also known as masterbatching. Manual weighing and filling of hoppers results in generation of large amounts of dust that can be reduced through the use of local exhaust ventilation. The materials are combined and loaded into banburies for mixing. In certain applications, the uncured rubber may be heated prior to mixing.

Other activities include the mixing of rubber with **solvents** to form cements for use in the manufacturing process. Up to the 1940s, solvents such as benzene, carbon disulfide, and carbon tetrachloride were used routinely. Currently, a wide variety of solvents are used in rubber cements and adhesives, including chlorinated, aliphatic, and aromatic hydrocarbons, ketones, and other petroleum derivatives. Mixers should be well sealed and provided with local exhaust ventilation to limit the release of solvent vapors into the workplace.

Milling, Extrusion, & Calendering

Rubber stock is heated and milled to confer softness and plasticity for further processing. The time and the temperature of the mills govern the chemical reactions within the batch, determining the properties of the finished material. During the formation of rubber sheets, the uncured rubber is coated with an antitack agent to reduce sticking. Talc was used extensively for this purpose in the past but has now largely been replaced by amorphous silica (kaolin) and liquid soaps. The rubber stock is cooled in dip tanks, generating steam.

In tire manufacturing, the milled rubber sheet is extruded through a die corresponding to the tread dimensions and weight. This is cut into specified lengths, and the ends are joined manually or automatically, using cement. Rubber sheet is also formed into ply stock by calendering onto steel cord and fabrics (nylon, rayon, polyesters, and fiberglass). Fabric may be pretreated using a phenol-formaldehyde solution to improve adhesion.

All of these operations result in potential exposure to the reaction products from the unvulcanized feedstock. In addition, there is potential exposure to dust (talc, kaolin) from the antitack agents and solvent vapors from the cements.

Product Fabrication

Many rubber products combine different materials. Tires are assembled on a drum combining ply stock, beads, sidewalls, and other components. The surface of the components may be treated with solvent (primarily naphtha) during the tire building process. Many rubber products, such as hoses, are already formed into their final shape prior to curing. Tires are sprayed with a mold release agent and placed in steel molds to impart the final shape and surface characteristics during the curing process.

Vulcanization

The application of heat and pressure initiates the cross-linking reactions that will define the shape and characteristics of the final product. Vulcanization may take place in heated molds, ovens, autoclaves, curing pans, or curing presses employing various heat sources. The main exposure is to curing fume, a complex mixture produced by the volatilization of rubber compounds, additives, and impurities.

Finishing Operations

After vulcanization, the final products may undergo further processing, such as grinding, trimming, painting, and assembly. Potential occupational health hazards in the finishing operations involve exposure to dusts and solvent vapors, repetitive trauma, and the use of sharp instruments and machinery.

HEALTH HAZARDS IN RUBBER MANUFACTURING

As in many other manufacturing industries, noise remains a major concern in the rubber industry. The extensive use of milling and mixing equipment, extruders, calenders, conveyers, and hydraulic tools in the tire industry results in noise levels exceeding 85 db throughout most operations. Other physical hazards include risk of thermal burns and heat stress.

DERMATITIS

A number of accelerators and other compounds used in the rubber industry—including thiurams, amines, and mercaptobenzothiazole—are skin sensitizers causing allergic contact dermatitis in both rubber workers and users of rubber products. Many of the common rubber sensitizers are included in patch test batteries employed by dermatologists and allergists. Cross-reactivity to similar substances may occur, and sensitized individuals generally need to be removed from further exposure.

Irritant dermatitis may be precipitated by contact with solvents, caustics, and acids. Phenols and hydroquinones can cause focal hypopigmentation (leukoderma).

Dermatitis can be prevented by avoidance of skin contact with these substances. Treatment with topical steroids and emollients is usually effective.

RESPIRATORY DISEASE

Several studies have demonstrated a high incidence of respiratory symptoms and pulmonary function abnormalities in rubber workers. Findings consistent with mucous hypersecretion and mild airway obstruction have been reported in workers exposed to carbon black and other additives, talc, and curing fumes. Symptoms reported by these workers have included cough and phlegm production, chest colds, and episodes of bronchitis. Spirometry has shown decrements in flow rates with preservation of lung volumes. In general, the effects of smoking and workplace exposures appear to be additive.

The long-term impact of exposures in the rubber industry on respiratory status is uncertain. Radiographic evidence of pulmonary fibrosis (talcosis, asbestosis) has been reported only rarely in rubber workers and has been related to specific materials and work practices. Mortality studies have not shown excess mortality rates from respiratory diseases.

If the primary pulmonary insult is the inhalation of particulates and mild irritants, then improved ventilation, material substitution, and better work practices should lessen these effects.

CANCER

Excess deaths from various cancers have been reported in rubber workers, and the International Agency for Research on Cancer (IARC) has classified exposures in the rubber industry as carcinogenic in humans. As might be expected based on the changes in materials, operations, and work conditions over the past 60 years, epidemiologic investigations have identified excesses of several different cancers in rubber workers depending on the time of the study and the population of interest. While in some instances specific causes have been identified, the factors contributing to cancer excess in rubber workers remain uncertain.

The first cancer identified in rubber workers was an excess in **bladder cancer** in Great Britain. The excess in the initial workers studied was ultimately attributed to the use of aromatic amines, primarily b-naphthylamine, as accelerators. This was discontinued in 1950, and excess bladder cancers have not been identified in other studies.

Several studies have identified an excess incidence of **gastrointestinal cancers** in rubber workers. The most consistent finding has been an increased risk of stomach cancer, with over half of the studies reporting excesses from 25% to over 100%. Excess mortality rates from cancer of the colon and esophagus have also been reported, although less consistently. Etiologic factors considered include carbon black and other particulates, nitrosamines, and curing fume, though none have been clearly implicated.

Some studies have also shown certain rubber workers to be at increased risk of developing **leukemia.** Solvents have been considered as the primary etiologic agents, particularly where an excess of myelogenous leukemia has been found related to use of benzene (a pliofilm process being the most publicized). Excess risks found in other studies include a risk of lymphocytic leukemia from exposure to solvents other than benzene. Limited studies of workers producing synthetic rubber (SBR) have also suggested an excess leukemia risk.

While rubber workers in general have not been found to be at an increased risk for developing **lung cancer,** excesses have been found in a variety of worker subpopulations. This has been associated with exposure to compounding, mixing and milling, and curing fume exposure, but the studies are inconsistent. Smoking, interactions of smoking with other exposures in the rubber industry, and chance clustering (given the extensive investigation of this industry) all remain possible explanations for the findings related to lung cancer to date.

MEDICAL SURVEILLANCE

Health surveillance programs for rubber workers should include periodic audiometry and spirometry. If possible, the information should be standardized to allow assessment of the effectiveness of controls in high-risk areas. Physical examinations should focus on the respiratory system as well as the skin. Despite many uncertainties regarding the true cancer risks in the rubber industry, screening for gastrointestinal cancer should be considered. These diseases are relatively common in the general population, and early detection can markedly improve the outcome, particularly for cancer of the colon.

PREVENTION

Reduction in the release of air contaminants into the work environment through the use of proper ventilation and material substitution presents a continuing challenge for the rubber industry. Comprehensive hearing conservation programs need to be in place and enforced. Given the potential risks of respiratory disease and cancer, workplace smoking restriction policies and smoking cessation programs may be extremely beneficial for rubber workers.

REFERENCES

Arp EW Jr, Wolf PH, Checkoway H: Lymphocytic leukemia and exposures to benzene and other solvents in the rubber industry. *J Occup Med* 1983;**25**:598.

Checkoway H et al: A case-control study of bladder cancer in the United States rubber and tyre industry. *Br J Ind Med* 1981;**38**:240.

Checkoway H et al: An evaluation of the associations of leukemia and rubber industry solvent exposures. *Am J Ind Med* 1984;**5**:239.

Delzell E, Andjelkovich D, Tyroler HA: A case-control study of employment experience and lung cancer among rubber workers. *Am J Ind Med* 1982;**3**:393.

Gooch JJ, Hawn WF: Biochemical and hematological evaluation of chloroprene workers. *J Occup Med* 1981;**23**:268.

Matanoski GM, Schwartz L: Mortality of workers in styrene-butadiene polymer production. *J Occup Med* 1987;**29**:675.

McKinnery WN, Heitbrink WA: *Control of Air Contaminants in Tire Manufacturing.* US Department of Health and Human Services (NIOSH) Publication 84-111, 1984.

Peters JM et al: Occupational disease in the rubber industry. *Environ Health Perspect* 1976;**17**:31.

The rubber industry. *IARC Monogr Eval Carcinog Risk Chem Hum* 1982;**28**:1.

Sorahan T et al: Mortality in the British rubber industry 1946–1985. *Br J Ind Med* 1989;**46**:1.

Weeks JL, Peters JM, Monson RR: Screening for occupational health hazards in the rubber industry. (Part 1.) *Am J Ind Med* 1981;**2**:125.

Pesticides

30

Jon Rosenberg, MD, MPH

As defined by the Federal Insecticide, Fungicide, and Rodenticide Act (FIFRA), the federal law that regulates the manufacture, sale, and use of pesticides in the USA, a pesticide is "any substance or mixture of substances intended for preventing, destroying, repelling, or mitigating any insects, rodents, nematodes, fungi, or weeds or any other forms of life declared to be pests; any substance or mixture of substances intended for use as a plant regulator, defoliant or desiccant."

There are over 1200 chemical compounds used as pesticides and marketed in over 30,000 formulations and under different brand names. The USA uses 35–45% of the total world supply of pesticides, or about 900 million pounds annually. The greatest recent increase has been in the use of herbicides, which now account for approximately 60% of pesticide sales. Prior to World War II, most pesticides were inorganic chemicals. Since then, most pesticides in use have come to be synthetic organic chemicals. Most of these can be divided into categories, or families, according to structure or use, with certain properties in common—including health effects on workers and others exposed to toxic quantities by various routes. The specific clinical discussions that begin on p 408 are organized in that way.

Information on identity, exposure, toxicity, and clinical management of specific pesticides is often difficult to obtain. It is therefore important to become familiar with the sources of such information that are available in any particular area of practice. These can include the county agricultural commissioner, county health officer, regional poison control center, state departments of health and agriculture, union officials, and local growers. The *Farm Chemical Handbook* is a useful source for identification of a pesticide by common name, chemical name, trade name, and manufacturer or marketer. The EPA booklet *Recognition and Management of Pesticide Poisonings* is a useful concise guide to diagnosis and treatment. *Pesticides Studied in Man* is a more definitive source of health-related information.

Although there have been regulatory requirements for toxicity testing of pesticides in the USA for a number of years, for most pesticides no data are available on which to base a complete or even partial health hazard assessment (see Regulation of Use of Pesticides, below).

USES OF PESTICIDES

Approximately 90% of all pesticides produced are used for commercial agriculture and the remainder for structural pest control, horticulture, and home and garden purposes. The principal goal of pesticide application in commercial agriculture and horticulture is to reduce crop loss or decrease growing or cultivation costs in order to enhance economic returns. Structural pesticides are applied to prevent or reduce structural damage from pests, such as termites, or reduce the impact of pest infestations, such as cockroaches, which may be a threat to public health. Certain pesticides may be used specifically for protection of public health, such as drinking and swimming water treatment, disinfectants for medical facilities, and control of carriers of disease such as mosquitoes and rodents. The public health benefits of pesticides are particularly noteworthy in developing countries.

OCCUPATIONAL & ENVIRONMENTAL PESTICIDE EXPOSURES

Typical occupational and nonoccupational pesticide exposure situations are listed in Table 30–1. The nature, extent, and route of exposure may vary among these different circumstances.

The nature of exposure depends on whether exposure is to the commercial formulation of a pesticide, as applied in a field or structure, or only to the active ingredient, as occurs in a manufacturing facility. A pesticide as applied consists of the technical grade chemical ("active" ingredient), formulated with diluents (often organic solvents), additives ("adjuvants"), and other "inert" ingredients, and then applied mixed or unmixed, as sprays, dusts, aerosols, granular or impregnated preparations, fumigants, baits, or systemics. "Inert" ingredients are not necessarily nontoxic; many are organic solvents such as methylene chloride. Systemic pesticides are water-soluble chemicals that are taken up by a plant and translocated to a part of the plant where a pest, usually an insect, feeds on plant juices and ingests the pesticide. The term is also used for animal systemics, or feed-through pesticides, when an animal is fed the pesticide and pests that feed on feces ingest the pesticide also. The use of systemic, granular, bait,

Table 30–1. Occupational and environmental pesticide exposure situations.

Occupational exposures
 Research and development
 Manufacturing: Technical grade material produced.
 Formulation: Technical grade material mixed with "inert" ingredients such as solvents, adjuvants.
 Transportation
 Pest control
 Mixing: Commercial material diluted with water or other material.
 Loading: Into tanks in planes, ground rigs, backpacks, or hand-held sprayers.
 Application
 Flagging: Standing at the end of fields to mark the rows to be sprayed by crop-dusting aircraft.
 Farm work: Field workers, pickers, sorters, packers, and others who come into contact with pesticide residues on leaves and fruit.
 Emergency and medical work: Personnel exposed to contaminated persons and equipment in the process of responding to spills, accidents, and poisonings.
Environmental and consumer exposures
 Accidents and spills: Especially ingestion by children
 Suicide and homicide
 Home use: House and garden
 Structural use: Residents and occupants of buildings
 Bystanders
 Contamination: Food, water, air

and impregnated pesticide formulations can result in significantly reduced exposure during application.

Pesticides used by consumers for home and garden are often nearly identical in formulation to those used by commercial applicators or differ only in reduced concentration of active ingredient. The most serious exposures occur from accidental or deliberate ingestions. Although pesticides account for a relatively small percentage of childhood ingestions, they account for a major proportion of serious illnesses and deaths from poisoning in this population.

PHARMACOKINETICS OF PESTICIDE TOXICITY

The highest exposures and highest incidence of poisonings occur in those involved in agricultural pest control operations: mixing, loading, applying, and flagging. Mixers and loaders are exposed to concentrated pesticides and large volumes, respectively. The use of closed systems for mixing and loading has reduced these exposure and poisonings considerably. The exposure of applicators varies with the type of application, from leaking backpack sprayers to enclosed-cab vehicles with filtered cooled air. Exposures in most manufacturing facilities are low because of the use of automated closed systems. Exposures in formulating facilities may be much higher, particularly if dusty formulations (dusts, powders, granules) are produced in open systems.

The most important route for most occupational exposures is dermal, though in some occupations such as manufacturing inhalation may be equally significant. A high percentage of pesticides are absorbed across intact human skin to a significant degree, since they must be absorbed through the coverings of insects or plants to be effective. The ratio of dermal LD50 to oral LD50—values that are available for most pesticides—can provide a rough indication of degree of dermal absorption. Other pharmacokinetic considerations vary considerably among pesticide families and so are discussed below according to family.

EFFECTS, PREVENTION, & TREATMENT OF PESTICIDE TOXICITY

Some toxic effects of pesticides, such as cancer, require consideration as a class, since the populations shown to be at increased risk are exposed to many different types. For some effects, such as acute poisoning, there are general principles of diagnosis, treatment, and prevention. After these general remarks, the individual pesticides will be considered.

Clinical Findings
A. Symptoms and Signs:

1. Acute exposure—The manifestations of acute toxicity vary among pesticide families. The vast majority of acute pesticide poisonings are due to organophosphates and carbamates. However, the diagnosis of acute pesticide poisoning in general relies upon the following features: (1) Signs and symptoms consistent with exposure to one or more chemical families of pesticides. (2) A temporal relationship to known exposure to pesticides, or field work, even in the absence of known recent pesticide application. Temporal relationships will vary depending on the type of pesticide, the route and duration of exposure, and the nature of the toxic effect. (3) Evidence of poisoning in other workers or family members.

Severe acute poisoning usually does not present a diagnostic challenge, since a history of high-level acute exposure is usually available and a full spectrum of clinical manifestations is usually present. However, mild acute intoxication or subacute poisoning may not be readily apparent, since the signs and symptoms are likely to be nonspecific and similar to some common illness, such as influenza, and a history of exposure may not be particularly remarkable or even known to the patient.

2. Chronic exposure—Specific organ-related chronic effects are discussed in later sections. Some general considerations regarding dermatologic effects, carcinogenicity, and the reproductive toxicity of pesticides are discussed here.

a. Dermatologic effects—Approximately one-third of all reported pesticide-related diseases are dermatologic—about the same percentage estimated for other chemicals. Pesticides may be primary skin irritants or skin sensitizers, resulting in irritant or allergic contact dermatitis. Sulfur and propargite

(Omite) are common causes of irritant dermatitis when used as fungicides on grapes, while the dithiocarbamates, phthalimides, and benomyl (Benlate)—all fungicides—are common causes of both irritant and allergic contact dermatitis. However, because of the lack of reporting and research in pesticide-related skin disease, any pesticide must be considered for its possible role in causation of rash in an exposed worker.

The diagnosis and management of dermatitis in a worker exposed to pesticides differs little from that for dermatitis in other workers except in the case of field workers. These workers usually do not know what pesticide residues are present on the plants they are in contact with, and they may be exposed to plants known to have primary irritant or allergic contact dermatitis. (For a discussion of plant-related dermatitis, see Chapter 17.) Diagnosis of irritant dermatitis is made on the basis of the history and by noting resolution of symptoms when further exposure is prevented. Reexposure with recurrence may confirm the diagnosis. Treatment consists of alleviation of symptoms with corticosteroids and moisturizers. Prevention of further exposure sufficient to cause recurrence is usually possible with protective clothing.

Diagnosis of allergic contact dermatitis is made on the basis of the history, physical presentation, and patch testing. Patch tests are available for a number of pesticides and plants known to be sensitizers and may be made for others. The distinction between pesticide and plant allergy is important for field workers, since a pesticide-related cause may mean transfer from the field for several days at one time during a season, while a plant-related cause may mean permanent avoidance of a particular crop for at least part of its growing cycle.

b. Cancer—No pesticides currently in use are recognized human carcinogens—with the exception of inorganic arsenic. Epidemiologic studies of cancer in farmers have shown a relatively consistent increase in certain cancers, notably leukemia, lymphoma, and multiple myeloma. Although these findings are suggestive of an increase in cancer due to pesticide exposure, specific pesticides could not be incriminated, and other causes related to farm work could not be ruled out.

Few studies have looked at cancer incidence in pesticide applicators. Two have indicated elevated risks for lung cancer and one for bladder cancer without being able to attribute carcinogenicity to specific pesticides. A number of studies have suggested (without proof) an association between phenoxy herbicides and soft tissue sarcoma. For a number of pesticides—most notably the halogenated hydrocarbons—there is evidence of carcinogenicity in animals. Table 30–2 lists pesticides known or preliminarily identified by the EPA to be associated with evidence for carcinogenicity in animals—recognizing that such evidence is often uncertain, controversial, and subject to reevaluation. It is important to realize that these and other toxicologic data were generated primarily by pesticide manufacturers

Table 30–2. Pesticides with evidence for carcinogenicity in animals.[1]

Pesticide	Comment
In current use	
Acephate	Weakly carcinogenic.
Alachlor	Used extensively on corn; may be restricted.
Aldrin	Most uses canceled.
Amitraz	Data uncertain.
Amitrole	Under United States EPA.
Arsenicals	Many no longer used, rest may be restricted.
Azinphosmethyl	Under EPA review.
Benomyl	Under EPA review.
Cacodylic acid	Studies being repeated.
Captafol	
Captan	Duodenal cancer by gavage.
Carbon tetrachloride	Cancellation of all uses likely.
Chlordane	Most uses except termiticide canceled.
Chlordimeform	Bladder cancer; restricted use on cotton.
Chlorbenzilate	Data uncertain.
Chlorthalonil	Under EPA review.
Cypermethrin	
Cyromazine	Metabolized to melamine, a potential carcinogen.
Daminozide	Metabolized to dimethylhydrazine, a carcinogen; used extensively on red apples; to be restricted and possibly phased out due to concern over consumer exposure.
Diallate	Weakly carcinogenic.

continued

Table 30–2 (con't). Pesticides with evidence for carcinogenicity in animals.[1]

Pesticide	Comment
Dichloropropane	Use restricted.
Dichloropropene	Use restricted.
Diclofop methyl	Pathologic nature of lesions controversial.
Dicofol	Contaminated with DDT; may itself be carcinogenic.
Dimethipin	Controversial; unresolved.
Dimethoate	Weakly carcinogenic.
Dinitramine	Under EPA review.
Dithiocarbamates (ethylene bis-)	Metabolized to ethylenethiourea, which causes thyroid dysfunction and thyroid tumors.
Ethafluralin	Under EPA review.
Ethylene dichloride	Use being phased out.
Ethylene oxide	Regulated by OSHA as carcinogen.
Folpet	
Glyphosphate	Controversial; unresolved.
Igran	Weakly carcinogenic.
Lindane	Mouse hepatomas; controversial, most uses canceled.
Linuron	
Maleic hydrazide	All uses canceled in USA.
Methanearsonic acid	
Methomyl	
Methyl bromide	Preliminary studies being repeated.
Mirex	Under EPA review, most uses canceled.
Monuron	Most uses voluntarily canceled.
Orazylin	
Oxadiazon	Weakly carcinogenic.
Oxyfluorfen	Under EPA review.
Paraquat	
PCNB	
Pentachlorophenol	Contaminated with carcinogenic dioxin.
Permethrin	Weakly carcinogenic.
o-Phenylphenol	
Profluralin	Weakly carcinogenic.
Pronamide	Weakly carcinogenic.
Propoxur	
Ronnel	Weakly carcinogenic.
Thiodicarb	
Thiophanate-methyl	Under EPA review.
Trifluralin	Carcinogenic contaminant to be kept below 1 ppm.
Triallate	Weakly carcinogenic.
Ziram	Under EPA review.

Little or no current use
  Aldrin
  Cadmium compounds
  Chlordecone
  Dibromochloropropane
  Dieldrin
  Endrin
  Ethylene dibromide
  Nitrofen
  Heptachlor
  OMPA
  Safrole
  Sulfallate
  Terpene polychlorinates
  Trichlorobenzoic acid
  Toxaphene	

[1]Data from United States EPA (1985) and California Department of Food and Agriculture (1987).

in response to regulatory requirements (see below) and are generally unpublished and usually unavailable to persons outside the companies and regulatory agencies.

A committee of the National Research Council of the National Academy of Sciences examined the issue of carcinogenic pesticides present as food residues. Using the same list of carcinogenic or potentially carcinogenic pesticides as in Table 30–2, they determined that—on the basis of pounds of pesticide applied 30% of insecticides, 90% of fungicides, and 60% of herbicides are suspected carcinogens. Carcinogenic risks from these residues were considered as well as alternative ways to regulate the residues.

c. Reproductive effects–No pesticides are recognized human teratogens or female reproductive toxins. However, there are few studies of reproductive outcome for women exposed to pesticides. Table 30–3 is a list of pesticides with some current evidence for female reproductive toxicity in animals.

In 1977, a number of male workers were discovered to have reduced or absent sperm, infertility or sterility, and testicular atrophy as a result of exposure to dibromochloropropane (DBCP) (see Chapter 24). Similar effects were observed in animals. A short time later, workers exposed to chlordecone (Kepone) in a manufacturing facility were found to have similar testicular changes, followed by confirmatory animal tests. These episodes prompted an increase in the screening of pesticides for male reproductive toxicity. Table 30–4 is a list of pesticides determined in animals to be male reproductive toxins.

B. Laboratory Findings: For acute pesticide poisoning, laboratory findings are usually specific and timely only for cholinesterase inhibition by organophosphate and possibly carbamate pesticides. Measurement of the pesticide or its metabolites in body fluids is usually helpful only in later confirmation of diagnosis, since the information is rarely available in time to aid in management. The use of biologic levels is not helpful in the diagnosis of chronic toxicity because adequate dose-response data are unavailable for most pesticides and because biologic levels at the time of diagnosis, if present at all, may not reflect those present during exposure.

Prevention

A. Work Practices: Manufacturing and formulation workers, mixers, loaders, applicators, and flaggers are all directly exposed to the concentrated or dilute product and so can only be protected by engineering controls and personal protective clothing and devices. Field-workers are exposed primarily to residues on plants and in soil. They are protected primarily by reentry intervals—the minimum time allowed between application of a pesticide on a field and entry into that field. The rate of degradation and the toxicity of the degradation products are important determinants of the extent and effect of exposure in this group. Pesticide degradation rates often vary among geographic regions, so that reentry intervals

Table 30–3. Pesticides with evidence of reproductive toxicity in female animals.[1]

Pesticide	Comments
Benomyl	Fungicide; teratogenic in rats at doses above 125 mg/kg/d; acceptable risk is dependent upon estimation of limited dermal absorption and is apparently adequate if protective clothing is used by applicators.
Bromoxynil	Herbicide; weakly teratogenic and embryotoxic in rats.
Captafol	Fungicide; suggestive evidence of teratogenic effects.
Captan	Fungicide; suggestive evidence of teratogenic effects.
Carbaryl	Insecticide; effects seen only in beagle dogs at relatively high doses; negative in a number of other species, so that risk to humans is questionable.
Cyanazine	Herbicide; teratogenic or fetotoxic in rats and rabbits at doses above 1 mg/kg.
Dimethoate	Insecticide; fetotoxic in rats.
Dinocap	Fungicide, acaricide; teratogenic in rabbits by oral but not dermal route.
Dinoseb	Nematocide; strongly teratogenic, all uses suspended.
Diuron	Herbicide; weakly teratogenic.
Endothall	Herbicide; teratogenic in rabbits.
Endrin	Insecticide; teratogenic, most uses canceled.
Ethylene bis dithio-carbamates (EBDCs): Maneb, Nabam, Zineb, Metiram	Fungicides; teratogenic in rats; a metabolite, ethylenethiourea, is also teratogenic in rats.
Folpet	Fungicide; suggestive evidence of teratogenicity.
Lindane	Insecticide; weakly teratogenic or fetotoxic; many uses canceled.
Naled	Insecticide; fetotoxic.
Oxydemetonmethyl	Insecticide; suggestive evidence of fetotoxicity.
Pentachlorophenol	Wood preservative; fetotoxic and possibly teratogenic; contaminated with tetrachlorodibenzodioxin, which is teratogenic; under review by EPA; restrictions being considered (see Chapter 26).
Thiram	Fungicide structurally related to EBDCs; teratogenic in mice above 250 mg/kg/d.
Triadimefon	Fungicide, replacement for sulfur on grapes; teratogenic at high doses, embryotoxic at lower doses; acceptable risk is dependent upon estimation of limited dermal absorption, and is apparently adequate.
Warfarin	Rodenticide; drug data indicate teratogenicity, not considered a risk to applicators.

[1]Adapted from California Department of Food and Agriculture (1987).

Table 30–4. Pesticides with evidence for reproductive toxicity in male animals.

Ethylene dibromide	Fumigant, nematocide, testicular toxin in a number of species; alkylating agent, mutagen, carcinogen; epidemiological study indicating decreased sperm count; almost all uses suspended.
Dibromochloropropane	Nematocide; testicular toxin in a number of species; alkylating agent, mutagen, carcinogen; number of reports and studies indicating infertility in formulating workers and applicators; almost all uses suspended.
Chlordecone	Insecticide; testicular toxin in a number of species; infertility in manufacturing and formulating workers; no longer manufactured.
Carbaryl	Insecticide: spermatotoxin in rodents; study in manufacturing and formulating workers indicating no effect at relatively low levels of exposure.
Triphenyltin	Fungicide; testicular toxin in rats; no human studies.
Ordram	Rice herbicide; spermatotoxin in rats, not other species; epidemiologic study of manufacturing and formulating workers indicating no effect at relatively low levels of exposure.
Chlorbenzilate	Insecticide; testicular toxin in rodents; inadequate human studies.
Fenchlorphos	Spermatotoxin in cattle.

may need to be specific to an area or climate. One of the most common causes of acute pesticide intoxication in agriculture is the too early entry of a group of field-workers into a field where an acutely toxic pesticide has been recently applied.

Since skin contamination is the most important route of most occupational exposures, the focus of prevention is to reduce dermal exposure, though the use of respirators by manufacturing or formulation workers or pesticide applicators is often necessary. Contamination of clothing, irritated skin, heat, and sweat are all factors common in agricultural work that promote absorption through the skin. The use of protective clothing in agriculture is usually impeded by the fact that most agricultural work takes place in hot and frequently humid environments. Therefore, the need for skin protection, which is difficult to quantify, must be balanced against the risk of heat-related disorders. The use of personal protective equipment for structural pest control is sometimes hampered by the need to work in tight areas, such as crawl spaces, but the confined nature of these spaces often makes their use necessary.

B. Medical Surveillance: Specific medical and biologic monitoring is available for cholinesterase-inhibiting organophosphate pesticides, as discussed below. For most other pesticides, surveillance is limited to general and occupational histories and

physical examinations, with available tests discussed under laboratory findings for each family.

Treatment

Treatment of pesticide poisoning in general proceeds in 3 steps, as described below.

A. Decontamination: Decontamination is the first priority unless life-saving measures are required. In the case of acute dermal overexposure, the skin and clothing are reservoirs for continued exposure, as is the gastrointestinal tract in the case of ingestion. All clothing should be removed and placed in double plastic bags for later analysis, decontamination, or disposal. The skin and, if necessary, the hair should be washed with soap. Contamination should be looked for under the fingernails. If the eyes have been contaminated, they should be irrigated. The need for gastrointestinal lavage or activated charcoal instillation should be determined on a case-by-case basis, ie, depending on the pesticide, on whether vomiting or diarrhea has occurred, and the level of consciousness. All procedures should be done in such a way as to minimize the contamination of medical personnel and equipment without compromising patient care.

B. Specific Antidotes: Specific antidotes are available only in the form of atropine and pralidoxime for cholinesterase-inhibiting pesticides, as discussed in detail below, and chelating agents for heavy metal pesticides such as arsenic and mercury, which rarely result in the need for treatment except for cases of ingestion.

C. Supportive Care: Supportive care may be the only treatment indicated and may be lifesaving. Assessment of respiratory status and provision of appropriate ventilatory support are critical, since most fatal or serious acute pesticide poisonings are mediated at least in part through respiratory embarrassment or arrest. Certain medications that might otherwise be given based on clinical diagnosis may be contraindicated once the diagnosis of a specific pesticide intoxication is known. An example is the use of morphine for pulmonary edema, which can precipitate cardiac arrhythmias in the presence of organophosphate poisoning.

REGULATION OF USE OF PESTICIDES

Pesticides are regulated differently from other chemicals in the USA and most other countries that have chemical regulatory systems. Prior to enactment of the Federal Insecticide, Fungicide, and Rodenticide Act (FIFRA) in 1970, there was little regulation and testing of pesticides in the USA. Since that time, the US Environmental Protection Agency (EPA) has applied an increasingly strict testing scheme for registration for sale and use of pesticides in the USA.

Since the discovery of irregularities and even fraud by certain commercial laboratories performing these tests under contract to manufacturers, greater attention has been paid to good laboratory practice and laboratory audits. The data required by EPA for registration of a pesticide are set forth in Table 30–5. Until recently, access to these data was completely restricted in accordance with trade secrecy laws.

In spite of these requirements for testing, there remain serious data gaps for both old and new pesticides. In 1984, the National Academy of Sciences (NAS)–National Research Council (NRC) published the results of a survey on toxicity testing for chemicals. Although testing was more complete for pesticides than for industrial chemicals (and less complete than for cosmetics and food additives), the toxicity data available for most pesticides can only be described as incomplete or inadequate.

The NAS–NRC survey identified 3350 pesticides and inert ingredients and selected 50 for evaluation. For 19 of those (38%), no toxicity information was available; for 13 (26%), there was less than minimal toxicity (acute and subchronic only) information; and for only 5 (10%) was there sufficient information to allow a complete health hazard assessment. By category of testing, 59% were studied for acute effects,

51% for subchronic effects, 23% for chronic effects, 34% for reproductive effects, and 28% underwent mutagenicity studies.

In the USA, the EPA regulates the registration, sale, and conditions of use of all pesticides and is responsible for the protection of agricultural workers exposed to pesticides. When a pesticide is approved for use, its use is specified as either general or restricted (to be applied only through permit to a licensed pest control operator) and it is registered and assigned an EPA registration number. The label information and use instructions, including hazard information and first-aid recommendations, are specified by EPA. Labels contain useful information, and use of a pesticide in any way other than as specified by the label is illegal. Each pesticide is assigned a toxicity category according to its acute toxicity. Table 30–6 shows the EPA labeling categories with their hazard signal words and precautionary statements.

The Occupational Safety and Health Administration (OSHA) is responsible for the protection of manufacturing and formulation workers. A criteria document for these exposures was published by the National Institute for Occupational Safety and Health (NIOSH) in 1978. State agriculture and health departments, along with county agriculture and health departments and other state and local agencies, along with OSHA, may have a variety of regulatory or advisory functions in regard to the use of pesticides. Structural pest control—the application of pesticides to commercial and residential buildings—may fall under one or another of these jurisdictions or often through cracks in the regulatory system.

PESTICIDES & ADDITIVES IN FOOD

There are over 300 pesticides (active ingredients) used on food in the USA. The EPA (in conjunction with the FDA) regulates the residues of pesticides and their breakdown products in foods by establishing tolerance levels, the legal limits for residues in foods. The regulation of pesticide residues in food is a complicated and controversial process.

Tolerances for raw agricultural commodities are established through field trials to determine the highest residues likely to occur in the course of normal agricultural procedures and practices. Tolerances for processed foods are established by determining the degree to which the residues might become concentrated during processing, such as milling or juicing. The risks to health of pesticide residues in food are considered only after the development of proposed tolerances, through a separate process. There are inconsistencies in the way in which health effects are considered. Tolerances for raw commodities may be arrived at by considering both health risks and economic benefits of pesticides, whereas tolerances for processed foods—which include all food additives such as artificial sweeteners, preservatives, chemical processing aids, animal drug residues, and packaging

Table 30–5. United States Environmental Protection Agency (EPA) requirements for pesticide registration.[1]

Product chemistry
  Production composition
  Physical and chemical characteristics
  Residue chemistry
  Environmental fate

Hazards to humans and domestic animals
  Acute studies
    Oral LD50: rat
    Dermal DL50: usually rabbit
    Inhalation LC50: rat
    Primary eye irritation: rabbit
    Primary dermal irritation: rabbit
    Dermal sensitization
    Acute delayed neurotoxicity: organophosphates
  Subchronic studies: Required depending on nature of
      exposure
    90-day feeding: rodent, nonrodent
    21-day dermal
    90-day dermal
    90-day inhalation: rat
    90-day neurotoxicity: if acute studies positive
  Chronic studies: required for pesticides with allowable
      food residues (tolerances), or if "significant" worker
      exposure
    Chronic feeding: 2 species, rodent and nonrodent
    Carcinogenicity: 2 species, rat and mouse preferred
    Teratogenicity: 2 species
    Reproduction: 2 generations
  Mutagenicity studies: A battery to include:
    Gene mutations
    Structural chromosomal aberrations
    Other genotoxic effects as appropriate
  Metabolism studies (pharmacokinetics)

Hazard to nontarget organisms
  Short-term studies
  Long-term and field studies
    Avian and mammalian testing
    Aquatic organism testing
    Plant protection
    Nontarget insect

[1]Source: US Environmental Protection Agency, 1983.

Table 30–6. Environmental protection agency (EPA) labeling toxicity categories.[1]

Hazard Indicators	Toxicity Categories			
	I	II	III	IV
Oral LD50	< 50 mg/kg	50–500 mg/kg	500–5000 mg/kg	> 5000 mg/kg
Inhalation LD50	< 0.2 mg/L	0.2–2 mg/L	2–20 mg/L	> 20 mg/L
Dermal LD50	< 200 mg/kg	200–2000 mg/kg	2000–20,000 mg/kg	> 20,000 mg/kg
Eye effects	Corrosive; corneal opacity not reversible within 7 days	Corneal opacity reversible in 7 days; irritation for 7 days	No corneal opacity; irritation reversible in 7 days	No irritation
Skin effects	Corrosive	Severe irritation at 72 hours	Moderate irritation at 72 hours	Mild or slight irritation at 72 hours
Signal word	"Danger"	"Warning"	"Caution"	"Caution"
Precautionary statements	Fatal (poisonous) if swallowed, inhaled, or absorbed through skin. Do not breathe vapor, dust, or spray mist. Do not get in eyes or on skin or clothing.	May be fatal if swallowed, inhaled, or absorbed through skin. Do not breathe vapor, dust, or spray mist. Do not get in eyes or on skin or clothing.	Harmful if swallowed, inhaled, or absorbed through skin. Avoid breathing vapor, dust, or spray mist. Avoid contact with skin, eyes, or clothing.	No precautionary statements required.

[1]US Environmental Protection Agency, 1983.

materials—are derived by considering only health risks. The Delaney Clause (see below) prohibiting tolerance for any additive found to cause cancer in humans or animals, applies to processed foods but not to raw foods. New tolerances are usually denied for pesticides known to be carcinogenic, but many older pesticides have been found to be carcinogenic only after food tolerances have been established. This is the case with daminozide (Alar), the growth regulator used in apples (see below). In these cases, pesticide use often continues while EPA proceeds through a regulatory process that often takes years, generating considerable controversy.

With the exception of the occurrence of high concentrations of acutely toxic pesticides in food, such as aldicarb in watermelon (see Organophosphates and Carbamates, below), the principal health concern regarding pesticide residues in food—given their usual low concentrations—is carcinogenic risk. Of approximately 8350 tolerances for raw commodities, about 2500 are for carcinogenic pesticides, as are 31 of 150 tolerances for processed foods. A committee of the National Research Council recently published *Regulating Pesticides in Food: The Delaney Paradox,* a report examining the issue of regulating carcinogenic pesticides in food. A small number of carcinogenic pesticides (mostly fungicides) present in a small number of foods were found to contribute most of the estimated carcinogenic risk from eating food containing residues of carcinogenic pesticides. The committee recommended a consistent standard for regulating pesticide residues in food rather than the current inconsistencies according to whether food was raw or in processed form and old versus new tolerances. They recommend a negligible risk standard rather than the zero risk of the Delaney Clause and a focus on those pesticides that contribute to a majority of the risk. These recommendations will

probably be implemented in some form by EPA and FDA in the future.

Monitoring for pesticide residues in food is performed by the US Department of Agriculture (USDA) in meat and poultry and by the FDA in domestic and imported raw and processed food. A number of states and private groups also analyze samples for pesticides. The amount of sampling performed and the analytical methods used have been subjects of further controversy. Most of the methods used detect only about 50% of food-use pesticides and are designed to detect levels at or near the tolerance level but not below that level. Thus, it is difficult on the basis of available sampling data to accurately judge the risk to consumers of current pesticide residues in food. There is increasing pressure to improve monitoring programs and to calculate risks based on a range of diets and for sensitive populations, particularly children.

MANAGEMENT OF TOXICITY DUE TO PESTICIDES

ORGANOPHOSPHATE & CARBAMATE CHOLINESTERASE-INHIBITING INSECTICIDES

Essentials of Diagnosis

Acute effects:
- Acetylcholinesterase inhibition-acetylcholine excess: parasympathetic nervous system hyperactivity, neuromuscular paralysis, central nervous system dysfunction, depression of red cell and plasma cholinesterase activity.

Chronic effects:

- Persistent CNS dysfunction (organophosphates): irritability, anxiety, mood lability, fatigue, impaired short-term memory, impaired concentration—for weeks or months after acute pesticide exposure.
- Organophosphate-induced delayed neuropathy: rapid onset of distal symmetric sensorimotor neuropathy.
- Dermatitis.

General Considerations

Organophosphates are esters of phosphoric acid that exist in 2 forms: -thion and -oxon, the latter shown in Fig 30–1B. Carbamates are esters of carbamic acid:

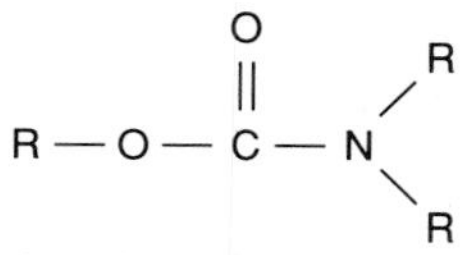

$$R - O - \overset{\overset{\displaystyle O}{\|}}{C} - N \overset{\displaystyle R}{\underset{\displaystyle R}{}}$$

The organophosphates and carbamates are considered here as a single class because they share a common mechanism of acute toxicity—cholinesterase inhibition—with similar signs and symptoms of acute poisoning. The thiocarbamates and dithiocarbamates do not inhibit cholinesterase and are considered separately under fungicides and herbicides.

The carbamates differ from organophosphates primarily in the transient and reversible nature of their cholinesterase inhibition, which results in a shorter duration of acute toxicity without persistent sequelae.

Together, these substances represent one of the largest and most important classes of pesticides. Commonly used compounds are listed according to acute toxicity in Table 30–7. They vary widely in their potency in inhibiting cholinesterase, as reflected in their LD50 values.

As a result of their widespread use and acute toxicity, the organophosphates and carbamates are the most common cause of acute pesticide intoxication. Cholinesterase inhibition produces a relatively stereotypical clinical presentation that, in conjunction with determination of cholinesterase levels, makes diagnosis more accurate than with other pesticides. Specific and nonspecific antidotes are available for treatment. A presumably small but uncertain percentage of patients acutely poisoned by organophosphates display persistent central nervous system dysfunction for weeks or months after acute poisoning. A small number of organophosphate pesticides also cause a delayed neuropathy that is correlated with inhibition of the enzyme neurotoxic esterase (Table 30–8). This is the only recognized human health effect of these compounds that is unrelated to cholinesterase inhibition.

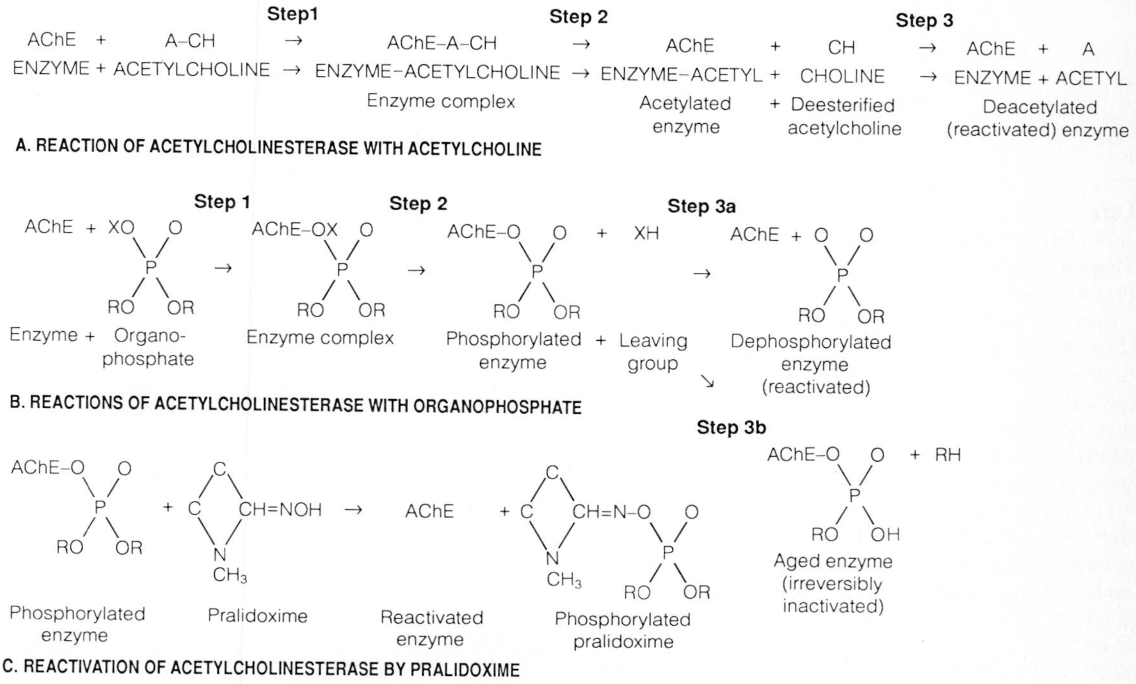

Figure 30–1. A: Reaction of acetylcholinesterase with acetylcholine. **B:** Reactions of acetylcholinesterase with organophosphate. **C:** Reactivation of acetylcholinesterase by pralidoxime.

Table 30–7. Some organophosphate and carbamate pesticides in common use in the USA.

Common Name	Trade Name	Oral LD50 (mg/kg)	Dermal LD50 (mg/kg)
Organophosphates: Category I			
Parathion		1–5	1–10
Mevinphos	Phosdrin	1–5	1–10
Methyl parathion		5–10	50–100
Carbophenothion	Trithion	5–10	20
EPN		5–10	20
Methamidophos	Monitor	10–20	100
Azinphos-methyl	Guthion	10–20	200
Methidathion	Supracide	20–30	400
Dichlorvos (DDVP)	Vapona	20–30	50–100
Organophosphates: Category II			
Chlorpyrifos	Dursban, Lorsban	50–150	2000
Diazinon	Spectracide	50–150	400
Phosmet	Imidan	50–150	3000
Dimethoate	Cygon	150–500	150
Fenthion	Baytex	150–500	300–400
Naled	Dibrom	150–500	1000
Trichlorfon	Diptarex	150–500	2000
Organophosphates: Categories III and IV			
Acephate	Orthene	500–1000	2000
Malathion		500–1000	4000
Stirofos	Gardona, Rabon	1000–5000	5000
Carbamates			
Aldicarb	Temik	1–5	1–10
Carbofuran	Furadan	5–10	10,000
Methomyl	Lannate	15–25	1000
Propoxur	Baygon	100	1000
Bendiocarb	Ficam	100–200	. . .
Carbaryl	Sevin	300–600	2000

Use

A. Organophosphates: Organophosphate pesticides were developed following World War II as a consequence of the synthesis of the organophosphate "nerve gases" sarin, soman, and tabun. Since then, they have largely replaced inorganic pesticides and organochlorines as the principal insecticides used in agriculture. A number are water-soluble, which enables them to be used as systemic insecticides. Many are highly toxic and therefore restricted but still used extensively in agriculture (eg, parathion). Others, such as malathion and diazinon, are of relatively low toxicity and are used commonly in home and garden. Dichlorvos has a very high vapor pressure and so is impregnated into pet collars and pest strips for slow release. Chlorpyrifos is perhaps the insecticide most frequently used by structural pest control operators against cockroaches and other structural pests.

B. Carbamates: The cholinesterase-inhibiting carbamates are all insecticides. Carbaryl has by far the largest use, owing to its low mammalian toxicity and relatively wide spectrum of activity. The others have more narrow spectrums. Aldicarb, carbofuran, and methomyl are highly water-soluble, which results in their being taken up into plants for use as systemic

Table 30–8. Commonly used organophosphate pesticides with evidence for delayed neuropathy in humans and animals.

	In Humans	In Animals
Trichlorphon	+	+
Merphos (Folex)	+	+
O-Ethyl-O-p-nitrophenyl ben-zene-thiooposphonate (EPN)	?	+
Methamidophos	?	+
Fenthion	?	?
Trichloronate	NR	+
S,S,S-Tributyl phosphorotrithioate (DEF)	NR	+
Diisopropylfluorophosphate (DFP)	NR	+
Dichlorvos	NR	?

? = uncertain; NR = not reported; + = reliably reported.

pesticides. Propoxur is used by structural pest control operators and in the home against cockroaches.

Occupational & Environmental Exposure

Organophosphates and carbamates are applied by a variety of techniques, from aerial spraying to hand application. Granular and bait formulations significantly reduce exposure.

These pesticides are generally rapidly degraded in the environment, though in hot, dry climates they persist to a greater degree, and longer reentry intervals (1–2 weeks) have been necessary to prevent acute poisoning of field-workers. Water contamination from organophosphates has not been a major problem to date.

Carbamates as a class were generally thought to be rapidly degraded in the environment and not to migrate into groundwater. However, aldicarb (Temik), the most acutely toxic carbamate, has been found in groundwater and drinking water. Since aldicarb is water-soluble, it concentrates in the watery parts of fruits and vegetables. An outbreak of acute aldicarb intoxication in hundreds of consumers of watermelons in the western United States occurred in 1985 as a result of the illegal use of aldicarb on some fields of the fruit. Similar but smaller episodes had taken place earlier following the instillation of aldicarb into the water of hydroponically grown tomatoes and cucumbers.

Pharmacokinetics & Mechanism of Action

Organophosphates and carbamates are well absorbed by inhalation, skin contact, and ingestion; the primary route of occupational exposure is dermal. They differ from each other in lipid solubility and therefore distribution in the body, particularly to the central nervous system.

Many commercial organophosphates are applied in the -thion or (sulfur-containing) form but readily undergo conversion to the -oxon (oxygen-containing) form (Fig 30–1B). Most of the -oxon forms have much greater toxicity than the -thion form. The conversion occurs in the environment, so that residues on crops field-workers are exposed to may be more toxic than the pesticide that was applied. Some of the sulfur is released in the form of mercaptans, which produce the typical odor of the -thion form of organophosphates. The mercaptans have very low odor thresholds, and the reactions to their noxious odor, including headache, nausea, and vomiting, are often mistaken for acute organophosphate poisoning.

The conversion from -thion to -oxon also occurs in vivo as a result of hepatic microsomal metabolism, so that the -oxon becomes the active form of the pesticide in both animal pests and in humans. Hepatic esterases rapidly hydrolyze organophosphate esters, yielding alkyl phosphates and phenols, which have little if any toxicologic activity and are rapidly excreted. Carbamates are also metabolized by the liver and excreted as metabolites in urine without evidence of significant accumulation.

Organophosphates and carbamates exert their effects on insects and mammals, including humans, by inhibiting acetylcholinesterase at nerve endings. The normal function of acetylcholinesterase is the hydrolysis and thereby inactivation of acetylcholine (Fig 30–1A). The reactions of organophosphates and acetylcholinesterase are shown in Fig 30–1B. The inhibition of acetylcholinesterase occurs through the formation of a pesticide-enzyme complex (step 1) and hydrolysis of the –X (leaving group), resulting in phosphorylation of the enzyme (step 2). The enzyme can then be spontaneously dephosphorylated and reactivated (step 3a) or aged through the hydrolysis of an alkyl (–R) group, resulting in irreversible inactivation. After irreversible inactivation, normal enzyme activity can only be restored by the synthesis of new acetylcholinesterase, a process that can take up to 60 days to complete.

Carbamates initially react with acetylcholinesterase in the same fashion as organophosphates, resulting in accumulation of acetylcholine in the same distribution as organophosphates. The carbamyl-enzyme product does not progress to an aging reaction but instead dissociates relatively rapidly. As a family, the carbamates have no known health effects other than those resulting from this acute reversible inhibition of cholinesterase and resulting overactivity of acetylcholine.

The clinical manifestations of acute organophosphate or carbamate poisoning depend upon the organs where acetylcholine is the transmitter of nerve impulses, as shown in Table 30–9.

The character, degree, and duration of acute illness produced by cholinesterase-inhibiting organophosphate and carbamate pesticides are all directly related to the degree and rate of acetylcholinesterase inhibition and subsequent accumulation of acetylcholine. Rapid rates of inhibition are associated with clinical illness at levels of inhibition that may not be associated with symptoms following slower rates of inhibition. Chronic inhibition of acetylcholinesterase appears to result in tolerance to some of the acute effects. Even if tolerance occurs, chronic inhibition of acetylcholinesterase results in a state in which exposure to a dose of an organophosphate that previously would have had no effect may now lower acetylcholinesterase levels below a critical threshold and result in clinical illness. Cumulative inhibition of acetylcholinesterase is unlikely to occur from carbamates owing to the rapidly reversible nature of the enzyme inhibition.

Organophosphate pesticides possess structural differences that result in differences in cholinesterase-inhibiting potency, in lipid solubility—and therefore distribution, particularly to the central nervous system—in rates of reversibility and aging, and in physical properties such as volatility. However, for both organophosphates and carbamates, cholinesterase-inhibiting potency is the only characteristic of

Table 30–9. Signs and symptoms of acute organophosphate poisoning by site of acetylcholine neurotransmitter activity.

System	Receptor Type	Organ	Action	Sign or Symptom
Parasympathetic	Muscarinic	**Eye** Iris muscle Ciliary muscle	Contraction Contraction	Miosis Blurred vision
		Glands Lacrimal Salivary Respiratory Gastrointestinal Urinary Sweat	Secretion	Tearing Salivation Bronchorrhea, pulmonary edema Nausea, vomiting, diarrhea Urination Perspiration
(Sympathetic)		**Heart** Sinus node AV node	Slowing Refractory period increased	Bradycardia Arrhythmias, heart block
		Smooth muscle Bronchial Gastrointestinal wall Sphincter	Contraction Contraction Relaxation	Bronchoconstriction Vomiting, cramps, diarrhea
		Bladder Fundus Sphincter	Contraction Relaxation	Urination, incontinence
Neuromuscular	Nicotinic	Skeletal	Excitation	Fasciculations, cramps, followed by weakness, loss of reflexes, paralysis
Central nervous		Brain	Excitation (early)	Headache, dizziness, malaise, apprehension, confusion, hallucinations, manic or bizarre behavior, convulsions
			Depression (late)	Depression of, then loss of consciousness; respiratory depression

practical clinical significance. For a large proportion of patients with acute intoxication, the clinician will not know the identity of the particular pesticide or pesticides at the time of initial presentation, and decisions regarding diagnosis and management will have to be made on the basis of clinical signs, symptoms, and laboratory data.

The only known systemic health effect of organophosphate pesticides that is entirely unrelated to cholinesterase inhibition is organophosphate-induced delayed neuropathy. The pathologic lesion consists of symmetric distal axonal degeneration in the distribution of the ascending and descending nerve fiber tracts in the central and peripheral nervous systems. The mechanism of action is unknown. Inhibition of an enzyme known as neurotoxic esterase (NTE), found in the central and peripheral nervous systems of various species, is an indicator of neurotoxic potential and a potential biologic monitor for exposure to neurotoxic organophosphates. Compounds that are neurotoxic not only must inhibit NTE but must do so irreversibly through an aging process similar to that responsible for cholinesterase inhibition. Animal studies indicate that irreversible inhibition of NTE to 75% of initial activity will be followed 10–14 days later by a rapidly progressive ascending peripheral neuropathy. However, NTE does not appear to play a direct role in the pathogenesis of the neuropathy. There is no relationship between cholinesterase and NTE inhibition. The commonly used organophosphate pesticides with evidence of neurotoxicity are shown in Table 30–8. Carbamates do not cause delayed neuropathy.

A number of organophosphates and carbamates are known to cause primary irritant dermatitis. Only a few, including malathion, parathion, dichlorvos, and naled, are known to cause allergic contact dermatitis.

Organophosphate and carbamate compounds are alkylating agents, though generally not strong ones. A few are mutagenic, but most if tested have not been found to be carcinogenic in animals, and none have been found—on the basis of animal studies—to pose a significant carcinogenic risk to humans. Many have not been adequately tested for reproductive toxicity. Although some are fetotoxic at doses near or at cholinesterase-inhibiting levels in maternal animals—and this is of some concern for women directly handling pesticides—none have been found (by animal studies) to pose a significant teratogenic risk to humans. Carbaryl is teratogenic to beagle dogs but not to a number of other animal species. It is spermatotoxic in animals but showed no evidence of that effect in one study of manufacturing workers (exposed to relatively low levels).

Clinical Findings

A. Symptoms and Signs: In spite of the popularity of mnemonics such as MUDDLES (miosis, urination, diarrhea, defecation, lacrimation, excitation, and salivation), the signs and symptoms of acute intoxication with organophosphates and carbamates are best learned on a neurophysiologic basis by grouping them according to cholinergic classification (Table 30–9). There is some variability in parasympathetic nervous system manifestations because they are opposed by the sympathetic nervous system, which has preganglionic cholinergic innervation. Thus, the heart rate may be slow, normal, or fast and the pupils may be small, normal, or large depending on which system predominates. In one large series of organophosphate-poisoned patients, 90% had at least muscarinic manifestations, 40% both muscarinic and nicotinic manifestations, 30% muscarinic and central nervous system manifestations, and 10% had all three. The number of systems involved increases with the severity of intoxication. Mild poisoning is usually manifested by mild muscarinic signs and symptoms only.

The onset of illness after acute overexposure is unpredictable but is related to dose and route of exposure. Mild symptoms generally precede more severe ones, often for periods of 6–8 hours, but following extreme overexposure severe symptoms and death can occur within minutes. Absorption through the skin is prolonged, so that onset and progression of symptoms are slower. Because pesticide absorbed at a site near a target organ may directly inhibit acetylcholinesterase there without undergoing systemic circulation, that organ may be affected early.

The cause of death in acute organophosphate poisoning is usually respiratory failure. Bronchorrhea or pulmonary edema, bronchoconstriction, and respiratory muscular paralysis all contribute to respiratory failure. Cardiac arrhythmias such as heart block and cardiac arrest are less common causes of death. Ventricular arrhythmias have been observed in some of these cases. Seizures are not uncommon in cases of severe poisoning but rarely persist long enough to require treatment. Severe poisoning from occupational exposure to carbamates is uncommon. Owing to the rapid spontaneous reactivation of acetylcholinesterase, workers who become ill on the job are often better by the time they are seen at a medical facility.

Organophosphate-induced delayed neuropathy was first identified following 2 massive outbreaks of paralysis from ingestion of the nonpesticidal organophosphate triorthocresyl phosphate. The first occurred in the USA in 1930 as a result of consumption of an adulterated alcoholic extract of ginger root known as Jamaica ginger, or Jake; the second occurred in Morocco in 1959 as a result of adulteration of cheap cooking oil with surplus airplane lubricant. A number of other smaller outbreaks have been reported between 1930 and 1978 as a result of contamination of food, and there is one report of exposure in an enclosed space during manufacture of triorthocresyl phosphate.

Most of the reported cases of human delayed neuropathy have been manifested initially by signs and symptoms of acute cholinergic excess, although following ingestion these have been predominantly gastrointestinal (nausea, vomiting, stomach cramps, diarrhea). An asymptomatic period of about 7–21 days generally follows, depending on the size of the dose and the duration of exposure. The first symptoms of neuropathy are usually cramplike pains in the calves and numbness and tingling in the feet. This is followed by increasing and ascending weakness, initially in the legs and followed, in many cases, by weakness in the arms. Loss of balance due to weakness is common. Examination reveals symmetric weakness—distal more so than proximal, lower more so than upper—and sensory loss that is generally of lesser degree than motor loss. Deep tendon reflexes are lost in a pattern corresponding to the degree of weakness, usually ankle but not knee or wrist.

B. Laboratory Findings:

1. Cholinesterase—A number of nonspecific laboratory findings may be present in an individual with acute poisoning, including leukocytosis, proteinuria, glycosuria, and hemoconcentration. However, changes in cholinesterase activity, along with the typical signs and symptoms, provide sufficient information for the diagnosis and management of most cases. Red cell cholinesterase is called "true" cholinesterase since it is the same enzyme present in nerve endings and its activity more closely parallels that in the nervous system than does plasma cholinesterase, particularly in the time course of recovery after inhibition. However, red cell cholinesterase is more difficult to measure and therefore more susceptible to analytic error than plasma cholinesterase. Organophosphates and carbamates may differentially inhibit one enzyme relative to the other, so that if one and not the other appears depressed, it is conservative to assume that neuronal cholinesterase more closely corresponds to the lower of the two. For example, the commonly used organophosphate chlorpyrifos (Dursban, Lorsban) preferentially depresses plasma cholinesterase, causing illness without significant depression of red cell cholinesterase.

Different types of analytic methods are used to measure both red cell and plasma cholinesterase, with results usually reported in different units. Results obtained by one method cannot be compared with results from another, even if the units expressed by each are the same. There is considerable variability in cholinesterase activity in unexposed persons, so that reports of results relative to "normal" are meaningless.

Individuals with a genetic trait for atypical plasma cholinesterase have lowered plasma but not red cell cholinesterase. They have prolonged muscular paralysis after administration of succinylcholine and other neuromuscular blocking agents that are normally metabolized by plasma cholinesterase, but they are not more susceptible to cholinesterase-inhibiting pesticides. Plasma cholinesterase will not be a reliable indicator of exposure or poisoning in these individuals, but red cell cholinesterase will remain so.

Plasma cholinesterase production may be lowered as a result of liver disease extensive enough to impair the production of proteins such as albumin. Albumin-losing conditions such as nephrotic syndrome may be accompanied by elevated levels of plasma cholinesterase as a result of increased hepatic protein synthesis. The only medical conditions known to influence red cell cholinesterase activity are those associated with reticulocytosis, such as recovery from hemorrhage, pernicious anemia, and some other anemias.

There are 2 circumstances in which cholinesterase determinations may be useful: (1) routine biologic monitoring of exposure to organophosphates and (2) diagnosis of acute poisoning by organophosphates. In each case, comparison of the current level to a preexposure baseline level is helpful, and for biologic monitoring it is essential. Biologic monitoring of exposure consists of determination of preexposure baseline levels followed by periodic determinations in intervals based upon the frequency and nature of exposure. If only one test is used, red cell cholinesterase should be monitored, since it is more specific for organophosphate pesticides and is an indicator of cumulative absorption of organophosphate over a relatively long period of time. Plasma cholinesterase is more immediately responsive to inhibition by acute doses and may be preferentially inhibited by some organophosphates, such as chlorpyrifos. Cholinesterase levels are of limited value in assessing exposure to carbamates because of the rapid reversal of inhibition, even in a test tube.

The appearance of symptoms is more dependent upon the *rate* of inactivation of cholinesterase than the absolute level of activity reached. For example, workers may reach a cholinesterase level of 40% of baseline (60% inhibition) over the course of a number of weeks without experiencing symptoms, but a previously unexposed person may develop symptoms

at a level of 70% of baseline activity (30% inhibition) following acute exposure.

An individual's baseline red cell cholinesterase activity may vary up to 22% from day to day when measured by the same method by the same laboratory. Therefore, 25–30% inhibition (70–75% of baseline) during periodic monitoring can be taken as a warning level of a biologic response to chronic exposure to organophosphate pesticides, approaching a level likely to produce intoxication.

Fig 30–2 shows a set of theoretic values for "Worker 1" being monitored routinely every 15 days during exposure by red cell and plasma cholinesterase measurements. In this case, both plasma and red cell cholinesterase levels are progressively declining and doing so in parallel fashion. For Worker 1, both cholinesterase levels have declined to about 70% of baseline on day 60, and removal from exposure on that day was followed by a return toward baseline— plasma level more rapidly than red cell level. Removal of workers at this level (70% of baseline) and prevention of further exposure until levels return to approximately baseline is likely to prevent the development of clinical signs and symptoms of toxicity. Examination of the workplace situation leading to this level of depression is indicated.

Severe poisoning is usually accompanied by cholinesterase levels well below normal for the laboratory. However, patients with mild to moderate poisoning often have cholinesterase levels reported as equivocal, normal, and even above normal. The diagnosis can be confirmed retrospectively by periodic (ie, weekly or biweekly) determinations of cholinesterase until levels fluctuate by no more than 30%. If the average level at this time—the "retrospective baseline"—is more than 30% higher than the level at the time of illness, exposure to cholinesterase-inhibiting pesticides was almost certainly present, and the illness may have been due to that exposure. The rate of recovery of red cell cholinesterase—in the absence of treatment with

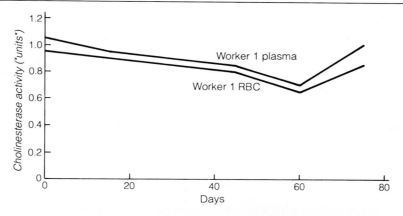

Figure 30–2. Cholinesterase monitoring for chronic organophosphate exposure.

pralidoxime and of further exposure—depends upon the rate of formation of new red cells, which is about 1% per day. Red blood cell cholinesterase levels will reach a plateau in about 60–70 days and plasma cholinesterase in 30–50 days.

Fig 30–3 shows theoretic values for cholinesterase levels for 2 workers taken every 15 days following acute organophosphate poisoning on Day 0. "Worker 2" has initial plasma and red cell cholinesterase values within normal, but for both types levels increase to about double the initial values, indicating a probable initial 50% depression from baseline for both. Plasma cholinesterase rises more rapidly and reaches a plateau sooner than red cell cholinesterase. "Worker 3" has an initial red cell cholinesterase value that is below the lower limit of normal and increases to about double the initial value, also indicating a probable initial 50% depression from baseline. Thus, even though Worker 3 has an initial cholinesterase level lower than normal and lower than Worker 2, the actual level of inhibition is similar for both.

2. Intact pesticides and metabolites—Measurement of the parent organophosphate or carbamate— or their metabolites—in blood or urine has been investigated to a limited extent. No such measurements are currently likely to be helpful in the diagnosis of acute intoxication. Measurement of alkyl phosphate metabolites in urine has not been of use in biologic monitoring of exposure because of its lack of specificity and instability. Measurement of *p*-nitrophenol in urine can be useful for monitoring exposure to parathion; 0.5 mg/L in a sample collected at the end of an exposure interval corresponds to exposure to parathion at the current TLV. Measurement of 1-naphthol in urine has been used to monitor exposure to carbaryl.

3. Neurotoxic esterase—Laboratory methods to measure neurotoxic esterase (NTE) activity are not available clinically. Limited research has indicated that determination of peripheral lymphocyte NTE

may be useful as a biologic marker of exposure to a neurotoxic organophosphate pesticide, particularly if its NTE-inhibiting potency is greater than its cholinesterase-inhibiting potency. However, there are at present no specific tests for the diagnosis of organophosphate-induced delayed neuropathy. If for some reason exposure to a neurotoxic organophosphate pesticide is uncertain, nerve conduction velocity studies may be of some help in distinguishing organophosphate-induced delayed neuropathy—with little to moderate slowing due to axonal loss—from Guillain-Barré syndrome (idiopathic acute symmetrical polyneuropathy), which is characterized by markedly diminished conduction velocities due to demyelination.

Differential Diagnosis

Mild acute poisoning from organophosphates or carbamates most closely resembles acute viral influenza, respiratory infections, gastroenteritis, asthma, or psychologic dysfunction. The most significant differential diagnosis is between severe organophosphate poisoning and acute cerebrovascular accident: Unequal pupils due to the local effect of an organophosphate in one eye of a comatose patient is a major source of misdiagnosis. Other conditions to be distinguished from acute organophosphate poisoning include heat stroke, heat exhaustion, and infections.

As noted above, the major disorder to be distinguished from organophosphate-induced delayed neuropathy is idiopathic acute symmetric polyneuropathy. Other toxic and disease-related neuropathies are generally insidious in onset and slowly progressive in course.

Treatment

Treatment that is otherwise indicated should never be delayed pending determination of cholinesterase levels. The initial diagnosis can be made on clinical grounds alone, samples sent to the laboratory, and a test dose of atropine delivered. Atropine blocks the

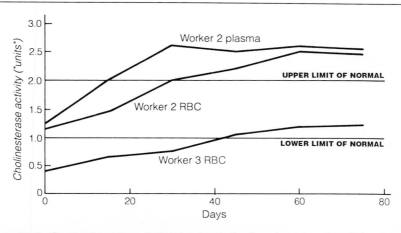

Figure 30–3. Cholinesterase monitoring for diagnosis of acute organophosphate exposure.

effects of acetylcholine at muscarinic receptors. A dose of atropine sulfate, 0.5 mg intravenously, produces signs of mild atropinization (dry mouth, dry eyes, increased heart rate, large pupils) in a normal adult; it has no effect in an individual with organophosphate poisoning. A dose of 1–2 mg intravenously will produce marked signs of atropinization in a nonpoisoned adult and may reverse the signs of cholinergic excess in a case of poisoning.

Samples must be sent for cholinesterase measurement before administration of pralidoxime, which will regenerate cholinesterase in red cells and plasma as well as nerves. Atropine has no effect on cholinesterase levels.

Treatment of acute intoxication must be predicated upon assessment of the severity of poisoning, which is largely dependent upon clinical judgment and experience. Assessment of severity should focus primarily on the respiratory system, since it is affected by all 3 types of cholinergic sites and is the critical one for survival and serious morbidity. The most commonly used severity rating defines mild toxicity as involving only muscarinic signs and symptoms, moderate toxicity as involving more than one system but not requiring assisted breathing, and severe toxicity as requiring ventilatory assistance.

Treatment modalities include the following:

(1) Decontamination, including bathing of skin, shampooing of hair, or emptying of stomach—as dictated by route of exposure.

(2) Atropine sulfate—in a dosage of 1–2 mg intravenously for mild to moderate poisoning, 2–4 mg intravenously for severe poisoning—as often as every 15 minutes as needed. There is no maximum dosage. Atropine blocks muscarinic activity but not the nicotinic (muscle paralysis) or central nervous system effects. Patients without evidence of muscle weakness or respiratory depression may be treated with atropine alone until one or more signs of mild atropinization appear, ie, tachycardia, flushing, dry mucous membranes, dilated pupils. Multiple doses may have to be administered over a prolonged time.

(3) For organophosphate poisoning only, give pralidoxime chloride (2-PAM, Protopam), 1 g intravenously slowly (no more than 0.5 g/min), repeated once in 1–2 hours, then at 10- to 12-hour intervals if needed. Pralidoxime acts by breaking the bond between acetylcholinesterase and organophosphate, reactivating the enzyme and restoring acetylcholine activity to normal (Fig 30–1C). Its advantages over atropine include acting at the neuromuscular junction to reverse muscular paralysis and possibly crossing the blood-brain barrier to reverse central nervous system depression. Overdosage is not a problem if the drug is administered slowly to avoid inducing hypotension. The decision to use pralidoxime must be made reasonably soon after diagnosis, since it is not effective once aging has occurred. A high incidence of atropine toxicity may result from the often recommended regimen of first using atropine until signs of atropinization appear and then using pralidoxime if necessary. This may be avoided by making the decision to use pralidoxime early.

(4) Artificial ventilation, ventilatory assistance, oxygen, and clearance of secretions.

The use of pralidoxime for carbamate poisoning is controversial. Fortunately, it is rarely indicated. There is experimental evidence that pralidoxime may be helpful in the management of poisoning by some rarely used carbamates, but for most of the commonly used carbamates this drug has not been studied. One animal study indicated that pralidoxime may be harmful in the treatment of carbaryl poisoning.

Morphine, aminophylline, and phenothiazines are contraindicated because of the increased risk of cardiac arrhythmias. Diuretics for pulmonary edema and fluids for hypotension are contraindicated also. It is recommended that atropine be withheld until adequate ventilation has reversed hypoxia, since atropine can be arrhythmogenic in the presence of hypoxia.

By the time the diagnosis of organophosphate-induced delayed peripheral neuropathy is made, the initial manifestations of cholinesterase inhibition, if present, have resolved. Administration of atropine or pralidoxime initially or later does not influence the course of neuropathy. Treatment of delayed neuropathy is supportive; in a few cases, mechanical ventilation has been required because of respiratory failure due to muscular paralysis.

Prognosis

If treatment for organophosphate or carbamate poisoning is initiated before hypoxia results in tissue damage, antidotal therapy and respiratory support should ensure complete recovery even in the most severe cases. Persistence of manifestations beyond 24 hours indicates the possibility of continued absorption of pesticide and the need to carefully consider and examine the skin, fingernails, eyes, and gastrointestinal tract as possible reservoirs.

Sudden death occurs in a small percentage of organophosphate-poisoned patients (2% in one series) 24–48 hours after apparent complete recovery from the acute phase of poisoning, due in at least some cases to ventricular arrhythmias. Sudden relapse of acute signs and symptoms within a few days after apparent recovery has been occasionally reported, perhaps as a result of mobilization of pesticide from fat following mobilization of the patient from bed.

Deaths have been reported as a result of accidental or deliberate ingestion of carbamates, as a result of large doses and prolonged gastrointestinal absorption, and perhaps as a complication of delayed or inadequate treatment. Intoxication from occupational exposure may be serious but is rarely fatal and usually is of brief duration. Poisoning from contaminated fruits and vegetables with high water content may also be serious but not persistent.

A number of reports have described persistent central nervous system symptoms in a small percentage of patients following well-documented incidents of acute poisoning from organophosphates but not carbamates. Typical symptoms include irritability, depression, mood lability, anxiety, fatigue, lethargy, difficulty in concentrating, and short-term memory loss. Limited studies have suggested that neurobehavioral test results and electroencephalograms may be different for such patients compared with controls. Symptoms may persist for weeks or months after the initial intoxication and are difficult to distinguish from psychologic reactions likely to occur after such an event. Sympathetic counseling and judicious use of antianxiety agents when appropriate will generally be more effective than intensive psychotherapy and antipsychotic medicine.

The rate and extent of recovery of delayed neuropathy appears to be related to the severity of the manifestations when they are maximal, usually within a few days to a week after the onset of weakness. At the rate of average axonal regeneration—approximately 1 mm/d—the longest axons affected may take up to a year to recover. Physical therapy appears to strongly influence the rate and perhaps the degree of recovery of strength and function. Long-term follow-up of survivors of Jamaica ginger paralysis indicated the development of an upper motor neuron syndrome that became apparent following recovery of peripheral nerve function. Continued disability was related to spasticity of the lower limbs, though muscle atrophy and weakness were present in some individuals.

ORGANOCHLORINE INSECTICIDES

Essentials of Diagnosis

Acute effects:
- Central nervous system excitation: irritability, excitability, dizziness, disorientation, paresthesias, tremors, convulsions.

Chronic effects:
- Cancer in animals.
- Aplastic anemia?

General Considerations

The organochlorine insecticides are chlorinated hydrocarbon compounds of cyclic structure and high molecular weight. In contrast to chlorinated hydrocarbon solvents and fumigants, they are of low volatility and are central nervous stimulants rather than general anesthetics. The prototype organochlorine chlorphenothane (DDT) was discovered in 1939, and until it was banned from most uses in the USA in 1973 over 4 billion pounds were applied, in agriculture and in control programs aimed at mosquitoes and other insects that transmit human disease such as yellow fever and malaria. From 1940 through the 1970s, a number of other organochlorine compounds were widely used as insecticides, but following recognition of their persistence in the environment, bioaccumulation in animals and humans, adverse

effects on some wildlife, and carcinogenicity in laboratory animals, most have been deregistered or severely restricted in use. Those compounds still in use in the USA are listed in Table 30–10. Since the acute toxicity of the remaining compounds is low and their use is currently limited, they rarely cause acute intoxication.

Use

Shortly after the development of DDT, hexachlorocyclohexane, better known as benzene hexachloride (BHC), was developed and became widely used. Only one isomer, gamma benzene hexachloride, was active, and this was developed into the insecticide lindane. Lindane currently has limited agricultural use, but it is marketed for human use as a scabicide as lindane (Kwell and others) lotion and shampoo. In some European countries, malathion is used instead for scabies.

After 1945, a group of organochlorine insecticides called cyclodienes were developed. These included aldrin, endrin, dieldrin, heptachlor, mirex, chlordecone, endosulfan, and chlordane. Because of environmental persistence and evidence of carcinogenicity of the first 6 compounds, only endosulfan and chlordane are currently registered and used. Endosulfan is still used in agriculture, while the use of chlordane is restricted to structural termite control. It is available to consumers for this purpose, though recent evidence of evaporation into the inside air of homes may lead to elimination of its use as a termiticide.

Occupational & Environmental Exposure

There is little information on current occupational exposure to organochlorines. Owing to their persistence and bioaccumulation, environmental exposure to organochlorines will continue for years even to compounds no longer in use, though there is evidence that levels are decreasing. Most of the world's population have measurable levels of DDT and other organochlorine compounds in fat and blood.

Pharmacokinetics & Mechanism of Action

The organochlorines are well absorbed by inhala-

Table 30–10. Organochlorine pesticides used in the USA.

	Oral LD50 (mg/kg)	Dermal LD50 (mg/kg)
Endrin	5–15	10–20
Endosulfan	20–40	75–150
Heptachlor	50–200	100–300
Benzene hexachloride (BHC), gamma BHC, lindane	100–200	500–1000
Chlordane	200–300	500–600
Methoxychlor	5000	3000

tion or ingestion and variably absorbed through the skin. Most are highly fat-soluble and are distributed to adipose tissue, the liver, and the nervous system. Most are metabolized by the liver and excreted in urine as metabolites. For some this is a slow process, so that accumulation in adipose tissue occurs during chronic exposure. DDT is metabolized and excreted slowly and is found in the fat of most persons; average DDT levels in the fat of Americans has been decreasing since cessation of its use in the USA.

Although the clinical picture of acute intoxication is similar for members of this family of compounds, their precise mechanism of action is unknown, and whether they share a common mechanism is for that reason uncertain. They cause central nervous system excitation and dysfunction with little pathologic change, presumably as a result of changes in the transmission of nerve impulses. They cause hepatocellular necrosis in high doses, hepatocellular hypertrophy and carcinomas—particularly in mice—at lower doses, and are inducers of hepatic microsomal enzymes.

Clinical Findings

A. Symptoms and Signs: Acute or subacute intoxication from organochlorines produces a picture of generalized nervous system excitability and dysfunction: apprehension, excitability, dizziness, headache, disorientation, confusion, disequilibrium, weakness, paresthesias, muscle twitching, tremor, convulsions, and coma. Nausea and vomiting are common after ingestion but not after dermal exposure, the primary route in the workplace. Most organochlorines are formulated with organic solvents, which may account for central nervous system depression, particularly after ingestion. Fever commonly occurs after seizures but may be a result of seizure activity rather than an effect of the pesticide. Chlordecone, no longer in use, caused a unique chronic intoxication.

There are a number of case reports and case series suggesting an association between aplastic anemia and exposure to organochlorine pesticides. These reports cannot exclude the possibility of coincidental occurrence of this rare condition with relatively common exposures.

B. Laboratory Findings: With the exception of measurement of parent compounds or metabolites in biologic samples, laboratory findings are nonspecific. Electroencephalography may show generalized seizure activity. For some compounds, a correlation between biologic levels and degree of poisoning is known, but such levels are rarely available in time to assist in management.

Differential Diagnosis

Severe organochlorine poisoning usually occurs following obvious overexposure and so does not present a problem in diagnosis. Other causes of central nervous system overactivity or seizures must be considered, particularly drug intoxications. Infec-

tions of the nervous system must be considered in the presence of seizures. Pneumonitis may be present as a result of aspiration of organic solvent.

Treatment

There are no antidotes, so treatment is supportive, directed primarily at maintenance of respiratory function and prompt management of seizures with anticonvulsant medication. Decontamination of the skin, hair, and gut (as appropriate) is important, as in all cases of acute intoxication. Cholestyramine has been shown to accelerate the elimination of chlordecone and recovery from chronic intoxication but has not been studied for use in management of poisoning with any other organochlorine.

Prognosis

Uncontrolled seizures may result in anoxic brain or other organ damage. If hypoxia is prevented, recovery should be complete.

FUMIGANTS & NEMATOCIDES (Table 30–11)

Essentials of Diagnosis

Acute effects:
- Respiratory tract irritation: burning eyes, nose, throat; cough, shortness of breath, pulmonary edema.

Table 30–11. Fumigants and nematocides used in the USA.

	Oral LD50 (mg/kg)
Halogenated hydrocarbon Ethylene dibromide	
Methyl bromide	200 ppm vapor inhalation
Ethylene dichloride	700–900 (1000 ppm vapor inhalation)
Carbon tetrachloride	2800 (8000 ppm vapor inhalation)
Dibromochloropropane	150–300
1,3-Dichloropropene	250
Chlorpicrin	250 (150 ppm vapor inhalation)
p-Dichlorobenzene	500
Sulfur and phosphorus compounds Sulfuryl fluoride	
Phosphine (aluminum and zinc phosphide)	
Sulfur dioxide	
Cyano compounds Hydrogen cyanide	<0.5
Oxides Ethylene oxide	
Propylene oxide	3000 ppm vapor inhalation
Aldehydes Formaldehyde	800
Glutaraldehyde	600
Acrolein	40–50

- Central nervous system depression: headache, nausea, vomiting, dizziness, drowsiness, fatigue, slurred speech, loss of balance, disorientation, loss of consciousness, respiratory depression.
- Encephalopathy (methyl bromide): tremors, seizures, elevated serum bromide level, late personality changes, cognitive dysfunction.

Chronic effects:
- Liver damage (halogenated hydrocarbons): anorexia, abdominal pain, jaundice, abnormal liver function tests.
- Peripheral neuropathy (methyl bromide): progressive distal symmetric sensorimotor neuropathy, ascending paresthesias, numbness, weakness.

General Considerations

Most of the fumigants are halogenated hydrocarbons and as such are lipid-soluble anesthetics and often alkylating agents. Most of the nematocides are soil fumigants. Ethylene oxide is a registered pesticide and is used to fumigate spices. However, it is used primarily for the sterilization of medical instruments, a nonagricultural use that is regulated by OSHA (see Chapter 26).

Use

Fumigants are used to kill insects, insect eggs, and microorganisms. Cultivated crops, herbs and spices, and packaged products such as dried fruits, beans, and medical materials are usually treated in fumigation chambers. Structures such as houses, warehouses, grain elevators, and greenhouses may be sealed, fumigated, and then aerated before being reoccupied. Fumigants are highly penetrating and will pass through most material. Soil is usually treated by application under a tarpaulin that provides a relatively tight seal. The nematocide vapors spread through soil and reach microscopic roundworms in the water that surrounds soil particles.

Occupational & Environmental Exposure

The fumigants are either gases at ambient temperatures or require heating to generate vapors. Exposure is primarily through inhalation of vapors. Since vapors can penetrate biologic tissue and protective clothing and pass through absorbent filters, opportunities for direct exposure must be minimized. Workmen applying fumigants may be exposed when leaks occur in equipment or when buildings are not adequately sealed and when checking for leaks and entering chambers or buildings before complete aeration without appropriate protective equipment. Exposure of applicators, field-workers, and bystanders to soil fumigant nematocides most commonly occurs when tarpaulins are disturbed, usually by wind. Phosphine is applied in solid formulations of aluminum or zinc phosphide, which liberate phosphine gas when in contact with water in the environment or after ingestion by pests such as rodents.

Zinc phosphide pellets that are ignited and dropped into animal burrows are also available. Poisoning has resulted from accidental ingestion of these preparations and from inhalation of gas following contact of the solid with water while in storage.

The high volatility and rapid environmental degradation of fumigants and nematocides provoked little concern in the past over food residues and water contamination. This changed following the discovery of residues of ethylene dibromide in raw and prepared foods and in water supplies, which led to phasing out of ethylene dibromide as a pesticide in most countries. The environmental fates of other fumigants and nematocides is of concern as a result but have been studied to a lesser extent.

Pharmacokinetics & Mechanism of Action

Most fumigants and nematocides are well absorbed by all routes of exposure and are rapidly excreted without significant bioaccumulation. Inhalation of vapors is the most common route of exposure, though dermal absorption of vapors or liquid can also occur. The vapors and liquids are usually primary irritants, in some cases quite potent. Most are general anesthetics (central nervous system depressants), while some such as methyl bromide have specific neurotoxic effects. The halogenated hydrocarbon fumigants share most of the effects of the halogenated hydrocarbon solvents, including cardiac sensitization, direct cellular toxicity to the liver and kidneys, and carcinogenicity in laboratory animals. The mechanism of multiple organ toxicity of phosphine and phosphides is unknown. Hydrogen cyanide is a metabolic poison that acts by inactivating cytochrome oxidase.

Most of the halogenated hydrocarbons are carcinogenic in animals. Ethylene dibromide, dibromochloropropane, and methyl bromide are alkylating agents positive in a number of short-term tests of genotoxicity, including mutagenicity. Ethylene dibromide and dibromochloropropane are potent carcinogens and spermatotoxins and have been banned from most uses for these reasons. Methyl bromide is currently being tested for carcinogenicity. Carbon tetrachloride is an animal carcinogen; liver cancer has been reported in workers following hepatic necrosis and cirrhosis from acute and chronic exposure.

Clinical Findings

A. Symptoms and Signs: Halogenated hydrocarbon exposure is marked by general anesthetic effects: initially, headache, nausea, vomiting, and dizziness, followed by drowsiness, fatigue, slurred speech, loss of balance, disorientation, and, in severe poisoning, loss of consciousness, respiratory depression, and death. Tremors, myoclonus, and generalized seizures may occur, particularly from methyl bromide poisoning. Acute and chronic poisoning from methyl bromide may be followed by prolonged and in some cases permanent organic brain damage marked by personality changes and cognitive dysfunction. Workers have been diagnosed as suffering from severe psychologic disorders until a source of methyl bromide exposure was recognized. Direct contact with liquid halogenated hydrocarbons may result in erythema and blisters. Damage to the skin can be severe if liquid is spilled on clothing and shoes, which retard evaporation.

Chronic exposure to halogenated hydrocarbons may cause liver damage manifested by anorexia, abdominal pain, nausea, vomiting, jaundice, dark urine, and light stools. Chronic exposure to methyl bromide can result in progressive peripheral neuropathy, with ascending paresthesias, numbness, and weakness, with or without depressed deep tendon reflexes.

Chloropicrin, formaldehyde, acrolein, and sulfur dioxide are strong mucosal irritants and are water-soluble, affecting exposed surfaces and the upper airway early. Acute exposure causes burning of the eyes, nose, and throat, tearing of the eyes, cough, hoarseness, and sometimes wheezing. Acute or chronic effects other than nosebleeds are unlikely from these potent acute irritants.

The halogenated hydrocarbons and phosphine are less soluble and less potent irritants and are therefore more likely to cause pulmonary edema, which may occur early or late after acute exposure. Many cases of acute phosphine poisoning result in death from pulmonary edema, seizures, and respiratory depression. Nonfatal cases have been marked by liver injury with abdominal pain, nausea, vomiting, jaundice, elevated hepatic enzymes, and coagulopathy with bleeding. The acute and chronic effects of sulfuryl fluoride are uncertain; this compound appears to be an acute irritant and may cause seizures and perhaps liver and kidney damage.

B. Laboratory Findings: For the most part, laboratory findings in cases of fumigant poisoning and overexposure are nonspecific and related to the organ affected, eg, abnormal liver function tests. Halogenated hydrocarbons can be measured in blood and exhaled air, but this is rarely helpful except in forensic cases. Methyl bromide is rapidly degraded to inorganic bromide, and measurement of serum bromide may be helpful in diagnosis of methyl bromide toxicity. A level of less than 50 mg/L is usually not associated with symptoms; a level above 50 mg/L is considered indicative of excessive exposure and a need for withdrawal from exposure; and levels above 100 mg/L are usually associated with symptoms and represent a serious threat to health. These levels are based on small numbers of cases in which exposure was both acute and chronic and analysis was performed at variable lengths of time following exposure. They should be used as diagnostic tools for evaluation of symptomatic individuals and not for routine monitoring of chronic exposure of applicators. They are different from the levels of inorganic bromide associated with poisoning by ingestion of inorganic bromide, a formerly popular sedative, which produces encephalopathy similar to that associated with methyl bromide but at much higher levels of serum bromide.

Differential Diagnosis

Anesthesia from halogenated hydrocarbons must be distinguished from exposure to other central nervous system depressants, including drugs and alcohol. The acute irritation produced by chloropicrin, formaldehyde, acrolein, and sulfur dioxide will be marked by the presence of their distinctive odors. Phosphine has a garliclike odor that can often be detected on a victim's breath. The encephalopathy and peripheral neuropathy from methyl bromide are similar to those from other organic causes of central or peripheral disease, such as alcohol, drugs, and other neurotoxins (see Chapter 22). Toxicity can occur from exposure to levels without a detectable odor, making diagnosis difficult without a history of exposure.

Treatment

Treatment of all fumigant poisoning except cyanide is symptomatic: respiratory support and anticonvulsants should be provided as indicated. Dimercaprol (BAL) has been used in early methyl bromide poisoning but without evidence of benefit; given its toxicity, it cannot be recommended. Treatment to increase the excretion of inorganic bromide has no rational basis.

Prognosis

Toxicity from the irritants chloropicrin, formaldehyde, acrolein, and sulfur dioxide is limited to their acute reversible effects. On the other hand, deaths have been reported from the use of most of the other fumigants and nematocides. Recovery from nonfatal poisoning of most is usually complete except for methyl bromide, which has caused permanent organic brain damage and a prolonged if not permanent peripheral neuropathy. Acute liver necrosis followed by cirrhosis and liver cancer has been reported from industrial solvent use of carbon tetrachloride but not from its use as an agriculture fumigant.

SUBSTITUTED PHENOLS
(Dinitrophenols, Chlorinated Phenols)

Essentials of Diagnosis

Acute effects:
- Uncoupling of oxidative phosphorylation: fever, flushing, sweating, thirst, tachycardia, hypertension, euphoria, anxiety, restlessness, hyperpnea, cyanosis, seizures.
- Yellow staining of skin, nails, conjunctiva.

Chronic effects:
- Uncoupling of oxidative phosphorylation: weight loss, fatigue, restlessness, anxiety, thirst.
- Dermatitis.

General Considerations

The substituted phenols are generally highly toxic compounds used for a variety of agricultural purposes. They act by uncoupling oxidative phosphorylation.

Use

The dinitrophenols include dinitro-*o*-cresol (DNOC), dinoseb, dinocap, and binapacryl and are used as insecticides, ovicides, fungicides, and herbicides. The use of dinoseb is being phased out followed discovery of its teratogenicity in animals. The chlorinated phenols are represented primarily by pentachlorophenol, which is used principally as a wood preservative and is discussed in Chapter 26.

Occupational & Environmental Exposure

Pentachlorophenol has been the subject of a relatively large number of occupational and environmental studies. It is known to be present throughout the food chain and can be found in biologic samples of most of the population in industrialized societies. In contrast, there is little quantitative information regarding exposure to nitrophenols.

Pharmacokinetics & Mechanism of Action

The mechanism of action of nitrophenols and chlorinated phenols in human poisoning and in some pests is uncoupling of oxidative phosphorylation, which results in increased oxygen consumption and heat production. The chlorinated phenols are strong irritants, while the nitrophenols are less so. All substituted phenols can directly damage the liver and kidneys by precipitating proteins. There are few chronic toxicity data for most members of these families.

These compounds are well absorbed by all routes of exposure and are primarily excreted in urine unchanged or bound to glucuronide, with a lesser degree of hepatic metabolism. Nitrophenols have been reported to be excreted within 3–4 days, while other substituted phenols may be excreted over longer periods of time due to deposition in fat.

Clinical Findings

A. Symptoms and Signs: Nitrophenols impart a yellow stain to tissues, so that yellow skin, nails, and hair are a result of contact and yellow scleras and urine are a sign of systemic absorption. Chlorinated phenols do not produce a stain. Systemic poisoning from any of the substituted phenols consists of a general hypermetabolic state. Profuse sweating, headache, thirst, malaise, and lassitude are common early signs, while fever, flushed skin, apprehension, anxiety, mania, tachycardia, and hypertension occur later with more serious degrees of intoxication. Altered consciousness, loss of consciousness, seizures, cyanosis, tachypnea, and dyspnea are signs of tissue anoxia, particularly cerebral. Liver and kidney injury are likely to be subclinical. Chronic intoxication is marked by weight loss and low-grade fever.

B. Laboratory Findings: The most common findings are nonspecific, due to dehydration and hypermetabolism, such as hemoconcentration and metabolic acidosis. Proteinuria, pyuria, hematuria, glycosuria, and elevated serum urea nitrogen and creatinine reflect renal injury; increased serum AST and bilirubin reflect liver injury. Anemia and leukopenia have been reported after exposure to both chlorinated phenols and nitrophenols and aplastic anemia after chlorinated phenols, though leukocytosis is more commonly seen as a nonspecific response to acute poisoning. Nitrophenols can be measured in blood and urine, but little is known of the relationship of levels to degree of intoxication; more information is available in this regard for pentachlorophenol (see Chapter 26).

Differential Diagnosis

Other hypermetabolic states to consider include hyperthyroidism, intoxication with stimulant drugs, and aspirin or salicylate poisoning, which also uncouples oxidative phosphorylation.

Treatment

Specific treatment should be directed at reducing body temperature; restoration of fluids and electrolytes, including glucose; and treatment of seizures or any increase in muscle activity, which will contribute to hyperthermia. Reduction of body temperature is similar to the treatment of heat stroke and can often be achieved with sponge baths or a fine spray mist. If this is ineffective, enteric lavage with iced saline solution should be considered. Drugs such as aspirin and other antipyretics and atropine and other anticholinergics should be avoided as they may further increase body temperature, with potentially disastrous results. Liberal amounts of glucose should be administered unless marked hyperglycemia is present, since glucose and glycogen stores may be depleted in spite of normal or high blood glucose levels. Hemodialysis and hemoperfusion have not been shown to be of benefit.

Prognosis

Deaths have occurred from acute intoxication from both nitrophenols and chlorinated phenols. Prolonged seizures and severe renal or liver damage are poor prognostic signs. Following recovery, reexposure should be avoided until metabolic processes have completely returned to normal and body weight has returned to baseline.

RODENTICIDES

Rats are the most important pest in many developing countries, consuming up to 20% of stored grain, and represent a significant threat to the food supply in developed countries as well. Other rodents and small mammals such as squirrels, gophers, and rabbits compete for food and act as reservoirs of diseases that affect humans and are considered pests for that reason.

Poisoning with rodenticides is the most widely used method of control of small mammals. To be effective, rodenticides must be attractive to a rat as food, which is difficult since they are fastidious eaters. They must also be delayed in action if used as bait, since rats will avoid returning to feed where another rat has died after eating. Unfortunately, what is attractive, edible, and ultimately lethal to a rat is usually those things also to pets and other animals and small children. Since application of baits results in negligible exposure to applicators, the primary human health hazard from most rodenticides is childhood poisoning from ingestion, though serious poisoning from single ingestions of warfarin is rare.

Rodenticides in current use are shown in Table 30–12. Yellow phosphorus and Vacor are no longer used because of their extreme human health hazard. Sodium fluoroacetate is similarly hazardous but may have some utility against coyotes and wolves. Strychnine may be useful against rats when anticoagulants are no longer effective, but it is toxic to all warm-blooded animals, is not always an effective rodenticide, and its use is controversial. ANTU is rarely used, since rodents quickly develop tolerance to it; it is also a possible bladder carcinogen.

The usefulness of rodenticides is limited primarily by the development of resistance in the target species.

Since anticoagulants are usually the only chemical used against rodents, the rest of this discussion will be confined to members of this class.

Use

The anticoagulants include 2 classes of closely related compounds: the coumarins, represented by warfarin; and the indandiones, represented by diphacinone. Warfarin is formulated as a dust (10 g of active ingredient per kilogram, or 1%) for use in holes and runs and as a powder (1 g and 5 g/kg, or 0.1% and 0.5%) for mixing with bait for a final concentration of 50–250 mg/kg (0.00005–0.00025%). Diphacinone is formulated as prepared baits in concentrations of 50–125 mg/kg (0.00005–0.000125%). Both warfarin and diphacinone have been used extensively therapeutically as oral anticoagulant medications.

Occupational & Environmental Exposure

There are no reports of harmful exposure from the manufacture, formulation, or application of dry anticoagulant rodenticides. There is one report of bleeding in a farmer following extensive and prolonged skin contact with a liquid warfarin solution. Childhood ingestion of these compounds is common, though bleeding as a result is uncommon.

Pharmacokinetics & Mechanism of Action

Warfarin is well absorbed from the gastrointestinal tract and to a lesser extent through the skin. Diphacinone is absorbed following ingestion, but there is no information regarding its dermal absorption. All the anticoagulants act through inhibition of hepatic synthesis of prothrombin (factor II) and factors VII, IX, and X, apparently through formation of an inactive form of vitamin K. In humans and rats, the half-lives of these factors are longer than the half-life of the anticoagulants, so that repeated doses are necessary before significant depression and bleeding occur. The indandiones appear to act in rats faster than the coumarins. Resistance to warfarin in humans and rats appears to be genetic and may be due to rapid metabolism.

The anticoagulants also produce capillary damage through an uncertain mechanism, though this too is reversed by administration of vitamin K. Skin necrosis and dermatitis have been reported as a rare complication of therapeutic use of warfarin but have not been reported as a result of exposure to rodenticides. The indandiones cause neurologic and cardiovascular toxicity in some animal species but these effects have not been reported in humans.

Clinical Findings

A. Symptoms and Signs: Most cases of accidental ingestion do not result in evidence of toxicity even without treatment, since doses are usually single and relatively small. Repeated doses could be followed by bleeding, primarily from the mucous membranes such as the gums and nasal passages and into the skin, joints, and gastrointestinal tract. Abdominal, flank, back, and joint pain reflect bleeding into those areas.

B. Laboratory Findings: Prolonged prothrombin time may appear 24–48 hours after ingestion of an anticoagulant and is often the only evidence of toxicity following a single exposure. Coagulation time will be increased in cases of significant poisoning, but bleeding time may be normal. Specific factors other than prothrombin may be depressed. Warfarin can be measured in plasma and its metabolites in urine, but these measurements have little utility.

Table 30–12. Rodenticides used in the USA.

	Oral LD50 (mg/kg)
Alpha-naphthylthiourea (ANTU)	6
Coumafuryl	25
Dicumarol	550
Diphacinone	3
Pindone	280
Strychnine	1–30
Warfarin	180
Zinc phosphide	50

Differential Diagnosis

Most cases of rodenticide ingestion are observed or reported episodes and do not result in significant toxicity. Failed suicidal or homicidal use may result in otherwise unexplained bleeding and depressed prothrombin time.

Treatment

Treatment of single acute ingestions is usually unnecessary, but patients should be observed (at home) for 4–5 days following ingestion. Vitamin K (phytonadione, AquaMephyton) can be administered orally in a dosage of 15–25 mg for adults and 5–10 mg for children with a history of ingestion, or intramuscularly in a dosage of 5–10 mg for adults and 1–5 mg (up to 0.6 mg/kg) for children with prolonged prothrombin time or with bleeding. Following treatment, prothrombin times should be determined every 6–12 hours and used as the basis for further treatment. If bleeding is severe, slow intravenous infusion can be considered but carries a risk of adverse reactions including flushing, dizziness, hypotension, dyspnea, cyanosis, and death. Transfusion and iron to replace blood loss should be considered.

Prognosis

Treatment is usually effective within 3–6 hours. The prognosis is determined by the extent and location of bleeding and is usually good.

FUNGICIDES (Phthalimides, Dithiocarbamates, Benomyl)

Pesticides classified as fungicides are active against fungi and a number of related plant pathogens, including bacteria, viruses, rickettsiae, and others. Most fungicides are distinct from other pesticides owing to the unique plant characteristics of fungi and the fact that the chemical must kill or inhibit the fungi without adversely affecting the host plant.

About 150 fungicides are available, mostly synthetic organic chemicals of relatively recent development. This discussion will be confined to the most commonly used compounds, the dicarboximides, dithiocarbamates, and benomyl. Others in common use are listed in Table 30–13.

The dicarboximides, or phthalimides, are structurally related to thalidomide but have not been found to share its teratogenicity. Disulfiram (Antabuse), used to treat alcoholism because of its ability to produce an adverse reaction in the presence of alcohol, is a dithiocarbamate and shares a number of properties with these compounds. The dithiocarbamates, which include the ethylenebisdithiocarbamates (EBDCs), are also used as accelerators in the vulcanization of rubber.

These compounds are not acutely toxic, the primary recognized health effect being dermatitis, both irritant and allergic. Animal studies have indicated their potential to cause chronic health effects, though there are few studies in humans. The dicarboximides are mutagenic and carcinogenic; the dithiocarbamates are mutagenic, carcinogenic, and teratogenic; and benomyl is teratogenic.

Use

A broad variety of crops are susceptible to fungi and related diseases. Frequent application of fungicides is often necessary owing to the rapid replication of many fungi. With the exception of a few systemics, fungicides are only active where they have been left as a residue on a plant, making uniform application necessary. They are applied as sprays or dusts, so that a film of residue is left on the plants. Many seeds are treated with fungicides. A limited number of general purpose lawn and garden fungicides are available for home use.

Occupational & Environmental Exposure

Field-workers and employees in greenhouses and nurseries are more apt to be exposed to fungicides than to other pesticides on a routine basis, since fungicides are only effective as long as a residue is present on plant surfaces and application is often necessary at the same time plants must be handled by these workers. Seed treatment facilities are an important site of exposure to fungicides.

Homeowners are exposed to lawn and garden treatments. Most fruits and vegetables have allowable residues (tolerances) for one or more fungicides.

Table 30–13. Some fungicides used in the USA.

	Oral LD50 (mg/kg)
Dicarboximides	
Captan	9,000
Folpet	10,000
Captafol	6,000
Dithiocarbamates (ethylenebisdithiocarbamates [EBDCs])	
Ferbam	1,000
Vapam	1,700
Maneb	7,000
Zineb	5,000
Thiram	800
Ziram	1,500
Substituted aromatics	
Chlorothalonil	10,000
Chloroneb	11,000
Pentachloronitrobenzene (PCNB)	12,000
Hexachlorobenzene	10,000
Pentachlorophenol (PCP)	200
Inorganic	
Sulfur	None
Copper compounds	200–10,000
Mercury compounds	1–200

Water contamination has not been a significant problem to date.

Pharmacokinetics & Mechanism of Action

Little is known of the pharmacokinetics of the phthalimides in humans; they are rapidly excreted unchanged in urine in animals. They are carcinogenic in animal feeding studies, causing gastrointestinal tumors, but are of uncertain risk via dermal and inhalation exposure. All the dithiocarbamates are metabolized to carbon disulfide (see Chapter 26), which may be the basis for their effects on fungi and the potential for chronic toxicity to humans. The EBDCs are further metabolized to ethylene thiourea, which may account for their antithyroid, mutagenic, carcinogenic, and teratogenic activity. All the dithiocarbamates have the potential to cause a reaction to alcohol (alcohol intolerance) similar to the disulfiram-alcohol reaction owing to inhibition of alcohol and aldehyde dehydrogenases. Thiram has been shown to potentiate the carcinogenicity of ethylene dibromide as a result of inhibition of alcohol dehydrogenase, which participates in the detoxification of ethylene dibromide. Benomyl is teratogenic in laboratory animals but is believed to be of low human hazard in this regard owing to limited dermal absorption.

Clinical Findings

A. Symptoms and Signs: The phthalimides, dithiocarbamates, and benomyl all cause allergic contact dermatitis, which is indistinguishable from other contact dermatitides. A few reports indicate that the phthalimides may also cause asthma. An alcohol-dithiocarbamate reaction is marked by headache, nausea, vomiting, flushing, dizziness, confusion, and disorientation.

B. Laboratory Findings: Confirmation of a hypersensitivity response to a fungicide is by patch testing for allergic contact dermatitis and inhalation challenge for asthma. Diagnosis of an alcohol-dithiocarbamate reaction is based on the history of concurrent exposures.

Differential Diagnosis

Fungicide-induced allergic contact dermatitis must be distinguished from contact dermatitis due to irritants and allergic contact dermatitis caused by other pesticides or plants. Asthma in a phthalimide manufacturing worker may be due to an intermediate in the manufacturing process.

Treatment

Allergic contact dermatitis is treated by withdrawal of the offending agent and local steroids. Asthma is treated by removal from exposure and symptomatic treatment as needed.

Prognosis

Fungicide-related allergies should resolve following cessation of exposure.

HERBICIDES

1. MISCELLANEOUS HERBICIDES OF LOW TOXICITY

Herbicides are pesticides that are intended to prevent or control the growth of unwanted plants or to kill them once they have appeared. They have largely replaced mechanical methods of weed control and are currently the largest category of pesticides used in agriculture, accounting for 60% of pesticide sales in the USA and 40% of sales worldwide in 1983. Included here are plant growth regulators that alter plant development, defoliants that cause leaves to drop prematurely, and desiccants that accelerate the drying of plant parts. Nonselective herbicides affect all plants; selective herbicides affect specific target weeds; contact herbicides affect plant parts that touch the chemical; and translocated herbicides are absorbed by the plant and act at distant sites.

The herbicides having serious recognized or suspected human health effects—the dipyridyls and the chlorophenoxyacetic acids—are considered separately in following sections. Substituted phenols used as herbicides were discussed above. The organophosphate defoliants are not toxicologically distinct from the organophosphate insecticides. The rest of the organic compounds in this class have few if any recognized human health effects. The inorganic herbicides are more hazardous and are being used with decreasing frequency. Some examples of the organic herbicides considered in this class are listed in Table 30–14.

Use

In addition to agriculture, herbicides are used to clear rights-of-way along roadsides, railroads, power lines, fence lines, and property lines; to reduce competition for seedlings in forests; and for fire prevention, by reducing the amounts of combustible grasses and brush available as fuel. They are usually sprayed in bands or strips, broadcast over an entire area, or focused on one area or group of weeds (spot or directed treatment). The timing of application may be preplanting (before planting crop), preemergence (after planting but before emergence of weeds or crop), and postemergence (after weeds or crops emerge).

Occupational & Environmental Exposure

Occupational exposure to herbicides occurs as a result of dermal exposure to spray applicators and flaggers, while environmental exposure occurs in the form of residues on crops and food. Although a few studies have suggested the possibility of health effects occurring in populations as a result of spray drift or other environmental contamination from herbicides, with the exception of cases of obvious spray drift with damage to nontarget plants, such exposure is difficult to document.

Table 30–14. Some herbicides with little or no known human health effects.

	Oral LD50 (mg/kg)
Alachlor	1,000
Amitrole	1,000
Ammonium sulfamate	4,000
Atrazine	3,000
Bifenox	6,500
Dalapon	6,500
Dicamba	1,000
Diuron	3,500
Ethfluralin	10,000
Glyphosphate	4,300
Linuron	1,500
Monuron	3,500
Oryzalin	10,000
Oxadiazon	3,500
Picloram	8,000
Prometon	3,000
Pronamide	5,500
Propham	9,000
Propanil	1,500
Simazine	5,000
Terbutryn	2,000
Trifluralin	3,500

Pharmacokinetics & Mechanism of Action

These compounds show little evidence of toxicity to mammals; consequently, there is little information on pharmacokinetics or mechanisms of action in humans. A few of the pesticides shown in Table 30–2 as having some evidence of carcinogenicity in animals are herbicides—most notably alachlor, whose use on grain crops makes it one of the most heavily applied pesticides in the USA—may be suspended or canceled as a result.

Clinical Findings

A. Symptoms and Signs: Some formulations of herbicides contain organic solvents, surfactants, emulsifiers, or other vehicles and additives that may cause eye, nose, or throat irritation in applicators exposed to spray mists or dermatitis in mixers and loaders as a result of prolonged skin contact. Otherwise, these compounds have no known human health effects.

B. Laboratory Findings: There is little or no information regarding measurement of parent compounds or metabolites in biologic media.

Differential Diagnosis

It is always possible that these compounds have effects in humans not yet appreciated, particularly from accidental or deliberate ingestion. The toxicity of "inert" ingredients should be considered in evaluating persons with symptoms following exposure.

Treatment

Since these compounds have little or no known human health effects, treatment of any symptoms resulting from their use should be symptomatic only. For evaluation of symptomatic patients, the manufacturer should be consulted, particularly for identification of the inert ingredients.

Prognosis

Acute irritation and dermatitis from herbicide formulations should resolve shortly after cessation of exposure.

2. CHLOROPHENOXYACETIC ACIDS

Essentials of Diagnosis

Acute effects:
- Irritation: redness of skin, burning, soreness in throat and chest, cough.
- Peripheral neuropathy (2,4-D): acute nausea, vomiting, diarrhea, abdominal pain, followed in 7–10 days by rapidly ascending numbness, paresthesias, and weakness, with normal to slightly decreased nerve conduction velocities.

Chronic effects:
- None known.

General Considerations

The principal herbicidal derivatives of phenoxyacetic acid include 2,4-dichlorophenoxyacetic acid (2,4-D), 2,4,5-trichlorophenoxyacetic acid (2,4,5-T), 2-methyl-4-chlorophenoxyacetic acid (MCPA), and their salts and ester derivatives. Silvex, kuron, and fenac are homologues of 2,4,5-T, while 2,4-DB and MCPB, MCPCA, and MCPP are homologues of 2,4-D and MCPA, respectively. They are translocated herbicides relatively selective for broad-leaf plants. 2,4,5-T and its homologues are no longer manufactured or used in the USA because of their combination with 2,3,7,8-tetrachlorodibenzo-*p*-dioxin (TCDD) and the controversy over its alleged health effects in environmentally exposed populations and Vietnam veterans. While certain batches of 2,4-D have been found to be contaminated with low levels of other lesser chlorinated dioxins, such as dichlorodibenzo-*p*-dioxin, none of its contaminants have been found to be of toxicologic importance. The toxicity of dioxins is discussed in Chapters 26 and 39.

Use

The chlorophenoxy herbicides have had a wide variety of uses, including control of undesirable perennial hardwood trees and plants for "release" of desirable evergreen softwood trees.

Occupational & Environmental Exposure

Occupational exposure occurs primarily as direct contact with liquid concentrate during mixing and loading and inhalation and contact with spray mist during application. Although concern has been expressed about environmental exposure of populations living near conifer forests where chlorophenoxy herbicides are applied, in the absence of obvious spray drift with nontarget crop damage such exposure is difficult to document. 2,4-D is rapidly degraded in the environment, and water contamination has not been a major problem.

Pharmacokinetics & Mechanism of Action

The herbicidal mechanism of action of chlorophenoxyacetic acids is uncertain but appears to involve a mimicking of plant auxins (growth hormones) and effects on plant metabolism. They are absorbed by inhalation, dermal contact, and ingestion and excreted rapidly unchanged in urine. The mechanisms of any health effects on humans other than irritation are uncertain. They are weak uncouplers of oxidative phosphorylation and may produce hyperthermia at extremely high doses as a result of increased heat production. A study reported to the EPA indicated that 2,4-D caused an increase in brain tumors in rats given 40 mg/kg/d by mouth. A study of cancer deaths in farmers in Kansas was reported in 1986 to show an association between lymphoma and the use of 2,4-D. 2,4-D is weakly teratogenic in mice.

Clinical Findings

A. Symptoms and Signs: Some formulations produce skin irritation following contact with liquid; irritation of the eyes, nose, throat, and respiratory tract, with burning and cough, from exposure to spray mist; and irritation of the gastrointestinal tract, with abdominal pain, nausea, and vomiting following ingestion. Ingestion of chlorophenoxyacetic acid herbicides has resulted in nausea, vomiting, abdominal pain, and diarrhea followed by muscle twitching, myotonia, metabolic acidosis, and a hypermetabolic state with fever, tachycardia, hypertension, sweating, convulsions, and coma.

Approximately 6 cases of peripheral neuropathy have been reported following relatively large dermal exposures to 2,4-D over the course of a few days. Clinically, these resembled idiopathic acute symmetric polyneuropathy (Guillain-Barré syndrome) and organophosphate-induced delayed neuropathy in that an initial influenzalike illness associated with nausea, vomiting, diarrhea, and myalgias was followed by an asymptomatic interval and then, 7–10 days later, by rapidly ascending loss of both motor and sensory nerve function. Respiratory function was spared in most cases.

Chloracne has been reported as a result of exposure to TCDD in 2,4,5-T manufacturing plant workers. A number of epidemiologic studies have suggested an association between exposure to chlorophenoxyacetic acid herbicides and soft tissue sarcomas. A registry of cases of such tumors has been established by NIOSH.

B. Laboratory Findings: Exposure to a chlorophenoxyacetic compound can be confirmed through analysis of blood or urine by gas-liquid chromatography. Urine samples should be collected as soon as possible after exposure because the chemical may be excreted completely within 24–72 hours. There is insufficient information to relate a spot urine level precisely to a level of exposure. However, since these compounds are excreted almost entirely unchanged in urine, a dose can be measured by collecting and analyzing all urine as long as collection is started promptly after exposure. Other laboratory findings in cases of acute intoxication are entirely nonspecific. In the few cases of peripheral neuropathy associated with exposure to 2,4-D where testing was done, nerve conduction velocities have been normal or slightly depressed, and spinal fluid analyses have been unremarkable.

Differential Diagnosis

Acute irritation following direct exposure or acute intoxication following ingestion present with obvious diagnoses. The differential diagnosis for a patient with peripheral neuropathy following exposure to 2,4-D includes idiopathic acute symmetric polyneuropathy and exposure to other neurotoxic compounds, including organophosphates.

Treatment

Treatment of acute irritation and peripheral neuropathy are entirely symptomatic. Since chlorophenoxyacetic compounds are weak organic acids, they are preferentially excreted in alkaline urine. In severe poisoning from ingestion of large doses, alkalinization of the urine can hasten elimination of the chemical and may improve the course of intoxication. Administration of large fluid volumes to achieve "forced" diuresis should be avoided owing to the risk of precipitating pulmonary edema.

Prognosis

Although death from ingestion of a chlorophenoxyacetic acid has been reported, severe intoxications have apparently been infrequent, and most victims have survived. In cases of peripheral neuropathy following exposure to 2,4-D, maximum paralysis lasted approximately 1 week or less. Recovery of function was usually prolonged for up to 1 year following exposure, with some residual weakness in most cases.

3. DIPYRIDYLS (Paraquat & Diquat)

Essentials of Diagnosis

Acute effects:
- Contact with skin, eyes, and respiratory tract: irritation and fissuring of skin of hands, cracking and discoloration of fingernails, conjunctivitis, sore throat, coughing.

- Ingestion of paraquat: early (1–4 days), oral and abdominal pain, nausea, vomiting, diarrhea; later (24–72 hours), liver injury (jaundice, elevated hepatocellular enzymes), and renal injury (proteinuria, hematuria, pyuria, elevated serum urea nitrogen and creatinine); late (3–4 days), pulmonary fibrosis (cough, dyspnea, tachypnea, cyanosis, respiratory failure).
- Ingestion of diquat: same as paraquat without late pulmonary fibrosis.

General Considerations

Paraquat is used extensively in the USA and worldwide, diquat to a lesser extent. They are nonselective contact herbicides.

Use

The dipyridyls are used extensively as general purpose herbicides owing to their ability to kill most plants on contact. They are also used as defoliants and desiccants, since the foliage of plants becomes dry and frostbitten in appearance, resulting in the premature dropping of leaves. Paraquat is used on cotton, potatoes, and soybeans, while diquat is used on alfalfa, clover, and soybeans.

Occupational & Environmental Exposures

The most important occupational exposures occur by direct contact of the skin with liquid concentrate during mixing and loading and inhalation and skin contact with spray mist during application. A case of acute paraquat intoxication was reported in a flagger who endured extensive dermal exposure to spray mist. Environmental exposure through field residues, food residues, and water contamination has not been a concern. The program of the United States Drug Enforcement Agency to spray marihuana fields with paraquat generated controversy over the possibility of inhalation of paraquat by marihuana smokers. Most of the paraquat probably undergoes thermal decomposition before it is inhaled, but the possibility of adverse effects from paraquat or its decomposition products has not been ruled out.

Pharmacokinetics & Mechanism of Action

The dipyridyls affect both plants and mammals by damaging tissue through the generation of free oxygen radicals. Their effect on plants requires the presence of sunlight. They are absorbed by inhalation, dermal contact, or ingestion. They damage epithelial tissues such as skin, nails, cornea, gastrointestinal tract, and respiratory tract and also the liver and kidneys.

Paraquat is more toxic to humans than diquat. A small sip of the liquid concentrate can kill an adult, which accounts for the hundreds of deaths reported worldwide from accidental and deliberate ingestion of this herbicide. An experimental trial that consisted of adding an emetic to formulations of paraquat was recently instituted in an attempt to reduce the frequency of fatal ingestions.

A relatively small number of cases of serious poisoning from paraquat have been reported as a result of large dermal exposures, while none have been reported from inhalation exposure in the absence of significant skin contact. Pulmonary injury from chronic dermal or inhalation exposure has not been reliably reported or found in the few epidemiologic studies performed with applicators. Neither paraquat nor diquat has been adequately tested for carcinogenicity.

Clinical Findings

A. Symptoms and Signs: Direct contact with concentrated liquid dipyridyls results in skin irritation and fissuring and in cracking, discoloration, and sometimes loss of the fingernails. Liquid splashed in the eye can cause conjunctivitis and opacification of the cornea. Inhalation of spray mist can irritate the nose and throat, causing nosebleeds and sore throat.

Ingestion of either paraquat or diquat can result in an early phase (1–4 days) of inflammation of the mouth and gastrointestinal tract, with soreness, ulceration, burning pain, nausea, vomiting, diarrhea, and sometimes hematemesis and melena. These symptoms can range from mild to severe, and their intensity may not predict the severity of the following phases. The second phase begins 24–72 hours after exposure and is marked by evidence of hepatic and renal injury. Hepatocellular injury is indicated by abdominal pain, nausea, and jaundice. Renal injury is usually asymptomatic unless oliguria or anuria develops. Renal and hepatic injury from ingestion of paraquat is common and frequently severe, while that from ingestion of diquat is less common and often milder.

A late phase (> 72–96 hours) of pulmonary fibrosis occurs from paraquat but not diquat, presumably because paraquat but not diquat becomes concentrated in pulmonary epithelial tissue. Pulmonary edema has occasionally occurred following ingestion of either paraquat or diquat. In cases of paraquat poisoning, pulmonary fibrosis is marked by cough, shortness of breath, and tachypnea. Advanced fibrosis is indicated by progressive cyanosis.

B. Laboratory Findings: In the early phase of acute poisoning, the findings are nonspecific, usually related to dehydration from nausea and diarrhea. In the later phase, liver injury is indicated by elevated bilirubin and hepatocellular enzymes. Renal injury, primarily tubular, is indicated by proteinuria, hematuria, pyuria, and elevated serum urea nitrogen and creatinine. Oliguric renal failure typical of acute tubular necrosis may occur. Laboratory evidence of pulmonary fibrosis from paraquat in the form of a progressive decline in arterial oxygen tension and diffusion capacity for carbon monoxide commonly precedes the appearance of pulmonary symptoms. Later, pulmonary function findings are typical of restrictive lung disease.

The diagnosis of acute intoxication from paraquat or diquat can be confirmed by analysis of either compound in blood and urine. Analyses and consultation are available from the Chevron Emergency Information Center (Environmental Health Center), Box 4054, Richmond, CA 94804; 24-hour telephone (415) 233–3737.

Differential Diagnosis

The early phase of acute intoxication from a dipyridyl may be mild and in the absence of a history of ingestion may be mistaken for gastroenteritis or ingestion of another irritant chemical. The combination of renal and hepatic injury could occur following exposure to a chlorinated hydrocarbon solvent such as carbon tetrachloride. In the absence of a history of paraquat exposure, the differential diagnosis of the pulmonary injury is the same as for acute pulmonary fibrosis (see Chapter 18).

Treatment

The primary treatment during any phase of intoxication from paraquat or diquat is supportive, particularly during periods of organ failure. Bentonite and fuller's earth have been found to be more effective absorbents for dipyridyls in the gastrointestinal tract than activated charcoal. If available, they should be administered as a 7 g/dL suspension in normal saline in quantities of at least 2 L to any patient suspected of ingesting any quantity of a dipyridyl within the preceding several days. If neither bentonite nor fuller's earth is available, a similar quantity of the usual concentration of activated charcoal should be administered.

Saline catharsis is then recommended, using sodium sulfate rather than magnesium salts because of the risk of magnesium retention in the presence of impaired renal function. This cycle may be repeated for several days. Given the high fatality rate following paraquat ingestion, this extreme degree of gut cleansing is probably worth the risk of fluid and electrolyte imbalance, which must be monitored closely.

The issue of enhanced excretion of dipyridyl is controversial. There is no basis for the recommendation that glucose and electrolyte infusions be given in large quantities to minimize toxicant concentrations in tissues and force diuresis of the compounds. Hemodialysis is clearly ineffective for removal of paraquat. Hemoperfusion with coated charcoal may be effective in removing paraquat from the blood if it is performed before the chemical has been distributed to tissues. However, few patients have a confirmed diagnosis and can be placed in a facility where the procedure can be performed early (24–48 hours after ingestion). The decision to perform hemoperfusion should be made by a physician with experience in the technique and familiar with the issues and risks involved.

A number of therapies are available to attempt to retard pulmonary fibrosis from paraquat. Increased levels of alveolar oxygen increase the rate of production of free oxygen radicals and accelerate the process of pulmonary fibrosis. Animal studies have shown increased survival in low oxygen atmospheres, but there are no comparable human studies. Early placement of a patient in an atmosphere of 15% oxygen has been recommended. Supplemental oxygen should be administered only as necessary to maintain minimally acceptable levels of oxygenation. Early experimental results with the free radical scavenger superoxide dismutase have been disappointing. Corticosteroids and cytotoxic agents such as azathioprine have been tried with uncertain results.

Prognosis

Once pulmonary fibrosis occurs as a result of paraquat ingestion, death from respiratory failure can be expected. Survival with disability from restrictive lung disease may also occur. Occasionally, recovery of lung function may take place over a course of weeks to months. Although death from liver and kidney necrosis may occur following diquat ingestion, recovery is more common than that following paraquat ingestion.

MISCELLANEOUS PESTICIDES

1. PYRETHRUM & SYNTHETIC PYRETHRIN (PYRETHROID) INSECTICIDES

Essentials of Diagnosis
Acute effects:
- None known

Chronic effects:
- Allergic contact dermatitis: erythema, vesicles, papules, itching.
- Allergic rhinitis: nasal congestion, sore throat.
- Asthma: wheezing, cough, chest tightness, dyspnea.

General Considerations

Pyrethrum is a partially refined extract of the chrysanthemum flower that has been used as an insecticide for more than 60 years. There are 6 known insecticidally active compounds in pyrethrum, 2 of which are esters known as pyrethrins. Synthetic pyrethrins (pyrethroids) are based structurally on the pyrethrin molecule but modified to improve stability.

Chrysanthemum and pyrethrum have long been recognized to be human allergens without other recognized adverse effects in humans. The pyrethroids have not been recognized as having significant human health effects, though a few—such as permethrin and resmethrin—may cause cancer in animals.

Use

There are several hundred commercial products

containing pyrethrum and pyrethroids, usually in combination with a synergist (see below) and often with an additional insecticide, such as a carbamate or organophosphate. Many are available for home use against flies, mosquitoes, and fleas. The usual household formulation contains about 0.5% active ingredient. The greater stability of the synthetic pyrethrins has made them useful in agricultural applications.

Occupational & Environmental Exposures

Their low toxicity has resulted in little interest in quantifying exposure levels. The application of indoor ''bug-bomb'' propellants in homes has resulted in some concern about hazards to small children from residues on interior surfaces, particularly with respect to the organophosphates and carbamates.

Pharmacokinetics & Mechanism of Action

The pyrethrins are apparently poorly absorbed from the gastrointestinal tract and through the skin, hydrolyzed in the gut and tissues, and rapidly excreted. The nervous system toxicity responsible for their efficacy as insecticides is not manifested in mammals. Pyrethrins are active inducers of liver microsomal enzymes, an effect that has not been studied in humans. The allergenicity of pyrethrum to humans has not been replicated in experimental animals.

Clinical Findings

A. Symptoms and Signs: The most common effect of pyrethrum exposure is allergic contact dermatitis, which is manifested by itching and an erythematous vesicular rash. Bullae, edema, and photosensitivity may also occur. Allergic rhinitis is not uncommon, with nasal congestion, sneezing, and sore throat. Asthma and hypersensitivity pneumonitis have been reported but are uncommon. Dyspnea, cough, and wheezing indicate asthma, while these manifestations plus fever, malaise, and pulmonary infiltrates are indicative of hypersensitivity pneumonitis. Anaphylaxis with bronchospasm, laryngeal edema, and shock have been reported occasionally after inhalation of pyrethrum. These allergic manifestations have not been reported from exposure to synthetic pyrethrins.

B. Laboratory Findings: Skin testing can aid in the diagnosis of sensitivity to pyrethrum. There are no biologic monitoring methods for exposure to pyrethrum or pyrethroids.

Differential Diagnosis

Allergy to other pesticides, plants or flowers, insect stings, and household products must be considered in the evaluation of one of the allergic manifestations of pyrethrum.

Treatment

The key to treatment of any allergy is removal from exposure to the allergen. Allergic contact dermatitis may be treated with application of topical steroid preparations. Allergic rhinitis may be treated with antihistamines, decongestants, and a steroid nasal spray if needed. Asthma is treated with bronchodilators and steroids as appropriate. Anaphylaxis may require epinephrine, aminophylline, or a parenteral corticosteroid.

Prognosis

If the diagnosis is correct, treatment prompt, and removal from exposure effective, recovery should be rapid and complete.

2. SYNERGISTS (Piperonyl Butoxide)

Although there are a few other examples, by far the most common synergistic insecticide combination is that of piperonyl butoxide with pyrethrins.

Use

Piperonyl butoxide is used as an insecticide synergist with pyrethrins in ratios of 5:1 or 20:1 in a variety of formulations, many available for home use. They are used primarily for flies, mosquitoes, and fleas, often in combination with a carbamate or organophosphate.

Occupational & Environmental Exposure

There is no information specifically on exposure to synergists.

Pharmacokinetics & Mechanism of Action

Piperonyl butoxide is poorly absorbed from the gastrointestinal tract and probably poorly absorbed dermally. It is metabolized but also retained unchanged to an uncertain degree in rodents. Its mechanism of action is inhibition of hepatic mixed-function oxidase enzymes.

Clinical Findings

A. Symptoms and Signs: There are no reports of clinical illness occurring as a result of exposure to piperonyl butoxide.

B. Laboratory Findings: There is no evidence of enzyme inhibition from piperonyl butoxide in humans. A single oral dose of 50 mg did not change the metabolism of antipyrine in 8 volunteers.

Differential Diagnosis

Any illness occurring in an individual exposed to a formulation containing piperonyl butoxide is probably due to another ingredient, such as allergy to pyrethrum or an effect of a carbamate or organophosphate, or to something other than the pesticide.

Treatment

Treatment if required would be symptomatic.

Prognosis

The outcome would depend upon actual diagnosis.

3. INORGANIC & ORGANOMETALLIC COMPOUNDS

Included in this group are sulfur, arsenicals, mercurials, cadmium compounds, lead compounds, antimony, and thallium—all of which have been used as insecticides, herbicides, and fungicides. Many, such as the inorganic lead and arsenic compounds and all forms of mercury and cadmium, are of limited use or have been banned because of human and environmental toxicity. Some of these compounds have been discussed elsewhere (see Chapter 25). They will be reviewed only briefly here.

Inorganic sulfur is used in large amounts as a fungicide and acaricide in the form of dusts, wettable powders, and pastes. It has no known systemic toxicity but is a common cause of irritant dermatitis in field-workers exposed to residues on foliage. Propargite (Omite) is an organophosphate compound used as a miticide that in some formulations also causes irritant dermatitis. The dermatitis from both sulfur and propargite can be severe and may result in significant lost time from work.

Inorganic arsenicals are no longer used as general insecticides and herbicides. Historically, the use of these compounds in agriculture was associated with skin lesions, skin cancer, and polyneuropathy. Liver toxicity in vineyard workers—including hepatitis, cirrhosis, and angiosarcoma—may have been due to ingestion of arsenic-contaminated wine. Remaining uses of inorganic arsenic are the wood preservatives chromate copper arsenate and acetocopper arsenite (Paris green) and a number of arsenate salts used as ant killers (eg, Antrol). The EPA is considering restrictions for arsenical wood preservatives because of concern over the carcinogenic risk to end-users such as carpenters, who are exposed to arsenic-containing dust. Childhood ingestion of arsenical ant poisons has required treatment with chelating agents such as dimercaprol and penicillamine but have been reduced in frequency following repackaging into child-resistant containers. Home use of arsenical and chlorinated phenol (pentachlorophenol) wood preservatives has been superseded to some extent by the use of copper-containing preservatives such as copper naphthenate and copper quinolate. Although copper itself has little toxicity unless ingested, these compounds have not been subjected to long-term toxicity testing.

Organotin compounds, particularly tributyltin, are fungicidal and are commonly used in marine antifouling bottom paints. Tributyltin does not show the neurotoxicity displayed by triethyltin, but it is toxic to some marine life and its use may be restricted on this basis. Triphenyltin is used as an agricultural fungicide. It caused marked testicular atrophy in rats fed 20 mg/kg/d for 20 days, and its use has been restricted in some locations as a result. There are no reports of systemic toxicity in humans from the pesticidal use of any organotin compounds.

Organomercury compounds were used extensively in the past in the treatment of seeds and as fungicides. These uses were severely curtailed following the disaster of Minamata Bay involving alkylmercury compounds. Cadmium once had uses similar to those associated with mercury, but it has largely been replaced by safer fungicides.

4. DISINFECTANTS & ALGICIDES

If one includes the use of chlorine and chlorine compounds for water treatment, these are the most heavily used pesticides worldwide. They include the halogens (chlorine, hypochlorites, chloramine, and iodine), the phenols, the aldehydes (formaldehyde and glutaraldehyde), and the detergents.

The use of chlorine in water treatment is generally not a toxic concern except for accidental releases. The use of hypochlorite in swimming pools has been associated with thinning of dental enamel in people who swim regularly when the acidity produced from the generation of chlorine and hydrochloric acid was not buffered properly. The substitution of chloramine for chlorine has raised concern for dialysis patients and aquarium fish.

The hazards of phenol were discussed in Chapter 27 and those of formaldehyde in Chapter 26. Glutaraldehyde is chemically similar to formaldehyde but has not been tested for carcinogenicity. It is commonly used in hospitals as a disinfectant (Cidex) and causes eye, nose, and throat irritation when an aerosol is created. It has not been reported to cause asthma.

5. REPELLENTS

The best-known repellents are insect repellents for human application. The most common is deet (diethyl toluamide), used primarily to repel mosquitoes. Its use has generally been without incident, with the exception of a single reported case of an acute neurologic reaction in a young child who underwent heavy aerosol exposure. However, some concern has been expressed regarding the heavy use of deet by personnel working outdoors in mosquito-infested areas.

GROWTH REGULATORS & BIORATIONAL PESTICIDES

Growth regulators are substances that alter the behavior of the target organism, most often a plant, through a physiologic effect, to hasten or retard growth or other biologic processes. They are generally without known or suspected adverse human health effects, but the discovery that the breakdown product of the plant growth regulator daminozide (Alar)—unsymmetrical dimethyl hydrazine (UDMH)—causes cancer in animals has generated considerable controversy. Daminozide restricts growth of apples so that they remain on the trees longer and become firmer, making them resistant to insects. UDMH is concentrated in processed or cooked apple products, further increasing any cancer risk from daminozide residues. Daminozide was used to a lesser extent on other crops—including fruit, peanut vines, and flowers—producing varied growth responses. The manufacturer of daminozide may voluntarily suspend sales in the US until the risk from residues in apples is resolved.

There are 6 classes of plant growth regulators. The **auxins** are plant growth hormones that include indoleacetic acid and the phenoxyacetic acids, the latter discussed above in the section on herbicides. The **giberellins** are represented primarily by giberellic acid, which has a variety of beneficial effects on fruit and no known adverse effects on humans. The **cytokinins** are naturally occurring compounds such as adenine, which are unlikely to affect humans in the amounts used as pesticides. Ethylene generators, including ethylene itself and etephon, initiate degreening and ripening of many fruits without affecting humans. Inhibitors range from simple organic acids of low toxicity, such as benzoic, gallic, and cinnamic acid, to maleic hydrazide, for which preliminary evidence of carcinogenicity in animals has been reported. Finally, growth retardants include newly developed substances such as chlorflurenol that are generally without known human health effects.

A number of insect growth regulators—chemical substances that disrupt the action of insect hormones, controlling molting and other stages of development—have been recently developed. Many of these are biorational pesticides, either naturally occurring organisms (such as *Bacillus thuringiensis*) or chemical analogues of naturally occurring biochemical substances (such as the sex attractant pheromones). To date, this class has not produced any evidence causing concern for human health.

REFERENCES

Committee on Scientific and Regulatory Issues Underlying Pesticide Use Patterns and Agricultural Innovation, Board of Agriculture, National Research Council: *Regulating Pesticides in Food: The Delaney Paradox.* National Press, 1987.

Coye MJ, Lowe JA: Biological monitoring of agricultural workers exposed to pesticides: I. Cholinesterase activity determinations. II. Monitoring of intact pesticides and their metabolites. *J Occup Med* 1986;**28**:619, 628.

Farm Chemicals Handbook. Meister Publishing Co., Published annually.

Hayes WJ Jr: *Pesticides Studied in Man.* Williams & Wilkins, 1982.

Morgan DP: *Recognition and Management of Pesticide Poisonings,* 3rd ed. US Government Printing Office, 1982.

Moses M: Pesticides. In: *Environmental and Occupational Medicine.* Rom WN (editor). Little, Brown, 1983.

NIOSH: *Criteria for a Recommended Standard for Occupational Exposure During the Manufacture and Formulation of Pesticides.* US Government Printing Office, 1978.

31

Gases

Charles E. Becker, MD

On December 3, 1984, more than 2500 people were killed and 200,000 injured in Bhopal, India, from the release of a highly noxious reactive gas, methyl isocyanate. Many health and safety issues have been raised by this tragedy and will be debated for years. The event has heightened our awareness of the danger of noxious gases to workers and to communities.

The composition of air is very complex in an industrialized society. Methyl isocyanate illustrates the overwhelming effect of one potent irritant gas. This chapter will review the noxious gases that pose a health risk to humans.

Harmful airborne materials may be suspended in the form of gases or in a particulate state. A liquid particulate is known as a mist, while a fine solid particulate is often called a fume. Toxic inhalations and resulting exposure to a wide variety of gases and fumes may occur in the ambient environment, at work, or in the home.

Gases and fumes pose a hazard of injury to the lung in 5 five ways:

(1) They may simply displace oxygen from the inspired air, causing asphyxia.

(2) They may be absorbed into the systemic circulation, interfering with the process of oxygen transport and utilization (chemical asphyxiants).

(3) They may cause systemic toxicity without affecting oxygen delivery.

(4) They may cause direct respiratory tract irritation or injury. The site of injury is related to the solubility of the gaseous material. The most water-soluble substances are absorbed onto conjunctiva and mucous membranes of the nose and upper respiratory tract (eg, ammonia); the less water-soluble substances exert their harmful effects especially in the lower respiratory tract (eg, oxides of nitrogen).

(5) They may cause allergic responses that damage the lung directly or impair gaseous exchange.

Table 31–1 lists the noxious gases that exemplify these 5 categories.

ASPHYXIANT NOXIOUS GASES

Some noxious gases, such as carbon dioxide, methane, and nitrogen, may cause sudden death by displacing oxygen from the inspired air. Onset is with sudden collapse. Rescuers may also be exposed to environments lacking sufficient oxygen. When inspired air contains less than 10% oxygen, death ensues quickly.

Carbon dioxide is heavier than air and is often present during fires or in poorly ventilated mine shafts. The patient must be removed from the environment and given oxygen. Carbon dioxide collects in the basement of a building in which there has been a fire and may extinguish flames by displacing oxygen. It may also be released in nature, as in the recent catastrophe at Cameroon Lake in Africa.

Methane is a product of decaying organic matter. Pockets of methane are classically found in coal mines. Methane is lighter than air and therefore tends to accumulate at higher work stations in explosive concentrations and thus poses a hazard for sudden combustion.

Nitrogen is the most abundant component of air. When oxygen is burned in a closed area, nitrogen and

Table 31–1. Mechanisms of noxious gas injury to the lung.

Substance	Source
Asphyxiant	
Carbon dioxide	Fires
Methane	Mining
Nitrogen	Diving
Chemical asphyxiants	
Carbon monoxide	Fires
Cyanide	Gold extraction; electroplating and fires
Hydrogen sulfide	Oil refining; decaying organic matter
Systemic toxicants	
Arsine gas	Microelectronics
Phospine	Microelectronics
Paraquat	Agriculture
Metal fume fever	Welding
Direct respiratory irritants	
Chlorine	Production of alkali, disinfectants, household cleaners
Ammonia	Fertilizer production, refrigeration
Oxides of nitrogen	Welding, auto exhaust
Sulfur dioxide	Paper manufacturing, oil refining
Hydrogen fluoride	Microelectronics
Allergic lung reactions	
Isocyanates	Polyurethane plastics and foams
Platinum salts	Catalysts and electroplating
Solder fumes and flux	Soldering

carbon dioxide remain, displacing the oxygen. Nitrogen collects in underwater worksites and in mine shafts. Oxygen must be supplied quickly to affected persons or brain death will ensue.

CHEMICAL ASPHYXIANTS

Chemical asphyxiants are absorbed through the lung without injuring lung function and are distributed to tissues, where they inhibit tissue oxygenation. The most common chemical asphyxiant is carbon monoxide.

CARBON MONOXIDE

Essentials of Diagnosis

Acute effects:
- Headache (10% carboxyhemoglobin [COHb]).
- Dizziness, dyspnea (20% COHb).
- Visual disturbances, impaired judgment (30% COHb).
- Syncope, coma, convulsions over 40–50% COHb.
- Precipitation of angina.

Chronic effects:
- Neurologic deficits.
- Cerebral infarction.
- Myocardial infarction.
- Fetal damage.

Exposure Limits
ACGIH TLV: 50 ppm TWA, 400 ppm STEL
OSHA PEL: 35 ppm TWA
NIOSH REL: 35 ppm TWA, 200 ppm ceiling

General Considerations
Carbon monoxide is an odorless, tasteless, nonirritating gas produced by the incomplete combustion of carbonaceous substances. It is formed in most fires and along with cyanide is a key factor in fire deaths. Carbon monoxide competes with oxygen for binding sites on hemoglobin and decreases the oxygen hemoglobin saturation and oxygen delivery to tissues.

Occupational & Environmental Exposure
Normal catabolic processes in the body generate small amounts of carboxyhemoglobin. Environmental sources include cigarette smoking, automobile exhaust, and home cooking or heating with charcoal. Some chemicals, eg, methylene chloride, are converted in the body to carbon monoxide.

Metabolism & Mechanism of Action
Carbon monoxide combines with hemoglobin to reduce the oxygen-carrying capacity of the blood. As the concentration of carboxyhemoglobin increases, the oxygen dissociation curve shifts to the left so that less oxygen is available to be given up to tissues. The partial pressure of oxygen in the blood remains near normal, with the result that the chemoreceptor responses do not stimulate rapid breathing. In addition, carbon monoxide competes directly with oxygen for binding sites on hemoglobin and may also bind to critical extravascular proteins such as myoglobin. In these ways, carbon monoxide causes tissue hypoxia.

The dose of carbon monoxide absorbed by an individual depends on the concentration in the environment and the minute ventilation. Length of exposure and metabolic demand may also be critical. A fire fighter working vigorously in an environment with only a slightly elevated carbon monoxide level may experience dramatically increased minute ventilation and oxygen requirements. The organs with the highest oxygen requirement are most likely to be affected first by carbon monoxide—particularly heart and brain.

Clinical Findings
A. Symptoms and Signs:
1. Acute exposure–Consciousness may be lost with few symptoms. The most prominent early symptoms are headache and subtle changes of mental function in the range of 10% carboxyhemoglobin. At 20% carboxyhemoglobin, there is typically a throbbing headache and loss of dexterity; at 30–40% carboxyhemoglobin, there may be syncope; and above 40–50%, coma and convulsions. Because carboxyhemoglobin imparts a bright red color to blood, cyanosis is not a common feature of carbon monoxide poisoning. The greater the workload and the higher the oxygen requirement and metabolic rate, the more sensitive the individual is to the effects of carbon monoxide. Birds—especially canaries—were used in mines to detect carbon monoxide because of their high metabolic rate. Follow-up testing of central nervous system function is crucial in order to detect subtle hypoxic damage.

2. Chronic exposure–The ECG may reflect injury to the cardiovascular system. In workers with preexisting cerebrovascular or cardiovascular disease, stroke syndromes, angina, or myocardial infarction may be precipitated with only slightly elevated carbon monoxide levels. Rare presentations of carbon monoxide poisoning may include skin bullae in non-pressure point areas or retinal hemorrhages. Chronic exposure to low levels of carbon monoxide may induce subtle neurologic changes, decreased exercise tolerance, increased hematocrit, and changes of the fetus in a pregnant patient.

B. Laboratory Findings: The most reliable means of documenting carbon monoxide poisoning is to measure the percentage of carboxyhemoglobin in venous blood by spectrophotometric methods. Arterial blood gases will indicate a metabolic acidosis with a relatively well maintained oxygen concentration. The ECG can assess the effect of carbon monoxide on the heart. Delayed central nervous system sequelae from carbon monoxide poisoning may require sophisticated neurobehavioral testing for full documentation of neurologic injury.

Differential Diagnosis

Other chemical asphyxiants such as cyanide and hydrogen sulfide must be excluded. Cyanide and carbon monoxide may both be present where fires have occurred. Hydrogen sulfide can be detected by its rotten egg odor. The Po_2 is usually normal in carbon monoxide poisoning, and arterial-venous oxygen differences are not altered—whereas increase in venous oxygen content is present with cyanide poisoning.

Prevention

A. Work Practices: A sufficient supply of oxygen for combustion of carbonaceous material will decrease carbon monoxide production. Ventilation of blast furnaces, engines, and other generators of carbon monoxide must be adequate to ensure that concentrations do not rise dangerously. Wherever fires occur, protective equipment with self-contained breathing apparatus must be utilized.

B. Medical Surveillance: There is no formal medical surveillance program for carbon monoxide, though NIOSH has recommended monitoring of workers exposed to methylene chloride. Industrial hygiene monitoring of the workplace is essential. Smokers have up to 10% carboxyhemoglobin in venous blood, which may make it difficult to detect occupational carbon monoxide poisoning.

Treatment

Treatment consists first of removal from exposure, then administration of oxygen. The half-life of carboxyhemoglobin in room air is almost 6 hours. In an atmosphere of 100% oxygen, the half-life falls to 1 hour. With oxygen under pressure of 3 atm, the half-life is about 20 minutes.

Hyperbaric oxygenation presents many problems of management. Oxygen toxicity, nitrogen narcosis, and decompression sickness may occur. If hyperbaric oxygenation is considered for carbon monoxide poisoning, it is essential that the patient receive 100% oxygen while being transported to the hyperbaric chamber.

Patients with carbon monoxide poisoning must be followed closely for severe cerebral edema, which may occur within hours. It is uncertain whether carboxyhemoglobin levels in the range of 5–7% are associated with health sequelae. Subtle injury to the nervous system, cardiac system, and fetus are likely if cellular hypoxia occurs.

Prognosis

The prognosis of carbon monoxide poisoning is difficult to assess without detailed baseline central nervous system and cardiovascular tests. In general, injury is proportionate to duration and intensity of exposure.

CYANIDE

Essentials of Diagnosis

Acute effects:
- Dizziness.
- Nausea.
- Rapid breathing (suffocation sensation).
- Loss of consciousness.

Chronic effects:
- Suppression of thyroid function.
- Neuropathy.
- Optic atrophy.
- Abnormal neuropsychologic effects and neurologic injury with extrapyramidal effects.

Exposure Limits

ACGIH TLV: 5 mg/m^3 TWA
OSHA PEL: 5 mg/m^3 TWA
NIOSH REL: 5 mg/m^3 ceiling (10 minutes)

General Considerations

Cyanide is one of the most rapidly lethal poisons known. Cyanide serves no useful purpose in the human body but may be found in the workplace, food, air, and water. Contamination of Tylenol medication and the mass suicide tragedy at Jonestown have focused attention on the importance of cyanide poisoning. Cyanide may also be released in fires, especially in aircraft and high-rise buildings.

Use

Cyanide is a common laboratory reagent that is used in photography and in the extraction of gold. Acrylonitrile is used in synthetic rubber manufacture.

Occupational & Environmental Exposure

Cyanide may be encountered in industry as sodium or potassium cyanate or as acrylonitrile. Exposure to inorganic cyanide salts may occur from gold extraction and in photographic laboratories or electroplating.

Cyanide is a very reactive, volatile nucleophile with a pKa of 9.2. It is normally found in low levels in the plasma, blood, and tissues of healthy individuals as a result of normal metabolism, eating certain foods, and cigarette smoking.

Metabolism & Mechanism of Action

Table 31–2 lists normal levels of cyanide and thiocyanate in smokers and nonsmokers. Because of the pronounced instability of cyanide in plasma, there has been great difficulty in interpreting blood cyanide and thiocyanate levels. Appropriate methods for detecting cyanide must be utilized.

Table 31–2. Blood levels of cyanide and thiocyanate in smokers and nonsmokers.

Cyanide			
Nonsmoker	Mean	0.02 μg/mL	Whole blood
Smoker	Mean	0.04 μg/mL	Whole blood
Toxic		>0.1 μg/mL	Whole blood
Fatal		>1.0 μg/mL	Whole blood
Thiocyanate			
Nonsmoker		1-4 μg/mL	Plasma
Smoker		3-12 μg/mL	Plasma

Cyanide causes chemical asphyxiation by inhibiting the terminal cytochrome oxidase of the mitochondrial respiratory chain. It is likely that more than a single biochemical lesion induced by cyanide accounts for the chemical hypoxia. There are also differences in cytochrome oxidase in various tissues. Cytochrome oxidase in the brain is the most susceptible to cyanide inhibition, making the central nervous system the target for cyanide's lethal effects.

Clinical Findings

A. Symptoms and Signs:

1. Acute exposure—Cyanide rapidly causes vertigo, convulsions, confusion, altered speech, coma, and death. There may also be nausea, vomiting, hypertension with a decreased heart rate, and abdominal and chest pain. Cyanide specifically stimulates respiration, so that patients hyperventilate and have an intense sense of suffocation.

The odor of bitter almonds may be detected if cyanide is present. Because cyanide inhibits the terminal oxidase of the cytochrome system, no arterial venous oxygen difference will be found. Acute ST segment elevations may indicate myocardial injury in poisoned individuals.

2. Chronic exposure—There has been speculation that chronic cyanide poisoning could result from occupational exposures or from eating foods containing large amounts of cyanide. Pernicious anemia or hypothyroid states may also complicate cyanide metabolism. Increased levels of cyanide due to tobacco smoke or occupational exposure may be associated with low birth weight in infants.

B. Laboratory Findings: Cyanide induces severe metabolic acidosis. The body is unable to utilize oxygen, so there is arterialization of venous blood. The ECG will show evidence of acute anoxic injury to the heart. Cyanide is unstable in plasma, and there is great difficulty in interpreting blood and plasma cyanide levels as well as thiocyanate levels. Thiocyanate levels are also elevated in cigarette smokers. Cyanide levels must be measured by specific assay systems immediately after exposure.

Differential Diagnosis

Differential diagnosis includes poisoning with carbon monoxide and hydrogen sulfide and any cause of severe shock. The diagnosis of cyanide poisoning should be suspected in any individual involved in a fire involving urethanes, especially if there are exposures to chemicals that could release cyanide. Carbon monoxide and hydrogen sulfide should also be monitored in patients exposed in a fire. Myocardial infarction, stroke, or seizure may present with sudden collapse and severe metabolic acidosis with shock.

Prevention

Workers chronically exposed to cyanide solutions must have skin protection. In addition to focusing attention on having antidotal treatments available, great care is required when handling cyanide products. Workers at risk of exposure to acrylonitrile and other cyanide-containing products should wear impermeable clothing.

Treatment Rationale

Table 31–3 lists the principles of cyanide antagonism. Oxygen, metabolic detoxification, and chelation have been proposed. Though there are doubts about the therapeutic rationale, many studies have shown that oxygen does enhance other antidotes in preventing cyanide toxicity. While oxygen does not enhance the protective effect of sodium nitrite alone, it does enhance the antidotal combination of sodium nitrite and thiosulfate.

The thiosulfate sulfur transferase in the liver, known as rhodanese, is able to convert cyanide to thiocyanate. Rhodanese is principally responsible for metabolizing cyanide to less toxic products. Administration of crystalline enzyme rhodanese may prove to be of value for treatment of acute cyanide poisoning. Sodium thiosulfate as a key sulfur donor to aid the enzyme rhodanese is useful.

Cyanide has a higher affinity for methemoglobin than for oxyhemoglobin. Creating methemoglobin with nitrites as a means of treatment of cyanide poisoning has been known for over 100 years and extensively studied for 50 years. However, recent studies suggest that methemoglobin formation by sodium nitrite may be only a partial explanation for the therapeutic benefit of nitrite in cyanide poisoning. Nitrites may act through effects on the cardiovascular system or changes in regional blood flow. Cobalt salts and hydroxocobalamin have been known to form stable complexes with cyanide. At this time, the cobalt salts have proved to be too toxic for use in humans. Although hydroxocobalamin is currently not available in the USA in doses sufficient to treat cyanide poisoning, it is a safe and reasonable alternative. In addition, cyanide has been found to interact with various carbonyl groups, such as pyruvate or α-ketoglutarate to form cyanohydrin. This may also be a useful antidote in the future.

Death from cyanide poisoning may be so rapid in the workplace or at the fire scene that the patient may be found without any evidence of trauma or burns. Cyanide stimulates the carotid body and peripheral chemoreceptors promoting stimulation of ventilation, which may worsen cyanide inhalation.

Because of the rapidity of poisoning with cyanide,

Table 31–3. Treatment of acute cyanide poisoning.

Antidote	Mechanism	Toxicity	Preparation	Efficacy
Nitrites	Induction of methemo-globin and perhaps other mechanisms	Tachycardia, vomiting, hypotension, hypoxia, shock	Cyanide antidote kit	+ +
4-Dimethylaminophenol	Induction of methemo-globin	Minor cardiocirculatory derangements	Experimental	+ +
Sodium thiosulfate	Sulfur donation	Nontoxic	Cyanide antidote kit from hospital pharmacy	+ + +
EDTA-cobalt	Chelation	Cardiovascular prob-lems, vomiting, diar-rhea, depletion of Mg^{2+} and Ca^{2+}, anaphylac-toid reactions	Kelacyanor	Uncertain
Hydroxocobalamin	Chelation	Nontoxic	4 g hydroxycobalamin plus 8 g of sodium thio-sulfate	+ + +
Oxygen	Uncertain (hyperbaric oxygenation not useful)	Pulmonary and neuro-logic problems after 24–48 hours if Fio_2 >50%	Assisted ventilation	+ + +
Sodium pyruvate and α-ketoglutarate	Reestablishment of cel-lular respiration	Large doses needed	Experimental	?
Ifenprodil	Stimulation of respira-tory function at mito-chondrial level	Being studied	Experimental	?
Rhodanese	Formation of thiocy-anate	Being studied	Experimental	?

it may be difficult to confirm the clinical diagnosis. This is especially important because traditional anti-dotes such as nitrites may worsen the patient's hypoxia and hypotension if the diagnosis is incorrect. The large variety of antidotes for cyanide poisoning has puzzled physicians about appropriate methods of treatment. It may be difficult to decide whether the patient survives because of or in spite of antidotal treatment. Some patients have survived massive doses of cyanide without apparent long-term sequelae even without treatment other than supportive care.

Treatment

Critical treatment objectives are to remove the victim from exposure, maintain the airway, and provide supportive measures. Supplemental oxygen may modify the outcome of cyanide poisoning. The use of hyperbaric oxygen in cyanide poisoning is not justified. The nitrite-thiosulfate combination has been long used but is now being called into question. The use of nitrite in a patient who may have carbon monoxide poisoning alone without cyanide poison-ing, would worsen the patient. Thiosulfate poses no hazard and can be administered, though proof of thiosulfate efficacy alone is lacking. Research into appropriate chelating agents with minimal toxicity would be beneficial, especially in fire victims. Cobalt EDTA chelation therapy is probably too toxic and should not be used.

Hydroxocobalamin has been shown to protect animals from cyanide poisoning. Lyophilized hy-droxocobalamin is now available in the USA. Ad-ministration of 4 g of hydroxocobalamin plus 8 g of thiosulfate will most likely be the antidote that will be commonly utilized in the future. The only docu-mented side effect of hydroxocobalamin has been occasional skin lesions, which may be related to the vehicle in which it is administered.

HYDROGEN SULFIDE

Essentials of Diagnosis

Acute effects:
- Severe eye and respiratory irritation.
- Pulmonary edema.
- Coma.
- Death.

Chronic effects:
- Keratitis.
- Chronic lung disease.

Exposure Limits

ACGIH TLV: 10 ppm TWA, 15 ppm STEL
OSHA PEL: 10 ppm TWA, 15 ppm STEL
NIOSH REL: 10 ppm ceiling (10 minutes)

General Considerations

Hydrogen sulfide is a potent inhibitor of the terminal oxidase of cytochrome oxidase. This nox-ious gas is well known because of its ''rotten egg'' smell. Olfactory fatigue develops quickly, diminish-ing one's ability to detect the odor.

Occupational & Environmental Exposures

Hydrogen sulfide is found in tanneries, coal mines, rubber manufacturing plants, petroleum refineries, and septic tanks. Of special interest is the release of hydrogen sulfide in geothermal energy and in drilling for natural gas and oil.

Clinical Findings

A. Acute Exposure: Sudden severe eye and respiratory irritation occurs with acute exposure. Massive inhalation may cause direct pulmonary injury or sudden death. Sudden death is probably due to the inhibition of cellular respiration.

B. Chronic Exposure: Chronic eye irritation leads to keratitis and worsening of lung problems.

Mechanism of Action

Hydrogen sulfide inhibits cellular respiration in a similar fashion to cyanide, blocking the utilization of oxygen. The brain is the most sensitive organ affected, with coma and death being the most abrupt presentation.

Treatment

The similarity between the acute effects of cyanide and hydrogen sulfide has led to the use of nitrites and thiosulfate in hydrogen sulfide poisoning. There are equivocal data in animals suggesting that nitrites may increase the dose of hydrogen cyanide required to cause death, but the clinical use of these agents to create sulfmethemoglobin (analogous to the creation of cyanomethemoglobin) requires further study. The use of thiosulfate in hydrogen sulfide poisoning is not justified, since hydrogen sulfide is not metabolized by the enzyme rhodanese; therefore, addition of this cofactor would not be of value.

Hyperbaric oxygen has also been proposed to be of value by enhancing competitive inhibition of sulfide cytochrome binding, by enhancing sulfide detoxification, or by minimizing hypoxic injury. Further research is required to study the value of hyperbaric oxygenation in hydrogen sulfide poisoning.

Systemic Toxicants; Methemoglobin Formers

Methemoglobin is created by release of nitrites in the workplace. Nitrites have been released in fires, causing fire fighters to develop methemoglobinemia. Methemoglobin is hemoglobin in which the normal ferrous (Fe^{2+}) iron of the heme moiety has been oxidized to the ferric (Fe^{3+}) state. Because of the additional positive charge, the methemoglobin molecule is unable to bind oxygen. Methemoglobin is formed continuously in some normal erythrocytes but never reaches levels exceeding 1–2% because of effective reductive mechanisms—principally the enzyme methemoglobin reductase. Methemoglobin can occur when there are abnormal hemoglobins or hereditary deficiencies of enzymes in the methemoglobin reductase system or where workers are exposed to drugs or chemicals that increase the rate of oxidation to methemoglobin.

Symptoms in individuals exposed to nitrites are related to the rapidity of the rise of the methemoglobin level and oxygen demand. Concentrations below 20% methemoglobin usually result in only a trace of cyanosis without harmful effects. At levels above 20%, dizziness, headache, fatigue, and exertional dyspnea may occur. Methemoglobin, like carboxyhemoglobin, not only decreases oxygen-carrying capacity but also increases the affinity of the unaltered hemoglobin for oxygen, thus shifting the oxygen dissociation curve and impairing further oxygen delivery. Workplace exposures to nitroglycerin and other organic nitrates may also be associated with creating methemoglobinemia. For a more detailed discussion of metheoglobinemia, see Chapter 14.

Treatment

If symptoms are pronounced and the methemoglobin level is elevated above 20%, the antidote methylene blue, 1–2 mg/kg, will reverse methemoglobinemia. If methylene blue fails to do so, a congenital deficiency of methemoglobin reductase is possible or a genetic deficiency of glucose-6-phosphate dehydrogenase (G6PD) may be present. In G6PD deficiency, methylene blue will not generate the appropriate metabolites necessary to reverse the methemoglobinemia.

SYSTEMIC TOXICANTS

ARSINE

Essentials of Diagnosis

Acute effects:
- Headache, malaise, weakness.
- Abdominal pain, nausea and vomiting.
- Hemolysis in 2–24 hours.
- Sudden death with heavy exposure.

Chronic effects:
- Uncertain risk of cancer.

Exposure Limits

ACGIH TLV: 0.05 ppm TWA
OSHA PEL: 0.05 ppm TWA
NIOSH REL: 2 μg/m^3 ceiling

General Considerations

Arsine (AsH_3) is a colorless nonirritating gas at room temperature and has a slight garlicky odor. Arsine will evolve whenever nascent hydrogen is generated in the presence of arsenic or when water acts on metallic arsenide. Arsine poisoning has occurred during smelting or refining and in other industrial settings, including galvanizing, etching, lead plating, sewage work, and closed-space cleaning of contaminated tanks or vats and accidental release of stored arsine gas.

Use

Arsine is utilized to provide arsenic as a dopant in the semiconductor industry. It is produced in smelting and refining of arsenic-containing ores, which are treated with acid. Arsine may also be generated from the combustion of fossil fuels.

Occupational & Environmental Exposure

Most exposures to arsine occur in the microelectronics industry, where arsine is used in the manufacture of semiconductor chips. Arsine may also be released in transportation accidents, natural disasters, or by industrial sabotage. Small quantities of arsine may also be released when ores are treated with acid.

Metabolism & Mechanism of Action

The pathogenesis of arsine poisoning is not well understood. Arsine dissolves in the plasma and forms a nondialyzable complex within the red blood cell. The hemolysis is multifactorial. The postulated pathways include the formation of elemental arsenic or arsenic dihydride, the inhibition of catalase, and the formation of irreversible complexes with sulfhydryl groups of essential enzymes within the red blood cell. Arsine exerts an oxidant stress like that of many different drugs in patients with G6PD deficiency. Renal biopsy of fatal cases has demonstrated hemoglobin casts, but renal failure may be a result of direct toxic effects on the renal tubule, hypoxia secondary to anemia, or precipitation of the arsine hemoglobin-haptoglobin complex in the tubular lumen. Biopsies of nonfatal cases initially demonstrate extensive tubular damage followed by regeneration of tubules and a subsequent interstitial fibrosis.

Clinical Findings

A. Acute Exposure: In small mammals the mean lethal dose of arsine is approximately 0.5 mg/kg. Arsine is the most acutely toxic form of arsenic. Exposures to 250 ppm are instantaneously lethal, and 25–50 ppm is lethal after 30 minutes. The interval between the onset of exposure and symptoms varies from 2 to 24 hours and depends on the level of exposure.

In humans, a triad of abdominal pain, hematuria, and jaundice is typical. Other symptoms include headache, malaise, weakness, and gastrointestinal distress accompanied by nausea and vomiting. The most important laboratory findings include severe hemolytic anemia with a peripheral blood smear that may show anisocytosis, red blood cell fragments, and ghost cells. Plasma free hemoglobin is elevated, and urinalysis shows hemoglobinuria with an initial unremarkable urinary sediment. Acute renal failure is an early and often fatal complication of arsine poisoning.

Arsine is toxic also to heart, lungs, liver, the gastrointestinal tract and central nervous system, and bone marrow. Skeletal muscle damage releases myoglobin, which may add to renal injury. Peripheral neuropathy and Mees's lines may develop later in the course of the illness and are thought to be related to tissue fixation of elemental arsenic.

B. Chronic Exposure: The chronic consequences of subclinical arsine exposure are uncertain. Trivalent arsenic resulting from arsine metabolism may be carcinogenic with long-term exposure.

Differential Diagnosis

Massive hemolysis may occur from selected drugs in susceptible individuals, especially those with G6PD deficiency. Massive hemolysis may also occur with inappropriate blood transfusion and following exposure to stibine gas, the hydride of antimony.

Prevention

Protection of metal cylinders for transportation and storage of arsine gas is essential. Disaster plans for environmental exposure must be prepared in advance.

Treatment

Exchange transfusions are the treatment of choice. If renal failure develops, hemodialysis is indicated until renal function resumes. Alkaline diuresis is recommended to minimize precipitation of hemoglobin in the kidney. Exchange transfusions are utilized since the arsine hemoglobin-haptoglobin complex is not dialyzable and patients who are not treated with exchange transfusions may continue to hemolyze.

Gases Used in Microelectronics

Catastrophic release of arsine could be fatal to large numbers of people. Arsine is widely used in the microelectronics industry. Table 31–4 illustrates other noxious gases that are widely used in the microelectronics industry. Table 31–5 illustrates the effects these gases might have if released into the community environment. The rapid changes occurring in the technology of the microelectronics industry raises concern about the hazards of transport, storage, use, and disposal of these noxious gases.

PHOSPHINE

Essentials of Diagnosis

Acute effects:
- Weakness, fatigue, headache, vertigo.
- Paresthesias.
- Cough and shortness of breath.

Chronic effects:
- Unknown.

Exposure Limits

ACGIH TLV: 0.3 ppm TWA, 1 ppm STEL
OSHA PEL: 0.3 ppm TWA, 1 ppm STEL

Table 31–4. Toxic gases used in microelectronics.

	Flammability	Pyrophoric	Immediate Danger to Life Levels (ppm)	Irritant Threshold (ppm)	Odor Threshold (ppm)	Approximate TLV, 8-Hour TWA (ppm)
Hydrogen chloride (HCl)	0	0	100	5	1	5
Silane (SiH$_4$)	+ + + +	+ + +	–	–	–	0.5
Phosphine (PH$_3$)	+ + +	+ + +	200	8	2	0.3
Ammonia (NH$_3$)	±	0	30,000	50	5	25
Arsine (AsH$_3$)	+ + +	±	250	0	0.5	0.05
Diborane (B$_2$H$_6$)	+ + +	+ + +	?160	?	3	0.1

General Considerations

Phosphine (hydrogen phosphide; PH$_3$) is produced whenever nascent hydrogen reacts with metallic phosphides. Phosphine is emitted during storage and transport of ferrous alloys, which often contain phosphides as impurities. Phosphine is a colorless gas with a disagreeable odor of decaying fish (at 2 ppm). Above 48 °C, phosphine can self-ignite and pose a threat of fire and explosion.

Occupational & Environmental Exposure

Phosphine is produced during hydrolysis of phosphides (eg, in gallium phosphide grinding) or during acetylene generation. Aluminum and zinc phosphide are used as fumigants in grain storage and can evolve phosphine by hydrolysis from moisture in wheat. Phosphine also evolves during the handling of hot phosphoric acid.

Mechanism of Action

The pathogenesis of the effects of phosphine poisoning is not well understood. In addition to phosphine's local irritative effects, it also has systemic effects, causing myocardial and central nervous system depression. Fatalities from phosphine are from pulmonary edema, central nervous system depression, or cardiac arrhythmias. Additional systemic effects on the kidney, liver, and muscle have been reported.

There is currently no information available on phosphine's chronic effects.

Clinical Findings

Symptoms of acute phosphine poisoning in humans include weakness, fatigue, headache, vertigo, anorexia, nausea, vomiting, paresthesias, abdominal pain, thirst, tenesmus, shortness of breath, and cough. In more severe cases, staggering gait, convulsions, and coma may occur. Death may occur from cardiac arrest or from pulmonary edema. Acetylene workers with phosphine exposure often have pulmonary edema.

Differential Diagnosis

Phosphine poisoning may often be confused with arsine and diborane toxicity, where there is only limited eye, nose, and throat irritation. Hydrogen chloride and ammonia cause severe eye and throat irritation and distinctive upper airway irritation. Arsine is associated with hematuria, abdominal pain, acute hemolysis, and renal failure. Diborane causes

Table 31–5. Toxic inhalation effects of gases used in microelectronics.

	Eyes	Nose and Throat	Upper Respiratory Tract	Lower Respiratory Tract	Other Signs and Symptoms
Hydrogen chloride (HCl)	+ + +	+ +	+ +	+ + +	Pulmonary edema
Silane (SiH$_4$)	–	–	–	–	Asphyxiant
Phosphine (PH$_3$)	–	±	±	+ +	Pulmonary edema, headache, diarrhea, nausea and vomiting, dizziness, possible CNS and myocardial depression.
Ammonia (NH$_3$)	+ + + +	+ + + +	+ + +	+ +	Pulmonary edema, nasal and oral ulcerations
Arsine (AsH$_3$)	±	–	–	+	Pulmonary edema, headache, nausea and vomiting, hematuria, jaundice, abdominal pain, acute hemolysis, hemoglobinuria, renal failure
Diborane (B$_2$H$_6$)	+	+ +	+ +	+ + +	Pulmonary edema, CNS effects (subacute), metal fume feverlike syndrome

more upper respiratory irritation than does phosphine and may also present with pulmonary edema and central nervous system depression. Diborane may be associated with signs and symptoms suggestive of fume fever syndromes.

Treatment

Treatment of phosphine poisoning is nonspecific and supportive. Patients should be removed from exposure and monitored for central nervous system and cardiorespiratory complications.

PARAQUAT

The herbicide paraquat, which is used throughout the world, has been associated with reports of severe lung damage. Although most reported cases occur from suicidal ingestion, occasional cases have been described following percutaneous absorption in agricultural workers.

Paraquat causes lung injury by creating free radicals within the lung parenchyma that cause lipid peroxidation. The type II pneumocytes of the lung concentrate paraquat and cause progressive fibrosis and permanent lung injury that can be predicted by measuring blood levels of the substance.

Paraquat is bound by clays and resins, which can be used in treatment if the material has been ingested. Charcoal hemoperfusion may remove paraquat from the blood, but rebound increase in paraquat from tissues may require continuous hemoperfusion.

Lung transplantation has been used to treat patients with massive paraquat poisoning, but leaving one lung in place causes injury to the transplanted lung from the paraquat released in the intact lung.

METAL FUME FEVER

Inhalation of oxides of various metals may produce a fever and flulike illness known as metal fume fever. Oxides of zinc, copper, and magnesium have been associated with fever usually associated with welding operations performed with inadequate ventilation. The disease associated with the oxides occurs 4–6 hours after exposure. During exposure, there may be a metallic taste in the mouth but no obvious symptoms. After a few days of exposure, the syndrome subsides.

Classically, metal fume fever occurs on the first day when an employee starts work on Monday morning after a weekend free of welding. There is no apparent latent period. High fever, myalgias, muscular weakness, headaches, mild dyspnea, and profuse sweating occur most frequently, resembling a flulike illness. Symptoms subside spontaneously within 24 hours. The diagnosis is confirmed by a careful work history and increased urine levels of zinc or copper.

No known specific mechanism accounts for the illness, though it is thought to be immunologic in nature.

The best treatment is prevention by improved ventilation. Drinking milk during welding has no proved efficacy. See Chapter 25 for a more detailed discussion of metal fume fever.

IRRITANT NOXIOUS GASES

Many gases pose potential injury to the lung by direct effects on the respiratory lining following exposure to sufficient doses. Irritant gases injure the lungs by causing acute bronchospasm or by inducing airway inflammation. Irritant gases may also block the upper airway by injuring the larynx.

Irritant gas effects depend on the solubility of the gas. Ammonia, a highly soluble gas, may cause severe injury to the conjunctiva and upper respiratory tract. Other soluble gases include sulfur dioxide, which is very irritating to mucous membranes in the upper airway. Relatively insoluble gases are those that cause less irritation to the upper airways. With these gases, the concentration and the duration of exposure may determine the severity of lung injury. Patients may present with a wide spectrum of pulmonary conditions ranging from shortness of breath to severe hypoxia and pulmonary edema. Oxides of nitrogen are insoluble and are released in the handling of fresh silage, arc welding, and the combustion of nitrogen-containing materials in a fire. Indoor gas stoves are a common cause of nitrous oxide residential exposure.

Phosgene ($COCl_2$), used as a weapon in World War I, is a heavy colorless gas with a faint odor of hay. It is only slightly irritating to mucous membranes, but when inhaled for prolonged periods it causes pulmonary capillary injury and ulcerative bronchitis and bronchiolitis. When chlorinated hydrocarbon solvents are used as degreasing agents in proximity to welding, the vapors may decompose at high temperatures, forming phosgene. Treatment of phosgene poisoning is supportive, including respiratory support with oxygen. Bronchodilatory agents and corticosteroids as well as careful management of fluid and electrolyte balance have been recommended.

CHLORINE

Essentials of Diagnosis

Acute effects:
- Eye and respiratory irritation.
- Cough, shortness of breath.

Chronic effects:
- Possible obstructive and restrictive lung disease.
- Possible anosmia.

Exposure Limits

ACGIH TLV: 1 ppm TWA, 3 ppm STEL (intended change: 0.5 ppm TWA, 1 ppm STEL)

OSHA PEL: 0.5 ppm TWA, 1 ppm STEL
NIOSH REL: 0.5 ppm ceiling (15 minutes)

General Considerations

Molecular chlorine (Cl_2) is a highly reactive and toxic element that was used in World War I as an agent of chemical warfare.

Use

Chlorine is frequently used as a chemical intermediate in plastics manufacturing and in the treatment of water and sewage. Chlorine may also be released from household cleaners.

Occupational & Environmental Exposure

Although millions of tons of chlorine are used annually in the manufacture of chemicals, plastics, and paper and in the purification of water and sewage, relatively few fatalities have been reported. Cases of poisoning have followed transportation or industrial accidents and mixing of acidic household cleansers with bleaches containing sodium hypochlorite. Chlorine has a pungent odor that can usually be detected at concentrations less than 0.5 ppm and does not lead to olfactory fatigue.

Metabolism & Mechanism of Action

The severity of the injury from chlorine gas is a function of the concentration of the gas, the duration of the exposure, and the water content of the tissue. The toxic element is molecular chlorine, which is a strong oxidizing agent and reacts widely with many functional groups in cells and tissues.

Clinical Findings

A. Symptoms and Signs:

1. Acute exposure–Chlorine is less soluble than ammonia and is therefore more likely to affect the entire respiratory tract than to just cause laryngeal edema. Chlorine gas itself is many times more irritating to the respiratory tract than hydrogen chloride gas. Acute symptoms include cough, dyspnea, chest pain, and pulmonary edema.

2. Chronic exposure–Long-term follow-up in survivors of chlorine exposure is limited. Pulmonary restrictive as well as obstructive defects have been reported in people who inhale sublethal amounts of chlorine, presumably because of interstitial edema, injury to the lung, and scarring. Some workers chronically exposed to chlorine may become anosmic. An eye examination involving fluorescein should be performed to rule out corneal defects.

B. Laboratory Findings:
Patients with chlorine exposure should have arterial blood gas determinations to make certain that adequate oxygen is delivered to the blood and a chest x-ray to rule out pulmonary edema.

Differential Diagnosis

Other irritant gases released in fires may also cause acute symptoms similar to those resulting from chlorine exposure.

Prevention

A. Work Practices: Patients exposed to large quantities of chlorine in the workplace should wear complete respiratory protection to prevent respiratory insult. Workers at risk of exposure to chlorine in the manufacture of alkalies, bleaches, and disinfectants should be monitored to ensure minimal chlorine exposure.

B. Medical Surveillance: No formal medical surveillance has been established for chlorine, though chest x-rays and pulmonary function tests may be required for individuals with chronic exposure.

Treatment

Removal from exposure to chlorine and provision of adequate oxygen and ventilation are the first steps. Maximal respiratory toilet and special attention to control of respiratory secretions is essential. Corticosteroids have been employed in the management of people with chlorine exposure, but their role is not established and prophylactic antibiotics have not been shown to be effective in preventing infection.

AMMONIA

Ammonia is a common upper airway tract irritant. It is a highly soluble alkaline gas that is widely used in industry as a refrigerant and in the manufacture of fertilizers, explosives, and plastics. It attacks the skin, the conjunctiva, and the mucous membranes of the upper respiratory tract. Edema of the larynx and pulmonary edema can occur with exposure to high concentrations and can cause death.

Management consists of removing the patient from exposure followed by supportive care with oxygen and attention to fluid and electrolyte homeostasis. Most patients gradually improve over time and make a full recovery without parenchymal lung damage except for bronchiectasis.

FORMALDEHYDE

Formaldehyde is a potent upper respiratory tract irritant that is used as a disinfectant and industrial cleaner and may off-gas from particle board. It is an animal carcinogen and may cause acute bronchial irritation in humans.

HYDROGEN FLUORIDE

Hydrogen fluoride is used in the microelectronics industry for etching silicon chips and is also used to etch glass. It is a potent upper respiratory tract acid irritant that causes pulmonary edema.

OZONE

Ozone is an important irritating gas produced by photochemical oxidation of automobile exhaust and is generated in arc welding. Ozone causes nose and eye irritation and is a potent respiratory tract irritant that causes cough, tightness in the chest, and shortness of breath.

INHALATION INJURY TO THE LUNG

Direct injury to the lung as a result of inhalation of heated steam and smoke is a major cause of death among fire victims. Injury to the upper respiratory tract may not be evident clinically. Synthetic materials now used extensively in building supplies may release noxious agents that alter the upper airway and may also release cyanide and other chemical asphyxiants.

Heat that is inhaled is generally dissipated in the upper airway, where the extent of injury is more readily estimated. Facial burns—especially if circumoral or if there are carbon products in the pharynx or nose—strongly suggest upper airway injury. Blood gases and a chest x-ray may appear normal early with airway injury. Laryngospasm may result from airway irritation as a protective mechanism against excessive exposure to noxious agents.

A noxious gas in the context of a fire will transport irritant chemicals on particles to the lower airway and in that way cause deep lung injury. Chemical injury to the lung is frequently underestimated. Particles in the larger airways are removed by the mucociliary action of the lung or by coughing, whereas small particles gain deep entrance to the lung and may injure the macrophage system or the lung parenchyma directly.

Even severe injury to the lung can be effectively treated with aggressive pulmonary care. Fiberoptic bronchoscopy will demonstrate ulcerated mucosa, and ventilation-perfusion lung scanning with xenon will detect early changes in the small airways.

Patients should be followed carefully after inhalation injury, even if the initial chest x-ray and blood gases are normal. If lung compromise occurs, positive-pressure ventilation may be required to maintain the patency of the small airways. Humidification of inspired air, appropriate use of bronchodilators to decrease bronchospasm, and judicious electrolyte management are required. Corticosteroids have not been found to be of value and may enhance toxicity.

Long-term sequelae after inhalation injury include asthma, bronchiolitis obliterans, bronchiectasis, and persistent cough. Therapy to prevent these sequelae requires further study.

REFERENCES

Carbon Monoxide

Goldfrank L et al: The inhaled agents and other disorders of oxygen transport. In: *Goldfrank's Toxicologic Emergencies.* Appleton & Lange, 1986.

Morgan WK, Seaton A: Toxic gases and fumes. In: *Occupational Lung Disease,* 2nd ed. Saunders, 1984.

Winter PM, Miller JN: Carbon monoxide poisoning. *JAMA* 1976;**236**:1502.

Cyanide

Becker CE: The role of cyanide in fires. *Vet Hum Toxicol* 1985;**27**:487.

Blanc P et al: Cyanide intoxication among silver-reclaiming workers. *JAMA* 1985;**253**:367.

Jones J et al: Toxic smoke inhalation: Cyanide poisoning in fire victims. *Am J Emerg Med* 1987;**5**:317.

Hydrogen Sulfide

Lundholm M, Rylander R: Work related symptoms among sewage workers. *Br J Ind Med* 1983;**40**:325.

Smilkstein MJ et al: Hyperbaric oxygen for severe hydrogen sulfide poisoning. *J Emerg Med* 1985;**3**:27.

Arsine

Hesdorffer CS et al: Arsine gas poisoning: The importance of exchange transfusions in severe cases. *Br J Ind Med* 1986;**43**:353.

Landrigan PJ, Costello RJ, Stringer WT: Occupational exposure to arsine: An epidemiologic reappraisal of current standards. *Scand J Work Environ Health* 1982;**8**:169.

Phosphine

Wald PH, Becker CE: Toxic gases used in the microelectronics industry. *State Art Rev Occup Med* 1986;**1**:105.

Wilson R et al: Acute phosphine poisoning aboard a grain freighter. *JAMA* 1980;**244**:148.

Chlorine

Chlorine poisoning. (Editorial.) *Lancet* 1984;**1**:321.

Morgan WK, Seaton A: Toxic gases and fumes. In: *Occupational Lung Disease,* 2nd ed. Saunders, 1984.

Inhalation

Cahalane M, Demling RH: Early respiratory abnormalities from smoke inhalation. *JAMA* 1984;**251**:771.

Herndon DN et al: Pulmonary injury in burned patients. *Surg Clin North Am* 1987;**67**:31.

Inhalation injury: No mere puff of smoke. (Editorial.) *Lancet* 1984;**2**:849.

Martin DW, Naughton JL, Smith LH: Smoke inhalation. *West J Med* 1981;**135**:300.

Smoking & Occupational Health

32

Neal L. Benowitz, MD

CIGARETTE SMOKING & DISEASE

The smoking of cigarettes and other tobacco products is the most significant preventable cause of sickness and death in civilized countries. In the USA, it is estimated that 350,000 deaths a year are a consequence of cigarette smoking. The major immediate causes of death attributable to cigarette smoking are coronary heart disease, lung cancer, and chronic obstructive lung disease. Other diseases related to cigarette smoking are listed in Table 32–1.

Cigarette Smoking as a Form of Drug Dependency

Cigarette smoking is a form of drug dependency that appears to be motivated by the desire to partake of the pharmacologic actions of nicotine. Nicotine has multiple psychologic effects, including euphoria, reduction of anxiety or tension, suppression of appetite, mood stimulation or relaxation, and improvement in performance and memory. The stimulant effects of tobacco use may be particularly useful for workers who perform repetitive tasks but need to remain vigilant. Smokers tend to regulate nicotine intake to maintain consistent levels from day to day.

Smokers often find it extremely difficult to quit smoking, even when the motivation to do so, such as illness or social pressure, is high.

Components & Toxicology of Tobacco Smoke

Tobacco smoke is a complex mixture of chemical substances in the form of gases and particulates (Table 32–2). Toxic gases include carbon monoxide, which binds hemoglobin preferentially to oxygen and results in reduced oxygen delivery to tissues (see Chapter 31). Other gases such as nitrogen oxides are oxidizing agents or irritants and may contribute to chronic obstructive lung disease. Hydrogen cyanide impairs ciliary function in the lung, which may predispose to pulmonary infection. Volatile nitrosamines and other gaseous substances such as formaldehyde may contribute to cancer formation.

The particulate phase of tobacco smoke includes the alkaloids—chiefly nicotine—and tar. Aside from its central nervous system actions, nicotine is a sympathetic nervous system stimulant that increases heart rate, blood pressure, and myocardial contractility and causes release of free fatty acids. Nicotine causes release of stress hormones such as cortisol and growth hormone as well as vasopressin and β-endorphin. As a consequence of the cardiovascular effects of nicotine, myocardial oxygen demand increases. Exposure to nicotine and carbon monoxide results in reduced exercise tolerance in patients with angina pectoris and enhances the risk of acute myocardial infarction and sudden death in persons with coronary heart disease. Nicotine induces vasoconstriction, directly or perhaps by inhibition of prostacyclin synthesis, and may contribute to coronary spasm as well.

Tar is a complex mixture of chemicals that includes most of the suspected carcinogens, cocarcinogens, and tumor promoters in tobacco smoke. These include benzo(*a*)pyrene and other polynuclear aromatic hydrocarbons, nicotine-derived nitrosamines, β-naphthylamine, polonium-210, and metals such as nickel, arsenic, and cadmium.

OCCUPATION & SMOKING BEHAVIOR

Currently in the USA, about 30% of adults smoke cigarettes. The distribution of smokers within various occupations is not homogeneous. Persons who are better educated and have white collar jobs are less

---

Table 32–1. Diseases related to cigarette smoking.

Chronic bronchitis and emphysema
Coronary heart disease
Peripheral arterial occlusive disease
Aortic aneurysm
Cancer, many types (see Table 32–3)
Peptic ulcer disease
Reproductive disorders: Spontaneous abortion, low-birth-weight deliveries, increased neonatal mortality rates
Fire injuries

Table 32–2. Major toxic components of cigarette smoke.

Nicotine	Carbon monoxide[1]
Catechols	Acetaldehyde[1]
N′-Nitrosonor-nicotine	Nitrogen oxides[1]
Phenol[1]	Hydrogen cyanide[1]
Polynuclear aromatic hydrocarbons[1]	Acrolein[1]
β-Naphthylamine[1]	Ammonia[1]
Nickel (carbonyl)[1]	Formaldehyde[1]
Cadmium[1]	Urethan[1]
Arsenic[1]	Hydrazine[1]
Polonium-210[1]	Nitrosamines

[1]Potential occupational and environmental exposures.

likely to smoke. Blue collar workers (not including farmers) are most likely to smoke, and their cigarettes are more likely to be high-tar cigarettes.

Rates of smoking in particular industries have been as high as 80% in some studies. In the USA today, about 45% of blue collar workers smoke. Unfortunately, this group is also the one most likely to be exposed to occupational chemical carcinogens.

Men were at one time considerably more likely to be smokers than women. By the early 1980s, this difference had all but disappeared.

The higher rate of smoking among blue collar workers is a potential confounding factor in understanding the relationship between smoking, occupation, and disease. Smoking as a marker for lower socioeconomic class may be associated with dietary differences, greater consumption of alcohol, and greater air pollution in the home environment—due both to industrial pollution related to geographic location of housing and higher probability of exposure to tobacco smoke in the home.

INTERACTIONS BETWEEN SMOKING & OCCUPATION

Cigarette smoking can interact with occupational exposures to cause disease in several ways:

(1) Contamination of tobacco products with toxic substances in the workplace. For example, toxic exposures might occur when cigarettes become contaminated with pesticides, lead, or other chemicals.

(2) Pyrolysis of workplace chemicals into toxic chemicals, which are then inhaled by the smoker. An example is polymer fume fever in workers who inhale fumes from heated Teflon in contaminated cigarettes. The syndrome can be quite severe, causing pulmonary edema and even death. Prevention of such diseases requires prohibiting smoking at work and encouraging hand washing before smoking.

(3) Additive exposures to toxic agents found both in the workplace and in tobacco smoke. Most of the chemicals in tobacco smoke, with the exception of nicotine, may be found in work environments, particularly where there is combustion of organic material. Carbon monoxide is an example of a toxin for which there may be additive contributions of workplace and smoking. Habitual heavy smokers have blood carboxyhemoglobin concentrations of 5–10%. Similar increments may follow occupational carbon monoxide exposure owing to the presence of combustion engines or furnaces or to exposure to methylene chloride (which is metabolized in the body to carbon monoxide). A blood level of 5–10% occurring after either smoking or occupational exposure may be well tolerated, but a level of 10–20% resulting from combined exposure can cause headache, impair psychomotor function, and, in high-risk patients, aggravate ischemic vascular disease.

(4) Additive or synergistic (multiplicative) effects of workplace and tobacco smoke toxins. Effects of pulmonary irritants and carcinogenic compounds from cigarettes and the workplace may increase the risks of chronic obstructive lung disease or cancer. Synergistic interactions, such as the increased risk of lung cancer with exposure to cigarette smoke and asbestos, are particularly important because most cancers result from combined exposures to smoking and occupational toxins. Control of smoking would prevent most such cancers.

(5) Accidental injury related to tobacco smoking. This includes injuries from fires produced from cigarettes as well as vehicular, machinery, and other accidents occurring at a higher rate in smokers than in nonsmokers.

In addition to specific interactions, as discussed above, smokers are also less well able to tolerate respiratory tract infections, such as influenza. Smokers have more severe illnesses and prolonged disability after such infections. From all causes, smokers have 50% more work loss days then nonsmokers.

It has been estimated—considering excess health insurance, fire loss, worker's compensation claims and workplace accidents, absenteeism, loss of productivity, and the health consequences of passive smoking—that each smoking employee costs the employer $485–880 a year (in 1986 dollars).

SMOKING & OCCUPATIONAL CANCER

It has been estimated that smoking is responsible for 30% of cases of cancer in the USA today. Eighty to 90 percent of lung cancers, 75% of oral, laryngeal, and esophageal cancers, and 30–40% of bladder and kidney cancers have been attributed to smoking (Table 32–3). Lung cancer incidence data most clearly illustrate the smoking-cancer connection. The incidence of most types of cancer has been relatively constant in the USA since 1900, but the lung cancer rate has been steadily rising. The rise in lung cancer rate parallels the average per capita consumption of cigarettes, with a lag of 20–30 years (Fig 32–1). Smoking prevalence for men peaked in 1950–1960, but because of the lag, the lung cancer rate is just reaching its peak in the 1980s. Women began smoking later than men, and as a result lung cancer rates have more recently begun to increase for women.

Table 32–3. Cancers related to cigarette smoking.[1]

Site	Relative Risk	% Deaths Attributable
Lung	10	90
Laryngeal	20[1]	
Oral	6[1]	} 75
Esophageal	4[1]	
Bladder	3	56
Kidney	2	–
Pancreatic	2	40
Stomach	1.4	–
Uterine Cervix	2	–

[1]Alcohol acts synergistically (Surgeon General, 1982).

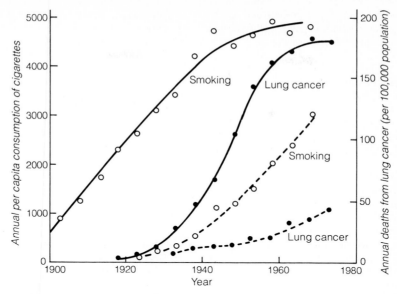

Figure 32–1. Temporal relationship between cigarette consumption and death rate from lung cancer. Solid lines represent men, dashed lines women. Data are for England and Wales. (Cairns, 1975.)

Lung cancer has now overtaken breast cancer as the leading cause of cancer deaths in American women.

How Does Cigarette Smoking Cause Cancer?

Tobacco smoke and smoke condensates produce cancer in experimental animals. The greatest contributors to the carcinogenesis of tobacco condensate appear to be the polyaromatic hydrocarbons, the most potent of which is benzo(*a*)pyrene.

Carcinogenesis is most likely when tumor initiators are delivered in high concentration to a target organ in the presence of tumor promoters. Tobacco smoking is an ideal model for carcinogenesis. Carcinogens and cocarcinogens are effectively delivered to the airways via inhaled cigarette smoke. A number of tumor promoters are also supplied to permit completion of the carcinogenesis process. Nonspecific pulmonary effects, including chronic inflammation with generation of oxygen-free radicals and impaired pulmonary clearance of carcinogens, may also contribute. Autopsy studies have shown that dysplastic lesions occur at the site of chronic inflammation. These dysplastic lesions are thought to be premalignant, preceding the development of squamous cell carcinoma. Inflammation may predispose to development of lung cancer; nitrogen oxides, acrolein, and other irritants are thought to contribute to carcinogenesis also.

Tobacco smoke carcinogens and occupational toxins may interact synergistically. If, as is currently thought to be the case, carcinogenesis depends on exposure to both initiators and promoters, smoking may provide the cocarcinogen or tumor promoter needed to compliment the actions of occupational carcinogens. Tobacco smoke may also be the vehicle for transmission of occupational carcinogens into the lung. Finally, cigarette smokers may be more tolerant to noxious substances in the air, allowing greater exposure to environmental carcinogens.

Asbestos, Smoking, & Lung Cancer

Lung cancer is a major type of cancer in asbestos workers. The interaction between smoking, asbestos exposure, and lung cancer is the best-studied example of the influence of smoking on occupational disease.

Studies of asbestos workers have indicated a substantially increased risk of lung cancer, but most lung cancers occur in persons exposed to both asbestos and cigarette smoke. For example, in analysis of data from a cohort of 12,051 asbestos installation workers with 450 cancer deaths, it appears that had there been no smoking but the same asbestos exposure, the cancer rate would have been only 10% of that observed (Table 32–4). Workers with lower levels of asbestos exposure have a correspondingly lower risk of lung cancer.

Table 32–4. Attributable risk of death of lung cancer from smoking and asbestos exposure.[1]

Total deaths	1946
Lung cancer deaths	450
Deaths attributable to:	
Cigarette smoking alone	94
Asbestos exposure alone	44
Smoking and asbestos	303
Deaths unrelated to smoking or asbestos	9

[1]Modified from Selikoff, 1981.

Several mechanisms of interaction between asbestos and smoking have been proposed: (1) Asbestos may act as a foreign body, resulting in chronic inflammation, with cell injury and repair. (2) Tobacco smoke acting as a tumor promoter might impair the capacity of cells to repair injury, leading instead to cancer. (3) Asbestos in the lung may attract pulmonary alveolar macrophages, which are capable of metabolizing polycyclic hydrocarbons to carcinogenic metabolites. (4) Asbestos fibers may adsorb, concentrate, and slowly release carcinogens from tobacco smoke.

The latency for lung cancer in asbestos workers is about 20 years. Although control of asbestos exposure has improved considerably in recent years, many workers have large body burdens of asbestos. The multiple-step carcinogenesis model strongly points toward smoking cessation as an intervention that could reduce the cancer risk prior to development of cancer. Thus, for workers already exposed to asbestos, the single most important way to decrease the risk of lung cancer is to stop smoking.

Smoking, Uranium Mining, & Cancer

Studies have shown a relationship between cumulative radiation exposure and the risk of bronchogenic cancer. Cigarette smoking substantially amplifies lung cancer rates, particularly at high radiation levels (Fig 32–2).

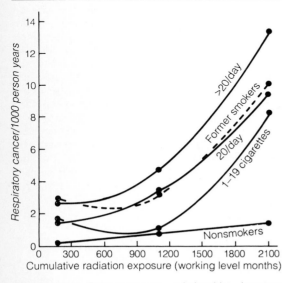

Figure 32–2. Dose-response relationship between cumulative radiation exposure (working level months) and respiratory cancer rate in uranium miners. Cigarette smoking amplifies the cancer rate, particularly at higher radiation exposure levels. (From Archer VE, Gillam JD, Wagoner JK: Respiratory disease mortality among uranium miners. *Ann NY Acad Sci* 1976;**271**:280.)

Uranium and other metal ores release radon gas, which decays to daughters, 2 of which are alpha-ray radiation emitters. The alpha-ray radiation, when present in close proximity to bronchial cells, causes local damage and ultimately neoplasm formation. Radioactive gases may adsorb onto particles which are then inhaled and deposited in the lung. Cigarette smoke may be an important source of particles for delivery of radiation to the lung. Tobacco itself is also a source of polonium-210. Therefore, smokers could have an additive radiation risk in addition to the risk from other sources of radiation. The carcinogenic effect of radiation could be promoted by toxic materials in tobacco smoke, which would explain shorter onset and latency times to cancer development in uranium miners who are smokers.

Chloromethyl Ethers: Can Smoking Protect Against Occupational Cancer?

Chloromethyl ether and bischloromethyl ether (a contaminant) are known to be carcinogenic in animals and humans. Chemical production workers exposed to chloromethyl ether experience a higher incidence of respiratory cancer, characterized by a short latency interval and a small cell histologic type. In a prospective study of 125 production workers, cancer was associated in a dose-related fashion to chloromethyl ether exposure but inversely related to the number of cigarettes smoked.

Chloromethyl ether and bischloromethyl ether are alkylating chemicals that are believed to produce cancer by actions on DNA. It is hypothesized that the presence of bronchorrhea due to smoking-related chronic bronchitis dilutes, degrades, or accelerates clearance of chloromethyl ethers.

An alternative explanation for the ''protective'' effect of smoking is self-selection, such that workers heavily exposed to chloromethyl ether, which produces respiratory irritation and dyspnea, are less likely to smoke.

Lung Cancer in Workers: Occupation Versus Smoking

There is convincing evidence in asbestos workers and uranium ore miners that smoking shifts the dose-response curve for occupational exposure, resulting in many more occupational cancers. Pastorino and coworkers (1984) attempted to determine the relative importance of occupation and smoking in causing lung cancer in a general population. In a study of all men in an industrial region of northern Italy, they identified 204 cases of lung cancer and 351 controls in whom occupational histories could be obtained. Subjects were classified as occupationally exposed if they worked with any of the following suspected respiratory carcinogens: asbestos, polycyclic aromatic hydrocarbons, arsenic, nickel, chromium, bischloromethyl ether, chloromethyl ether, and vinyl chloride. About 80% of the population were cigarette smokers. The relative risk of lung cancer was increased in workers with occupational exposure—and in a dose-dependent manner for cigarette smokers (Fig 32–3). At all smoking levels, the risk for exposed workers was 2-fold, indicating a multiplicative effect. Overall, 33% (95% confidence interval, 19.1–46.9%) of cases were attributable to occupational exposure (without modifying tobacco exposure) and 81% (95% confidence interval, 68.8–93.2%) to smoking (without modifying occupation).

This study indicates that in a general industrial worker population, occupational exposure to chemicals is a significant cause of cancer but that most of it would be prevented by smoking control. It also illustrates how an association between occupational chemical exposure and lung cancer risk might easily be missed where there is a high proportion of cigarette smokers in the work force unless very large worker populations are studied.

SMOKING & OCCUPATIONAL LUNG DISEASE

The major occupational chronic lung diseases are bronchitis, pneumoconiosis (fibrotic disease of the lung parenchyma), and occupational asthma. Cigarette smoking is clearly the major cause of chronic bronchitis and chronic obstructive lung disease and may also produce airway constriction in asthmatics. The net impairment of pulmonary function in workers is the sum of the influences of cigarette smoking, occupational exposures, and other factors such as genetic deficiency of α_1-antitrypsin.

Pathology & Pathophysiology of Smoking-Related Lung Disease

Chronic bronchitis—characterized by increased size of mucous glands, increased numbers of goblet cells, and mucous hypersecretion—is a nonspecific response to chronic irritant exposure. It may result either from cigarette smoking or exposure to a variety of chemicals or dusts. The risks of chronic bronchitis from smoking and occupational exposure to dusts are in most studies additive, with the largest percentages of cases today attributable to cigarette smoking. Chronic bronchitis may be associated with reduced airflow at high lung volumes, consistent with large airway disease.

Chronic obstructive lung disease is the lung disease most specific for cigarette smoking. Small airway injury is common in smokers even without symptoms. Pulmonary function tests in smokers commonly reveal reduction of maximum midexpiratory flow rates, a manifestation of small airway disease.

Emphysema is a more advanced stage of smoking-related chronic lung disease in which destruction of alveolar walls results in airflow obstruction, increased lung compliance and total lung capacity, and decreased diffusing capacity for carbon monoxide. The pathophysiology of smoking-related emphysema is believed to involve exposure to oxidant gases with concomitant impairment of antioxidant protective mechanisms such as α_1-antitrypsin activity.

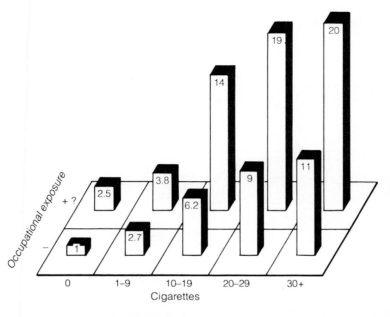

Figure 32–3. Risk of lung cancer in men in the Lombardy region of Italy as a function of occupational exposure (to chemicals known to cause lung cancer in humans) and daily cigarette consumption. Risks of occupational exposure and smoking are multiplicative. (Pastorino et al, 1984.)

Migration of neutrophils into the lung, which may be mediated in part by the effects of nicotine, may contribute to oxidant injury of membranes. Typically, the pattern of smoking-related emphysema is centrilobular.

Exposure to mineral dusts, such as coal or silica, may also produce small airway disease, with fibrosis of small airways and, later, focal emphysema. Typically, such disease is asymptomatic. Parenchymal lung disease with diffuse fibrosis may occur with asbestosis, silicosis, or coal miner's pneumoconiosis. Chest x-rays usually show parenchymal opacities ranging in size from less than 1 cm to massive fibrosis that involves large portions of the lung, and pulmonary function tests reveal severe restrictive disease, though there may be an element of obstructive disease as well. Findings of advanced pneumoconiosis are generally distinguishable from those associated with tobacco-related emphysema.

Cigarette smoking, including passive smoke exposure, may increase the degree of airway obstruction in asthmatics. Smoking increases the risk of sensitization to occupational allergies and would be expected to aggravate occupational asthma from any cause. Specific examples of interactions between occupational exposures and cigarette exposures in causing disease are shown in Table 32–5.

A good example of the interaction between smoking and occupation in causing acute respiratory disease is byssinosis in textile workers exposed to cotton dust. Some workers develop bronchitis or chest tightness after exposure to cotton dust, typically following a weekend or holiday when they have not been exposed. Pulmonary function tests indicate acute bronchoconstriction resembling asthma. The severity of symptoms is related both to the magnitude of cotton dust exposure and to whether or not the worker is a cigarette smoker. The symptoms and the magnitude of the pulmonary function test abnormalities are greatest in workers with higher dust exposure. Symptoms and manifestations are much more severe with the same level of cotton dust in smokers.

Although controversial, there are also reports of chronic airway disease in cotton textile workers, most severe in smokers but occurring also in nonsmokers. The interaction between smoking and cotton dust exposure has provoked debate concerning workers' compensation and regulatory issues; clearly, control of both risk factors should be goals of occupational health programs.

PASSIVE SMOKING

Mainstream Versus Sidestream Cigarette Smoke

On average, 75% of the smoke generated in smoking a cigarette is released into the environment. Sidestream smoke—that which is released into the environment—comes from tobacco burned at a higher temperature with less oxygen compared to mainstream smoke. Concentrations of various toxic chemicals, including polyaromatic hydrocarbons, are higher in sidestream compared to mainstream smoke. Sidestream smoke condensate is more carcinogenic than mainstream smoke condensate. Irritant gases

Table 32–5. Interactions between occupation and cigarette smoking in causing disease.

Occupation	Exposure	Disease	Smoking-Occupation Interaction
Asbestos workers	Asbestos	Lung cancer	Multiplicative
		Chronic lung disease (restrictive, obstructive)	Additive
Aluminum smelter workers	Polynuclear hydrocarbons	Bladder cancer	Additive or multiplicative
Cement workers	Cement dust	Chronic bronchitis, obstructive lung disease	Additive
Chlorine manufacturing	Chlorine	Chronic obstructive lung disease	Additive
Coal miners	Coal dust	Chronic obstructive lung disease	Additive
Copper smelter workers	Sulfur dioxide	Chronic obstructive lung disease	Additive
	Arsenic	Lung cancer	Additive or multiplicative
Grain workers	Grain dust	Chronic bronchitis, obstructive lung disease	Additive
Rock cutters, foundry workers	Silica dust	Obstructive lung disease	Additive
Textile workers	Cotton, hemp, flax dust	Acute airway obstruction (byssinosis)	Possibly multiplicative
		Chronic bronchitis	Additive
Uranium miners	Alpha radiation	Lung cancer	Additive or multiplicative
Welders	Irritant gases, metal fumes, dusts	Chronic bronchitis, obstructive lung disease	Additive

such as formaldehyde, ammonia, and volatile nitrosamines are present in far greater concentration in sidestream than in mainstream smoke.

Evidence That Nonsmokers Inhale Cigarette Smoke

Several studies have provided evidence of tobacco smoke components in the environment and in biologic fluids of nonsmokers. Biochemical measures have included plasma and urinary nicotine and cotinine (the latter a metabolite of nicotine) and increased carboxyhemoglobin and plasma thiocyanate (the latter a metabolite of cyanide, which is present in tobacco smoke). Cotinine excretion in the urine of nonsmokers exposed to other cigarette smokers in the home and in the urine of those exposed in the workplace are equivalent. Exposure in both places results in an additive increase in cotinine excretion (Fig 32–4). From urinary cotinine data, it is estimated that nonsmokers may consume tobacco smoke equivalent to as much as 1–2 cigarettes per day. There is overlap in the intake of heavily passively exposed nonsmokers and light primary smokers.

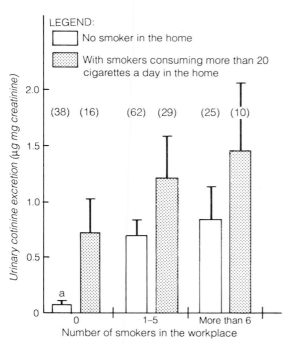

Figure 32–4. Intake of environmental tobacco smoke by nonsmokers as a function of number of smokers in the workplace. Cotinine is a metabolite of nicotine. Urinary cotinine is an indicator of nicotine intake. Intake after workplace and home exposures are additive. Figures in parentheses indicate numbers of subjects in each group. Bars indicate SEM. (Matsukura S et al: Effects of environmental tobacco smoke on urinary cotinine excretion in nonsmokers: Evidence for passive smoking. *N Engl J Med* 1984;**311**:828.)

Health Hazards of Passive Smoking

A number of studies have indicated that passive cigarette smoke exposure may present health hazards. Exposure of a nonsmoker to cigarette smoke is well known to be a source of annoyance, primarily because of eye irritation, nose irritation, and malodor. That passive smoking may affect pulmonary function is supported by observations in children whose mothers smoke, ie, a higher incidence of respiratory infection during the first year of life, exacerbation of asthma, and evidence of reduced pulmonary function. In adults, passive smoke exposure may aggravate angina pectoris or asthma and may result in mild impairment of small airway pulmonary function, although the lifelong significance of the latter is unclear.

Cancer & Passive Smoke Exposure

Several studies have reported an increased risk of lung cancer in nonsmokers who are passively exposed to cigarette smoke. The first report was of a study of 142,800 women in Tokyo, of whom 91,500 were nonsmoking wives. In a 14-year follow-up prospective study, there were 346 cases of lung cancer, including 174 in nonsmoking wives. The relative risk for lung cancer in women who were smokers compared with women who neither smoked nor had a spouse who smoked was 3.8. The relative risk of lung cancer in nonsmoking wives with husbands who smoke was 1.6 if husbands smoked less than 20 cigarettes a day and 2.1 if husbands smoked more than 20 cigarettes a day. Since most men in Japan at the time of the study smoked cigarettes and most women did not, passive smoke exposure appeared to be the most important cause of lung cancer in Japanese women.

A number of criticisms of the Japanese study have been voiced, including questions about statistical methods and comments about cultural differences between Japanese and American wives, raising a question about relevance of the results for American women. Subsequently, 2 prospective and 15 case-control studies from many countries have been published. All but 4 of these studies have found an increased risk of lung cancer in nonsmokers married to smokers compared with those not married to smokers.

A problem in many of these studies is the difficulty of measuring the extent of passive smoke exposure. The studies also suffer from the absence of occupational and other environmental tobacco smoke exposure data. This is a more significant problem in the American studies because a larger percentage of American women—compared with women from other countries where studies were conducted—work outside the home where they might be exposed to tobacco smoke or other chemical toxins.

The conclusion suggested by these studies with all their limitations is that there is a small but real increase in lung cancer rate, with a relative risk of about 1.3, in passive smokers. The question that must then be asked is whether the magnitude of that risk is biologically plausible. Since there is a clear-cut dose-response relationship between number of cigarettes smoked per day and the risk of lung cancer, a relative risk of 1.3 is quite plausible if one assumes that passive smoke exposure is equivalent to smoking ½–1 cigarette per day.

In addition to lung cancer, there are reports indicating an increased risk of cervical and other smoking-related cancers in nonsmoking spouses of smokers.

Passive Smoking & Workplace Cancer

Workplace exposure to cigarette smoke can result in significant smoke intake, and passive smoke exposure may be related to impaired respiratory function and an increased risk of lung cancer in nonsmokers. For nonsmokers sharing a work environment with cigarette smokers, the workplace must be considered hazardous independently of any specific industrial toxic exposure. This risk is particularly important when a high percentage of the workers smoke or where smokers and nonsmokers work in poorly ventilated areas.

Another concern is that passive smoke exposure may act synergistically—as does primary smoking—with toxic industrial materials to amplify the dose-response curve for those substances. Although there is no empiric evidence to support this hypothesis at present, the possibility must be considered.

CONTROL OF SMOKING IN THE WORKPLACE

If the goal of an occupational health program is to prevent illness and disability, the most effective way to do so is by control of cigarette smoking. The importance of controlling exposure to potentially toxic industrial chemicals is obvious, but total elimination of exposure is often impossible. An optimal employee health program should include simultaneous control of toxic exposures and smoking. A smoking control program should include both programs to encourage smoking cessation and environmental control measures to protect nonsmokers from tobacco smoke of their colleagues.

Smoking Cessation Strategies

Three general strategies are available for control of workplace smoking. The first is development of programs to encourage employees to quit smoking by physician counseling, educational activities, and either offering smoking cessation programs on the job or by paid referral of workers to outside smoking cessation programs such as those made available through the American Cancer Society or the Ameri-

can Lung Association. Some businesses also offer various incentives for employees to quit smoking. Despite the importance of smoking as a health problem, smoking control programs are offered by only about 8–15% of companies in various surveys. Optimally, smoking cessation programs should be sponsored jointly by management and labor.

A second strategy is restricting or prohibiting smoking in the workplace. Many companies restrict smoking in certain work areas; however, the motives have usually been related to protecting products or equipment, pleasing clients, or minimizing explosion risks. Some companies, such as the Johns-Manville Corporation, have restricted smoking in asbestos operations because of the potential synergistic effects between smoking and asbestos exposure. Such restriction seems to be the minimum that high-risk industries should undertake.

A third strategy is not to hire cigarette smokers. When the risks of smoking and occupational exposure are clearly synergistic, such as with asbestos exposure or uranium mining, not hiring smokers seems quite sensible.

Control of Passive Smoke Exposure

The concentration of tobacco smoke in a room depends upon the size of the room, the number of smokers, the extent of ventilation, and other factors such as the nature of wall surfaces. Ventilation with outside air or the use of high-efficiency filtration systems substantially reduces smoke concentrations and is required at a minimum for workplace control of cigarette smoke. But even with good ventilation, such as with central air conditioning systems, substantial concentrations of carbon monoxide and particulates are found in the workplace. Ventilation alone is not adequate.

Segregation of smokers and nonsmokers by space alone is partially effective, but primarily for particulates. The greater the ratio of smoking to nonsmoking areas, the less effective the segregation. Placing physical barriers between smoking and nonsmoking areas may be more effective, but the effectiveness depends on the air flow between the segregated areas. If it is not possible to place smokers and nonsmokers in separate rooms, barriers are better than nothing.

Prohibition of smoking at the work site is the most effective way to reduce environmental smoke concentrations. Restricting workplace smoking so as to provide a smoke-free workplace for nonsmokers has been mandated legislatively in a number of communities. Compliance with such local ordinances has been good, and enforcement has not been a major problem.

Air quality standards and permissible occupational exposure levels relevant to tobacco smoke components should be developed, monitored, and enforced. This may be an important area of activity for the Occupational Safety and Health Administration (OSHA).

Finally, where there is not adequate environmental control of cigarette smoke, nonsmoking workers should be advised of and given the opportunity to accept or reject the health risks of passive smoke exposure, as would be the case for workers in other hazardous environments.

REFERENCES

Cigarette Smoking & Disease: General Considerations

Benowitz NL: Pharmacologic aspects of cigarette smoking and nicotine addiction. *N Engl J Med* 1988; **319:**1318.

Pollin W, Ravenholt RT: Tobacco addiction and tobacco mortality: Implications for death certification. *JAMA* 1984;**252:**2849.

Surgeon General of the United States: *The Health Consequences of Smoking: Cancer and Chronic Lung Disease in the Workplace.* US Department of Health and Human Services, 1985.

Surgeon General of the United States: *The Health Consequences of Smoking: Nicotine Addiction.* US Department of Health and Human Services, 1988.

Workers' health: Occupational or personal? (Editorial.) *Lancet* 1984;**1:**1390.

Wynder EL, Hoffmann D: Tobacco and health: A societal challenge. *N Engl J Med* 1979;**300:**894.

Occupation & Smoking Behavior

Covey LS, Wynder EL: Smoking habits and occupational status. *J Occup Med* 1981;**23:**537.

Harris JE: Cigarette smoking among successive birth cohorts of men and women in the United States during 1900–1980. *J Natl Cancer Inst* 1983;**71:**473.

Sachs DP: Smoking habits of pulmonary physicians. (Letter.) *N Engl J Med* 1983;**309:**799.

Interactions Between Smoking & Occupation

Aronson MD et al: Association between cigarette smoking and acute respiratory tract illness in young adults. *JAMA* 1982;**348:**181.

Blake GH, Abell TD, Stanley WG: Cigarette smoking and upper respiratory infection among recruits in basic combat training. *Ann Intern Med* 1988;**109:**198.

Kark JD, Lebiush M, Rannon L: Cigarette smoking as a risk factor for epidemic A(H1N1) influenza in young men. *N Engl J Med* 1982;**307:**1042.

Kristein MM: How much can business expect to profit from smoking cessation? *Prev Med* 1983;**12:**358.

Luce BR, Schweitzer SO: Smoking and alcohol abuse: A comparison of their economic consequences. *N Engl J Med* 1978;**298:**569.

Sterling TD: Does smoking kill workers or working kill smokers? or The mutual relationship between smoking, occupation, and respiratory disease. *Int J Health Serv* 1978;**8:**437.

Van Tuinen M, Lond G: Smoking and excess sick leave in a department of health. *J Occup Med* 1986;**28:**33.

Surgeon General of the United States: Interaction between smoking and occupational exposures. In: *Smoking and Health: A Report of the Surgeon General.* US Department of Health and Human Services, 1979.

Wilson RW: Cigarette smoking, disability days and respiratory conditions. *J Occup Med* 1973;**15:**236.

Smoking & Occupational Cancer

Archer VE, Gillam JD, Wagoner JK: Respiratory disease mortality among uranium miners. *Ann NY Acad Sci* 1976;**271:**280.

Auerbach O, Hammond EC, Garfinkel L: Changes in bronchial epithelium in relation to cigarette smoking, 1955–1960 vs 1970–1977. *N Engl J Med* 1979; **300:**381.

Hammond EC, Selidoff IJ, Seidman H: Asbestos exposure, cigarette smoking and death rates. *Ann NY Acad Sci* 1979;**330:**473.

Hillerdal G, Karlén E, Aberg T: Tobacco consumption and asbestos exposure in patients with lung cancer: A three-year prospective study. *Br J Ind Med* 1983; **40:**380.

Hoffmann D, Hecht SS, Wynder EL: Tumor promoters and cocarcinogens in tobacco carcinogenesis. *Environ Health Perspect* 1983;**50:**247.

Loeb LA et al: Smoking and lung cancer: An overview. *Cancer Res* 1984;**44:**5940.

Pastorino U et al: Proportion of lung cancers due to occupational exposure. *Int J Cancer* 1984;**33:**231.

Selikoff IJ: Two comments on smoking and the workplace. (Letter.) *Am J Public Health* 1981;**71:**92.

Selikoff IJ, Seidman H, Hammond EC: Mortality effects of cigarette smoking among amosite asbestos factory workers. *J Natl Cancer Inst* 1980;**65:**507.

Surgeon General of the United States: *Health Consequences of Smoking: Cancer.* US Department of Health and Human Services, 1982.

Weiss W: Chloromethyl ethers, cigarettes, cough and cancer. *J Occup Med* 1976;**18:**194.

Whittemore AS, McMillan A: Lung cancer mortality among US uranium miners: A reappraisal. *J Natl Cancer Inst* 1983;**71:**489.

Wynder EL, Goodman MT: Smoking and lung cancer: Some unresolved issues. *Epidemiol Rev* 1983;**5:**177.

Smoking & Occupational Lung Disease Other Than Cancer

Elmes PC: Relative importance of cigarette smoking in occupational lung disease. *Br J Ind Med* 1981;**38:**1.

Kilburn KH: Particles causing lung disease. *Environ Health Perspect* 1984;**55:**97.

Smoking, occupation, and allergic lung disease. (Editorial.) *Lancet* 1985;**1:**965.

Wegman DH, Levenstein C, Greaves IA: Byssinosis: A role for public health in the face of scientific uncertainty. *Am J Public Health* 1983;**73:**188.

Passive Smoking

Collishaw NE, Kirkbride J, Wigle DT: Tobacco smoke in the workplace: An occupational health hazard. *Can Med Assoc J* 1984;**131:**1199.

Fielding JE, Phenow KJ: Health effects of involuntary smoking. *N Engl J Med* 1988;**319:**1452.

Hirayama T: Nonsmoking wives of heavy smokers have a higher risk of lung cancer: A study from Japan. *Br Med J* 1981;**282**:183.

Kabat GC, Wynder EL: Lung cancer in nonsmokers. *Cancer* 1984;**53**:1214.

Matsukura S et al: Effects of environmental tobacco smoke on urinary cotinine excretion in nonsmokers: Evidence for passive smoking. *N Engl J Med* 1984;**311**:828.

National Research Council, Committee on Passive Smoking: *Environmental Tobacco Smoke: Measuring Exposures and Assessing Health Effects*. National Academy Press, 1986.

Olshansky SJ: Is smoker/nonsmoker segregation effective in reducing passive inhalation among nonsmokers? *Am J Public Health* 1982;**72**:737.

Surgeon General of the United States: *Health Conse-quences of Involuntary Smoking*. U.S. Department of Health and Human Services, 1986.

White JR, Froeb HF: Small-airways dysfunction in nonsmokers chronically exposed to tobacco smoke. *N Engl J Med* 1980;**303**:720.

Control of Smoking in the Workplace

Sutton S, Hallett R: Randomized trial of brief individual treatment for smoking using nicotine chewing gum in a workplace setting. *Am J Public Health* 1987;**77**:210.

Walsh DC: Corporate smoking policies: A review and an analysis. *J Occup Med* 1984;**26**:17.

Walsh DC, McDougall V: Current policies regarding smoking in the workplace. *Am J Ind Med* 1988;**13**:181.

Building-Associated Illness

33

Michael L. Fischman, MD, MPH

The Clean Air Act, passed in the mid 1960s, focused national attention on cleaning up outdoor air but directed little interest toward improving the quality of indoor air—even though people spend only 10–20% of their time out of doors and the rest of their time indoors at home or at work. Until recently, buildings and homes were thought to pose little hazard to occupants from pollutants trapped inside structures. Recent studies are confirming that concentrations of pollutants inside buildings may greatly exceed standards established for outdoor concentrations.

Indoor air contamination has been linked to a wide variety of building materials and consumer products. The entire problem is exacerbated by concerns about energy conservation that have led to decreasing air turnover within homes and other buildings.

TYPES OF BUILDING-ASSOCIATED ILLNESSES & HEALTH CONCERNS

It is possible to divide building-associated illnesses into 2 categories: (1) acute short-latency illnesses and (2) potential chronic long-latency ones. The nature of the exposures that may give rise to each type differs substantially. The term ''building-associated illnesses'' is reserved for health problems that develop in settings customarily considered nonhazardous, eg, homes and offices. A classification scheme for building-associated illness is presented in Table 33–1.

The short-latency illnesses include closed building syndrome, mass psychogenic illness, specific illnesses resulting from identifiable sources of noxious materials, certain infectious diseases, and building-associated hypersensitivity pneumonitis. These conditions are characterized by a relatively acute onset,

Table 33–1. Types of building-associated illness.

Short-latency illnesses
  Closed building syndrome
  Mass psychogenic illness
  Building-associated hypersensitivity pneumonitis
  Building-associated infections
    Legionnaires' disease
    Pontiac fever
    Q fever
  Illnesses associated with specific contaminants
Possible long-latency illnesses
  Lung cancer
  Chronic nonmalignant respiratory disease

---

closely related in time to the individual's presence within the building and often relieved by removal from further exposure.

In contrast, the long-latency illnesses include cancer and chronic pulmonary diseases perhaps resulting from long-term low-level exposure to contaminants of indoor air. Because of the long induction-latency periods for these conditions and their multifactorial origin, it is much more difficult to establish a causal link to the building exposure. Agents in indoor air that may be responsible for such illnesses include cigarette smoke, asbestos, radon gas, oxides of nitrogen, polycyclic aromatic hydrocarbons, and chlorinated hydrocarbon insecticides.

The relationship of these long-latency illnesses to indoor air pollution is generally speculative. Estimates of incidence are predicated—often on the basis of mathematical extrapolations—on high-dose industrial or animal experimental exposures to substances encountered in lower doses in building environments.

There are more data suggesting a problem with cigarette smoke than with the other agents (see Chapter 32). Indoor asbestos exposure occurs at very low levels unless the insulation materials are disturbed or improperly removed. Exposure to low levels of radioactivity occurs in the form of radon gas from building materials and soil underlying basements or foundations. Polycyclic aromatic hydrocarbons are released into indoor air from wood-burning fireplaces and other sources. Based on the increased risk of lung cancer in much more heavily exposed asbestos workers, uranium miners, and coke oven workers, respectively, there is some concern about the impact of these agents on lung cancer incidence in the general population.

Certain products of combustion, such as oxides of nitrogen from unvented gas appliances, may pose long-term health risks. There is limited epidemiologic evidence suggesting increased respiratory infections and reduced performance on pulmonary function testing associated with exposure to gas stove emissions.

NATURE, SOURCES, & CONCENTRATIONS OF EXPOSURES

Potential sources of indoor air contaminants can be classified as follows: (1) contaminants released from the building or its contents, including asbestos, form-aldehyde, and radon; (2) contaminants generated by such diverse human activities as cooking, heating, cigarette smoking, and cleaning; and (3) infiltrated contaminants—agents that enter the house or building along with the outside air but in lower concentration (typically by 25–75%).

The concentration of contaminants is influenced not only by the source of exposure but also by the exchange rate between indoor and outdoor air. The introduction of outdoor air into a home or building occurs either by implemented ventilation or by infiltration. **Infiltration** occurs through cracks or other leaks in the structure or through open doors and windows. The amount of infiltration is dependent on the type of building, the amount of insulation and other weather-proofing, and climatic conditions. **Implemented ventilation**—eg, forced-air heating or air conditioning systems—may provide substantial amounts of outdoor air but may also be designed to recirculate preconditioned air with minimal fresh air intake.

The amount of air exchange is often expressed in air changes per hour (ACH). ACH may vary from 0.2 in tightly sealed homes to 0.7 in an average home to 60 or more in some industrial settings with implemented ventilation. Alternatively, with implemented ventilation, the amount of outdoor air supplied may be expressed in cubic feet per minute (cfm) or cfm per occupant.

The concentration of contaminants at any location within a building will be influenced by the location of the source and the degree of air mixing. In the case of reactive or particulate contaminants, the concentration will be affected by the rate of chemical reaction or the rate of deposition, respectively.

EVALUATION OF BUILDING ASSOCIATED ILLNESS
(See also Table 33–2.)

Proper assessment of illnesses relating to indoor air quality involves both evaluation of the symptoms, usually by a physician, and assessment of the work environment, preferably by an industrial hygienist. A symptom questionnaire may be helpful in establishing the nature, chronology, and frequency of complaints, the locations at which complaints arise, any incidents or activities that preceded the complaints, and the coexistence of any medical problems or risk factors that might account for some of the symptoms. Personal interviews and targeted physical examinations of affected employees may be indicated, depending upon the results from analysis of the questionnaires.

Industrial hygiene evaluation should begin with gathering of background information on the building, such as its age, type of construction, ventilation system design, and history of renovations and repairs. A walk-through survey will permit an appre-

ciation of the floor plan and the physical locations at which symptoms have occurred as well as inspection of the ventilation system and any possible point sources of air contaminants, eg, blueprint machines, cleaning supplies, and cafeteria equipment.

Limited environmental monitoring may be helpful in assessing the adequacy of ventilation—including the extent of fresh versus recirculated air—and temperature and humidity control. Minimal equipment is required for this monitoring—a room thermometer and relative humidity meter, smoke tubes to assess air movement, and direct-reading carbon dioxide colorimetric detector tubes.

Because carbon dioxide is a product of respiratory metabolism, its accumulation in office buildings reflects a balance between generation by building occupants and removal through ventilation and introduction of fresh outdoor air. Measurement of CO_2 levels aids in evaluating whether sufficient quantities of fresh air are being introduced into the building. The outdoor concentration of CO_2 varies typically from 250 to 350 ppm. The presence of CO_2 in concentrations above 1000 ppm inside the building suggests inadequate fresh air ventilation. In prior building investigations, levels above 1000 ppm are often associated with complaints of headache and mucous membrane irritation. Though the CO_2 itself is clearly not responsible for these symptoms, a high concentration suggests that other air contaminant levels are likely to be increased; in other words, the CO_2 level serves as a surrogate measure for the presence of other as yet unidentified contaminants likely to be the cause of these symptoms. Increasing the fresh air ventilation to lower the CO_2 concentration to below 600 ppm usually results in subsidence of symptoms.

Guidelines for temperature and humidity control to achieve a "comfort zone" for the majority of occupants have been issued by the American Society of Heating, Refrigerating, and Air-Conditioning Engineers (ASHRAE). For slightly active or sedentary individuals in office buildings, this zone lies between 73 and 77 °F and between 20% and 60% relative humidity. Relative humidity levels below 20% often result in drying of mucous membranes, with associated discomfort. Depending upon the ventilation system design, there may be localized areas within buildings that fall outside the comfort zone even though the rest of the building is adequately controlled.

ASHRAE has also issued guidelines for provision of adequate amounts of fresh outside air. For general office areas in which smoking is not allowed, outside air should be provided at a rate of 5 cubic feet per minute (cfm) per occupant. In areas where smoking is allowed, a minimum of 20 cfm of outside air per occupant should be provided.

Further and more specific air sampling should be performed if significant sources of air contaminants are identified or suspected. In the absence of such point sources, however, it is quite unlikely that

Table 33–2. Indoor air quality consultation services.[1]
If further evaluation or technical expertise is needed to resolve the problems discussed in this chapter, on-site assistance is available from the following sources.

1. Local or state health departments or consulting programs (availability and expertise vary with locality and state).
2. Private consultants (availability and expertise vary):
   a. A list of industrial hygiene consultants who are members of the American Industrial Hygiene Association (AIHA) is available from that organization:
      American Industrial Hygiene Association
      475 Wolf Ledges Parkway
      Akron, OH 44311-1087
   b. A list of engineering firms certified by the National Environmental Balancing Bureau (NEBB) is available from that organization:
      National Environmental Balancing Bureau
      8224 Old Courthouse Road
      Vienna, VA 22180
3. NIOSH Health Hazard Evaluation Program
   National Institute for Occupational Safety and Health
   Hazard Evaluation and Technical Assistance Branch
   4676 Columbia Parkway
   Cincinnati, OH 45226

[1]Reproduced from *Guidance for Indoor Air Quality Investigations.* NIOSH, 1987.

extensive untargeted industrial hygiene sampling will identify an unrecognized contaminant in concentrations sufficient to cause symptoms. Moreover, such sampling will invariably be expensive.

RESULTS OBTAINED FROM BUILDING INVESTIGATIONS

Investigators at the National Institute for Occupational Safety and Health have reported the results of their evaluations, through December 1986, of 446 buildings with indoor air quality problems. Although they recognized that some of the problems may have had multiple causes, they were able to classify the results by the primary identified cause. In 52% of the evaluations, building ventilation was found to be inadequate, as evidenced by inadequate fresh air intake, poor air distribution and mixing, draftiness, poor temperature and humidity control, pressure differences between office spaces, or air filtration problems. Inside contamination accounted for 17% of the problems, eg, from various types of wet copiers, improper pesticide application, improper use of cleaning agents such as rug shampoo, tobacco smoke, and combustion gases (eg, from cafeterias). Such contaminants were present at levels above the normal background but far below any permissible exposure limits. Outside contamination sources were the primary factor in 11% of their investigations, generally due to entrainment of contaminated outside air as a result of improperly located exhaust and intake vents or contaminant generation near intake vents. One of the most common identified sources was the entrainment of vehicle exhaust fumes from parking garages into the air intake vent. Other contaminants included boiler gases, previously exhausted air, and asphalt from roofing operations. Microbiologic contamination accounted for 5% of the problems, resulting from standing water in ventilation system components or from water damage to carpets or other furnishings. A variety of disorders—hypersensitivity pneumonitis, humidifier fever, allergic rhinitis, and conjunctivitis—can arise from microbial contaminants. Building materials were the source of contaminants in 3% of their investigations, including such things as particle board, plywood, urea-formaldehyde foam insulation, and some glues and adhesives. In 12% of their investigations, the factor or factors involved remained unknown.

Though they did not list it as a primary cause, the NIOSH investigators indicated that tobacco smoke may be a major contributor to indoor air quality problems, largely because it contains numerous irritant compounds. The significance of environmental tobacco smoke in the induction of closed-building syndrome or other building-related illness remains a hotly debated subject. There is no question that heavy cigarette use, when combined with poor ventilation, can result in high levels of environmental tobacco smoke that may result in irritant symptoms, eg, in cafeterias or crowded lobbies. In the more typical office building environment, the extent to which tobacco smoke contributes to indoor air quality problems is less clear and probably depends on ventilation and fresh air intake rates as well as on smoker density. Some investigators have demonstrated significant increases in respirable particulate concentrations in buildings where smoking is permitted relative to comparable nonsmoking buildings. Urinary levels of cotinine, a metabolite of nicotine, increase in a clear dose-response relationship with increasing exposure to environmental tobacco smoke in a variety of settings. Survey results indicate that many office workers feel that smoke generated by co-workers impairs their productivity. Other surveys suggest that contact lens wearers and allergic individuals may be more susceptible to irritant effects of tobacco smoke.

SHORT-LATENCY ILLNESSES

CLOSED BUILDING SYNDROME

The term closed building syndrome (also called tight building syndrome) denotes a characteristic set of symptoms, typically headache and mucous membrane irritation, recognized recently among occupants of buildings tightly sealed to prevent the infiltration of outside air. The syndrome has occurred principally in new buildings with centrally controlled ventilation systems and without openable windows. Many sealed structures have been built recently in accordance with ventilation engineering standards designed to conserve energy.

Occurrence & Etiology

The incidence of closed building syndrome is unknown, but reported outbreaks of illnesses consistent with this diagnosis have increased dramatically in recent years. Thirteen percent of requests to NIOSH for health hazard evaluations are to investigate health complaints attributed to the building (in nonindustrial workplaces). Outbreaks have occurred chiefly in government offices, business offices, and schools or colleges.

The contaminants responsible for this syndrome have not been identified. Despite extensive measurements for a wide variety of possible contaminants, no substances have been found to be consistently present in concentrations judged sufficient to induce symptoms. One common feature present in virtually all afflicted buildings is a central ventilation system that depends on a significant proportion of recirculated air. The most widely held theory is that this ventilation design permits the accumulation of low levels of many substances—cigarette smoke, aldehydes, solvents, etc—which together induce the symptoms.

There are a number of potential sources for such substances in the office environment. Formaldehyde is present in and will evaporate from resins in particle boards and plywood (used in furniture and construction materials), furnishings (including carpets and draperies), and urea-formaldehyde foam insulation. Other sources include cigarette smoke and unvented gas appliances. Organic solvents may evaporate from carpet glues and drying paints. Releases from photocopiers and other office equipment may also contribute to the symptoms.

Clinical Findings

The most common symptoms are those associated with mucous membrane irritation and headaches. Eye irritation, difficulty in wearing contact lenses, nasal and sinus irritation and congestion, throat irritation, chest tightness or burning, nausea, headache, dizziness, and fatigue are common complaints. Some symptoms may be psychophysiologic in origin.

Symptoms typically occur shortly after entering the building and are relieved soon after leaving. Physical findings are minimal, consisting perhaps of mild injection of the oropharyngeal or conjunctival mucous membranes. Laboratory studies, including spirometry and chest x-rays, are normal. Atopic subjects, with a history or findings consistent with allergic rhinitis or asthma, seem in general to be more prone to develop symptoms in association with indoor air quality problems.

Treatment & Prevention

For the individual patient, treatment consists of reassurance, with explanation of the apparent source and benign nature of symptoms and temporary removal from the environment if necessary. Since a group of workers is typically affected, meetings with the group as a whole may be useful, providing ample opportunity for questioning of the investigators. Successful ''treatment'' of the building typically involves increasing the ventilation rate and particularly the fresh air intake. Such alterations, even without prior knowledge by building occupants, have often resulted in resolution or diminution of symptoms. Depending upon the nature of the problem identified, other changes may be necessary also, such as relocation of air intake vents or alteration in cleaning or pesticide application practices.

Prevention would appear to require balancing energy conservation concerns with the need to provide adequate fresh air intake rates when designing ventilation systems.

MASS PSYCHOGENIC ILLNESS

Mass psychogenic illness is an illness of psychophysiologic origin occurring simultaneously in a group of individuals. Less satisfactory terms include ''mass hysteria'' and ''behavioral contagion.''

Occurrence & Etiology

Episodes felt to represent building-associated mass psychogenic illness have occurred in office buildings, light industrial facilities, and electronics plants. The incidence of these illnesses is unknown. The precise cause, though unknown, would appear to involve the occurrence of an appropriate stimulus or trigger in a psychologically susceptible population. The trigger is often an unexplained odor, concern about which may initiate psychophysiologic symptoms in some individuals. Since the trigger may be low levels of a respiratory irritant or an irritating odor, symptoms of closed building syndrome may occur concurrently. Thus, closed building syndrome and mass psychogenic illness may occur simultaneously or sequentially in the same building incident.

Episodes of mass psychogenic illness have occurred in groups of workers in low-paying jobs they perceive as stressful, often with repetitive work and physical stress from such factors as poor lighting.

Clinical Findings

Symptoms commonly reported in NIOSH investigations of outbreaks felt to represent mass psychogenic illness have included headaches, dizziness or lightheadedness, nausea, dry mouth and throat; eye, nose, and throat irritation; drowsiness, weakness, numbness or tingling, and chest tightness. It may be difficult to attribute particular symptoms in any given incident to mass psychogenic illness as opposed to closed building syndrome. Headache, dizziness, nausea, and numbness tend to predominate over symptoms of mucous membrane irritation in mass psychogenic illness when compared with symptom profiles in closed building syndrome. In mass psychogenic illness, symptoms are diverse in individuals in the group and occur or recur when the group is together, both inside and outside the building. The attack rate is generally higher among women than among men. There are few or no physical or laboratory findings. Some subjects may be observed to hyperventilate.

Certain features strongly suggest the diagnosis of mass psychogenic illness. The symptoms are difficult to explain on an organic basis and are not consistent with the toxicologic properties of any suspected contaminants. There is a visual or auditory chain of transmission. In other words, subjects typically do not become ill unless they see or hear that others are becoming ill. The illness in the index cases may be due to actual exposure to an unpleasant odor or noxious substance or to a nonoccupational cause, eg, a viral syndrome. Despite severity and sudden onset of illness, the illnesses are consistently benign without sequelae.

Treatment

Treatment involves primarily reassurance in a supportive environment away from the site at which symptoms developed. As in the management of groups suffering from closed building syndrome, emphasis should be placed on the lack of physical findings and other abnormalities and the absence of evidence suggesting a significant toxic exposure. Some investigation of the building is indicated to exclude the presence of significant contaminants. The scope of such an investigation will depend upon the potential sources of exposure, which are limited in an office setting. An exhaustive search for every measurable chemical substance is a costly, low-yield effort.

Early intervention with the group is essential, reporting to them the absence of significant exposures or hazards and the benign nature of the symptoms.

BUILDING-ASSOCIATED HYPERSENSITIVITY PNEUMONITIS

Hypersensitivity pneumonitis is a form of interstitial lung disease—characterized pathologically by lymphocytic and granulomatous infiltration of alveolar walls—that results from inhalation of a variety of organic dusts. The prototype of this disease is farmer's lung, which results from inhalation of bacterial spores and antigens from stored moist hay. However, hypersensitivity pneumonitis has been described in a variety of occupational and avocational settings.

Recently, hypersensitivity pneumonitis has been reported in a number of individuals in homes or offices where mold had been allowed to grow on humidifiers or air conditioners. Attack rates in such outbreaks have varied from 1% to 71% of the exposed population.

Occurrence & Etiology

Hypersensitivity pneumonitis is an immunologic disorder triggered by repeated inhalation exposures to a foreign antigen, which probably results from a combination of immunopathogenic mechanisms. There is evidence to suggest a type III immunologic reaction with precipitating or complement-fixing antibodies to the offending antigen and positive intermediate skin test reactivity. Some antigens may be capable of direct complement activation. Type IV cell-mediated immune responses probably play a role in disease development, particularly in chronic hypersensitivity pneumonitis. In building-associated hypersensitivity pneumonitis, a number of agents and antigens have been implicated, including bacteria (thermophilic actinomycetes, such as *Thermoactinomyces vulgaris, Micropolyspora faeni*), fungi (*Aspergillus, Penicillium, Alternaria,* and others) and perhaps amebas (*Naegleria* and *Acanthamoeba*). The source of antigens has usually been contaminated ventilation systems. Less commonly, persistently moist carpets, furnishings, and surfaces in occupied areas from water leaks have been implicated.

Clinical Findings

There are both acute and chronic forms of hypersensitivity pneumonitis. The acute form presents typically with fever, chills, shortness of breath, nausea, myalgia, malaise, and cough—without wheezing—usually developing 4–6 hours after exposure to the antigen. Symptoms may erroneously be attributed to an influenzalike illness. With the acute form, avoidance of exposure results in resolution of symptoms, and reexposure will result in recurrence of symptoms. The chronic form of hypersensitivity pneumonitis is typically manifested by the insidious onset of fatigue, progressive dyspnea, nonproductive cough, and weight loss. A history of acute bouts of illness, as described above, may not be present.

Physical findings may include fever, tachypnea, dyspnea, and bibasilar rales.

Diagnosis

Laboratory features may include leukocytosis with a leftward shift in acute bouts and chest x-ray and pulmonary function test abnormalities. Chest x-rays may be normal or may show increased interstitial markings or patchy ill-defined densities. Pulmonary function tests may reveal a restrictive pattern, with reductions in vital capacity and total lung capacity. However, ventilatory abnormalities are not always present. The most consistent pulmonary function abnormality is reduction of diffusing capacity for carbon monoxide.

The presence of serum precipitating antibodies to suspected antigens is of limited usefulness in that it documents exposure but does not indicate the presence of clinical pulmonary disease. Such antibodies may be seen in asymptomatic individuals, and some individuals with hypersensitivity pneumonitis may have negative precipitin tests. Gallium lung scans, bronchoalveolar lavage, and ultimately lung biopsy may be useful in confirming a diagnosis.

In a study of hypersensitivity pneumonitis in office workers exposed to a contaminated air cooling system, a respiratory questionnaire was found to be the most sensitive method by which to detect possible cases among the large group of potentially exposed workers. Shortness of breath and fever were present in all of the affected individuals. If the onset of these 2 symptoms was in close temporal association with exposure to the workplace, this finding was even more suggestive of hypersensitivity pneumonitis. Chest x-rays and assays for precipitins were of limited value, while pre- and postexposure measurements of FEV_1, FVC, and diffusing capacity were quite helpful in confirming a diagnosis.

Treatment

Avoidance of further exposure by removal from the environment usually results in resolution of symptoms and abnormalities. If symptoms fail to resolve following removal, a short course of corticosteroids—typically prednisone in high doses—is indicated. In some outbreaks, extensive clean-up efforts, including removal of contaminated items and alteration of ventilation systems, have allowed the return of affected workers without recurrence of symptoms.

OTHER BUILDING-ASSOCIATED ILLNESSES

Certain infectious diseases that are noncommuni-

cable may be transmitted in indoor air. Legionnaires' disease—a multisystem disease dominated by pneumonia—is caused by the recently identified bacterial organism *Legionella pneumophila*. Most commonly, building-associated outbreaks have resulted from contaminated aerosols from cooling towers, evaporative condensers, and air-conditioning systems.

Pontiac fever, also caused by *L pneumophila*, is an influenzalike illness characterized by fever, chills, headache, myalgias, and sometimes cough and sore throat. The sources are again, typically, contaminated air-conditioning systems.

Finally, Q fever, caused by the rickettsial organism *Coxiella burnetii*, has been responsible for several building-associated outbreaks. The animal reservoirs for this infection are sheep, goats, and cattle. Airborne transmission of organisms from animal excreta to humans has occurred via ventilation systems in animal-handling and medical research facilities.

Certain hazardous materials whose presence is not routinely suspected in nonindustrial buildings have been linked to building-associated symptoms or illnesses. Elevated levels of formaldehyde have been found in mobile homes and trailers—in which large quantities of urea-formaldehyde wood products are used—and in conventional homes to which urea-formaldehyde foam insulation has been applied. One study of residences whose occupants had reported symptoms found median levels of 0.35 ppm of formaldehyde, with some levels as high as 2–4 ppm (the ACGIH threshold limit value for 8-hour occupational exposures is 1 ppm TWA). Commonly reported symptoms included eye irritation and burning, runny nose, dry or sore throat, headache, and cough.

Finally, carbon monoxide in buildings may be the cause of mild symptoms, such as headache and nausea, or more severe, potentially life-threatening intoxication. Incomplete combustion in defective gas furnaces or unvented gas stoves and other appliances may occasionally be the source of significant indoor emissions of carbon monoxide. Less commonly, carbon monoxide may be entrained from the outside via air intakes in the vicinity of vehicle loading docks.

REFERENCES

Arnow PM et al: Early detection of hypersensitivity pneumonitis in office workers. *Am J Med* 1978;**64**:236.

Boxer PA: Occupational mass psychogenic illness: History, prevention, and management. *J Occup Med* 1985;**27**:867.

Cone JE, Hodgson MJ (editors): Problem buildings: Building-associated illness. *State Art Rev Occup Med* 1989;**4**:(entire issue).

Dally KA et al: Formaldehyde exposure in nonoccupational environments. *Arch Environ Health* 1981;**36**:277.

Esmen NA: The status of indoor air pollution. *Environ Health Perspect* 1985;**62**:259.

Fielding JE, Phenow KJ: Health effects of involuntary smoking. *N Engl J Med* 1988;**319**:1452.

Kreiss K, Hodgson M: Building-associated epidemics. In: *Indoor Air Quality*. Walsh PJ, Dudney CS, Copenhaver ED (editors). CRC Press, 1984.

National Institute for Occupational Safety and Health: *Guidance for Indoor Air Quality Investigations*. NIOSH, 1987.

Repace JL, Lowrey AH: Environmental tobacco smoke and indoor air quality in modern office environments. (Editorial.) *J Occup Med* 1987;**29**:57.

Spengler JD, Sexton K: Indoor air pollution: A public health perspective. *Science* 1983;**221**:9.

Sterling TD, Collett CW, Sterling EM: Environmental tobacco smoke and indoor air quality in modern office work environments. *J Occup Med* 1987;**29**:57.

Biologic Monitoring

34

David M. Rempel, MD, MPH, Jon Rosenberg, MD, MPH, & Robert J. Harrison, MD, MPH

Biologic monitoring is the measurement of a chemical, its metabolite, or a nonadverse biochemical effect in a biologic specimen for the purpose of assessing exposure. The term may also be used to denote drug abuse monitoring and other types of medical surveillance, but to avoid confusion it should be restricted to exposure monitoring. Typically, specimens are blood, urine, or exhaled air. For example, exposure to organophosphorus insecticides can be confirmed by measuring the metabolite—alkyl phosphates—in the urine or by measuring a biochemical effect—the activity of the enzyme cholinesterase—in the blood. Most often, however, exposure is assessed by measuring the chemical or its metabolite in a body fluid.

Environmental monitoring is measurement of the ambient (external) exposure of a chemical in the workplace. Typically, samples are taken from the air or from surfaces at the workplace. Environmental monitoring provides information about potential exposure primarily from one route of exposure (eg, air or workplace surfaces), whereas biologic monitoring provides a measure of the quantity of a chemical absorbed regardless of route of absorption (eg, inhalation, skin contact, or ingestion). Total exposure is measured, rather than only workplace exposure.

The biologic level may not correlate well with environmental measurements (Fig 34–1). This variability occurs for several reasons: (1) actual work practices vary among employees doing identical work—eg, one worker may have more skin contact or may inhale more of a chemical than another worker; (2) a high respiratory rate can increase pulmonary absorption of solvents by a factor of 3–4; (3) the rate of metabolism and excretion will vary between individuals even when hepatic or renal function is normal; and (4) lipid-soluble chemicals may accumulate to a greater extent in a person with excess adipose tissue.

Workplace exposure to more than 100 different chemicals can be estimated in an individual by measuring the chemical in the blood, urine, or exhaled air. Depending on the pharmacokinetics of the target substance, the body fluid sampled, and the time of sampling, the measured level will reflect the duration of exposure ranging from acute recent exposure or accumulated lifetime exposure (body burden).

The purpose of this chapter is to give the clinician practical information on biologic monitoring.

Because some chemicals are rapidly cleared from the blood, interpretation of biologic levels depends on accurate timing of sample collection. Because significant errors can be introduced in the sampling process, following standard methods of sample collection will improve the clinician's ability to interpret a biologic level.

HOW TO USE BIOLOGIC MONITORING

Biologic monitoring of workers exposed to toxic agents has gained increasing acceptance as a means of accurately determining exposure. It should be used to augment other sources of exposure assessment, such as occupational history and environmental monitoring. Like environmental monitoring (see Chapter 38), biologic monitoring assesses the extent of exposure of workers and thus only indirectly the risk of health effects as a result of that exposure. Moreover, any action arising out of abnormal biologic monitoring levels should be based not on a single measurement but on multiple measurements.

It cannot be assumed that a biologic level necessarily represents a more accurate reflection of dose than an environmental level. All occurrences of elevated levels judged to be due to excessive workplace exposure should be evaluated with the assistance of an industrial hygienist.

Table 34–1 is useful in 2 different situations. The first is the routine monitoring of a healthy employee

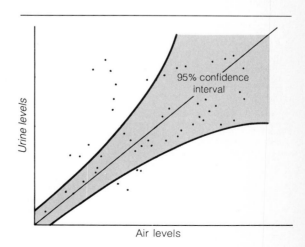

Figure 34–1. Relationship of levels of a substance measured in the breathing zone of workers to levels measured in urine.

Table 34–1. Chemicals for which there are reliable data for determining reference biologic monitoring levels.

Chemical *Determinant*[1]	Media (units)	Levels Without Occupational Exposure	No Adverse Effect Level	Clinical Effect Level	Timing of Sample[2]	Terminal Half-Time ($t_{1/2}$)	Comments
Inorganics: Metals							
Arsenic	Urine (μg/L)	< 30	100–300	> 300	EWW	1–2 d	No seafood for 48 hours before collection.
Cadmium	Urine (μg/g Cr)	0.02–4	10	20	NC	10–30 y	Reflects chronic exposure (years) after 1 year of exposure.
	Blood (μg/L)	0.4–1	10	20	NC	10–15 y	Reflects recent exposure (months). Smokers may have blood levels of 1.4–4.5 μg/L.
Chromium	Urine (μg/g Cr)	< 5	30	. . .	EOS, EWW	15–40 h	Exposure from welding stainless steel.
Lead	Blood (μg/dL)	2–9	25	80	NC	. . .	Use lead-free needles and tubes. BEI, blood 50 μg/dL.
	Urine (μg/g Cr)	10–65	150	. . .	NC	. . .	$t_{1/2}$ for soft tissue is 1 month; for skeleton, 20 years.
Zn protoporphyrin (ZPP)	Blood (μg/dL)	16–35	100	. . .	NC	2–4 wk	Useful after 1 month of exposure. Reflects total body burden. Free erythrocyte protoporphyrin (FEP) is interpreted similarly to ZPP.
Mercury (inorganic)	Urine (μg/L)	< 20	50	200	NC	60 d	Reflects prior 2–4 months' exposure.
Nickel	Urine (μg/L)	< 5	70	. . .	EOS	17–39 h	Corrected to SG of 1.018. Measures only soluble nickel.
	Plasma (μg/dL)	0.2–0.4	0.7	. . .	EOS	. . .	
Selenium	Plasma (μg/dL)	5–18	. . .	. . .	. . .	. . .	
	Urine (μg/g Cr)	7–79	25	. . .	. . .	100–150 d	
Vanadium	Urine (μg/g Cr)	< 1	50	. . .	. . .	20–40 h	
Inorganics: Other							
Carbon disulfide *TTCA*	Urine (mg/g Cr)	0	5	. . .	EOS	2–3 d	TTCA is 2-thiothiazolidine-4-carboxylic acid. Carbon disulfide is a metabolite of disulfiram (Antabuse) and dithiocarbamates.
Carbon monoxide *COHb*	Blood (%)	0.4–0.7	8	10	EOS	1–8 h	Blood COHb following: Cigarettes 1 ppd = 5–6% 2–3 ppd = 7–9% Driving on urban highways = 5%
Cyanide *Thiocyanate*	Urine (mg/24 h)	0.11	6.5	. . .	. . .	. . .	
Fluorides	Urine (mg/L)	< 0.4	3	. . .	PNS	4–7 h	In unexposed persons, varies with drinking water fluoride, use of dental products.
		. . .	10	. . .	EWW	. . .	
Organics: Aliphatics and alicyclics							
Acetone	Urine (mg/g Cr)	< 2	20	46	DS	. . .	
	Blood (mg/dL)	< 0.2	2	. . .	DS	6 h	Elevated during diabetic or fasting ketoacidosis.
	Alveolar air (mg/m³)	. . .	53	. . .	DS	4 h	
Cyclohexane *Cyclohexanol*	Urine (mg/L)	. . .	3.2–5.5	. . .	L4H	. . .	
	Blood (μg/dL)	. . .	46–52	. . .	DS	. . .	

continued

Table 34–1 (cont'd). Chemicals for which there are reliable data for determining reference biologic monitoring levels.

Chemical Determinant[1]	Media (units)	Levels Without Occupational Exposure	No Adverse Effect Level	Clinical Effect Level	Timing of Sample[2]	Terminal Half-Time ($t_{1/2}$)	Comments
Cyclohexane	End-exhaled air (mg/m³)	. . .	780–880	. . .	DS	. . .	
Dioxane β-Hydroxyethoxy-acetic acid	Urine (mg/L)	. . .	36.5	. . .	EOS	1 h	
Dioxane	Blood (mg/L)	. . .	12	. . .	DS	. . .	
Ethylene glycol Oxalic acid	Urine (mg/g Cr)	< 100	. . .	0.3–4.3 g/l	. . .	2–6 h	
Ethylene glycol monoethyl ether Ethoxyacetic acid	Urine (mg/L)	< 0.07	6	. . .	PNS	21–24 h	
n-Hexane 2,5-Hexanedione	Urine (mg/L)	0.1–0.8	5	. . .	EOS	. . .	Large individual variability. Correlates best with air concentration.
n-Hexane	End-exhaled air (ppm)	. . .	40	. . .	DS	1–2 h	Large individual variability.
Methanol	Urine (mg/L)	0.3–2.6	15	. . .	EOS	1.5–2 h	
Formic acid	Urine (mg/g Cr)	5–50	80	. . .	PNS, EWW	. . .	
Methyl ethyl ketone	Urine (mg/L)	. . .	2	. . .	EOS	. . .	Large individual variability.
2-Methyl pentane 2-Methyl-2-pentanol	Urine (mg/L)	. . .	< 0.1–5.5	. . .	EOS	. . .	
3-Methylpentane 3-Methyl-3-pentanol	Urine (mg/L)	0	< 0.1–1	. . .	EOS	. . .	
Propylene glycol monoethyl ether (PGME)	End-exhaled air (ppm)	0	4	. . .	EOS	. . .	
Organics: Aromatic Benzene Total phenol	Urine (mg/L)	0–20	50	. . .	EOS	28 h	Large individual variability.
Benzene	Mixed-exhaled air (ppm)	< 0.03	0.08	. . .	PNS	30 h	
	End-exhaled air (ppm)	< 0.03	0.12	. . .	PNS	30 h	
	Blood (µg/dL)	. . .	. . .	1–20	PNS	1–3 h	
Ethyl benzene Mandelic acid	Urine (g/g Cr)	< 0.005	1.5	. . .	EOS	5 h	Large individual variability.
Ethyl benzene	End-exhaled air (ppm)	< 0.03	2	. . .	PNS, EWW	2 d	
Phenol	Urine (mg/g Cr)	0–20	250	. . .	EOS	3.5 h	Large individual variability.
	Urine (mg/h)	. . .	15	. . .	L2H		
Styrene Mandelic acid	Urine (g/g Cr)	< 0.005	0.8	. . .	EOS	25 h	Large individual variability.
Styrene	Mid-exhaled air (ppm)	0	0.04	. . .	PNS	3 d	
		0	18	. . .	DS		
	Blood (mg/L)	0	0.55	. . .	EOS	3 d	
		0	0.02	. . .	PNS		

continued

Table 34–1 (cont'd). Chemicals for which there are reliable data for determining reference biologic monitoring levels.

Chemical Determinant[1]	Media (units)	Levels Without Occupational Exposure	No Adverse Effect Level	Clinical Effect Level	Timing of Sample[2]	Terminal Half-Time ($t_{1/2}$)	Comments
Phenylglyoxylic acid	Urine (mg/g Cr)	. . .	240	. . .	EOS	7–10 h	
Toluene *Hippuric acid*	Urine (g/g Cr)	< 1.5	2.5	. . .	EOS	1–2 h	Large individual variability.
	Urine (mg/min)	< 0.4	3	. . .	L4H		
Toluene	Blood (mg/L)	<0.015	1	> 1	EOS	3–4 h	
	End-exhaled air (ppm)	0	< 20	. . .	DS	3.7 h	
Xylene *Total methylhip-puric acid*	Urine (g/g Cr)	0	1.5	. . .	EOS	30 h	
	Urine (mg/min)	0	2	. . .	L4H		
Xylene	Blood (mg/L)	0	. . .	3–40	EOS	20–30 h	Fatalities reported at 3–40
Organics: Haloge-nated Methyl bromide *Bromide*	Blood (mg/dL)	0.05–0.2	1.1	5	. . .	. . .	
Methylene chloride *Carboxyhemo-globin*	Blood (%)	0.4–0.7	2.5	> 10	EOS	10–12 h	Smoking and CO exposure additive in COHb levels. Longer $t_{1/2}$ than with CO exposure.
			1	. . .	PNS	. . .	
	End-exhaled air (ppm)	< 2	3–6	8–13	EOS	10–12 h	
Methylene chlo-ride	Blood (mg/dL)	0	0.08	0.3–1.2	EOS	. . .	
Perchloroethylene	End-exhaled air (ppm)	0	18	30	EOS	. . .	
			10	. . .	PNS, EWW	64 h	
	Blood (mg/dL)	0	1	. . .	PNS, EWW	. . .	
Trichloroacetic acid	Urine (mg/g Cr)	0	7	. . .	EOS	80 h	
Polychlorinated biphenyl *Total chloro-biphenyl*	Blood (µg/L)	0–30	150	600	NC	3–7 y	Method of analysis critical. Results differ depending on specific PCB isomer.
1,1,1-Trichloro-ethane	End-exhaled air (ppm)	0	40	. . .	PNS, EWW	. . .	
	Blood (mg/dL)	0	0.5	. . .	EOS	. . .	
Trichloroethanol	Urine (mg/L)	0	30	. . .	EOS, EWW	10–15 h	
	Blood (mg/L)	0	1	. . .	EOS, EWW		
Trichloroacetic acid	Urine (µg/L)	0	10	. . .	EWW	70–100 h	
Trichloroethylene *Free trichloro-ethanol*	Blood (mg/L)	0	4	. . .	EOS, EWW	12 h	
Trichloroethylene	End-exhaled air (ppm)	0	0.5	. . .	PNS, EWW	30 h	
Trichloroacetic acid	Urine (mg/L)	0	100	200	EWW	50–100 h	Wide individual variability.
Trichloroacetic acid and tri-chloroethanol	Urine (mg/L)	0	300	. . .	EOS, EWW	. . .	

continued

Table 34–1 (cont'd). Chemicals for which there are reliable data for determining reference biologic monitoring levels.

Chemical Determinant[1]	Media (units)	Levels Without Occupational Exposure	No Adverse Effect Level	Clinical Effect Level	Timing of Sample[2]	Terminal Half-Time ($t_{1/2}$)	Comments
Organics: Nitrogen-containing							
Aniline *p-Aminophenol*	Urine (mg/L)	0	50	. . .	EOS	. . .	Wide individual variability.
Methemoglobin	Blood (%)	1–2	5	. . .	EOS	. . .	
Dimethylformamide *N-Methylform- amide*	Urine (mg/g Cr)	0	40	. . .	EOS	12 h	
Dinitrobenzene *Methemoglobin*	Blood (%)	1–2	5	. . .	EOS	. . .	
Ethylene glycol dini- trate	Blood (μg/L)	0	0.2	. . .	DS	30 min	
Nitrobenzene *p-Nitrophenol and p-amino- phenol*	Urine (mg/g Cr)	0	5	. . .	EOS	60 h	
Methemoglobin	Blood (%)	1–2	5	. . .	EOS	. . .	
Organics: Pesticides							
Organophosphates *RBC cholines- terase*	Blood (% depression)	< 20	< 30	> 40	NC	20–30 d	Levels are % depression from baseline. Symptoms depend on rate of decline in addition to absolute level.
Parathion *RBC cholines- terase*	Blood (% depression)	< 20	< 30	> 40	NC	20–30 d	Reflects chronic exposure.
p-Nitrophenol	Urine (mg/L)	0.01–0.03	0.5	2	EOS	4 h	Reflects recent exposure.
Carbamates *RBC cholines- terase*	Blood (% depression)	< 20	< 30	> 40	EOS	1–2 h	Cholinesterase is reactivated very quickly.
Carbaryl *RBC cholines- terase*	Blood (% depression)	< 20	< 30	> 40	EOS	1–2 h	Cholinesterase is reactivated very quickly.
1-Naphthol	Urine (mg/g Cr)	1.5–4	10	. . .	EOS	. . .	
Chlordane	Blood (μg/L)	0	6	3000	. . .	. . .	
Dieldrin	Blood (μg/L)	. . .	150	200– 1000	. . .	. . .	
Endrin	Blood (μg/L)	0	50		EOS	. . .	
Anti-12-hydroxy- endrin	Urine (mg/g Cr)	0	130	. . .	EOS	. . .	
Hexachlorobenzene	Blood (mg/L)	. . .	3	. . .	NC	2 y	
Lindane	Serum (μg/L)	0	20–30	500	. . .	20 h	

[1]If the laboratory determinant is other than the material itself, it is listed below in italics.
[2]NC not critical; DS during shift; EOS end of shift; EWW end of work week; L2H last 2 hours of shift; L4H last 4 hours of shift; PNS prior to next shift; · · · insufficient data.

who works with a toxic chemical. The clinician must determine whether the exposure is significant and potentially harmful. If the biologic level measured is below the "no adverse health effect level" or if it is within the range "levels in unexposed," the exposure is probably not harmful. This situation is analogous to measuring airborne concentrations of a chemical and comparing them to recommended levels. For a few chemicals, biologic monitoring of exposed workers is mandated by law. In the case of an employee

who works with lead, if the blood lead concentration is above a certain level, that worker must be transferred to an area where he or she is not exposed to lead.

Table 34–1 is useful also in the clinical assessment of an ill employee who has been exposed to a toxic chemical. Is it possible that the employee's abnormal symptoms, signs, or laboratory tests are due to exposure to that chemical? The "clinical effect level" is one that has been associated with illness typically caused by that chemical. If an employee has signs and symptoms consistent with those caused by the chemical and if the measured level is at or above the "clinical effect level," there is a high probability that the chemical is causing the illness. However, samples from ill individuals are usually taken at variable and often unspecified times following exposure and therefore reflect an uncertain duration of exposure. A biologic level—no matter how high—still only reflects exposure and a given probability of illness and is never diagnostic of illness.

Between the "no adverse health effect level" and the "clinical effect level" there often lies a gray zone. These concepts are illustrated in Fig 34–2. If the employee's level falls into this zone, the clinician may repeat the measurement, use other indices of exposure, or do further reading of the primary literature to refine the evaluation.

Individuals differ in their response to chemicals; one worker may develop peripheral neuropathy from n-hexane exposure whereas another worker with the same exposure will not. This difference in sensitivity to a chemical may be due to variable rates of metabolism or excretion, different sensitivity of end organ receptors, different tolerance to discomfort, a preexisting illness, or simultaneous exposure to drugs or other toxins. Because of these differences between individuals, within a group of exposed workers the biologic level associated with symptoms will usually follow a bell-shaped distribution.

METHODOLOGY

Ideally, the biologic level of a chemical is determined by its rate of absorption, elimination, and metabolism. Unfortunately, many other factors affect the measured level and are potential sources of error.

Timing of Collection

The timing of the sample collection relative to the exposure is usually the most critical methodologic

factor and may be the greatest source of error. For chemicals with a short half-time, the difference between sampling 15 minutes versus 1 hour after the end of exposure may alter the results by as much as a factor of 10.

Collection Methods

Before taking a specimen, it is advisable to consult the laboratory about proper collection methods. Errors in sampling will occur if standard collection methods are not followed. Once collected, chemicals may deteriorate if not analyzed rapidly. The specimens often must be centrifuged or frozen soon after collection. An improper container may bind (adsorb) the chemical of interest or contaminate the specimen (eg, lead-free glass tubes should be used for measuring blood lead levels). A urine collection can be contaminated from unwashed hands or clothing.

Body Site Sampled

The most frequent sites sampled are blood, urine, and exhaled air. Other body sites that are sampled but for which there is little scientific information about are hair and adipose tissue. The utility of hair analysis is limited by the unpredictable absorption of many chemicals by the hair root.

A. Blood: Blood is usually considered to provide the most accurate assessment of exposure. However, for volatile substances with short half-times, the variation in blood level can be considerable.

Unless otherwise indicated, blood sampling calls for whole venous blood. If the plasma-erythrocyte distribution ratio is not near unity, sampling may call for a serum specimen. The venous sample of a chemical that easily penetrates the skin—eg, nitroglycerin—may reflect skin absorption distal to the sampling site and not total body exposure.

B. Urine: Urine is the easiest fluid to sample. A 24-hour urine collection provides the most accurate assessment of exposure, but for practical reasons in the workplace setting the sample usually collected is the spot urine—a single sample collected at a specified time relative to exposure. Unfortunately, significant variation can occur in spot urine levels owing to fluctuation in urine concentrations. This variability may be reduced by adjusting levels to urine specific gravity (SG 1.014) or urine creatinine (1 g creatinine). This type of standardization should be done on a case-by-case basis. For example, while correcting for urinary creatinine will decrease variability in the assessment of mercury exposure, it appears to have no effect on variability when one is assessing cadmium exposure. In Table 34–1, urine values refer to spot urine levels and where appropriate are corrected for specific gravity or creatinine. Highly concentrated (SG > 1.030 or Cr > 3 g/L) or highly dilute spot urine specimens (SG < 1.010 or Cr < 0.3–0.5 g/L) are usually not suitable for monitoring, and a new specimen should be collected. Urine monitoring may not be appropriate for workers with advanced renal disease.

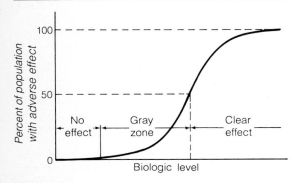

Figure 34–2. Percentage of population demonstrating adverse clinical effects from increasing biologic levels of the chemical.

C. Exhaled Air: Measurements of chemicals in exhaled air are noted in the "comments" column of Table 34–1 to be either mid-exhaled or end-exhaled air. In general, the concentrations in end-exhaled air during exposure are smaller than in mixed-exhaled air, and during postexposure the concentrations in mixed-exhaled are smaller than in end-exhaled air. Workers with emphysema should not be monitored by exhaled air sampling. Sampling must be performed in an area free of the chemical being measured. The process usually involves breathing into a Saran bag that is then exhausted through a charcoal-containing tube.

Selecting a Laboratory

Selection of a laboratory for analysis of specimens is generally the responsibility of the medical supervisor of a biologic monitoring program. Selection should be on the basis of analytic accuracy, convenience, turnaround time, and cost. Analytic accuracy is the most important factor but is often difficult if not impossible to assess. The only true assessment of accuracy is an independent intra- and interlaboratory program of quality assurance. This is accomplished by submitting blind samples to laboratories and comparing the results with those of a reference laboratory, followed by certification of laboratories meeting minimum standards. Certification in this way has been implemented on a national basis in the USA only for blood lead determinations.

Determination of cholinesterase levels for state-mandated monitoring of pesticide handlers must be done by state-certified laboratories in California, the only state with such a program. The World Health Organization recently conducted an international quality assurance program for blood lead and urine cadmium determinations.

Initial feedback from these testing and certification programs indicates that even the most experienced laboratories can fail to meet minimum standards and that without a regular quality assurance program analytic quality cannot be assured. The practitioner responsible for a monitoring program should request data on the laboratory's testing and certification status. It is more common, however, for the practitioner to rely on the use of "experienced" laboratories to produce reliable monitoring results. Analysis of a random sample of "split" specimens by another—preferably a reference—laboratory is an alternative to an internal quality assurance program.

For a number of compounds, the use of specific collection equipment is critical. Many laboratories provide such equipment as a service and may deliver and pick up samples on site. The laboratory should provide information on methods of sample collection, containers, and sources of contamination. Some laboratories have collected biologic specimens from unexposed populations and generated a range of "normal" or "background" levels. Careful attention must be paid to the definition of "normal," which may be different for workers than for nonoccupa-

tional populations. The amount of assistance and accuracy of information provided should help to indicate the level of experience and expertise of the laboratory in analyzing the compounds of interest.

HOW TO USE TABLE 34–1

Selection of Chemicals

Only agents for which there have been adequate biologic monitoring studies to date have been included in Table 34–1. Chemicals are arranged in the table first by major chemical group (metals, other inorganics, organics, etc). Within each major group, the chemicals are arranged alphabetically.

Under each chemical name are listed the body media (blood, urine, breath) in which the chemical or its metabolite can be measured and in what units. Only those media that have been adequately studied are included. The body fluids to be sampled are ranked so that the one with the greatest scientific validity is listed first. For practical reasons, the one ranked highest may not always be the measurement of choice.

Levels in Unexposed Populations

Biologic levels in populations without occupational exposure to that agent usually follow a poison distribution (skewed bell shape). The ranges listed in this column will include the majority, or 90%, of the unexposed population. The 5% of the population with the highest levels would be expected to be above this range.

No Adverse Health Effect Level

This is the level at which almost all workers will be free of symptoms, signs, and adverse clinical laboratory test results. An adverse result is one that reflects end organ damage. For example, an elevated serum AST would be considered an adverse laboratory result, whereas an abnormal serum ALA synthetase level would not. A very small number of people with biologic levels below the "no adverse health effect" level may have clinical findings. Unless otherwise noted, reproductive or carcinogenic effects of chemicals are not considered in calculating this level.

Only a limited number of chemicals have been studied for the purpose of determining the biologic level associated with absence of adverse health effects. If such data do not exist, the "no adverse health level" may be based on extrapolation from limit values of environmental monitoring recommended by ACGIH or NIOSH. For example, almost all workers exposed to perchloroethylene (a cleaning solvent) below ambient air levels of 100 ppm will fail to experience the irritant and central nervous system depressant properties of perchloroethylene. The corresponding perchloroethylene blood or exhaled air level would be the biologic "no adverse health effect" level. This does not take into account the theoretic risk of cancer from animal cancer data. "No adverse health effect" levels that have been arrived at by extrapolation from recommended environmental levels are identified with an asterisk.

Biologic exposure indices (BEI) are reference biologic monitoring levels established by the ACGIH. A BEI is a level that corresponds to the level measured in a worker exposed to a substance at the threshold limit value-time weighted average (TLV-TWA) (see Chapter 38). Where a BEI has been established, it is in essential agreement with Table 34–1 unless otherwise noted in the comments to that table.

Clinical Effect Level

This is the level that is commonly associated with symptoms, signs, or abnormal laboratory tests. This level is most useful for diagnostic purposes, ie, for evaluating a worker with an abnormal clinical presentation whose degree of exposure is uncertain. For example, the differential diagnosis of a worker exposed to pentachlorophenol includes salicylate poisoning, hyperthyroidism, and pentachlorophenol poisoning. The latter would be confirmed by a blood pentachlorophenol level near or above the "clinical effect" level.

Timing of Sample Collection

The interpretation of a biologic level is critically dependent on the timing of sample collection. The following abbreviations are standard times for biologic sample collections and should be considered relative to standard work days and work weeks. For example, PNS ("prior to next shift") means sampling 16 hours after the last shift, and EOS ("end of shift") means sampling 15–30 minutes after last exposure. The time recommendations are most important for the number that appears in the "no adverse health effect level" column.

NC not critical
DS during shift
L2H last 2 hours of shift
L4H last 4 hours of shift
EOS end of shift
PNS prior to next shift
EWW end of work week

Terminal Half-time

The rate of elimination of an agent—its terminal half-time—is useful for interpreting measured levels relative to the timing of sample collection. If the half-time is short (minutes to hours), the timing of collection is critical. If the half-time is long (days to weeks), the timing of collection is not critical.

Most organic chemicals have 2 half-times—an initial short half-time and a terminal longer one. The short half-time is usually a measure of the rate at which the solvent equilibrates from the blood to other tissues (fat, muscle, brain) and may be very rapid. The terminal half-time more accurately reflects the rate of elimination of the bulk of the chemical from the body.

Biologic levels of chemicals with short half-times should be interpreted with caution when they are evaluated using an average elimination half-time. The rates of metabolism and elimination may vary significantly between individuals. For example, the average half-time of carboxyhemoglobin is about 5 hours, with a range of 1–8 hours. A carboxyhemoglobin level obtained 1 hour after exposure will therefore represent somewhere between 50% and 95% of the end-of-shift level depending on the individual's elimination half-time.

REFERENCES

Aitio A, Järvisalo J: Biological monitoring of occupational exposure to toxic chemicals: Collection, processing, and storage of specimens. *Ann Clin Lab Sci* 1985;**15**:121.

Alessio L et al (editors): *Biological Indicators for the Assessment of Human Exposure to Industrial Chemicals.* Commission of the European Communities, 1984.

Alessio L et al (editors): *Human Biological Monitoring of Industrial Chemicals Series.* Commission of the European Communities, 1983.

Baselt RC (editor): *Disposition of Toxic Drugs and Chemicals in Man,* 2nd ed. Biomedical Publications, 1982.

Documentation of the Threshold Limit Values and Biological Exposure Indices, 5th ed. American Conference of Governmental Industrial Hygienists, 1986.

Fowler BA et al: Arsenic. In: *Handbook of Toxicology of Metals.* Friberg L, Nordberg G, Vour VB (editors). Elsevier/North-Holland, 1978.

Fukuchi Y: Nitroglycol concentrations in blood and urine of workers engaged in dynamite production. *Int Arch Occup Environ Health* 1981;**48**:339.

Groeseneken D, Veulemans H, Masschelein R: Urinary excretion of ethoxyacetic acid after experimental human exposure to ethylene glycol monoethyl ether. *Br J Ind Med* 1986;**43**:615.

Hayes AW (editor): *Principles and Methods of Toxicology.* Raven Press, 1982.

Lauwerys R: *Industrial Chemical Exposure: Guidelines for Biological Monitoring.* Biomedical Publications, 1983.

Perbellini L, Brugnone F, Faggionato G: Urinary excretion of the metabolites of n-hexane and its isomers during occupational exposure. *Br J Ind Med* 1981;**38**:20.

Perbellin L, Brugnone F, Pavan I: Identification of the metabolites of n-hexane, cyclohexane, and their isomers in men's urine. *Toxicol Appl Pharmacol* 1980;**53**:220.

Recommended Health-Based Limits in Occupational Exposure to Heavy Metals. WHO Technical Report No. 647. World Health Organization, 1980.

Roi R et al (editors): *Occupational Health Guidelines for Chemical Risk.* Commission of the European Communities, 1983.

Occupational Stress

35

James P. Seward, MD, MPP

Stress is an increasingly important occupational health problem and a significant cause of economic loss. While "stress" remains a broad, somewhat ill-defined concept, research efforts have led to a clearer understanding of the problem, its causes, and its consequences. Occupational stress may produce both overt psychologic and physiologic disability; however, it may also cause more subtle manifestations of morbidity that can affect personal well-being and productivity.

Although many of the factors in the workplace that may cause stress have been studied, the ability to predict a stress response in any given individual remains poor. The control of occupational stress is best accomplished in a preventive way by recognizing problem situations as well as early clinical or behavioral signs. Although the treatment of stress in the individual case depends on the clinical manifestations, rehabilitation must include a consideration both of the work environment and of the individual's coping mechanisms.

STRESS CONCEPT & MODELS

Hans Selye defined stress in general terms as a syndrome that involves a nonspecific response of the organism to a stimulus from the environment. In framing the concept to make it applicable to the occupational setting, stress might be defined as a *perceived* imbalance between occupational demands and the individual's ability to perform when the consequences of failure are important. The element of individual perception introduces subjectivity into the definition of stress, and this perceptual component has become very important for the evaluation of stress in the workers' compensation system.

Models of stress attempt to integrate individual and environmental factors into a working scheme of how stress is generated. An ideal model for occupational stress would be useful both in ongoing theoretic research and in practical problem-solving. Such a model would have to meet many criteria. It should offer a clear definition of how stress develops and allow for differentiation of stressful and nonstressful situations. The model should help to explain why certain events produce stress in some individuals but cause no detectable stress in others—and why stress may lead to varying degrees of pathologic or even beneficial effects according to the circumstances.

All of the major factors that determine the stress response should be considered in the model. In general terms, these factors would include occupational, social, familial, and individual characteristics. If such a conceptual framework were developed, it would help to integrate the results of past research and suggest new areas for inquiry. It would also allow accurate predictions. Unfortunately, none of the available models meet these stringent criteria.

Several good efforts have been made that reflect different viewpoints on the genesis of occupational stress. Different models or partial models reflect the lack of consensus about weighing the etiologic factors. The main question is whether stress results primarily from the nature of the stimulus, the manner in which the stimulus is perceived, or the way in which the individual responds to the stimulus.

One simple explanatory model has been proposed by McLean (Fig 35–1). Overlapping circles represent the environmental context, individual vulnerability, and the initiating situation or condition, called the stressor. The stressor is able to produce stress only

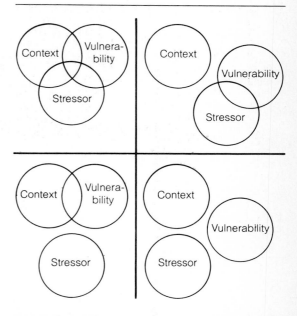

Figure 35–1. Symptomatic relationships between context, vulnerability, and stressors. (From McLean AA: *Work Stress.* Addison & Wesley, 1980.)

when all circles overlap, indicating a symptomatic response to a concurrence of these factors.

This basic model makes no attempt to weigh environmental versus individual factors in causing stress; however, it implies that favorable individual characteristics (low vulnerability) might prevent a symptomatic stress response when the environmental context and the presence of a stressor would otherwise facilitate one. Similarly, favorable environmental context alone might avoid a stressful outcome.

A more complex paradigm to explain the causation of stress is called the Person-Environment Fit Model (Fig 35–2). In this model, a distinction is made between the objective and subjective evaluations of the individual and the environment. Stress is produced by the subjective Person-Environment Fit, which is mediated ultimately by the individual's perceptions of the self and the environment. In this system, good mental health in the working situation depends on the outcome of 4 interactions: the objective environment-objective person, the objective environment-subjective environment, the objective person-subjective person, and the subjective environment-subjective person. A simple example will clarify these concepts:

> A garment worker may be expected to produce 40 pieces per hour (objective environment), whereas she believes she is required to produce 50 (subjective environment). She may actually be capable of producing 45 pieces (objective individual), but she thinks she can only produce 40 pieces (subjective individual).

In this case, there is a good match between the objective environmental demands (40 garments) and the objective person's ability (45 garments). However, the worker's perception that 50 garments are demanded (subjective environment) and undervaluation of her own abilities (subjective person) lead to a stressful situation. Given this scenario, the worker might experience stress based on a poor subjective Person-Environment Fit despite an adequate objective fit.

The Person-Environment Fit Model is fairly comprehensive and clearly places much emphasis on the individual's subjective interaction with the environment. Another model places more emphasis on the work environment and the extent to which it may allow individuals to modify the stress response. The Job Decision Control Model concept holds that stress results from an imbalance between demands on a worker and the worker's ability to modify those demands (Fig 35–3). This model focuses on the adaptive response of the individual to a potentially stressful stimulus. When the worker can modify the response or alter the circumstances, less stress may result. Low decision-making control coupled with high job demands leads to high strain or to a stressful situation. Proponents of the Job Decision Control Model have tended to focus on work tasks, but other aspects of the work environment such as organizational features or opportunities for creativity and independent thought might be as important.

These 2 models have been chosen as examples from many competing theories of occupational stress because they have different emphasis. They are not mutually exclusive, and neither one meets the criteria of completeness and universal applicability of an ideal model. The Person-Environment Fit Model has

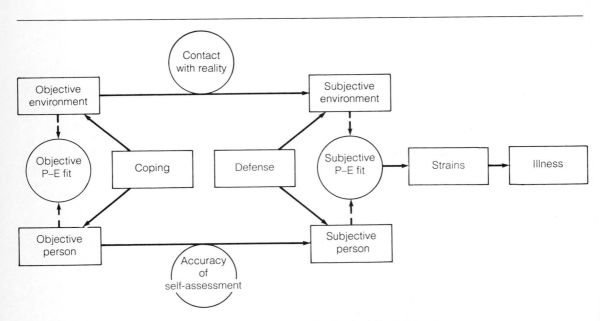

Figure 35–2. Effects of psychosocial stress in terms of fit between the person and the environment. Concepts within circles are discrepancies between the 2 adjoining concepts. Solid lines indicate causal effects. (From Harrison RV: Person-environment fit and job stress. In: *Stress at Work.* Cooper C, Payne R [editors]. Wiley, 1978.)

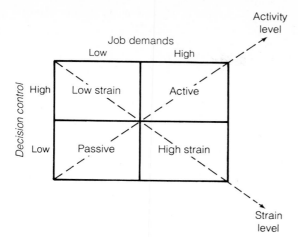

Figure 35–3. The job-demand control model, indicating the effects of job demands and decision latitude on strain. (From Baker DB: The study of stress at work. *Annu Rev Pub Health* 1985;**6:**367.)

Table 35–1. Common workplace stressors.

Organizational
  Change
  Inadequate communication
  Interpersonal conflict
  Conflict with organizational goals
Career development
  Lack of promotional opportunity
  New responsibilities beyond level
  Unemployment
Role
  Role conflict
  Role ambiguity
  Inadequate resources to accomplish job
  Inadequate authority to accomplish job
Task
  Quantitative and qualitative overload
  Quantitative and qualitative underload
  Responsibility for the lives and well-being of others
  Low decision making latitude
Work environment
  Poor aesthetics
  Physical exposures
  Ergonomic problems
  Noise
  Odors
  Safety hazards
Shift work

gained much acceptance in the USA and Great Britain, where explanations of stress have tended to focus on the individual. The Job Decision Control Model and others that examine stress-modifying mechanisms built into the work environment have a growing audience, especially in some Scandinavian nations.

An important consideration is the predictive accuracy of any given model. While neither of these 2 models has been well tested in a prospective manner, the predictive value of the Person-Environment Fit Model has been fairly low. However, there are many variables involved in this model that may be inherently difficult to measure. The Job Decision Control Model has had reasonably good predictive value in several investigations. Methodologic and theoretic issues make rigorous comparison of these 2 limited models difficult.

Despite the lack of theoretic consensus regarding occupational stress, a great deal can still be said regarding specific workplace and environmental conditions that produce stress, the effects of stress on the individual and the organization, and methods that may control or alleviate stress in the work setting. Subsequent sections will consider these issues.

WORKPLACE STRESSORS

Various characteristics of working life may contribute to occupational stress (Table 35–1). These characteristics may be grouped with much overlap into 5 general categories: organization and organizational relationships, career development, role of the individual, job task or assignment, and working environment and conditions. The following sections will discuss the contribution of each of these areas to the genesis of occupational stress.

Organization & Organizational Relationships

Most people in industrialized societies are now employed in some organizational context and are subject to fallout from factors that affect the organization as a whole. Issues inherent in organizational life such as political conflict, communication difficulties, delegation of tasks, decision-making authority, and regulations may be sources of conflict and stress. Relationships with supervisors are particularly important determinants of subjective well-being.

Stressful conditions are often produced when organizations undergo change. The situations encountered in producing new products or services, reorganizing institutional structure, and expanding or contracting operations often challenge the individual's ability to adapt. Increased levels of anxiety and diminished job satisfaction and morale have been shown in companies during the process of introducing new product lines. Thus, the process of change may disrupt an individual's equilibrium within an organization and place him or her at increased risk of a stress response.

Poor communication within organizations and a sense of not being consulted by managers can similarly lead to stress as manifested by low job satisfaction. Conversely, good interpersonal support from colleagues—but especially from supervisors—may alleviate stress. Conflict with a supervisor or coworker is a powerful stressor. Moral or ideologic conflict between the individual and the goals of the organization can also produce psychologic strain. The salesperson required to promote what is perceived to be a shabby or socially irrelevant product and the manager forced to fire a respected older employee will both experience substantial stress.

Table 35–2. Personal factors influencing possible increased risk from shiftwork.

Sleep disorders
Gastrointestinal disorders
Advanced age
Some chronic diseases
Psychologic problems
Family and social situations

Table 35–3. Workplace factors affecting possible increased risk to shift workers.

Shift scheduling
Location and transportation
Physical exposures
Heat
Others
Chemical exposures
Safety factors, eg, lighting
Availability of meals
Social environment
Access to medical care

Career Development

Many transitions in working life are recognized as stressful situations. A change in jobs, getting a promotion or being passed over, and being laid off or fired are all high-risk events.

Studies of workers undergoing periods of unemployment have shown increased rates of mental illness and alcohol and drug use. There is also a suggestion of increased rates of disease such as peptic ulcer and hypertension.

Retirement as such, on the other hand, does not seem to be the cause of significant mental or physical ill health. Several longitudinal studies of morbidity and mortality rates in retired workers have shown no substantial age-adjusted increase in mortality rates. There is no strong evidence for an overall adverse impact of retirement on mental well-being with the possible exception of a reduced sense of usefulness.

Promotion is a potential stressor. New job responsibilities, especially when calling for skills not previously exercised, can result in anxiety and psychologic decompensation. Promotion to a position beyond one's abilities has the potential for inducing behavioral disorders. Frustrated career goals and underpromotion have been associated with increased rates of mental hospitalization, as documented in a study of United States Navy enlisted men who achieved officer status. Thus, symptomatic stress may result both from the frustration of thwarted ambition and from the inability to cope with new demands.

Role in the Organization

Role conflict exists when 2 or more competing expectations make simultaneous satisfaction of both difficult. Role ambiguity implies insufficient information or guidance on which to base decisions and behavior. In one survey, approximately half of the work force reported having role conflicts, and over a third were disturbed by ambiguous expectations and duties.

Role conflict often occurs at interface positions. For example, a production supervisor occupies a position between management and staff, with an interest in keeping both sides happy without compromising production. Other examples of role conflict include differing opinions over what a given job should entail, contradictory job demands, and managing disputes between colleagues. Correlations have been observed between role conflict and increased heart rate as well as job dissatisfaction.

Role ambiguity may occur as a result of specific ill-defined responsibilities, unclear expectations of personal image, or hazy organizational objectives. The source of stress in these situations may be the lack of clarity itself or inability to assess one's own performance.

Another type of role-related stress may result when individuals experience discrepancies between their supervisors' expectations and the resources available to meet them. Insufficient time, personnel, or funding put a strain on the responsible individual who lacks the power to increase the availability of resources or to change expectations.

Task

Work overload and underload, decision-making ability, and level and type of responsibility are important task-related issues with relevance for occupational stress. Both quantitative and qualitative overload have been implicated in stress disorders. In quantitative overload, the individual is overwhelmed by the amount of work. In qualitative overload, the expected functional level is too high—ie, the work is too difficult. High quantitative workload has been associated with coronary artery disease in several studies; there is also a relationship to alcohol and tobacco use, lost work time, poor motivation, and poor self-image.

Qualitative overload also has adverse physiologic effects. Blood cholesterol levels have been shown to rise in medical students under conditions of qualitative overload during an evaluation process. Tax accountants had higher cholesterol levels at deadlines. University professors with personal expectations of very high quality work scored poorly in terms of one stress indicator: self-esteem.

Qualitative and quantitative underload may also cause stress. One study of disease indicators in a large executive population showed higher rates of disease among individuals at the 2 extremes of the spectrum—the overworked and the underworked. Mental difficulties may be induced by understimulation and excessively routinized activities; workers become bored and alienated and lose initiative.

Job responsibilities are significant sources of stress; work that involves responsibility for the lives of others is particularly stressful. Physicians, air traffic controllers, and first-line supervisors who make decisions affecting the lives of others may have higher rates of peptic ulcer; myocardial infarction and hypertension may also be related to work involving responsibility for others.

Several studies have shown a beneficial effect of higher job autonomy on stress indicators. Greater latitude to make basic decisions regarding performance of one's work has been associated with fewer myocardial infarctions and fewer job-related injuries. Conversely, low decision-making autonomy has been related to higher levels of stress.

Work Environment

The physical environment of the workplace may present many potential stressors. Most environmental hazards are identified with specific health effects they may cause, such as hearing loss from noise exposure. However, these exposures may also contribute to stress in a variety of ways. Physical exposures, chemical exposures, crowding, and ergonomic problems may function independently or collectively as stressors.

Noise provides a good example of a multifaceted stressor. In addition to its cumulative effect on the cochlea, noise may acutely raise blood pressure. In addition, high levels of sound isolate workers by preventing conversation and drowning out other auditory cues to events near the worker. In one experiment, many of the physiologic and psychologic changes associated with excessive noise were eliminated by providing a button that could be used to control sound levels. The beneficial effect occurred whether or not the control option was used.

Other physical exposures such as excessive heat or cold, extremes of lighting or glare, and vibration may produce ill effects. While the magnitude of these effects may not themselves be disabling, the associated discomfort can contribute to mental distress and to secondary physiologic changes characteristic of stress.

Physical comfort and pleasant surroundings have been correlated with mental health. Ergonomic factors in tool and work station design also play a role in worker frustration, morale, and ultimately productivity.

Chemical exposures may also induce stress through a variety of mechanisms. There may be direct irritating or intoxicating effects. Anxiety may arise regarding personal welfare subsequent to potentially hazardous exposures. Unpleasant chemical odors—regardless of toxicity—may be powerful stressors by themselves.

Safety hazards inherent in some workplaces, such as risks of explosion or falls, add the element of fear to other work concerns. Welding on a thousand-foot-high tower is clearly more stressful than welding at ground level.

The assumption should be made—even though good documentation is not available—that the effects produced by stressful conditions are additive. Combined environmental stressors may even operate synergistically in some situations. Any given job is likely to have a complex array of potential stressors acting in a variety of ways. More research is needed, specifically on the cumulative effects of environmental stressors.

Shift Work

Rotating work shifts are a common stressor that affect a growing proportion of the working population worldwide. Estimates are that between 15% and 20% of the United States work force do some form of shift or night work. Rotating shifts usually involve regularly changing work hours. Employees' shifts change periodically (eg, every 2–30 days), so that time spent working day, evening, and night shifts will be shared fairly equally by the work force. These schedule changes have consequences for mental and physical well-being. Much has been learned in recent years about the physiologic effects of shift rotation, and there have been some practical applications (Tables 35–2 and 35–3). Many of the issues faced by shift workers are shared by individuals who have permanent night work schedules.

There have been numerous studies of the physiologic and health consequences of shift work and the relationship of shift work to accidents, social well-being, productivity, and absenteeism. Despite these investigations, there is uncertainty regarding both long-term health effects and the role of personal factors in adaptation to shift work. Some points of general agreement provide the bases for evaluating work schedules and advising shift workers.

Circadian Rhythms

Many physiologic systems in the human body display a regular circadian rhythm. In a free-running state unregulated by clocks, sunlight, or the regular pattern of daily activity, many of the major human circadian rhythms follow a 25-hour cycle. The usual 24-hour day thus requires a daily adjustment backward of about 1 hour in our "natural" rhythm. In changing our daily schedules, it is generally more difficult to arise progressively earlier than to delay awakening by an hour, since earlier awakening increases the adaptation required (shifting the internal clock back), whereas later awakening is a more natural adjustment. The same theory may explain why adjustment to time zone changes after air travel usually takes longer in the west-east direction; adapting to a more easterly time zone is essentially the same process as awakening earlier.

When this information is applied to rotating shift work, it becomes apparent, from a theoretical standpoint, that successful shift rotation should proceed from night to day to evening shifts rather than the reverse order. By following a "clockwise" progression to later shifts, the rotation order puts less strain on the adaptive ability of the internal clock. Application of the forward rotation principle to a mining company in the USA resulted in increased productiv-

Table 35–4. Preplacement and follow-up examinations for shift workers.

Health and functioning at work
Sleep quality and quantity
    Sleep environment, noise
    Chronic fatigue, naps
Gastrointestinal disease
Chronic diseases
Use of medication
Use of alcohol, caffeine, tobacco, drugs
Accidents on and off the job
Psychologic problems
Social and family problems

ity and subjective well-being as well as less job turnover.

A second issue related to circadian rhythms is incomplete entrainment of the normal diurnal cycle following shift rotation. With change from a day to a night schedule, the various physiologic circadian rhythms begin to readjust; however, each one adapts at its own rate, with resulting dyssynchrony. In theory, all the rhythms would reach a new homeostasis if the new schedule were perfectly maintained. In practice, there is seldom complete readjustment, because the individual tends to resume daytime schedules on days off and because of inadequate numbers of days on a given schedule.

There are at least 2 schools of thought regarding the preferred way to schedule shift work based on a knowledge of circadian rhythms. One approach is to assign shifts that rotate slowly so that workers have at least 5 days and often much longer on a given schedule. In theory, workers have a longer time to adapt to the schedule both physiologically and socially. The other viewpoint advocates a short rotation length of 1–3 days on a given schedule. Proponents of these fast rotations argue that workers never fully adapt to night shifts and that short night rotations cause less chaos with circadian rhythms. Physiology notwithstanding, the acceptability of a shift schedule will depend to a significant extent on environmental, social, and recreational factors.

The physical and mental exertion involved in the work, the social and family support systems available, and the opportunities to eat well at the workplace should also be considered in scheduling decisions.

Health Effects of Shift Work

Both short- and long-term health effects have been anticipated as a result of shift work. However, the case for short-term effects is much stronger. One factor influencing the long-term studies is bias through self selection of individuals who tolerate shift work. The tendency of individuals who experience ill effects to cease shift work may lead to underestimates of the medical consequences.

Among the short-term or immediate problems related to shift work, sleep disorders, gastrointestinal disturbances, and effects on underlying medical problems are of greatest concern.

Sleep is affected in several ways. Studies have shown that there is a tendency to fewer hours of sleep while on night shift. Sleep may be interrupted by street noise, family activity, the telephone, or other causes. The quality of sleep may also be altered, with changes in the sleep cycles and less REM sleep.

Gastrointestinal complaints are increased in rotating shift workers. There are changes in appetite and increased constipation. Alimentation is often adversely affected by poor availability or poor quality of food for night shift employees. Studies have shown a high incidence of peptic ulcer among shift workers and an even higher incidence among workers who dropped out of shift work. A contributing factor to the gastrointestinal problems may be the increased consumption of caffeine and tobacco among rotating shift workers.

There is concern and some documentation that rotating shift work exacerbates chronic medical conditions. Insulin-dependent diabetes mellitus may be more difficult to control, in part because of the irregularity of meals. The alternation of the sleep cycle may cause increased seizure frequency in epileptics.

There is conflicting information regarding cardiovascular morbidity and mortality in shift workers. Although some studies have shown more absence due to cardiovascular disease, there is no clear indication of increased mortality from this cause.

While psychiatric disorders are not elevated overall, there are clearly social and familial stresses resulting from shift work. A shift worker will often have difficulty maintaining normal social contacts and community involvement. Altered sleep and leisure schedules can result in periods of low interaction with children and spouses.

Despite the wide-ranging impacts on an individual's life and the many ways in which health may be affected, shift work does not appear to change overall mortality. Several studies have examined longevity of rotating shift workers in relation to daytime workers without showing a significant difference.

Special considerations should be given to concerns of safety for night workers. Especially with boring and repetitive work, there is increased likelihood of reduced attention and increased errors. In situations where safety risk is high, alertness monitors, extra measures to protect against injury, and perhaps shorter shifts should be recommended.

Medical Advice to Shift Workers

Medical evaluation for shift work should include particular attention to a history of gastrointestinal problems, sleep disorders, epilepsy, difficulty with night vision, or other chronic disorders that might be affected by night work and rotating schedules. In shift work, the timing of medication and the quality of nutrition for people with chronic diseases is of concern.

While it may be theoretically possible to predict which individuals are well or poorly suited to shift work based on their circadian rhythms or sleep-wake cycles, practical criteria for selection do not yet exist. As a result, there is an enormous amount of self-selection that occurs after experiencing shift work. An important role for the occupational practitioner is to advise shift workers regarding possible health concerns and how best to adapt to them. It is important to cover social and familial concerns as well as sleeping habits, diet, and caffeine and other stimulant use (Table 35–4). The clinician should offer periodic evaluations to check for maladaptation or for specific medical problems related to shift work.

Individual & Social Factors in Stress

Both personality traits and stressors from outside the workplace can influence the likelihood of work-induced stress. According to the Person-Environment Fit Model, individual response to a stressor is an important determinant of the outcome. Any comprehensive model of stress must help to explain why workers exposed to the same stressors will exhibit different responses. When attempting to reduce occupational stress, more emphasis should be placed on workplace stressors than on individual predisposition; however, the latter should not be ignored—especially as a precipitating factor.

Many variables may affect individual vulnerability to occupational stress. Personality structure, family life, stage in life, and social support systems are among the most important factors affecting the stress response. Many cases of occupational stress are precipitated by factors in the personal sphere. In addition to a thorough inquiry about stressors at work, physicians should always inquire about events in an individual's nonworking life when evaluating patients with stress symptoms.

The Holmes-Rahe Scale (Table 35–5) of recent life events (both "positive" and "negative") is an effort to rate the difficulty of change and adjustment associated with stressful occurrences. In studies of several different groups, there was a correlation between higher total cumulative scores over a 1-year period and higher frequency and severity of illness. It is reasonable to infer that high scores on personal life stressors might also predispose a population to greater impact from workplace stressors.

Personality factors may also predispose certain individuals to a greater risk of stress-related disease. A case has been made for increased incidence of heart disease in individuals with aggressive, achievement-oriented personalities. Individuals with obsessive personality traits may depend on the structure of their jobs and undergo stress when changes occur. Preexisting psychiatric disorders as well as passive-aggressive, antisocial, and other maladaptive personality traits may impact on the worker's ability to cooperate and be productive.

Changes in the workplace affect individuals differently according to their age and stage in life. According to the theory of life stages, adults undergo developmental changes that result in new needs and expectations from working life. Phases such as choosing a career, struggling for advancement, and reaching a high level of maturity and experience can be stressful depending on the individual's underlying personality organization and whether they are accompanied by appropriate recognition and reward. A transfer to very different job duties may be less taxing to a new employee who is just acquiring skills than to an established one who is trying to gain recognition for accomplishments in a specific area.

Social support by individuals outside the workplace can be an important mitigating factor in development of stress. The spouse is usually the most important person in this regard, but other family members and friends can also play an important role in supporting individuals in stressful occupations. An important concern here is that families often bear the

Table 35–5. The Holmes-Rahe schedule of recent life events.[1]

Rank	Event	Value
1	Death of spouse	100
2	Divorce	73
3	Marital separation	65
4	Jail term	63
5	Death of close family member	63
6	Personal injury or illness	53
7	Marriage	50
8	Fired from work	47
9	Marital reconciliation	45
10	Retirement	45
11	Change in family member's health	44
12	Pregnancy	40
13	Sex difficulties	39
14	Addition to family	39
15	Business readjustment	39
16	Change in financial status	38
17	Death of close friend	37
18	Change to different line of work	36
19	Change in number of marital arguments	35
20	Mortgage or loan of over $10,000	31
21	Foreclosure of mortgage or loan	30
22	Change in work responsibilities	29
23	Son or daughter leaving home	29
24	Trouble with in-laws	29
25	Outstanding personal achievement	28
26	Spouse begins or stops work	26
27	Starting or finishing school	26
28	Change in living conditions	25
29	Revision of personal habits	24
30	Trouble with boss	23
31	Change in work hours, conditions	20
32	Change in residence	20
33	Change in schools	20
34	Change in recreational habits	19
35	Change in church activities	19
36	Change in social activities	18
37	Mortgage or loan under $10,000	17
38	Change in sleeping habits	16
39	Change in number of family gatherings	15
40	Change in eating habits	15
41	Vacation	13
42	Christmas season	12
43	Minor violation of the law	11

[1]Reproduced, with permission, from Holmes TH, Rahe RH: Social Readjustments Rating Scale. *J Psychosomat Res* 1967;**11**:213.

burden for alleviating stress originating in the work-place. The deterioration of family or social support relationships may precede decompensation from stress at work.

STRESS & DISEASE

Those who study occupational stress have been attempting to clarify the links between stress and disease. While there is good epidemiologic evidence relating occupational stress to a number of disease states, the pathophysiologic mechanisms often remain obscure.

The question of how stress produces disease is frequently debated. One theory holds that certain kinds of stress are consistently likely to produce given physiologic responses and, consequently, specific pathologic states. Another viewpoint is that stress is "nonspecific" and that personal factors such as conditioning and heredity determine which organ system, if any, will be affected by a variety of stressors. A given individual may have a specific susceptible organ that will be the target of a variety of stresses; thus, some people are gastrointestinal reactors, and others are cardiac or muscle tension reactors. Finally, stress may also be viewed as a nonspecific force that exacerbates existing disease states.

The stress response has been associated with a variety of physiologic changes that may be postulated as mediators in the development of disease. The hypothalamic-pituitary axis, the autonomic nervous system, and the catecholamine response are often cited as stress-sensitive systems. These and other neurologic and endocrine systems may be important actors in the chain of events leading to cardiovascular, gastrointestinal, endocrine, and other stress-related disorders.

Mental Illness

The mental health effects of stress exist on a continuum ranging from subjective symptoms that have a relatively mild effect on daily life to significant psychiatric disease with impairment of functions (Table 35–6). Subjective reports regarding personal well-being constitute some of the earliest measures of stress. Frequently noted symptoms include anxiety, tension, anger, irritability, poor concentration, apathy, and depression. These manifestations of stress interfere with a sense of well-being and may be precursors of more severe illness.

Behavioral changes may also occur in response to occupational stress. Diminished participation in family activities, increased marital discord, and reduced participation in club activities have been attributed to stress. Rates of substance abuse are often increased. Studies have shown increased rates of alcohol abuse among individuals with high levels of stress and job dissatisfaction. Tobacco consumption is elevated among people with heavy workloads and tends to increase near deadlines. Other behavioral changes

may include alterations in appetite and eating behavior, risk-taking (eg, when driving), and reduced interest in recreational activities.

Overt psychologic dysfunction is frequently attributed to stress. Examples of such diagnoses include clinical depression, anxiety disorders, somatoform disorders (eg, hypochondriasis, psychogenic pain), and exacerbation of existing physical conditions by psychologic factors. While these disorders are frequently observed in stressed individuals, no clear model has emerged to adequately explain the genesis of these disorders as related to stress. A statistical association between a stressor and such overt psychiatric disease has been shown in several instances; unemployment and lack of opportunity for promotion have both been related to increased psychiatric hospitalizations and suicide rates.

However, there is no good analysis of the specific types of psychiatric disorders that occur most frequently among stressed workers seeking medical attention. The theoretic question again arises whether stress nonspecifically increases the incidence of all psychiatric problems or whether certain diagnoses result with greater frequency. Anxiety disorders (eg, panic disorder, agoraphobia), somatoform disorders, and depression are 3 types of problems frequently discussed in the literature on stress.

Two specific conditions—posttraumatic stress disorder and mass psychogenic illness—are related to stress and deserve specific mention. Posttraumatic stress disorder usually follows a specific psychologically traumatic episode of significant severity which, in the occupational setting, is often an accident affecting the patient or a coworker. The patient subsequently reexperiences the traumatic event and develops symptoms of reduced responsiveness to the external world. Anxiety, depression, avoidance of activities that evoke the memory, emotional lability, and other symptoms often accompany the syndrome. This disorder is often a complicating factor in the rehabilitation of injured workers and may be respon-

Table 35–6. Examples of mental manifestations of stress.

Mild subjective
  Anxiety
  Tension
  Anger
  Depression
  Decreased concentration
  Irritability
Mild behavioral
  Decreased participation in family
  Marital discord
  Reduced social activity
  Risk taking
Clinical psychiatric disorders
  Adjustment disorders
  Affective disorders
  Anxiety disorders including posttraumatic stress disorders
  Somatoform disorders and psychophysiologic disorders
  Exacerbation of existing medical and psychiatric conditions
  Substance abuse

sive to brief psychotherapy and antianxiety medication.

Mass psychogenic illness is the collective occurrence of physical symptoms among 2 or more persons without evidence for an identifiable source. Symptoms are usually subjective, such as nausea, headache, dizziness, and neurasthenia. There are usually few, if any, objective findings. They generally resolve spontaneously with time or supportive care. There is usually a triggering event such as a strange odor or unexplained or rumored illness in one coworker. Factors associated with many of the industrial outbreaks have included boring, routine work, heavy production demands, physical stressors, poor communication opportunities, and poor labor-management relations. Many of these factors are also implicated in the stress response; it may be theorized that mass psychogenic illness is a particularly dramatic manifestation of occupational stress.

Cardiovascular Disease

There is growing evidence for the designation of occupational stress as a risk factor for cardiovascular disease. Coronary artery disease and myocardial infarction are mediated in part by known risk factors of serum cholesterol, smoking, hypertension, and sedentary lifestyle. If stress is a contributor to cardiovascular disease, it may operate independently or through other risk factors.

Although causality is difficult to establish, a great number of retrospective and prospective studies have implicated workplace stressors in the etiology of coronary artery disease. Excessive workload has been associated with increased myocardial infarction rates; workers with more than one job or excessively long work hours had more heart disease than a control group with fewer work hours. Role conflict and coronary artery disease are associated for some white collar workers. The studies regarding cardiovascular disease and occupational level are conflicting; some indicate higher rates of disease for high-status employees, whereas others indicate that lower level employees have a higher prevalence. This disparity makes it likely that factors other than occupational level will explain the phenomenon better and that future research should examine specific job components.

An inverse relationship between job satisfaction and coronary artery disease has been well demonstrated. This factor seems most strongly predictive for white collar workers. Self-esteem, which may be related to satisfaction, is also negatively correlated with coronary artery disease. These factors may in turn be related to another proposed predictor of coronary artery disease—job decision-making latitude. Many studies have shown that coronary artery disease mortality and morbidity are increased among individuals with demanding jobs that allow little decision-making latitude.

Occupational stress may clearly influence behavioral and physiologic risk factors for coronary artery disease. Serum cholesterol has been shown to rise in tax accountants near deadlines, students taking exams, and shift workers. Statistically significant rises in blood pressure have been found with some stressful jobs such as telephone switchboard operators and air traffic controllers. Increased serum and urine catecholamine levels have been found in workers in competitive situations or those with high work loads. Tobacco use increases among some stressed workers. Some epidemiologic studies have implicated sedentary work in increasing the risk of coronary artery disease.

One of the interesting controversies in cardiovascular medicine concerns the issue of personality type as a risk factor for coronary artery disease. Several studies have shown that individuals with "type A" personalities have an increased incidence of coronary artery disease. The traits shared by type A individuals are aggressive, ambitious behavior, competitiveness, and a sense of time urgency. While the type A hypothesis has its detractors, it is nonetheless interesting because of its implications for occupational stress. Such individuals may bring a personal predisposition to stress with them to the workplace; when encountering specific stressors that particularly frustrate or upset them, increased rates of coronary artery disease may result. Alternatively, some work environments may reinforce such maladaptive behavior.

Gastrointestinal Disease

Gastrointestinal disease, particularly peptic ulcer disease, has long been associated with stress and emotional changes. However, advances in diagnostic ability during the last several decades have allowed an improved understanding of this subject.

While some evidence has pointed to peptic ulcer disease as an ailment of executives and managers, stronger epidemiologic evidence shows an elevated prevalence of peptic ulcer disease among foremen. The explanation for this finding may be that foremen assume responsibility for the behavior and safety of others; they also occupy an interface role between workers and management. Other occupations that involve responsibility for others—physicians and air traffic controllers—also have high rates of peptic ulcer disease. Workers anticipating plant shutdowns also experienced an increase in ulcer disease, as do rotating shift workers. The incidence of duodenal ulcer—but not gastric ulcer—has also been shown to be related to workload as measured by energy expenditure. The incidence of ulcer disease may be modified by good social support networks both at home and at work.

There are several possible physiologic mechanisms responsible for the relationship of stress to ulcer disease. Autonomic nervous system activity plays a part in gastric acid secretion. Serum pepsinogen levels are often elevated in individuals predisposed to ulcers. Gastric acid secretion in response to catecholamine stimulation may also be a contributing factor.

Other gastrointestinal problems such as eating disorders, ulcerative colitis, functional bowel disease, and constipation have been related to stress. However, there is generally very little information regarding their association with occupational factors. One exception is rotating shift work, where appetite disturbances and constipation have frequently been noted.

Other Diseases

The general model of stress as a stimulus producing a wide variety of physiologic adaptations suggests the possibility that many human diseases may be precipitated or aggravated by occupational stress. The great frequency with which some disorders—such as back pain—occur in the work setting makes them logical candidates for study. Although stress may exacerbate muscular spasm and the experience of pain, there is no formal evidence linking stress to this common occupational ailment. Other diseases such as diabetes, headaches, asthma, and thyroid disease have been recognized also as having a psychophysiologic component in some individuals, and it is probable that occupational factors can contribute to their pathogenesis. There is suggestive evidence that air traffic controllers have higher rates of non-insulin-dependent diabetes.

Concern for the effects of stress on reproduction have been raised. Among stressed workers, there is evidence for an increase in cigarette, alcohol, and other substance abuse—each of which can produce ill effects on the fetus. Direct adverse impact of stress on fetal well-being is possible through transplacental hormonal mechanisms; however, there is no proof of poor reproductive outcomes as a result of stress.

The role of occupational stress in the causation of a wide range of diseases from cancer to eczema is not adequately confirmed or defined. Based on existing evidence for some specific illnesses such as coronary artery disease and peptic ulcer disease, such associations are more than speculative. Many potential pathophysiologic mechanisms are stimulated by occupational stress. The task remains to study the magnitude and clinical significance of these relationships.

Accidents

There is a multifactorial relationship between occupational stress and accidents in the workplace. The stress of high workload demands may lead to compromise of safety measures in order to attain higher productivity. Workers paid on a piecework basis have increased numbers of accidents. Attention span may be altered by low levels of stimulation and long periods without breaks; inattention can lead to accidents. Changes of shift are associated with higher rates of injury on the first days of new shifts. There is mounting evidence to relate shift changes and sleeplessness to airplane pilot and air traffic controller errors. There may also be a relationship between job decision latitude and frequency of injury. The contri-bution of stress to substance abuse also leads to accidents; a large proportion of motor vehicle accidents on the job involve alcohol.

Some authors have noted a relationship between stressful events in an employee's life and subsequent occupational accidents. The possibility exists that stress from work or personal factors may contribute to the likelihood of an accident. Stressors should be assessed in evaluating injured employees; treatment of the physical impairment alone may not result in successful return to work.

Sickness, Absence, & Productivity

A clear relationship exists between sickness, absence from work, and lost productivity. Stress may be an independent variable influencing each of these 3 factors. The case for stress as a contributor to sickness has already been made. However, absence from work is a complex phenomenon involving not just organic disease but also mental health, motivation, satisfaction with employment, and other personal and work-related factors. True malingering probably represents only a small part of the problem. Occupational stress probably contributes to the problem of absence due to illness, but the problem is compounded by sources of stress in the personal sphere.

In most organizations, a small number of employees account for a large proportion of the absences. Stressful situations frequently underlie these illnesses either as a proximate cause or as an exacerbating factor. The illness may provide a justification for escaping the work situation. In these cases, the ulcers may be a manifestation of the worker's feelings of alienation from the work environment. Observation in several industries has shown that wage dissatisfaction is not the primary explanation for such absences; pay raises have not altered attendance records in these situations. Stress evaluation and referral for assistance can have an impact on the rate of illness absence.

Productivity on the job is, similarly, a stress-sensitive function. Reduced output, production delays, and poor performance may be manifestations of stress. Declining productivity of an organization or individual should prompt a search for occupational stressors. A stress management program may promote increases in attendance and productivity. This has been demonstrated by experiments that increase employee decision-making participation as well as by revisions of workers' rotating shifts according to psychologic principles.

Stress & Workers' Compensation
(See also Chapter 3.)

While representing only a small portion of the costs of stress, workers' compensation claims for mental injuries are rapidly increasing. Most states in the USA recognize mental stress as a compensable disorder. In California, the number of reported stress claims increased by 500% between 1980 and 1988.

While stress claims represent only about 2.5% of the nation's occupational disease (as opposed to injury) claims, the proportion has been growing.

Several legal developments have permitted the increase in compensated stress cases. In the 1960 case of *Carter v General Motors* (361 Mich 577, 106 NW 2d), the Michigan State Supreme Court awarded workers' compensation benefits to a man with paranoid schizophrenia on the grounds that his illness had been caused by his work with the corporation although no physical injury or single traumatic event was involved. The legal definition of causation used in this and other cases is different from scientific causality. In the legal sense, psychiatric disability may be caused by work if the employment substantially contributed to its development.

The states have developed different criteria for evaluating these claims. In 1982, Michigan enacted a law authorizing payment only when stress resulted from significant work-related causes. Approximately 20 states award benefits for disability only when produced by sudden, shocking events or unusual stresses. While a few states do not require compensation for stress at all, most have no specific legal limitations on the nature of the stresses that may be compensated.

A second legal trend that has increased the compensability of occupational stress has been the cumulative injury claim. The concept of cumulative trauma argues that prolonged or repeated small injuries lead to disability over time. This legal approach has existed for many years but has recently been broadened in some states. Even though most cumulative trauma claims involve orthopedic injury or cardiovascular disease, a substantial minority involve psychologic impairment.

The number of claims for psychologic stress arising as a result of physical injury is also increasing. Given this increase both in numbers and costs of postinjury stress claims, efforts to identify such grounds for claims and intervene early to correct the problems may be beneficial both to workers and to the organization. Several factors associated with better outcomes include early psychiatric referral (especially after multiple surgical procedures), early contact by the immediate supervisor after injury, and early return to work even with light duty restrictions.

Prevention & Management of Stress

The prevention and management of occupational stress is a great challenge. Although there is often insufficient understanding of the genesis of stress in any given situation, it is frequently possible to apply existing knowledge to control this problem. Control begins with recognition—increased awareness on the part of health professionals is essential. Approaches to management and prevention may be organizational or individual in focus. Historically, stress management programs in the USA have tended to focus on solutions at the individual level by instruction in coping and adaptive techniques. Growing evidence

and experience point to the need for solutions that improve the relationship of the individual to the workplace. These solutions usually involve organizational changes that health professionals may help to accomplish.

Role of the Health Professional

Occupational health physicians and other health professionals must monitor their patients and, when possible, the entire organization for signs of adverse consequences of stress. Many possible indicators should be considered. Individuals or clusters of patients may present with symptoms including mild mental distress, frequent absences from work, substance abuse, or severe mental impairment. Productivity may fall. Rates of injury may increase. Physical symptoms may be out of proportion to the type of injury.

Once alerted to the problem, the clinician may take steps to counsel individuals and offer assistance in stress reduction. The availability of programs designed for this purpose is a great asset; however, the clinician must take primary responsibility for helping the patient gain insight into the problem and often for providing concrete advice on its management (see next section).

The role of health professionals in effecting organizational change is often more difficult. Managers will often seek help for the individual employee with stress-related problems. They usually expect the clinician to deal with the situation on an individual level; they do not often expect or welcome intervention at the source of the problem when that involves changes in the workplace. The challenge for occupational health professionals is to bridge the gap from the traditional medical model to a more comprehensive model of stress control as well as to convince employers to cooperate. Managers may be caught between conflicting objectives of economic gain and employee well-being. Although stress reduction may increase productivity and reduce costs from employee illness, the potential for conflict between these 2 goals remains an obstacle to many organizational innovations proposed by health professionals.

Ideally, the health professional will not wait for signs of stress to be manifested in the employees; primary prevention of stress-related symptoms is a far more desirable objective. The development of preventive programs requires the commitment of management, access to the work site, and a good understanding of the stressors operating in a given situation. While there is no proof that such efforts are cost-effective, certain positive outcomes have been demonstrated. Improved morale, increased sense of well-being, and less use of sick days have resulted from some interventions. There is a need for controlled studies comparing the impact of different approaches to stress prevention and management.

Individual Approaches

Most stress management approaches focus on the

individual and attempt to teach skills for the management or reduction of stress. These programs may be offered to all employees of an organization or to targeted groups or individuals.

A great variety of approaches have been developed. Information may be transmitted through methods ranging from simple self-study brochures to intensive individual counseling. Most programs rely on group training sessions.

The objectives of work site stress programs are usually to educate employees about stress and its effects, to increase awareness of stress in their lives and jobs, and to teach skills for managing or reducing the problem. These programs aim to identify people in the early stages of stress before it has become a significant health problem. By teaching the skills to minimize the ill effects of stress, these programs may limit the long-term sequelae of occupational stress.

Educational efforts may involve the distribution of written materials, lectures, seminars, poster campaigns, and a variety of other methods. Self-assessment questionnaires may help educate employees about stressors and personal levels of stress compared to a norm. The stress assessment questionnaire may also be a way for clinicians to determine where stress is most prevalent within an organization.

It is usually insufficient to increase awareness of occupational stress without teaching specific skills to improve the individual's ability to respond to the stressful situation. These skills may be broadly classified as stress management and stress reduction techniques. Management techniques focus on methods to help the individual deal with physiologic and psychologic reactions to stress. By contrast, stress reduction techniques are skills and interpersonal strategies that aim to reduce stress in the work environment.

Most stress management techniques involve relaxation or meditation exercises (Table 35–7); some emphasize physical activity; and others teach the individual to be aware of emotions related to stressful situations and to discharge them in a safe way. The role of social support from spouses, friends, and coworkers is emphasized in some programs.

Evaluation of stress management efforts in occupational settings is difficult; studies of these programs have tended to show improvements in perceived stress, stress-related symptoms, and a variety of other end points such as muscle tension, use of health services, and interference with job performance. However, the benefits of stress management programs have tended to fade with time, and few long-term (1 year or more) follow-up evaluations have been done. There is little information comparing the effectiveness of the various stress management techniques.

Stress reduction programs usually educate the individual to make a variety of adaptations (Table 35–8). Some of these stress reduction methods involve strategies for coping with stressful situations; time management, priority setting, improved planning abilities, and decision-making skills may all be helpful to the individual whose job allows their implementation. Interpersonal skills such as assertiveness training, conflict resolution, and relationship building may also be useful. Another method of stress reduction involves teaching cognitive skills to help individuals recognize what personal beliefs, perceptions, expectations, and internal dialogues lead to stress.

Research has been done to identify the characteristics of the stress-resistant individual who remains healthy in stressful circumstances that might produce illness in coworkers. One study of executives found several personal qualities associated with low illness rates under stressful life conditions. Control over one's life, commitment to one's goals and work, and an attitude of challenge when confronted by change distinguished these individuals. While these personal traits may be predictors of resistance to stress, it is unclear whether they can be taught to individuals experiencing stress-related problems.

The potential exists that these stress reduction programs could result in work site benefits (such as increased productivity) as well; however, few evaluations of these kinds of stress interventions have been done. The role of the programs in stress reduction itself remains to be demonstrated.

Another type of intervention at the individual level involves counseling or psychotherapy; this type of treatment is usually reserved for individuals with significant stress-related problems who have been identified through employee assistance programs or by health care providers. Personal counseling in these situations may also make use of the other stress management and reduction techniques. Short-term therapy involving a few sessions may be sufficient to ameliorate the individual's condition; however, periodic follow-up is advised. For some workers, group psychotherapy may be more appropriate and acceptable. Others may experience symptoms of depression

Table 35–7. Stress management techniques.

Autogenic training
Biofeedback
Deep breathings
Exercise
Leisure activities
Massage
Meditation
Progressive relaxation exercise
Social support
Yoga

Table 35–8. Stress reduction techniques.

Assertiveness training
Conflict resolution
Decision-making and problem-solving skills
Goal and priority setting
Interpersonal skills training
Time management
Psychotherapy
Psychopharmacologic treatments

or anxiety amenable to a course of antidepressant or antianxiety medication.

Organizational Approaches

Although a great number of employers have introduced stress control programs directed at individuals, there have been few such efforts at the organizational level. In this type of approach, the objective is to reduce the stressors resulting from the organization itself. Interventions may be directed at the organization's structure, communication style, decision-making processes, corporate culture, work roles, characteristics of work tasks, physical environment, and methods of selecting and training employees (Table 35–9).

In most situations, the design of an appropriate type of stress reduction program depends on an accurate assessment of the origin of the problem. An evaluation involving surveys and analysis of illness and other data often helps to localize problems. Frequent employee concerns that may be the basis for stress reduction efforts include improved communications, increased employee participation in decisions regarding work, and improved environmental safety conditions. The level of variety and stimulation in job tasks should also be considered. Efforts need to be directed at physical needs (eg, ergonomics, comfort, rest areas) as well as psychologic needs (eg, interesting work, recognition and advancement, relationships with coworkers). Since there have been few evaluations of organization-based stress reduction efforts, new programs should ideally be set up as experiments. Positive effects can then be assessed before widespread application of the interventions.

Although many types of stress reduction programs have been introduced in recent years, one innovation with an organizational focus has been the Quality Circle. This program involves a regular meeting of a

Table 35–9. Examples of potential organizational interventions in stress reduction.

Reorganizing job tasks to increase employee decision-making and creativity
Improving organizational communication
Developing employee assistance programs and supervisor awareness of stress
Quality circles and peer support groups
Environmental, ergonomic, and safety improvements at work sites

small production unit to discuss problems and solutions related to the work process. In addition to resulting in increased self-esteem, morale, and job satisfaction, these meetings can increase employee participation in the work process; new ideas and productivity gains have sometimes resulted. Alternatives to the traditional assembly line production method have also been proposed to increase employee involvement; a team approach to production has been tried in some industries.

Apart from efforts initiated within an organization, there are increasing signs of societal and governmental attempts to deal with the problem of occupational stress. Both Norway and Sweden have laws requiring that work be organized in such a way as to satisfy the physical and psychologic needs of the workers. Employee organizations are given the statutory right to review and influence decisions on work processes.

Organizational level approaches to stress may be more difficult for the health professional to initiate than personal level programs. There is a need for research to demonstrate their stress reduction potential as well as other gains in health and productivity. While this is a largely uncharted area, the field is developing rapidly, and analysis of specific organizational interventions will be available in the future.

REFERENCES

Stress Concept & Models

Baker DB: The study of stress at work. *Annu Rev Public Health* 1985;**6:**367.

Hall EM, Johnson JV: A case study of stress and mass psychogenic illness in industrial workers. *J Occup Med* 1989;**31:**243.

Harrison RV: Person-environment fit and job stress. In: *Stress at Work.* Cooper CL, Payne R (editors). Wiley, 1978.

Karasek R et al: Job decision latitude, job demands, and cardiovascular disease: A prospective study of Swedish men. *Am J Public Health* 1981;**71:**694.

McLean AA: *Work Stress.* Addison-Wesley, 1979.

Organization & Organizational Relationships

House JS, Wills JA: Occupational stress, social support and health. In: *Reducing Occupational Stress.* McLean AA (editor). NIOSH, 1977.

McLean AA: *Work Stress.* Addison-Wesley, 1979.

Career Development

Arthur RJ, Gunderson EK: Promotion and mental illness in the Navy. *J Occup Med* 1965;**7:**452.

Institute for Social Research: *Termination: The Consequences of Job Loss.* Univ of Michigan Press, 1977.

Role in the Organization

Kahn RL: Conflict, ambiguity, and overload: Three elements in job stress. In: *Occupational Stress.* McLean AA (editor). Thomas, 1974.

Miles RH: Organization boundary roles. In: *Current Concerns in Occupational Stress.* Cooper CL, Payne R (editors). Wiley, 1980.

Task

Frankenhaeuser M, Gardell B: Underload and overload in working life: Outline of a multidisciplinary approach. *J Hum Stress* 1976;**2:**35.

Murphy LR, Harrell JJ: Machine pacing and work stress. In: *New Developments in Occupational Stress.* Schwartz R (editor). Institute of Industrial Relations, 1979.

Weiman CG: A study of occupational stressor and the incidence of disease/risk. *J Occup Med* 1977;**19:**119.

Work Environment

Levi L: *Preventing Work Stress.* Addison-Wesley, 1981.

Shift Work

Johnson LC et al: *Biological Rhythms, Sleep, and Shift Work.* Spectrum, 1979.

Moore-Ede MC et al: *The Clocks That Time Us.* Harvard Univ Press, 1982.

Rutenfranz J et al: Biomedical and psychosocial aspects of shift work: A review. *Scand J Work Environ Health* 1977;**3:**165.

Zeisler C, Moore-Ede M, Coleman R: Rotating shift work schedules that disrupt sleep are improved by applying circadian principles. *Science* 1982;**217:**30.

Individual & Social Factors in Stress

Holmes TH, Rahe RH: Social readjustment rating scales. *J Psychosom Res* 1967:**11:**213.

House JS: *Work Stress and Social Support.* Addison-Wesley, 1980.

Levenson H, Hirschfeld ML, Hirschfeld AH: Industrial accidents and recent life events. *J Occup Med* 1980; **22:**53.

Levinson DJ: *The Seasons of a Man's Life.* Knopf, 1978.

Mental Illness

Colligan MJ, Murphy LR: Mass psychogenic illness in organizations: An overview. *J Occup Psychol* 1979; **52:**77.

Kasl SV: Epidemiological contributions to the study of work stress. In: *Stress at Work.* Cooper CL, Payne R (editors). Wiley, 1978.

Cardiovascular Disease

Buring JE et al: Occupation and risk of death from coronary heart disease. *JAMA* 1987;**258:**791.

Dorian B, Taylor CB: Stress factors in the development of coronary artery disease. *J Occup Med* 1984; **26:**747.

Karasek R et al: Job decision latitude, job demands, and cardiovascular disease: A prospective study of Swedish men. *Am J Public Health* 1981;**71:**694.

Gastrointestinal Disease

Dunn JP, Cobb S: Frequency of peptic ulcer among executives, craftsmen and foremen. *J Occup Med* 1982;**24:**343.

Sonnenberg A, Sonnenberg GS: Occupational factors in disability pensions for gastric and duodenal ulcer. *J Occup Med* 1986;**28:**87.

Susser M: Causes of peptic ulcer: A selective epidemiologic review. *J Chronic Dis* 1967;**20:**435.

Other Diseases

Kagan A, Levi L: Health and environment—psychosocial stimuli: A review. *Soc Sci Med* 1974;**8:**225.

Accidents

Levenson H, Hirschfeld ML, Hirschfeld AH: Industrial accidents and recent life events. *J Occup Med* 1980; **22:**53.

Tasto D: The health consequences of shift work. In: *Occupational Stress.* Schwartz R (editor). Institute of Industrial Relations, 1978.

Sickness, Absence, & Productivity

Seamonds C: Stress factors and their effect on absenteeism in a corporate employee group. *J Occup Med* 1982;**24:**393.

Stress & Workers' Compensation

LaDou J: Cumulative injury in workers' compensation. *State Art Rev Occup Med* 1988;**3:**611.

London DB et al: Workers' compensation and psychiatric disability. *State Art Rev Occup Med* 1988;**3:**595.

Sprehe DJ: Workers' compensation: A psychiatric follow-up study. *Int J Law Psychiatry* 1984;**7:**165.

Prevention & Management of Stress

Benson H: *The Relaxation Response.* Morrow, 1975.

Carrington P et al: The use of meditation: Relaxation techniques for management of stress in a working population. *J Occup Med* 1980;**22:**221.

Jaffe D, Scott C: *From Burnout to Balance.* McGraw-Hill, 1985.

Kobasa SC: Stressful life events, personality, and health: An inquiry into hardiness. *J Pers Soc Psychol* 1979;**37:**1.

McElroy K et al: Assessing the effects of health promotion in worksites: A review of the stress program evaluations. *Health Educ Q* 1984;**11:**379.

Newman J, Beehr T: Personal and organizational strategies for handling job stress: A review of research and opinion. *Personnel Psychol* 1979;**32:**1.

Warshaw LJ: *Stress Management.* Addison-Wesley, 1980.

Organizational Approaches

Crocker O, Chice J: *Quality Circles.* Facts on File, 1984.

Gardell B: *Legislative and Regulatory Programs: The Scandinavian Experience in Reducing Occupational Stress.* NIOSH, 1978.

Levi L: *Preventing Work Stress.* Addison-Wesley, 1981.

Murphy LR, Schoenburn TF: Stress management in work settings. DHHS (NIOSH) Publication No. 87–111, May 1987.

Newman J, Beehr T: Personal and organizational strategies for handling job stress: A review of research and opinion. *Personnel Psychol* 1979;**32:**1.

Substance Abuse & Employee Assistance Programs

36

Charles E. Becker, MD, & Robert C. Larsen, MD

Chemical agents are used recreationally by workers to alter mood, thoughts, feelings, and performance. Some employees ignore well-established dosing and timing of these agents, leading to behavior that is indicative of chemical dependency.

The term "chemical dependency," as now broadly defined, denotes both physical and psychologic reliance on a chemical. Chemical dependency poses a major health problem for industry and has become a proper subject for intervention by the occupational physician. The annual cost of alcohol and drug abuse programs alone is well in excess of $1 billion. Concerns for individual and public safety, productivity, absenteeism, and rising health care costs require employers and employees to face and solve the problem of chemical dependency in the workplace.

The term "substance abuse" is often thought to include only chemical dependency that leads to significant signs and symptoms when chemicals are abruptly stopped or the dose reduced. The term in fact has a broader meaning that includes signs and symptoms of physical dependency, tolerance, and behavioral abnormalities. Thus, in broadest terms, substance abuse is best defined as physical and psychologic reliance on chemicals associated with characteristic symptoms and recognized prognoses.

ALCOHOL ABUSE

The largest and best-studied chemical dependency problem in the workplace involves alcohol consumption. The consumption of alcohol by workers has increased by 30% in the past 20 years. Currently, more than 200,000 workers die annually from alcohol-related deaths.

About 20% of our total national expenditure for health care is for problems related to alcohol. Alcohol dependency as a cause of death has been estimated to reduce life expectancy by an average of 15 years. Two-thirds of all incidents of domestic violence and one-third of cases of child abuse are alcohol-related. About 50% of traffic fatalities, fire deaths, rapes, and suicides are thought to involve alcohol. One out of every 2 Americans will be in an alcohol-related traffic accident during his or her lifetime; and on an average weekend night, one out of every 10 drivers on the road is under the influence of alcohol.

The total cost to industry of alcohol consumption is in the billions of dollars. Accidents, loss of productivity, and absenteeism in the workplace can all be related to the use of alcohol.

The average American worker consumes 2–3 drinks a day, yet about three-fourths of the alcohol consumed by the work force is accounted for by only 10–15% of the workers. The mortality risk from alcohol begins to increase with consumption of 3–5 drinks a day and rises sharply with consumption of 6 or more drinks a day.

In a nontolerant worker, impairment of motor coordination, sensory perception, and cognitive function usually occurs at a blood level between 30 mg/dL and 60 mg/dL.

Little is known about the extent of alcohol-related cognitive decrements in the working population or the threshold for these effects. Computer tomography, brain scanning, and more sophisticated neuropsychologic testing methods are expected to provide new methods to study alcohol- and solvent-related defects at work. Few studies to date adequately control for nutritional factors, other workplace exposures, drug abuse, and use of medications.

Medical Consequences of Alcoholism

Alcohol can injure the esophagus, stomach, small intestine, pancreas, and liver directly. Short- and long-term alcohol consumption results in direct injury to the mucosa of the upper gastrointestinal tract. The liver is the key organ in metabolism of alcohol and is easily damaged by prolonged consumption of alcoholic beverages. Because the mechanism by which alcohol causes fatty liver, alcoholic hepatitis, or cirrhosis is currently not known, it is difficult to estimate the total dose of alcohol required to produce these changes and any enhancement of these changes that may occur as a result of exposure to workplace chemicals. As little as 60 g a day of alcohol (about 6 drinks) will suffice to cause liver dysfunction in male workers and as little as 20 g a day (approximately 2 drinks) in women. Acetaldehyde and superoxide anion have been suggested to be mediators for the advanced features of alcohol-induced liver diseases. Because the liver is essential in the detoxification of many workplace substances, it is also theoretically possible that alcohol alters basic liver function and that other toxic agents are the primary cause of the liver disease.

DRUG ABUSE

Licit drugs are prescription medications, over-the-counter drugs, alcohol, caffeine, and nicotine. These agents may pose risks—especially the use of prescription sedative-hypnotic drugs by individuals required to perform skilled activities. Illicit drugs are nonprescription agents such as narcotics, stimulants, and hallucinogens.

All drugs of abuse may cause acute intoxication and organic brain syndromes. Certain classes of drugs cause panic reactions (eg, stimulants), withdrawal symptoms (eg, depressants), or flashbacks (eg, hallucinogens) (Table 36–1). Central nervous system depressants include the barbiturates and antianxiety agents. The physician must be aware of the patient's occupation and work schedule when prescribing such medications. Even in the service-oriented work force, where machinery is not involved, the use of benzodiazepines by office staff is frequently associated with an increased error rate and inattention to details.

Both licit and illicit narcotics and other analgesics are being used in today's workplace. Given that musculoskeletal injuries represent the most common form of occupational injury, narcotic analgesics (eg, codeine, meperidine, pentazocine) and nonnarcotic analgesics may be used by a worker with back pain or other musculoskeletal complaints. Workers taking opiates or sedatives may have decreased response time and impaired manual dexterity.

Cannabis is the most common illicit drug in the workplace. A recent study of airline pilots indicates the potential for an increased error rate for the 24 hours following marihuana use. Less dramatic examples have become common in virtually all work settings.

In the past, central nervous system stimulants in the workplace were chiefly amphetamines and their derivatives. The behavioral effects of amphetamines have been used as a model for understanding psychotic disorders such as schizophrenia. While acute intoxication can be associated with inappropriate behavior and poor judgment, chronic use can lead to frank paranoid delusions.

The illegal importation of cocaine into the USA has increased dramatically in recent years. Use of this stimulant substance was not thought to be physiologically addictive in the past. Cocaine abuse is now found among all levels of workers from the executive suite down through middle management to the blue collar level. The route of administration is important to elicit in taking a history. The employee who moves from intranasal means of administering the drug to "free basing" markedly increases the risk of severe medical consequences. The "free base" referred to is the cocaine alkaloids separated from the hydrochloride salt, allowing the cocaine to be smoked without chemical decomposition. Crack cocaine is a free-base preparation using baking soda as reagent. This form of cocaine has become extremely common in recent years. It is sold in small quantities, giving the user the impression that it is inexpensive, but in fact by weight of the active drug it is twice as expensive as cocaine in powdered form. The word "crack" is from the cracking sound made when the material is heated. An intense rapid drug effect is achieved by both free-base and crack forms of the drug. Addiction resulting from use of crack and free-base cocaine is a more rapid process than occurs with intranasal use. The smoking of cocaine is frequently associated with violent behavior, paranoid ideation, labile mood, and depression.

Polydrug abuse in the workplace complicates medical assessment and intervention. As the drug epidemic widens in American society, the abuse in industry becomes more common. It is estimated that 20% of workers engage in some form of drug and alcohol abuse. Table 36–2 gives 1988 estimates of drug use among Americans of working age. It is clear that drug use as a whole poses a major occupational health problem.

Table 36–1. Clinically most significant drug problems by class.[1]

	Panic	Flashbacks	Toxicity	Psychosis	OBS[2]	Withdrawal
Depressants	−	−	+ +	+ +	+ +	+ +
Stimulants	+	−	+ +	+ +	+	+
Opiates	−	−	+ +	−	+	+ +
Cannabinols	+	+	+	−	+	−
Hallucinogens	+ +	+ +	+	−	+	−
Solvents	+	−	+ +	−	+ +	−
Phencyclidine (PCP)	+	?[3]	+ +	[3]	[3]	?[3]
Over-the-counter	+	−	+	−	+ +	−

[1]From Schuckett MA: *Drug and Alcohol Abuse: A Clinical Guide to Diagnosis and Treatment,* 3rd ed. Plenum, 1989.
[2]OBS = organic brain syndrome
[3]Most PCP problems appear to be related to a toxic reaction and the subsequent stages of recovery.

Table 36–2. 1988 estimates of drug use among Americans of working age.[1,2]

	Any Drugs	Cannabis	Cocaine
1985 NIDA Household Survey (self-report last 30 days)	19%	11%	2%
Tractor-trailer drivers on the road (urinary drug screening)	29%	15%	2%
Applicants, Georgia Power Co. (urinary drug screening)	15%	5.2%	1.6%
Armed Forces examinees (urinary drug screening)	5%	3%	1.5%
Southern Pacific Railroad employees (urinary drug screening)	5%	2.5%	1%
New Post Office employees (urinary drug screening)	11%	6%	2%

[1]From Wright C: Occupational chemical dependency programs: The business of alcohol and drug dependency. *State Art Rev Occup Med* 1989;4:195.
[2]Within the last 30 days by self-report or by positive urinary drug screen.

In a position statement adopted by the American Psychiatric Association and amending the Association's previously stated position on marihuana and cocaine, the psychiatric concerns involving cannabis are noted to include acute adverse reactions, flashbacks, and both psychotic and nonpsychotic prolonged reactions. Chronic anxiety, depression, and behavioral changes, including an antimotivational syndrome, are described. Psychiatric complications of cocaine use include euphoria, sleep disturbance, hyperexcitability, dysphoria, anxiety, and cognitive difficulties. Panic attacks, paranoia, and persecutory delusions also occur. The onset of dependency is most rapid with the use of crack cocaine. Cocaine withdrawal syndrome is characterized by depression, lethargy, fatigue, anxiety, and suicidal ideation lasting 12–36 hours.

The industrial solvents represent another large category of abuse potential the occupational physician must be aware of. Though the worker exposed to solvents does not intentionally seek a drug high, a good rule to keep in mind is that if a substance can be used to alter the state of consciousness, it will be so used by some workers.

CHEMICAL DEPENDENCY: WORKPLACE CONSIDERATIONS

It is desirable and sometimes mandatory to make certain that a prospective employee does not have a problem of chemical dependency. The employer should inform job applicants about any screening that will be done and how the company intends to deal with altered performance or impaired function on the job. This raises concerns about monitoring chemical dependency. Workers whose performance affects public safety—eg, bus drivers, police officers, airline pilots, and physicians—may soon have mandatory requirements for screening.

The job itself may enhance the likelihood of chemical dependency. This is especially true in some health professionals and in workers assigned to lonely duty stations that provide and sanction consumption of alcoholic beverages. Corporate policies that may include inexpensive alcoholic beverages or encourage drinking at business meetings will enhance the likelihood of chemical dependency. The individual's support system or cultural bias may encourage or proscribe use of alcohol or other substances.

Chemical dependency in the workplace may lead to impaired function that may be reflected in absenteeism or poor job performance. It may also increase the risk of accident and pose a danger to fellow workers and in some circumstances to public safety.

A long period free of drug or alcohol abuse is one critical factor in determining the prognosis for recovery from chemical dependency. Chemical dependency treatment often involves creation of a monitoring contract, in which job performance and specialized toxicologic laboratory testing are provided by the employer. Workers who consume alcohol and are exposed to certain chemical agents may experience adverse health effects, such as nausea, dizziness, headache, and even liver damage. Amides, oximes, thiurams, and carbamates have all been shown to be effective inhibitors of the enzymes involved in alcohol metabolism. These agents cause symptoms similar to those of "acetaldehyde syndrome" or disulfiramlike syndromes when alcohol has been consumed at work. Alcohol enhancement of the toxicity of halogenated hydrocarbons, such as carbon tetrachloride, has also been observed in industry. Interactions of industrial chemicals with alcohol to enhance toxicity have been described with methylene chloride, cobalt, manganese, and mercury.

DRUG SCREENING

Chemical dependency poses risks to employers and employees. Five methods have been traditionally used to predict chemical dependency in employee applicants, none of which have proved completely reliable: (1) observation by trained personnel; (2) checking medical records and references; (3) direct voluntary history of the patient; (4) medical examination for needle marks or physical signs and symptoms of chemical dependency; and (5) urine or blood screening for chemical agents.

Each of these 5 methods has weaknesses. Applicants for employment should be told in advance that past records will be reviewed and results made available. Tests of suspected drug use vary according to drug class.

Preemployment urine screening has been advocated, but there is no proof that the results have been more valuable than observation, checking references, obtaining medical histories, or physical examination. In addition, there are technical problems concerning urine or blood testing—eg, the urinary test for marihuana may remain positive for many weeks after a single exposure.

Chromatographic or immunoassay testing is usually done on thin-layer plates or by immunoassay and then confirmed by quantitative tests. Confirmatory tests are necessary to reduce the number of false-positive results.

Unfortunately, screening tests disclose only the presence or absence of a chemical agent and not the pattern of use, and they may not be specific for the chemical agents involved (eg, abuse of anesthetic gases by hospital personnel). If screening is performed, someone must observe the collection of the urine sample to ensure its authenticity, and the worker must sign an informed consent statement.

It is important that a questionnaire be taken at the same time a urine or blood sample is obtained to ensure that abnormal test results are not due to prescription drugs. The chain of custody in sample handling requires initials of all the parties. Specificity and sensitivity of screening methods must be known. Methods of storage must be checked. Confidentiality must also be guaranteed. Of primary importance, the risk of a false-positive result must be considered.

Bus drivers and airline pilots are often required to report specialized prescription drug therapy and any prior treatment for chemical dependency. It is appropriate in such a setting to ask for volunteered information from driving records that may indicate chemical dependency-related driving behavior.

Where chemical dependency of an employee has been documented, a monitoring contract must be established and periodic screening tests performed. A policy of drug screening of workers involved in motor vehicle accidents is common in the transportation industry. Workers with histories of drug use should be monitored on a random time schedule. Under these circumstances, a drug-free environment can be established.

Screening techniques for chemical dependency may involve psychologic screening for behavior and personality, using psychometric testing. Some resulting diagnostic categories are seen with increased frequency in predicting chemical dependency. These include increased anxiety, depression, and antisocial behavior. No single chemical dependency risk is predicted by these tests. Neuropsychologic tests may also be useful as a baseline should individuals later be exposed to neurotoxicologic substances.

When public safety is a factor, such as with drivers, pilots, and physicians, chemical dependency is a risk to the public, sometimes leading to accidents and safety investigation. Assessment of accidents and injuries on the job should include a written policy of excluding substance abuse as a work-related contributory factor. Records of drug and alcohol testing should be thoroughly documented and maintained in strict conformity with written guidelines.

EMPLOYEE ASSISTANCE PROGRAMS & THE CHEMICALLY DEPENDENT WORKER

The employee assistance program (EAP) is a service sponsored by the employer or union designed to assist employees—and in some cases their families—in finding help for mental or emotional, family, drug, health, or other personal problems. EAPs are considered employee benefits with value to the employer through improvements in productivity and reduced employee turnover. The programs vary greatly, some dealing solely with the drug abuse problems, others primarily with family counseling. Because of extreme urgency to control drug and alcohol abuse in industry, the following discussion of EAPs will emphasize that element of their activities.

Chemical dependency may present in the workplace as intoxication. A corporate policy should be prepared and given to all employees concerning the method of assessment of intoxication on the job. This should include medical evaluation, recording of mental status and performance, and documentation by urine or blood testing. The most important element of the corporate policy statement is that pertaining to treatment and job consequences. It is essential to emphasize that testing is done for the purpose of introducing the worker to a treatment program and not in order to develop a record that will support termination. Although the job can and should be used to provide a strong incentive for behavioral change on the part of the worker, it is the primary goal of a detection program to keep the worker performing successfully on the job.

When chemicals are taken regularly and the dose is then decreased or stopped abruptly, a sequence of events occurs that is determined by the dose of chemical abused, the duration of abuse, and the specific chemical agent taken. Thus, with withdrawal from alcohol, patients may present on a job with only a tremor of the hands or with a progression of symptoms all the way through agitation, sweating, hypertension, and seizures.

Chemical dependency in the workplace may also present as accelerated medical complications such as liver disease. It is much more likely, however, that the presentation of chemical dependency in the workplace will be more subtle, involving frequent absenteeism—especially on Monday—and impaired job performance.

IMPORTANCE OF EARLY IDENTIFICATION

The key to intervening and treating the substance abuser is early identification and institution of care.

As an outgrowth of occupational alcoholism programs, the majority of Fortune 500 companies now have some form of employee assistance program (EAP).

EAP programs can either be internally based within a corporate setting or be located externally, ie, provided on a contractual basis by arrangement with an outside service. Companies with fewer than 3000 employees almost invariably elect the latter option. The occupational health physician involved in planning such services should be sure the program accommodates a range of concerns, including personal problems of the worker that might affect productivity, consultation with management and union representatives regarding EAP policies, confrontations between managers and employees regarding declining job performance, and referral of employees to cost-effective treatment services in the community. The program should provide for informational interaction with various departments of the company and should have as one of its main goals worker education about chemical dependency and emotional dysfunction as treatable medical problems.

One of the crucial tasks of these programs is helping the chemically dependent worker, whether self-referred or management-referred, to enter into a program of behavior modification. Because of the tendency for the troubled employee to deny the extent of drug or alcohol abuse, intervention techniques have been developed to direct the worker into a program. Denial may go beyond the affected individual to involve coworkers, supervisors, and family. An effective intervention makes clear to the chemically dependent worker that his health as well as his occupational and economic welfare are at stake. The clinician conducting the intervention may use family members and coworkers familiar with the troubled employee's deteriorating physical and emotional status to help the worker recognize the damaging pattern of behavior and the need for treatment. The goal of intervention is to have the affected individual commit to treatment immediately.

Chemical Dependency: Instituting Treatment

After an appropriate clinical evaluation is made by either a member of the company's EAP or a consulting clinician, the next step is directing the substance-abusing individual into treatment. In some case evaluations, what is perceived as a behavioral problem associated with possible drug use may be the clinical manifestation of a primary emotional disorder such as depression. If chemical dependency is diagnosed, the employee might be referred to a 28-day inpatient drug treatment program; and if a primary emotional disorder is diagnosed, referral may be made for outpatient psychotherapy. Treatment for emotional disorder will not be effective unless chemical dependency is also treated.

Twenty-eight-day inpatient treatment programs have become the standard for treatment of chemical dependency. However, the cost of such programs is high, and for some employees with less than optimal health insurance coverage, a shorter period of inpatient care followed by halfway house or residential treatment setting can be utilized.

Types of Treatment

Many models exist for the treatment of chemical dependency. The need for self-participation is stressed by Alcoholics Anonymous (AA) and Narcotics Anonymous (NA), though outcome studies have not been done. For the recovering alcoholic or drug abuser, this group self-help approach is often crucial in maintaining a state of sobriety. Most treatment programs utilize some form of group psychotherapy in addition to the 12-step approach of AA. Other psychotherapeutic modalities may include individual and family therapy.

The chemically dependent worker usually requires a defined structure, guidelines, and rules. The inpatient treatment model is often the best means for initially creating such a framework. A medical history and physical examination with appropriate laboratory testing are necessary upon entry into treatment. The greatest chance of success with a chemically dependent worker emphasizes total abstinence. Some individuals will require pharmacologic support with disulfiram or naltrexone to decrease their chance of recidivism. However, even with such measures, "slips" do occur. The chemically dependent adult must understand that "cure" consists of being "in the process of recovery" on an indefinite basis.

Medical evaluation may indicate the need for an antidepressant medication or lithium for treating an associated affective disturbance. The prognosis for any one individual is improved by early entry into treatment and by support from the family, the employer, and fellow workers. Crucial to effective treatment is follow-up care after inpatient treatment. While for some individuals AA or NA alone may be sufficient, for others a more structured monitoring program including urine screening may be necessary.

The occupational medicine physician should be a contributor to the design of EAP programs in the industrial and business communities served. The options involve whether to situate the EAP within the company or outside the company as a contracted service.

All EAPs should provide evaluation, treatment referral, follow-up, and employee education. Other services include short-term treatment, management training, drug monitoring, and consultation to departments in the company. A properly run program maintains confidentiality in self-referral cases and spells out the loss of confidentiality when management must intercede in treatment or in job safety. Other planning functions of the medical consultant include a review of health insurance benefits for treatment of substance abuse and psychiatric illness.

THE ROLE OF PSYCHIATRY IN MANAGEMENT OF CHEMICAL DEPENDENCY

Psychiatrists and other mental health professionals are often called upon to play a consultative or treatment role in managing problems of disturbances of mood, thoughts, perceptions, and behavior in the workplace. Various clinical approaches to the patient with such a problem are advocated by psychiatrists. The psychiatrist is trained to assess the psychologic underpinnings for an individual's maladaptive use of substances as well as the biologic, social, cultural, and family factors important to the diagnosis and treatment of addictive diseases.

Before implementing any treatment plan— psychotherapy, drug therapy, biologic monitoring, etc—accurate diagnosis is necessary. As in any other area of medicine, one must take a careful history and attend to current complaints and the presenting problem. Special attention to patterns of use and abuse of habituating substances at work is important. Because of the tendency for the chemically dependent worker to avoid, deny, repress, and misrepresent the true extent of his or her problem, it is essential in the evaluative process to obtain collateral data from many sources. Information from supervisors, coworkers, and family members can be invaluable.

In assessing the worker with potential alcohol or drug abuse behavior, a phenomenologic approach can be useful in categorizing the pattern of substance use. The *Diagnostic and Statistical Manual of Mental Disorders* breaks down the use of alcohol and other drugs into 2 groupings. **Abuse** is exemplified by a pattern of maladaptive use involving impairment in social, occupational, psychologic, or physical functioning. Hazardous behavior may be associated with recurrent use. The history will contain references to binges, drinking at particular times of day, amnesic episodes, inability to cut back "social drinking," and the use of drugs to perform certain tasks. Job loss, increased use of sick leave, involvement in motor vehicle accidents, arrests for impaired driving, marital disruption, and physical confrontations in social settings will also be noted.

Alcohol and other types of drug **dependency** not only meet the criteria for abuse but add the elements of tolerance, an increase in time devoted to obtaining and using the substance, and withdrawal. Withdrawal symptoms that may range from "a bad hangover" to frank delirium tremens are found with the reduction or cessation of drug use.

In recent years, the use of cocaine has increased dramatically in the workplace. Cocaine intoxication can mimic manic type clinical presentations. Dependence on this central nervous system stimulant is accompanied by drug craving and severe health and economic consequences to the individual. Depression is a frequent component of drug withdrawal, and mood instability and suicidal ideation are especially common after stopping free base or crack cocaine.

The occupational physician must be aware of the trends in drug abuse in the society in general and within particular industries. The psychiatric professional is best equipped to identify aspects of the chemically dependent worker's personality structure that underlie the overt drug abuse patterns. Dependent, passive-aggressive, and avoidant personality traits are commonly seen in this population.

The frequency of abuse is important information. Regular daily use of an increasing amount of substance is far different from infrequent episodic binging. The use of licit or illicit drugs (including alcohol) in particular settings, such as when a supervisor is or is not present or when an employee is or is not on vacation, should be noted.

When the clinician feels that enough information has been gathered for diagnostic purposes, treatment planning can follow. The acuity of the problem will have a major influence on whether inpatient or outpatient care is involved. The chemically dependent individual will often choose outpatient treatment, claiming that disruption of life by hospitalization is too great to be faced. However, the outpatient option is not possible when monitoring of withdrawal symptoms requires a supervised setting. In addition, the structure of such a setting ensures that the individual will not act out behaviorally and resume use of the involved substances. Many clinicians have been made humble by treatment failures in working with addictive individuals where the doctor-patient relationship alone is not enough to prevent recidivism. This is an area in medicine where the physician requires the ancillary services of other health professionals and paraprofessionals in order to optimize the treatment response.

The various elements of drug treatment by phase of treatment and according to the patients' responsibilities have recently been outlined by Washton (Table 36–3). Not every employer is willing to stand by and support an employee during a period of drug withdrawal and treatment. While the threat of termination can be a very powerful motivating force for the entry and continued commitment to treatment, actual termination can have a devastating effect on the individual in the early stages of a treatment program. Fear of such retribution can add to the delay in the troubled employee's seeking appropriate treatment measures. Corporate policies for the chemically dependent worker must address this issue.

PSYCHIATRIC CONDITIONS ASSOCIATED WITH CHEMICAL DEPENDENCY

While all forms of chemical dependency may be considered a primary psychiatric condition with disturbances of emotions, behavior, and thinking, there are other specific types of psychiatric illness that must be considered in association with chemical dependency. While many individuals who present with alcoholism and drug abuse may not have a separate treatable psychiatric disorder, the proportion of substance abusers with other psychiatric illnesses is felt to be greater than in the general population. Studies of the prevalence of psychiatric illness in the general population indicate that anxiety disorders are the most frequent in our society. Generalized anxiety and paniclike symptoms may lead the frightened and worried employee to turn to increased use of alcohol and central nervous system depressants. This is commonly seen in situational or adjustment problems with the threat of job loss, demotion, or even impending promotion. The use of alcohol or antianxiety agents, while initially serving to quell the apprehension of the anxious employee, may with time become the primary problem.

The association of depression and alcohol has been debated for some time. Individuals with family histories of affective disturbance have a higher prevalence of alcohol abuse among their family members. Addictionologists argue that substance abuse is a primary disorder and depression a secondary factor. Psychiatrists have described the maladaptive use of alcohol and other drugs in a self-medicating fashion by the individual with a primary affective disorder.

Workers who have developed chronic pain not uncommonly present with disturbance of mood, sleep difficulty, and disruption of normal activities. Rather than labeling such individuals as malingerers, it behooves the occupational physician to take a careful history about the behavior associated with pain. Changes in the use of analgesic medication can come from placing the employee on a time-contingent versus a pain-contingent schedule. Other treatment approaches to chronic pain such as biofeedback, autohypnosis, and increasing exercise can assist in reducing the use of potentially addictive medications.

Marked disturbances in behavior and cognition do show up in the workplace. These are less frequent than the depressive or anxiety presentations. Certainly the differential diagnosis must include the acute or chronic use of substances when a presentation of delirium is found in the workplace. An individual with an altered state of consciousness who is disoriented and agitated may not be the appropriate historian at that moment. Once the medical emergency has been appropriately handled, the health professional's duty is to uncover the cause of the acute organic brain syndrome. Again, coworkers and family members must be relied upon in addition to any biologic testing to determine the form of substance abuse. While hallucinogenic substances and phencyclidine can result in psychotic presentations, such states are more frequently the result of central nervous system stimulants in the working population.

Finally, severe character disorders are frequently

Table 36–3. Stages of treatment of cocaine addiction.[1]

STAGE 1
Stabilization and Crisis Intervention (First 2 Weeks)
Immediately stop all drug and alcohol use.
Break off contact with dealers and users.
Recover from acute aftereffects and drug "withdrawal."
Stabilize daily functioning.
Stabilize or resolve immediate crisis situations.
Establish a positive connection to the treatment program.
Formulate a treatment plan.

STAGE 2
Early Abstinence (Months 1 and 2)
Learn about addictive disease.
Admit that the addiction exists.
Establish a support system.
Begin involvement in self-help.
Achieve stable abstinence for at least 2 weeks.

STAGE 3
Relapse Prevention (Months 3 Through 6)
Progress from verbally admitting to emotionally accepting that the disease exists.
Learn about the relapse process, relapse warning signs, relapse risk factors, and how to counteract them.
Make positive, lasting changes in life-style.
Learn how to deal effectively with problems, adjustments, and setbacks.
Learn how to identify and handle negative feelings.
Learn how to have fun without drugs.
Deepen involvement in self-help.
Maintain stable abstinence for at least 6 months.

STAGE 4
Advanced Recovery (Open-Ended)
Achieve more lasting changes in attitude, lifestyle, and behavior.
Change addictive thinking styles and personality traits.
Address issues of arrested maturity.
Solidify adaptive coping and problem-solving skills.
Work through emotional, relationship, and self-esteem problems.
Continue and deepen involvement in self-help.

[1]From Washton AMK: *Cocaine Addiction: Treatment, Recovery, and Relapse Prevention.* Norton, 1989.

associated with the maladaptive use of substances. The individual who has few healthy adult defenses for coping with anxiety and uncertainty will turn to an external means for coping with such effects.

In a study of 511 patients seeking treatment for substance abuse, overall lifetime prevalence rates for mental disorders were found to be 78%; a 65%

prevalence rate for mental disorders was found at the time of the study. The most common lifetime disorders included antisocial personality, phobias, psychosexual dysfunction, and depression. Sedative-hypnotic, amphetamine, and alcohol abusers have the highest prevalence rates for psychiatric illness aside from their substance abuse problems.

REFERENCES

Gawin FH, Ellinwood EH: Cocaine and other stimulants: Actions, abuse, and treatment. *N Engl J Med* 1988; **318**:1173.

Kaufman E et al: Committee on Drug Abuse: Position statement on psychoactive substance use and dependence: Update on marijuana and cocaine. (American Psychiatric Association Official Actions.) *Am J Psychiatry* 1987;**144**:698.

Lawton B: The EAP and workplace psychiatric injury. *State Art Rev Occup Med* 1988;**3**:695.

Ross HE, Glaser FB, Germanson T: The prevalence of psychiatric disorders in patients with alcohol and other drug problems. *Arch Gen Psychiatry* 1988;**45**:1023.

Saxon AJ et al: Clinical Evaluation and Use of Urine Screening for Drug Abuse. *West J Med* 1988;**149**:296.

Schuckit MA: Drug and alcohol abuse: A clinical Guide to Diagnosis and Treatment, 3rd ed. Plenum, 1989.

Spicer J: *The EAP Solution: Current Trends and Future Issues*. Hazeldon Foundation, 1987.

Washton AM: *Cocaine Addiction: Treatment, Recovery, and Relapse Prevention*. Norton, 1989.

Wright C (editor): Alcoholism and chemical dependency in the workplace. *State Art Rev Occup Med* 1989;**4**:195.

Occupational Safety

37

Franklyn G. Prieskop, MS, CSP

The occupational health physician—whether employed directly by a company, retained on a consulting basis, or working in an occupational medicine clinic serving the industrial community—will be called upon to work with safety professionals. In very large organizations, the physician and the safety professional may be part of a loss control team or may even work in the same department. In smaller organizations, the internal safety professional will often be the point of contact for the outside occupational physician.

The physician's interactions with the safety professional will occur in the following spheres, among others:

1. Cooperating in the establishment of emergency medical facilities or services.
2. Performing individual medical monitoring of employees potentially exposed to occupational health hazards.
3. Designing and implementing medical screening programs for potential employees.
4. Participating in employee training programs on health hazards, chemical safety, and the use of personal protective equipment.
5. Evaluating the effectiveness of personal protective equipment.
6. Serving on management oversight committees reviewing the safety program's effectiveness.
7. Assisting in accident investigations or reviews.
8. Providing medical expertise in the areas of ergonomics or appropriate design of work stations.
9. Providing consultant services to management to interpret safety analyses.

Whatever the level of contact between the occupational health physician and the safety professional, it will be useful for the physician to understand that individual's background, role, and concerns.

THE SAFETY PROFESSION

In the first half of the 1900s, safety professionals were called either "safety engineers" or "safety inspectors" to reflect their primary functions. The job was restricted to discovering and correcting unsafe machinery or conditions. In those days, the hazards were fairly obvious and the controls were unsophisticated but effective (eg, barrier guards, personal protective equipment, warning signs). The basically untrained "safety inspector" went around the plant looking for hazards, warning of dangers, and investigating accidents. The "safety engineer," who had a mechanical or electrical engineering degree, designed guards for machinery or supervised the installation of guardrails, exits, or material handling equipment.

By the 1960s, the most obvious and easily corrected gross hazard conditions had been recognized and, for the most part, controlled or eliminated from the workplace. Federal and state governments then began to regulate the workplace to ensure a safe place to work for all employees.

Society's increasing concern for the health and safety of workers reflected itself also in product liability lawsuits against manufacturers of unsafe equipment. Government regulatory agencies focused attention of employers on unsafe conditions and work practices they had previously allowed to exist. The result was that the "safety inspector" and "safety engineer" were no longer sufficient to meet the demands of industry.

The real task today for the safety professional consists of enlisting management support, motivating supervisors, and educating workers. To accomplish these enabling objectives, the safety professional must be able to discuss highly technical issues in nontechnical terms for management and relate loss control to financial or production goals. The professional must also be able to understand and use trade vocabularies and draw upon relevant experience when communicating with craftsmen or specialists.

Precise conformity with government safety standards is not always a solution to industrial safety problems. The safety professional must sometimes negotiate for implementation of safer work practices that are acceptable both to management and to the workers yet comply in substantial terms with government regulations. Obviously, if there is no safe alternative to full compliance with regulations, the safety professional must be able to withstand the pressure to compromise worker safety.

Professional Qualifications

The modern safety professional usually has a bachelor's degree but is no longer necessarily an engineer (fewer than 40% have engineering degrees). More valuable today than engineering expertise are degrees in management, business administration, or systems analysis. Several universities offer baccalaureate, masters, and even doctoral degrees specifically in occupational safety and health or safety management, with a few state and community colleges now offering associate degrees or technical certification in the field.

Almost half of all safety professionals are employed in the industrial manufacturing environment. Another 35-40% are employed either by insurance companies or government compliance authorities and in those capacities either oversee or assist the industrial safety professionals. The remaining professionals work in research or education.

Registered Professional Engineer (Safety) certificates are granted by some states. Professional associations in the various disciplines are now providing recognition through nationwide testing for certification of their practitioners. Certification is now available for safety professionals, industrial hygienists, fire protection engineers, and others.

POSITION WITHIN THE ORGANIZATION

Most commonly, the safety professional works in the personnel department. Because the goal is to protect the worker, the position is considered a human resources feature conferring benefit on the employee. Personnel is always a staff function, so one has the advantage of being outside the direct line of authority, which makes it easier to communicate with the whole organization. The drawbacks are that the personnel department is often looked upon by management as an overhead function, representing a loss area on the balance sheet. However, a well-run safety program should be considered a loss control or cost containment function that operates to the *advantage* of the organization's balance sheet.

The second traditional organizational placement of the safety professional is within the security department, which again means that the safety professional has the independence of a staff function; and it often gives one access to the security guards, a fairly large pool of underutilized personnel who can be profitably employed to conduct routine inspections and monitoring. The drawback is that the security department usually is located far down within the organizational hierarchy, resulting in limited access to upper management and with numerous layers of authority between.

Occasionally, the safety professional is placed in the quality assurance or quality control department. This positioning usually occurs only if products liability or systems safety responsibilities are incorporated into the normal duties associated with employee safety.

Including the safety professional within a manufacturing or operations function is usually disastrous to the safety effort, since the department manager will have a conflict of interest. The manager's major goal is to produce the maximum product or service with the minimum interruption or cost, and the safety program could be viewed as detrimental to this effort. Furthermore, being in a line department (as opposed to serving a staff function) severely restricts communications with other manufacturing functions. The safety professional's communications often must follow chain-of-command procedures rather than being allowed the direct access of most staff functions.

Occasionally, the safety professional is located in the finance department and subordinated to the risk manager. This is an excellent position because it has the advantages of being a staff department and yet is viewed favorably by the top management. The safety professional also benefits from the accessibility of the financial data and can utilize this information in choosing where to direct the loss control efforts and convince middle management of the need to initiate safety efforts. Obviously, this location also assists the safety efforts with accountability programs that utilize budgetary pressures on department managers to achieve progress toward greater worker safety. The single greatest problem with this location is that middle and lower management personnel tend to look at the safety professional in an adversarial relationship, considering it to be an audit function.

The best position of all is almost never achieved—that of an independent staff function reporting directly to top management. The obvious power of this relationship is not lost on other managers, who recognize the ease of access to top management. The communication lines from this position are optimized, and of course management would be listening directly to safety concerns. The safety professional in this position must be aggressive, professional, and efficient because failures as well as successes will be clearly obvious to top management.

SAFETY PROGRAM ORGANIZATION & DOCUMENTATION

Large companies are too vast and complex to operate their day-to-day business activities by direct personal supervision by the proprietors. Therefore, these organizations produce documents that communicate the basic intentions of top management and delegate authority for carrying out those functions. These documents are meant to be expressions of basic philosophy and guidelines to provide the large organization with a unified approach to fundamental areas of concern.

The documents of primary importance to the safety professional are the Corporate Safety Policy and Corporate Directive on Safety. From these documents, the safety program receives its direction and authority to exist. It is upon these documents that the safety professional must rely to obtain the necessary cooperation from the other individuals within the organization.

The occupational health physician, when working as part of the safety program in conjunction with the safety professional, will also rely upon these documents to obtain the necessary cooperation from other departments within the organization. When the physician is functioning beyond the scope of the safety program, the physician may very well feel the need to draw up similar documentation to cover such areas as "Employee Health Programs" or "Medical Services."

Corporate Safety Policy

The corporate safety policy should be set forth in a clear declaration of management's intention to eliminate or control hazardous exposures. To achieve its purpose, the policy should be in writing and communicated to all employees, particularly to all supervisory personnel.

Corporate Directive on Safety

The corporate safety policy is the organization's expression of general philosophy and management support. The corporate directive on safety will achieve the following goals:

1. Establish the authority of the responsible department.
2. Serve as a reference, by outlining the major program elements.
3. Define the responsibilities of the major departments and individuals expected to be involved with the program.
4. State the program audit functions, by which the safety department intends to ensure that the various program elements are being initiated and pursued.
5. Review the basic reporting responsibilities by which the safety department will keep management informed.

Safety Practices

While many large organizations do not carry their formal documentation programs beyond the policy and directive stages, most will require the safety professional to write program element descriptions. These descriptions in more formal organizations are often known as "company practice" documents.

The purpose of a safety practice document is to provide a detailed description of the workings of a specific program element (eg, forklift training, eye protection programs, safety committees). In the case of a training program, it would define who is to be trained, what the training is to consist of, how and where it is to be administered, who will conduct the training, and what documentation of the training will be made. It might also review such items as who will develop the training program, how often it will be given, and what is to be done with new employees until such training is given.

Contracts & Purchase Orders

Some safety programs will require the safety professional to write or modify existing purchase orders or contracts for certain products. For example, when safety glasses are provided to employees for eye protection, the safety professional may find it necessary to be quite specific in the standards to be adhered to in obtaining these items.

Record-Keeping

The safety professional is responsible for keeping safety records. Among the most common of these are the following:

1. National, state, or locally required accident records.
2. Accident or incident investigation reports.
3. Monitoring and sampling results for chemicals or physical hazards.
4. Minutes of meetings of safety and other related committees.
5. Employee training records.
6. Physical inspection logs.
7. Audit evaluations performed to ensure compliance with programs.

ELEMENTS OF THE SAFETY PROGRAM

Training

The safety professional is primarily concerned with the prevention of accidents. This can be accomplished to a large extent through proper training of employees. The primary cause of accidents in the workplace is not unsafe machinery or dangerous chemicals—it is the lack of understanding by employees about the nature or severity of the hazards surrounding them.

A prudent employer will provide employees with adequate training to warn them of hazards peculiar to their jobs and instruct them in safe operating practices.

The Occupational Safety and Health Act (OSHA) requires that workers be warned about hazardous materials through the use of warning labels and similar devices. OSHA also requires that workers be made aware of the relevant symptoms of overexposure and of emergency treatment procedures. But the most important feature of the law is that which requires employers to make workers understand appropriate precautions.

Since the passage of OSHA, many other federal and state hazard communications have been promulgated. These require the employer to train workers to understand the labeling of hazardous materials and to use the Material Safety Data Sheets (MSDS) that must be maintained for all chemicals and other hazardous substances to which the worker may be exposed.

Various OSHA standards also require specialized training for employees operating specific types of equipment (forklifts, cranes, powered punch presses, etc). These laws require that numerous training programs be established for workers in various job categories or working conditions.

Communication

Safety committees draw together individuals from throughout the work force so they can pool their experience and efforts to achieve greater safety. Several types of safety committees may be formed to fulfill various needs within the organization. The company physician may be asked to serve on an executive committee functioning as an oversight committee for the safety department or on a general planning committee. Other safety committees might include supervisory committees, joint union-management committees, and shop workers committees.

Safety suggestion boxes are a form of communication. To make them effective however, management—often through its delegated representative, the safety professional—must demonstrate that it listens to all serious suggestions and responds in a timely and serious manner.

Safety posters, placards, and signs are also forms of communication. They are effective only insofar as they are kept relevant to the hazards and, in the case of posters, if they are frequently changed to stimulate safety awareness.

Emergency Response Programs

The safety professional must recognize the need to prepare for a disaster or emergency situation.

A. Evacuation Planning: Federal, state, and local authorities now require that businesses establish emergency evacuation plans. Items to consider in an evacuation plan include the following:

1. Who can authorize evacuation?
2. How will the employees be instructed to evacuate?
3. What other notifications are necessary—medical, fire department, police, etc?
4. Who will be responsible to see that evacuation is carried out?
5. Where should evacuated employees go?
6. How will it be determined that all employees are out?
7. Have all contractor personnel, and visitors, been evacuated?
8. What medical facilities are likely to be needed?
9. Will electrical and gas services be shut down also?
10. Are there manufacturing processes that should be shut down in emergencies?
11. Who will do the shutdowns? How? Are they trained?

B. Chemical Response Teams: Plants that use large quantities of toxic or dangerous chemicals will often form specialized teams of employees to contain or control exposures to the employees, the general public, or the environment resulting from accidental discharge. The occupational physician will often be asked to help in the planning and training stages when these teams are formed.

C. Fire Brigades: Industries or operations located at remote sites or with special fire hazards often require the formation of fire-fighting teams. These trained employees are responsible for ensuring swift reaction to the outbreak of fire and for containing the fire until professional help arrives.

D. Emergency Medical Facilities: State regulations now require almost all places of employment to provide a minimum level of emergency medical capability. Depending upon the exposures involved, the safety professional, in concert with the occupational physician, might wish to significantly improve on this minimum requirement.

For an office building with no special hazards, the Red Cross Multi-Media training certifications for 2 or 3 employees, perhaps with CPR training added, might very well be sufficient. However, a hazardous chemical processing plant would require at least several EMT-1 level trained personnel and perhaps even an occupational health nurse or an on-site occupational physician.

Personal Protective Equipment

One method of providing for employee safety in hazardous conditions is the use of personal protective equipment. These devices are intended to protect employees in case an accident occurs or to insulate the employee from a hazardous condition (noise, dusts, fumes, etc) that is part of the normal operation.

The basic problem with personal protective devices is that the individual must understand the need to wear the protection, must wear it properly, and must maintain the device in good working condition. In situations where engineering or administrative controls are not yet effective in eliminating the hazard, protective devices must be issued as a last line of defense to prevent injury to the employee.

The occupational health physician may be called upon by the safety professional to consult about the appropriateness of the device chosen or to assist in educating employees about the necessity for the device.

Any program that provides personal protective equipment to employees must follow the same basic procedures. First, the hazards must be evaluated to ensure that the equipment will be appropriate. Second, the equipment itself must be checked to see that it meets all applicable government standards of manufacture. Employees must be informed of the hazards involved and be trained in how to wear protective equipment and maintain it properly. Supervisors must be trained to ensure that the protection is worn at all times when it is needed. Warnings must be posted to inform everyone of the need for protection.

Inspections & Monitoring

The safety professional, especially in the industrial environment, is responsible for numerous inspections and periodic monitoring. The principal monitoring techniques are measurement of airborne chemical contamination levels and physical exposure levels to noise, vibration, and ionizing and nonionizing radiation. While monitoring is usually performed by an industrial hygienist, the safety professional is often required to perform some routine monitoring. Individual medical monitoring is also required under certain conditions. Again, while monitoring and testing are usually done under the direction of the occupational health physician, the safety professional is often charged with the administrative and record-keeping details of the program.

Physical inspections are the direct responsibility of the safety professional. Federal and state regulations now require periodic inspections of the work environment designed to recognize hazard potentials. Often this type of inspection is actually performed as part of the safety committee's duties, so that various points of view are brought to bear in the attempt to identify accident potentials. However, even when this is the case, the safety professional must review the results and recommendations.

Various pieces of equipment also require periodic inspection to ensure that they are in place, fully functional, certified, and suitable for their intended purposes.

Chemical Safety

Specific hazards to employees must be recognized and detailed for each chemical or process. Where feasible, engineering controls such as containment, automated processing, or ventilation systems should be installed. Administrative controls such as job rotation or multistationed work processes should be used to control exposures. Where applicable, personal protective equipment must be issued. Periodic monitoring of environmental chemical exposures should be established. Chemical safety training specific to the processes involved must be given to all employees. With certain chemicals, employee health monitoring may be required to discover exposure levels or hazard conditions. Safe chemical handling rules and process instructions must be initiated. Emergency containment or evacuation systems must be initiated. Emergency shutdown and protection equipment must be installed and employees trained in their use. Finally, all of the above procedures and equipment must be periodically reviewed to ensure proper functioning of control measures and to see that controls are adequate. Material safety data sheets must be obtained and reviewed on all chemicals used in the work setting.

Accident Investigations

Accident investigation is the responsibility of the safety professional. However, depending upon the frequency of occurrence of accidents and the distances involved, the safety professional is not always able to personally investigate all accidents. Furthermore, in most routine accidents, it is helpful if the supervisor or manager conducts the accident investigation in order to learn from the experience, though the safety professional will have to instruct the supervisors or managers in how to proceed and should review the results.

Accidents almost never have just one cause but are the result of chains of events and circumstances. Finding the causes of an accident calls for more than simply reviewing the injured employee's actions at the scene; the physical conditions and all equipment must be scrutinized to determine what could be done to prevent recurrences. Such items as work flow patterns, environmental conditions, and stress levels must also be considered.

One of the main purposes of accident investigation is to initiate changes or preventive measures to prevent repetitions.

OTHER SAFETY PROGRAM ELEMENTS

Fire Protection

Safety professionals are usually required to take charge of fire protection activities of the organization as well as employee safety functions. In fact, only organizations with extraordinary casualty exposure will employ a fire protection engineer.

The primary duty is of course to prevent fires. The fire safety program follows much the same pattern as has been outlined for the employee safety program, which was designed to keep injuries from occurring: (1) training, (2) communications, (3) emergency protective equipment, (4) chemical safety, and (5) accident investigation.

The safety professional should be involved in the construction and remodeling of facilities as well as occupancy plans in order to create a relatively fire-protected office or plant environment.

Once the facility has been constructed, fire prevention activities are usually limited to monitoring of hazardous areas, fire emergency planning, training, and monitoring of the adequacy of fire suppression equipment.

Vehicle Fleet Safety

Management usually does not realize the severity of its losses to vehicular accidents unless the company happens to operate an unusually large number of vehicles or is in the transportation industry. The safety professional should gain control of this area of responsibility, as it frequently represents one of the major sources of injury within an organization.

The safety professional would begin with documentation to obtain clear-cut authority for a control program through the company's safety policy and directives.

Employee or applicant screening is probably the major loss control available to the employer. This is one of the few cases where there is sufficient legal precedent to allow medical and driver history screening of drivers. Therefore, the safety professional will rely upon the occupational health physician to devise an adequate and responsible medical screening program to meet the employer's needs.

The second element of the fleet vehicle safety program must be a preventive maintenance program on all vehicles. This program must be meticulously documented in order to be of any value in dealing with insurers or the government agencies that monitor them.

The remaining fleet vehicle safety program elements again are training, communications, emergency planning, accident investigation, and inspections or monitoring.

Product Safety & Product Liability

Manufacturers—especially those whose products end up in the hands of the private consumer or in high-technology systems (eg, nuclear reactors, commercial aircraft, or aerospace modules)—are vitally concerned with the safety of their products. It is not uncommon for the organization's safety professional to become involved in product safety or product liability reviews.

A product safety review must consider first the intended uses and foreseeable misuses of the product. The aim of the review is to provide the most painstaking analysis—often using the techniques known as systems safety analysis (see below)—to ensure the product's correct and safe functioning under the most adverse foreseeable usage.

The product liability review is performed to determine how to assess or limit (to the extent possible) the legal liability of any unsafe operation of the product that might occur. From this review, the manufacturer—or its product liability insurance carrier—can determine the probable extent to which the manufacturer may be held liable in litigation for product operations or failures that cause personal injury or property damage.

MANAGEMENT APPROACHES TO ACCIDENT PREVENTION

Systems Safety

Systems safety analysis is not a single technique or process but rather a group of analytic techniques wherein operations (such as manufacturing a printed circuit board) or machines (such as punch presses) are viewed as if they were a single system. That system should in turn have each of its discrete parts, steps, or functions analyzed for potential hazards. All of this must be limited by practical considerations of operational effectiveness, time availability, and cost-effectiveness.

The traditional approach to safety is called the "fly-fix-fly" method, wherein an operation is initiated or a machine designed and put into use and then, when the operation or machine breaks down, causes an accident, or generally does not perform as

expected, it is redesigned, reengineered, or otherwise changed. The operation or machine is then put back into use again until another problem is found with it.

In our modern world, however, we have discovered certain systems for which we cannot afford the first accident, such as the following:

1. Core meltdown of a nuclear reactor.
2. Accidental nuclear weapons explosion.
3. Crash of a commercial airliner.
4. Loss of a manned space shuttle.
5. Release of a toxic gas cloud in an urban area.

This is not to say that these catastrophes cannot happen but rather that the manufacturers and operators involved must approach these potentials *as if* they cannot be allowed to happen.

A. Failure Modes and Effects Analysis: One of the earliest "systems safety" approaches was developed by reliability engineers to identify problems that could arise from machinery malfunctions. The technique analyzes each of the components, subassemblies, and subsystems, to find out how each might fail and what effect its failure would have on the system as a whole.

B. Fault Hazard Analysis: This refinement of the foregoing considers only those failure modes that could cause an accident, ignoring all other failures or failure modes. This allows analysis of larger systems while not requiring the reviewer to be bogged down in extraneous detail.

Criticality ratings are used to see which components or subsystems need design changes, tighter production controls, more comprehensive testing, specialized safeguards, monitoring, shielding, etc.

C. Fault Tree Analysis: Unlike the first 2 techniques, which consider all possible individual failures in order to find out what they would do to the system as a whole, fault tree analysis takes a single undesirable event (such as leakage of a toxic gas from a process) and works backward, trying to establish what could cause leakage to occur. Quantitative values are assigned to individual failure points to show the likelihood that failure will occur. The use of flow charting clearly demonstrates the relationships between the various components and thus encourages the analyst to consider cumulative failure possibilities (ie, 2 or more simultaneous component failures that cause the event).

D. Human Factors Analysis: This technique was developed to fit the human operator into the system with the maximum safety. Most machinery is designed for the convenience of the work flow or operation, and the operator is required to adapt to the machine's requirements. Because the human being is the most adaptable component in the system, it is relatively easy to make the system fit the "average" physical form. This leads designers and engineers to ignore the human element. Recognition that the "average" human physique and operating limits did not meet all the needs of industry gave emphasis to this discipline.

The most common need is for adjustability of work stations to fit the operator. The occupational health physician can be useful in this systems safety technique by providing consultation and physical data on body mobility, environmental stresses, repetitive motion effects, and sensory inputs.

More challenging still is the fitting of the operator's psychologic and cultural differences into the work environment. The fact that blue instead of red may be the color associated with "stop" or "emergency" in some cultures has cost the lives of workers.

Employee Operations & Management Reviews

Systems safety analysis was initially concerned only with equipment failures because it grew out of the quality control discipline. Later, it was realized that the operator is more than just a physical element in the system. The human decisions and actions were in fact a major risk factor and therefore had to be considered as part of the system. Finally, systems safety practitioners began applying the techniques of this discipline to human organizations.

A. Job Safety Analysis: This technique was developed during World War II when large numbers of inexperienced workers had to be integrated into the work force quickly and safely.

By systematic observation and detailed analysis, one uncovers the inherent hazards in the work environment. This task can be performed by supervisors, who in turn gain great understanding and appreciation of the areas under their control. The employees who participate develop a better recognition of the hazards they face. Finally, this system develops an effective teaching tool and documentation upon which personnel departments may effectively base their physical hiring requirements for certain jobs.

B. Techniques for Human Error Rate Prediction: This technique is primarily a method of quantifying what has been called "pilot error" in the broad sense of that term to determine probabilities of occurrence. Since it is solely directed toward human errors, it is often used in conjunction with fault tree analysis or failure modes and effects analysis.

In their analysis, all human tasks are broken down into the smallest possible discrete actions. Each component task is referenced to a set of tables reflecting basic human tasks with the probability of functioning correctly considered for each of 9 potential error states. A "basic error rate" can be obtained, expressed as errors per million operations. These values are obtained through detailed clinical research.

C. Management Oversight Risk Tree: This technique was developed to combine the systems safety analysis techniques with modern management techniques. The result was a large analytic diagram or flow chart portraying the operation of a safety management program in a logical and orderly manner, with the actual safety program compared with an idealized system. The evaluator can thus detect omissions, oversights, and ineffective programs. The defects might be as diverse as poor training or employee misconduct, and the effective diagnosis of these problems provides the evaluator with a tool for loss control.

D. Techniques of Operation Review: This is a system for analyzing the root causes of accidents or other undesired events. The examiner starts with an undesired event and cross-references it on a chart with a large number of organizational processes (training, supervision, management, etc). The technique provides a simplistic but systematic method of examining potential causes of causes within an organization in relation to any specific failure event.

WORKING WITH OTHER PROFESSIONALS

Loss Control

When the organization includes other professionals (such as industrial hygienists, occupational physicians, occupational health nurses, fire protection engineers, etc), the safety professional has obvious responsibilities toward those individuals, as follows:

1. To cooperate in establishing and maintaining joint loss control activities.
2. To provide constant resource information and advice to these functions.
3. To constantly review plans and activities of all of these functions to ensure coordinated action and maximum efficiency.

Additionally, where the loss control functions have been gathered together in a single department, it is often the safety professional who functions as the department manager.

In addition to the loss control functions, the safety professional must become directly involved with at least 5 other departments: facilities, maintenance, purchasing, personnel, and finance.

Facilities

The facilities department within a large organization determines the occupancy of various buildings, purchases or constructs new facilities, and usually is responsible for major remodeling or modifications of existing plants. The safety professional must maintain a close relationship with this department.

New and revised occupancy plans must be reviewed to make certain that incompatible processes are not in the same areas and that the buildings are suitable for occupancy by the intended operations. In reviewing construction or remodeling plans, the safety professional must ensure that proper consideration be given to providing environmental controls such as ventilation or sound barriers. Additionally, the plans must provide for adequate safety systems such as fire suppression systems, routes of exit, and the ability to seal off or contain areas where spills or releases of toxic chemicals might occur.

The facilities department usually oversees the work being performed within the facilities by outside contractors. The safety professional must ensure that these contractors are aware of and will conform with the basic elements of the safety program applicable to their activities when in the facility. Furthermore, their work should not produce additional hazards to either the contractor's employees or the internal employees who must work around them. Certificates of insurance should be obtained from all contracting companies to make certain that adequate insurance is being maintained.

Maintenance

The maintenance department is separate from the facilities department in most organizations. One is an engineering and planning unit, whereas the other handles the day-to-day repairs and minor modifications constantly required in a large facility.

The safety professional is always closely involved with the maintenance function. Maintenance personnel must correct any physical safety deficiencies discovered. It therefore must be kept informed about safety problems. A priority system must be arranged with the maintenance manager so that more important modifications are made quickly and efficiently.

The maintenance department may perform or contract for routine inspections and monitoring of equipment such as cranes, forklifts, fire extinguishing systems, ventilation systems, and alarm systems.

Purchasing

The purchasing department obtains from outside suppliers all the production equipment, supplies, component parts, and raw materials used by an organization. In the purchasing of equipment, the safety professional must be sure the purchasing department obtains only such equipment as meets the current government safety and manufacturing standards. If this department is performing the contract negotiations for obtaining subcontractors, it must be certain to include provisions requiring minimum safety standards while the work is being performed. When purchasing raw materials, component parts, or process materials, this department must ensure that any substitutions are approved by the appropriate departments to be certain unforeseen hazards are not being introduced into the work areas or end products produced.

The safety professional must be sure that all chemical purchases are being routed through this department and that deliveries of chemicals not authorized by that department are not accepted.

When a new chemical is ordered from suppliers, the purchasing department must request that a material safety data sheet be included with the order. These sheets list the composition of the chemical and the hazards that might be encountered with its use, recommend proper handling and control procedures, and give precise emergency treatment and containment instructions. New MSDSs should be obtained periodically in order to keep up with changes that might occur.

Personnel

The interface between the safety professional and the personnel department is generally limited to 2 main areas, providing (1) the information on which applicant screening programs are based and (2) the safety evaluations on which manager and supervisor accountability programs are based.

The employer using a physical screening program must prove that the job function for which applications are being taken requires the potential employee to have a certain level of mobility, strength, or sensory perception. This can usually be accomplished by the performance—by a safety professional—of a detailed job safety analysis. The job safety analysis breaks down the individual job functions into their component operations, analyzing each for its hazard potentials and physical requirements. The analysis must then be reviewed by an occupational physician to establish the actual minimum physical abilities an employee must have to perform these functions on a day-to-day basis. It is only when this has been done that the personnel department can draw up an enforceable applicant screening program.

Many organizations today are attempting to focus greater attention on making sure that individual managers and supervisors are carrying out the wishes of the organization as expressed in the corporate policy statements. In the area of safety, this usually takes the form of either financial chargeback programs to the individual departments or accountability reviews being made on safety performance as part of the individual manager's or supervisor's personnel review. Both of these systems are effective because they hold the individual managers or supervisors directly accountable for safety in their departments.

Within this accountability system, the safety professional is charged with maintaining the records, comparisons, and accident evaluations upon which the individual managers or supervisors will be judged. The safety professional must therefore maintain and organize the various reporting systems in such a way as to provide the personnel or finance departments with complete and accurate information on which to base its decisions.

Finance

The safety professional's input to the finance department concerns accountability of managers and supervisors to ensure maximum compliance with the safety goals of the organization. In this case, the safety professional is required to maintain departmental breakdowns of accident and safety-related costs (such as insurance, multiple department training, and large capital items related to worker safety). These charges must also be indexed in some manner so as to provide an accurate picture of the actual expenditures for each major department. The charge system must take into account such items as long-term capital improvements, total costs of long-term injuries, operating levels, and actual responsibility. Once figures have been established for each department, they must be charged back to the respective departments. Thus, the department manager's budget versus performance will reflect either a credit or debit depending on the department's performance during the fiscal period. This has the effect of requiring managers to justify to their superiors large budgets for expected accident losses or poor performance due to those same accident losses. On the other hand, it also allows the department to take credit for savings occurring through improved safety performance within their own area.

SOURCES OF OUTSIDE HELP

Safety professionals have many outside sources to which they can turn when they need assistance.

Consulting Physicians & Occupational Injury Clinics

The safety professional often calls upon either the consulting physician or the occupational injury clinic physician when medical advice is needed for training, for evaluations, or for emergency medical planning. The prudent industrial safety professional will also request the physician who will treat an organization's employees to tour the facility and become familiar with the work environment and job functions. It is hoped that this will provide the physician with a basis upon which to make decisions about physical restrictions on injured workers or on return to work after injury.

Government Agency Consulting Services

The federal government, some states, and some local governments have established numerous large administrative bodies to deal with issues of occupational safety and health. Many of these are compliance agencies whose primary thrust is standards or codes enforcement. Most of these same agencies offer free consulting services so that interested parties can ask specific questions about those regulations and their applicability. Many consulting services also have field agents who will visit the place of employment if asked to do so to review specific situations and give advice.

Employers are reluctant to ask for assistance from these consulting branches of government agencies because they are afraid that information received by the consulting service might be transferred to the compliance enforcement personnel of that same agency. This appears to be an unfounded concern, since there is no evidence of this sort of transfer of information having occurred unless there is an imminent hazard condition that may cause serious injury or death.

Governmental agency consulting is limited by regulations. They will not assist with problems not covered by or related to their regulations, and they are often unwilling or unable to become involved in complex issues or numerous minor problems.

Insurance Industry Consulting

Various lines of insurance coverage (workers' compensation, general liability, fleet, property, and products liability) include consultant services as a benefit to the client intended to minimize claims. Many insurance companies merely have a few generalized safety personnel available to their clients. Some of the larger companies, however, provide the services of fully formed loss control teams.

Private Consulting Firms

There are numerous private consulting firms offering their services to industrial concerns in need of assistance. Some of these firms are highly specialized, providing specific services such as radiation control and testing, industrial hygiene services, or training courses. Other consulting firms try to be more generalized in their approach. Many firms are also available to provide specialized assistance in the area of litigation by furnishing legal advice, expert witnesses, claims defense services, and even total program reviews.

Private consulting firms are expensive. It is important to check into the qualifications, experience, and professionalism of any consultant firm.

Sales Organizations

Safety equipment sales personnel are often quite knowledgeable within their own limited fields of expertise and have a vested interest in providing reliable service and advice.

Local offices of the National Safety Council serve as a resource to companies who are members of the organization. While membership is based on corporate size, it is fairly expensive. However, the Council does sell a good product line of films, videos, books, and training courses.

Hot Lines

Industry and trade associations and various government agencies have established telephone "hot lines" to provide information to industry or the public about safety and health issues. For example, the chemical industry has its Chemical Referral Center Hotline (1-[800]-262-8200) and its CHEM-TREC number (1-[800]-424-9300), which can be called to find out the basic properties, toxic effects, and treatments available for most widely available chemical substances. This service was set up to provide information in chemical emergencies, but the personnel will refer nonemergency requests to local members of the organization. These members frequently have experience with acute and chronic effects of chemicals they use or manufacture and are aware of preferred treatments.

Professional Contacts

Personal contacts with other safety professionals made at conferences, training classes, trade associa-tion meetings, and the like are invaluable as a source of assistance, advice, and practical examples.

REFERENCES

General Safety

National Safety Council: *Accident Prevention Manual For Industrial Operations,* 9th ed. National Safety Council, 1988.

Petersen D: *Analyzing Safety Performance.* Garland STPM Press, 1980.

Tarrants W: *The Measurement of Safety Performance,* 2nd ed. Garland STPM Press, 1984.

Safety Management

Asfahl CR: *Industrial Safety and Health Management.* Prentice-Hall, 1984.

Grimaldi J, Simonds R: *Safety Management,* 2nd ed. Irwin, 1989.

Petersen D: *Safety Management: A Human Approach,* 2nd ed. Aloray, 1988.

Petersen D: *Techniques of Safety Management.* McGraw-Hill, 1971.

Slote L: *Handbook of Occupational Safety and Health.* Wiley-Interscience, 1987.

Accident Investigation

Ferry T: *Modern Accident Investigation and Analysis: An Executive Guide,* 2nd ed. Wiley, 1988.

Safety Training

Strasser M et al: *Fundamentals of Safety Education,* 3rd ed. Macmillan, 1981.

Safety Engineering

Brown D: *Systems Analysis and Design for Safety.* Prentice-Hall, 1978.

Burch C: *Strength of Materials for Technology.* Wiley, 1978.

Gloss D, Wardle M: *Introduction to Safety Engineering.* Wiley-Interscience, 1984.

Hammer W: *Occupational Safety Management and Engineering.* Prentice-Hall, 1985.

Life Safety Code Handbook, 4th ed. National Fire Protection Association, 1988.

Winburn DC: *Practical Electrical Safety.* Marcel Dekker, 1988.

Chemical & Environmental Safety

Dux J, Stalzer R: *Managing Safety in the Chemical Laboratory.* Van Nostrand Reinhold, 1987.

National Institute for Occupational Safety and Health: *The Industrial Environment: Its Evaluation and Control.* US Government Printing Office, 1973.

Laser & Optical Safety

Sliney D, Wolbarsht M: *Safety With Lasers and Other Optical Sources: A Comprehensive Handbook.* Plenum Press, 1980.

Compressed Gas Safety

Effects of Exposure to Toxic Gases: First Aid and Medical Treatment, 3rd ed. Matheson Gas Products, 1988.

Guide to Safe Handling of Compressed Gases. Matheson Gas Products, 1983.

Handbook of Compressed Gases, 2nd ed. Compressed Gas Association, 1980.

Products Liability & Systems Safety

Bass L: *Products Liability: Design and Manufacturing Defects.* McGraw-Hill, 1986.

Brown D: *Systems Analysis and Design for Safety.* Prentice Hall, 1976.

Hammer W: *Product Safety Management and Engineering.* Prentice Hall, 1972.

Fleet Vehicle Safety

Bierlein L: *Red Book on Transportation of Hazardous Materials,* 2nd ed. Van Nostrand Reinhold, 1988.

Motor Fleet Safety Manual. National Safety Council, 1979.

Fire Protection

Fire Protection Handbook, 16th ed. National Fire Protection Association, 1986.

Industrial Hygiene

38

Douglas P. Fowler, PhD, CIH

The 3 definitive elements of industrial hygiene are the recognition, evaluation, and control of occupational health hazards. The recognition of health hazards has primacy, since it must take place before proper evaluation or (if needed) control can take place. Upon recognition of a health hazard, the industrial hygienist should be able to identify measures necessary for proper evaluation. Upon completion of the evaluation, the industrial hygienist then is in a position—in consultation with other members of the occupational health and safety team—to recommend and implement controls needed to reduce exposures to tolerable limits.

Recognition of Health Hazards in the Workplace

Recognition of health hazards is the first step in the process leading to evaluation and control and entails the identification of materials and processes that have the potential for causing harm to workers. Sources of information about health hazards include clinical data about health problems in exposed populations; information in scientific journals, bulletins of trade associations, and reports of government agencies; conversations with peers; and direct reports from workers, union representatives, supervisors, or employers.

Inspection of the workplace is the best source of directly relevant data about health hazards. There is no substitute for observation of work practices, use of chemical and physical agents, and apparent effectiveness of control measures. The physician should be able to recognize major and obvious health hazards and distinguish those that require formal evaluation by the industrial hygienist.

The Walk-Through Survey

The "walk-through survey" in the company of the occupational physician is the first and most important technique for recognition of occupational health hazards.

The survey should begin with a proper introduction to plant management and discussion of the purpose of the survey and inquiry about any relevant recent complaints. If appropriate, a simplified process flow diagram should be prepared at this time.

Following the process flow through the plant is most productive. The survey might thus begin at the loading dock, where materials entering the plant can be examined. Warning labels, descriptive language about the chemical composition of materials, and the packaging of incoming materials should be noted. Questions should then be asked regarding the handling of unknown materials or materials about which insufficient information is available. The incoming materials should then be followed into the process flow stream, and each of the processes of interest in the plant should be observed in action. Of interest throughout the survey will be the methods used for materials handling as well as the labeling of materials, particularly at points where they are transferred from manufacturers' containers into vessels for use within the plant.

Observations to Be Made

At each point in the process, the industrial hygienist should observe handling procedures as well as any protective measures that are employed. Controls that may be appropriate are listed below in the discussion of control of health hazards. Use of respiratory protection and protective clothing should be recorded, as well as other common-sense observations such as the apparent effectiveness of engineering controls—as indicated by absence of characteristic odors, visible dust accumulations, and loud noise. The survey should continue through to the final product produced by the plant and its packaging.

The industrial hygienist should also follow the pathway of any waste materials and determine their disposal sites.

The numbers of employees at each process step should be noted, as well as any relevant data on gender, ethnicity, or age that might affect employees' sensitivity to chemicals in the workplace. It is also important to look for obvious stigmas such as drying and roughening of the skin, as might be expected where exposure to solvents occurs. It is usually appropriate to discuss work practices with the personnel directly involved, since the perception of those practices is often very different on the shop floor from what it is in the executive offices.

The Industrial Hygiene Survey Checklist on p 500 summarizes the steps in evaluation.

Data Review

An important part of the industrial hygienist's role in recognition of health hazards in the workplace will be data review. Such data may include reports from physicians on clinical findings that may be related to exposures in the workplace as well as a review of company records on materials coming into the work-

AN INDUSTRIAL HYGIENE SURVEY CHECKLIST

Determine purpose and scope of study:
  Comprehensive industrial hygiene survey?
  Evaluation of exposures of limited group of workers to specific agents?
  Determination of compliance with specific recognized standards?
  Evaluation of effectiveness of engineering controls?
  Response to specific complaint?

Discuss purpose of study with appropriate representatives of management and labor.

Familiarize yourself with plant operations:
  Obtain and study process flow sheets and plant layout.
  Compile an inventory of raw materials, intermediates, by-products, and products.
  Review relevant toxicologic information.
  Obtain a list of job classifications and the environmental stresses to which workers are potentially
    exposed.
  Observe the activities associated with job classification.
  Review the status of workers' health with medical personnel.
  Observe and review administrative and engineering control measures used.
  Review reports of previous studies.
  Determine subjectively the potential health hazards associated with plant operations.
  Review adequacy of labeling and warning.

Prepare for field study:
  Determine which chemical and physical agents are to be evaluated.
  Estimate, if possible, ranges of contaminant concentrations.
  Review—or develop if necessary—sampling and analytic methods, paying particular attention to the
    limitations of the methods.
  Calibrate field equipment as necessary.
  Assemble all field equipment.
  Obtain personal protective equipment as required (hard hat, safety glasses, goggles, hearing protection,
    respiratory protection, safety shoes, coveralls, gloves, etc).
  Prepare a tentative sampling schedule.
  Review specific applicable OSHA regulations.

Conduct field study:
  Confirm process operating schedule with supervisory personnel.
  Advise representatives of management and labor of your presence in the area.
  Deploy personal monitoring or general area sampling units.
  For each sample, record the following data:
    1. Sample identification number.
    2. Description of sample (as detailed as possible).
    3. Time sampling began.
    4. Flow rate of sampled air (check frequently).
    5. Time sampling ended.
    6. Any other information or observation that might be significant (eg, process upsets, ventilation
      system not operating, use of personal protection).
  Dismantle sampling units.
  Seal and label adequately all samples (filters, liquid solutions, charcoal or silica gel tubes, etc) that
    require subsequent laboratory analyses.

Interpret results of sampling program:
  Obtain results of all analyses.
  Determine time-weighted average exposures of job classifications evaluated.
  Determine peak exposures of workers.
  Determine statistical reliability of data—eg, estimate probable error in determination of average
    exposures.
  Compare sampling results with applicable industrial hygiene standards and regulations.

Discuss survey results with appropriate representatives of management and labor.

Implement corrective action comprised of, as appropriate:
  Engineering controls (isolation, ventilation, etc).
  Administrative controls (job rotation, reduced work time, etc).
  Personal protection.
  Biologic sampling program.
  Medical surveillance.
  Education and training.

Determine whether other safety and health considerations warrant further evaluation:
  Air pollution?
  Water pollution?
  Solid waste disposal?
  Safety?
  Health physics?

Schedule return visit(s) to evaluate effectiveness of controls:
  Walk-through and observation.
  Measurements.

place that may represent significant health hazards. The current OSHA ''Workers' Right-to-Know'' regulation has made explicit (and subject to governmental investigation) the common-sense duty of the employer to inform workers of the nature and hazards of materials to which they may be exposed. Where exposures are to materials purchased from a third party, data on materials and their hazards will usually be derived from Material Safety Data Sheets (MSDSs).

Value & Limitations of MSDSs

The industrial hygiene review of MSDSs and other forms made available by law from suppliers, should include attention to identifiable health hazards as well as recommended control measures. While MSDSs have been far more informative recently than in the past, there are still substantial differences between the information provided by different manufacturers for the same (generic) materials. In addition, the MSDSs provided may be prepared by people without substantial health science backgrounds and represent merely a reprinting of data from conventional sources, often outdated and sometimes inappropriate. The industrial hygienist must therefore compare and balance the recommendations made by various manufacturers in order to provide a unified program for control of materials of similar sorts, regardless of their commercial sources.

As chemical manufacturers have grown more sophisticated, the available MSDSs have tended to stress protective measures more completely than in the past. This has come about both from manufacturers' concerns that their materials were in some cases being misused and from fear of litigation. In some cases, recommended personal protective measures are unnecessarily complex—particularly where the chemicals are used in very small quantities. The industrial hygienist may be able to recommend less restrictive protection if the combination of quantities used, inherent toxicity, process controls, and other engineering control measures combine to reduce exposures to acceptable levels.

Materials of Uncertain Toxicity

In some cases, the industrial hygienist must assess the potential for harm of chemicals for which no reliable human toxicologic data are available. This need arises most often in research and development settings but also wherever chemical intermediates are produced.

An important consideration is that the worker must be protected at all cost. If uncertainty exists, it should be resolved in favor of a higher standard of concern.

Upon completion of the walk-through survey, the industrial hygienist will ordinarily have a closing conference with the plant management, at which time obvious concerns can be discussed and follow-up measures agreed upon. Where the industrial hygienist is a regulatory agency representative, follow-up surveys may require special notices and interaction with agency officials as well as plant officials. In any case, a report on the walk-through survey, together with conclusions and recommendations, should be completed for the record.

EVALUATION OF HEALTH HAZARDS

Evaluation of health hazards within the plant will include measurement of exposures (and potential exposures), comparison of those exposures to existing standards, and recommendation of controls if needed.

Exposure Measurements

Exposure measurements are intended to be determinations of doses delivered to the individual. The mere existence of chemicals in the workplace—or even in the workplace atmosphere—does not necessarily imply that the chemicals are being delivered to a sensitive organ system. The effective dose will depend upon such things as particle sizes of dusts in the air, the use of protective devices (respirators, protective clothing), and the existence of other contaminants in the workplace. The task of determining the dose delivered to the worker may be complicated by the existence of multiple pathways of absorption and metabolism. Such contaminants as lead are absorbed readily both through inhalation and ingestion, and both routes of intake must be considered in evaluation of the potential for harm. Similarly, many solvents are readily absorbed through the skin, and mere determination of airborne levels is not sufficient to determine the complete range of potential exposures.

Sampling & Analysis of Airborne Contaminants

Inhalation of airborne contaminants is the major route of entry for systemic intoxicants. Thus, evaluation and control of airborne contaminants is an important part of any occupational health program.

Sampling and analysis of airborne contaminants is the definitive function of the industrial hygienist. While it is the joint responsibility of the hygienist and physician to interpret the results of such measurements, measurement alone makes a contribution to the awareness of hazards as well as to their evaluation. Recent developments in instrumentation have made it possible to measure very low concentrations, with the result that previously unsuspected contamination is now being discovered.

In some cases, these more sophisticated measurements, coupled with evaluations of the health status of those exposed, have led to discoveries of connections between relatively low levels of airborne contaminants and health effects. The field of "indoor air quality" is one such general case. The determination of exposures to occupants of buildings (office workers) has not received substantial attention in the past, but health effects are now being found at concentrations of contaminants well below established occupational standards.

Maximum acceptable exposure limits have typically been lowered as both our ability to discern clinical effects and our expectations of no detectable health effects have increased in recent years. An example is concerns about asbestos in buildings. The hygienist should attempt to ensure that there is no avoidable exposure to asbestos, since there is no definitive evidence that a threshold exists below which harmful effects do not occur. Thus, measurements of asbestos concentrations down to and including ambient levels have become relatively commonplace.

General Approaches to Air Monitoring

There are 2 major approaches to air sampling for determination of airborne contaminant levels. In personal, or breathing zone, sampling, the hygienist places a collection device near to the breathing zone of the worker. The collection device may either be active, requiring that air be drawn through it; or passive, requiring no pump or other suction source (a "dosimeter"). The second approach (area sampling) employs fixed or mobile sampling stations in the work area.

A. Personal Breathing Zone Sampling: Personal breathing zone sampling is usually preferred, since exposures are measured at the point nearest to the actual entry of airborne contaminants and the sampling system moves with the worker. Thus, measurements are more likely to represent actual potential exposures. An example of a worker with a breathing zone (personal) sampler in place is shown in Fig 38–1.

B. Area Monitoring: There are disadvantages to the personal breathing zone approach, however. First, the volume of air sampled is limited by the capacity of the battery-operated pumps used (or the diffusion coefficient of a passive collection device), so that trace contaminants may be difficult to measure. Second, where complex evaluations are required, the number of collection devices may be too cumbersome for practical installation in the worker's breathing zone. In these circumstances—or when direct-reading instruments (usually larger and often requiring line power) are to be used—area monitoring by means of fixed monitoring stations may be employed. Fixed monitoring stations may also be used to measure emissions from sources; to measure background concentrations; or to measure concentrations in several areas simultaneously in order to evaluate the effectiveness of controls. Fig 38–2 shows the application of both area sampling and personal sampling inside a work area.

Time-Weighted Average Exposures

The time course of exposure potential should be identified before beginning the sampling process, so that all times during which exposure is possible will be appropriately sampled. Time-weighted average exposure determinations should be made for the entire period of work to be evaluated. In a continuous ("assembly line") process, the period of exposure will usually be the entire work shift. In other cases, exposures may only occur for a relatively short time within the work shift. The time-weighted average exposure throughout the workday is usually required for determination of compliance with relevant standards (see below) and may be useful also for comparison of exposures at various points within the plant.

The Time Course of Exposure

Although chronic diseases are usually the result of long-continued exposures, peak exposure levels can be important in evaluating acute effects and may be more directly relevant even in long-term exposures than their relative contribution on a time-weighted

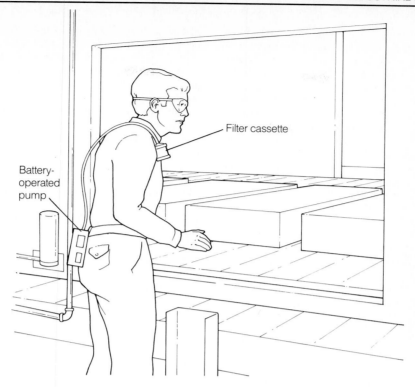

Battery-operated pump

Filter cassette

Figure 38–1. Worker wearing personal breathing zone monitor. The monitor samples air near enough to the nose and mouth to catch the same type of air the worker is breathing.

average would indicate. In other words, peak exposures may overwhelm such defenses as the mucociliary pathway for removal of contaminants and may occur at times of maximal exertion and maximal intake of airborne contaminants. Peak exposures may be determined by taking an integrated sample for a relatively short period (for performance of a specific operation, or for 10–15 minutes at a time when maximum exposure is expected) or by using direct-reading instruments for real-time measurements.

SAMPLING FOR SPECIFIC CONTAMINANTS

The general approaches introduced above may be applied to determination of individual agents or groups of agents. In general, sampling analytic methods are divided into those for gases and vapors and those for airborne particles.

1. GAS & VAPOR SAMPLING

Gas and vapor sampling may be accomplished by any of 5 methods: (1) active collection, by drawing a measured volume of air through a collection system that is then analyzed; (2) passive collection, with a dosimeter that attracts gas or vapor molecules by diffusion from the atmosphere; (3) collection in a color-sensitive medium in a device in which color change is proportionate to concentration of the contaminant and which can be read directly; (4) collection in an evacuated container used to carry a sample of air to a convenient site for analysis; and (5) collection in direct-reading instruments sensitive to one or several atmospheric gases or vapors.

In general, the first method—using active collection devices with subsequent laboratory analysis—is more sensitive and can be used to determine lower concentrations than the other approaches listed. However, the direct-reading devices (both instrumental [5] and color change [3]) provide a more rapid (immediate) result and are useful when an immediate hazard must be assessed. Passive dosimeters offer the advantage of not requiring a suction source to draw air through the collection device and are thus more acceptable to workers since the need for carrying a pump is avoided.

Collection Media

Collection media for gases and vapors may be either solid or liquid.

A. Solid Sorbents: The most commonly used solid sorbent is activated charcoal, which can be used for collection of many low-molecular-weight hydrocarbons as well as some inorganic gases and vapors. The most common analytic procedure employed in determining concentrations from the gases and vapors collected on the charcoal is gas chromatography. The collected sample, with the molecules of gas or vapor adsorbed to the surface of the charcoal, is usually desorbed with a solvent (often carbon disulfide) compatible with those to be determined. The solvent extract of the charcoal is then either injected directly into the gas-liquid chromatograph column or the volume of the extract is reduced to provide greater sensitivity, followed by injection.

In some cases, particularly for oxygenated hydrocarbon species, silica gel is used. Desorption is often accomplished with distilled water or oxygenated solvents, again followed by analysis by either gas chromatography or other analytic approaches. Another group of sorbents are less commonly used for routine industrial hygiene sampling but are finding increasing utilization in evaluation of indoor air quality and for collection of samples for analysis of higher molecular weight species. These are the solid sorbents that were initially developed as gas chromatographic column packings. Examples are Tenax and the variously numbered Chromosorb materials. Some of these sorbents can be characterized as "molecular sieves" and find particular use in collection of samples in environments where compounds that may irreversibly bind to charcoal are found. Desorption is often conveniently accomplished by heating the sample collection tube while injecting a carrier gas (nitrogen or other inert gas) through the sample tube during heating. This approach, coupled with analysis of the desorbed gas by gas chromatography or mass spectrometry or some other analytic method, is often useful where a complex environment with many trace components is suspected.

B. Liquid Media: Gases and vapors may also be

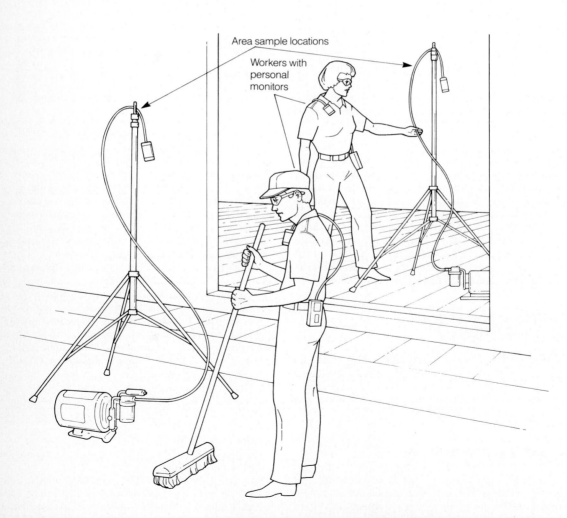

Figure 38–2. Worker wearing personal monitor. Industrial hygienist is gaining additional information by installing an area monitoring device.

effectively collected from the atmosphere using various liquids as the collection media. The air is drawn through the measured volume of the liquid into a device that may be called an "impinger" or "bubbler" or a "gas washing bottle." Sampling in liquid for gases and vapors has several disadvantages when personal breathing zone concentrations are to be determined. Some of the liquids that have been recommended are themselves toxic, and placing a glass vial on a worker's lapel may add to the risk in the workplace. There is a danger also of spillage from any liquid container, and the liquid may evaporate—either of which will complicate evaluation of the results.

C. Evacuated Containers: Collection of samples of air in evacuated containers such as bags, glass bottles, stainless steel cylinders, or other containers is appropriate only if it is certain that the samples will be analyzed before analytes of interest have had a chance to either degrade or react. In most cases, this limits the utility of the technique to relatively stable gases and vapors. The technique is particularly useful for inorganic and nonreactive gases such as carbon monoxide. Reactions may include those with the walls of the container (or simple sorption to the walls) as well as reactions with other airborne contaminants held within the container. In addition, care must be taken to avoid exposure of the collected gas to sunlight or other sources of artificial light that may initiate photochemical reactions. However, the technique is very useful when such analytic procedures as gas-phase infrared spectrometry appear to be useful approaches and a laboratory-based instrument offers advantages in sensitivity or precision over field direct-reading instruments.

Direct-Reading Instruments

A variety of direct-reading battery-powered instruments are now available, so that direct measurements of "real time" concentrations can be made. Some of these units measure oxygen concentrations also, making them useful for evaluating the safety of entry into enclosed spaces. Others measure only one or 2 contaminants but are useful where the suspected contamination is relatively well known.

A. Data Loggers: With the recent advent of portable "data loggers" from which data may be down-loaded to computer systems, it has become feasible to record the real-time output from these small direct-reading instruments. This makes it possible to construct individual exposure profiles over time. An important application of this approach has been in indoor air quality studies, where the relative contributions of various sources to overall exposures to CO have become much better understood recently.

Other available direct-reading instruments are less portable but more accurate and more easily and permanently calibrated. The detection principles employed are often the same as those in the small instruments, but the detection systems and associated electronics are often more reliable. Output may be to either digital or analog meters, strip chart recorders, or data loggers.

B. Portable Chromatographs: A recent development in industrial hygiene instrumentation has been the adaptation of chromatographs to portable field use. With these instruments, a bolus of air may be drawn directly into the instrument through a gas sampling valve, or an evacuated container (often a syringe) may be used to collect a small sample of air that is then injected directly into the instrument. These instruments share the advantages (specificity and sensitivity) of laboratory gas chromatographs but have the disadvantage that a relatively extensive calibration effort may be required in order to obtain quantitative results. The detectors used may be selected to measure only the family of airborne contaminants of interest.

C. Infrared Spectrophotometers: These instruments (an example is the family of MIRAN instruments manufactured by Foxboro-Wilks) can be used to measure concentrations of several hundred gases and vapors at or near the 1 part per million level.

D. Fixed Monitors: Any of the direct-reading instruments described above can be made substantially more reliable if installed permanently with line power. Such installations have been used for many years where potential for exposure to highly toxic gases exists.

E. A measured volume of air is drawn through a glass tube containing a reagent (usually adsorbed onto a solid support) that reacts with specified chemicals in the air. The degree of color change in the reagent—either the shade of coloration or the "length of stain" along the tube length—is proportionate to the concentration of contaminant and can be compared to standard charts. The major danger in their use is that they may not be reliable—they should not, generally speaking, be considered any more accurate or precise than about half of the indicated value. In addition, their lower limit of sensitivity may be near to the level at which controls should be implemented.

2. PARTICULATE MATERIAL SAMPLING

Measurement of airborne particulate contamination can be done either by collection of integrated samples with subsequent analysis or by use of direct-reading instruments. Integrated sample collection and analysis is by far the more common modality of evaluation, both because of certain inherent difficulties associated with direct-reading measurements and because of the greater precision associated with laboratory analysis.

Filter Sampling

Modern airborne particle sampling is ordinarily done with filters. The filter selected for use must collect and retain the particles of interest; must not offer so much resistance to flow that pumps cannot draw air through it at a useful rate; and must be compatible with the analytic method of choice.

Size-Selective Sampling

Inhalation and retention of particulate material in the lung is dependent upon the "aerodynamic equivalent diameter" of the particles. That is, only particles within a specific size range (which is dependent upon the specific gravity and shape of the particles) will both penetrate to and be retained within the alveolar and lower bronchiolar (unciliated) air spaces. Thus, sampling to evaluate hazards associated with crystalline silica is done with the aid of a size-selective sampling device (a "cyclone") preceding the filter upon which the material is to be collected for analysis. Only particles small enough to both penetrate to and be retained within the deep lung space will pass through the selective device and be captured on the filter for analysis. This "respirable dust sampling" by cyclone is the method of choice for evaluation of the pneumoconiosis-causing dusts, with the exception of asbestos. (See also Impingers and Impactors, below.)

Total Particulate Sampling

In circumstances where a biologically active material may be absorbed readily at many portals of entry, total particulate sampling may be the approach of choice. This is the case, for example, where such biologically active compounds as pesticides require evaluation. Such chemicals may be absorbed in the upper respiratory tract, when inhaled into the deep lung, or indeed even upon skin contact. In addition, clearance mechanisms (the mucociliary elevator) may remove the contaminant from the ciliated portion of the respiratory tract and yet not fully clear the contaminant from the body because of the swallowing of saliva. It is therefore important to collect all airborne particles if the full extent of the hazard is to be evaluated.

Impingers & Impactors

Other devices used in particulate material sampling include direct inertial collectors such as impingers and impactors. The former utilizes a wet collection system, where a jet of air is directed against a collecting surface within a liquid bath. Impingers are now used mainly for gas and vapor collection. While impingers are effective for the collection of large particles, they are not particularly suitable for collection of very small particles owing to the limitations of the inertial forces employed for such collection. They should thus be used with caution when particles less than 1 μm in diameter are potentially important in health effects.

Impactors use a dry collection system, wherein particles are directed in a jet of air against a dry (or sometimes greased) collection surface. Impactors are often used in a stacked-plate array, with the plates pierced with equal numbers of holes that decrease in size from inlet to exit. The jets thus formed increase in velocity (in inverse proportion to their diameters), and successively smaller particles are removed from the gas stream. The final stage of the impactor is usually a filter, where the remaining (small) particles are collected. Size-selective sampling with greater detail than offered by the cyclone is thus provided.

Analysis of Particulate Material Samples

Analysis of collected samples may be by any of a variety of techniques appropriate to the analyte of interest. The evaluation of exposures to asbestos is by microscopy.

A. Analysis by Microscopy: In the case of materials such as asbestos, where the numerical concentration of particles is the most important toxicity factor, a sample is taken by drawing air through a filter and the number of particles on the filter is counted by microscopic techniques.

The most common analytic procedure used for evaluation of asbestos is that involving optical phase-contrast microscopy as specified by NIOSH and OSHA. The procedure is relatively simple but has the disadvantages that not all airborne asbestos fibers are visualized or counted and that other (nonasbestos) fibers are counted. However, since the fibers most often considered to be harmful—those longer than 5 μm—are counted, the method gives an index of exposure to all asbestos fibers.

Where more detailed information on the total airborne fiber population is desired, transmission electron microscopy is used. This method, which is capable of visualizing all airborne asbestos fibers (and differentiating asbestos fibers from other fibers) is much more complex and costly. (The analytic cost of the phase-contrast method is typically in the range of $25 per sample, while transmission electron microscopy typically costs from $250 to $1500 per sample depending upon the level of detail required in the results (and the speed of analysis).

B. Other Analytic Approaches: Other commonly used analytic approaches are atomic absorption or emission spectroscopy for analysis of elements in the particles, x-ray diffraction for identification of crystalline materials, and (where appropriate) any of the aforementioned organic analysis modalities where organic compounds exist in particulate form.

3. COMBINED COLLECTION DEVICES

In some environments, it may be appropriate to use combined particulate and gaseous (or vapor) collection devices. This may be the case where a substance exists in particulate form in the atmosphere but has an appreciable vapor pressure, so that substantial amounts may evaporate following collection on a filter. In this case, a vapor-sorbing material would be used behind the filter to ensure complete collection. Such a combined sampling approach is often used for collection of pesticides and polynuclear aromatic hydrocarbons.

4. SURFACE EVALUATION
(Wipe Sampling)

Evaluation of surface contamination can be a useful supplementary technique for evaluation of exposure potential and particularly for evaluation of the effectiveness of control measures. Wipe sampling is useful also for identifying contaminated areas where a spill of toxic material has occurred. As an example, wipe sampling is routinely used to evaluate the extent of contamination resulting from spills of such materials as PCBs, pesticides, and other materials for which absorption through the skin may be an important route of entry.

Wipe sampling may also be a useful adjunct to programs used to evaluate the effectiveness of housekeeping measures, particularly in manufacturing facilities where separation of manufacturing areas from cafeterias, offices, or dressing rooms is important. A typical program would call for the wipe sampling of identical areas once a month or quarterly.

Wipe sampling must be done according to a well-defined protocol if it is to have any significant utility for long-term evaluations. Most commonly, a template of a defined size (usually 10×10 cm) is prepared, and wiping is done within the exposed area of the template for the sake of uniformity. Any suitable substance may be used to perform the wiping, but filter papers (usually the low-ash, "quantitative" type of papers) are most commonly used.

Other methods of surface evaluation are also sometimes useful. For example, the polynuclear aromatic hydrocarbons fluoresce readily when irradiated with ultraviolet light, and this characteristic can be used to make qualitative surveys of areas where contamination is feared.

PHYSICAL AGENT EVALUATION

Evaluation of physical agents requires specialized equipment that is often not routinely available (except for sound level meters). Evaluation of ionizing or nonionizing radiation requires specialized training, but many industrial hygienists have developed expertise in these evaluations.

Noise Exposure Evaluation

Evaluation of exposures to noise is a traditional industrial hygiene function. The equipment used is of 2 principal types.

A. Sound Level Meters: Sound level meters consist of a microphone and associated electronic circuitry, with a meter that gives a readout in decibels. The circuitry typically contain filtering circuits that permit evaluation of exposures to components of the noise spectrum weighted in accordance with their effects upon hearing. The "A weighting" network has been adopted as the standard for determination of occupational noise exposure. In this weighting scheme, the very low and very high frequencies are

suppressed, and the middle frequencies (1000–6000 Hz) are slightly accentuated. This gives primacy to the "speech frequencies."

Noise level meters may be fitted with filtering circuits for determination of noise levels within specified band widths. One octave or (less commonly) one-third octave band width circuits are often employed. With such devices, it is possible to isolate and identify the specific frequencies of occurrence of the noise. This identification of sources is essential to control in complex noise environments.

A sound level meter is shown in use in Fig 38–3. Note that the instrument is used to measure noise intensity in an area.

B. Noise Dosimetry: Noise dosimeters employ a recording circuit consisting of a small microphone placed close to the ear of the worker to record noise exposure. The devices may either give an overall integrated average exposure for the course of the measurement period or a readout showing exposure as a function of time. Dosimetry is the preferred approach, since the exposures measured are specific and unique to the individual, and offers the same advantage over area sampling as indicated above for breathing zone sampling for airborne contaminants. Fig 38–4 shows the use of a dosimeter. Note that the microphone is located close to the worker's ear.

OBSERVATIONS OF WORK PRACTICES & PROCESS VARIABLES

Exposures often vary substantially from time to time during a day, week, month, or year. The work practices employed by workers whose exposures are measured should be observed during the monitoring period. The description of the workplace must include personal protective devices so that an estimation of "true exposure" (actual intake of chemical into the worker's body) can be derived.

Ventilation equipment and other engineering controls must also be evaluated, so that sampling results are placed in a sensible context.

Workers and supervisors will ordinarily be able to estimate how closely conditions during the survey period approximate "usual" conditions.

General conditions in the workplace, including such things as whether windows and doors are open or closed, must also be evaluated and recorded.

The ideal industrial hygiene report will be detailed enough so that another industrial hygienist entering the workplace later will be able to determine whether conditions are the same as or different from those that existed during the survey period.

COMPARISON WITH STANDARDS

The industrial hygienist must determine whether exposures measured are likely to cause harm to those exposed. If such harm seems likely, action must be taken to reduce exposures to tolerable levels. (See Control of Health Hazards, below.) In most cases,

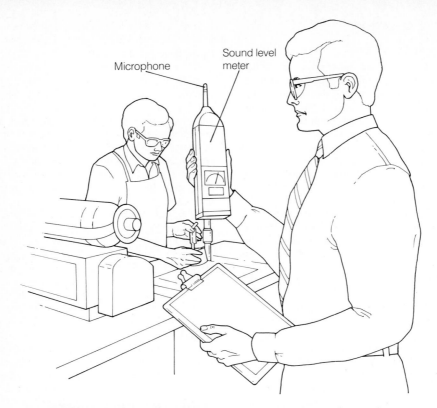

Figure 38–3. Industrial hygienist using a sound level meter in a work area.

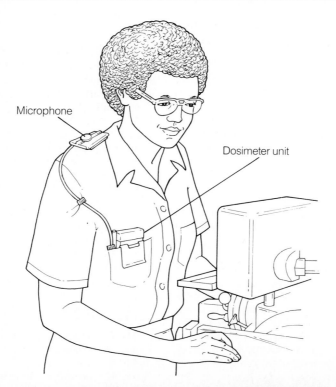

Figure 38–4. Worker wearing a noise dosimeter with a microphone located close to the ear.

the industrial hygienist will refer to a set of standards for various individual chemical contaminants or physical agents. Exposures are acceptable (1) if the measured concentrations are less than the allowable upper limit and (2) if exposures are unlikely to rise above that allowable limit.

Occupational Exposure Standards for Airborne Contaminants

Lists of occupational exposure standards for airborne contaminants have been available for over 50 years. The first standards were for a few widely recognized health hazards, such as lead, mercury, and benzene. Currently, hundreds of chemicals and physical agents are either regulated (eg, by federal or state OSHA programs) or have recommended control limits (from NIOSH or voluntary organizations). In the USA, standards are derived from the following sources:

(1) The American Conference of Governmental Industrial Hygienists Threshold Limit Values (TLVs) (*Threshold Limit Values and Biological Exposure Indices for 1988–1989,* American Conference of Governmental Industrial Hygienists, 6500 Glenway Avenue, Bldg. D-7, Cincinnati, OH 45211–4438.)

(2) The Recommended Exposure Levels (RELs) of the National Institute for Occupational Safety and Health *(NIOSH Recommendations for Occupational Safety and Health Standards, 1988, Morbidity and Mortality Weekly Report* (Supplement) August 26, 1988/Vol. 37/No. 5–7, Centers for Disease Control, Atlanta, GA 30333.)

(3) The Permissible Exposure Limits (PELs) of the Occupational Safety and Health Administration. *(Air Contaminants–Permissible Exposure Limits* [OSHA Publication 3112, available from OSHA Regional Offices; see Chapter 2.] Full text of standards published in the Federal Register, January 19, 1989, Vol. 54, No. 12, pp 2332–2983.)

Only the OSHA PELs (and similar lists prepared by some state OSHA programs) are legally enforceable. The TLVs and RELs should be considered advisory.

Threshold Limit Values

Of the sets of standards to which industrial hygienists have reference in this regard, the most important (in the USA) is the table of "threshold limit values" (TLVs) published annually by the Threshold Limit Values Committee of the American Conference of Governmental Industrial Hygienists (ACGIH). This listing has been published annually since the mid 1940s and is used not only in the USA but in other countries as well. In 1970, upon enactment of OSHA, the 1968 TLVs were adopted and given the status of law. In their incarnation as OSHA regulations, they have been named "permissible exposure limits" (PELs). ACGIH also publishes a loose-leaf binder (updated periodically) in which are set forth the data on which the TLVs are based.

The TLVs include values for chemical substances, physical agents (heat, ionizing radiation, lasers, noise and vibration, radio frequency and microwave radiation, ultraviolet and infrared radiation, and visible light). A section added recently sets forth biologic exposure indices for a few chemicals for which well-established acceptable levels of the parent chemical or its metabolites in body fluids have been documented. The ACGIH Biological Exposure Indices (BEIs) are discussed in Chapter 34.

Despite warnings to the contrary in the ACGIH booklet, many people improperly consider TLVs (and PELs) as "safe levels." However, TLVs have always been intended only as guidelines for control of workplace atmospheres by personnel with adequate training and experience in industrial hygiene. The following is quoted (bold emphasis in the original) from the ACGIH publication, *TLVs: Threshold Limit Values and Biological Exposure Indices for 1988–1989:*

> These limits are intended for use in the practice of industrial hygiene as guidelines or recommendations in the control of potential health hazards and for no other use, eg, in the evaluation or control of community air pollution nuisances, in estimating the toxic potential of continuous, uninterrupted exposures or other extended work periods, as proof or disproof of an existing disease or physical condition, or adoption by countries whose working conditions differ from those in the United States of America and where substances and processes differ. These limits *are not* fine lines between safe and dangerous concentration nor are they a relative index of toxicity, and *should not* be used by anyone untrained in the discipline of industrial hygiene.

Too many personnel (both industrial hygienists and others) interpreting occupational exposure measurements have implied that exposures just beneath the TLVs are acceptable. In fact, it has always been considered good practice to hold exposures to the minimum practically possible—ie, no unnecessary exposure to any toxic material should be tolerated. In some cases it is necessary, because of economic or engineering factors, to expose workers to levels greater than zero (ambient) levels. In such cases, the TLVs should be used as a guide to the *maximum* tolerable exposure levels. (The equivalent German values are in fact entitled, in English translation, Maximum Allowable Concentrations, which was the title of the threshold limit values for several years in the past.) It is emphasized again that the TLVs—or the OSHA PELs and the NIOSH RELs—represent *maximum allowable* exposure levels. The industrial hygienist or physician should attempt to hold exposures to the lowest level practically possible or to a level at which risk is "acceptable."

There is no environment which is risk-free; a "safe" environment is one in which the level of risk is acceptable.

It should also be recognized the OSHA PELs were not significantly modified between 1970 and 1989.

Only a few substances have been added to those regulated, and for a few more the allowable exposures were reduced. Substantial and significant changes were made in the TLVs in that period. Thus, certain exposures that were generally agreed to be potentially harmful were acceptable to OSHA during the 1970s and 1980s.

Because some of those exposed may develop disease as a consequence of lifetime exposures at the TLV level, many organizations have adopted a policy of setting standards at some fraction of the TLV. Ten percent, 25%, or 50% of the TLV may be designated the internal control level. Some companies have gone so far as to attempt to remove all contamination from workplace atmospheres. In such cases, any detectable odor or irritation is considered to be unacceptable, and control measures are instituted to reduce exposures when any process effluvia are detected.

Other Sources of Standards

Several other sources of recommended exposure limits are available to the industrial hygienist. Among these are the Workplace Environmental Exposure Limits promulgated by the American Industrial Hygiene Association for several chemicals not listed by the TLV Committee. Another set of references of value in determining allowable exposures are the various "Criteria Documents" of NIOSH. In this set of documents, NIOSH has provided an evaluation of the literature, recommended control measures, and recommended upper limits for exposures. Many of the allowable exposure recommendations of NIOSH are lower than the recommended TLVs for the same chemicals.

Industrial experience, new developments in technology, and available scientific data clearly indicate that in many instances those adopted limits are now obsolete and inadequate. Furthermore, many new toxic materials commonly used in the workplace are not covered. These inadequacies are evidenced by the lower allowable exposure limits recommended by many technical, professional, industrial, and government organizations in the United States and elsewhere. In addition, these organizations have identified many other substances for which allowable exposure limits are needed to supplement the existing OSHA PELs with their own internal corporate guidelines.

Although many countries outside the USA have adopted the ACGIH TLVs without substantial modification, several have active committees evaluating allowable exposure limits. The International Labor Office has published, in tabular form, the occupational exposure limits for airborne toxic substances from all countries (ILO, 1980). This tabulation is very useful in identifying substances for which exposure limits lower than the TLVs might reasonably be established.

Where no established standards are available for guidance, in-house research may be necessary to establish guidelines. Where a chemical not previously used is being widely adopted in a particular industry, a trade association study of the effects of that chemical may be an appropriate venue for such research. Because of the potential risks associated with subtle health effects not easily foreseen, such control limits should be established only with great caution.

The monitoring process is, in the statistical sense, a "sampling" process. If there is no systematic bias in the measurements made, it can be presumed that the measurements are accurate.

However, all industrial hygiene measurements are subject to imprecision and inaccuracy because of sampling and analytic errors. Therefore, it is prudent to construct confidence intervals about the sample means, so that the range within which the true average concentration may be expected to fall is known. The upper 95% confidence limit should fall below the allowable exposure limit before it can be stated that the concentration is probably below that standard.

A precautionary note is in order. Because of the inherently great dispersion of environmental data, it should be presumed that the data are log-normally distributed and the logarithmic transformation of individual data points should be performed before the data are evaluated. The "geometric mean" (the inverse log of the average of the logarithms of the data points) is usually an appropriate measure of central tendency when evaluating environmental data.

CONTROL OF HEALTH HAZARDS

Upon completion of the evaluation, the industrial hygienist should be in a position to recommend appropriate controls, if needed. Recommendations should take into account not only the conditions found during the survey but also those that may be expected to prevail in the future. Controls should be adequate to prevent unnecessary exposure during accidents and emergencies as well as during normal operating conditions. Planned process modifications should be taken into account, and recommendations should be adaptable to future needs.

Consideration must be given to "fail-safe" operation of controls—ie, recommended controls should always operate to protect workers regardless of process fluctuations.

Substitution

All possibilities for substitution of a nontoxic for a toxic material or agent should be explored. If a toxic material can be dispensed with and a less harmful material substituted, that should be done. Substitution can of course only be done if a useful substitute is available—one that is suitable for existing processes or for which the processes can be relatively easily adapted.

This obvious approach must be undertaken with caution, however, since several instances have been known where an apparently harmless substitute for an obvious hazard was later found to be harmful in and of itself.

Engineering Controls

Engineering controls on toxic exposures consist mainly of enclosure (building structures around the sources of emissions), isolation (placing hazardous process components in areas with limited human contact), and ventilation.

A. Ventilation: Local exhaust ventilation conforms to the principle that control should be implemented as near to the source as practically possible. Thus, application of a local exhaust inlet on a specific tool (such as a grinder) would be inherently more desirable than performing the grinding operation in a ventilated hood, which in turn would be more desirable than installing general ventilation in the room where the grinding is performed. In a situation where a very toxic substance is being manipulated in such a way that exposure is possible, all 3 ventilation systems might be reasonable to use. Thus, the operator would be protected by ventilation of the specific tool, nearby workers (as well as the operator) would be protected by the hood and the remainder of the building would be protected by the general ventilation system. Fig 38–5 is a conceptual model of a "typical" operation, showing the 3 zones of control required.

Design of ventilation systems for contamination control should ordinarily not be left to engineers without specific background or experience. Similarly, an industrial hygienist without engineering training and experience in the processes to be controlled may produce an unsatisfactory design.

ACGIH publishes a biennial document on industrial ventilation that provides guidance on the principles of ventilation control.

B. Other Engineering Controls: In addition to ventilation, enclosure, and isolation, some specific engineering controls may be appropriate in the specific process environment. It is, for example, often necessary to design process pipelines and valves to minimize splashes and ejection of toxic chemicals. Control systems that will permit safe and orderly shutdown of the process to avoid runaway reactions may also be of substantial benefit.

Controls on Human Behavior

These can be subdivided into the general categories of administrative controls and work practice controls.

A. Administrative Controls: Control of behavior patterns within the process environment includes such things as establishment of prohibited areas, areas where smoking and eating are either prohibited or allowed, and safe pathways through the work environment. Administrative controls will also include work scheduling in such a way that dangerous operations are carried out when the fewest workers are present.

Less desirable is the practice of scheduling individual workers to perform tasks for short periods, where excessive exposures would be incurred over an extended period of time. This practice was at one time common in the nuclear power industry, where temporary employees were used to perform maintenance tasks in high radiation environments. These "jumpers" were employed and paid by the day, although their actual work period may have been as short as 15 minutes. Such practices, where exposure to carcinogenic or genotoxic agents is spread across a larger population group although individual exposures are lower, is entirely unacceptable. While the individual risk may be relatively low, the effect of distributing an exposure with potential genetic effects to many members of the population is inherently unsound.

On the other hand, administrative controls that include scheduling are usually essential to control of the work environment. An example is prohibiting personnel who do not have adequate training from entry into spaces where health or safety hazards exist.

B. Work Practices Control: Control of work practices implies control over the behavior of individual workers on the job. Such details as handling of contaminated tools and appliances are included. Education (on the hazards to be avoided) and training (on the desired practices) are of course required. Close supervision of workers is needed in order to enforce compliance with proper work practices. Controls on work practices are particularly important where engineering controls are either not adequate or not possible and where there is significant potential for generation of airborne contaminants outside of controlled spaces.

Personal Protection

Personal protective equipment use, though often essential, is less desirable than other approaches because of the difficulty in ensuring that it is both used and effective. Examples on construction sites are "hard hats" and "safety shoes." In laboratory environments, the use of protective eyewear is common, as is the use of protective garments, such as laboratory coats.

However, there are significant complexities in both design and function of the protective devices used to reduce exposures.

A worker who is issued and is wearing a "respirator," for example, may feel adequately protected from all potential hazards in the workplace and may therefore neglect the use of engineering controls, may violate administrative control guidelines, and may ignore required work practices. In fact, without substantial attention to selection, fitting, training, and maintenance of respirators, exposures during their use may be nearly as high as for those of "unprotected" workers.

Respirators are often handed out without adequate attention to any of these precautions. It is common, for example, to see workers with beards wearing air-purifying respirators in areas where contaminants are present in the air. The devices are of course useless unless they fit tightly, which is impossible if the wearer has a lot of facial hair.

Similarly, gloves protect against exposure to solvents and other toxicants only if chosen with knowledge of what materials are suitable in each case. (See Table 17–3 for some examples.) In addition, prolonged wearing of gloves into which skin hazardous materials have either leached or leaked through holes may result in substantial exposure to the worker (sometimes higher than would occur without the gloves).

Integrated Control

A well-regulated control program in a company with diverse operations will usually employ all of the modes mentioned above plus adequate housekeeping and disposal of waste materials. It is emphasized

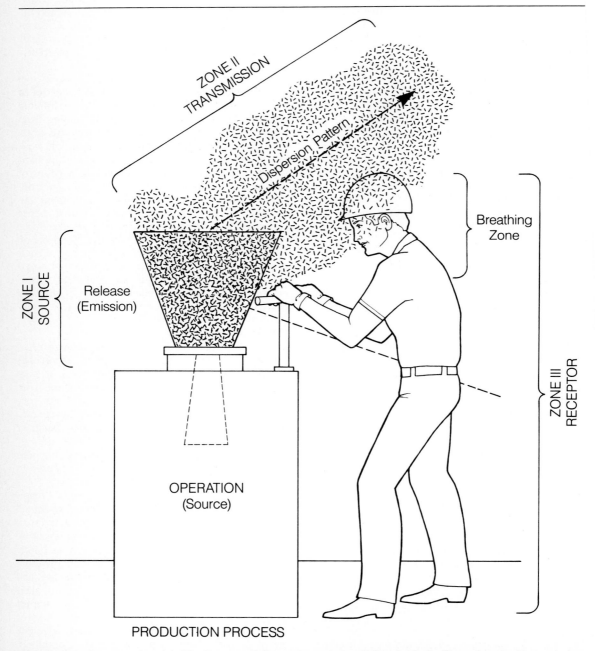

Figure 38–5. Conceptual model of the 3 zones of influence to control workplace hazards. (Reproduced, with permission, from Corn M: The role of control technologies in preventing occupational disease. *Arch Environ Health* 1984;**39**:235.)

again that substitution should be the first consideration. Where substitution cannot be rationally adopted, isolation of workers from exposure and enclosure of sources should be next considered. If no substitute material is readily available and if complete isolation and enclosure are not possible, local exhaust ventilation should be next considered. General exhaust ventilation is a useful supplement to local exhaust ventilation and should be part of the ventilation design.

When none of these engineering controls can completely abate the hazard, administrative controls, work practices controls, and personal protection may be necessary.

The controls process must be viewed as a continuing one in which existing controls are continually evaluated for their effectiveness. Equipment ages, personnel change, processes evolve, and the level of management attention to control varies with time. All of these forces act to change the effectiveness of a given control. The evaluation of effectiveness is the province of the industrial hygienist, who must involve managers, engineers, and workers in the evaluation.

REFERENCES

General Industrial Hygiene

*Clayton GD, Clayton FE (editors): *Patty's Industrial Hygiene and Toxicology,* 3rd ed. Vol 1: *General Principles;* Vols 2 A–C: *Toxicology;* Vol 3A: *The Work Environment.* Vol 3B: *Biological Responses.* Mosby, 1978–1985.

Parmeggiani L (editor): *Encyclopedia of Occupational Health and Safety,* 3rd ed. 2 vols. International Labor Office, 1983.

*Plog BA (editor): *Fundamentals of Industrial Hygiene,* 3rd ed. National Safety Council, 1989.

Occupational Exposure Standards

Air contaminants. In: *General Industry OSHA Safety and Health Standards.* OSHA Publication No. 2206. US Government Printing Office, 1983.

Documentation of the Threshold Limit Values and Biological Exposure Indices. ACGIH, 1986.

NIOSH *Recommendations for OSHA Standards.* HHS Publication No. (CDC) 86-8017.

Threshold Limit Values for Chemical Substances and Physical Agents in the Work Environment and Biological Exposure Indices. ACHIG (annual).

Sampling & Analysis

Air Sampling Instruments, 7th ed. ACGIH, 1990.

NIOSH *Manual of Analytical Methods,* 3rd ed. USD-HHS (NIOSH) Publication No. 84-100. US Government Printing Office, 1985.

Chemical Processes

*Cralley L, Cralley L: *Industrial Hygiene Aspects of Plant Operations.* Vol 1: *Process Flows;* Vol 2: *Unit Operations and Product Fabrication;* Vol 3: *Engineering Considerations.* Macmillan, 1982–1985.

*Grayson M (editor): *Kirk-Othner's Concise Encyclopedia of Chemical Technology,* 3rd ed. 24 vols. Wiley, 1985.

Kirk-Othner's Encyclopedia of Chemical Technology, 3rd ed. 24 vols. Wiley, 1978–1984.

*Available from: American Conference of Governmental Industrial Hygienists, 6500 Glenway Avenue, Building D-7, Cincinnati, OH 45211. (513) 661–7881.

39

Environmental Health

Joseph LaDou, MD

Beginning with the industrial revolution in England in the late 18th century, environmental contamination has increased steadily throughout the world—and radically so since World War II. The technologic advances of the past 40 years have resulted in toxic hazards that proliferate each year as new materials and new methods of production are introduced.

Government at all levels, as well as the public, are becoming increasingly concerned about contamination of the environment. Widely publicized disasters such as those at Bhopal, Chernobyl, and Minamata Bay have emphasized these concerns, and similar events not so widely publicized are equally important.

Occupational physicians are today increasingly concerned with problems of environmental health. The physician must be concerned with contamination outside the workplace as well as within and knowledgeable about disposal of toxic wastes emanating from the workplace. The general practice physician must also understand the effects of toxic environmental exposures, and the requirement for greater awareness in this area extends also to public health officials and environmentalists.

To control all naturally occurring contaminants in the environment would be an impossible task. To control the toxic hazards we ourselves introduce into the environment is at least theoretically possible given sufficient resources and the will to do so.

THE MAGNITUDE OF ENVIRONMENTAL CONTAMINATION

All industrialized nations are faced with serious problems of environmental contamination, and Third World countries will have to deal with the same difficulties as their industrialization progresses. Since one-fourth of the world's population live in industrialized societies where most environmental contaminants are produced, 1.25 billion people may be exposed on a daily basis to contaminants in the air, water, and soil.

USA industries produce more than 250 million tons of hazardous wastes each year, or approximately 1 ton per person, and this figure may double by the end of the century. To compound the problem, in the USA there are over 500,000 hazardous waste dump sites and contaminated pits, ponds, and lagoons.

The air in urban areas is heavily polluted by the annual release of 440 million pounds of xylene and 1.37 billion pounds of toluene as automotive exhaust gases. Even the water we drink may be unhealthful, as indicated by the fact that water samples from 16.8% of systems serving fewer than 10,000 persons and 28% of those supplying more than 10,000 persons contain at least one volatile organic compound.

Rural areas become contaminated because of the injudicious use of pesticides and herbicides in agriculture. Forests and fisheries are decimated by sulfur and nitrogen emissions carried by wind and rain from industrial centers.

The vast size of the subject population and the proliferation of new materials with unknown effects introduced by advancing technology have made it critical that we find some means of controlling the possible deleterious health effects of environmental contaminants. Unfortunately, we know little about what these effects will be, particularly over the long term, and epidemiologic studies—our primary source of information—cannot answer many of our questions.

PRIMARY SOURCES OF CONTAMINATION

Chemical manufacturing is one of the main sources of environmental contamination. Others include pulp and paper milling, petroleum production, smelting, textile manufacturing, and mining. All these activities produce particulates or dusts that contaminate air or water.

Internal combustion engines using gasoline as fuel also contribute heavily to air pollution. Federal and state restrictions on automotive output of particulates have reduced the problem somewhat, but there are still older motor vehicles in use, so that contaminants continue to be discharged into the environment in unacceptable quantities.

Agriculture is a major contributor to environmental contamination through the extensive use of pesticides and herbicides. As insects adapt to survive contact with currently used pesticides, new and more potent ones are produced. These substances contaminate not only surface and underground waters but also the land itself as well as the food it produces.

MAJOR ENVIRONMENTAL CONTAMINANTS

Of all the contaminants that human commercial ingenuity has introduced into the environment, probably the most publicized are asbestos, lead, dioxins, and polychlorinated biphenyls (PCBs). All are highly toxic and persist for long periods in the environment.

ASBESTOS

The mineral asbestos is a family of fibrous hydrated silicates that is one of the most pervasive environmental hazards in the world. Asbestos occurs naturally in the form of serpentine rock. It contaminates drinking water both through the natural erosion of surface rock formations and by the breakdown of asbestos-containing products made by humans. Because of its resistance to thermal and corrosive destruction and the tensile strength asbestos confers, it has been used in more than 100,000 miles of water mains and sewage pipes in the USA.

Asbestos is found in the drinking water of most Americans, usually less than 1 million fibers per liter. Some water supplies contain over 1 billion fibers per liter, and where water flows through natural areas of asbestos, the concentrations in drinking water are over 10 billion fibers per liter.

Asbestos is present in over 3000 manufactured products, and more than 30 million tons of asbestos in its various forms have been mined since the turn of the century. To many, its perceived benefits outweigh the importance of preventing further asbestos contamination of the environment. Many countries have considered a ban on the mining and uses of asbestos only to begin a long process of granting exceptions to maintain competitive positions in world trade.

Major Health Effects

Asbestos is inhaled in dust particles that lodge in the lungs and usually remain there. It can result in asbestosis, a chronic reaction of the lungs accompanied by fibroid induration; lung cancer; and mesothelioma, a tumor arising in the membranes lining the pleural and peritoneal cavities. By the 1930s, asbestosis was generally regarded as a hazard to persons working with asbestos fibers in manufacturing. Although the risk of lung cancer was suspected at that time, it was not until the mid 1950s that the causal link was firmly established. Mesothelioma resulting from asbestos exposure was not demonstrated until 1960. The danger of this mineral is exemplified by the experience of 8–11 million shipyard workers from World War II into the 1960s. Approximately 50% of all deaths among this group resulted from lung cancer or other asbestos-related diseases. At present, there are questions about whether cancer of the gastrointestinal or genitourinary tract may result from ingestion of asbestos fibers.

Sources of Exposure

Asbestos fibers enter the body either by inhalation or by ingestion. Not only are asbestos workers at risk from inhaling the fibers, but a large proportion of the population is at the same risk from the breakdown of manifold products in which it has been incorporated. They are in our homes, our schools, and our public places in the form of insulation products and other structural materials and even in paving materials for parking areas and paved playgrounds.

Ingestion of the fibers comes primarily from drinking water contaminated either from natural sources or from asbestos-reinforced concrete water pipes as they gradually deteriorate. It has recently been demonstrated that asbestos fibers are present in a number of foods—particularly processed foods—and other ingestible items. Sizeable numbers of fibers have been found in everything from aspirin tablets to chewing gum. They occur also in mayonnaise, lard, catsup, sticky rice, and many other foods that have been shown to contribute more than a million fibers a day to the typical diet.

Epidemiologic studies to date that compare populations drinking high concentrations of asbestos in water with low-exposure groups have failed to demonstrate an increased rate of gastrointestinal and genitourinary cancers in the high exposure groups. But the studies are seriously flawed because the fibers in foods were not taken into account. Future studies will be difficult to conduct because there is no readily available technique for assaying the asbestos content of various foods. Asbestos in drinking water and foods may be a carcinogen of major significance, but in the absence of a control group it will be difficult to measure the effects in humans.

The level of exposure that produces asbestosis can be determined with relative reliability, but it has not been possible to determine a dose level that produces a finite risk of cancer in humans. It is known, however, that a far smaller dose is required for developing cancer than for developing asbestosis. Unfortunately, occupational standards for asbestos exposure have until very recently dealt only with risk estimates for asbestosis. Variation in state and federal protection standards for workers reflect this inherent problem.

Controlling the Problem

It may not ever be possible to fully control asbestos exposure. Asbestos is ubiquitous in our environment, and there is no way in which the enormous quantities already used can be removed. In many instances, experts agree that methods of containment are far more practical than efforts at removal.

The Environmental Protection Agency (EPA) has directed all schools to inspect their facilities for the presence of asbestos-containing products and to inform parents and school employees of the possibility of exposure. The agency has not provided information about the risks of exposure.

Asbestos exposure in the ambient air of many urban areas is higher than it is in buildings containing asbestos products. One study of the risk to students exposed to an average asbestos concentration of 0.001 fiber/mL of schoolroom air for an average enrollment period of 6 school years is about 5 lifetime excess cancers per million students.

LEAD

Lead is a highly toxic heavy metal that contaminates all of the environment but especially urban centers. Lead is used in the manufacture of storage batteries, gasoline additives, printing, radiation shielding, cable covering, solder, foil, paint (though this use has been considerably reduced), and numerous alloys. Workers may carry lead dust into their homes on their clothing, thus exposing their families. One estimate is that the average city dweller discards into the trash over 40 lb of lead annually. Lead contaminates the environment through emissions from older motor vehicles that burn lead-containing gasoline, and an estimated 45% of gasoline sold in the USA contains lead. Little progress is being made in the reduction of lead from smelting emissions. Worldwide, atmospheric lead emissions have increased 2000-fold since the pre-Roman era, when lead was already being mined.

Major Health Effects

Lead is highly toxic by inhalation or ingestion of either dust or fumes. The toxicology of lead exposure in adults is discussed in Chapter 25. In pregnant women, such exposure is associated with a wide range of reproductive problems.

Children are particularly susceptible to the toxic effects of lead. Excessive absorption of lead dust is one of the most prevalent and preventable of debilitating childhood health problems. Each year in the USA, 200 children die from lead poisoning. Of the 12,000–16,000 who are treated and survive, 25% suffer permanent damage to the central nervous system. Many studies support the finding that moderate elevations of blood lead in children (40–70 μg/dL) result in significant impairment of cognitive, verbal, perceptual, and fine motor skills.

Sources of Exposure

There are many sources of lead exposure in the home and environment. Homes built before 1940 contain lead in a variety of construction products including insulation, paint, interior woodwork, and wallpaper. Many common household items also contain significant quantities of lead. Brightly colored magazine pages may be significantly contaminated with lead. Printed food wrappers, handles of kitchen utensils, and the seals on bottles of wine may serve as exposure opportunities for both adults and children.

Acid foods and beverages dissolve lead from improperly glazed earthenware pottery. Copper pipes conveying drinking water through lead-soldered joints are a common source of lead exposure.

The average body burden of lead among children and adults in the USA is 100 times greater than the "natural burden," and the rate of lead absorption is now roughly 30 times greater than in preindustrial societies. Epidemiologic studies of children and adults living in urban areas reveal that the amount of lead in the body is directly proportionate to the amount of lead in the air. Between 10% and 50% of urban children demonstrate a chronic body lead burden (> 40 μg/dL of blood lead). The more than 500,000 children between the ages of 6 months and 5 years in this country with blood lead concentrations of at least 30 μg/dL—considered by the Centers for Disease Control to represent excessive lead absorption—indicate the extent of the environmental health issue presented by this pervasive toxin. The current definition of "elevated blood lead" in whole blood of children is 25 μg/dL or more. Lead toxicity occurs when an elevated blood lead is accompanied by an erythrocyte protoporphyrin (EP) level in whole blood of 35 μg/dL or greater.

Controlling the Problem

The control of lead dusts and fumes in the environment is a large undertaking. To date, some important steps have been taken in that direction, notably (1) the concerted effort to restrict lead-containing emissions from motor vehicle exhausts, (2) the restriction on use of lead in paint, and (3) the requirement that smelters and other lead-related industries install equipment to control their emissions. Companies that work with lead are also required to install exhaust equipment that will protect workers from exposure to hazardous levels of the toxin. Furthermore, because of known reproductive effects, women of child-bearing age are no longer permitted to work in lead products operations. Workers should be required to shower and change clothes after their shifts so as not to carry lead dust out of the workplace.

There are circumstances that tend to frustrate control efforts. First, the nation has thousands of older homes where lead is inherent in the structure—in paint, woodwork, insulation, and water systems that contain lead pipe. Second, older motor vehicles continue to emit lead into the atmosphere. Finally, the emission control devices used on smelters and other industrial emitters of lead dusts and fumes are not totally effective. It is unfortunately true also that managers in industry are not in all cases committed to the idea of controlling the problem.

DIOXIN

Dioxin (see 2,3,7,8-TCDD in Chapter 26) is a trace contaminant of the chlorinated hydrocarbon

2,4,5-trichlorophenoxyacetic acid (2,4,5-T). After the neurotoxin botulin and some nerve gases and other weapons of chemical warfare, it is the most toxic substance known. Moreover, it is highly stable in the environment. It has been widely distributed in herbicides throughout the USA and was a contaminant of the defoliant Agent Orange (a mixture of equal parts of 2,4-D and 2,4,5-T), used on rice paddies, trails, and jungles during the Vietnam War. Dioxin's contamination of products used in this country to control weeds in lawns, along highways, and in utility and railroad right-of-ways—and in commercial forests—may have adverse health effects.

Major Health Effects

The known near-term effect of exposure to dioxin is chloracne, a severe form of acne that persists for long periods. In 1976, an explosion at a chemical factory in Seveso, Italy, exposed the nearby town to a cloud of dioxin and other contaminants. Four percent of the population, including many children, suffered chloracne. The long-term effects of this exposure remain to be determined.

Although dioxin has been found to produce carcinogenic and teratogenic effects in some laboratory animals at uniformly low doses and has been lethal to some species at doses of less than 1 µg/kg of body weight, little has been determined about the long-term effect in humans.

The many Vietnamese exposed to dioxin from Agent Orange would be an excellent subject population for epidemiologic studies, but the difficulty of conducting such studies is obvious. However, thousands of US service personnel were also exposed and are currently the subject of numerous studies. To date, this group has shown no increased risks of fathering children with birth defects, but early findings will continue to be challenged. Similarly, the population of Seveso will continue to be monitored.

Determining the health effects of dioxin exposure is made difficult by differences in interpretation of epidemiologic data. For example, one expert interpreted the Seveso findings as demonstrating "only mild cases of chloracne, and no significant change in the incidence of spontaneous abortions, congenital malformations, or postnatal development." Another noted "a sharp increase in spontaneous abortions during the first trimester of 1977, followed by a slow decrease to 1976 levels and a significant increase in the risk of malformation." Interpretations of Seveso data on reproductive effects is complicated by the number of abortions that were permitted by Catholic Church and government authorities after the accident.

Sources of Exposure

Exposure to dioxin is possible wherever the substance has been indiscriminately used as a herbicide. In Times Beach, Missouri, for example, 10 years before the danger of dioxin was fully recognized, waste oils containing dioxin were sprayed on roads to control dust. This created such outrage in the community—with extensive media coverage—that the EPA ordered the area closed and the federal government actually paid for the deserted houses in the evacuated area.

Aside from areas of large accidental release or deliberate spraying, as in Seveso and Vietnam, the most important source of exposure is in the use or manufacture of herbicides and in the combustion products of low-temperature incineration. Many older incinerators in Europe and the USA have been closed because of dioxin emissions even though there is no American standard for incinerator emissions or human exposure.

Controlling the Problem

The only means of controlling the problem of dioxin contamination of the environment is to outlaw its further presence in plant hormones, herbicides, and defoliants and to control its emissions in waste burning operations.

POLYCHLORINATED BIPHENYLS

Polychlorinated biphenyls (PCBs) are biphenyls extracted from petroleum and chlorinated in the presence of a catalyst, usually iron. PCBs were manufactured in the USA between 1929 and 1977. Because of their stability, high boiling point, and low electrical conductivity, they were used primarily as coolants for electrical transformers; as dielectrics for electrical capacitors; and in stone-cutting oils, hydraulic fluids, and heat transfer fluids. They were also used as plasticizers, in carbonless multicopy office forms, and as constituents of paints and objective immersion oils for microscopes. Although their manufacture is no longer permitted, total PCBs currently in the environment exceed 500 million pounds, and 750 million pounds are still in use in capacitors and transformers. PCBs are thus a continuing danger in the environment.

Health Effects

PCBs are stored in body fat, and it is believed that exposure has been widespread in industrialized nations. In the USA, almost everyone has detectable amounts of PCBs in the body.

Pregnant women working in low-exposure areas produce premature infants of significantly lower birth weight. Newborn infants whose mothers consumed moderate quantities of lake fish contaminated with PCBs had lower birth weights and smaller head circumferences. Lactating mothers have been shown to transmit the toxins in milk.

PCBs cause hepatocellular carcinoma in rats. Although carcinogenic effects to date have not been established in humans, numerous other deleterious health effects have been determined. Much of what is known about the toxicity of PCBs in humans resulted from an incident in Japan in 1968, when an accidental leak in a rice oil processing plant caused high levels of PCBs (and furans) in the cooking oil. In a matter of weeks, consumers of the oil were ill and exhibited mild to severe chloracne; hyperpigmentation of the skin, nails, conjunctiva, and mucous membranes; liver disease, including necrosis; fatigue; headache; menstrual disorders; palpebral edema and meibomian gland hypersecretion; and birth defects, usually hyperpigmentation. Nursing infants who had not ingested the oil also showed symptoms, indicating that the mother's milk may have transmitted the toxin.

A similar event occurred in Taiwan in 1979. Rice cooking oil was contaminated by polychlorinated dibenzofurans and PCBs as well as a wide variety of other chemicals and their isomers. By the end of 1980, there were a reported 1843 cases of PCB poisoning from 4 counties in central Taiwan. The latent period from time of ingestion to the manifestation of clinical symptoms was approximately 3–4 months. After 3.5 years, 2061 persons were determined to have PCB poisoning. Thirty-nine infants born to PCB-exposed mothers showed hyperpigmentation. In the Taiwan case, the fatality rate was relatively high. By the end of 1980, eight of the exposed group had died; and by the end of 1983, twenty-four more had died. Almost half had died from hepatomas, liver cirrhosis, or liver disease with hepatomegaly.

Children born to affected women were shorter and lighter than controls. Delays of developmental milestones were observed, along with abnormalities noted on behavioral and developmental testing. The findings of growth abnormalities and hyperpigmentation, persistent conjunctival swelling, and abnormalities of nails, hair, teeth, and gums are generally consistent with an acquired neuroectodermal dysplasia.

It is not yet known whether the health effects of such major exposures are similar to those of long-term, low-level exposures that are occurring in many areas. Over prolonged periods, the moderate consumption of contaminated fish may show similar effects.

Sources of Exposure

Accidental leaks of PCBs are the primary source of exposure. Such leaks can contaminate surface and groundwaters and contaminate freshwater fish. We have seen the devastating health effects of leaks in Japan and Taiwan.

Controlling the Problem

Solving the problem of PCB contamination of the environment will require the efforts of both the government and the electrical utilities—the government in locating the dangerous discards, and the utilities in carefully monitoring units still in use and discarding others properly. Further study will be needed on health effects of PCBs and on safe and effective means of disposing of these contaminants.

THE PROBLEM OF AIR POLLUTION

Clean air is a mixture of gases with tiny particles contained in it. It consists of approximately 78% nitrogen and 21% oxygen, less than 1% of carbon dioxide and argon, and trace amounts of other gases. This is the air we breathe on clear days in the high mountains. Air that is blown in from the ocean may contain minute particles of salt, and air blown over land usually contains fine sand, pollen, plant spores, and other inorganic and organic substances not usually harmful to plants, animals, or humans.

Human societies have added other deleterious substances to the air primarily through the burning of fossil fuels and gasoline. Polluted air contains sulfur dioxide, oxides of nitrogen, hydrocarbons, lead, ozone, and carbon monoxide, among other noxious substances. The chief sources of these contaminants are from vehicle exhausts, domestic heating, forest fires and other open burning, industry, and solid waste disposal. Pollutants are harmful to plants and animals, humans, and property. Although steps have been taken to reduce emissions from both factories and motor vehicles and to restrict outdoor burning, the problem continues as the population increases, with more cars and more use of home heating fuels. The problem is greatest in industrial and urban areas but may be carried to rural areas by winds just as the contamination from Chernobyl was carried around the world. Thus, weather, season, and topography play important roles in acute air pollution. When cooler surface air is trapped under a layer of warmer air (inversion) and cannot rise, the effects of air pollution are compounded. These conditions occur most frequently during the fall and winter and are persistent on the West Coast of the USA. When these inversions occur in combination with a high level of air pollution, the results can be life-threatening because of high concentrations of sulfur dioxide and various particulates.

Weather plays a key role in air pollution effects. Fog and rain can exacerbate the problem, and wind can carry pollutants to cleaner areas.

Health Effects of Air Pollution

Pollutants in air can affect both the skin and the gastrointestinal tract but chiefly cause problems in the respiratory system. Pollutants may be particulates or gases and are taken in with the 10,000–20,000 L of air inspired by a person each day. Each liter of inspired air may contain several million suspended particles. Particles produced by industry and internal combustion engines are the most hazardous: Because of their light weight, they remain in the air for long periods, are easily inhaled, and are liable to contain toxic chemicals.

The possibility of gastrointestinal toxicity from air pollution stems from the methods by which the lungs are cleared of particulates. Virtually all particulates will adhere to any surface they touch. Highly soluble particles, however, will pass into the bloodstream to be metabolized and excreted. This clearance process occurs at 3 areas in the respiratory system: the upper respiratory tract (nasopharynx), the tracheobronchial tree, and the pulmonary alveoli.

In the nasopharynx, particles are deposited on the fine hairs and the walls of narrow passages of the nose. These are cleared by nose blowing, sneezing, coughing, mucociliary action, and swallowing. Less soluble particles that touch the ciliated areas of the nasopharynx are deposited on a mucous blanket that covers the airways and moves particles toward the pharynx, where they mix with saliva and are swallowed. The mucous blanket is critical to clearing particulates from this area of the respiratory system. Particles in the air stream in the tracheobronchial tree are removed by sedimentation and diffusion. Those that are deposited are cleared by coughing or mucociliary action or absorbed into the bronchial blood flow. Particles that are deposited on the pulmonary alveoli are transported to the ciliated epithelium by alveolar macrophages, cells designed to limit particles from penetrating the alveolar wall. These cells have both good and bad effects. Although they are useful in their primary purpose, when they are damaged or die they emit proteolytic enzymes which are thought to contribute to the development of emphysema and other pulmonary diseases. They also tend to aggregate particulates into groups so that their deleterious effects are emphasized.

Particles that are not cleared by the foregoing means may be transported to the lymph circulation and bloodstream. Although they are no longer a threat to the respiratory system, they may cause health problems in other organs.

Air Pollution & Respiratory Disease

The considerable literature on photochemical smog comparing the death rates of persons living in high-risk urban areas to those of persons living in cleaner rural areas has failed to prove a relationship between such exposures and deaths resulting from lung cancer, respiratory failure, or other disorders. Nonetheless, exposure to air pollutants can cause or exacerbate chronic obstructive pulmonary disease, bronchial asthma, acute respiratory disease, and cardiovascular problems.

A. Chronic Obstructive Pulmonary Disease: Chronic obstructive pulmonary disease (COPD) includes emphysema, chronic bronchitis, pneumonia, and a variety of other respiratory problems. Epidemiologic studies relating degrees of air pollution to the incidence of these diseases have been conducted in most industrialized countries. In many, morbidity rates were adjusted for such factors as age, sex, smoking, and occupation, and most have compared the incidence of morbidity in high- and low-pollution areas. Studies of specific pollutants indicated that the sulfur dioxide-particulate combination was the most

damaging. It is not yet clear, however, whether air pollution causes this class of disease or whether it simply compounds preexisting health problems.

B. Bronchial Asthma: Although bronchial asthma is a chronic disease, attacks occur intermittently and may vary in intensity and duration, ranging from mild to severe and even resulting in death. Increased air pollution levels can contribute to acute asthmatic attacks. An early study of the Donora (Pennsylvania) tragedy—see below—revealed that 87.6% of asthmatic individuals in that area experienced symptoms. Most studies of the correlation between increased air pollution and asthmatic attacks have used subjective reports from sufferers or emergency room statistics. The problem of identifying specific causes of such attacks is complicated by a number of other factor: time of day and day of week, temperature, humidity, and emotional stress.

C. Acute Respiratory Infections: Acute respiratory infections in humans have been linked to air pollution by several studies. Animal studies suggest that air pollution (with SO_2, NO_2, and ozone) impairs resistance to such infections. In both children and adults, increased air pollution has been linked with pneumonia and bronchitis.

Second-grade school children exposed to high levels of sulfur dioxide and smoke pollution show diminished ventilatory volumes and a higher incidence of acute respiratory diseases than controls. Children exposed to parental smoking demonstrate symptoms of coughing, wheezing, and sputum production. Children in homes using gas cooking fuel have more coughs than children in homes where electricity is used.

Air Pollution & Cardiovascular Disease

There is little question that airborne pollutants—particularly carbon monoxide—exacerbate cardiovascular problems and may even cause death in individuals with impaired coronary circulation. The incidence of anginal attacks rises during high levels of air pollution. The National Academy of Sciences has estimated that 4000 premature deaths from cardiovascular disease occur annually as a result of exposure to automobile exhausts.

Air Pollution & Lung Cancer

Conclusions about the correlation between air pollution and lung cancer are complicated by the existence of contributory factors such as cigarette smoking and occupational exposure to carcinogens. Although the results of studies have been contradictory, a connection has been suggested by the higher rates of lung cancer in urban as opposed to rural areas. Furthermore, certain carcinogens are known to be present in polluted air. Benzo(a)pyrene, in particular, has been implicated as an ambient pulmonary carcinogen. Nonetheless, the question of a direct causative link between air pollution and cancer remains unsettled.

Other Health Effects of Air Pollution

Industrial communities where manufacturing facilities emit heavy metals, hydrocarbons, asbestos, or radionuclides may face other health problems. For example, smelters emit high levels of airborne lead, which can cause severe neurologic damage in residents, especially children. Extensive study and enhanced emission controls are needed in these areas.

SPECIFIC AIR CONTAMINANTS

A number of contaminants are known to pollute the air, including ozone, carbon monoxide, sulfur dioxide, oxides of nitrogen, hydrocarbons, lead, and other heavy metals such as cadmium. Other substances such as halogenated compounds and pesticides could be added to this list. The major pollutants and their effects are listed in Table 39–1.

Ozone

Ozone is a major component of smog in today's cities. Like peroxyacetal nitrate, formaldehyde, and peroxides, ozone is not emitted directly into the air but is formed in the air by chemical reaction of hydrocarbons and nitrogen oxide. Since sunlight is needed to complete the reaction, ozone content in the air is higher during the day than at night. At current levels of pollution, this substance can irritate the respiratory system and cause histologic changes in the lung, including infiltration of alveolar macrophages and thickening of the alveolar wall. Severe exposure can cause fibrosis and pulmonary edema.

Carbon Monoxide

Carbon monoxide, a colorless, odorless, poisonous gas, results from the incomplete combustion of carbon-containing fuels. Understandably, it is the most plentiful air pollutant because of the millions of vehicles in use. It usually does not persist in the air, however, because it is converted to carbon dioxide fast enough to prevent heavy accumulation. It is estimated that 85 million metric tons of carbon monoxide are emitted annually in the USA. This substance affects the central nervous system and the cardiovascular system. At high concentration it is an asphyxiant, and it is the component of automobile exhaust producing death in suicides.

Sulfur Dioxide

Sulfur dioxide is usually classified with suspended particulates, such as dust, soot, smoke, and chemical residues, because the 2 are commonly found together in urban areas and because sulfur dioxide is converted in the air to a particulate, sulfate aerosol. The sulfur dioxide-particulate complex results chiefly from the burning of fossil fuels. Exposure can cause irritant and toxic effects on the human airways and result in bronchoconstriction. It also can aggravate existing pulmonary or cardiac problems. The mortality rates from both cardiac and respiratory problems are higher during severe air pollution occurrences.

Nitrogen Dioxide

Nitrogen dioxide is a component of automobile exhaust fumes and consequently a major air pollutant. Although it is not as toxic as ozone and is not present in the environment in concentrations as high as ozone, acute exposure can cause bronchoconstriction in persons with respiratory problems. Furthermore, nitrogen dioxide may add to the toxic action of ozone. Animals chronically exposed have exhibited histopathologic changes, suggesting that chronic exposure may make humans more susceptible to respiratory infections.

Lead

Lead also pollutes environmental air as a result of the use of leaded gasoline in vehicles and emissions

Table 39–1. Major pollutants associated with adverse pulmonary effects.[1]

Pollutant	Outdoor Sources	Indoor Sources	Possible Adverse Effects
Sulfur oxides	Power plants, oil refineries, smelters	Kerosene space heaters	Bronchoconstriction
Oxides of nitrogen	Automobile exhaust, power plants, oil refineries	Gas stoves and furnaces, kerosene space heaters	Airway injury, impaired lung defenses (pulmonary edema, bronchiolitis)
Ozone	Automobile exhaust	Aircraft cabins, electrical appliances, ozone generators	Airway injury, impaired lung defenses (pulmonary edema, bronchiolitis)
Polycyclic hydrocarbons	Diesel exhaust	Cigarette smoke	Lung cancer
Asbestos	Asbestos processing plants	Insulation, building materials, workers' clothing	Mesothelioma (lung cancer, pulmonary fibrosis)
Ionizing radiation	Cosmic rays	Building materials	Lung cancer
Arsenic	Smelters	Cigarette smoke	Lung cancer
Allergens	Pollen	Animal dander, house dust, mites	Exacerbations of asthma

[1]Reproduced, with permission, from Boushey HA, Sheppard D: Air pollution. Chapter 70 in: *Textbook of Respiratory Medicine.* Murray JF, Nadel JA (editors). Saunders, 1988.

from lead and copper smelters. In 1975, vehicle emissions accounted for 90% of lead in the atmosphere, but federal regulations restricting the use of leaded gasoline have reduced this figure to about 60%.

Hydrocarbons

Hydrocarbons, some of which are known carcinogens, contribute to air pollution as a product of incomplete combustion or evaporation of gasoline. In addition to gasoline-powered vehicles, other major sources of the 28 million metric tons of hydrocarbons emitted in the USA each year include gasoline, vehicle exhausts, solvents, paints, and dry-cleaning fluids. Some hydrocarbons also contribute to the formation of photochemical smog.

Other Atmospheric Pollutants

The atmosphere is further polluted by a number of other substances, including asbestos, mercury, beryllium, vinyl chloride, arsenic, benzene, and radionuclides as well as cadmium, pesticides, and other toxic chemicals emitted by any number of industrial sources.

ACID RAIN & ACID FOG

Under clear air conditions, rain and fog are not acidic—they become so only when they combine with polluted air. In the presence of moisture, the sulfur dioxide in polluted air forms sulfuric acid, a reaction catalyzed by the oxides of nitrogen in the air, which themselves are converted to nitric acid. The resultant sulfuric and nitric acids are carried by the winds and deposited on forests, lakes, and streams. Acid rain is a hazard to natural resources, destroying vegetation and fouling lakes and streams, with resultant loss of wildlife. It also leaches nutrients from the soil and releases toxic metals into streams and lakes. Both acid rain and acid fog also deposit toxic metals, such as lead, cadmium, and mercury; and organic pollutants, such as alkanes, PCBs, and polycyclic aromatic hydrocarbons, some of which are known carcinogens. Acid fog combined with thermal inversion has been the cause of a number of air pollution disasters in this century.

In December 1930, Belgium was blanketed by thick fog for an entire week. Inhabitants of the heavily industrialized Meuse River Valley suffered severe health problems from the acid fog. The thermal inversion and fog trapped pollutants that stagnated day after day. Thousands became ill and 63 died, mostly the elderly and those with cardiorespiratory disease. Those who did not become seriously ill complained of coughing and shortness of breath. This episode raised concern throughout the industrialized world.

During October of 1948, thermal inversion and acid fog brought tragedy to Donora, Pennsylvania, in the industrialized Monongahela River Valley. Six thousand inhabitants became ill and 20 died, again primarily the high-risk groups consisting of the elderly and those with cardiorespiratory diseases.

Both London and New York have experienced several such episodes. The one in London in December 1952 was by far the most severe. Coal smoke from hundreds of residential fireplaces became admixed with fog and locked-in industrial emissions during a 5-day thermal inversion. Four thousand people are estimated to have died, and morbidity more than doubled. Again, the 2 high-risk groups—the elderly and those with respiratory disorders—accounted for most of the deaths. Prior to this episode, London had experienced 6 similar tragedies dating back to 1873 with a combined total of 2500 dead. Subsequently, in December 1962, another such episode occurred in which 750 people died. New York City had 4 such episodes in 1953, 1962, 1963, and 1966. Epidemiologic studies indicate that there were 200 excess deaths in the 1953 episode, 405 in 1963, and 168 in 1966; the lower death rate in 1966 was attributed to the fact that the inversion occurred during a Thanksgiving weekend when emission-contributing facilities were not in operation and certain previously imposed pollution restrictions.

Controlling the Problem

Unfortunately, it is extremely difficult to trace wind-borne acid rain from the area of deposition back to the source. For example, Ohio, Indiana, and Illinois, the main coal-burning states, are responsible for the greatest acid precipitation and toxic heavy metal deposition in the USA. These states produce almost one-quarter of the total sulfur dioxide emissions and one-sixth of the nitrogen oxide emissions in this country. Although they have created a pool of acid air pollution over the entire northeastern region of the continent, the vast number of emission sources in those states makes it impossible to pinpoint a specific site that is responsible. Furthermore, the argument by industry that acid rain comes from natural sources succeeds in further complicating an already difficult identification problem, but 90–95% of the acid rain downwind from this area comes from man-made sources.

Controls such as higher smokestacks and electrostatic precipitators have not been effective. Higher smokestacks only spread the pollutants to a wider geographic area, and removal of ash (an alkali) by some precipitators only makes the acids stronger. Thus, the primary contributors—the electric utilities and other fossil fuel-burning industries (emitting sulfur dioxide) and motor vehicles (emitting nitrogen oxides)—continue to foul the air and contribute to acid rain.

The overall results of efforts to control the quantity of air pollution in the USA have been encouraging. Total suspended particulates, sulfur dioxide, carbon monoxide, and lead have all decreased over the past decade. Ozone pollution has shown a reduction in peak levels in several urban areas. Nitrogen dioxide is the only major pollutant to continue an upward trend in several urban areas.

WATER POLLUTION

Improper waste management and hazardous substances used either industrially or in homes and gardens are the main causes of water contamination in the USA and other industrialized nations. Both surface water and groundwater have been contaminated by chemical manufacture and use, petroleum operations, mining and smelting, and agriculture as well as by disposal of household and human and animal wastes.

Surface water contamination has become a national issue in recent years as lakes, rivers, and streams have been heavily—and visibly—contaminated. Efforts to return surface waters to an uncontaminated status have met with some success, while contamination of groundwater is emerging as the more difficult issue. This problem is much more serious because the sources of contamination are often difficult to locate and because contamination may continue for years before it is discovered.

Water falling as snow or rain filters down through layers of earth into geologic formations called aquifers, which may be close to or far beneath the earth's surface. There the water is held until pumped to the surface. This water is vital to agriculture, accounting for about 40% of all water used in crop irrigation. About 30 trillion gallons of groundwater are removed from the earth each year. About 50% of the US population—and over 90% of rural Americans—rely on aquifers for their drinking water.

Health Effects of Water Pollution

The primary health concern related to water pollution is the growing number of reproductive toxins and carcinogens that are occurring in drinking water. Other hazardous substances in water may also present health risks to communities. Both the EPA and the public have become increasingly aware that the nation's drinking water, from either surface water or groundwater sources, often contains substances that are hazardous to health. With rare exceptions, the levels of water contamination with synthetic organic chemicals are small in comparison to the levels of similar chemicals in food.

Outbreaks of waterborne disease have increased in recent years. One explanation is the overloading of water treatment plants with source water of increasingly poor quality. Many rivers used for potable water supplies now contain 10% or more of sewage effluent. Consequently, about 100 million persons throughout the world are consuming water that contains significant amounts of effluents.

Many epidemiologic studies have attempted to quantify the health risks of drinking contaminated water. This large literature is characterized by studies that assumed well water was clean and that populations drinking water from aquifers could be used as controls for comparison with populations drinking surface waters. There was often no attempt to control for the many intervening variables in such studies. For example, urban centers typically drink chlorinated surface waters. Rural populations drink water from aquifers almost exclusively—often without chlorination. After many of these studies failed to demonstrate significant differences in cancer rates or evidence of impact on reproductive health, groundwater was often found to be contaminated by the same chemicals as surface waters and in similar concentrations. In fact, other assumptions about the safety of groundwater should have been studied before attempts to interpret the data were made. It is increasingly clear that the deeper the source of aquifer water, the more likely it is that the water is contaminated by naturally occurring heavy metals and by radioactive minerals.

The entire epidemiologic literature has been reviewed by many investigators. From this large body of scientific endeavor, it is virtually impossible to draw any reliable clinical conclusions regarding risk to health from pollution of drinking water. Nowhere is there more ample evidence of the limitations of epidemiologic studies to determine risk to the public health than in the recent attempts to quantify the risk of water contamination.

Sources of Groundwater Pollution

Groundwater can be contaminated by the agricultural application of fertilizers and pesticides; leaking storage tanks containing chemicals, petroleum products, or other toxic wastes; improperly managed landfills; industrial impoundments; municipal wastewater discharges; deep well disposal; and accidental spills of toxic materials. Synthetic organic contaminants may constitute a major hazard to human health. Many toxic chemicals cannot be broken down by microorganisms in the earth or filtered out by the soil before reaching underground aquifers. Among the most persistent and dangerous wastes are biorefractory chlorinated hydrocarbons, such as trichloroethylene, tetrachloroethylene, and carbon tetrachloride, which are used widely in some industries. Trapped in the aquifers, these volatile solvents remain in the water.

The rate of movement of contaminants into groundwater aquifers depends on the types of soil involved—ie, unconsolidated sand and gravel or consolidated materials such as various types of rocks. Aquifers that are not surmounted by impermeable materials and thus are supplied by water seeping through the soil are at greatest risk of contamination. Depending on hydraulic gradients and the permeability of the aquifer, the flow rate may range from a fraction of an inch to a few feet per day. This slow rate of flow prevents the natural purging of contaminants that can be accomplished by rivers and streams.

The degree of hazard from contaminated aquifers depends on the volume and toxicity of the contaminant, its concentration in the aquifer, the life span of the chemical or mineral, and the length of time humans ingest the contaminated water. It is thought that only a small percentage of the nation's groundwater is already contaminated, but the reality is probably much higher because many groundwater sources have never been tested. Twenty-five percent of public wells tested to date in California show evidence of organic chemical contamination.

Landfills

Landfills are a primary source of groundwater contamination, since a large proportion of toxic wastes generated each year are dumped there. The EPA has estimated that there are 75,000 industrial landfills and 15,000 municipal landfills, of which 30,000 sites are thought to be abandoned—but abandoned or not, they may still contaminate groundwater systems because of the slow rate at which leaching occurs. It is further believed that companies are dumping industrial wastes in closed sites owned in most cases by the companies themselves. These closed sites have been the repository over time of more than 1 billion tons of industrial wastes. Improper waste management at landfills, together with the action of rainfall and snow, make both active and inactive landfills continuing sources of groundwater contamination. In an attempt to offset this growing problem, the EPA established a close-off date (November 8, 1985) by which operators of toxic dumps had to close down unless they were able to certify that they were monitoring nearby groundwater for pollution and had insurance or assets to compensate for environmental damages. Environmentalists and industry officials contend that the EPA is so ill-informed about the nation's toxic waste sites and inspects them so infrequently that many facilities will continue to operate even though they do not meet EPA requirements.

Surface Impoundments

Another threat to groundwater purity stems from surface impoundments (pits, ponds, or lagoons) used to store, treat, or dispose of industrial, municipal, agricultural, mining, and oil and gas-brine wastes. By 1980, more than 170,000 of these impoundments existed throughout the USA, and 90% were unmonitored. Seventy percent were unlined, permitting seepage through the soil; 30% were not only unlined but also located directly above usable groundwater sources; and 10% were unlined and within a mile of drinking water wells. These figures, however, may represent only the tip of the iceberg, because in this EPA survey, only state-permitted impoundments were surveyed and particularly those for which extensive data were available. Non-state permitted impoundments, which may represent a much more threatening situation, were omitted from the survey.

Underground Storage Tanks

There are at least 3.5 million underground storage tanks throughout the nation to store petroleum products, chemicals, and hazardous wastes such as solvents and other liquids. Many of them may be leaking because of fatigue, improper location, or other factors. The resultant leakage is a serious danger to groundwater sources and over time may result in extensive contamination. For example, over a period of 18 months, a 6000-gallon fiberglass storage tank in California leaked 58,000 gallons of solvent into the groundwater, contaminating 3 aquifers and wells providing drinking water for a large community. But even much smaller discharges—on the order of one-half gallon per day—have caused major damage to drinking water supplies.

Despite this very hazardous situation, only one-third of the states have legislation specifically intended to protect surface and groundwater from pollution. Regulatory programs include requirements for permits to install a tank, inventory controls, tank testing and monitoring, and leak detection equipment. There are also regulations pertaining to equipment and procedures for closing down storage tanks. EPA has estimated that at least 10% of the tanks are leaking. Consequently, the possibility exists that groundwater contamination may occur from more than 300,000 underground tanks, but the actual number may be much higher since few states have begun to do widespread testing.

Asbestos Contamination of Water

The contamination of drinking water with asbestos has become a major concern since the discovery in 1973 of large amounts of amphibole asbestos fibers in Lake Superior, which served as a source of municipal water supplies for the city of Duluth, Minnesota. Asbestos can contaminate drinking water through geologic erosion, pollution (logging and construction), or from the asbestos-cement pipes that transmit the water. Data on concentrations of asbestos fibers in drinking water indicate that asbestos contamination of drinking water is very common.

Controlling the Problem
A. Conventional Water Treatment Processes:
Treatment of municipal drinking water with chlorine and charcoal filtering—along with wider use of bottled water for drinking—have not reduced the possibility of exposure to toxic chemicals. Chlorine treatment enhances the amount of chloroform in the water, raising it from a few micrograms to several hundred micrograms per liter. Chlorine also produces chlorinated hydrocarbons or enhances the toxicity of those already present and produces other compounds, such as chlorinated phenols. The resultant products can be more toxic or carcinogenic than the originals. Although treatment of water by filtering through

deionizing charcoal reduces the concentration of chloroform and benzene, filtered water has been found to contain higher concentrations of tetrachloroethylene, methylmethacrylate, and styrene than does unfiltered water. Analyses of commercially bottled artesian water have shown the presence of acetaldehyde, benzene, bromodichloromethane, dichloropropane, diethyl ether, ethyl acetate, and toluene.

Conventional water treatment processes in many cases also add biorefractory chemicals to the drinking water. The National Academy of Sciences has estimated that more than 90% of the total organic content of drinking water is not identified by typical gas chromatography-mass spectrophotometric analysis. Concentrates of nonvolatile organics in drinking water are mutagenic in bacterial and mammalian cells and can induce cellular transformations in human and mouse fibroblasts. The amount of total organic materials in water is characterized by its biochemical oxygen demand (BOD). The BOD is the amount of dissolved oxygen decrease in a water sample over a 5-day period. Identification of all the organics would entail high-powered liquid chromatography (HPLC), an expense beyond the budgetary resources of most public health agencies. Sadly, much of the commercial effort to sell expensive water to the public is founded on misinterpretation of water analyses.

B. Water Softening: Water softening removes calcium from water and replaces it with sodium. This may result in an increase in the incidence of deaths from heart disease. Early onset of hypertension has also been found in populations of youths drinking water with sodium chloride concentrations over 100 mg/L. Many municipal and commercial sources of water have salt concentrations in this range. Water softening increases the level of sodium in water already high in sodium chloride.

The significance of these studies is challenged on the basis that drinking water provides only a small percentage of the usual daily intake of dietary minerals.

AGRICULTURAL CONTAMINATION: PESTICIDES & FERTILIZER

The agricultural use of pesticides (including herbicides) and fertilizers is treated separately here because it contaminates more than one aspect of the environment. Both materials run off or leach into the soil through the action of rain and irrigation. As a result, they contaminate the soil itself, enter the food chain, and poison both surface water and groundwater, destroying natural resources and endangering human health.

Since the introduction of DDT in 1939 and its successful use against mites, ticks, and mosquitoes during World War II, the production and number of pesticides has proliferated in the USA. Faced with a continuing problem of insects and weeds that became resistant to current products, the chemical industry has concentrated on developing more and more new products. Between 1945 and 1975, pesticide production (including herbicides) in the USA rose from 100 million pounds to 1.6 billion pounds. Herbicide use is increasing dramatically as the savings in fuel costs for plowing and cultivating is added to the savings in human labor costs. In 1981, about 625 million pounds of herbicides—more than the total amount of insecticides—were applied to US soils. The USA is the largest producer and user of these products in the world. The Federal Office of Technology Assessment reports that 260,000 tons of active ingredients in the pesticides and 42 million tons of fertilizer are spread annually over the equivalent of 280 million acres across the country.

Health Effects

The impact of toxic agricultural agents on human health has become a growing concern as their residues increasingly enter drinking water sources and the food chain. Continuing exposure to low levels of pesticides places farm workers at risk of cancer, reproductive disorders, birth defects, and many long-term illnesses. Especially disturbing are the residues of pesticides that affect infants and children. It is believed that pesticide residues will continue in the food chain and be concentrated in the fatty tissues of almost all Americans for the foreseeable future. One recent study found that imported fruits and vegetables contained twice the levels of residual pesticides found in domestic foods.

Controlling the Problem

The use of pesticides has significantly altered agricultural processes that previously helped control pests. First, crop rotation—a method for ensuring that more pest-resistant crops would alternate with less resistant ones—no longer appeals to farmers, who would rather use the readily available chemical controls. Second, tilling agricultural waste acreage to eliminate out-of-season support of pests has decreased considerably. Third, the use of natural predators of the pests has declined.

However, the ever-growing resistance of pests has led to research to determine whether the former methods should not be combined with the use of less toxic chemical agents to solve the problem. This outcome would be preferable to deluging the environment with a continuous flow of newer and ever more toxic chemicals.

Finally, restrictions on chemical agricultural products will need to be more stringent, and black markets for these chemicals will have to be eliminated. Controlling the problem will not be easy in a contracting agricultural economy.

IONIZING RADIATION

Ionizing radiation is electromagnetic radiation that has sufficient energy to separate electrons from their atomic or molecular orbits. Exposure to ionizing radiation poses a severe threat to humans and animals.

Although natural background radiation from both cosmic and terrestrial sources has always been part of the environment, technology has added numerous other potential sources of exposure to ionizing radiation, particularly in the field of medicine. Moreover, humans also carry internally trace amounts of radioactive isotopes, such as carbon 14 and potassium 40.

Health Effects

From the beginning of this century, cases have been seen of severe radiation burns in physicists and medical personnel working with unshielded x-ray tubes and with radionuclides, especially radium. After appropriate latency periods, an unusual incidence of various cancers was also observed among these early researchers and practitioners. So great was the toll among this group that a Monument to the Martyrs of Radiology has been erected in Hamburg, Germany.

Very early, it was recognized that radiation exposure caused eye irritation, cataracts, dermatitis, loss of hair, and cancerous ulcers. Laboratory animals also exhibited—in addition to the effects seen in humans—evidence of bone growth inhibition, bone abnormalities, and sterility. Later findings in both humans and animals have identified additional effects, including cell death, genetic defects, cancer, impairment of the immune system, and shortening of life.

Evidence of the severe hazards of radiation exposure continue to mount. For example, a recent retrospective study found that 10 years after patients were treated with x-ray for gastric ulcer—a procedure used between 1948 and 1960—those patients showed a higher mortality rate from stomach cancer and other diseases than did matched untreated controls.

A number of factors affect the severity of radiation damage, including age, individual physiologic variations, and differences between species. The usually long latency period of cancer development may mask other health effects when research objectives concentrate strictly on carcinogenic effects. For example, when the immune repair mechanism is damaged by radiation, exposed individuals may die much earlier from infectious diseases, particularly pneumonia, so that the cancer incidence would appear only in the strongest individuals.

Present knowledge of the health effects of radiation has been derived from 2 primary sources: atomic bomb survivors in Japan and medical patients who have undergone radiation diagnostic studies or radiation therapy. Both of these groups received high-level exposure. Consequently, the health risk level of low-dose exposure is not entirely clear and remains a major issue of environmental protection today.

Sources of Exposure

A. Natural Background Radiation: Levels of natural background radiation differ with geographic location. The type of soil in an area and the radionuclides present in soil affect the exposure rate, or dose-equivalent rate. For example, the Colorado Plateau area has a higher dose-equivalent rate (75–140 mrem/y) than do either the Atlantic and Gulf Coastal plains (15–35 mrem/y) or the remainder of the coterminous United States (35–75 mrem/y).

Cosmic radiation that descends to earth consists of extraterrestrial particles that pass through the earth's atmosphere and additional particles created by the passage. The dose-equivalent rate increases as the earth's atmospheric shield becomes thinner. The dose-equivalent rate from extraterrestrial sources is higher at higher altitudes, being twice as high at 1800 m as it is at sea level. It is also affected by solar changes. Overall, the dose-equivalent rate for the US population is estimated to be approximately 31 mrem/y.

B. Radiation Generated by Health Services: The Bureau of Radiological Health has determined that x-rays used in patient diagnosis or treatment are the chief source of radiation exposure of the US population. More than 300,000 x-ray units exist in the various health services, and an estimated 129 million people are exposed annually through medical and dental x-rays. Those most at risk are the people who work with the equipment daily. The EPA has estimated that these people receive about 50 mrem/y.

Another important source of radiation exposure in health services is the use of radiopharmaceuticals, which more than 10,000 physicians in the USA are licensed to administer. Ten to 12 million doses of the radionuclides are administered annually for diagnosis or treatment involving the brain, liver, bone, lung, thyroid, kidney, and heart. According to EPA estimates, this represents about 20% of the total radiation resulting from health services.

C. Exposure From Nuclear Weapons Tests: Prior to 1963, when most nuclear tests were performed in the atmosphere, large amounts of radioactive material were released to be carried by the wind and brought to earth by rains. The first explosion at Bikini Atoll in 1954 exposed many in the area to radioactive fallout, including the inhabitants of surrounding islands and 23 Japanese fishermen who were downwind. It was estimated that the fishermen themselves received an average of approximately 200 R of total body radiation, and all suffered from acute radiation syndrome. One subsequently died from a transfusion complication. The catch of tuna was also severely contaminated, and other catches contaminated via the waterborne route were detected intermittently over several months. Among the Marshall

Islanders, an unusual incidence of benign and malignant thyroid nodules, hypothyroidism, and growth retardation has been documented secondary to radioiodine exposure. Both groups suffered from acute beta irradiation burns to the skin.

This and related episodes indicate that significant harmful exposure occurs outside the prescribed "danger area," in part because of the unpredictability of atmospheric dispersion. Moreover, radionuclides can enter the food chain by means of rainfall on croplands as well as via contaminated fish and drinking water. Atmospheric tests conducted in Nevada during the 1950s and 1960s produced excessive levels of radioactivity in food and dairy products in many parts of the USA.

D. Radiation Exposure From Nuclear Power: Several hundred nuclear reactors now exist in the USA for power production, scientific study, and other uses. Because of public indignation over the Three Mile Island and Chernobyl accidents and because of the accelerating costs involved, the building of additional nuclear reactors remains in question. However, the existing reactors pose a risk not only to their workers but also to populations in the area. Short of a full-scale "meltdown" with breach of the containment vessel, the major concern with possible reactor accidents relates to the emission of radioactive isotopes of iodine and their potential effect on the thyroid. Radioiodines, particularly ^{131}I, are the major public health risks following a reactor accident, because they are readily volatilized and dispersed and rapidly taken up by the thyroid gland.

The mining and milling of uranium to feed the reactors pose a steady-state risk to the inhabitants of several southwestern states in the USA, where 140 million tons of radon-emitting uranium mill tailings lie exposed to the atmosphere. Further risks are related to the disposal of radioactive wastes and to the flow of cooling water containing tritium, carbon 14, and krypton 85 into streams and rivers. These elements are nearly impossible to contain or remove and are capable of contaminating fish, drinking water, and the crops used for human consumption or animal feed that are irrigated with the water.

E. Other Sources of Radiation: Additional sources of potential radiation include a number of products, some of which are in widespread use. Products that either contain radioactive materials or generate x-rays during operation include luminous dial watches, dental prostheses, smoke detectors, cardiac pacemakers, tobacco products, fossil fuels, and some building materials. Air flight also is a source of radiation from the x-ray inspection systems at airports to cosmic radiation exposure during flight. Further exposure may occur if the flight is transporting radioactive materials.

Controlling the Problem

Since all possibilities cannot be included in any radiation research project, no reliable permissible dose equivalent has yet been established. Rather, the problem has been approached from risk-benefit considerations—ie, How much radiation exposure are we willing to accept to achieve the benefits of nuclear energy? Most scientists would agree that no level of ionizing radiation is entirely safe or can ever be made so. Man-made radiation sources have already doubled the level of exposure in the past hundred years.

HAZARDOUS WASTE MANAGEMENT

United States industry produces 250 million metric tons of hazardous wastes per year. The majority of these wastes are derived from industries that produce (1) organic chemicals and pesticides and (2) explosives and primary metals. These 2 together account for twice the amount of wastes produced by the next most common sources: electroplating and inorganic chemicals. About 75% of the wastes are disposed of on the company property where they are generated; the remainder usually is transported to licensed disposal facilities. The mid-Atlantic and Midwestern states have the highest amounts of hazardous toxic wastes in the nation. The rest of the states are also at risk, especially those with high population growth and extensive new home development.

Before concern over toxic waste contamination became an issue, companies dumped them into rivers, at municipal dumps, or as landfill in then uninhabited areas. These practices resulted in widespread surface and groundwater contamination. With the growing population and demand for housing, developers began to build houses and schools on toxic waste landfill areas that had been closed down or abandoned. The result has been that many people are living above buried toxic wastes that can gradually surface. Since a large number of the wastes are not biodegradable and can persist for several decades or even longer, there is a vital need to protect the health of the exposed population through proper methods of waste management and control of existing hazards. This section concentrates, therefore, on various approaches to that problem.

Government Response

In the face of public concern over protecting the environment and public health, Congress passed 2 important bills: (1) the Resource Conservation and Recovery Act of 1976 (RCRA) and (2) the Comprehensive Environmental Response, Compensation and Liability Act of 1980 (CERCLA, known as the Superfund). RCRA regulates the management of toxic wastes being produced at present. Superfund provides leadership and funding for the clean-up of abandoned hazardous waste disposal sites.

Until a recent amendment to RCRA, much more toxic waste was exempt from federal control than was regulated. In the USA, under the small quantity exemption, 700,000 companies were not required to dispose of hazardous wastes at licensed facilities. But these small companies represent 92% of all toxic waste producers. Another regulatory loophole, the boiler exemption, allows more than 1000 boilers to burn hazardous wastes as fuels with virtually no government monitoring of the efficiency of destruction of the materials. The irony is that government rushed to create the climate for boiler burning in the early years of rising energy costs. Now that fuel costs are more stable, the boiler industry continues to provide an environmentally unsound method of waste removal.

Only about 10% of all hazardous wastes are disposed of in a manner consistent with federal regulations. Nearly 50% is disposed of by lagooning in unlined surface impoundments; 30% in nonsecure landfills; and about 10% by dumping into sewers, spreading on roads, injection into deep wells, and incineration under uncontrolled conditions.

The Superfund

The Superfund legislation created a fund to clean up hazardous wastes contaminating the environment and to seek out and clean up abandoned dumping sites that harbor hazardous materials. Many of these locations are not known at this time, and others are up to 100 years old. The amount of money actually needed to accomplish the goals of Superfund can hardly be imagined. The Office of Technology Assessment estimates that dealing with the most critical 10,000 sites will cost $100 billion.

The Superfund concept is a slow process and subject to political maneuvering. To date, only about 900 sites have been identified for priority attention, of which 6 have been totally cleaned up. One of these—the Butler mine tunnel in Pittston, Pennsylvania—poured millions of gallons of polluted water from the tunnel when rain from Hurricane Gloria flooded it in September of 1985. Others may also be questionable, and it may well be that no cleanup will ever be complete.

If the level of contamination from wastes is significant, we should be able to measure their health effects using the methods of epidemiologic analysis. Yet even with communities located close to hazardous waste dump sites, the impact on public health is interpreted with caution. Of the 900 hazardous waste dump sites receiving priority attention by the EPA, only 20 have been studied for effects on human health. No prospective study has yet been initiated among affected populations.

Federal laws and most state laws do not provide a mechanism for compensating individuals who have developed illnesses from environmental exposures to hazardous waste sites. Instead, individuals must bring personal injury actions against firms shown to have caused disposal of the waste and must prove that this particular waste caused the illness. Even though these suits are difficult to win, thousands of plaintiffs are pressing such claims in the USA and many other countries.

Landfilling

The government favors a new type of landfill and has provided guidelines for its construction. The recommended landfill consists of a pit 60 feet deep sealed in a plastic liner. Liquid that passes to the bottom is collected by a perforated collection pipe and pumped again to the surface for treatment. Exterior monitors check for chemicals migrating into the groundwater. The arguments against this design are as follows:

(1) The plastic liner can easily be breached by external forces such as the bulldozer used to cover the liner with clay, sand, and gravel.

(2) The waste materials disintegrate the liner, sometimes within months.

(3) The weight of the waste may crush the collection pipes, or sludge may clog the perforations.

(4) The protective cover may be damaged by external forces or erosion, permitting rainwater to penetrate to the wastes, overloading the collection system or causing the landfill to overflow.

The consensus is that no landfill system can be entirely secure. Chemical wastes may persist in the environment for decades or even centuries, while the most carefully designed landfill may begin to leak within months.

Alternatives to Landfilling

A. Incineration: There are more effective means of hazardous waste disposal than dumping. West Germany, Denmark, and a number of other countries have utilized other means of coping with such wastes for more than a decade. Denmark, for example, burns up to 50% of its waste in high-temperature kilns. The USA is only beginning to consider such alternatives to landfilling even though the technology is available. Consequently, only a small number of high-temperature kilns are now operating in the USA. Although incineration cannot destroy all organic constituents of hazardous waste, the important consideration is optimal burning temperature and air mixture so that a minimum of products of incomplete combustion are discharged into the atmosphere.

The principal concern to date has centered on the quantities of dibenzodioxins and dibenzofurans measured from the stacks of incinerators. There are also problems with fine particulate matter, hydrogen halide gases, metal aerosols, and other materials that escape the incineration process. Incineration can be done aboard specially equipped vessels in areas of the ocean at some distance from land, but there is concern that the ocean will not be able to buffer the high acidity of emissions from these ships. The incineration practices of early ships equipped for this purpose have been criticized.

Another argument against incineration by ships at sea is that the oceans are already put at risk by the millions of tons of waste being discharged into them each year. Sewage can be discharged into the ocean at less than a quarter of the cost of land disposal. At present, 17 million tons of sewage sludge are dumped into the oceans off US shores annually. Most fish species in these dumping areas demonstrate contamination with PCBs. The occurrence of fin erosion and fish neoplasms appears to reflect water contamination by chemicals contained in sewage and its bioconcentration by the fish harvested in the region. DDT and pentachlorophenol have been found in the fish of many countries.

Other examples of toxic contaminants found in marine animals include plastics, plasticizers, detergents, chlorinated styrenes, phenols, components from pulp industries, and lubricating oil. Mercury contamination of marine animals occurs through bioconcentration and storage. Large predatory fish, such as tuna and swordfish, and other fish-eating species, such as seals and many seabirds, can accumulate mercury in high concentrations. However, most commercial fish species are less than 10 years old at marketable size, with no evidence of harmful mercury accumulation except in areas of high mercury input.

Unfortunately, in the absence of alternative methods of treatment, to be overly protective of ocean waters is to encourage the dumping of wastes in soil or their burning in inadequate and unregulated facilities. At present, treatment methods for detoxifying even the worst poisons are at a standstill in laboratories because there is little market for them and federal regulations do not encourage their use.

B. Recycling: EPA believes that waste recycling could reduce the toxic waste burden in the environment by 20% and that doing so would benefit both the disposer and the recipient. The disposer would avoid fines and the high costs of other methods of proper disposal; the recipient would benefit because the recycled materials could be made purer and cheaper than some new materials. Substances most apt to be dealt with successfully in this manner are solvents and oils, paper, wood, scrap metals, and surplus chemicals.

The main problem with this approach is that many companies prefer not to disclose the identities of materials used in their processes. This objection can be overcome by marketing the recycled product without revealing its source. Forty of these exchanges have been established, but many have failed to survive, primarily—according to EPA—because state and local governments participated and many companies are reluctant to divulge information about their products to so broad a group. Moreover, ineffective management of the exchanges contributed to a number of failures.

C. Detoxification: Wastes that cannot be recycled may be suitable for detoxification by chemical treatment to render them harmless or reduce their volume to manageable amounts. Chemical treatment frequently can be more efficient when performed by outside contractors rather than by the generator of the waste. With this approach, disposal is accomplished at less cost, since one company's waste sometimes can be used to neutralize another's. Regional waste disposal centers in West Germany, for example, neutralize one company's acid wastes with the alkaline wastes of another.

1. Neutralization—Neutralization is the most commonly used chemical treatment. Residues from electroplating and other metal finishing processes are frequently neutralized because they are too acidic to be released into the environment. They are often neutralized by the addition of lime or other inexpensive alkaline materials. In many cases, they become safe to release. Certain forms of neutralization also precipitate heavy metal ions in liquids as insoluble hydroxide salts. When these ions are removed, the liquid becomes safe for disposal and the much smaller volume of ions can be disposed of more readily in another way. The iron and steel industry, as well as metal-finishing operations, often use this method.

2. Oxidation and evaporation—Cyanide is oxidized by sodium hypochlorite or a combination of sodium hydroxide and chlorine to produce carbon dioxide and nitrogen. Other chemicals may be treated in the same manner, but the oxidizers will differ depending on the chemical to be treated. Water in wastes can be evaporated in properly constructed holding ponds to reduce the amount to be disposed of or while materials wait for additional treatment. The pulp and paper industry, for example, evaporates black and sulfate liquors from papermaking by exposing the liquors to hot flue gases before incinerating them.

D. Biologic Treatment: Incorporating wastes into soil and allowing microorganisms to biodegrade them is an approach that is acceptable to the EPA under certain conditions. The procedure consists of 4 steps: (1) applying the wastes on or turning them into the soil; (2) mixing the wastes with surface soil to aerate the mass and permit soil microorganisms to reach the wastes; (3) adding nutrients as needed; and (4) mixing the waste and soil mass periodically to maintain aerobic conditions. This approach, commonly known as "land farming," was developed primarily by the petroleum industry.

Although the EPA has accepted the concept of land farming, it has laid down strict regulations as to how it is to be accomplished:

(1) The farmed area must be 1.5 m above the historically recorded highest groundwater level.

(2) It must be at least 150 m from any water supply.

(3) It should have minimal erosion potential.

(4) It should be located in an area with very low annual rainfall to prevent formation of an anaerobic mine.

(5) It must be monitored regularly to a depth of 1 m to detect any downward movement of trace metals or other contaminants.

This concept has 2 very important disadvantages: It is not suitable for substances such as heavy metals that are not biodegradable; and the large areas of land required can make it very costly.

Recent Developments in Disposal Methods

Despite serious gaps in waste management regulations, such as the omission of small waste producers and lack of encouragement, some universities, research organizations, and private companies are still searching for new techniques for disposing of hazardous wastes. Advancing technology has contaminated our environment, but it may also serve to reduce or perhaps eliminate the contaminants.

A hot bath of **molten salt** is known to destroy DDT and is now believed capable of destroying toxic solvents and acids as well. This process consists of injecting the waste into a pool of sodium salt heated to 900 °C (1650 °F), which is lower than the heat required for incineration. Hydrocarbons burn at once, being converted to carbon dioxide and water. Other chemicals, such as sulfur and chlorine, react with the molten salt by becoming inorganic ash, which is readily disposed of. Because of the lower temperature, the production of nitrous oxide, a product of high-temperature incineration, is minimized, as is the potential for acid rain. Following molten salt incineration, less than 1% of the original volume remains.

Of the many chemicals used too widely before their hazards were fully known, PCBs are a prime example. When the extreme danger of PCBs was finally recognized, more than 1 billion gallons of PCB-contaminated oil existed in various electrical components, both in use and dumped. Although production was halted in 1977, there still remains a staggering amount throughout the USA. In 1980, a new method for disposing of these wastes appeared that used chemical means of detoxification. The wastes are pumped into a "chemical soup" containing metallic sodium. The sodium removes the chlorine from the PCBs and combines with it to form sodium chloride. The biphenyls are reduced to a harmless residue. The oil itself may be reused or disposed of without creating any health hazard.

Microwave plasma arc detoxification appears to offer a highly satisfactory means of coping with hazardous wastes since it is capable of reducing them to residues in the parts per trillion range. In this process, a powerful bolt of electricity is sent between 2 electrodes, raising the temperature of air molecules to 25,000 °C (45,000 °F) and transforming them into **plasma,** a cloud of high-energy particles, creating a highly effective conductor of electricity. In the present approach, toxic waste is fed continuously into the chamber where high-energy electrons bombard the material, break molecular bonds, and reduce the material to its basic element—usually carbon, hydrogen, oxygen, or chlorine. The gases that result are pumped to a scrubber where they are neutralized.

Plasma devices can detoxify chemicals 6 million times faster than incineration. They also seem capable of detoxifying almost any toxic chemical. The expense of these devices will hamper their development and use.

Regulatory Procedures & Controls

As public and government concern grew over contamination of the environment, Congress passed a number of statutes directed toward the problem of containment. The EPA was assigned responsibility for establishing acceptable standards for disposal of hazards, monitoring adherence to those standards, and initiating legal action for enforcement. The statutes protecting the environment include the Clean Air Act, the Clean Water Act, and the Safe Drinking Water Act. Those regulating hazardous substances are the Resource Conservation and Recovery Act and the Comprehensive Environmental Response, Compensation, and Liability Act.

A. Air Pollution Statutes: The Clean Air Act, which was passed in 1963, evolved from the Air Pollution Control Act of 1955 and exemplified a trend toward legislative control over this subject matter by the federal government. The 1955 statute delegated primary responsibility for controlling air pollution to the states, with the federal government to provide technical assistance to state and local governments through support of research, training, and demonstration projects. The 1963 Clean Air Act, in addition to authorizing the federal government to provide grants to state air pollution control agencies, authorized it to intervene legally in the control of interstate air pollution. With passage of the Air Quality Act in 1967, the federal government assumed a distinctly regulatory role. Amendments to this act in 1970 and 1977 enlarged the federal government's regulatory role.

Under the 1970 amendments, the EPA was directed to establish "National Ambient Air Quality Standards" (NAAQS) for protecting human life and welfare. Standards have already been established for particulate matter, sulfur oxides, nitrogen oxides, carbon monoxide, photochemical oxidants, and lead. The standards apply to all states alike regardless of geographic location. Each state must submit an implementation plan detailing how it will handle each pollutant for which standards are devised.

The 1970 amendments included a provision for the establishment of National Emission Standards for Hazardous Air Pollutants (NESHAPS) and authorized EPA to establish nationally uniform standards for air pollutants ". . . to which no ambient air quality standard is applicable and which in the judgment of the Administrator causes, or contributes to, air pollution which may reasonably be anticipated to result in an increase in mortality or an increase in serious irreversible, or incapacitating reversible, illness." NESHAPS standards have been established for beryllium, asbestos, mercury, and vinyl chloride. Inorganic arsenic, radionuclides, and benzene have been listed as hazardous air pollutants though standards governing them have not yet been established. Acrylonitrile, formaldehyde, nickel, and polycyclic organic matter are also subject to listing as hazardous air pollutants.

The Clean Air Act as now constituted provides the following penalties for noncompliance:

(1) A $25,000 fine for each day of violation.

(2) Enforced compliance by court order.

(3) Enforced compliance by EPA order.

(4) Criminal penalties of $25,000 per day of noncompliance as well as imprisonment for up to 1 year for the first conviction and $50,000 and imprisonment for up to 2 years for subsequent convictions.

(5) Automatic noncompliance penalties based on the economic value of the violation.

(6) Exclusion from participation in federal procurement contract bidding.

Vehicle pollution is controlled by the Clean Air Act. Vehicles are the major contributors to air pollution (34% of hydrocarbons, 75% of carbon monoxide, and 29% of nitrogen oxides). To control these emissions on the nation's highways, the Clean Air Act authorizes the EPA to establish standards for pollutants and particulates and requires vehicle manufacturers to adhere to them. Manufacturers may apply for waivers from the standards for each specific case. Waivers have been granted for carbon monoxide and nitrogen oxide emissions. No vehicle may be offered for sale until the EPA has issued a certificate of conformity for that particular vehicle. Certification requires that the manufacturer must provide several prototype vehicles of each engine type for testing by the EPA. Under the Clean Air Act, the EPA either tests the vehicles for emissions or requires the manufacturer to do so. The EPA may also test production vehicles as they leave the assembly line. When the number of vehicles not meeting emission standards reaches 40%, the EPA has the authority to revoke or suspend the certificate of conformity and may also recall vehicles already on the market when a substantial number do not perform appropriately. Other EPA responsibilities authorized by the Clean Air Act include (1) the regulation of lead and other additives used in gasoline and (2) requiring the states to monitor vehicles with catalytic converters for compliance with emission standards.

B. Water Pollution Statutes: Like the Clean Air Act, the Clean Water Act evolved over a long period, with each step showing increasing federal control. The original Federal Water Pollution Control Act was passed in 1948. It was amended 5 times and finally rewritten. In this complex area, the 5 amendments established state water quality requirements for intrastate waters but established such a time-consuming and inefficient method of implementation that further legislation was needed. In 1970, Congress passed the Refuse Act Permit Program amendment, which prohibited discharge of any refuse into navigable waters unless permitted by the Secretary of the Army. This requirement remained in effect until 1977, when the entire Clean Water Act was revised. It was amended at that time to provide more time for compliance and to broaden the scope to include toxic contaminants. The Act provides for federal grants to construct publicly owned sewage treatment plants, regulation of the discharge of toxic pollutants, and regulation of oil spills and accidental discharges of toxic contaminants. The EPA was assigned responsibility for establishing standards for permissible manufacturing and effluent discharges.

The Clean Water Act is directed primarily at controlling pollution of waterways. In 1974, the federal government focused on the problem of drinking water and the Safe Drinking Water Act was passed, becoming effective on December 1, 1974. The Act required that piped water systems serving the public provide drinking water as free of contaminants as humanly possible. It provided for (1) identifying toxic contaminants that are dangerous to health, and (2) establishing maximum contaminant levels (MCLs) for each contaminant identified. To date, the following contaminants to drinking water have been identified and MCLs established for them: arsenic, barium, cadmium, lead, mercury, selenium, silver, endrin, lindane, methoxychlor, toxaphene, 2,4-D, 2,4,5-T, silvex, trihalomethanes, nitrates, coliform bacteria, fluoride, and radionuclides.

The Safe Drinking Water Act divides drinking water quality into 2 areas of standards: primary and secondary. The primary drinking water regulations are concerned with protecting human health; the secondary regulations are concerned with protecting human welfare and specifying standards for taste, odor, appearance, or any factor that would impair the water-drinking pleasure of consumers. The first is federally enforced; the second is not. The Act also required EPA to establish regulations restricting underground injection of hazardous wastes that would contaminate drinking water sources. These regulations became effective in 1980.

States can assume primary responsibility for compliance with the Act if EPA determines that the state's regulations are as stringent as the federal requirements and that it is enforcing those regulations. If the state does not perform these tasks adequately, EPA can bring suit against it in federal court. Owners and operators of public water systems must notify their consumers whenever the system is unable to meet federal requirements. Variances are permitted in areas where the quality of the raw water is such that bringing it up to established standards would be impossible. Applications for variance must include a schedule for compliance—and it should be noted that very few such requests have been granted except for new water systems.

Exemptions to the regulations may be granted (1) if there are good reasons why the utility cannot comply; (2) a satisfactory alternative source of drinking water is unavailable; and (3) no undue health consequences will result.

When a drinking water hazard exists and the state

has not properly attempted to comply, the EPA is empowered to take action by issuing administrative orders or by initiating a civil action against the utility. Fines of up to $5000 per day of violation can be levied.

The EPA also may assume an advisory role when public health is at risk. Such advisories to the states and regional offices have no legal effect and are usually concerned with levels of contaminants that have not previously been covered by MCLs. They are developed administratively by the EPA and are known as "Suggested No Adverse Response Levels (SNARL)."

C. Statutes Controlling Hazardous Substance Disposal or Handling:

In 1976, Congress passed the Resource Conservation and Recovery Act (RCRA)—actually an amendment to the Solid Waste Disposal Act of 1965. This Act has been amended not only by the RCRA but also by the Resource Recovery Act of 1970, the Quiet Communities Act of 1978, and the 1980 amendments to the Solid Waste Disposal Act. The RCRA was designed to meet needs not covered by clean air or water legislation. It is not concerned with regulating air or water pollution per se but is directed at any medium contaminated or threatened by hazardous wastes. It applies to all wastes (except uncontained gaseous material), although such wastes are inappropriately termed "solid wastes" in the statute. "Hazardous wastes" would be a more appropriate term since that is what the statutes apply to.

Under the RCRA, the EPA is responsible for identifying and listing hazardous wastes by individual contaminant, its source, and the process in which it is used. The agency is also responsible for establishing criteria for identifying hazardous wastes, not only at present but in the future. The criteria the agency has developed are as follows:

(1) Is it ignitable?
(2) Is it corrosive, damaging to human tissue, interacting unfavorably with other toxic wastes, dangerous when mixed with other wastes, harmful to aquatic life, or corrosive to metal?
(3) Is it explosive or capable of violent reaction?
(4) Is it toxic?

From the time of inception to disposal, hazardous materials require meticulous bookkeeping under the RCRA. Every instance of production, transportation, treatment, storage, or disposal of such wastes must be reported to EPA, which then assigns an identification number to each reporting so that the hazardous material can be tracked.

The waste generator is the most important factor in the tracking system, since individuals acting as agents of the generator must determine whether or not the material in question is hazardous and, if it is hazardous, must properly pack and label it. Furthermore, appropriate manifests must be prepared to ensure that the material reaches its intended destination if it is to be treated, stored, or disposed of at another location. If a shipment does not reach its destination, that fact must be reported to the EPA (or state official). Consequently, careful records must be maintained on all shipments of hazardous materials, since the generator is responsible for appropriate disposition. It should be noted that this responsibility cannot be contracted out or delegated to anyone else.

Transportation of hazardous wastes is regulated jointly by the EPA and the Department of Transportation (DOT). To meet EPA requirements, the transporter must have an identification number; deliver the load to the designated treatment, storage, or disposal facility; and comply with the EPA manifest requirements for tracking and transporting hazardous wastes. To meet DOT requirements, the transporter must report any spills and clean up any hazardous wastes discharged during the journey.

Treatment, storage, and disposal facilities are issued only interim operating permits until they satisfy the stringent standards and conditions governing issuance of permits. The EPA may delegate responsibility for these facilities to the states provided that their requirements are at least as strict as federal requirements. Nonetheless, initially, the states receive only interim authorization until they prove themselves qualified to grant final authorization.

EPA may bring suit against anyone improperly disposing of hazardous wastes and force them to assume the cost of cleanup. But locating the financially responsible disposers—sometimes after many years—can be difficult. The EPA has established a list of hazardous substances and the quantities of substances that must be reported. Anyone storing, treating, disposing of, or transporting the substances must report to the EPA. Failure to do so can result in severe sanctions. Those responsible for release of hazardous substances listed by the EPA are subject to a fine of up to $5000 a day and punitive damages up to 3 times the cost of cleanup.

REFERENCES

Asbestos

Craighead JE: Asbestos: An environmental reality. *JAMA* 1984;**252**:3292.

Davis DL, Mandula B: Airborne asbestos and public health. *Annu Rev Public Health* 1985;**6**:195.

Davis JM et al: Low level exposure to asbestos: Is there a cancer risk? *Br J Ind Med* 1988;**45**:505.

Edelman DA: Exposure to asbestos and the risk of gastrointestinal cancer: A reassessment. *Br J Ind Med* 1988;**45**:75.

Hughes JM, Weill H: Asbestos exposure: Quantitative assessment of risk. *Am Rev Respir Dis* 1986;**133:**5.

Marsh GM: Critical review of epidemiologic studies related to ingested asbestos. *Environ Health Perspect* 1983;**53:**49.

Nicholson WJ: Human cancer risk from ingested asbestos: A problem of uncertainty. *Environ Health Perspect* 1983;**56:**111.

Peto J et al: Relationship of mortality to measures of environmental asbestos pollution in an asbestos textile factory. *Ann Occup Hyg* 1985;**29:**305.

Weill H: Asbestos-associated diseases: Science, public policy, and litigation. *Chest* 1983;**84:**601.

Lead

Amitai Y et al: Hazards of ''deleading'' homes of children with lead poisoning. *Am J Dis Child* 1987; **141:**758.

Chisolm JJ Jr: The continuing hazard of lead exposure and its effects in children. *Neurotoxicology* 1984; **5:**23.

Johnson BL, Mason RW: A review of public health regulations on lead. *Neurotoxicology* 1984;**5:**1.

Needleman HL, et al: The long-term effects of exposure to low doses of lead in childhood. *N Engl J Med* 1990; **322:**83.

Wedeen RP: *Poison in the Pot: The Legacy of Lead.* Southern Illinois Univ Press, 1984.

Dioxin

Erickson JD et al: Vietnam veterans' risks for fathering babies with birth defects. *JAMA* 1984;**252:**903.

Evans RG et al: A medical follow-up of the health effects of long-term exposure to 2,3,7,8-tetrachlorodibenzo-*p*-dioxin. *Arch Environ Health* 1988;**43:**273.

Fara GM, Del Corno G: Pregnancy outcome in the Seveso area after TCDD contamination. In: *Prevention of Physical and Mental Congenital Defects.* Marois M (editor). Liss, 1985.

Friedman JM: Does Agent Orange cause birth defects? *Teratology* 1984;**29:**193.

Hoffman RE et al: Health effects of long-term exposure to 2,3,7,8-tetrachlorodibenzo-*p*-dioxin. *JAMA* 1986; **255:**2031.

Kahn PC et al: Dioxins and dibenzofurans in blood and adipose tissue of Agent Orange-exposed Vietnam veterans and matched controls. *JAMA* 1988; **259:**1661.

Mastroiacovo P et al: Birth defects in the Seveso area after TCDD contamination. *JAMA* 1988;**259:**1668.

Tschirley FH: Dioxin. *Sci Am* (Feb) 1986;**254:**29.

Webb K et al: Results of a pilot study of health effects due to 2,3,7,8-tetrachlorodibenzodioxin contamination: Missouri. *JAMA* 1984;**251:**1139.

PCBs

Drotman DP et al: Contamination of the food chain by polychlorinated biphenyls from a broken transformer. *Am J Public Health* 1983;**73:**290.

Fein GG et al: Prenatal exposure to polychlorinated biphenyls: Effects on birth size and gestational age. *J Pediatr* 1984;**105:**315.

Hsu ST et al: Discovery and epidemiology of PCB poisoning in Taiwan: A four-year follow-up. *Environ Health Perspect* 1985;**59:**5.

Kuratsune M, Shapiro RE: PCB poisoning in Japan and Taiwan. (Symposium.) *Am J Ind Med* 1984;**5:**1. [Entire issue.]

Rogan WF et al: Congenital poisoning by polychlorinated biphenyls and their contaminants in Taiwan. *Science* 1988;**241:**334.

Schwartz PM et al: Lake Michigan fish consumption as a source of polychlorinated biphenyls in human cord serum, maternal serum, and milk. *Am J Public Health* 1983;**73:**293.

Taylor PR et al: Polychlorinated biphenyls: Influence on birthweight and gestation. *Am J Public Health* 1984;**74:**1153.

World Health Organization: Assessment of health risks in infants associated with exposure to PCBs, PCDDs and PCDFs in breast milk. *Environmental Health,* No. 29, 1988.

Air Pollution

Andrews C et al: Guidelines as to what constitutes an adverse respiratory health effect, with special reference to epidemiologic studies of air pollution. *Am Rev Respir Dis* 1985;**131:**666.

Bethel RA et al: Effect of exercise rate and route of inhalation on sulfur dioxide-induced bronchoconstriction in asthmatic subjects. *Am Rev Respir Dis* 1983; **128:**592.

Boushey HA, Sheppard D: Air pollution. In: *Textbook of Respiratory Medicine.* Murray JF, Nadel JA (editors). Saunders, 1988.

Chameides WL et al: The role of biogenic hydrocarbons in urban photochemical smog: Atlanta as a case study. *Science* 1988;**241:**1473.

Goldstein E, Dungworth D, Ricci PF: Photochemical air pollution. (Part 2.) *West J Med* 1985;**142:**523.

Holland WW et al: Health effects of particulate pollution: Reappraising the evidence. *Am J Epidemiol* 1979;**110:**527.

Russell M: Ozone pollution: The hard choices. *Science* 1988; **241:**1275.

Sheppard D et al: Exercise increases sulfur dioxide-induced bronchoconstriction in asthmatic subjects. *Am Rev Respir Dis* 1981;**123:**486.

Speizer FE: Ozone and photochemical pollutants: Status after 25 years. *West J Med* 1985;**142:**377.

Whittemore AS: Air pollution and respiratory disease. *Annu Rev Public Health* 1981;**2:**397.

Water Pollution

Crump KS, Guess HA: Drinking water and cancer: Review of recent epidemiological findings and assessment risks. *Annu Rev Public Health* 1982;**3:**339.

Folsom AR, Prineas RJ: Drinking water composition and blood pressure: A review of the epidemiology. *Am J Epidemiol* 1982;**115:**818.

Frye RS et al: *Clean Water Act Update.* Executive Enterprises Publications Company, 1987.

Holden P: *Pesticides and Groundwater Quality.* National Academy Press, 1986.

Kraybill HF: Global distribution of carcinogenic pollutants in water. *Ann NY Acad Sci* 1978;**298:**80.

National Research Council: *Drinking Water and Health.* Vol 4. National Academy Press, 1982.

Rice RG, Gomez-Taylor M: Occurrence of by-products of strong oxidants reacting with drinking water contaminants: Scope of the problem. *Environ Health Perspect* 1986;**69:**31.

Sun M: Groundwater ills: Many diagnoses, few remedies. *Science* 1986;**252:**1490.

Ionizing Radiation

Becker DV: Reactor accidents: Public health strategies and their medical implications. *JAMA* 1987;**258:**649.

Crawford M: Mill tailings: A $4-billion problem. *Science* 1985;**229:**537.

Gale RP: Immediate medical consequences of nuclear accidents: Lessons from Chernobyl. *JAMA* 1987: **258:**625.

Hamilton TE et al: Thyroid neoplasia in Marshall Islanders exposed to nuclear fallout. *JAMA* 1987;**258:**629.

National Research Council: *The Effects on Populations of Exposure to Low Levels of Ionizing Radiation.* National Academy Press, 1980.

US House of Representatives Committee on Interstate and Foreign Commerce: *The Forgotten Guinea Pigs.* US Government Printing Office, 1980.

Whalen JP, Balter S: Radiation risks associated with diagnostic radiology. *DM* (March) 1982:**28:**1.

Toxic Waste Management

Dawson GW, Mercer BW: *Hazardous Waste Management.* Wiley, 1986.

Deibler PM: *Poisoning Prosperity: The Impact of Toxics on California's Economy.* California Commission for Economic Development, 1985. (Copies of this report may be obtained from: Office of the Lieutenant Governor, State Capitol, Room 1208, Sacramento, CA 95814.)

Findley RW, Farber DA: *Environmental Law.* West Publishing Co., 1983.

Firestone DB, Reed FC: *Environmental Law for Nonlawyers.* Ann Arbor Science, 1983.

Freeman HM: *Standard Handbook of Hazardous Waste Treatment Disposal.* McGraw-Hill, 1988.

Grisham JW: *Health Aspects of the Disposal of Waste Chemicals.* Permagon Press, 1986.

Maugh TH II: Toxic waste disposal: A growing problem. *Science* 1979;**204:**819.

Appendix: Biostatistics & Epidemiology

Susan T. Sacks, PhD, & Marc B. Schenker, MD, MPH

It is apparent to anyone who reads the medical literature today that some knowledge of biostatistics and epidemiology is a necessity. Research has become more rigorous in the area of study design and analysis, and reports of clinical and epidemiologic research contain increasing amounts of statistical methodology. The purpose of this Appendix is to provide a brief introduction to some of the basic principles of biostatistics and epidemiology.

I. BIOSTATISTICS

DESCRIPTIVE STATISTICS

Types of Data

Data collected in medical research can be divided into 3 types: nominal (categorical), ordinal, and interval (continuous).

Nominal (categorical) data are those that can be divided into 2 or more unordered categories, eg, sex, race, religion. In occupational medicine, for example, many outcome measures such as cancer rates are considered separately for different sex and race categories.

Ordinal data are one step up from nominal data, the difference being a predetermined ordering underlying the categories. Examples of ordinal data are clinical severity, socioeconomic status, or ILO (International Labor Office) profusion category for pneumoconiosis on chest x-rays.

Both nominal and ordinal data are examples of discrete data. They take on only integer values.

Interval data, also called **continuous data,** are data measured on an arithmetic scale. Examples include height, weight, blood lead, and forced expiratory volume. The accuracy of the number recorded depends on the measuring instrument, and the variable can take on an infinite number of values within a defined range. For example a person's height might be recorded as 72 inches or 72.001 inches or 72.00098 inches, depending on the accuracy of the measuring instrument.

Summarizing Data

Once research data have been collected, the first step should be to summarize them. The 2 most common ways of summarizing data are measures of location, or central tendency, and measures of spread, or variation.

A. Measure of Central Tendency:

1. Mean–The mean ($\bar{x}$) is the average value of a set of interval data observations. It is computed using the following equation:

$$\bar{x} = \frac{\sum_{i=1}^{n} x_i}{n}$$

where n = sample size and
  x_i = random variable, such as height, with
    i = 1,...,n.

The mean is strongly affected by extreme values in the data. If a variable has a fairly symmetric distribution, the mean is used as the appropriate measure of central tendency.

2. Median–The median is the "middle" observation, or 50th percentile—ie, half the observations lie above the median and half below. It can be applied to interval or ordinal data. When there are an odd number (n) of observations, the median equals the (n + 1)/2 observation; when there are an even number of observations, the median is halfway between the (n/2) observation and the (n/2) + 1 observation. The median does not have the mathematical niceties of the mean, but it is not as susceptible as the mean to extreme values. If the variable being measured has a distribution that is asymmetric or skewed—ie, if there are a few extreme values at one end of the distribution—the median is a better descriptor than the mean of the "center" of the distribution.

3. Mode–The mode is the most frequently occurring observation. It is rarely used except when there are a limited number of possible outcomes.

4. Frequency distribution–In discussing measures of location or spread, we often refer to the frequency distribution of the data. A frequency distribution consists of a series of predetermined intervals (along the horizontal axis) together with the number (or percentage) of observations whose values fall in that interval (along the vertical axis). An example of a frequency distribution is presented in Fig 1.

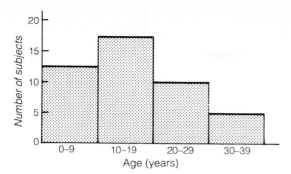

Figure 1. Frequency distribution of subjects by age category.

Table 1. Calculation of mean, median, mode, variance, and standard deviation. (n = 10 workers.)

x_i = number of years of exposure to asbestos.

Worker	x_i	$(x_i - \bar{x})$	$(x_i - \bar{x})^2$
1.	x_1 = 4.0	−2.2	4.84
2.	x_2 = 4.5	−1.7	2.89
3.	x_3 = 5.0	−1.2	1.44
4.	x_4 = 5.0	−1.2	1.44
5.	x_5 = 6.0	−0.2	0.04
6.	x_6 = 6.5	+0.3	0.09
7.	x_7 = 7.0	+0.8	0.64
8.	x_8 = 7.5	+1.3	1.69
9.	x_9 = 8.0	+1.8	3.24
10.	x_{10} = 8.5	+2.3	5.29
Total:	Σx_i = 62.0		$\Sigma(x_i - \bar{x})^2$ = 21.6

Mean: $\bar{x} = \frac{62.0}{10} = 6.2$

$\quad$ **Variance** $= \Sigma(x_i - \bar{x})^2/(n-1) = 21.6/9 = 2.4$
$\quad$ **Standard deviation** $= \sqrt{2.4} = 1.55$

Median:
1. Order the observations from lowest to highest.
2. Median $= \frac{1}{2} \left(\left[\frac{n}{2} \right] \text{ observation} + \left(\left[\frac{n}{2} \right] + 1 \right) \right.$
$\quad$ $\left. \text{observation} \right) = \frac{1}{2}$ (5th observation + 6th observation)
3. Therefore, median $= \frac{1}{2}$ (6.0 + 6.5) = 6.25

Mode:
Most commonly occurring observation is 5.0, since it occurs twice and all other observations occur once.

B. Measures of Variation:

1. Range–The range is the simplest measurement of variation and is defined as the difference between the highest and lowest values. One disadvantage of the range is its tendency to increase in value as the number of observations increases. Furthermore, the range does not provide information about distribution of values within the set of data.

2. Variance–The sample variance (s^2) is a measure of the dispersion about the mean arrived at by calculating the sum of the squared deviations from the mean and dividing by the sample size minus one. The equation for deriving sample variance is as follows:

$$s^2 = \frac{\sum\limits_{i=1}^{n} (x_i - \bar{x})^2}{n-1}$$

Variance can be thought of as the average of squared deviations from the mean.

3. Standard deviation–The sample standard deviation (s) is equal to the square root of the sample variance.

$$s = \sqrt{\frac{\sum\limits_{i=1}^{n} (x_i - \bar{x})^2}{n-1}}$$

See Table 1 for examples of the calculation of mean, median, mode, variance, and standard deviation.

Sample Versus Population Descriptive Statistics

The descriptive statistics discussed thus far are sample estimates of true population values or parameters. Because we usually do not have the resources to measure variables of interest on entire populations, we instead select a sample from the population of interest and then estimate the population mean from the sample mean or the population variance from the sample variance. The population mean is usually represented by the Greek letter μ and the population variance by the Greek letter σ^2. One almost never knows the true population values for these parameters and is almost always conducting sample surveys to estimate them.

The Normal Distribution

The most important continuous probability distribution is the normal or Gaussian distribution, also known as the bell-shaped curve. Many quantitative variables follow a normal distribution, and it plays a central role in statistical tests of hypotheses. Even when one is sampling from a population whose shape departs from the normal distribution, under certain general conditions it forms the basis for statistical testing of hypotheses.

We often transform data to make them more normal in distribution. For example, in occupational exposure studies, the log dose is used rather than the dose because the log dose more closely approximates a normal distribution. A particular normal distribution is defined by its mean and variance (or standard deviation). Two normal distributions with different means but the same variance will differ in location but not in shape (Fig 2). Two normal distributions with the same mean but different variances will have the same location but different shapes or "spreads" about the mean value (Fig 3). Note that the normal distribution is unimodal, bell-shaped, and symmetric about the mean.

The normal distribution has several nice properties

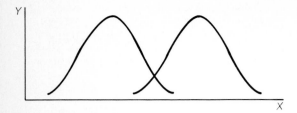

Figure 2. Two normal distributions with different means but identical standard deviations.

that make it amenable to statistical analysis, and variables that follow a normal distribution are for that reason preferred. Thus, data are often transformed to make them more normal, eg, log dose.

The population encompassed by 1 standard deviation (s) on either side of the mean in a normally distributed population will include approximately 67% of the observations in that population (Fig 4); the population between 2 s on either side of the mean will include approximately 95% of the observations; and that between 3 s on either side of the mean encompasses more than 99% of the observations in the population (Fig 4). This property of the normal distribution is particularly useful when a researcher or clinician is trying to identify patients with high or low values in response to a certain test. If one knows the mean for that particular test and has some idea of what the standard deviation is, the range within which one would expect (let us say) 95% of patients to fall can be determined, and a patient with values outside this range might need to be examined further.

To utilize this property of the normal distribution, the sample should be large enough—eg, 20 observations or more—to provide reasonably certain estimates of mean and standard deviation.

> **Example I:** If the mean hematocrit in a clinical population is 42% with a standard deviation of 3%—and assuming hematocrit follows a normal distribution—one would expect 95% of the clinic population to have hematocrits between 42% ± (2 × 3%) or (36, 48)%. A patient falling outside this range could be identified for further testing.

Another principle relevant to normal distribution is the **central limit theorem,** which holds that no matter what may be the underlying distribution of x, the particular variable of interest, the sample mean (x̄) will have a normal distribution if the sample size (n) is large enough. Thus, if x itself comes from a population with a mean value μ and population standard deviation σ, then x̄ (calculated from a sufficiently large sample of size n) will have a normal distribution with the same population mean μ and a smaller population standard deviation equal to ($\sigma/\sqrt{n}$). One can then test hypotheses concerning the sample mean x̄, because it is known to have a normal distribution and its mean and standard deviation are also known. The standard deviation of x̄ is called the standard error of the mean (SEM).

Since one is usually concerned with estimating the true population mean from the sample mean x̄, it is important to know how good an estimate the sample mean is of the true mean. Every time a sample of size n is selected from the population and x̄ is calculated, a different value for x̄ will be obtained and thus a different estimate of μ. If this were done over and over again and many x̄'s were generated, the x̄'s themselves would have a normal distribution centered on μ with standard deviation equal to ($\sigma/\sqrt{n}$). In practice, one does not calculate several x̄'s to estimate μ—only one is calculated. The SEM quantifies the certainty with which this one sample mean estimates the population mean. The certainty with which one estimates the population mean increases with sample size, and it can be seen that the standard error decreases as n increases. Furthermore, the more variability in the underlying population, the more variable will be the estimate of μ. It can also be seen that the standard error increases as σ increases. The "true" SEM is $\sigma/\sqrt{n}$, and the sample estimate of the standard error of the mean is $s/\sqrt{n}$, where s is the sample standard deviation.

Many investigators summarize the variability in their data with the standard error because it is smaller in value than the standard deviation. However, the standard error does not quantify variability in the population; it quantifies the uncertainty in the estimate of μ, the population mean. An investigator describing the population sampled should use the standard deviation to describe that population. The standard error of the mean is used in testing hypoth-

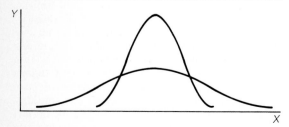

Figure 3. Two normal distributions with identical means but different standard deviations.

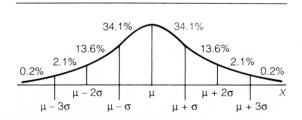

Figure 4. Standard normal distribution.

eses about the population mean—as will be discussed later.

Example II: Suppose blood lead is measured on 20 patients. Assume the sample mean ($\bar{x}$) equals 20 μg/dL and the sample standard deviation (s) equals 5 μg/dL with sample size (n) of 20. If blood lead has a normal distribution in this sample, one would expect 95% of the population to lie within 2 s of the mean. Thus, if the investigator's sample was a representative one, 95% of the population will have blood leads between 20 ± (2 × 5) (ie, between 10 and 30 μg/dL). These numbers quickly summarize the distribution and give the readers a range against which to compare their own patients. However, investigators often summarize their data with the mean and the standard error of the mean and report that "blood lead in this sample population was 20 ± (2 × (5/ $\sqrt{20}$))." This would lead a reader to believe that 95% of blood leads would be expected to fall between 17.8 and 22.2 μg/dL if one did not know the difference between the standard deviation and the standard error of the mean. In reality, 17.8 and 22.2 μg/dL describe a quantity known as the 95% confidence interval for the true mean blood lead μ: it does not describe a range of expected values. The reader of the report usually wishes to compare a patient's blood lead with an expected range of values for blood lead, ie, the mean ± 2 s.

INFERENTIAL STATISTICS

In general, there are 2 steps to be followed in data analysis. The first is to describe the data using descriptive statistics such as the mean, median, variance, and standard deviation. The second step is to test specific hypotheses that were formulated *before* conducting the research project. This is done by formulating a **null hypothesis** and an **alternative hypothesis,** wherein the null hypothesis is "no difference exists" and the alternative hypothesis is "difference exists."

An example of a null hypothesis might be, "There is no difference in pulmonary function between groups of underground miners and surface miners." The alternative hypothesis would be, "There is a difference between the 2 groups."

Once the hypotheses are formulated, the appropriate statistical test can be performed. Some of the most commonly used methods will be discussed below.

The Case of Two Groups: The t-Test

In many instances an investigator is interested in comparing 2 groups to determine whether they differ on average for some continuous variable. For example, an investigator might be interested in determining whether exposure to organic solvents has an effect on psychomotor performance such as reaction time. To do this, one would select a sample of a group of industrial painters who are exposed to such solvents and compare their test performances with those of a group of workers not exposed to such solvents. Obviously, even if there are truly no differences between 2 employee groups in how they perform on such a test, the sample mean test scores will probably be unequal simply because of random fluctuation.

The main question is, "Are the differences larger than one would expect by chance if there truly is no difference in the reaction times?"—ie, do the samples come from one underlying population, not two? The null hypothesis in this situation is that the true mean reaction time in the painter group equals the true mean reaction time in the nonpainter group.

The alternative hypothesis is that the underlying true means are unequal. This is usually called a 2-sided alternative hypothesis, because we are not specifying the direction of the inequality. In the example, average reaction time in the painter group might be faster or slower than average reaction time in the nonpainter group. Differences in either direction are examined in testing the null hypothesis.

The appropriate statistical test in this situation is the 2-sample *t*-test. Two independent samples have been drawn—ie, the individuals in one sample are independent of the individuals in the other. The *t*-test has the following form:

$$t = \frac{\bar{x}_1 - \bar{x}_2}{SE(\bar{x}_1 - \bar{x}_2)}$$

where $\bar{x}_1$ = sample mean group 1 and
$\bar{x}_2$ = sample mean group 2.

Note that the numerator is the difference of sample means and the denominator is the standard error of this quantity. Dividing by the SE standardizes the difference in sample means by the variability present in the data. If the difference in the means was very large but the data from which it was calculated was highly variable, the *t*-statistic would reflect this and would be adjusted accordingly. The *t*-statistic reduces down as shown below:

$$t = \frac{\bar{x}_1 - \bar{x}_2}{\sqrt{\left(\frac{s_1^2}{n_1}\right) + \left(\frac{s_2^2}{n_2}\right)}}$$

where s_1^2 = variance in group 1 and
s_2^2 = variance in group 2.

Use of the *t*-statistic assumes that the 2 samples have the same underlying population variance σ^2. Thus, a pooled estimate of the variance is calculated and substituted into the *t*-statistic. This pooled estimate s_p^2 has the following form:

$$s_p^2 = \frac{(n_1 - 1)s_1^2 + (n_2 - 1)s_2^2}{(n_1 + n_2 - 2)}$$

Therefore, the 2-sample t-statistic is as follows:

$$t = \frac{\overline{x}_1 - \overline{x}_2}{\sqrt{\left(\dfrac{s_p^2}{n_1}\right) + \left(\dfrac{s_p^2}{n_2}\right)}}$$

Note that the pooled estimate of the variance is simply a weighted average of the variances from sample 1 and sample 2. Thus, if one sample is much larger than the other, more weight is given to its estimate of σ^2 because it is assumed to be more reliable since based on a larger sample size. Note further that if the 2 samples are of equal size, the pooled variance is simply the sum of the 2 sample variances divided by 2. From the format of the t-test, one can see that if the 2 sample means are similar in value, the numerator of t will be close to zero—and, consequently, the value of t would be small, leading to the conclusion that the null hypothesis is true and that there is probably only one underlying distribution from which the 2 samples come. If one obtains a large value for the t-statistic, it is likely that the 2 samples come from 2 different underlying distributions, and one would therefore want to reject the null hypothesis.

How large does t have to be to reject the null hypothesis? Tables of the t statistic indicate what value of t would cause the null hypothesis to be rejected. Even when the null hypothesis is true and there really is no difference between the groups being compared, there is the possibility that a large value of t might occur owing to random chance alone. One would like the probability of this occurrence to be small, ie, less than 5%.

To find the proper value of t for a particular study, a quantity known as the **degrees of freedom** is necessary. The degrees of freedom are equal to $(n_1 + n_2 - 2)$. Once the degrees of freedom are known, the value of t may be obtained from the t table and compared to the t statistic calculated in the study. If the study t statistic is larger than the tabled cutoff value, one can conclude that this is unlikely to have happened under the null hypothesis, which is therefore rejected.

Bear in mind that the alternative hypothesis was the 2-sided alternative, meaning that the 2 group means were simply *different* but not specifying the direction of the difference. Consequently, in the t-table, 2 cutoff points are actually obtained, since both very large negative and very large positive values of t are of interest. The t-distribution is symmetric, so that the 2 cutoff points are simply $\pm (t)$. If the study t-value is larger than $+t$ or smaller than $-t$, the null hypothesis is rejected.

An example problem is worked below to give the flavor of the t-test and how it is used.

Example III: Two-sample t-test. The following tabulation presents the mean change in plasma cholines- terase concentration from baseline levels for 15 pesticide applicators and 14 unexposed controls.

	N	Mean Decline (%)	Standard Deviation
Applicators	15	25	11
Controls	14	10	6

Do the data present sufficient evidence from which to conclude that the mean decline in cholinesterase is different for the 2 groups?

The null hypothesis is that there is no difference in cholinesterase change between the 2 groups. The alternative hypothesis is that there is a difference in cholinesterase change between the 2 groups.

First calculate s_p^2:

$$s_p^2 = \frac{(n_1 - 1) s_1^2 + (n_2 - 1) s_2^2}{(n_1 + n_2 - 2)}$$

$$= \frac{(15 - 1)\, 11^2 + (14 - 1)\, 6^2}{(15 + 14 - 2)}$$

$$= 80.07$$

Substitute into the formula for t:

$$t = \frac{\overline{x}_1 - \overline{x}_2}{\sqrt{\left(\dfrac{s_p^2}{n_1}\right) + \left(\dfrac{s_p^2}{n_2}\right)}}$$

$$= \frac{25 - 10}{\sqrt{\left(\dfrac{80.07}{15}\right) + \left(\dfrac{80.07}{14}\right)}}$$

$$= \frac{15}{\sqrt{11.06}}$$

$$= 4.51$$

Therefore, $t = 4.51$ and $df = n_1 + n_2 = 27$.

The study t-value of 4.51 with 27 degrees of freedom is compared with the tabled t value of ± 2.05, which has a 5% chance of occurring when the null hypothesis is true. Since $+4.51$ is larger than $+2.05$, the null hypothesis is rejected—ie, there is a statistically significant difference in the mean change in plasma cholinesterase from baseline between the 2 study groups.

Paired t-Test

The above discussion concerns the 2-sample *t*-test and is appropriate for the situation in which 2 independent groups are being compared. Another common situation occurs when there are paired samples—ie, the 2 observations are not independent of one another.

For example, suppose a researcher is measuring change in pulmonary function (eg, FEV_1) over a workshift and there are 20 subjects in the study. (See example below.) The researcher would measure FEV_1 among the subjects before and after the workshift. Clearly, the before and after measurements are not independent, and one would like to take advantage of the fact that all individual (nonexposure) characteristics have been controlled. To do this, the *difference* in FEV_1 (before-after) is calculated for each subject. Since the *difference* is the only observation made per subject, the data set has now gone from 40 observations (2 per subject) to 20 observations (one per subject). If there is no effect of workshift on FEV_1, one would expect the difference in FEV_1 for each subject to be small in value or close to zero. If the null hypothesis is not true and workshift exposure does change FEV_1, the differences will not be close to zero. The *t*-statistic calculated in this situation is known as the paired *t*-statistic and has the following form:

$$t = \frac{\bar{D}}{(s_D/\sqrt{n})}$$

where $\bar{D} = \dfrac{\sum D_i}{n}$ = average difference and

s_D = standard deviation of differences

$$= \sqrt{\frac{\displaystyle\sum_{i=1}^{n}(D_i - \bar{D})^2}{n-1}}$$

The appropriate null hypothesis is that the true mean of the differences is zero, and the appropriate alternative hypothesis is that the true mean of the differences is not zero. Again, it is a 2-sided alternative, and one is looking for large positive as well as large negative differences. Small absolute values of the *t*-statistic would indicate that the null hypothesis is probably true, and large absolute values of *t* would lead to rejection of the null hypothesis. One goes to the *t*-table to determine how large a value of *t* is needed to reject the null hypothesis. To enter the table, one needs to know the appropriate degrees of freedom. In the paired *t* situation, there are $n-1$ degrees of freedom, or the number of pairs minus one.

Common Errors in Use of the t-Test

A common mistake made with the *t*-test is known

EXAMPLE: Paired t-test

A study of painters involved measuring pulmonary function (FEV_1; liters) at the beginning (A) and end (B) of a workshift. The results were as follows:

Case #	A_i	B_i	$D_i=(A_i-B_i)$	$(D_i-\bar{D})$	$(D_i-\bar{D})^2$
1	3.14	3.01	0.13	0.10	0.010
2	2.85	2.80	0.05	0.02	0.000
3	2.50	2.30	0.20	0.17	0.029
4	3.01	3.15	−0.14	−0.17	0.029
5	1.55	1.55	0.00	−0.03	0.001
6	2.21	2.15	0.06	0.03	0.001
7	2.81	2.68	0.13	0.10	0.010
8	3.25	3.34	−0.09	−0.12	0.014
9	2.66	2.56	0.10	−0.07	0.029
10	1.95	1.90	0.05	−0.02	0.000
11	3.50	3.46	0.04	0.01	0.000
12	3.95	4.06	−0.11	−0.14	0.020
13	4.10	3.90	0.20	0.17	0.029
14	3.60	3.56	0.04	0.01	0.000
15	2.80	2.90	−0.10	−0.13	0.017
16	2.50	2.50	0.00	−0.03	0.001
17	2.10	2.16	−0.06	−0.09	0.008
18	3.70	3.61	0.09	0.06	0.004
19	2.92	2.86	0.06	0.03	0.001
20	3.31	3.42	−0.11	−0.14	0.020
			0.54		0.198

$$\bar{D} = \frac{\sum D_i}{n} = \frac{0.54}{20} = 0.027$$

Degrees of freedom = n − 1 = 19

$$s_D = \sqrt{\frac{\displaystyle\sum_{i=1}^{n}(D_i - \bar{D})^2}{n-1}}$$

$$= \sqrt{\frac{0.198}{19}} = 0.102$$

$$t = \frac{\bar{D}}{(s_D/\sqrt{n})} = \frac{0.027}{0.102/\sqrt{20}} = 1.18$$

Compare the calculated *t* of 1.18 to the tabled *t* of 2.093. Since the calculated *t* is less than the *t* in the table, the null hypothesis (of no change in function over workshift) is not rejected.

---

as the multiple comparison problem. The problem arises when an investigator has several groups to compare and proceeds to compare them 2 at a time, using the *t*-test each time. In other words, group 1 is compared with group 2 with the *t*-test, then group 2 with group 3, then group 1 with group 3, etc. Each time the null hypothesis is rejected, the computed value of *t* is likely to occur less than 5% of the time under the null hypothesis. The problem with proceeding in this fashion is that overall there is more than a 5% chance of mistakenly rejecting the null hypothesis—even though there is only a 5% chance of making this mistake with each individual comparison. This increased probability of making a mistake occurs because the comparisons are not independent of one another—the same sample group appears in more than one comparison. There are many ways of adjusting for this situation, known as **multiple comparison procedures.** What is important to remember is that if one does enough of such 2-group comparisons, the probability of rejecting the null hypothesis incorrectly at least once increases with the number of such comparisons made and can be quite a bit greater than 5%.

Analysis of Variance

When the variables under study are of the interval (continuous) type and there are more than 2 groups under study, the investigator is usually concerned with whether the means in the groups are different from one another. The appropriate statistical method to use in this situation is analysis of variance. A typical analysis of variance situation can now be described.

Suppose one were studying 3 groups of workers occupationally exposed to 3 different gases. One might want to test whether the particular gases affected mean FEV_1 levels differently in the 3 groups. In this example, individual FEV_1 values would be adjusted for nonexposure determinants (age, sex, height, race). In this situation, the null hypotheses is that the group means for FEV_1 are equal, ie, that a particular exposure has no effect on FEV_1 values. Obviously, there will be differences between the sample means in each group owing to random fluctuations in FEV_1 among individuals.

Are the differences observed in the sample means due merely to random fluctuations or are they due to true differences in FEV_1 caused by the gas exposures. To answer this question, one proceeds under the assumption that the gas exposure has no effect and that the 3 groups are really random samples from the same underlying population. This assumes that the null hypothesis is true, except that the samples are expected to have different means and standard deviations since they are samples of the underlying population. The null hypothesis assumes that such differences are due simply to random sampling. Analysis of variance tests this null hypothesis by estimating the true population variance in 2 different ways and comparing these 2 estimates of the variance. If the 3 samples do indeed come from the same underlying population, these 2 estimates of the variance will be very close in value. If the 3 samples do not all come from the same underlying population, these 2 estimates will be further apart in value, and this separation is what one hopes to detect.

Certain statistical assumptions are made when an analysis of variance test is performed on a set of data: (1) It is assumed that there has been random assignment to treatment groups and that the groups are independent; (2) the underlying variance σ^2 in each group is assumed to be the same (even though the true group means may be different and the sample variances may differ slightly); and (3) the random variable under study—eg, FEV_1—has a normal distribution. Conceptually, the method of analysis of variance proceeds as follows:

Once the null hypothesis is formulated, the sample variance is computed within each exposure group. Each of these estimates, computed within an exposure group, is unaffected by differences among the group means. Each "within" group estimate of the variance is estimating σ^2. These estimates are averaged to obtain one "within" group variance estimate. The values of the individual exposure group means are then used to arrive at a second estimate of σ^2. In this second case, differences (or variability) among the group means will affect the estimate of σ^2. If a particular gas exposure has no effect on FEV_1, both estimates of σ^2 should be similar. To test the null hypothesis, a statistic known as the F statistic is calculated. The "F" is simply the ratio of the "between" group variance estimate to the "within" group variance estimate. Since both numbers estimate the same parameter (σ^2), if the null hypothesis is true, the value of F should be close to 1. If F is significantly larger than 1, one is led to reject the null hypothesis and must conclude that the exposure groups are different in levels of FEV_1.

How does one determine how large F must be in order to reject the null hypothesis? Because of random fluctuations in the data, it is possible that a large F-statistic might result even when the null hypothesis is true. However, one would like the chance of this happening to be very small. Tables of the F statistic are available to assist the investigator in selecting a value of F against which the F-statistic calculated from the data can be compared. The tabled value of F is one that would occur less than about 5% of the time if the null hypothesis were true. If the F-statistic calculated from the researcher's data is larger than the one in the table, the results are known to occur less than 5% of the time just by random chance, even when the null hypothesis (no difference in sample groups) is true. Since the observed results are therefore very unlikely to happen under the null hypothesis, the researcher can reject the null hypothesis and say that there is a difference among the groups. A 5% cutoff point is an arbitrary one, and, depending on the individual situation, one could set the cutoff at 1% or 10%. The conventional cutoff point is 5%.

When one is studying *more than 2 groups* and the data involved are continuous (eg, FEV, blood lead) and the question of interest is whether the groups all come from the same underlying population—ie, have the same mean value—the most appropriate *first test* of the null hypothesis is the analysis of variance. If one fails to reject the null hypothesis with the F-statistic, no further investigation of this null hypothesis is necessary. There are no differences among groups. One does not need to start comparing the mean of group 1 with the mean of group 2, etc. On the other hand, if one performs an analysis of variance on the data and rejects the null hypothesis, then there exist some differences in FEV_1 among the study groups resulting from particular gas exposure. One can then use procedures known as multiple comparison tests to identify exactly which group or groups differ significantly from the others.

This is an oversimplified discussion of analysis of variance meant only to develop the concept of this important statistical method. Not enough details have been provided for the reader to be able to perform this test. The purpose is to convey the flavor of the method so that situations in which analysis of variance is the appropriate first analytic procedure will be recognized. The bibliography includes references to texts in which the method is described in greater detail.

Analyzing Rates & Proportions: The Chi Square Test

In the previous sections, the discussion concerned the analysis of continuous type data. This section begins a discussion of the analysis of categorical data. An example of a situation in which categorical data appear is the following table from a hypothetical newspaper account of a "Bay to Breakers" footrace that takes place every year in San Francisco:

	Males	Females
Finished race in < 45 minutes	20,000	5,000
Finished race in $\geq$ 45 minutes	10,000	15,000
	30,000	20,000

Without doing any statistical tests on these data, one can see that the men finished the race faster than the women—so there is a relationship between the sex of the runner and how quickly he or she finished the race—ie, there is a relationship between the row variable (time) and the column variable (sex).

But suppose the results of the race had been as follows:

	Males	Females
Finished race in < 45 minutes	15,000	10,000
Finished race in $\geq$ 45 minutes	15,000	10,000
	30,000	20,000

The results of the race are not related to the sex of the runner, since half the men finished in less than 45 minutes and half the women finished in less than 45 minutes. Now one would say that there is no association between the row variable (time) and the column variable (sex).

Most situations with categorical data are not as clear-cut as these 2 examples. In most cases, one cannot simply "eyeball" the data to determine whether the 2 variables are or are not independent of one another. The statistical test one uses to determine whether or not there is an association in such data is known as the chi square test. An example of a situation in which the chi square test is applied is shown below.

Example IV: Three groups of farm workers are studied for the occurrence of new skin rashes during the growing season. The 3 groups are involved in growing and harvesting of (1) grapes, (2) citrus crops, and (3) tomatoes. The workers are followed for the growing season, and the occurrence of new rashes in the 3 groups is compared to determine if there is an association between exposure (crop) and outcome (rash).

Crop 1 N = 100
Crop 2 N = 200
Crop 3 N = 200

Response	Exposure (Crop)			
	1	2	3	
Rash	30	40	32	102
No rash	70	160	168	398
	100	200	200	500

The null hypothesis in this situation is again the hypothesis of "no difference"—only it is phrased as no association between the row variable (rash) and the column variable (crop). In the Bay to Breakers example, the null hypothesis was that there was no association between running time and sex of the runner.

One can quickly compute from the table that the percentage working on crop 1 with a rash is 30%; on crop 2, it is 20%; and on crop 3, it is 16%. By just eyeballing the data, one would probably think that crop 1 is different from crops 2 and 3. The null hypothesis is there is no association between what crop a worker worked on and whether or not a rash developed. The question is whether the differences in response are due simply to random variation in the data or whether they are larger than one would expect by chance alone if the null hypothesis were true. To test this, the chi square statistic is calculated. As with the t-test and F-test, one determines whether this chi square is unlikely to have occurred by chance alone under the null hypothesis. The calculation of the chi square involves first determining an "expected" value for each cell in the table. The expected value is the value one would "expect" to see in the cell if there were no association between row (rash) and column (exposure) variables—ie, that value one would "expect" to see if the null hypothesis were true. The expected value is obtained as follows:

According to the null hypothesis, there are no differences among exposures, so we would expect the same proportion to develop a rash in each group. If this is true, the best estimate of the expected proportion with rashes in each exposure group comes from the overall information given by the row total number with rashes divided by the total number of workers in the study. That would be 102/500 = 0.204. Then, for exposure 1, one expects that 0.204 of the 100 people in exposure group 1 will develop rashes, ie, 20.4 people; for exposure 2, one expects that 0.204 of the 200 people working with crop 2 will develop rashes, ie, 40.8 people; and for crop 3, one expects that 0.204 of the 200 people will develop rashes, ie, 40.8 people. In other words, since under the null hypothesis there is no association between exposure and percentage developing a rash, one expects the same percentage to respond favorably (or unfavorably) in each group. The expected proportion of workers not developing rashes is obtained in the same manner. The best estimate of the proportion not developing a rash in each group is the total number not developing a rash divided by the total number of workers, which equals $398/500 = 0.796$. This gives an expected frequency of $100 \times 0.796 = 79.6$ working with crop 1 not developing rashes, 159.2 working with crop 2 not developing rashes, and 159.2 working with crop 3 not developing rashes. Putting the expected values in parentheses alongside the observed values, the table now looks like this:

Response	Exposure (Crop)			
	1	2	3	
Rash	30 (20.4)	40 (40.8)	43 (40.8)	102
No rash	70 (79.6)	160 (159.2)	168 (159.2)	398
	100	200	200	500

To test the null hypothesis, one looks at the observed and expected numbers in each cell to see how close together the 2 values are. If the values are close together, one may decide that the null hypothesis is true. If they are very different, one may decide that the null hypothesis is not true. To decide whether the observed and expected values are close together, the chi square statistic is calculated. It has the following form:

$$\chi^2 = \sum_{i=1}^{n} \left[\frac{(O_i - E_i)^2}{E_i} \right]$$

where E_i = expected value in cell i,
O_i = observed value in cell i,
i = l,...,n, and
n = number of cells in the table.

Large values of chi square indicate a lack of agreement between observed and expected values; small values of chi square indicate close agreement.

How does one determine what is a large chi square? Just as in the preceding discussions about continuous data, one goes to a table of chi square values. The chi square value that would occur less than 5% of the time if the null hypothesis (no association) were true is identified in the table and compared to the study chi square value. If the study chi square is larger than the table cutoff value, the null hypothesis is rejected, since this is known to occur less than 5% of the time when the null hypothesis is true. If the study chi square value is smaller than the table cutoff value, the null hypothesis is not rejected, since this is known to happen more than 5% of the time when the null hypothesis is true. Alternatively, one could calculate the exact p (probability) value of the study chi square statistic. To use the chi square tables, the degrees of freedom are needed to enter the proper point in the table. The degrees of freedom in the chi square situation are equal to (number of rows $-$ 1) times (number of columns-1). When there are 2 rows and 3 columns in a table, the degree of freedom is $(2-1)$ times $(3-1)$, which equals 2 degrees of freedom. One thing to remember is that the chi square statistic works only when the sample is sufficiently large. A rule of thumb is that the chi square is a good approximation when all *expected* values are equal to or greater than 5.

Calculating the chi square statistic for the preceding example, the following results are obtained.

$$\begin{aligned} X^2 &= \frac{(70-79.6)^2}{79.6} + \frac{(160-159.2)^2}{159.2} \\ &+ \frac{(168-159.2)^2}{159.2} + \frac{(30-20.4)^2}{20.4} \\ &+ \frac{(40-40.8)^2}{40.8} + \frac{(32-40.8)^2}{40.8} \\ &= 8.08 \end{aligned}$$

The tabled value of chi square to which the calculated value is compared is 5.99. Since 8.08 is larger than 5.99, the null hypothesis is rejected.

Calculating the chi square statistic is only one method for analyzing categorical data. It is, however, one of the most common statistical tests found in the medical literature.

The *P*-Value & Statistical Significance

An important quantity in all statistical tests of hypothesis is the *P*-value. The *P*-value is the probability of observing a particular study result (eg, *t*-statistic calculated from study data) by chance alone when the null hypothesis is really true. In the examples thus far, the *P*-value of the test statistic has actually been used without calculating its exact value. The procedure has been to calculate, for example, a *t*-statistic from the study data. One then goes to a table of *t*-values and looks up that value of *t* that will occur less than 5% of the time by chance alone when the null hypothesis is true—ie, one looks up the tabulated *t*-statistic that has a *P*-value of 5%. If the value of the *t*-statistic computed for the sample is smaller than the one in the table, the null hypothesis is not rejected, since that is known to occur more than 5% of the time when the null hypothesis is true—ie, it has a *P*-value greater than 5%. When the computed sample *t*-statistic has a value larger than the one in the table, the null hypothesis is rejected, since that is known to occur less than 5% of the time when the null hypothesis is true. In other words, the sample *t*-statistic has a *P*-value less than 5%, so the null hypothesis is rejected. The exact *P*-value of the sample *t*-statistic can also be obtained from tabulated values, so that one can report *P*-values less than other cutoff values, eg, 1% ($P < 0.01$). When the *P*-value is less than 5%, the result is commonly referred to as being "statistically significant." However, "statistical significance" may not be the same as clinical or public health significance, since the former is affected by the size of the study population but may reflect differences that have no biologic importance.

The researcher in a typical study is interested in comparing an exposed group to a control group and using the observed difference in proportions or mean values to estimate the effect of the exposure. For example, one is interested in determining delta (δ), where δ equals the true mean value of sperm concentration among exposed workers minus the true mean value of sperm concentration in unexposed workers. One then wishes to test whether $\delta = 0$; one may wish to determine or whether the (true) proportion with disease from one exposure is equal to the (true) proportion with disease under a second exposure or control. One can then calculate δ as the difference between these 2 proportions, again testing to see whether $\delta = 0$.

Even if the treatment and control groups in the study are truly being sampled from one underlying population (ie, if there is no real difference between treatment and control) some differences between the 2 groups will occur by chance alone. If the observed difference in sample means or proportions has a small probability of occurring by chance alone (assuming no true underlying difference), then the null hypothesis that $\delta = 0$ is rejected. The "rule" for deciding how small that probability has to be before rejecting the null hypothesis is known as the **level of significance** of the statistical test and is designated as alpha (α).

Thus, the procedure in a typical study is to formulate a null hypothesis (H_0), and, usually,

H_0: $\mu_1 = \mu_2$
also written as H_0: $\delta = \mu_1 - \mu_2 = 0$

eg, H_0: mean sperm concentration with exposure 1 = mean sperm concentration with exposure 2.

or,

H_0: $p_1 - p_2 = 0$
also written as H_0: $\delta = p_1 - p_2 = 0$

ie, H_0: proportion with disease in exposure 1 = proportion with disease in exposure 2.

The (2-sided) alternative hypothesis is,

H_A: $\mu_1 \neq \mu_2$
also written as H_A: $\delta = \mu_1 - \mu_2 \neq 0$

ie, H_A: the mean sperm concentrations are not equal under treatments 1 and 2

or

H_A: $p_1 \neq p_2$
also written as H_A: $\delta = p_1 - p_2 \neq 0$

ie, H_A: the proportions with disease are not equal under treatments 1 and 2

After the study has been completed, sample estimates of μ or p are calculated for the 2 exposure groups. The probability is calculated that a difference as large as the one observed in the study would occur if the null hypothesis were true. This probability is the P-value of the test. If the P-value is less than α (the significance level), the null hypothesis is rejected. If the P-value is not less than α, the null hypothesis is not rejected.

THE TYPES OF MISTAKES ONE CAN MAKE IN DOING A RESEARCH STUDY

There are 2 types of errors one can make in deriving inferences from a typical research study. They are known as type I and type II errors.

Type I Error

If one decides to reject the null hypothesis and declare the 2 groups different when in fact they really are from the same underlying population, this is a type I error. The type I error is equal to the significance level α, and the significance level is *established before* the study is done. Thus, α equals the probability that one will reject the null hypothesis when the null hypothesis is true, ie, when the investigator decides what chance of making this kind of mistake is acceptable and sets the α level accordingly. For example, an investigator may decide that it is extremely important not to declare that a disease (eg, cancer) is associated with an exposure unless there is overwhelming evidence of an association from the study. In this case, the α level might be set at 1% instead of 5%, where 5% is the usual value for α used in most studies.

Type II Error

If a researcher decides not to reject the null hypothesis when, in fact, there is a difference between the 2 groups, a type II error has been made—ie, a true difference between the 2 groups has been missed. The type II error is usually designated with β.

In a research study, the type II error is not a single value. If the null hypothesis is false, this means that exposure does not equal control, ie, δ is not equal to 0. There are an infinite number of values that this difference could take on. For each different value of the difference δ between exposed and control, there is a different value for the type II error. If one is interested in determining the probability that one would miss a true difference between exposure and control groups, the exact value of the difference being examined must be specified. Once this is done, the probability that one would fail to reject the null hypothesis given the true nonzero difference between the 2 groups can be calculated.

The Power of a Study

One of the most important quantities calculated for a research study is the power of a particular study. The power is the probability that one will correctly reject the null hypothesis when the null hypothesis is truly false. In other words, the power is the probability of correctly recognizing a true difference between the 2 groups. The power of a study is actually the complement of the type II error β, ie, power $= 1 - \beta$. Thus, the power of a study is different for every different value of δ that occurs. To calculate the power, one must specify a particular alternative. Power is particularly important when one is evaluating a negative study—a study that finds no difference between the groups.

Suppose the power of a study is 40%. This means that the researcher had a 40% chance of finding a true difference between the exposure groups. If no difference between the exposure groups was found and the power of the study was reported as 40%, the reader might wonder whether that study even had a chance of finding a difference between exposures if the exposures were truly associated with different outcomes.

The power of a statistical test is determined or affected by 3 quantities: (1) the magnitude of the type I error α; (2) the size of the exposure effect δ the researcher is interested in detecting; and (3) the sample size of the study. Quantities (1) and (2) can be used to estimate the sample size needed in a study for a specified study power.

As the size of the type I error becomes smaller, the power of the study likewise becomes smaller. The type I error is the probability of incorrectly declaring a difference when there really is none. If it becomes harder to make this mistake (ie, α is smaller), it becomes harder to reject the null hypothesis in general, and power involves correctly rejecting the null hypothesis.

When a study is set up to look for a very large exposure effect δ, it is relatively easy to detect this large effect, and the chances are great that the null hypothesis will be correctly rejected. The opposite occurs when one is looking for a very small δ. Thus, power increases as δ increases.

As sample size increases, the variability of the measure of exposure effect decreases. Consequently, the test statistic increases in value, making it easier to exceed the cutoff point for rejecting the null hypothesis. This increases the chances of correctly rejecting the null hypothesis, and so power increases as sample size increases.

A handy table for remembering the quantities discussed in this section is shown below:

	H_0 true (no difference)	H_0 false (difference exists)
H_0 study (declare no difference)	Correct decision	Type II error β
H_0 reject (declare a difference)	Type I error α	Power $1-\beta$

REFERENCES

The 3 books listed below are excellent introductory texts for clinicians who wish to learn the basic concepts and vocabulary of biostatistics. All 3 cover the elementary descriptive and analytic statistical methods useful for understanding today's medical literature. Examples in these texts are taken from actual published studies.

Colton T: *Statistics in Medicine.* Little, Brown, 1974.
Glantz SA: *Primer of Biostatistics.* McGraw-Hill, 1987.
Ingelfinger JA et al: *Clinical Biostatistics.* Macmillan, 1983.

The following 4 books are also introductory statistical textbooks but are more technically difficult than the preceding group; they cover more statistical procedures in greater depth. The books differ somewhat in the amount of mathematics used, but nothing beyond college algebra is required to cover the material as presented.

Armitage P: *Statistical Methods in Medical Research.* Blackwell, 1971.
Brown BW Jr: Hollander M: *Statistics: A Biomedical Introduction.* Wiley, 1977.
Wonnacott RJ, Wonnacott TH: *Introductory Statistics,* 3rd ed. Wiley, 1977.
Zar JH: *Biostatistical Analysis.* Prentice-Hall, 1983.

II. EPIDEMIOLOGY

Epidemiology is the study of the distribution and determinants of health- and disease-related conditions in populations. It is concerned with both epidemic (excess of normal expectancy) and endemic (always present) conditions.

The basic premise of epidemiology is that disease is not randomly distributed across populations. Not only is it important to know what sort of disease a particular person has—it is necessary also to know what sort of person has a particular disease. While the practice of much of occupational medicine is concerned with the pathogenesis of disease and the treatment of individuals with diseases, the focus of occupational epidemiology is on groups of individuals—with or without diseases—in an attempt to infer the causes that precede specific diseases and to determine what occupational or other lifestyle factors can be manipulated to eliminate specific diseases or reduce the prevalence of the disease.

There are 3 major types of epidemiologic studies: descriptive, analytic, and experimental.

Descriptive epidemiologic studies characterize person, place, and time. (1) Person: What are the personal characteristics of people who get a particular disease?—eg, age, race, sex, occupation, socioeconomic status, immune status. (2) Place: Where do they live or work or travel?—eg, international, national, and local comparisons, urban/rural, climate, altitude. (3) Time: When does the illness occur?—eg, temporal variation, seasonal fluctuations.

Analytic studies attempt to determine the etiologic factors associated with a disease by calculating estimates of risk: (1) What exposures do people with the disease have in common?—eg, smoking, exogenous hormone use, diet, radiation, asbestos. (2) How much is risk increased by such exposures (using relative risk as the measure of excess risk)? (3) How many cases could be avoided if the exposure were eliminated (using attributable risk as the appropriate measure)?

Experimental studies involve a search for strategies for altering the natural history of disease. Examples of experimental studies are intervention trials to reduce risk factors, screening studies aimed at identifying the early stages of disease, and clinical trials of different treatment modalities to improve prognosis.

MORTALITY & MORBIDITY

The 2 basic measures of disease in a population are mortality rates and morbidity rates. Examples of different types of mortality rates and how each is calculated are given in Table 2. Morbidity is measured by calculating either prevalence or incidence rates. Prevalence is the number of existing cases of a disease at a given time divided by the population at

risk for that disease at that time. This result is usually multiplied by 100,000 to derive the prevalence rate per 100,000 population.

For purposes of etiology, the incidence rate is a more important measure of morbidity and is equal to the number of *new cases* of a disease occurring over a defined interval divided by the midinterval population at risk for that disease (multiplied by 100,000).

While mortality data are available throughout the world—with varying completeness depending on the quality of death registration systems—incidence rates can be calculated only for those diseases for which there are population-based registries of disease or for which special studies have been conducted. The National Cancer Institute has a program of cancer registries around the USA that provides information on cancer incidence covering approximately 10% of the United States population. Accurate enumeration of the population at risk—available from census data—is vital for deriving valid estimates of both mortality and morbidity rates. Rates can be specific to any subgroup of interest, defined by age, sex, race, or other characteristics. For example, the incidence rate for endometrial cancer among white women aged 50–54 in the USA in 1976 was 30 per 100,000, compared to 13.6 per 100,000 among black women of the same age. One must remember that in calculating a rate, the events in the numerator must be drawn from the population specified in the denominator—ie, those in the denominator must be at risk for the disease. Thus, for endometrial cancer, men would not be included in the denominator.

Some problems to keep in mind about current disease data include the following:

(1) The only complete registry for all causes is for deaths, and the cause-of-death assignment on the

Table 2. Measures of mortality.

$$\text{Crude death rate} = \frac{\text{Number of deaths in year (all causes)}}{\text{Total population}} \times 1000$$

eg, U.S. 1977 = 8.8 ÷ 1000 population or 878.1 ÷ 100,000 population

$$\text{Cause-specific death rate} = \frac{\text{Number of deaths from specific cause in year}}{\text{Total population}} \times 100,000$$

eg, Cancer in U.S. 1977 = 178.7 ÷ 100,000 population

$$\text{Age-specific death rate} = \frac{\text{Number of deaths among persons of specified age group in year}}{\text{Population in specified age group}} \times 100,000$$

eg, Cancer in age group 1–14 = 4.9 ÷ 100,000

$$\text{Infant mortality rate} = \frac{\text{Number of deaths among children less than 1 year of age in year}}{\text{Number of births in year}} \times 1000$$

eg, U.S. 1977 = 14.1 ÷ 1000 live births (12.3 for whites; 21.7 for black and other) death certificate is often inaccurate. In addition, for a disease whose case-fatality ratio is low (ie, a disease unlikely to result in death when it occurs), the death rate is a gross underestimate of the incidence of the condition in the community. An example of this would be nonmelanoma skin cancer.

(2) Morbidity reporting, even when it is legally mandated, as is the case for certain infectious diseases (eg, tuberculosis, sexually transmitted diseases), often results in severe under-reporting.

(3) Complete and accurate population-based morbidity registries are limited in geographic coverage.

ADJUSTMENT OF RATES

In attempting to compare disease rates across population groups or to assess changes in rates over time, the effect of differential age distribution in the 2 populations whose rates are being compared should be taken into account. Disease risk is almost always a function of age; differences in crude rates (ie, rates not adjusted for age) across populations may reflect age differences rather than differences in occupational or environmental factors of interest.

Age-specific rates are not subject to that shortcoming, provided the range in each age group is relatively narrow. It is cumbersome, however, to compare rates among populations across many age strata. Age adjustment or standardization provides a summary measure of disease risk for an entire population that is not influenced by variations in age distribution.

There are 2 methods for age-adjustment: a direct method, which applies observed age-specific rates to a standard population; and the indirect method, which applies age-specific rates from a standard population to the age distribution of an observed population. In discussing the methods for adjusting rates, cancer will be used as the disease being studied.

The **direct method** of age adjustment is appropriate when each of the populations being compared is large enough to yield stable age-specific rates. For example, the direct method is used for comparison of cancer rates over time in the USA. Crude mortality rates showing a dramatic increase in cancer over the past few decades would seem to provide strong evidence of a cancer epidemic. It needs to be ascertained, however, to what extent the aging of the country's population has contributed to the apparent epidemic or to what extent other factors, such as an increase in cancer-causing agents in the environment, might be responsible.

The first 3 columns of Table 3 show the actual age distributions of the United States population in 1940 and 1970, the percentage of the population in each group in the 2 periods, the corresponding number of actual cancer deaths, and the age-specific death rates. Crude death rates per 100,000 population were 120.2 for 1940 and 163.2 for 1970, an increase of over 30%. Comparison of the age-specific rates, however, shows only minor increases between the 2 time periods. It should be noted that the percentage of the population in all age groups over 40 was higher in 1970 than in 1940.

To remove the variable effect of age using the direct method of adjustment, a "standard" population is chosen. The number of people in each age group of the standard population is then multiplied by the appropriate age-specific rate in each of the study populations. This generates the number of deaths one

Table 3. Age adjustment by direct method, using cancer mortality data for the USA, 1940 and 1970.[1]

Age Group	Actual Population (1)	(2)	Number of Cancer Deaths (3)	Age-Specific Death Rates Per 100,000 (4)	Standard Population (5)	Expected Number of Cancer Deaths (6)
1940						
<40	87,737,829	66.7	10,283	11.72	217,093,330	25,443
40–49	17,053,068	13.	18,071	105.97	41,149,961	43,607
50–59	13,100,511	10.	33,279	254.03	34,177,557	86,821
60–69	8,534,997	6.5	43,686	511.85	24,143,606	123,579
70–79	4,073,514	3.1	38,160	936.78	13,352,179	125,080
80 +	1,139,143	0.9	14,721	1,292.29	4,934,355	63,766
Totals	131,639,062	100.	158,200[3]		334,850,988	468,296[3]
1970						
<40	129,355,501	63.7	16,096	12.44	217,093,330	27,006
40–49	24,096,893	11.9	26,075	108.21	41,149,961	44,528
50–59	21,077,046	10.4	61,143	290.09	34,177,557	99,146
60–69	15,608,609	7.7	90,099	577.24	24,143,606	139,367
70–79	9,278,665	4.6	88,826	957.31	13,352,179	127,821
80 +	3,795,212	1.9	49,333	1,299.87	4,934,355	64,140
Totals	203,211,926	100.	331,572[2]		334,850,988	502,008[2]

[1]Public Health Service, Vital Statistics of the United States, 1940 and 1970 (National Center for Health Statistics, Rockville, MD).
[2]Crude death rate = [sum of column 3 ÷ sum of column 1] × 10^5 = 163.2 per 100,000. Age-adjusted death rate = [sum of column 6 ÷ sum of column 5] × 10^5 = 149.9 per 100,000.
[3]Crude death rate = [sum of column 3 ÷ sum of column 1] × 10^5 = 120.2 per 100,000 population. Age-adjusted death rate = [sum of column 6 ÷ sum of column 5] × 10^5 = 139.8 per 100,000 population.

would expect in each age group if the populations had similar age distributions. The expected number of deaths is then summed over all age groups; the sum is divided by the total standard population; and the result is multiplied by 100,000. The choice of a standard population is arbitrary; it might be the combined population of the 2 groups whose rates are being compared, only one of those populations, or any other population.

In our example, the standard was the combined population of the USA in 1940 and 1970, shown in column 5 of Table 3. The age-specific rates for each period (column 4) were applied for each age group to the standard population, yielding the expected number of deaths shown in column 6. Age-adjusted rates are then calculated by dividing the sum of expected deaths for each period by the total standard population. The resulting adjusted rates are 139.8 per 100,000 for 1940 and 149.9 per 100,000 for 1970. Thus, the magnitude of the increase in the crude rates has been reduced from about 30% to 7%. It can be concluded that age is an important factor in the increased cancer rates in the United States, though age alone does not entirely explain changes over time.

When the group of interest is relatively small and thus likely to have unstable age-specific rates, it is more appropriate to use the indirect than the direct method of age adjustment. The **indirect method** is frequently employed to compare the cancer incidence or follow-up experience of a study group with that expected based on the experience of a larger population or patient series. With the indirect method, the age-specific rates from a standard population are multiplied by the number of person-years at risk in each group in the study series. The number of observed deaths is then compared with the number expected by means of a ratio.

The **standardized mortality ratio (SMR)** is an example of indirect standardization. In calculating an SMR, the age-specific rates from a standard population (eg, county, state, country) are multiplied by the person-years at risk in the study population (eg, industry employees) to give the expected number of deaths. The observed number of deaths divided by the expected number (times 100) is the SMR (see example in Table 4). An SMR may also control for

time-specific mortality rates by indirect standardization.

Thus, the equation for an SMR is as follows:

$$ SMR = \left[\frac{\Sigma\, a_i}{\Sigma\, E(a_i)} \right] \times 100 $$

$$ = \left[\frac{Observed}{Expected} \right] \times 100 $$

where a_i = the number of people with a specific death in the ith stratum of age (and time), and

$E(a_i)$ = the expected number of deaths based on the age-specific (and time-specific) rates in the reference population.

The result is multiplied by 100, so that when observed deaths equal expected deaths, the SMR is 100, and the differences from 100 represent the percentage difference in mortality in the study compared with that of the reference population.

Indirect standardization may also be used to adjust incidence rates for age or other factors. Thus, incident cases of a disease within a workplace could be expressed as the **standardized incidence ratio (SIR),** as follows:

$$ SIR = \left[\frac{Observed\ number\ of\ new\ cases}{Expected\ number\ of\ new\ cases} \right] \times 100 $$

Although it is most common to adjust rates for age and time, the direct and indirect methods of adjustment can be used to adjust for population differences in other factors as well, such as sex, race, socioeconomic status, or stage of disease.

Design Strategies for Analytic & Experimental Studies

Descriptive epidemiology provides disease rates for different groups. It identifies segments of the population—by age, sex, time, occupation, marital status, geographic area of residence, or other parameters—whose unique experience suggests etiologic hypotheses worthy of pursuit through rigorous analytic studies. Descriptive epidemiology tells *who* gets the disease *where* and *when* and is the basis of analytic epidemiology, which in turn focuses on specific questions, such as the following:

What exposure do people with the disease have in common, compared with people without the disease?

Why does exposure induce or promote disease?

How much is risk increased by such exposure?

How many cases might be avoided were the exposure eliminated?

The last question addresses the ultimate objective of epidemiologic research: to identify risk factors so that intervention might either prevent the occurrence of the disease (primary prevention) or lead to early detection (secondary prevention).

Table 4. Age adjustment by indirect method in computation of standardized mortality ratio (SMR).

Age	Observed Deaths (1)	Person Years (2)	US Population Rates (per 10^6) (3)	Expected Deaths = (2) × (3)
20–29	1	5,000	20.6	0.1
30–39	0	15,000	22.7	0.3
40–49	4	60,000	45.3	2.7
50–59	2	40,000	94.3	3.8
60–69	12	70,000	224.4	15.7
Σ Obs = 19				Σ Exp = 22.6

SMR = [Σ Obs/Σ Exp] × 100 = [19/22.6]100 = 84

The 3 basic strategies for analytic epidemiology are (1) the cohort study, (2) the case-control study, and (3) the experimental study (clinical trial).

Cohort and case-control studies are observational: the investigator does not control exposure or modify behavior of the study subjects. In the experimental study, the investigator intervenes by introducing treatment or other exposures to study their impact on the disease experience.

TYPES OF EPIDEMIOLOGIC STUDIES

THE COHORT STUDY

In the design of a cohort study, a disease-free group of individuals characterized by a common experience or exposure is identified and followed forward over time, or prospectively, to determine whether disease occurs at a rate different from that in a cohort without the exposure. The **relative risk** (RR) of disease associated with the exposure can then be calculated:

$$RR = \frac{Incidence\ rate\ in\ the\ exposed\ group}{Incidence\ rate\ in\ the\ nonexposed\ group}$$

A frequently cited example of the prospective cohort design is the follow-up study of British physicians whose smoking habits were ascertained by means of a mailed questionnaire. The doctors were grouped according to smoking habits, and their deaths were subsequently monitored. Lung cancer rates for those exposed to various levels of smoking were then compared with the rates for nonsmokers by means of the relative risk. Other examples of cohort studies include investigations of long-term cancer incidence among atomic bomb survivors exposed to varying degrees of radiation and deaths among British coal miners.

Theoretically, the prospective cohort study is ideal because the hypothesized cause or exposure precedes the effect—ie, disease—and because disease rates and relative risks can be calculated directly provided that a suitable comparison group is built into the study or otherwise available for calculation of rates in the nonexposed population. In addition, the exposure of interest can be accurately recorded at the time of exposure: it is not based on recall of past events. This approach has been popular in occupational studies in which the disease experience of workers exposed to putatively hazardous substances has been compared with that of other workers without the exposure or with that of the general population.

In practice, however, because of the expense, the time involved, and the number of subjects required,

the model prospective cohort study is relatively rare. To avoid some of these constraints, a **historical cohort study** might be done whereby a group of persons who in the past experienced an exposure of interest is identified and their disease record up to the present is investigated. An example is the follow-up of mortality among insulation workers exposed to asbestos. The population of union insulation workers in the 1940s was identified, and their cause-specific mortality rate through the 1970s was determined. Mortality rates for lung cancer and other causes in this population were tabulated and compared with those expected on the basis of mortality rates for all United States men. Because the historical cohort study is really a retrospective approach, the terms cohort study and prospective study should not be used synonymously.

Measures of Association in a Cohort Study

Three measures of association will be discussed using the symbols and numbers provided in Tables 5 and 6. Let us assume that one is doing a study of smokers and nonsmokers and following them to see who develops lung cancer over some defined period of time.

A. The First Measure of Association Is Relative Risk (RR): Relative risk is the risk of disease in people exposed to a factor relative to the risk in people not exposed and is a measure of the strength of association between an exposure and a disease.

$$RR = \frac{Disease\ rate\ in\ the\ exposed\ population}{Disease\ rate\ in\ the\ nonexposed\ population}$$

$$= \frac{\dfrac{a}{a+b}}{\dfrac{c}{c+d}} = \frac{\dfrac{63}{10^5}}{\dfrac{7}{10^5}} = 9$$

A relative risk greater than 1 implies a positive association of the disease with exposure to the factor; a relative risk less than 1 implies a negative association (protective effect) of exposure to the factor with disease.

The results in the above example suggest that the risk of lung cancer among smokers is 9 times greater than the risk for nonsmokers.

Relative risk is important for testing etiologic hypotheses. The second measure of risk is attributable risk.

Table 5. Presentation of data from a cohort study.

| | | Disease | | |
		Present	Absent	
Exposure {	Yes	a	b	a+b
	No	c	d	c+d

Table 6. Example of data collected in a cohort study of lung cancer and smoking.

	Develop Lung Cancer	Do Not Develop Lung Cancer	
Smokers	63	99,937	100,000
Nonsmokers	7	99,993	100,000

B. Attributable Risk (AR): Attributable risk is the rate in the exposed population minus the rate in the nonexposed population.

$$AR = \frac{a}{a+b} - \frac{c}{c+d}$$

$$= \frac{63}{10^5} - \frac{7}{10^5} = \frac{56}{10^5}$$

ie, 56 of the 63 lung cancer deaths that occur annually among 100,000 smokers (ie, 89%) are attributable to smoking. This calculation of attributable risk assumes (usually naively) a single-factor etiology.

Attributable risk is important for counselling individuals with risk factors. The third measure of risk is population attributable risk percentage.

C. Population Attributable Risk (PAR) Percentage: PAR percentage is the proportion of a disease in a population related to (or "attributable to") a given exposure.

$$PAR = \frac{P_e (RR - 1)}{P_e (RR - 1) + 1}$$

where P_e = the proportion of the population exposed to the risk factor and
RR = relative risk.

Assuming that 40% of the population smokes (P_e) and that the relative risk (RR) of lung cancer associated with smoking is 9, then

$$= \frac{0.4 (9 - 1)}{0.4 (9 - 1) + 1} = \frac{3.2}{4.2} = 76.2\%$$

That is to say, 76% of cases of lung cancer in the general population are attributable to smoking. Population attributable risk is important for public health policy and planning, ie, in estimating what percent of cases in a population could be eliminated by removing an exposure.

CASE-CONTROL STUDY

The case-control study is the most frequently used design in analytic epidemiology. It determines the risk factors associated with a particular disease by comparing a group of subjects (cases) who have the disease with one or more control groups composed of subjects who do not have the disease. Risk factors studied may be permanent, such as eye color; they may be current, such as present drug use; or they may be historical, such as previous employment. The difference in the frequency distribution of the risk factors between the case and control groups is examined, and the magnitude of the effect of these factors on the disease under study is estimated.

The case-control study is always retrospective. The investigator starts by identifying diseased and nondiseased individuals (ie, the effect) and looks backward for the presence or absence of attributes or exposures (ie, the causes) in these individuals.

For example, to study the relationship between asbestos exposure and mesothelioma, a case-control study would compare the history of asbestos exposure in a group of mesothelioma patients with the history of asbestos exposure in a group of subjects who do not have mesothelioma. The cohort study, in contrast, first identifies a group of disease-free individuals classified for absence or presence of the risk factor or exposure of interest and then follows these individuals over time to compare the incidence of disease in the exposed and unexposed groups. A cohort study of the relationship between asbestos and mesothelioma would first classify a group of nondiseased persons according to their asbestos exposure and follow them to determine whether the asbestos-exposed subjects had a higher incidence of mesothelioma over time than the nonexposed subjects.

Case-control studies generally can be done more rapidly and less expensively than cohort studies. The time required to complete the study is the time needed to assemble the necessary data; the investigator does not need to wait for cases of the disease to appear. This usually results in lower personnel costs. The study is also less costly because fewer subjects are necessary to test a hypothesis.

For example, suppose half of the general population is exposed to a risk factor (eg, cigarette smoking) and half is not. If a disease has an annual incidence rate of 100 per 100,000 in the exposed and 10 per 100,000 in the nonexposed population, a study of 100 cases and 100 controls would probably reveal the increased risk of disease associated with exposure to the factor. Uncovering 100 cases of disease in a cohort study would mean following 10,000 exposed people for 10 years. The more rare the disease, the greater the relative advantage of the case-control study.

Source & Selection of Cases

In defining a case, the diagnostic criteria should be clear and permit selection of a homogeneous group of cases. For example, in cancer studies, microscopic confirmation of disease and clearly defined criteria for classification by histologic type of cancer greatly enhance the validity and generalizability of the study findings. The case group is usually composed of (1) all persons with the disease seen at a particular medical facility or group of facilities in a specified period, or (2) all persons with the disease found in a community or in the general population in a specified period. Whatever the source of the cases, they should be newly diagnosed (or incident) cases of the disease. Inclusion of prevalent (diagnosed in the past) cases will increase the sample size but will complicate analysis and interpretation of results. Prevalent cases are "survivors" and are therefore not representative of all people who develop a disease. Inclusion of prevalent cases may identify factors that result from the disease rather than factors that are causally related to its development.

Source & Selection of Controls

The 4 most common sources of the control group are (1) the general population, (2) hospital patients, (3) relatives of cases, and (4) associates or friends of cases.

The **general population** control group is appropriate if all or most cases occur in a specific geographic area—eg, a county—in which event the controls represent the same target population as the cases. Using general population controls presents certain problems: potentially lower response rates than from other types of control groups and from the case group, varying quality of information if the interview setting differs for the cases and the controls, and higher costs.

The **hospital patient** control group is selected from patients at the same hospital or clinic that the cases attended. This control group may share the selective factors that influenced the cases to come to a particular hospital or clinic, eg, ethnicity or income. These patients (the controls) are readily available, have time to spare, and are more cooperative. The disadvantage of the hospital control group is that it is composed of people who are ill and who will differ from the general population with regard to factors often associated with disease, such as smoking habits and drug use. In addition, the factors that cause patients to attend a particular hospital may not be the same for all diseases. For example, a hospital with a national reputation for treating Hodgkin's disease may have patients with this disease from all over the country, whereas its population of coronary disease patients may come only from the region surrounding the hospital; thus, the 2 patient groups will differ greatly. Similarly, healthy people attending a hospital screening clinic may differ markedly in ethnic, socioeconomic, or other factors from the inpatient population of that hospital. One consideration in selecting controls is whether to draw them from the hospital's entire patient population or to exclude patients who have diseases related to factors under study. For example, in a case-control study of the relationship between lung cancer and smoking, it would seem logical to exclude from the control group persons who have emphysema, because emphysema is related to smoking, the factor under study. There is also the problem of not knowing whether factors being studied are related to diseases present in hos-

pital controls. Selecting controls from many diagnostic categories would minimize this problem.

Spouses and siblings are the relatives most commonly used as controls because of similarity in ethnicity and environment with the case group. Moreover, sibling controls are genetically similar to the cases. Spouses as controls are appropriate if there is an approximately equal number of male and female cases and the age range of cases is such that a high proportion of spouses are likely to be alive. When siblings are the controls, one sibling should be selected per case. Using all available siblings would result in the control group's having many characteristics related to large family size, and these factors may confound any observed associations. Similarly, cases who have no siblings must be excluded so that the case group is not weighted with the characteristics of one-child families.

A control group of **associates of cases** such as neighbors, coworkers, friends, or schoolmates has the advantage of being composed of generally healthy individuals who are similar to the case group in life-style characteristics—eg, neighborhood controls are usually of the same socioeconomic status as the cases. However, such associates might be more similar to cases than members of the general population with respect to risk factors under investigation, thus impairing the ability of the study to detect true differences in exposure between people with and without disease. Other disadvantages of associates as controls are the effort necessary to identify them, a response rate different from that of cases, and probable variations in the quality of information obtained from cases and controls.

Sampling

Once the source of the control group has been determined, one must decide on the method of selecting the controls. Either all eligible individuals are selected from a specific group—though this is usually not required—or a sample is selected. Whenever sampling is employed, its protocol should be defined and adhered to throughout the sampling. Examples of common sampling strategies are (1) random sampling, (2) systematic sampling, and (3) paired sampling.

In **random sampling,** each member of the source group has an equal chance of being represented in the control group. For example, all individuals might be assigned a number, and the sample would be selected using a table of random numbers.

In **systematic sampling,** the source group for controls is assumed to have an ordered sequence, and every nth individual is selected. As long as the sequence of the source group is not related to an important study variable, the resulting characteristics of a systematic sample are similar to those of a random sample.

In addition to random or systematic sampling, a popular method of selecting controls is **paired sampling.** In paired sampling, one or several controls are selected for each case based on a defined relationship to the case. For example, if we use hospital controls, the person who was admitted immediately before or after the case might be chosen for the control group. The investigator may choose to select for each case one or more controls who are individually matched with the case on characteristics such as sex, age, or socioeconomic status—which, if not controlled, might lead to spurious associations in the final results. For example, as a neighborhood control, the resident of the nearest dwelling to the right of the case's house who is of the same sex and age ($\pm$ 5 years) as the case might be selected. Such matching at the outset of the study is one way of taking into account any variables known to be associated with both the disease and the exposure of interest.

Sources of Bias

Bias is defined as deviation from the truth of results or of inferences or processes leading to such deviation.

While bias is more common in case-control studies, it may occur also in cohort studies—eg, outcome measures may be obtained differently in exposed and unexposed subjects. The principle is the same: Any difference in the way information is obtained from the study groups may bias the results of the study.

A. Selection Bias: The appropriate control group should be judiciously chosen to avoid selection bias. Under the null hypothesis, cases and controls have been equally "exposed" to the study factor. Therefore, the cases and controls must be comparable and representative of the same underlying population, so that if we reject the null hypothesis and determine that cases differ from controls on the study factor, it is not because we selected them to be different by using a biased procedure. Since the case group is usually chosen first, selection bias is avoided by a careful choice of the appropriate control group.

As an example of how selection bias can occur, suppose we are studying the relationship between endometrial cancer and menopausal estrogen use. We choose our case group from the inpatient population of a private hospital and our control group from the outpatient clinic of the same hospital. Once we have selected our cases and controls, we discover that they differ dramatically with respect to socioeconomic status—the inpatient population being predominantly upper middle class and the clinic population predominantly lower class. Thus, if we find that the cases and controls differ in terms of menopausal estrogen use, we would not know whether this is a true difference or whether the difference is due to other factors related to socioeconomic status.

Selection bias can also occur if the control group is composed of people who volunteer for the study, since volunteers differ in significant ways from nonvolunteers, eg, they may be more educated, more active in community affairs, less likely to be smokers.

B. Interviewer (Data Collection) Bias: In inter-viewing study subjects about past exposures or events, the interviewer who knows the disease status of the individual (case or control) may unconsciously pose questions or probe for answers in a different manner. For example, in a case-control study of factors related to lung cancer, an interviewer might pursue in greater depth questions concerning asbestos exposure when obtaining work or environmental histories from cases than from controls.

To avoid this bias, the procedure used to collect information should be identical for cases and controls. The data collector should ideally be unaware of the hypotheses being tested and whether the subject is a case or control; however, in collecting information of a medical or personal nature, it is often difficult to avoid learning of the person's disease status. Every effort must therefore be made to keep interviews as comparable as possible (eg, place, length, and format of questionnaire, attempts to gain cooperation and accurate information, and other aspects of the interview). Each interviewer should see an equal number of cases and controls.

C. Recall Bias: When a study subject is asked to recall past exposures or events, recall might depend on the person's current disease status. For example, a woman with diagnosed breast cancer may be more likely to remember past trauma to her breast than a control woman. To minimize recall bias in this instance, one might try to interview women before biopsy—or before the results of the biopsy are known. It is advantageous to use information recorded before the time of diagnosis wherever possible. In using data from interviews in which the case has a serious illness and the control has not, the items on which cases and controls can be compared with the greatest confidence are those least subject to recall bias. For example, marital history is a more objectively reported event than drug use during past pregnancy.

Confounding

The phenomenon of confounding is another explanation for an apparent association between an exposure and a disease and may also cause no association to be observed when a true association actually exists. As with bias, confounding may occur in any type of analytic epidemiologic study. When confounding occurs, an extraneous factor is associated with the exposure and is an independent cause of the disease being studied. In this situation, an observed association between an exposure and a disease is in fact due wholly or in part to the association of the exposure with the confounding factor, which in turn is a cause of the disease. If the confounding factor is not differentially associated with the exposed subjects or is not a cause of the disease, it cannot be a confounding factor.

An example of a confounding factor would be cigarette smoking in a study of an occupational exposure and lung cancer. Cigarette smoking is a known cause of lung cancer. If the cigarette smoking prevalence were greater (or less) in the population exposed to the agent, failure to control for smoking in the study design or analysis would lead to an apparently greater (or lesser) association between the exposure and lung cancer.

ANALYSIS OF CASE-CONTROL STUDIES

Data from the case-control study are conventionally arrayed so that cases and controls can be compared on exposure to a hypothesized etiologic factor:

		Disease Status	
		Cases	Controls
Exposure {	Yes	a	b
	No	c	d
		a + c	b + d

The **incidence** of disease among the exposed and nonexposed cannot be calculated using case-control data because the cases and controls in the study rarely reflect the true proportions of diseased and nondiseased persons in the population. (The investigator usually selects roughly equal numbers of cases [a + c] and controls [b + d] in the study, whereas there are many more nondiseased than diseased people in the population.) Therefore, relative risk of disease associated with exposure cannot be calculated directly in a case-control study, as it was for the cohort study. However, an estimate of the relative risk, known as the **odds ratio**, can be calculated if the proportion of diseased people in the general population is small compared with the proportion of nondiseased (almost always true). Recall that the true relative risk using data from a cohort or incidence study is as follows:

$$RR = \frac{\dfrac{a}{a + b}}{\dfrac{c}{c + d}}$$

where a = the number of cases among the exposed group in a cohort study,
    b = the number of noncases among the exposed group,
    c = the number of cases among the nonexposed group, and
    d = the number of noncases among the nonexposed group.

In a cohort study, as in the general population, "a" is *very* small relative to "b." Similarly, "c" is *very* small relative to "d." Thus, in the general population (and the usual cohort study), a/(a + b) $\simeq$ a/b and c/(c + d) $\simeq$ c/d. Consequently, the formula for relative risk reduces to

$$\frac{\dfrac{a}{b}}{\dfrac{c}{d}} = \frac{ad}{bc} = \textit{odds ratio (estimated relative risk)}$$

Example
100 men with lung cancer and 100 controls are interviewed regarding smoking history:

	Cases	Controls
Smokers	80	30
Nonsmokers	20	70
	100	100

$$\text{Odds ratio} = \frac{ad}{bc} = \frac{80 \times 70}{30 \times 20} = \frac{5600}{600} = 9.3$$

Since the odds ratio is an estimate of relative risk, one can conclude that these data show a 9-fold increased risk of lung cancer in smokers compared to nonsmokers.

Population attributable risk (PAR) (ie, the proportion of all instances of the disease in the population that can be attributed to the exposure of interest) can be estimated from case-control studies, using the following equation:

$$PAR = \frac{p\,(OR - 1)}{p\,(OR - 1) + 1}$$

where p = the proportion of the population with exposure of interest (estimated from controls as b ÷ [b + d]), and
    OR = the estimated relative risk (odds ratio) associated with the characteristic.

Matched Case-Control Studies
Controls are frequently selected in a case-control study so as to be individually matched to the cases as to characteristics such as age, sex, race, or socioeconomic status that are known to be related to the disease. Matching helps make the 2 groups similar with respect to factors other than the exposure of interest in the study and thus serves to reduce the likelihood of spurious associations. The investigator must be careful, however, not to overmatch, ie, to match cases and controls on factors related to the exposure of interest; overmatching can artificially reduce—may even eliminate—true exposure differences between diseased and nondiseased individuals in the study. It should be obvious that cases and controls cannot be compared in the analysis with respect to any characteristics on which they have been matched.

The data in a matched pairs analysis are organized as shown below:

		Controls	
			Not
		Exposed	exposed
Cases	Exposed	r	s
	Not exposed	t	u

where r = the number of pairs in which both case and control are exposed to the factor (concordant),

s = the number of pairs in which the case but not the control is exposed to the factor (discordant),

t = the number of pairs in which the control but not the case is exposed to the factor (discordant), and

u = the number of pairs in which both case and control are not exposed to the factor (concordant).

To compute the **odds ratio** (estimated relative risk) for a matched pairs study, only the discordant pairs enter into the calculation:

$$\text{Odds ratio} = \frac{s}{t}$$

$$\text{where } t \neq 0$$

Example

One hundred and seventy-five women aged 15–44 admitted to hospital in 1968 with thromboembolism were matched on age, sex, race, and date of admission to 175 controls. All women in the study were interviewed regarding use of oral contraceptives during the month preceding admission. The results regarding oral contraceptive use (OC) were as follows:

		Controls		
		Yes OC	No OC	Totals
Cases	Yes OC	10	57	67
	No OC	13	95	108
		23	152	175

$$\text{Odds ratio} = \frac{s}{t} = \frac{57}{13} = 4.4$$

These data show that women who have recently used oral contraceptives have a 4.4 times greater risk of admission for thromboembolism than nonusers of oral contraceptives.

THE EXPERIMENTAL STUDY

The experimental study is the type of design most familiar to clinical investigators, but it is rarely encountered in occupational epidemiology. Unlike the cohort and case-control studies, which are observational in nature—ie, the investigator observes exposed individuals for the development of disease or diseased individuals for past exposures—in an experimental study the investigator manipulates exposures and studies the impact upon disease. The intervention can occur at different points in the natural course of the disease. Subjects are normally randomly assigned to the different interventions in an experimental study. Ideally, study outcomes should also be determined by individuals blind to the exposure status of the subjects.

Experimental clinical trials are often undertaken among individuals with the same disease who are assigned to different treatment groups. An example is the Surgical Adjuvant Breast Cancer Study, in which women with breast cancer were randomly assigned to receive either radical mastectomy (the standard treatment) or modified radical surgery plus radiation therapy (the experimental treatment). The study was undertaken to determine whether survival among the modified surgery group was similar to that associated with the long-established standard radical surgical procedure.

Alternatively, intervention might occur in the form of a screening program offered to one group of people at risk of disease and not to another similar group.

An example of this type of intervention study is the National Cancer Institute's Cooperative Screening for Early Lung Cancer Program. Men aged 45 and older with a history of heavy cigarette smoking were assigned to a dual screened group receiving chest x-rays and sputum cytologies or to a group receiving only chest x-rays. The objective was to determine whether the addition of sputum cytology to regular chest radiography resulted in earlier detection and improved lung cancer survival.

Another intervention is to alter a risk factor before frank disease develops in the hope of reducing subsequent incidence of the disease. For example, in the area of coronary heart disease, the Multiple Risk Factor Intervention Trial was undertaken to determine the effectiveness of programs to reduce weight, end smoking, and lower blood pressure among middle-aged men at high risk for the disease. Participants were randomized into special intervention or normal care groups, and the later incidence rates of coronary heart disease in the 2 groups were compared.

CAUSAL ASSOCIATION

An epidemiologic study may demonstrate an association that is not statistically valid because of chance, bias, or confounding, as previously discussed. If the association is felt to be valid—ie, the disease occurrence is in fact not equal among the exposed and unexposed subjects—and the association cannot be explained by chance, bias, or confounding, the investigator must consider whether the data support a cause and effect association.

This process involves consideration of the study itself and all existing data on the subject. Factors that should be considered in evaluating whether an association is causal include (1) the strength of the association, ie, whether dose-response relationships are present; (2) consonance with existing knowledge;

(3) biologic credibility, ie, whether there is a proposed biologic mechanism; and (4) the time sequence, ie, whether cause precedes effect.

While uncertainties will always exist following an epidemiologic study, action on the findings of a study will depend in part on how strongly the data support a causal association and on the need for action versus the consequences of obtaining more data.

REFERENCES

Epidemiology

The books listed below are excellent general introductory texts in epidemiology and cover basic descriptive and analytic methods. Examples provided throughout are drawn from classic epidemiologic studies.

Checkoway H, Pearce N, Crawford-Brown DJ: *Research Methods in Occupational Epidemiology.* Oxford Univ Press, 1989.

Fletcher RH, Fletcher SW, Wagner EH: *Clinical Epidemiology: The Essentials.* Williams & Wilkins, 1982.

Hennekens CH, Buring JE: *Epidemiology in Medicine.* Little, Brown, 1987.

Kelsey JL, Thompson WD, Evans AS: Methods in Observational Epidemiology. Oxford Univ Press, 1986.

Last JM (editor): *A Dictionary of Epidemiology,* 2nd ed. Oxford Univ Press, 1988.

Lilienfeld AM, Lilienfeld DE: *Foundations of Epidemiology,* 2nd ed. Oxford Univ Press, 1980.

MacMahon B, Pugh TF: *Epidemiology: Principles and Methods.* Little, Brown, 1970.

Mausner JS, Kramer S: *Epidemiology: An Introductory Text,* 2nd ed. Saunders, 1984.

Monson RR: *Occupational Epidemiology,* 2nd ed. CRC Press, 1990.

Case-Control Studies

The following references describe in detail the methodologic issues and statistical theory underlying the design and analysis of case-control studies as used in epidemiologic research. Many examples drawn from published studies are presented.

Breslow NE, Day NE: *The Analysis of Case-Control Studies.* Vol 1 of: *Statistical Methods in Cancer Research.* IARC Scientific Publications, 1980.

Fleiss JL: *Statistical Methods for Rates and Proportions.* Wiley, 1981.

Schlesselman JJ: *Case Control Studies: Design, Conduct, Analysis.* Oxford Univ Press, 1981.

Index

and wipe sampling, 507
and work practices controls, 511
and work practices and process
variables, 507
Infections, **170–181**. *See also specific type*
and approach to suspected disease
outbreak, 180*t*
biologic surveillance and, 179–180
cutaneous, 219
exposure evaluation and, 180
exposure to infected humans and,
170–178
immunization and, 179
prophylaxis and, 179
and reproductive toxicity in
female, 285*t*
travel-associated, 177–178
zoonoses, 178–181
Inferential statistics, **537–543**
analysis of variance, 540–541
chi square test, 541–542
errors and, 543–544
p-value, 542–543
significance and, 542–543
t-test, 537–540
Inferior rectus muscle, entrapment of
in orbital floor fracture, 78
Infertility. *See also* Female reproductive toxicology; Male reproductive toxicology
relation of semen parameters to,
291–293
Infiltration, outdoor air introduced
by, 454
Inflammation, nonimmune activation
of, 147
Influenza vaccination, occupational
preexposure, 179*t*
Informed consent, in disability evaluation, 30
Infrapatellar bursitis, 68
Infrared radiation, injuries caused by,
119
to eye, 93, 119
Infrared spectrophotometers, in gas
and vapor sampling, 505
Inhalation challenge tests, 224*i*. *See
also* Bronchial provocation
tests
in hypersensitivity reactions,
152–153
Inhalation injury to lung, 442
Inhaled materials, deposition of, 221
Initiators, in carcinogenesis, 182–183
promoters differentiated from, 183*t*
Injuries. *See* Occupational injuries
Inorganic haptens, hypersensitivity
pneumonitis caused by, 228*t*
Insect repellents, 430
Insecticides. *See also* Pesticides
arsenical. *See* Arsenic; Arsenical
insecticides
carbamate. *See* Carbamate insecticides
organochlorine. *See* Organochlorine insecticides

organophosphate. *See* Organophosphate insecticides
toxic thrombocytopenia associated
with, 167*t*, 168
Inspiratory capacity, 223*i*
Inspiratory reserve volume, 223*i*
Insurance
compulsory, and workers' compensation law, 19
malpractice, for physician in workplace, 34
Intermaxillary fixation
in mandibular fracture, 75
in maxillary fracture, 77
in orbital floor fracture, 78
Internal combustion engines
as source of environmental contamination, 514
standards for emissions from, 530
International Commission on Occupational Health, 15
International Labor Office, 15
Intertrigo, 111
Interval data, 534
Intervertebral disks
cervical, degenerative disease of,
58–59
lumbar, degenerative disease of,
62–64
spinal stenosis and, 64
Interviewer bias, in epidemiologic
studies, 551
Intralipid, in thermal burns, 115
Intraocular foreign body, 88–89
Intraocular pressure
measurement of, 83
in ruptured or lacerated globe, 87
Intrauterine growth retardation, 277
Invasion of privacy, and liability of
workplace physician, 35
Ionizing radiation, **525–526**
as air pollutant, 520*t*
aplastic anemia associated with, 166
cancer associated with, 189*t*
and cigarette smoking in lung cancer caused by, 446, 448*t*
control of, 526
as environmental contaminant,
525–526
and exposure limits
external, 124*t*
organ-specific internal, 124*t*
health effects of, 525
high-dose, delayed effects of, 125
injuries caused by, **121–125**
acute localized, 125
and acute radiation syndrome,
122–124
clinical effects of, 123*t*
to eye, 92
and radionuclide contamination,
125
leukemia associated with
etiology of, 197–198
laboratory findings in, 199
pathophysiology of, 198–199
prevention of, 199

symptoms and signs of, 199
low-dose, effects of, 125
multiple myeloma associated with,
167
myelodysplasia associated with,
166–167
occupational exposure to, 122*t*
and reproductive toxicity in
female, 284*t*
skin tumors associated with,
195–196
sources of exposure to, 525–526
units of, 124*t*
Iridoplegia, 86
Iris, 80, 81*i*
injuries to, 86
Iron, in hexachlorobenzene-induced
porphyria, 161–162
Iron foreign bodies, in eye, 89
Iron and steel founding, cancer associated with, 189*t*
Irrigation of eye, in chemical burns,
85
Irritant chemicals
acute irritant contact dermatitis
caused by, 209–211
suitability of gloves for handling,
210*t*
Irritant noxious gases, **440–442**
Irritant respiratory syndrome, TMA
exposure and, 150
IRV. *See* Inspiratory reserve volume
Ischemic heart disease, nonatheromatous, toxic agents causing, 327*t*
Isocyanates
asthma caused by, 225–226, 394
health hazards of exposure to, 394
source of, 432*t*
Isoniazid
in silicosis with positive PPD, 231
for tuberculosis prophylaxis, 173
Isooctyl alcohol, 360*t*, 376
Isopropyl alcohol, 360*t*, 375–376
manufacture of, cancer associated
with, 189*t*
sinonasal cancer associated with,
206
Isosorbide dinitrate, in nitrate withdrawal ischemia, 242

Jaundice
acute cholestatic, 251
aromatic amines causing, 334–335
"Epping," 251, 334
Jaw, fracture of, 74–75
Job Decision Control Model of
stress, 468, 469*i*
Job design
approach to, 38
improvement of, 38–42
poor, physical stress due to, **38–42**

**Kallikrein, in immediate hypersen-
sitivity, 143**
action of, 143*t*
Kaloin, lung disease caused by, 235